P9-DEI-267

Introductory Clinical Pharmacology

EIGHTH EDITION

Sally S. Roach, MSN, RN, AHN-BC

Associate Professor
University of Texas at Brownsville
and Texas Southmost College
Brownsville, Texas

Susan M. Ford, MN, RN, OCN

Associate Dean for Nursing
Tacoma Community College
Tacoma, Washington

 Wolters Kluwer | Lippincott Williams & Wilkins
Health
Philadelphia · Baltimore · New York · London
Buenos Aires · Hong Kong · Sydney · Tokyo

Acquisitions Editor: Elizabeth Nieginski
Managing Editor: Betsy Gentzler
Director of Nursing Production: Helen Ewan
Senior Managing Editor / Production: Erika Kors
Production Editor: Mary Kinsella
Art Director: Brett MacNaughton
Design Coordinator: Holly Reid McLaughlin
Cover Designer: Anthony Groves
Interior Designer: Leslie Haimes
Manufacturing Coordinator: Karin Duffield
Senior Manufacturing Manager: William Alberti
Indexer: Gaye Tarallo
Compositor: TechBooks
Printer: R. R. Donnelley & Sons, Willard

8th Edition

Library of Congress Cataloging-in-Publication Data

Roach, Sally S.
   Introductory clinical pharmacology / Sally S. Roach, Susan M. Ford. —8th ed.
      p. ; cm.
   Includes index.
   ISBN-13: 978-0-7817-7595-3
   ISBN-10: 0-7817-7595-7
 1.   Clinical pharmacology. 2.   Nursing. I. Ford, Susan M. II. Title.
   [DNLM: 1. Pharmacology, Clinical—Nurses' Instruction. 2.   Drug Therapy—Nurses'
Instruction. 3.   Pharmaceutical Preparations—administration & dosage—Nurses'
Instruction. QV 38 R628i 2008]
   RM301.28.S34 2008
   615.5'8—dc22   2006030586

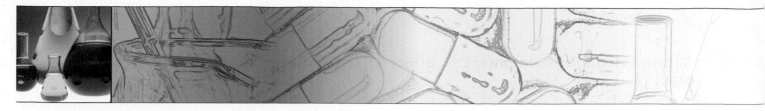

Reviewers

Mary Barrow Norris, MSN, RN, CCRN
Nursing Instructor
Lurleen B. Wallace Community College
MacArthur Campus
Opp, Alabama

Nicholle Bierberdorf, BAN, RN
Practical Nursing Instructor
Northwest Technical College
Bemidji, Minnesota

Kathy Bode, MS, RN
Chair, Division of Health
Flint Hills Technical College
Emporia, Kansas

Lisa Bridges, BSN, MBA, RN
Program Director
Dekalb Technical College
Covington, Georgia

Karen Briza, BSN, RN
Department Chair of Vocational Nursing
Alvin Community College
Alvin, Texas

Sister Marie Buckley, CIJ, MS, RCPT, MT (ASCP), RRT
Director of the Cardiovascular Technology
Program
Molloy College
Rockville Center, New York

Sheila Burcham, BSN, ASN
Nursing Educator
Northwest Mississippi Community College
Senatobia, Mississippi

Patricia Conejo, MSN, RN, WHNP
Assistant Professor of Nursing
Avila University
Kansas City, Missouri

Mary Davis, MSN, RN
Faculty
Valdosta Technical College
Valdosta, Georgia

Doreen DeAngelis, MSN, RN
Associate Professor
Community College of Allegheny County,
    South Campus
West Mifflin, Pennsylvania

Denise Doliveira, MSN, RN
Assistant Professor
Community College of Allegheny County,
    Boyce Campus
Monroeville, Pennsylvania

Judy Donnelly, MBA, BSN, RN
Instructor, Practical Nursing
Lancaster County Career and Technical
    Center
Willow Street, Pennsylvania

Melissa Falkenrath, BSN, RN
Practical Nurse Coordinator
Waynesville Technical Academy
    School of Practical Nursing
Waynesville, Missouri

Madeline V. Garcia, MSN, RN
Associate Professor
Victoria College
Victoria, Texas

Carly Hall, BSN, RN
Instructor, Practical Nursing Program
Camosun College
Victoria, BC, Canada

Lutricia Harrison, MSN, RN, APRN-BC
ADN Nursing Instructor
Kingwood College
Kingwood, Texas

Preface

The eighth edition of *Introductory Clinical Pharmacology* reflects the ever-changing science of pharmacology and the nurse's responsibilities in administering pharmacologic agents. All information has been updated and revised according to the latest available information to prepare nurses to safely administer medications. The text prepares the nurse to meet the challenges of the 21st century by promoting critical thinking and problem solving when administering medications.

Purpose

This text is designed to provide students with a clear, concise introduction to pharmacology. The basic explanations presented in this text are *not* intended to suggest that pharmacology is an easy subject. Drug therapy is one of the most important and complicated treatment modalities in modern health care. Because of its importance and complexity and the frequent additions and changes in the field of pharmacology, it is imperative that health care professionals constantly review and update their knowledge.

Current Drug Information

The student and practitioner should remember that information about drugs, such as dosages and new forms, is constantly changing. Likewise, there may be new drugs on the market that were not approved by the Federal Drug Administration (FDA) at the time of publication of this text. The reader may find that certain drugs or drug dosages available when this textbook was published may no longer be available. For the most current drug information and dosages, the practitioner is advised to consult references such as the most current *Physician's Desk Reference* or *Facts and Comparisons* and the package inserts that accompany most drugs. If reliable references are not available, the hospital pharmacist or physician should be contacted for information concerning a specific drug, including dosage, adverse reactions, contraindications, precautions, interactions, or administration.

Special Features

A number of features have proven useful for students in their study of basic pharmacology. The following features appear in the eighth edition:

- **Key Terms** listed at the beginning of each chapter highlight the important words defined in each chapter.
- **The Nursing Process** is used as a framework in most chapters for presenting care of the patient as it relates to the drug and the drug regimen.
- **Nursing Alerts** identify urgent nursing considerations in the management of the patient receiving a specific drug or drug category.
- **Gerontologic Alerts** alert the nurse to specific problems for which the older adult is at increased risk. As the number of the older adults in our society increases, it becomes imperative that nurses recognize the necessity of specialized care.
- **Contraindications, Precautions, and Interactions** of the most commonly used drugs in the category under discussion are included in each chapter. While space prevents every contraindication, precaution, and interaction to be listed, the more common ones are included in the text.
- **Home Health Care Checklists** highlight specific issues that the patient or family may encounter while undergoing drug therapy in the home setting. As more and more patients are cared for outside the hospital, it becomes increasingly important for the nurse to know what information the patient or family needs to obtain an optimal response to the drug regimen.
- **Patient and Family Teaching Checklists** highlight teaching points relating to specific pharmacologic techniques and must-know information for the patient undergoing drug therapy. This information empowers the family to participate knowledgeably and accurately in the patient's drug regimen.
- **Summary Drug Tables** contain commonly used drugs representative of the class of drugs discussed in the chapter. Important drug information is provided,

including the generic name, pronunciation guide for generic names, trade names, adverse reactions, and dosage ranges. In these tables, generic names are followed by trade names; when a drug is available under several trade names, several of the available trade names are given. When a drug is available only by its generic name, of course, no trade name is given. The most common or serious adverse reactions associated with the drug are listed in the table's adverse reaction section. It should be noted that any patient may exhibit adverse reactions not listed in this text. Because of this possibility, the nurse, when administering any drug, should consider any sign or symptom as a *possible* adverse reaction until the cause of the problem is determined by the primary health care provider.

The adverse reactions are followed by the dosage ranges for the drug. In most cases, the adult dosage *ranges* are given in these tables because space does not permit the inclusion of all possible dosages for various types of disorders. Likewise, space limitation does not permit an inclusion of pediatric dose ranges due to the complexity of determining the pediatric dose of many drugs. Many drugs given to children are determined on the basis of body weight or body surface area and have a variety of dosage schedules. When drugs are given to the pediatric patient, the practitioner is encouraged to consult references that give complete and extensive pediatric dosages.

- **Review Questions** at the end of each chapter are written in NCLEX-PN format and provide the student an opportunity to answer questions specifically about the drugs covered in the chapter. These questions enable the student to practice answering questions concerning medication therapy and administration of drugs. Answers to these questions are provided in Appendix G.

- **Medication Dosage Problems** provide the student an opportunity for immediate application in medication administration. Because calculation of medication dosage is an important aspect of medication administration, Chapter 3 reviews the mathematics involved in dosage calculation and formulas used in the calculate medication dosages. To ensure the student's understanding and application of this type of problem, two or more medication dosage problems are included at the end of most chapters and deal with specific medications discussed in the chapter. Answers to these questions are provided in Appendix G.

- **Critical Thinking Exercises** provide realistic patient care situations that help the student apply the material contained in the chapter by exploring options and making clinical judgments related to the administration of drugs.

- A **Glossary** at the end of the book lists and defines key terms and other drug-related terms.

- **Herbal** or **Health Supplement Alerts** provide important information on common herbs and supplements not regulated under the auspices of the Federal Drug Administration. **Appendix B** lists select herbs and natural products with examples of their common and scientific name(s). While not all of the common or scientific names are given, the most common names (both common and scientific) are included. With more and more individuals using herbs as a part of their health care regimen, it is critical that the nurse be aware of the more common herbs currently in use. The nurse must consult appropriate sources when patients indicate they are using herbs as part of their health care regimen.

- **Appendix F: Key to Abbreviations** provides a list of abbreviations used in this text, particularly the Summary Drug Tables.

New Features

- **Pediatric Alerts** identify significant pediatric considerations. While the text does not deal specifically with administration of medication to children, it is important to recognize some of the common precautions or considerations when administering medications to children.

- **Chronic Care Alerts** alert the nurse to situations that may arise during drug therapy for patients with chronic illnesses, such as diabetes, hypertension, or epilepsy.

- **Interactions Tables** present interactions of the most commonly used drugs in a table format so that the student can see at a glance how interactions with other drugs or even foods may affect a patient's progress.

Organization

The text contains 58 chapters, which are divided into 11 units. Organization of the text in this manner allows the student to move about the text when these general areas are covered in the curriculum. While pharmacologic agents are presented in specific units, a disease may be treated with more than one type of drug, which may require consulting one or more units. Each unit begins with an overview of the unit content.

Unit I presents a foundation for the study of pharmacology in five chapters that cover general principles of pharmacology, the administration of drugs, a review of arithmetic and calculation of drug dosages, a discussion of the nursing process as applicable to pharmacology, and a review of the teaching–learning process and general areas of consideration when educating the patient and family.

Unit II contains 11 chapters that present the anti-infective drugs, grouped according to classification. These shorter chapters allow for more inclusive coverage of the different types of anti-infectives and the appropriate nursing considerations for each classification.

Unit III includes four chapters covering the various types of drugs used to manage pain: the non-opioid analgesics (salicylates, nonsalicylates, and nonsteroidal anti-inflammatory drugs), the opioid analgesics, and the opioid antagonists.

Unit IV has been reorganized to include 14 chapters covering the various drugs of the neuromuscular system. The unit begins with the anesthetic drugs, followed by the antianxiety drugs, sedatives and hypnotics, antidepressants, central nervous system stimulants, and the antipsychotic drugs. The remaining chapters of this unit cover the adrenergic drugs, adrenergic blocking drugs, the cholinergic drugs, the cholinergic blocking drugs, anticonvulsants, antiparkinsonism drugs, and the cholinesterase inhibitors. The last chapter of Unit IV deals with drugs used to treat disorders of the musculoskeletal system.

Unit V has three chapters concerning drugs that affect the respiratory system. The first chapter in this unit discusses antitussives, mucolytics, and expectorants; the second chapter in the unit covers antihistamines and decongestants; and the last chapter of the unit deals with bronchodilators and antiasthma drugs.

Unit VI covers drugs that affect the cardiovascular system. This unit is divided into five chapters: cardiotonics and miscellaneous inotropic drugs, antiarrhythmic drugs, antianginal and peripheral dilating drugs, antihypertensives, and antihyperlipidemics.

Unit VII consists of two chapters dealing with drugs that affect the hematological system: anticoagulants and thrombolytic drugs, and agents used in the treatment of anemia.

Unit VIII has been expanded to cover drugs that affect both the upper and lower gastrointestinal tract and the urinary system. The unit consists of four chapters: diuretics; urinary tract anti-infectives, antispasmodics, and other urinary drugs; drugs that affect the upper gastrointestinal system; and drugs that affect the lower gastrointestinal system.

Unit IX discusses drugs that affect the endocrine system and consists of five chapters: antidiabetic drugs, pituitary and andrenocortical hormones, thyroid and antithyroid drugs, male and female hormones, and drugs acting on the uterus.

Unit X discusses drugs that affect the immune system. The unit consists of two chapters: immunologic agents and antineoplastic drugs.

Unit XI consists of three chapters that discuss types of drugs not previously discussed or that are not members of a particular class or group. Chapters in this unit include topical drugs used in the treatment of skin disorders, otic and ophthalmic preparations, and fluids and electrolytes.

Chapter Content

Each chapter opens with learning objectives and a listing of key terms used and defined in the chapter. Less commonly used medical terms are also defined within the chapter and may be found in the Glossary. Chapters 1 through 5 provide introductory information concerning general principles of pharmacology, medication administration, a review of arithmetic and calculation of drug dosages, the nursing process, and patient and family teaching. Each chapter ends with critical thinking questions and several chapter review questions.

The remaining chapters discuss specific drug classifications and follow a common format. In addition to the learning objectives and key terms, the remaining chapters contain a table indicating the drug classifications and drugs discussed in the chapter. The body of each chapter contains the actions, uses, adverse reactions, contraindications, precautions, and interactions of the class or type of drug being discussed, followed by a section devoted to the nursing process. These chapters end with critical thinking questions, several chapter review questions, and two or more medication dosage problems. To promote easy retrieval of information, each area is identified by a large type heading.

- **Actions**—a basic explanation of how the drug accomplishes its intended activity.

- **Uses**—the common uses of the drug class or type are provided. No unlabeled or experimental uses of drugs are given in the text (unless specifically identified as an unlabeled use) because these uses are not approved by the FDA. Students should be reminded that, under certain circumstances, some physicians may prescribe drugs for a condition not approved by the FDA or may prescribe an experimental drug.

When discussing the use of antibiotics, this text does not list specific microorganisms. Microorganisms can become resistant to antibiotic drugs very rapidly. Because of this, the author feels that listing specific microorganisms or types of infections for an antibiotic may be misleading to the user of the text. Instead, when antibiotics are needed, the author recommends consulting culture and sensitivity studies to indicate which antibiotic has the most potential for controlling the infection.

- **Adverse Reactions**—the most common adverse drug reactions are listed under this heading

- **Contraindications**—contraindications for administration of the drug or drugs discussed in the chapter

- **Precautions**—precautions to take before, during, or after administration

- **Interactions**—more common interactions between the drug(s) discussed in the chapter and other drugs

- **Nursing Process**—with a few exceptions, the nursing process is used in every chapter of the book and is geared specifically to the administration of the drugs discussed in the chapter. The assessment phase is divided into two distinct parts to include a preadministration and ongoing assessment. This division assists the reader in determining what assessments to perform before administration of specific drugs in various drug categories and what important assessments to perform during the entire time the drug is administered. Nursing diagnoses related to the administration of the drug are highlighted in a nursing diagnoses checklist. Under "Implementation," three sections are included when applicable: "Promoting an Optimal Response to Therapy," "Monitoring and Managing Patient Needs," and "Educating the Patient and Family." These sections provide invaluable information to ensure that the drug is properly administered and that effective nursing interventions are used when certain adverse reactions occur.

Comprehensive Teaching/Learning Package

- **Student Study Guide**—*Study Guide to Accompany Introductory Clinical Pharmacology*, 8th Edition, correlates with the textbook chapter by chapter. For every chapter in the textbook, the study guide contains a corresponding chapter, each with the following three sections: Assessing Your Understanding, Applying Your Knowledge, and Practicing for NCLEX. In Assessing Your Understanding, students are provided with matching and fill-in-the-blank questions while in Applying Your Knowledge, students are asked to complete more application-based exercises, such as short-answer questions and dosage calculations. Practicing for NCLEX gives students the opportunity to engage in that very activity: our NCLEX-style multiple-choice questions are presented in the same format as that used in the NCLEX examinations and provide students with at least five questions per chapter, complete with full rationales.

- **Student CD-ROM**—Free and bound in the book, this learning tool supplies an NCLEX alternate format tutorial, **WATCH LEARN** videos on preventing medication errors, **CONCEPTS** in action **ANIMATION** 3-D animated depictions of pharmacology concepts, a Spanish-English audio glossary, and monographs of the 100 most commonly prescribed drugs.

- **Instructor's Resource CD-ROM**—This CD-ROM contains additional information and activities that will help you engage your students from the semester's beginning to its end. To begin, the CD-ROM gives you and your students even more NCLEX-style questions, this time presented within a test generator that allows you to create and edit your own exams. Additionally, the Instructor's Resource CD-ROM supplies an image bank, PowerPoint presentations to accompany each chapter, and the Answers to the Review Questions and Medication Dosage Calculations from the textbook.

- **thePoint** http://thepoint.lww.com—This web-based course and content management system provides every resource instructors and students need in one easy-to-use site. Advanced technology and superior content combine at thePoint to allow instructors to design and deliver on-line and off-line courses, maintain grades and class rosters, and communicate with students. ThePoint offers a sample syllabus and an extensive collection of materials for each chapter, which consists of the following five components: Pre-Lecture Quizzes and Answers, which are quick, knowledge-based assessments that allow you to check students' reading; PowerPoint presentations; Guided Lecture Notes, which walk you through the chapters, objective by objective, and provide you with corresponding PowerPoint slide numbers; Discussion Topics (and suggested answers), which can be used as conversation starters and are organized by objective; and Assignments (and suggested answers), which are broken up into four categories—written, group, clinical, and web—and also map back to the chapters' learning objectives. Students can visit thePoint to practice for the NCLEX with five additional NCLEX-style review questions per chapter, access supplemental multimedia resources to enhance their learning experience, check the course syllabus, download content, upload assignments, and join an on-line discussion. ThePoint . . . where teaching, learning, and technology click!

Acknowledgments

I wish to thank everyone involved in the creation of this eighth edition of *Introductory Clinical Pharmacology*. A special thanks to Elizabeth Nieginski, Acquisitions Editor, for her guidance and support during the preparation of the manuscript. My heartfelt gratitude goes to Betsy Gentzler, Associate Managing Editor, and Deedie McMahon, free-lance development editor, for their support and editorial assistance with manuscript preparation and development. My gratitude to all those who worked in any way on the design, production, and preparation of this book: Mary Kinsella, Production Editor; Brett MacNaughton, Art Director; and Holly Reid McLaughlin, Design Coordinator.

Special Acknowledgment

A very special thank you to Sue Ford for her contribution and commitment to the eighth edition of this pharmacology text. Her input from the very beginning of the revision was invaluable and her willingness to devote many hours to the revision of the chapters is deeply appreciated.

Sally S. Roach, MSN, RN, AHN-BC

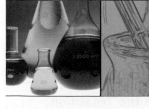

Contents

Foundations of Clinical Pharmacology

This unit provides a foundation for our study of pharmacology by discussing the general principles of pharmacology, reviewing the administration of medication and the arithmetic involved in dosage calculation, illustrating the nursing process, and discussing patient and family teaching.

Drugs are categorized as prescription (those given under the supervision of a licensed health care provider) or nonprescription (those obtained over the counter and designated as safe when taken as directed). Controlled substances are the most carefully monitored of all drugs and have the potential for abuse. Administration of a drug is a fundamental responsibility of the nurse.

Nurses have the responsibility for correctly administering the medication prescribed by the primary health care provider. The nurse administering a drug to a patient must consider the "six rights" of administration: right patient, right drug, right dose, right time, right route, and right documentation.

The nursing process is used to help members of the health care team provide effective patient care. This process is used to develop an individualized teaching plan for the patient. It is crucial that the patient understand the important information about the medication prescribed, including the dosage, how to take the medication, the expected effect, and adverse reactions.

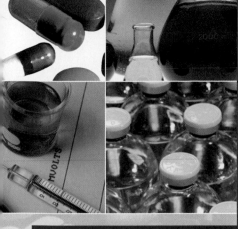

General Principles of Pharmacology

Learning Objectives

On completion of this chapter, the student will:

- Define pharmacology.
- Discuss drug development in the United States.
- Identify the different names assigned to drugs.
- Distinguish between prescription drugs, nonprescription drugs, and controlled substances.
- Discuss the various types of drug reactions produced in the body.
- Identify factors that influence drug action.
- Define drug tolerance, cumulative drug effect, and drug idiosyncrasy.
- Discuss the types of drug interactions that may be seen with drug administration.
- Discuss the nursing implications associated with drug actions, interactions, and effects.
- Discuss the use of botanical medicines.

Pharmacology is the study of drugs and their action on living organisms. A sound knowledge of basic pharmacologic principles is essential if the nurse is to administer medications safely and monitor patients who receive these medications. This chapter gives a basic overview of pharmacologic principles that the nurse must understand when administering medications. The chapter also discusses drug development, federal legislation affecting the dispensing and use of drugs, and the use of botanical medicines as they relate to pharmacology.

Drug Development

Drug development is a long and arduous process that can take from 7 to 12 years, and sometimes longer. The U.S. Food and Drug Administration (FDA) has the responsibility for approving new drugs and monitoring drugs currently in use for adverse or toxic reactions. The development of a new drug is divided into the pre-FDA phase and the FDA phase (Fig. 1-1). During the pre-FDA phase, a manufacturer discovers a drug that looks promising. In vitro testing (testing in an artificial environment, such as a test tube) using animal and human cells is done. This testing is followed by studies in live animals. The manufacturer then makes application to the FDA for Investigational New Drug (IND) status.

With IND status, clinical testing of the new drug begins. Clinical testing involves three phases, with each phase involving a larger number of people. All effects, both pharmacologic and biologic, are noted. Phase 1 involves 20 to 100 individuals who are healthy volunteers. If Phase 1 studies are successful, the testing moves to Phase 2, in which tests are performed on people who have the disease or condition for which the drug is thought to be effective. If those results are positive, the testing progresses to Phase 3, in which the drug is

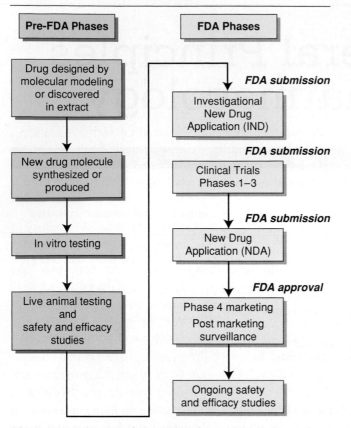

Figure 1.1 Phases of drug development. (Adapted from *PharmPhax*, 3[2], 2.)

given to large numbers of patients in medical research centers to provide information about adverse reactions. Phase 3 studies offer additional information on dosing and safety.

A New Drug Application (NDA) is submitted after the investigation of the drug in Phases 1, 2, and 3 is complete and the drug is found to be safe and effective. With the NDA, the manufacturer submits all data collected concerning the drug during the clinical trials. A panel of experts, including pharmacologists, chemists, physicians, and other professionals, reviews the application and makes a recommendation to the FDA. The FDA then either approves or disapproves the drug for use. After FDA approval, continued surveillance is done to ensure safety.

Postmarketing surveillance (Phase 4) occurs after the manufacturer places the drug on the market. During this surveillance, an ongoing review of the drug occurs with particular attention given to adverse reactions. Health care professionals are encouraged to help with this surveillance by reporting adverse effects of drugs to the FDA by using MedWatch (Display 1-1).

Display 1.1 How to Report Adverse Reactions

A drug must be used and studied for many years before all of the adverse reactions are identified. To help in identifying adverse reactions the nurse must be aware of reporting mechanisms. The FDA established a reporting program called MedWatch by which nurses or other health care professionals can report observations of serious adverse drug effects by using a standard form (see Appendix A). The FDA protects the identity of those who voluntarily report adverse reactions. This form also is used to report an undesirable experience associated with the use of medical products (e.g., latex gloves, pacemakers, infusion pumps, anaphylaxis, blood, blood components). It is important to submit reports, even if there is uncertainty about the cause–effect relationship.

Nurses play an important role in monitoring for adverse reactions. The FDA considers serious adverse reactions those that may result in death, life-threatening illness, hospitalization, or disability or those that may require medical or surgical intervention.

Adverse drug reactions may be reported to the FDA by completing the MedWatch form and sending it to:

MedWatch

5600 Fishers Lane

Rockville, MD 20852-9787

Reports may be faxed to the following number:

1-800-FDA-0178

Forms are available online and can be downloaded, completed, and returned via mail, fax, or electronic mail. See the following website:

www.fda.gov/medwatch/index.html

Special FDA Programs

Although it takes considerable time for most drugs to get FDA approval, the FDA has special programs to meet different needs. Examples of these special programs include the orphan drug program and accelerated programs for urgent needs.

Orphan Drug Program

The Orphan Drug Act of 1983 was passed to encourage the development and marketing of products used to treat rare diseases. The act defines a "rare disease" as a condition affecting fewer than 200,000 individuals in the United States or a condition affecting more than 200,000 persons in the United States but for which the cost of producing and marketing a drug to treat the condition would not be recovered by sales of the drug. The National Organization of Rare Disorders reports that there are more than 6000 rare disorders that affect approximately 25 million individuals. Examples of rare disorders include Tourette's syndrome, ovarian cancer, amyotrophic lateral sclerosis (ALS, also called Lou Gehrig's disease), Huntington's disease, and certain forms of leukemia.

The act provides for incentives, such as research grants, protocol assistance by the FDA, and special tax credits, to encourage manufacturers to develop orphan drugs. If the drug is approved, the manufacturer has 7 years of exclusive marketing rights. More than 100 new drugs have received FDA approval since the law was passed. Examples of orphan drugs include thalidomide for leprosy, triptorelin pamoate for ovarian cancer, and tetrabenazine for Huntington's disease.

Accelerated Programs

Accelerated approval of drugs is offered by the FDA as a means to make promising products for life-threatening diseases available on the market, based on preliminary evidence and before formal demonstration of patient benefit. The approval that is granted is considered a "provisional approval," with a written commitment from the pharmaceutical company to complete clinical studies that formally demonstrate patient benefit. This program seeks to make life-saving investigational drugs available before granting final approval to treat diseases that pose a significant health threat to the public. One example of a disease that qualifies as posing a significant health threat is

acquired immunodeficiency syndrome (AIDS). Because AIDS is so devastating to the individuals affected and because of the danger the disease poses to public health, the FDA and pharmaceutical companies are working together to shorten the IND approval process for some drugs that show promise in treating AIDS. This accelerated process allows primary care providers to administer medications that indicate positive results in early Phase 1 and 2 clinical trials, rather than wait until final approval is granted. If the drug continues to prove beneficial, the process of approval is accelerated.

Drug Names

Throughout the process of development, drugs may have several names assigned to them: a chemical name, a generic (nonproprietary) name, an official name, and a trade or brand name. This can be confusing, and the nurse must have a clear understanding of the different names used. For example, a drug can have several trade names. To avoid confusion, it is best to use the generic name. Table 1-1 identifies the various names and provides an explanation of each.

Drug Categories

After approval of a drug, the FDA assigns the drug to one of the following categories: prescription, nonprescription, or controlled substance.

Table 1.1 Drug Names

Drug Name and Example	Explanation
Chemical name (scientific name) Example: ethyl 4-(8-chloro-5,6-dihydro-11*H*-benzo[5,6] cyclohepta[1,2-*b*]-pyridin-11-ylidene)-1-piperidinecarboxylate	Gives the exact chemical makeup of the drug and placing of the atoms or molecular structure; the chemical name is not capitalized.
Generic name (nonproprietary) Example: loratadine	Name given to a drug before it becomes official; may be used in all countries, by all manufacturers; the generic name is not capitalized.
Official name Example: loratadine	Name listed in *The United States Pharmacopeia-National Formulary*; may be the same as the generic name.
Trade name (brand name) Example: Claritin©	Name that is registered by the manufacturer and is followed by the trademark symbol; the name can be used only by the manufacturer; a drug may have several trade names, depending on the number of manufacturers; the first letter of the trade name is capitalized.

Prescription Drugs

Prescription drugs are designated by the federal government as potentially harmful unless their use is supervised by a licensed health care provider, such as a nurse practitioner, physician, or dentist. Although these drugs have been tested for safety and therapeutic effect, prescription drugs may cause different reactions in some individuals.

In institutional settings the nurse administers the drug and monitors the patient for therapeutic effect and adverse reactions. Some drugs have the potential to be **toxic** (harmful). The nurse plays a critical role in evaluating the patient for toxic effects. When these drugs are prescribed to be taken at home, the nurse provides patient and family education about the drug.

Prescription drugs, also called *legend drugs*, are the largest category of drugs. Prescription drugs are prescribed by a licensed health care provider. The prescription (Fig. 1-2) contains the name of the drug, the dosage, the method and times of administration, and the signature of the licensed health care provider prescribing the drug.

DEA # _____

CHARLES FULLER M.D.
SUSAN LUNGLEY R.N., A.N.
1629 TREASURE HILLS
HOUSTON, TX 79635

NAME _____

ADDRESS _____ DATE _____

R$_x$

☐ Label

Refill _____ times PRN NR

_____ M.D.

To ensure brand name dispensing, prescriber must write 'Dispense As Written' on the prescription.

Figure 1.2 Example of a prescription form.

Nonprescription Drugs

Nonprescription drugs are designated by the FDA as safe (when taken as directed) and can be obtained without a prescription. These drugs are also referred to as over-the-counter (OTC) drugs and may be purchased in a variety of settings, such as a pharmacy, drugstore, or the local supermarket. Over-the-counter drugs include those given for symptoms of the common cold, headaches, constipation, diarrhea, and upset stomach.

These drugs are not without risk and may produce adverse reactions. For example, acetylsalicylic acid, commonly known as aspirin, is potentially harmful and can cause gastrointestinal bleeding and salicylism (see Chapter 17). Labeling requirements give the consumer important information regarding the drug, dosage, contraindications, precautions, and adverse reactions. Consumers are urged to read the directions carefully before taking OTC drugs.

Controlled Substances

Controlled substances are the most carefully monitored of all drugs. These drugs have a high potential for abuse and may cause physical or psychological **dependency**. **Physical dependency** is a compulsive need to use a substance repeatedly to avoid mild to severe withdrawal symptoms; it is the body's dependence on repeated administration of a drug. **Psychological dependency** is a compulsion to use a substance to obtain a pleasurable experience; it is the mind's dependence on the repeated administration of a drug. One type of dependency may lead to the other.

The Controlled Substances Act of 1970 regulates the manufacture, distribution, and dispensing of drugs that have abuse potential. Drugs under the Controlled Substances Act are divided into five schedules, based on their potential for abuse and physical and psychological dependence. Display 1-2 describes the five schedules.

Prescriptions for controlled substances must be written in ink and include the name and address of the patient and the Drug Enforcement Agency number of the primary health care provider. Prescriptions for these drugs cannot be filled more than 6 months after the prescription was written or be refilled more than five times. Under federal law, limited quantities of certain schedule C-V drugs may be purchased without a prescription, with the purchase recorded by the dispensing pharmacist. In some cases state laws are more restrictive than federal laws and impose additional requirements for the sale and distribution of controlled substances. In hospitals or other agencies that dispense controlled substances, the scheduled drugs are counted every 8 to 12 hours to account for each ampule, tablet, or other

Display 1.2 Schedules of Controlled Substances

Schedule I (C-I)
- High abuse potential
- No accepted medical use in the United States
- Examples: heroin, marijuana, LSD (lysergic acid diethylamide), peyote

Schedule II (C-II)
- Potential for high abuse with severe physical or psychological dependence
- Examples: narcotics such as meperidine, methadone, morphine, oxycodone; amphetamines; and barbiturates

Schedule III (C-III)
- Less abuse potential than schedule II drugs
- Potential for moderate physical or psychological dependence
- Examples: nonbarbiturate sedatives, nonamphetamine stimulants, limited amounts of certain narcotics

Schedule IV (C-IV)
- Less abuse potential than schedule III drugs
- Limited dependence potential
- Examples: some sedatives and anxiety agents, non-narcotic analgesics

Schedule V (C-V)*
- Limited abuse potential
- Examples: small amounts of narcotics (codeine) used as antitussives or antidiarrheals

*Under federal law, limited quantities of certain schedule V drugs may be purchased without a prescription directly from a pharmacist if allowed under state law. The purchaser must be at least 18 years of age and must furnish identification. All such transactions must be recorded by the dispensing pharmacist.

form of the drug. Any discrepancy in the number of drugs must be investigated and explained immediately.

Drug Use and Pregnancy

The use of any medication—prescription or nonprescription—carries a risk of causing birth defects in the developing fetus. Drugs administered to pregnant women, particularly during the first trimester (3 months), may have teratogenic effects. A **teratogen** is any substance that causes abnormal development of the fetus, often leading to severe deformation. Some drugs are teratogens.

In an effort to prevent teratogenic effects, the FDA has established five categories suggesting the potential of a drug for causing birth defects (Display 1-3). Information regarding the pregnancy category of a specific drug is found in reliable drug literature, such as the inserts accompanying drugs and approved drug references. In general, most drugs are contraindicated during pregnancy and lactation unless the potential benefits of taking the drug outweigh the risks to the fetus or the infant.

Display 1.3 Pregnancy Categories

Pregnancy Category A
- Controlled studies show no risk to the fetus.
- Adequate well-controlled studies in pregnant women have not demonstrated risk to the fetus.

Pregnancy Category B
- There is no evidence of risk in humans.
- Animal studies show risk, but human findings do not.
- If no adequate human studies have been done, animal studies are negative.

Pregnancy Category C
- Risk cannot be ruled out.
- Human studies are lacking, and animal studies are either positive for fetal risk or lacking.
- The drug may be used during pregnancy if the potential benefits of the drug outweigh its possible risks.

Pregnancy Category D
- There is positive evidence of risk to the human fetus.
- Investigational or postmarketing data show risk to the fetus.
- However, potential benefits may outweigh the risk to the fetus. If needed in a life-threatening situation or a serious disease, the drug may be acceptable if safer drugs cannot be used or are ineffective.

Pregnancy Category X
- Use of the drug is contraindicated in pregnancy.
- Studies in animals or humans or investigational or postmarketing reports have shown fetal risk that clearly outweighs any possible benefit to the patient.

Regardless of the pregnancy category or the presumed safety of the drug, no drug should be administered during pregnancy unless it is clearly needed and the potential benefits outweigh potential harm to the fetus.

During pregnancy, no woman should consider taking any drug, legal or illegal, prescription or nonprescription, unless the drug is prescribed or recommended by the primary health care provider. Smoking or drinking any type of alcoholic beverage also carries risks, such as low birth weight, premature birth, and fetal alcohol syndrome. Children born of mothers using addictive drugs, such as cocaine or heroin, often are born with an addiction to the drug abused by the mother. Women who are pregnant should also be very careful about the use of herbal supplements because these products can act like drugs. No woman should take a herbal supplement without discussing it first with her primary health care provider.

Drug Activity Within the Body

Drugs act in various ways in the body. Oral drugs go through three phases: the pharmaceutic phase, pharmacokinetic phase, and pharmacodynamic phase. Liquid and parenteral drugs (drugs given by injection) go through the latter two phases only.

Pharmaceutic Phase

In the **pharmaceutic** phase, dissolution of the drug occurs. Drugs must be soluble to be absorbed. Drugs that are liquid or drugs given by injection (parenteral drugs) are already dissolved and are absorbed quickly. A tablet or capsule (solid forms of a drug) goes through this phase as it disintegrates into small particles and dissolves into the body fluids in the gastrointestinal tract. Tablets that have an enteric coating do not disintegrate until they reach the alkaline environment of the small intestine.

Pharmacokinetic Phase

Pharmacokinetics refers to activities within the body after a drug is administered. These activities include absorption, distribution, metabolism, and excretion. Another pharmacokinetic component is the half-life of the drug. **Half-life** is a measure of the rate at which drugs are removed from the body.

CONCEPTSin action **ANIMATION**

Absorption

Absorption follows administration and is the process by which a drug is made available for use in the body. It occurs after dissolution of a solid form of the drug or after the administration of a liquid or parenteral drug. In this process the drug particles in the gastrointestinal tract are moved into the body fluids. This movement can be accomplished in several ways:

- Active transport—cellular energy is used to move the drug from an area of low concentration to one of high concentration
- Passive transport—no cellular energy is used as the drug moves from an area of high concentration to an area of low concentration (small molecules diffuse across the cell membrane)
- Pinocytosis—cells engulf the drug particle (the cell forms a vesicle to transport the drug into the inner cell).

As the body transfers the drug from the body fluids to the tissue sites, absorption into the body tissues occurs. Several factors influence the rate of absorption, including the route of administration, the solubility of the drug, and the presence of certain body conditions. Drugs are most rapidly absorbed when given by the intravenous route. Absorption occurs more slowly when the drug is administered orally, intramuscularly, or by the subcutaneous route because the complex membranes of the gastrointestinal mucosal layers, muscle, and skin delay drug passage. Bodily conditions such as lipodystrophy, the atrophy of subcutaneous tissue from repeated subcutaneous injections, inhibit absorption of a drug given in the lipodystrophic site.

The **first-pass effect** may also affect absorption. When a drug is absorbed by the small intestine it travels to the liver before being released to circulate to the rest of the body. The liver may metabolize a significant amount of the drug before releasing it again into the body. When the drug is released into the circulation the remaining amount of active drug may not be enough to produce a therapeutic effect, and the patient will need a higher dosage.

Distribution

The systemic circulation distributes drugs to various body tissues or target sites. Drugs interact with specific receptors during distribution. Distribution of an absorbed drug in the body depends on protein binding, blood flow, and solubility.

When a drug travels through the body it comes into contact with proteins such as the plasma protein albumin. The drug can remain free or bind to the protein. Only free drugs can produce a therapeutic effect. Drugs bound to protein are pharmacologically inactive. Only when the protein molecules release the drug can the drug diffuse into the tissues, interact with receptors, and produce a therapeutic effect. A drug is said to be highly protein bound when it is more than 80% bound to protein.

A drug is distributed quickly to areas with a large blood supply such as the heart, liver, and kidneys. In other areas such as the internal organs, skin, and muscle, distribution of the drug occurs more slowly.

Solubility or the drug's ability to cross the cell membrane affects its distribution. Lipid-soluble drugs easily cross the cell membrane, whereas water-soluble drugs do not.

Metabolism

Metabolism, also called **biotransformation**, is the process by which the body changes a drug to a more or less active form that can be excreted. Usually the resulting form is a **metabolite** (an inactive form of the original drug). In some drugs one or more of the metabolites may have some drug activity. Metabolites may undergo further metabolism or may be excreted from the body unchanged. Most drugs are metabolized by the liver, although the kidneys, lungs, plasma, and intestinal mucosa also aid in the metabolism of drugs.

Excretion

The elimination of drugs from the body is called *excretion*. After the liver renders drugs inactive, the kidney excretes the inactive compounds from the body. Also, some drugs are excreted unchanged by the kidney without liver involvement. Patients with kidney disease may require a dosage reduction and careful monitoring of kidney function. Children have immature kidney function and may require dosage reduction and kidney function tests. Similarly, older adults have diminished kidney function and require careful monitoring and lower dosages. Other drugs are eliminated in sweat, breast milk, or breath, or by the gastrointestinal tract through the feces.

Half-Life

Half-life refers to the time required for the body to eliminate 50% of the drug. Knowledge of the half-life of a drug is important in planning the frequency of dosing. For example, drugs with a short half-life (2 to 4 hours) need to be administered frequently, whereas a drug with a long half-life (21 to 24 hours) requires less frequent administration. It takes five to six half-lives to eliminate approximately 98% of a drug from the body. Although half-life is fairly stable, patients with liver or kidney disease may have problems excreting a drug. Difficulty in excreting a drug increases the half-life and increases the risk of toxicity. For example, digoxin (Lanoxin) has a long half-life (36 hours) and requires once-daily dosing. However, aspirin has a short half-life and requires frequent dosing. Older patients or patients with impaired kidney or liver function require frequent diagnostic tests measuring renal or hepatic function.

Onset, Peak, and Duration

Three other factors are important when considering a drug's pharmacokinetics:

- Onset of action—time between administration of the drug and onset of its therapeutic effect

- Peak concentration—when absorption rate equals the elimination rate (not always the time of peak response)
- Duration of action—length of time the drug produces a therapeutic effect.

Pharmacodynamic Phase

Pharmacodynamics is the study of the drug mechanisms that produce biochemical or physiologic changes in the body. Pharmacodynamics deals with the drug's action and effect in the body. After administration, most drugs enter the systemic circulation and expose almost all body tissues to possible effects of the drug. All drugs produce more than one effect in the body. The primary effect of a drug is the desired or therapeutic effect. Secondary effects are all other effects, desirable or undesirable, produced by the drug.

Most drugs have an affinity for certain organs or tissues and exert their greatest action at the cellular level on those specific areas, which are called *target sites*. A drug exerts it action by two main mechanisms:

1. Alteration in cellular function
2. Alteration in cellular environment

Alteration in Cellular Function

Most drugs act on the body by altering cellular function. A drug cannot completely change the function of a cell, but it can alter its function. A drug that alters cellular function can increase or decrease certain physiologic functions, such as increasing heart rate, decreasing blood pressure, or increasing urine output.

RECEPTOR-MEDIATED DRUG ACTION Many drugs act through drug–receptor interaction. The function of a cell alters when a drug interacts with a receptor. This occurs when a drug molecule selectively joins with a reactive site—known as a **receptor**—on the surface of a cell. When a drug binds to and interacts with the receptor, a pharmacologic response occurs.

An **agonist** is a drug that binds with a receptor and stimulates the receptor to produce a therapeutic response. An **antagonist** is a drug that joins with receptors but does not stimulate the receptors. The therapeutic action in this case consists of blocking the receptor's function.

There are two types of antagonists: competitive antagonists and noncompetitive antagonists. A competitive antagonist competes with the agonists for receptor sites. Because competitive agonists bind reversibly with receptor sites, administering larger doses of an agonist can overcome the antagonist effects. The noncompetitive antagonist binds with receptor sites and always blocks the effects of the agonists. Administering larger doses of the agonists will not reverse the action of the noncompetitive antagonist.

RECEPTOR-MEDIATED DRUG EFFECTS The number of available receptor sites influences the effects of a drug. When only a few receptor sites are occupied, although many sites are available, the response will be small. When the drug dose is increased, more receptor sites are used and the response increases. When only a few receptor sites are available, the response does not increase when more of the drug is administered. However, not all receptors on a cell need to be occupied for a drug to be effective. Some extremely potent drugs are effective even when the drug occupies few receptor sites.

Alteration in Cellular Environment

Some drugs act on the body by changing the cellular environment, either physically or chemically. Physical changes in the cellular environment include changes in osmotic pressure, lubrication, absorption, or the conditions on the surface of the cell membrane. An example of a drug that changes osmotic pressure is mannitol, which produces a change in the osmotic pressure in brain cells, causing a reduction in cerebral edema. A drug that acts by altering the cellular environment by lubrication is sunscreen. An example of a drug that acts by altering absorption is activated charcoal, which is administered orally to absorb a toxic chemical ingested into the gastrointestinal tract. The stool softener docusate is an example of a drug that acts by altering the surface of the cellular membrane. Docusate has emulsifying and lubricating activity that lowers the surface tension in the cells of the bowel, permitting water and fats to enter the stool. This softens the fecal mass, allowing easier passage of the stool.

Chemical changes in the cellular environment include inactivation of cellular functions or alteration of the chemical components of body fluid, such as a change in the pH. For example, antacids neutralize gastric acidity in patients with peptic ulcers.

Other drugs, such as some anticancer drugs and some antibiotics, have as their main site of action the cell membrane and various cellular processes. They incorporate themselves into the normal metabolic processes of the cell and cause the formation of a defective final product, such as a weakened cell wall, which results in cell death, or produce a lack of a needed energy substrate that leads to cell starvation and death.

Drug Reactions

Drugs produce many reactions in the body. The following sections discuss adverse drug reactions, allergic drug reactions, drug idiosyncrasy, drug tolerance, cumulative drug effect, and toxic reactions. Pharmacogenetic reactions can also occur. A pharmacogenetic reaction is a genetically determined adverse reaction to a drug.

Adverse Drug Reactions

Patients may experience one or more adverse reactions or side effects when they are given a drug. **Adverse reactions** are undesirable drug effects. Adverse reactions may be common or may occur infrequently. They may be mild, severe, or life-threatening. They may occur after the first dose, after several doses, or after many doses. Often, an adverse reaction is unpredictable, although some drugs are known to cause certain adverse reactions in many patients. For example, drugs used in treating cancer are very toxic and are known to produce adverse reactions in many patients receiving them. Other drugs produce adverse reactions in fewer patients. Some adverse reactions are predictable, but many adverse drug reactions occur without warning.

Some texts use both terms *side effects* and *adverse reactions*, using *side effects* to explain mild, common, and non-toxic reactions and *adverse reactions* to describe more severe and life-threatening reactions. For the purposes of this text, only the term *adverse reactions* is used, with the understanding that these reactions may be mild, severe, or life-threatening.

Allergic Drug Reactions

An **allergic reaction** is also called a **hypersensitivity** reaction. Allergy to a drug usually begins to occur after more than one dose of the drug is given. On occasion, the nurse may observe an allergic reaction the first time a drug is given because the patient has received or taken the drug in the past.

A drug allergy occurs because the individual's immune system views the drug as a foreign substance called an **antigen**. When the body views the drug as an antigen, a series of events occurs in an attempt to render the invader harmless. Lymphocytes respond by forming **antibodies** (protein substances that protect against antigens). Common allergic reactions occur when the individual's immune system responds aggressively to the antigen. Chemical mediators released during the allergic reaction produce symptoms ranging from mild to life-threatening.

Even a mild allergic reaction produces serious effects if it goes unnoticed and the drug is given again. Any indication of an allergic reaction is reported to the primary health care provider before the next dose of the drug is given. Serious allergic reactions require contacting the primary health care provider immediately because emergency treatment may be necessary.

Some allergic reactions occur within minutes (even seconds) after the drug is given; others may be delayed for hours or days. Allergic reactions that occur immediately often are the most serious.

Allergic reactions are manifested by a variety of signs and symptoms observed by the nurse or reported by the patient. Examples of some allergic symptoms include itching, various types of skin rashes, and hives (urticaria). Other symptoms include difficulty breathing, wheezing, cyanosis, a sudden loss of consciousness, and swelling of the eyes, lips, or tongue.

Anaphylactic shock is an extremely serious allergic drug reaction that usually occurs shortly after the administration of a drug to which the individual is sensitive. This type of allergic reaction requires immediate medical attention. Symptoms of anaphylactic shock are listed in Table 1-2.

All or only some of these symptoms may be present. Anaphylactic shock can be fatal if the symptoms are not identified and treated immediately. Treatment is to raise the blood pressure, improve breathing, restore cardiac function, and treat other symptoms as they occur. Epinephrine (adrenalin) 0.1 to 0.5 mg may be given by subcutaneous injection in the upper extremity or thigh and may be followed by a continuous intravenous infusion. Hypotension and shock may be treated with fluids and vasopressors. Bronchodilators are given to relax the smooth muscles of the bronchial tubes. Antihistamines and corticosteroids may also be given to treat urticaria (hives) and angioedema (swelling).

Table 1.2 Symptoms of Anaphylactic Shock

Respiratory	Bronchospasm Dyspnea (difficult breathing) Feeling of fullness in the throat Cough Wheezing
Cardiovascular	Extremely low blood pressure Tachycardia (heart rate >100 bpm) Palpitations Syncope (fainting) Cardiac arrest
Integumentary	Urticaria (hives) Angioedema Pruritus (itching) Sweating
Gastrointestinal	Nausea Vomiting Abdominal pain

Angioedema (angioneurotic edema) is another type of allergic drug reaction. It is manifested by the collection of fluid in subcutaneous tissues. Areas that are most commonly affected are the eyelids, lips, mouth, and throat, although other areas also may be affected. Angioedema can be dangerous when the mouth is affected because the swelling may block the airway and asphyxia may occur. Difficulty in breathing and swelling in any area of the body are reported immediately to the primary health care provider.

Drug Idiosyncrasy

Drug idiosyncrasy is a term used to describe any unusual or abnormal reaction to a drug. It is any reaction that is different from the one normally expected from a specific drug and dose. For example, a patient may be given a drug to help him or her sleep (e.g., a hypnotic). Instead of falling asleep, the patient remains wide awake and shows signs of nervousness or excitement. This response is idiosyncratic because it is different from what the nurse expects from this type of drug. Another patient may receive the same drug and dose, fall asleep, and after 8 hours be difficult to awaken. This, too, is abnormal and describes an over-response to the drug.

The cause of drug idiosyncrasy is not clear. It is believed to be due to a genetic deficiency that makes the patient unable to tolerate certain chemicals, including drugs.

Drug Tolerance

Drug tolerance is a term used to describe a decreased response to a drug, requiring an increase in dosage to achieve the desired effect. Drug tolerance may develop when a patient takes certain drugs, such as narcotics and tranquilizers, for a long time. The individual who takes these drugs at home increases the dose when the expected drug effect does not occur. The development of drug tolerance is a sign of drug dependence. Drug tolerance may also occur in the hospitalized patient. When the patient receives a narcotic for more than 10 to 14 days, the nurse suspects drug tolerance (and possibly drug dependence). The patient may also begin to ask for the drug at more frequent intervals.

Cumulative Drug Effect

A **cumulative drug effect** may be seen in those with liver or kidney disease because these organs are the major sites for the breakdown and excretion of most drugs. This drug effect occurs when the body is unable to metabolize and excrete one (normal) dose of a drug before the next dose is given. Thus, if a second dose of the drug is given, some drug from the first dose remains in the body. A cumulative drug effect can be serious because too much of the drug can accumulate in the body and lead to toxicity.

Patients with liver or kidney disease are usually given drugs with caution because a cumulative effect may occur. When the patient is unable to excrete the drug at a normal rate, the drug accumulates in the body, causing a toxic reaction. Sometimes, the primary health care provider lowers the dose of the drug to prevent a toxic drug reaction.

Toxic Reactions

Most drugs can produce **toxic** or harmful reactions if administered in large dosages or when blood concentration levels exceed the therapeutic level. Toxic levels build up when a drug is administered in dosages that exceed the normal level or if the patient's kidneys are not functioning properly and cannot excrete the drug. Some toxic effects are immediately visible; others may not be seen for weeks or months. Some drugs, such as lithium or digoxin, have a narrow margin of safety, even when given in recommended dosages. It is important to monitor these drugs closely to detect and avoid toxicity.

Drug toxicity can be reversible or irreversible, depending on the organs involved. Damage to the liver may be reversible because liver cells can regenerate. However, hearing loss from damage to the eighth cranial nerve caused by toxic reaction to the anti-infective drug streptomycin may be permanent. Sometimes drug toxicity can be reversed by administering another drug that acts as an antidote. For example, in serious instances of digitalis toxicity, the drug Digibind may be given to counteract the effect of digoxin toxicity.

Nurses must carefully monitor the patient's blood level of drug to ensure that the level remains within the therapeutic range. Any deviation should be reported to the primary health care provider. Because some drugs can cause toxic reactions even in recommended doses, the nurse should be aware of the signs and symptoms of toxicity of commonly prescribed drugs.

Pharmacogenetic Reactions

A **pharmacogenetic disorder** is a genetically determined abnormal response to normal doses of a drug. This abnormal response occurs because of inherited traits that cause abnormal metabolism of drugs. For example, individuals with glucose-6-phosphate dehydrogenase (G6PD) deficiency have abnormal reactions to a number of drugs. These patients exhibit varying degrees of hemolysis (destruction of red blood cells) when these drugs are administered. More than 100 million people are affected by this disorder. Examples of drugs that cause hemolysis

in patients with a G6PD deficiency include aspirin, chloramphenicol, and the sulfonamides.

Drug Interactions

It is important for the nurse administering medications to be aware of the various drug interactions that can occur, especially drug–drug interactions and drug–food interactions. This section gives a brief overview of drug interactions. Specific drug–drug and drug–food interactions are discussed in subsequent chapters.

Drug–Drug Interactions

A drug–drug interaction occurs when one drug interacts with or interferes with the action of another drug. For example, taking an antacid with oral tetracycline causes a decrease in the effectiveness of the tetracycline. The antacid chemically interacts with the tetracycline and impairs its absorption into the bloodstream, thus reducing the effectiveness of the tetracycline. Drugs known to cause interactions include oral anticoagulants, oral hypoglycemics, anti-infectives, antiarrhythmics, cardiac glycosides, and alcohol. Drug–drug interactions can produce effects that are additive, synergistic, or antagonistic.

Additive Drug Reaction

An **additive drug reaction** occurs when the combined effect of two drugs is equal to the sum of each drug given alone. For example, taking the drug heparin with alcohol will increase bleeding. The equation $1 + 1 = 2$ is sometimes used to illustrate the additive effect of drugs.

Synergistic Drug Reaction

Drug **synergism** occurs when drugs interact with each other and produce an effect that is greater than the sum of their separate actions. The equation $1 + 1 = 4$ may be used to illustrate synergism. Drug synergism is exemplified when a person takes both a hypnotic and alcohol. When alcohol is taken simultaneously or shortly before or after the hypnotic is taken, the action of the hypnotic increases. The individual experiences a drug effect that is greater than if either drug was taken alone. On occasion, the occurrence of a synergistic drug effect is serious and even fatal.

Antagonistic Drug Reaction

An antagonistic drug reaction occurs when one drug interferes with the action of another, causing neutralization or a decrease in the effect of one drug. For example, protamine sulfate is a heparin antagonist. This means that the administration of protamine sulfate completely neutralizes the effects of heparin in the body.

Drug–Food Interactions

When a drug is given orally, food may impair or enhance its absorption. A drug taken on an empty stomach is absorbed into the bloodstream more quickly than when the drug is taken with food in the stomach. Some drugs (e.g., captopril) must be taken on an empty stomach to achieve an optimal effect. Drugs that should be taken on an empty stomach are administered 1 hour before or 2 hours after meals. Other drugs—especially drugs that irritate the stomach, result in nausea or vomiting, or cause epigastric distress—are best given with food or meals. This minimizes gastric irritation. The nonsteroidal anti-inflammatory drugs and salicylates are examples of drugs that are given with food to decrease epigastric distress. Still other drugs combine with a food, forming an insoluble food–drug mixture. For example, when tetracycline is administered with dairy products, a drug–food mixture is formed that is unabsorbable by the body. When a drug is unabsorbable by the body, no pharmacologic effect occurs.

Factors Influencing Drug Response

Certain factors may influence drug response and are considered when the primary health care provider prescribes and the nurse administers a drug. These factors include age, weight, sex, disease, and route of administration.

Age

The age of the patient may influence the effects of a drug. Infants and children usually require smaller doses of a drug than adults. Immature organ function, particularly of the liver and kidneys, can affect the ability of infants and young children to metabolize drugs. An infant's immature kidneys impair the elimination of drugs in the urine. Liver function is poorly developed in infants and young children. Drugs metabolized by the liver may produce more intense effects for longer periods. Parents must be taught the potential problems associated with administering drugs to their children. For example, a safe dose of a nonprescription drug for a 4-year-old child may be dangerous for a 6-month-old infant.

Elderly patients may also require smaller doses, although this may depend on the type of drug administered. For example, the elderly patient may be given the same dose of an antibiotic as a younger adult. However, the same older adult may require a smaller dose of a drug that depresses the central nervous system, such as a narcotic. Changes that occur with aging affect the pharmacokinetics (absorption, distribution, metabolism, and excretion) of a drug. Any of these processes may be altered because of the physiologic changes that occur with aging. Table 1-3 summarizes the changes that occur with aging and their possible pharmacokinetic effects.

Polypharmacy is the taking of numerous drugs that can potentially react with one another. When practiced by elderly patients in particular, polypharmacy leads to an

Table 1.3 Factors Altering Drug Response in the Elderly

Age-Related Changes	Effect on Drug Therapy
Decreased gastric acidity; decreased gastric motility	Possible decreased or delayed absorption
Dry mouth and decreased saliva	Difficulty swallowing oral drugs
Decreased liver blood flow; decreased liver mass	Delayed and decreased metabolism of certain drugs; possible increased effect, leading to toxicity
Decreased lipid content of the skin	Possible decrease in absorption of transdermal drugs
Increased body fat; decreased body water	Possible increase in toxicity of water-soluble drugs; more prolonged effects of fat-soluble drugs
Decreased serum proteins	Possible increased effect and toxicity of highly protein-bound drugs
Decreased renal mass, blood flow, and glomerular filtration rate	Possible increased serum levels, leading to toxicity of drugs excreted by the kidney
Changes in sensitivity of certain drug receptors	Increase or decrease in drug effect

Adapted from Eisenhauer, L., Nichols, L., Spencer, R., & Bergan, F. (1998). *Clinical pharmacology and nursing management* (5th ed., p. 189). Philadelphia: Lippincott-Raven. Used with permission.

increase in the number of potential adverse reactions. Although multiple drug therapy is necessary to treat certain disease states, it always increases the possibility of adverse reactions. The nurse needs good assessment skills to detect any problems when monitoring the geriatric patient's response to drug therapy.

Weight

In general, dosages are based on a weight of approximately 150 lb, which is calculated to be the average weight of men and women. A drug dose may sometimes be increased or decreased because the patient's weight is significantly higher or lower than this average. With narcotics, for example, higher or lower than average dosages may be necessary, depending on the patient's weight, to produce relief of pain.

Sex

The sex of an individual may influence the action of some drugs. Women may require a smaller dose of some drugs than men. This is because many women are smaller and have a different body fat-to-water ratio than men.

Disease

The presence of disease may influence the action of some drugs. Sometimes disease is an indication for not prescribing a drug or for reducing the dose of a certain drug. Both hepatic (liver) and renal (kidney) disease can greatly affect drug response.

In liver disease, for example, the ability to metabolize or detoxify a specific type of drug may be impaired. If the average or normal dose of the drug is given, the liver may be unable to metabolize the drug at a normal rate. Consequently, the drug may be excreted from the body at a much slower rate than normal. The primary health care provider may then decide to prescribe a lower dose and lengthen the time between doses because liver function is abnormal.

Patients with kidney disease may exhibit drug toxicity and a longer duration of drug action. The dosage of drugs may be reduced to prevent the accumulation of toxic levels in the blood or further injury to the kidney.

Route of Administration

Intravenous administration of a drug produces the most rapid drug action. Next in order of time of action is the intramuscular route, followed by the subcutaneous route. Giving a drug orally usually produces the slowest drug action.

Some drugs can be given only by one route; for example, antacids are given only orally. Other drugs are available in oral and parenteral forms. The primary health care provider selects the route of administration based on many factors, including the desired rate of action. For example, the patient with a severe cardiac problem may require intravenous administration of a drug that affects the heart. Another patient with a mild cardiac problem may experience a good response to oral administration of the same drug.

Nursing Implications

Many factors can influence drug action. The nurse should consult appropriate references or the hospital pharmacist if there is any question about the dosage of a drug, whether other drugs the patient is receiving will interfere with the drug being given, or whether the oral drug should or should not be given with food.

Drug reactions are potentially serious. The nurse should observe all patients for adverse drug reactions, drug idiosyncrasy, and evidence of drug tolerance (when applicable). It is important to report all drug reactions or any unusual drug effect to the primary health care provider.

The nurse must use good judgment about when to report adverse drug reactions to the primary health care provider. Accurate observation and evaluation of the circumstances are essential; the nurse should record all observations in the patient's record. If there is any question regarding the events that are occurring, the nurse can withhold the drug but must contact the primary health care provider.

National Center for Complementary and Alternative Medicine

The National Center for Complementary and Alternative Medicine (NCCAM) is one of the 27 institutes and centers that make up the National Institutes of Health (NIH). NIH is one of eight agencies in the Public Health Service in the U.S. Department of Health and Human Services (DHHS). NCCAM explores complementary and alternative healing practices through scientific research. It also trains complementary/alternative medicine (CAM) scientists and disseminates the information gleaned from the research it conducts. Among the various purposes of the NCCAM, one is to evaluate the safety and efficacy of widely used natural products, such as herbal remedies and dietary and food supplements. The Center is dedicated to developing programs and encouraging scientists to investigate CAM treatments that show promise. The NCCAM budget has steadily grown from $2 million in 1993 to more than $123 million in 2005. This funding increase reflects the public's interest and need for CAM information that is based on rigorous scientific research.

The NCCAM defines CAM as a "group of diverse medical and health care systems, practices, and products that are not presently considered to be part of conventional medicine." Examples of complementary therapies are therapies such as relaxation techniques, massage, aromatherapy, and healing touch. Complementary therapies are often used with traditional health care to "complement" conventional medicine. Alternative therapies, on the other hand, are therapies used in place of or instead of conventional or Western medicine. The term *complementary/alternative therapy* often is used as an umbrella term for many therapies from all over the world. NCCAM is the federal government's leading agency for scientific research on CAM. NCCAM uses rigorous science to explore CAM therapies, train researchers, and disseminate information on CAM.

Herbal Therapy and Dietary Supplements

Botanical medicine or herbal therapy is a type of complementary/alternative therapy that uses plants or herbs to treat various disorders. Individuals worldwide use herbal therapy and dietary supplements extensively. According to the World Health Organization (WHO), 80% of the world's population relies on herbs for a substantial part of their health care. Herbs have been used by virtually every culture in the world throughout history. For example, Hippocrates prescribed St. John's wort, currently a popular herbal remedy for depression. Native Americans used plants such as coneflower, ginseng, and ginger for therapeutic purposes. Herbal therapy is part of the group of nontraditional therapies commonly known as CAM.

Dietary Supplement Health and Education Act

Because herbs cannot be sold and promoted in the United States as drugs, they are regulated as nutritional or dietary substances. *Nutritional* or *dietary substances* are terms used by the federal government to identify substances that are not regulated as drugs by the FDA but purported to be effective for use to promote health. Herbs, as well as vitamins and minerals, are classified as dietary or nutritional supplements. This means that they do not have to meet the same standards as drug and over-the-counter medications for proof of safety and effectiveness and what the FDA calls "good manufacturing practices."

Because natural products cannot be patented in the United States, it is not profitable for drug manufacturers to spend the millions of dollars and the 7 to 12 years to study and develop these products as drugs. In 1994, the U.S. government passed the Dietary Supplement Health and Education Act (DSHEA). This act defines substances such as herbs, vitamins, minerals, amino acids, and other natural substances as "dietary supplements." The act permits general health claims such as "improves memory" or "promotes regularity" as long as the label also has a disclaimer stating that the supplements are not approved by the FDA and are not intended to diagnose, treat, cure, or prevent any disease. The claims must be truthful and not misleading and supported by scientific evidence. Some manufacturers have abused the law by making exaggerated claims, but the FDA has the power to enforce the law, which it has done, and these claims have decreased.

Educating Clients About Herbs and Dietary Supplements

The use of herbs and dietary supplements to treat various disorders is common. Herbs are used for various effects, such as boosting the immune system, treating depression, and promoting relaxation. Individuals are becoming more aware of the benefits of herbal therapies and dietary supplements. Advertisements, books, magazines, and Internet sites concerning these topics are prolific. People eager to cure or control various disorders take herbs, teas, megadoses of vitamins, and various other natural products. Although much information is available on dietary supplements and herbal therapy, obtaining the correct information can be difficult at times. Medicinal herbs and dietary substances are available at supermarkets, pharmacies, health food stores, specialty herb stores, and through the Internet. The potential for misinformation abounds. Because these substances are "natural products," many individuals incorrectly assume that they are without adverse effects. When any herbal remedy or dietary supplement is used, it should be reported to the nurse and the primary health care provider. Many of these botanicals have strong pharmacologic activity, and some may interact with prescription drugs or be toxic in the body. For example, comfrey, an herb that was once widely used to promote digestion, can cause liver damage. Although it may still be available in some areas, it is a dangerous herb and is not recommended for use as a supplement.

When obtaining the drug history, the nurse must always question the patient about the use of herbs, teas, vitamins, or other dietary supplements. Many patients consider herbs as natural and therefore safe. Some also neglect to report the use of an herbal tea as a part of the health care regimen because they do not think of it as such. The nurse should explain to the patient that just because an herbal supplement is labeled "natural," it does not mean the supplement is safe or without harmful effects. Herbal supplements can act the same way as drugs and can cause medical problems if not used correctly or if taken in large amounts. Display 1-4 identifies teaching points to consider when discussing the use of herbs and dietary supplements with patients.

Although a complete discussion about the use of herbs is beyond the scope of this book, it is important to remember that the use of herbs and dietary supplements is com-

monplace in many areas of the country. To help the student become more aware of herbal therapy and dietary supplements, Appendix B gives an overview of selected common herbs and dietary supplements. In addition, "alerts" related to herbs and dietary supplements appear throughout this text to alert the student to valuable information and precautions.

Critical Thinking Exercises

1. Judy Martin, a student nurse, has just administered an antibiotic to Mr. Green. When she returns to the room about 30 minutes later, she finds Mr. Green flushed, reporting a lump in his throat, and experiencing difficulty breathing. Determine what actions the student nurse should take.

2. Jenny Davis, aged 25 years, is pregnant. Jenny's primary health care provider tells her that she may not take any medication without first checking with the health care provider during the pregnancy. Jenny is puzzled and questions you about this. Discuss how you would address Jenny's concerns.

3. Ms. James, 80 years of age, is receiving a low dose of meperidine (Demerol), a narcotic analgesic, for postoperative pain. Her family questions the use of such a low dose. Determine what information you would give her family when they voice concerns that the dosage will not adequately relieve their mother's pain. Analyze what patient assessment, if any, you would need to make before talking with the family.

Display 1.4 Teaching Points When Discussing Herbal Therapy

- If you regularly use herbal therapies, invest in a good herbal reference book such as *Guide to Popular Natural Products*, edited by Ara DerMarderosian (Facts and Comparisons 2005).
- Store clerks are not experts in herbal therapy. Your best choice is to select an herbal product manufactured by a reputable company.
- Check the label for the word "standardized." This means that the product has a specific percentage of a specific chemical.
- Some herbal tinctures are 50% alcohol, which could pose a problem to individuals with a history of alcohol abuse.
- Use products with more than six herbs cautiously. It is generally better to use the single herb than to use a diluted product with several herbs.
- Do not overmedicate with herbs. The adage "If one is good, two must be better" is definitely not true. Take only the recommended dosage.
- Herbs are generally safe when taken in recommended dosages. However, if you experience any different or unusual symptoms, such as heart palpitations, headaches, rashes, or difficulty breathing, stop taking the herb and contact your health care provider.
- Inform your primary health care provider of any natural products that you take (e.g., herbs, vitamins, minerals, teas). Certain herbs can interact with the medications that you take, causing serious adverse reactions or toxic effects.
- Allow time for the herb to work. Generally, 30 days is sufficient. If your symptoms have not improved within 30 to 60 days, discontinue use of the herb.

Adapted from Fontaine, K. L. (2000). *Heating practices: Alternative therapies for nursing* (pp. 126–127). Upper Saddle River, NJ: Prentice Hall. Used with permission.

Review Questions

1. Mr. Carter has a rash and pruritus. You suspect an allergic reaction and immediately assess him for other more serious symptoms. What question would be most important to ask Mr. Carter?

   A. Are you having any difficulty breathing?

   B. Have you noticed any blood in your stool?

   C. Do you have a headache?

   D. Are you having difficulty with your vision?

2. Mr. Jones, a newly admitted patient, has a history of liver disease. In planning Mr. Jones' care, the nurse must consider that liver disease may result in a(n) _____.

   A. increase in the excretion rate of a drug

   B. impaired ability to metabolize or detoxify a drug

   C. need to increase the dosage of a drug

   D. decrease in the rate of drug absorption

3. Under the Controlled Substances Act, schedule V drugs are classified with a limited abuse potential. Which of the following are examples of schedule V drugs?

A. Narcotics

B. Antidiarrheals with codeine

C. Nonbarbiturate sedatives

D. Marijuana

4. A patient asks the nurse to define a hypersensitivity reaction. The nurse begins by telling the patient that a hypersensitivity reaction is also called a(n) _____ _____.

A. synergistic reaction

B. antagonistic reaction

C. drug idiosyncrasy

D. allergic reaction

5. In monitoring drug therapy, the nurse is aware that a synergistic drug effect may be defined as _____.

A. an effect greater than the sum of the separate actions of two or more drugs

B. an increase in the action of one of the two drugs being given

C. a neutralizing drug effect

D. a comprehensive drug effect

To check your answers, see Appendix G.

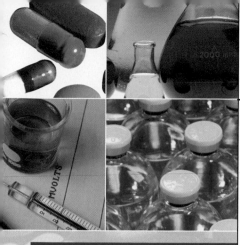

Administration of Drugs

Learning Objectives

On completion of this chapter, the student will:

- Discuss the six rights of drug administration.
- Discuss ways the nurse can avoid drug errors.
- Identify the different types of medication orders.
- Discuss the 2006 National Patient Safety Goals.
- Describe the various types of medication dispensing systems.
- Discuss general principles of drug administration.
- Describe general guidelines the nurse should follow when preparing a drug for administration.
- Discuss the administration of oral and parenteral drugs.
- Discuss the administration of drugs through the skin and mucous membranes.
- Discuss nursing responsibilities before, during, and after a drug is administered.

The administration of a drug is a fundamental responsibility of the nurse. An understanding of the basic concepts of administering drugs is critical if the nurse is to perform this task safely and accurately. In addition to administering the drug, the nurse monitors the therapeutic response (desired response) and reports adverse reactions. In the home setting, the nurse is responsible for teaching the patient and family members the information needed to administer drugs safely in an outpatient setting.

The Six Rights of Drug Administration

The nurse preparing and administering a drug to a patient assumes responsibility for this procedure. Responsibility entails preparing and administering the prescribed drug. There are six "rights" in the administration of drugs:

- Right patient
- Right drug
- Right dose
- Right route
- Right time
- Right documentation

Right Patient

When administering a drug, the nurse must be certain that the patient receiving the drug is the patient for whom the drug has been ordered. It is important to use two methods to identify the patient before administering the medication. This is accomplished by checking the patient's name on his or her wristband (Fig. 2-1). If

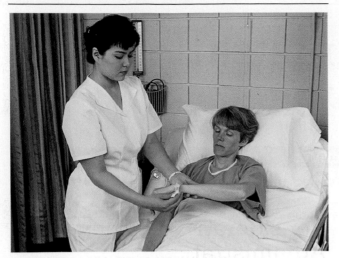

Figure 2.1 In following the "six rights" of medication administration, the nurse always verifies that the "right patient" is receiving the medication by using two identifiers, one of which is checking the patient's identification bracelet. (Photograph © B. Proud.)

there is no written identification verifying the patient's name, the nurse obtains a wristband or other form of identification before administering the drug. The nurse may also ask the patient to identify himself. However, the nurse should not ask, "Are you Mr. Jones?" Some patients, particularly those who are confused or have difficulty hearing, may respond by answering "yes" even though that is not

their name. Some nursing homes or extended care facilities have pictures of the patient available, which allows the nurse to verify the correct patient. If pictures are used to identify patients, it is critical that they are recent and bear a good likeness of the individual.

Right Drug

Drug names are often confused, especially when the names sound similar or the spellings are similar. Nurses who hurriedly prepare a drug for administration or who fail to look up questionable drugs are at increased risk for administering the wrong drug. Table 2-1 identifies examples of drugs that can easily be confused. The nurse should compare medication, container label, and medication record (Fig. 2-2).

Right Dose, Route, and Time

The nurse should obtain a primary care provider's written order for the administration of all drugs. The primary care provider's order must include the patient's name, the drug name, the dosage form and route, the dosage to be administered, and the frequency of administration. The primary care provider's signature must follow the drug order. In an emergency, the nurse may administer a drug with a verbal order from the primary care provider. However, the primary care provider must write and sign the order as soon as the emergency is over.

Any order that is unclear should be questioned, particularly unclear directions for the administration of the

Table 2.1 Examples of Drugs That Are Easily Confused With Other Drugs

Drug Name	Confused With	Drug Name	Confused With
acctohexamide	acctazolamide	K-Dur	Imdur
albuterol	atenolol	Klonopin	clonidine
Alupent	Atrovent	lamivudine	lamotrigine
Amikin	Amicar	Nicobid	Nitro-Bid
bretylium	Brevibloc	nifedipine	nicardipine
chlorpropamide	chlorpromazine	prednisolone	prednisone
Cefzil	Ceftin	Prilosec	Prozac
clonidine	clonazepam	Retrovir	ritonavir
DiaBeta	Zebeta	Taxol	Paxil
dobutamine	dopamine	TobraDex	Tobrex
Elavil	Mellaril	Versed	VePesid
Flomax	Fosamax	Zocor	Zoloft
Inderal	Isordil	Zyvox	Vioxx

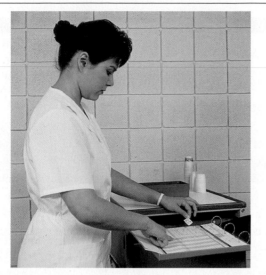

Figure 2.2 Before administering the medication, the nurse compares the medication, the container label, and the medication record to ensure that the patient received the "right drug" and the "right dose." (Photograph © B. Proud.)

drug, illegible handwriting on the primary care provider's order sheet, or a drug dose that is higher or lower than the dosages given in approved references.

Right Documentation

After the administration of any drug, the nurse records the process immediately (Fig. 2-3). Immediate documentation is particularly important when drugs are given on an as-needed (PRN) basis. For example, most analgesics require 20 to 30 minutes before the drug begins to relieve pain. A patient may forget that he or she received a drug for pain,

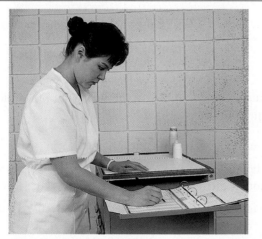

Figure 2.3 The nurse always documents the medication immediately after the drug is administered. (Photograph © B. Proud.)

may not have been told that the administered drug was for pain, or may not know that pain relief is not immediate, and may ask another nurse for drugs. If the administration of the analgesic was not recorded, the patient might receive a second dose of the analgesic shortly after the first dose. This kind of situation can be extremely serious, especially when narcotics or other central nervous system depressants are administered. Immediate documentation prevents accidental administration of a drug by another individual. Proper documentation is essential to the process of administering drugs correctly.

Considerations in Drug Administration

National Patient Safety Goals

The Joint Commission on Accreditation of Healthcare Organizations (JCAHO), the accrediting body for hospitals, approved the 2006 National Patient Safety Goals. These goals are established to help accredited organizations address specific areas of concern with regard to patient safety. Several of these goals directly affect medication administration. For example, there are new requirements to improve the accuracy of patient identification. At least two methods must be used to identify the patient (other than the patient's room number) when administering medication or blood products. Another important new standard that institutions desiring accreditation must follow is to compile a list of abbreviations, symbols, and acronyms *not* to be used throughout the institution. JCAHO has developed its own list of abbreviations that may no longer be used in any written medical documents (e.g., care plans, medical orders, nurses' notes). This list is referred to as the "minimum list." See Table 2-2 for the official "Do Not Use" list. Table 2-2 also lists additional abbreviations, acronyms, and symbols for possible addition to the official "Do Not Use" list in the future. Facilities accredited by JCAHO are required to be in compliance with the National Patient Safety Standards. Additional information on these standards can be found at the JCAHO website (www.jointcommission.org/Standards/NationalPatientSafetyGoals/).

Drug Errors

Drug errors include any event or activity that can cause a patient to receive the wrong dose, the wrong drug, an incorrect dosage of the drug, a drug by the wrong route, or a drug given at the incorrect time. Errors may occur in transcribing drug orders, when the drug is dispensed, or in

Table 2.2 JCAHO Official "Do Not Use" List

Abbreviation	Potential Problem	Use Instead
Official "Do Not Use" List*		
U (unit)	Mistaken as 0 (zero), 4 (four), or "cc"	Write "unit"
IU (international unit)	Mistaken as IV (intravenous) or 10 (ten)	Write "international unit"
Q.D., QD, q.d., qd (daily) Q.O.D., QOD, q.o.d, qod (every other day)	Mistaken for each other The period after the "Q" can be mistaken for an "I" and the "O" can be mistaken for "I"	Write "daily" and "every other day"
Trailing zero (X.0 mg)† Lack of leading zero (.X mg)	Decimal point is missed	Write X mg Write 0.X mg
MS MSO₄ and MgSO₄	Can mean morphine sulfate or magnesium sulfate Confused for one another	Write "morphine sulfate" or "magnesium sulfate"
Additional Abbreviations, Acronyms, and Symbols (For Possible Future Inclusion in the Official "Do Not Use" List)		
> (greater than) < (less than)	Misinterpreted as the number "7" or the letter "L"; confused with one another	Write "greater than" or "less than"
Abbreviations for drug names	Misinterpreted because of similar abbreviations for multiple drugs	Write drug names in full
Apothecary units	Unfamiliar to many practitioners; confused with metric units	Use metric units
@	Mistaken for the number "2" (two)	Write "at"
cc (cubic certimeter)	Mistaken for U (units) when poorly written	Write "mL" for milliliters
μg (microgram)	Mistaken for mg (milligrams), resulting in one thousand–fold overdose	Write "mcg" or "micrograms"

*Applies to all orders and medication–related documentation that is handwritten (including free-test computer entry) or on preprinted forms.
†Exception: A "trailing zero" may be used only where required to demonstrate the level of precision of the value being reported, such as for laboratory results, imaging studies that report size of lesions, or catheter/tube sizes. It may not be used in medication orders or other medication-related documentation.
©Joint Commission Resources: *Official "Do Not Use " List—2006 National Patient Safety Goals.* www.jointcommission.org/Patient Safety/DoNotUseList/. Last accessed, June 5, 2006. Reprinted with permission.

administration of the drug. Nurses serve as the last defense against drug errors. When a drug error occurs, it must be reported immediately so that any necessary steps to counteract the action of the drug or any observation can be made as soon as possible. In most institutions, the nurse must complete an incident report and notify the primary care provider. It is important to report errors even when the patient suffers no harm.

Drug errors occur when one or more of the six rights has not been followed. Each time a drug is prepared and administered, the six rights must be a part of the procedure. In addition to consistently practicing the six rights,

the nurse should adhere to the following precautions to help prevent drug errors:

- Confirm any questionable orders.
- When calculations are necessary, verify them with another nurse.
- Listen to the patient when he or she questions a drug, the dosage, or the drug regimen.
- Never administer the drug until the patient's questions have been adequately researched.
- Concentrate on only one task at a time.

Most errors are made during administration of the drug. Errors most commonly occur because of a failure to administer a drug that has been ordered, administration of the wrong dose or strength of a drug, or administration of the wrong drug. Two drugs often associated with errors are insulin and heparin.

The United States Pharmacopeia (USP) in cooperation with the Institute of Safe Medication Practices instituted a program called the Medication Errors Reporting Program. This program is designed to identify the number and type of drug errors occurring around the country. The goal of this voluntary reporting system is to collect data and disseminate information that will prevent such errors in the future. A copy of the report form is included in Appendix C. Nurses are urged to participate in this important program as a means of protecting the public by identifying ways to make drug administration safer.

The Medication Order

Before a medication can be administered in a hospital or other agency, the nurse must have a physician's order. Medications are ordered by the primary health care provider, such as a physician, dentist, or in some cases a nurse practitioner. Common orders include the standing order, the single order, the PRN order, and the STAT order. See Display 2-1 for an explanation of each.

Once-a-Week Drugs

Soon, many drugs will be available for once-a-week, or even once-a-month, administration. The doses are designed to replace daily doses of drugs. One of the first is alendronate (Fosamax), a drug used to treat osteoporosis

(see Chapter 34). In 2001, the U.S. Food and Drug Administration (FDA) approved two strengths for this drug to be given once a week: 70-mg and 35-mg tablets. The 70-mg tablet is used to treat postmenopausal osteoporosis and the 35-mg tablet for preventing postmenopausal osteoporosis. In clinical trials, once-a-week dosing showed no greater adverse reactions than the once-daily regimen. Once-a-week dosing may prove beneficial for those experiencing mild adverse reactions in that the reactions would be experienced once a week, rather than every day.

Drug Dispensing Systems

Several drug dispensing systems can be used by the nurse to dispense medication after it has been ordered for the patient. A brief description of three methods follows.

Computerized Dispensing System

Automated or computerized dispensing systems (Fig. 2-4) are used in most hospitals or agencies dispensing drugs. Drugs are dispensed in the pharmacy from drug orders that are sent from the individual floors or units. Each floor or unit has a medication cart in which medications are placed for individual patients. Medication orders are filled in the hospital pharmacy and placed in the drug dispensing cart. When orders are filled, the cart is delivered to the unit. To administer the drugs, nurses enter the patient's name and the drug to be administered. The drug is dispensed and automatically recorded into the computerized system. After drugs are dispensed and the cart is almost empty, it goes back to the pharmacy to be refilled and for new drug orders to be placed.

Display 2.1 Types of Medication Orders

Standing Order: This type of order is given when the patient is to receive the drug as prescribed on a regular basis. The drug is administered until the physician discontinues the drug's use. Occasionally a drug may be ordered for a specified number of days, or in some cases a drug can be given only for a specified number of days before the order needs to be renewed.

Example: Lanoxin 0.25 mg PO qd.

Single order: An order to administer the drug one time only.

Example: Valium 10 mg IVP @ 10:00 am.

PRN order: An order to administer the drug as needed.

Example: Demerol 100 mg IM q4h PRN for pain.

STAT order: A one-time order given as soon as possible.

Example: Morphine 10 mg IV STAT.

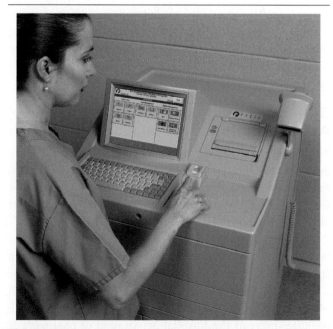

Figure 2.4 A computerized medication system.

Unit Dose System

The **unit dose** system is a method of dispensing medications in which drug orders are filled and medications dispensed to fill each patient's medication orders for a 24-hour period. The pharmacist dispenses each dose (unit) in a package that is labeled with the drug name and dosage. The drugs are placed in drawers in a special portable medication cart with a drawer for each patient. Many drugs are packaged by their manufacturers in unit doses—that is, each package is labeled by the manufacturer and contains one tablet or capsule, a premeasured amount of a liquid drug, a prefilled syringe, or one suppository. Hospital pharmacists also may prepare unit doses. The pharmacist restocks the cart each day with the drugs needed for the next 24-hour period. The nurse takes the drug cart into each patient's room.

Some hospitals use a bar code scanner in the administration of unit dose drugs. To use this system, a bar code is placed on the patient's hospital identification band when the patient is admitted to the hospital. The bar codes, along with bar codes on the drug unit dose packages, are used to identify the patient and to record and charge routine and PRN drugs. The scanner also keeps an ongoing inventory of controlled substances, which eliminates the need for narcotic counts at the end of each shift.

Floor Stock

Some health care agencies, such as nursing homes or small hospitals, use a floor stock method to dispense drugs. Some special units in hospitals, such as the emergency department, may use this method also. In this situation, drugs most frequently prescribed are kept on the unit in containers in a designated medication room or at the nurses' station. The nurse takes the medication from the appropriate container, administers the drug to the patient, and records the drug in the patient's administration record.

General Principles of Drug Administration

The nurse must have factual knowledge of each drug given, the reasons for use of the drug, the drug's general action, the more common adverse reactions associated with the drug, special precautions in administration (if any), and the normal dose ranges.

Some drugs may be given frequently; the nurse becomes familiar with pharmacologic information about a specific drug. Other drugs may be given less frequently, or a new drug may be introduced, requiring the nurse to obtain information from reliable sources, such as the drug package insert or the hospital department of pharmacy. It is of utmost importance to check current and approved references for all drug information.

The nurse also needs to take patient considerations, such as allergy history, previous adverse reactions, patient comments, and change in patient condition, into account before administering the drug. Before giving any drug for the first time, the nurse should ask the patient about any known allergies and any family history of allergies. This includes allergies not only to drugs but to food, pollen, animals, and so on. Patients with a personal or family history of allergies are more likely to experience additional allergies and must be monitored closely.

If the patient makes any statement about the drug or if there is any change in the patient, these situations are carefully considered before the drug is given. Examples of situations that require consideration before a drug is given include:

- Problems that may be associated with the drug, such as nausea, dizziness, ringing in the ears, and difficulty walking. Any comments made by the patient may indicate the occurrence of an adverse reaction. The nurse should withhold the drug until references are consulted and the primary caregiver contacted. The decision to withhold the drug must have a sound rationale and must be based on knowledge of pharmacology.

- Comments stating that the drug looks different from the one previously received, that the drug was just given by another nurse, or that the patient thought the primary care provider discontinued the drug therapy.

- A change in the patient's condition, a change in one or more vital signs, or the appearance of new symptoms. Depending on the drug being administered and the patient's diagnosis, these changes may indicate that the drug should be withheld and the primary care provider contacted.

Preparing a Drug for Administration

When preparing a drug for administration, the nurse should observe the following guidelines:

- Always check the health care provider's written orders and verify any questions with the primary health care provider.

- Wash hands immediately before preparing a drug for administration.

- Always check and compare the label of the drug with the Medication Administration Record (MAR) three times: (1) when the drug is taken from its storage area, (2) immediately before removing the drug from the container, and (3) before returning the drug to its storage area.

- Never remove a drug from an unlabeled container or from a package whose label is illegible.

- Do not let hands touch capsules or tablets.

- Be alert for drugs with similar names. Some drugs have names that sound alike but are very different (see Table 2-1). To give one drug when another is ordered could have serious consequences.

- Never give a drug that someone else has prepared. The individual preparing the drug must administer the drug.

- Return drugs requiring special storage to the storage area immediately after they are prepared for administration. This rule applies mainly to drugs that need refrigeration, but may also apply to drugs that must be protected from exposure to light or heat.

- Never crush tablets or open capsules without first checking with the pharmacist. Some tablets can be crushed or capsules can be opened and the contents added to water or a tube feeding when the patient cannot swallow a whole tablet or capsule. Some tablets have a special coating that delays the absorption of the drug. Crushing the tablet may destroy this drug property and result in problems such as improper absorption of the drug or gastric irritation. Capsules are gelatin and dissolve on contact with a liquid. The contents of some capsules do not mix well with water and therefore are best left in the capsule. If the patient cannot take an oral tablet or capsule, consult the primary care provider because the drug may be available in liquid form.

- When using a unit dose system, do not remove the wrappings of the unit dose until the drug reaches the bedside of the patient who is to receive it. After administering the drug, the nurse charts immediately on the unit dose drug form. The method of administering drugs by the unit dose system is widely used.

WATCH & LEARN

Administration of Drugs by the Oral Route

The oral route is the most frequent route of drug administration and rarely causes physical discomfort in patients. Oral drug forms include tablets, capsules, and liquids. Some capsules and tablets contain sustained-release drugs, which dissolve over an extended period. Administration of oral drugs is relatively easy for patients who are alert and can swallow.

Nursing Responsibilities

The nurse should observe the following points when giving an oral drug:

- Verify that the patient is able to swallow and is not nauseated or vomiting. Place the patient in an upright position. It is difficult, as well as dangerous, to swallow a solid or liquid when lying down.

- Assess the patient's need for assistance in holding the tablet or capsule or holding a glass of water. Some patients with physical disabilities cannot handle or hold these objects and may require assistance.

- Make sure that a full glass of water is readily available. Advise the patient to take a few sips of water before placing a tablet or capsule in the mouth.

- Instruct the patient to place the pill or capsule on the back of the tongue and tilt the head back to swallow a tablet or slightly forward to swallow a capsule. Encourage the patient first to take a few sips of water to move the drug down the esophagus and into the stomach, and then to finish the whole glass.

- Give the patient any special instructions, such as drinking extra fluids or remaining in bed, that are pertinent to the drug being administered.

- Never leave a drug at the patient's bedside to be taken later unless there is a specific order by the primary care provider to do so. A few drugs (e.g., antacids and nitroglycerin tablets) may be ordered to be left at the bedside.

- Patients with a nasogastric feeding tube may be given their oral drugs through the tube. Dilute and flush liquid drugs through the tube. However, crush tablets and dissolve them in water before administering them through the tube. Before administration, check the tube for placement. Flush the tube with water after the drugs are placed in the tube to clear the tubing completely.

- Instruct the patient to place **buccal** drugs against the mucous membranes of the cheek in either the upper or lower jaw. These drugs are given for a local, rather than systemic, effect. They are absorbed slowly from the mucous membranes of the mouth. Examples of drugs given buccally are lozenges and troches.

- Certain drugs are also given by the **sublingual** (placed under the tongue) route. These drugs must not be swallowed or chewed and must be dissolved completely before the patient eats or drinks. Nitroglycerin is commonly given sublingually.

Administration of Drugs by the Parenteral Route

Parenteral drug administration entails giving a drug by the **subcutaneous** (SC), **intramuscular** (IM), **intravenous** (IV), or **intradermal** route (Fig. 2-5). Other routes of parenteral administration that may be used by the primary

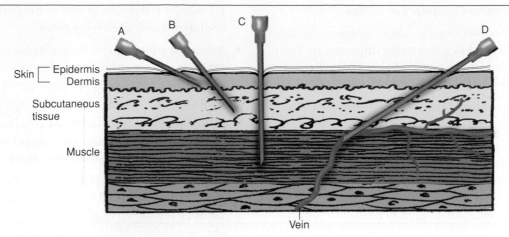

Figure 2.5 Needle insertion for parenteral drug. (**A**) Intradermal injection: a 26-gauge, 3/8-inch long needle is inserted at a 10-degree angle. (**B**) Subcutaneous injection: a 25-gauge, ½-inch long needle is inserted at an angle that depends on the size of the patient. (**C**) Intramuscular injection: a 20- to 23-gauge, 1- to 3-inch long needle is inserted into the relaxed muscle at a 90-degree angle with a dart-throwing type of hand movement. (**D**) Intravenous injection: the diameter and length of the needle used depend on the substance to be injected and on the site of injection.

care provider are intralesional (into a lesion), intra-arterial (into an artery), intracardiac (into the heart), and intra-articular (into a joint). In some instances, intra-arterial drugs are administered by a nurse. However, administration is not by direct arterial injection but by means of a catheter that has been placed in an artery.

Nursing Responsibilities

The nurse should observe the following points when giving a drug by the parenteral route:

- Wear gloves for protection from the potential of a blood spill when giving parenteral drugs. The risk of exposure to infected blood is increasing for all health care workers. The Centers for Disease Control and Prevention (CDC) recommends that gloves be worn when touching blood or body fluids, mucous membranes, or any broken skin area. This recommendation is referred to as **Standard Precautions**, which combine the Universal Precautions for Blood and Body Fluids with Body Substance Isolation guidelines.

- After selecting the site for injection, cleanse the skin. Most hospitals have a policy regarding the type of skin antiseptic used for cleansing the skin before parenteral drug administration. Cleanse the skin with a circular motion, starting at an inner point and moving outward.

- After inserting the needle for IM administration, pull back the syringe barrel to aspirate the drug. Aspirate for 5 to 10 seconds. If blood is in a small vessel, it takes time for the blood to appear. If blood appears in

the syringe, remove the needle so the drug is not injected. Discard the drug, needle, and syringe and prepare another injection. If no blood appears in the syringe, inject the drug. Aspiration is not necessary when giving an intradermal injection.

- After removing the needle from an IM, SC, or IV injection site, place pressure on the area. Patients with bleeding tendencies often require prolonged pressure on the area.

- Do not recap syringes, and dispose of them according to agency policy. Discard needles and syringes into clearly marked, appropriate containers to prevent needle-stick injuries. Most agencies have a "sharps" container located in each room for immediate disposal of needles and syringes after use. Proper disposal protects the nurse and others from injury and contamination.

- Most hospitals use needles designed to prevent sticks. This needle has a plastic guard that slips over the needle and locks in place as it is withdrawn from the injection site. Other models are available as well. These newer methods for administering parenteral fluids provide a greater margin of safety for nurses.

Administration of Drugs by the Subcutaneous Route

An SC injection places the drug into the tissues between the skin and the muscle (see Fig. 2-5B). Drugs administered in this manner are absorbed more slowly than IM injections. Heparin and insulin are two drugs commonly given by the SC route.

WATCH & LEARN

Nursing Responsibilities

The nurse should observe the following points when giving a drug by the SC route:

- A volume of 0.5 to 1 mL is used for SC injection. Larger volumes (e.g., >1 mL) are best given as IM injections. If a volume larger than 1 mL is ordered through the SC route, the injection is given in two sites, with separate needles and syringes.

- The sites for SC injection are the upper arms, the upper abdomen, and the upper back (Fig. 2-6). Rotate injection sites to ensure proper absorption and minimize tissue damage.

- When giving a drug by the SC route, insert the needle at a 45-degree angle. However, to place the drug in the SC tissue, select the needle length and angle of insertion based on the patient's body weight. Obese patients have excess SC tissue, and it may be necessary to give the injection at a 90-degree angle. If the patient is thin or cachectic, there usually is less SC tissue. For such patients, the upper abdomen is the best site for injection. Generally, a syringe with a 23- to 25-gauge needle that is 3/8 to 5/8 inch in length is most suitable for an SC injection.

- When administering an SC medication, aspirate by pulling back on the plunger of the syringe. If blood appears in the syringe, withdraw the needle, discard the syringe, and prepare a new injection. If blood does not appear, continue to inject the medication by depressing the plunger with a slow, even pressure. Heparin administration requires a different technique. Aspiration is

not recommended when administering heparin. For more detail on heparin administration, see Chapter 43.

Administration of Drugs by the Intramuscular Route

An IM injection is the administration of a drug into a muscle (see Fig. 2-5C). Drugs that are irritating to SC tissue can be given by IM injection. Drugs given by this route are absorbed more rapidly than drugs given by the SC route because of the rich blood supply in the muscle. In addition, a larger volume (1 to 3 mL) can be given at one site.

WATCH & LEARN

Nursing Responsibilities

The nurse should observe the following points when giving a drug by the IM route:

- If an injection is more that 3 mL, divide the drug and give it as two separate injections. Volumes larger than 3 mL will not be absorbed properly.

- A 22-gauge needle that is 1½ inches in length is most often used for IM injections.

- The sites for IM administration are the deltoid muscle (upper arm), the ventrogluteal or dorsogluteal sites (hip), and the vastus lateralis (thigh; Fig. 2-7). The vastus lateralis site is frequently used for infants and small children because it is more developed than the gluteal or deltoid sites. In children who have been ambulating for more than 2 years, the ventrogluteal site may be used.

- When giving a drug by the IM route, insert the needle at a 90-degree angle. When injecting a drug into the ventrogluteal or dorsogluteal muscles, it is a good idea to place the patient in a comfortable position, preferably in a prone position with the toes pointing inward. When injecting the drug into the deltoid, a sitting or lying-down position may be used. Place the patient in a recumbent position for injection of a drug into the vastus lateralis.

CONCEPTS in action **ANIMATION**

Z-Track Technique

The **Z-track** method of IM injection is used when a drug is highly irritating to SC tissues or has the ability permanently to stain the skin. The nurse should adhere to the following procedure when using the Z-track technique (Fig. 2-8):

- Draw the drug up into the syringe.

- Discard the needle and place a new needle on the syringe. This prevents any solution that may remain in the needle (that was used to draw the drug into the syringe) from contacting tissues as the needle is put into the muscle.

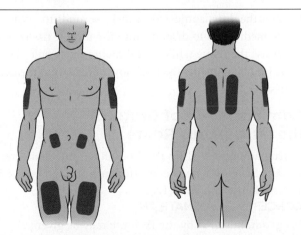

Figure 2.6 Sites on the body at which subcutaneous injections can be given.

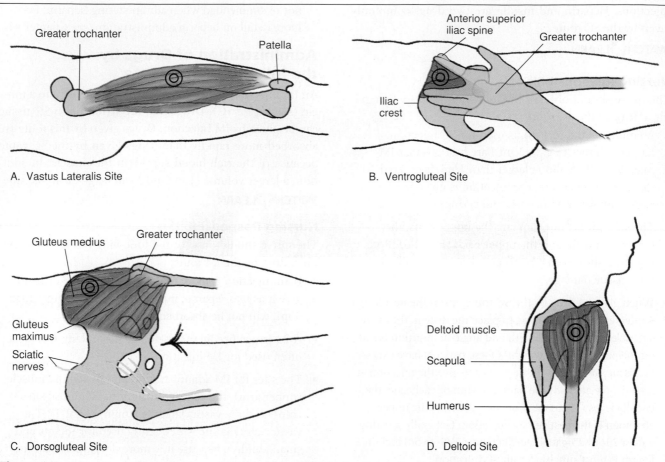

A. Vastus Lateralis Site

B. Ventrogluteal Site

C. Dorsogluteal Site

D. Deltoid Site

Figure 2.7   Sites for intramuscular administration. (**A**) Vastus lateralis site: the patient is supine or sitting. (**B**) Ventrogluteal site: the nurse's palm is placed on the greater trochanter and the index finger is placed on the anterior superior iliac spine; the injection is made into the middle of the triangle formed by the nurse's fingers and the iliac crest. (**C**) Dorsogluteal site: to avoid the sciatic nerve and accompanying blood vessels, an injection site is chosen above and lateral to a line drawn from the greater trochanter to the posterior superior iliac spine. (**D**) Deltoid site: the mid-deltoid area is located by forming a rectangle, the top of which is at the level of the lower edge of the acromion, and the bottom of which is at the level of the axilla; the sides are one third and two thirds of the way around the outer aspect of the patient's arm.

- Pull the plunger down to draw approximately 0.1 to 0.2 mL of air into the syringe. The air bubble in the syringe follows the drug into the tissues and seals off the area where the drug was injected, thereby preventing oozing of the drug up through the extremely small pathway created by the needle.

- Place the patient in the correct position for administration of an IM injection.

- Cleanse the skin.

- Pull the skin, SC tissues, and fat (that lie over the injection site) laterally, displacing the tissue to the side (approximately 1 inch).

- While holding the tissues in the lateral position, insert the needle at a 90-degree angle and inject the drug.

- After the drug is injected, wait 10 seconds to permit the medication to disperse into the muscle tissue, then release the tissue while withdrawing the needle. This technique prevents the backflow of drug into the SC tissue.

Administration of Drugs by the Intravenous Route

A drug administered by the IV route is injected directly into the blood by a needle inserted into a vein. Drug action occurs almost immediately.

CONCEPTS in action **ANIMATION**

Drugs administered by the IV route may be given:

- Slowly, over 1 or more minutes

- Rapidly (IV push)

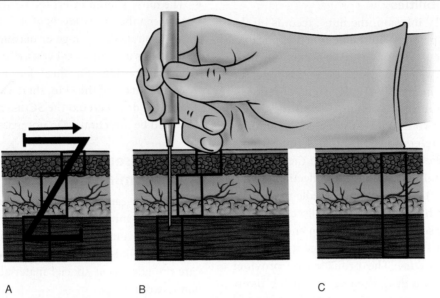

Figure 2.8 Z-track injection. (**A**) The tissue is tensed laterally at the injection site before the needle is inserted. This pulls the skin, subcutaneous tissue, and fat planes into a "Z" formation. (**B**) After the tissue has been displaced, the needle is thrust straight into the muscular tissue. (**C**) After injection, tissues are released while the needle is withdrawn. As each tissue plane slides by the other, the track is sealed.

- By piggyback infusions (drugs are mixed with 50 to 100 mL of compatible IV fluid and administered during a period of 30 to 60 minutes piggybacked onto the primary IV line)

- Into an existing IV line (the IV port)

- Into an intermittent venous access device called a *heparin lock* (a small IV catheter in the patient's vein; the catheter is connected to a small fluid reservoir with a rubber cap through which the needle is inserted to administer the drug)

- By being added to an IV solution and allowed to infuse into the vein over a longer period

WATCH & LEARN

When administering a drug into a vein by venipuncture, the nurse should place a tourniquet above the selected vein. It is important to tighten the tourniquet so that venous blood flow is blocked but arterial blood flow is not. The nurse should allow the veins to fill (distend) and then should pull the skin taut (to anchor the vein and the skin) and insert the needle into the vein, bevel up, and at a low angle to the skin. Blood should immediately flow into the syringe if the needle is properly inserted into the vein.

Performing a venipuncture requires practice. A suitable vein for venipuncture may be hard to find, and some veins are difficult to enter. The nurse should never repeatedly and unsuccessfully attempt a venipuncture. Depending on clinical judgment, three unsuccessful attempts on the same patient warrant having a more skilled individual attempt the procedure.

Some drugs are added to an IV solution, such as 1000 mL of dextrose 5% in water. The drug is usually added to the IV fluid container immediately before adding the fluid to the IV line. Whenever a drug is added to an IV fluid, the bottle must have a label attached indicating the drug and drug dose added to the IV fluid. In some hospitals, a pharmacist is responsible for adding specific drugs to IV fluids.

Intravenous Infusion Controllers and Pumps

Electronic infusion devices are classified as either infusion controllers or infusion pumps. The primary difference between the two is that an infusion pump adds pressure to the infusion, whereas an infusion controller does not. An infusion pump may be used to deliver the desired number of drops per minute. An alarm is set to sound if the rate of infusion is more or less than the preset rate.

Controllers and pumps have detectors and alarms that alert the nurse to various problems, such as air in the line, an occlusion, low battery, completion of an infusion, or an inability to deliver the preset rate. When any problem is detected by the device, an alarm is activated to alert the nurse. Potential complications in IV therapy with controllers and pumps are the same as those with a peripheral line.

Nursing Responsibilities

After the start of an IV infusion, the nurse records on the patient's chart the type of IV fluid and, when applicable, the drug added to the IV solution. It is important to check the infusion rate every 15 to 30 minutes. At this time, the nurse also inspects the needle site for signs of redness, swelling, or other problems. Swelling around the needle may indicate one of two things: extravasation or infiltration. **Extravasation** refers to the escape of fluid from a blood vessel into surrounding tissues while the needle or catheter is in the vein. **Infiltration** is the collection of fluid in tissues (usually SC tissue) when the needle or catheter is out of the vein. Both events necessitate discontinuation of the infusion and insertion of an IV line in another vein. Some drugs may cause severe tissue damage if extravasation or infiltration occurs. The primary care provider should be contacted if a drug capable of causing tissue damage, such as norepinephrine (Levophed), has escaped into the tissues surrounding the needle insertion site.

Nursing Alert

Use of an infusion pump or controller still requires nursing supervision and frequent monitoring of the IV infusion. Infiltration can progress rapidly because with the increased pressure, the infusion will not slow until considerable edema has occurred. Therefore, it is important to monitor frequently for signs of infiltration, such as edema or redness at the site. Careful monitoring of the pump or controller is also necessary to make sure the flow rate is correct.

Administration of Drugs by the Intradermal Route

Drugs given by the intradermal route are usually those for sensitivity tests (e.g., the tuberculin test or allergy skin testing; see Fig. 2-5A). Absorption is slow and allows for good results when testing for allergies or administering local anesthetics.

Nursing Responsibilities

The nurse observes the following points when administering drugs by the intradermal route:

- The inner part of the forearm and the upper back may be used for intradermal injections. The area should be hairless; areas near moles or scars or pigmented skin areas should be avoided. The nurse should cleanse the area in the same manner as for SC and IM injections.

- A 1-mL syringe with a 25- to 27-gauge needle that is 1/4 to 5/8 inch long is best suited for intradermal injections. Small volumes (usually <0.1 mL) are used for intradermal injections and administered with the bevel up.

- The nurse should insert the needle at a 15-degree angle between the upper layers of the skin. The nurse should not aspirate the syringe or massage the area. Injection produces a small wheal (raised area) on the outer surface of the skin. If a wheal does not appear on the outer surface of the skin, there is a good possibility that the drug entered the SC tissue, and any test results would be inaccurate. Do not massage the area.

Other Parenteral Routes of Drug Administration

The primary care provider may administer a drug by the intracardial, intralesional, intra-arterial, or intra-articular routes. The nurse may be responsible for preparing the drug for administration. The nurse should ask the primary care provider what special materials will be required for administration.

Venous access ports are totally implanted ports with a self-sealing septum that is attached to a catheter leading to a large vessel, usually the vena cava. These devices are most commonly used for chemotherapy or other long-term therapy and require surgical insertion and removal. Drugs are administered through injections made into the portal through the skin. These drugs are administered by the primary care provider or a registered nurse.

Administration of Drugs Through the Skin and Mucous Membranes

Drugs may be applied to the skin and mucous membranes using several routes: topically (on the outer layers of skin), transdermally through a patch on which the drug has been implanted, or inhaled through the membranes of the upper respiratory tract.

Administration of Drugs by the Topical Route

Most topical drugs act on the skin but are not absorbed through the skin. These drugs are used to soften, disinfect, or lubricate the skin. A few topical drugs are enzymes that have the ability to remove superficial debris, such as the dead skin and purulent matter present in skin ulcerations. Other topical drugs are used to treat minor, superficial skin infections. The various forms of topical applications and locations of use are described in Display 2-2.

Nursing Responsibilities

The nurse considers the following points when administering drugs by the topical route:

Administration of Drugs

Display 2.2 Topical Applications and Locations of Use

- Creams, lotions, or ointments applied to the skin with a tongue blade, gloved fingers, or gauze
- Sprays applied to the skin or into the nose or oral cavity
- Liquids inserted into body cavities, such as fistulas
- Liquids inserted into the bladder or urethra
- Solids (e.g., suppositories) or jellies inserted into the urethra
- Liquids dropped into the eyes, ears, or nose
- Ophthalmic ointments applied to the eyelids or dropped into the lower conjunctival sac
- Solids (e.g., suppositories, tablets), foams, liquids, and creams inserted into the vagina
- Continuous or intermittent wet dressings applied to skin surfaces
- Solids (e.g., tablets, lozenges) dissolved in the mouth
- Sprays or mists inhaled into the lungs
- Liquids, creams, or ointments applied to the scalp
- Solids (e.g., suppositories), liquids, or foams inserted into the rectum

---

- The primary care provider may write special instructions for the application of a topical drug—for example, to apply the drug in a thin, even layer or to cover the area after application of the drug to the skin.

- Other drugs may have special instructions provided by the manufacturer, such as to apply the drug to a clean, hairless area or to let the drug dissolve slowly in the mouth. All of these instructions are important because drug action may depend on correct administration of the drug.

Administration of Drugs by the Transdermal Route

Drugs administered by the **transdermal** route are readily absorbed from the skin and provide systemic effects. This type of administration is called a *transdermal drug delivery system.* The drug dosages are implanted in a small, patch-type bandage. The backing is removed and the patch is applied to the skin, where the drug is gradually absorbed into the systemic circulation. This type of drug system maintains a relatively constant blood concentration and reduces the possibility of toxicity. In addition, the administration of drugs transdermally causes fewer adverse reactions, and administration is less frequent than when the drugs are given by another route. Nitroglycerin (used to treat cardiac problems) and scopolamine (used to treat dizziness and nausea) are two drugs given frequently by the transdermal route.

Nursing Responsibilities

The nurse observes the following points when administering drugs by the transdermal route:

- Apply transdermal patches to clean, dry, nonhairy areas of intact skin.

- Remove the old patch when the next dose is applied in a new site.

- Rotate sites for transdermal patches to prevent skin irritation. The chest, flank, and upper arm are the most commonly used sites. Do not shave the area to apply the patch; shaving may cause skin irritation.

- Ointments are sometimes used and come with a special paper marked in inches. Measure the correct length (onto the paper), place the paper with the drug ointment side down on the skin, and secure it with tape. Before the next dose, remove the paper and tape and cleanse the skin.

Administration of Drugs Through Inhalation

Drug droplets, vapor, and gas are administered through the mucous membranes of the respiratory tract using a face mask, nebulizer, or positive-pressure breathing machine. Examples of drugs administered through **inhalation** include bronchodilators, mucolytics, and some anti-inflammatory drugs. These drugs primarily produce a local effect in the lungs.

Nursing Responsibilities

The primary nursing responsibility with drugs administered by inhalation is to provide the patient with proper

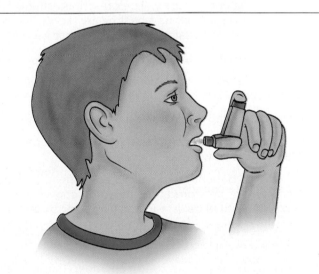

Figure 2.9 A respiratory inhalant is used to deliver a drug directly into the lungs. To deliver a dose of the drug, the patient takes a slow, deep breath while depressing the top of the inhaler's canister.

instructions for administering the drug. For example, many patients with asthma use a metered-dose inhaler to dilate the bronchi and make breathing easier. Without proper instruction on how to use the inhaler, much of the drug can be deposited on the tongue, rather than in the respiratory tract. This decreases the therapeutic effect of the drug. Instructions may vary with each inhaler. To be certain that the inhaler is used correctly, the patient is referred to the instructions accompanying each device. Figure 2-9 illustrates the proper use of one type of inhaler.

Nursing Responsibilities After Drug Administration

After the administration of any type of drug, the nurse is responsible for the following:

- Recording the administration of the drug. The nurse should complete this task as soon as possible. This is particularly important when PRN drugs (especially narcotics) are given.

- Recording (when necessary) any information concerning the administration of the drug. This includes information such as the IV flow rate, the site used for

parenteral administration, problems with administration (if any), and vital signs taken immediately before administration.

- Evaluating and recording the patient's response to the drug (when applicable). Evaluation may include such facts as relief of pain, decrease in body temperature, relief of itching, and decrease in the number of stools passed.

- Observing the adverse reactions. The frequency of these observations depends on the drug administered. The nurse must record all suspected adverse reactions and report them to the primary care provider. The nurse must report immediately serious adverse reactions to the primary care provider.

Administration of Drugs in the Home

Often, drugs are not administered by the nurse but in the home setting by the patient or family members serving as caregivers. When this is the case, it is important that the patient or caregivers understand the treatment regimen and are given an opportunity to ask questions concerning the drug therapy, such as why the drug was prescribed, how to administer the drug, and adverse reactions of the

Home Care Checklist

Administering Drugs Safely in the Home

For most patients, drugs will be prescribed after discharge to be taken at home. Because the home is not as controlled an environment as a health care facility, the nurse should assess the patient's home environment carefully to ensure complete safety. It is important to keep in mind the following when making a home safety assessment:

☑ Does the home have a space that is relatively free of clutter and easily accessible to the patient or a caregiver?

☑ Do any small children live in or visit the home? If so, is there a place where drugs can be stored safely out of their reach?

☑ Does the drug require refrigeration? If so, does the refrigerator work?

☑ If the patient needs several drugs, can the patient or caregiver identify which drugs are used and when? Do they know how to use them and why?

☑ Does the patient need special equipment, such as needles and syringes? If so, where and how can the equipment be stored for safety and convenience? Does the patient have an appropriate disposal container? Will the refuse be safe from children and pets?

- Suggest using plastic storage containers with snap-on lids or clean, dry glass jars with screw tops for needle disposal.

- Advise the patient to use an impervious container with a properly fitting lid, such as a coffee can, for safe disposal of needles. A plastic milk jug with a lid or a heavy-duty, clean, cardboard milk or juice carton may be used if necessary.

- Explain the importance of taking precautions to make sure discarded needles do not puncture the container.

drug (see Chapter 5 for information concerning patient and family education). The Home Care Checklist: Administering Drugs Safely in the Home gives some guidelines to follow when drugs are administered in the home by the patient or caregiver, rather than by the nurse.

Critical Thinking Exercises

1. Ms. Benson, a nurse on your clinical unit, tells you that the head nurse is upset with her because she has not been recording the administration of narcotics immediately after they are given. Discuss the rationales you could give to Ms. Benson to stress the importance of recording the administration of narcotics immediately after they are given.

2. After administering a drug to a patient, you find that the incorrect dosage was given. The dose that you administered was two times the correct dosage. Analyze what action, if any, you would take.

3. Discuss why the sixth right, right documentation, is important in drug administration.

4. Discuss the importance in participating in the Med-Watch program (see Chapter 1) and the Medication Errors Reporting Program.

Review Questions

1. The nurse correctly administers an IM injection by _____.

   A. displacing the skin to the side before making the injection

   B. using a 1-inch needle

   C. inserting the needle at a 90-degree angle

   D. using a 25-gauge needle

2. When preparing a drug for SC administration, the nurse is aware that the usual volume of a drug injected by the SC route is _____.

   A. 2 to 5 mL

   B. 3 to 4 mL

   C. 0.5 to 1 mL

   D. less than 0.5 mL

3. The nurse explains to the patient receiving an IV injection that the action of the drug occurs _____.

   A. in 5 to 10 minutes

   B. in 15 to 20 minutes

   C. within 30 minutes

   D. almost immediately

4. When administering a drug, the nurse _____.

   A. checks the drug label two times before administration

   B. is alert for any drugs with a similar name

   C. may administer a drug prepared by another nurse

   D. may crush any tablet that the patient is unable to swallow

5. When monitoring a patient with an IV line, the nurse observes that the area around the needle insertion site is swollen and red. The first action of the nurse is to _____.

   A. check the patient's blood pressure and pulse

   B. check further for possible extravasation

   C. ask the patient if the IV site has been accidentally injured

   D. immediately notify the primary health care provider

To check your answers, see Appendix G.

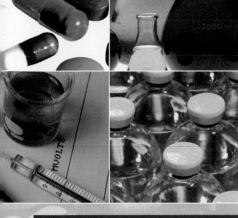

Chapter 3

Review of Arithmetic and Calculation of Drug Dosages

Key Terms

apothecaries' system
Celsius (C)
centigrade
decimal
decimal fraction
denominator
diluent
dimensional analysis
dividend
divisor
drams
Fahrenheit (F)
fluid drams
fluid ounces
grains
gram
household measurements
improper fraction
liter
meter
metric system
mixed decimal fraction
minim
mixed number
numerator
ounce
proper fraction
quotient
ratio
remainder
solute
solvent

Learning Objectives

On completion of this chapter, the student will:

- Accurately perform mathematical calculations when they are necessary to compute drug dosages.

Review of Arithmetic

Fractions

The two parts of a fraction are the **numerator** and the **denominator**.

$$\frac{2}{3} \begin{array}{l} \leftarrow \text{numerator} \\ \leftarrow \text{denominator} \end{array}$$

A **proper fraction** may be defined as a part of a whole or any number less than a whole number. An **improper fraction** is a fraction having a numerator the same as or larger than the denominator.

$$\text{proper fraction } \frac{1}{2}$$

$$\text{improper fraction } \frac{7}{3}$$

The numerator and the denominator *must be of like entities or terms*, that is:

Correct (like terms)	Incorrect (unlike terms)
$\dfrac{2 \text{ acres}}{3 \text{ acres}}$	$\dfrac{2 \text{ acres}}{3 \text{ miles}}$
$\dfrac{2 \text{ grams}}{3 \text{ grams}}$	$\dfrac{2 \text{ grams}}{5 \text{ milliliters}}$

Mixed Numbers and Improper Fractions

A **mixed number** is a whole number and a proper fraction. A whole number is a number that stands alone; 3, 25, and 117 are examples of whole numbers. A proper fraction is a fraction whose numerator is *smaller than* the denominator; 1/8, 2/5, and 3/7 are examples of proper fractions.

These are mixed numbers:

2 2/3 2 is the whole number and 2/3 is the proper fraction

3 1/4 3 is the whole number and 1/4 is the proper fraction

When doing certain calculations, it is sometimes necessary to change a mixed number to an improper fraction or change an improper fraction to a mixed number. An improper fraction is a fraction whose numerator is *larger than* the denominator; 5/2, 16/3, and 12 3/2 are examples of improper fractions.

To change a *mixed number to an improper fraction,* multiply the denominator of the fraction by the whole number, add the numerator, and place the sum over the denominator.

EXAMPLE Mixed number 3 3/5

1. Multiply the denominator of the fraction (5) by the whole number (3) or $5 \times 3 = 15$:

$$3 \,_\times\nwarrow \frac{3}{5}$$

2. Add the result of multiplying the denominator of the fraction (15) to the numerator (3) or $15 + 3 = 18$:

$$3 \,_\times\swarrow \frac{3}{5}$$

3. Then place the sum (18) over the denominator of the fraction:

$$\frac{18}{5}$$

To change an *improper fraction to a mixed number,* divide the denominator into the numerator. The **quotient** (the result of the division of these two numbers) is the whole number. Then place the remainder over the denominator of the improper fraction.

EXAMPLE Improper fraction 15/4

$$\frac{15}{4} \begin{array}{l} \leftarrow \text{numerator} \\ \leftarrow \text{denominator} \end{array}$$

1. Divide the denominator (4) into the numerator (15) or 15 divided by 4 ($15 \div 4$):

$$\begin{array}{r} 3 \leftarrow \text{quotient} \\ 4\overline{)15} \\ \underline{12} \\ 3 \leftarrow \text{remainder} \end{array}$$

2. The quotient (3) becomes the whole number:

$$3\frac{3}{4}$$

3. The **remainder** (3) now becomes the numerator of the fraction of the mixed number:

$$3\frac{3}{—}$$

4. And the denominator of the improper fraction (4) now becomes the denominator of the fraction of the mixed number:

$$3\frac{3}{4}$$

Adding Fractions With Like Denominators

When the denominators are the *same,* fractions can be added by adding the numerators and placing the sum of the numerators over the denominator.

EXAMPLES

$$2/7 + 3/7 = 5/7$$
$$1/10 + 3/10 = 4/10$$
$$2/9 + 1/9 + 4/9 = 7/9$$
$$1/12 + 5/12 + 3/12 = 9/12$$
$$2/13 + 1/13 + 3/13 + 5/13 = 11/13$$

When giving a final answer, fractions are *always* reduced to the lowest possible terms. In the examples above, the answers of 5/7, 7/9, and 11/13 cannot be reduced. The answers of 4/10 and 9/12 can be reduced to 2/5 and 3/4.

To reduce a fraction to the lowest possible terms, determine if any number, which always must be the same, can be divided into both the numerator and the denominator.

4/10: the numerator *and* the denominator can be divided by 2

9/12: the numerator *and* the denominator can be divided by 3

$$\text{For example: } \frac{4 \div 2 = 2}{10 \div 2 = 5}$$

If when adding fractions the answer is an improper fraction, it may then be changed to a mixed number.

2/5 + 4/5 = 6/5 (improper fraction)
6/5 changed to a mixed number is 1 1/5

Adding Fractions With Unlike Denominators

Fractions with *unlike denominators* cannot be added until the denominators are changed to like numbers or numbers that are the same. The first step is to find the *lowest common denominator,* which is the lowest number divisible by (or that can be divided by) all the denominators.

EXAMPLE Add 2/3 and 1/4

$$\left.\begin{array}{c} \frac{2}{3} \\ \frac{1}{4} \end{array}\right\}$$ The lowest number that can be divided by these two denominators is 12; therefore, 12 is the lowest common denominator.

1. Divide the lowest common denominator (which in this example is 12) by each of the denominators in the fractions (in this example 3 and 4):

$$\frac{2}{3} = \frac{}{12} \quad (12 \div 3 = 4)$$

$$\frac{1}{4} = \frac{}{12} \quad (12 \div 4 = 3)$$

2. Multiply the results of the divisions by the numerator of the fractions (12 ÷ 3 = 4 × the numerator 2 = 8 and 12 ÷ 4 = 3 × the numerator 1=3) and place the results in the numerator:

$$\frac{2}{3} = \frac{}{12} \quad \frac{8}{12}$$

$$\frac{1}{4} = \frac{}{12} \quad \frac{3}{12}$$

3. Add the numerators (8 + 3) and place the result over the denominator (12):

$$\frac{8}{12}$$
$$\frac{3}{12}$$
$$\frac{11}{12}$$

Adding Mixed Numbers or Fractions With Mixed Numbers

When adding two or more mixed numbers or adding fractions and mixed numbers, the mixed number is first changed to an improper fraction.

EXAMPLE Add 3 3/4 and 3 3/4

$$3\frac{3}{4} \text{ changed to an improper fraction} \rightarrow \frac{15}{4}$$

$$3\frac{3}{4} \text{ changed to an improper fraction} \rightarrow \frac{15}{4}$$

$$\text{The numerators are added} \rightarrow \frac{30}{4} = 7\ 2/4 = 7\ 1/2$$

The improper fraction (30/4) is changed to a mixed number (7 2/4) and the fraction of the mixed number (2/4) changed to the lowest possible terms (1/2).

EXAMPLE Add 2 1/2 and 3 1/4

$$2\frac{1}{2} \text{ changed to an improper fraction} \frac{5}{2}$$

$$3\frac{1}{4} \text{ changed to an improper fraction} \frac{13}{4}$$

In the example above, 5/2 and 13/4 cannot be added because the denominators are not the same. It will be necessary to find the lowest common denominator first.

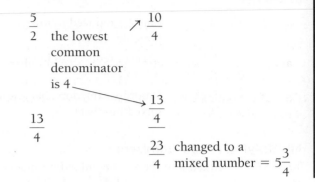

Comparing Fractions

When fractions with *like* denominators are compared, the fraction with the *largest numerator* is the *largest* fraction.

EXAMPLES

Compare: 5/8 and 3/8 Answer: **5/8** is larger than **3/8**.

Compare: 1/4 and 3/4 Answer: **3/4** is larger than **1/4**

When the denominators are *not* the same, for example, comparing 2/3 and 1/10, the lowest common denominator must first be determined. The same procedure is followed when adding fractions with unlike denominators (see above).

EXAMPLE Compare 2/3 and 1/10 (fractions with unlike denominators)

$$\frac{2}{3} = \frac{20}{30}$$
$$\frac{1}{10} = \frac{3}{30} \quad \text{lowest common denominator}$$

The largest numerator in these two fractions is 20; therefore, 2/3 is larger than 1/10.

Multiplying Fractions

When fractions are multiplied, the numerators are multiplied *and* the denominators are multiplied.

EXAMPLES

$$\frac{1}{8} \times \frac{1}{4} = \frac{1}{32} \qquad \frac{1}{2} \times \frac{2}{3} = \frac{2}{6} = \frac{1}{3}$$

In the above examples, it was necessary to reduce one of the answers to its lowest possible terms.

Multiplying Whole Numbers and Fractions

When whole numbers are multiplied with fractions, the numerator is multiplied by the whole number and the product is placed over the denominator. When necessary, the fraction is reduced to its lowest possible terms. If the answer is an improper fraction, it may be changed to a mixed number.

EXAMPLES

$$2 \times \frac{1}{2} = \frac{2}{2} = 1 \quad \text{(answer reduced to lowest possible terms)}$$

$$2 \times \frac{3}{8} = \frac{6}{8} = \frac{3}{4} \quad \text{(answer reduced to lowest possible terms)}$$

$$4 \times \frac{2}{3} = \frac{8}{3} = 2\frac{2}{3} \quad \text{(improper fraction changed to a mixed number)}$$

Multiplying Mixed Numbers

To multiply mixed numbers, the mixed numbers are changed to *improper fractions* and then multiplied.

EXAMPLES

$$2\frac{1}{2} \times 3\frac{1}{4} = \frac{5}{2} \times \frac{13}{4} = \frac{65}{8} = 8\frac{1}{8}$$

$$3\frac{1}{3} \times 4\frac{1}{2} = \frac{10}{3} \times \frac{9}{2} = \frac{90}{6} = 15$$

Multiplying a Whole Number and a Mixed Number

To multiply a whole number and a mixed number, *both* numbers must be changed to improper fractions.

EXAMPLES

$$3 \times 2\frac{1}{2} = \frac{3}{1} \times \frac{5}{2} = \frac{15}{2} = 7\frac{1}{2}$$

$$2 \times 4\frac{1}{2} = \frac{2}{1} \times \frac{9}{2} = \frac{18}{2} = 9$$

A whole number is converted to an improper fraction by placing the whole number over 1. In the above examples. 3 becomes 3/1 and 2 becomes 2/1.

Dividing Fractions

When fractions are divided, the *second* fraction (the divisor) is inverted (turned upside down) and then the fractions are multiplied.

EXAMPLES

$$\frac{1}{3} \div \frac{3}{7} = \frac{1}{3} \times \frac{7}{3} = \frac{7}{9}$$

$$\frac{1}{8} \div \frac{1}{4} = \frac{1}{8} \times \frac{4}{1} = \frac{4}{8} = \frac{1}{2}$$

$$\frac{3}{4} \div \frac{1}{2} = \frac{3}{4} \times \frac{2}{1} = \frac{6}{4} = 1\frac{1}{2}$$

In the above examples, the second answer was reduced to its lowest possible terms and the third answer, which was an improper fraction, was changed to a mixed number.

Dividing Fractions and Mixed Numbers

Some problems of division may be expressed as (1) fractions and mixed numbers, (2) two mixed numbers, (3) whole numbers and fractions, or (4) whole numbers and mixed numbers.

MIXED NUMBERS AND FRACTIONS When a mixed number is divided by a fraction, the whole number is first changed to a fraction.

EXAMPLES

$$2\frac{1}{3} \div \frac{1}{4} = \frac{7}{3} \div \frac{1}{4} = \frac{7}{3} \times \frac{4}{1} = \frac{28}{3} = 9\frac{1}{3}$$

$$2\frac{1}{2} \div \frac{1}{2} = \frac{5}{2} \div \frac{1}{2} = \frac{5}{2} \times \frac{2}{1} = \frac{10}{2} = 5$$

MIXED NUMBERS When two mixed numbers are divided, they are both changed to improper fractions.

EXAMPLE

$$3\frac{3}{4} \div 1\frac{1}{2} = \frac{15}{4} \div \frac{3}{2} = \frac{15}{4} \times \frac{2}{3} = \frac{30}{12}$$

$$= 2\frac{6}{12} = 2\frac{1}{2}$$

WHOLE NUMBERS AND FRACTIONS When a whole number is divided by a fraction, the whole number is changed to an improper fraction by placing the whole number over 1.

EXAMPLE

$$2 \div \frac{2}{3} = \frac{2}{1} \div \frac{2}{3} = \frac{2}{1} \times \frac{3}{2} = \frac{6}{2} = 3$$

WHOLE NUMBERS AND MIXED NUMBERS When whole numbers and mixed numbers are divided, the whole number is changed to an improper fraction and the mixed number is changed to an improper fraction.

EXAMPLE

$$4 \div 2\frac{2}{3} = \frac{4}{1} \div \frac{8}{3} = \frac{4}{1} \times \frac{3}{8} = \frac{12}{8} = 1\frac{4}{8} = 1\frac{1}{2}$$

Ratios

A **ratio** is a way of expressing *a part of a whole* or *the relation of one number to another.* For example, a ratio written as 1:10 means 1 in 10 parts, or 1 to 10. A ratio may also be written as a fraction; thus 1:10 can also be expressed as 1/10.

EXAMPLES

1:1000 is 1 part in 1000 parts, or 1 to 1000, or 1/1000

1:250 is 1 part in 250 parts, or 1 to 250, or 1/250

Some drug solutions are expressed in ratios, for example 1:100 or 1:500. These ratios mean that there is 1 part of a drug in 100 parts of solution or 1 part of the drug in 500 parts of solution.

Percentages

The term *percentage* or *percent* (%) means *parts per hundred.*

EXAMPLES

25% is 25 parts per hundred
50% is 50 parts per hundred

A percentage may also be expressed as a fraction.

EXAMPLES

25% is 25 parts per hundred or 25/100
50% is 50 parts per hundred or 50/100
30% is 30 parts per hundred or 30/100

The above fractions may also be reduced to their lowest possible terms:
25/100 = 1/4, 50/100 = 1/2, 30/100 = 3/10.

Changing a Fraction to a Percentage

To change a fraction to a percentage, divide the denominator by the numerator and multiply the results (quotient) by 100 and then add a percent sign (%).

EXAMPLES

Change 4/5 to a percentage

$$4 \div 5 = 0.8$$
$$0.8 \times 100 = 80\%$$

Change 2/3 to a percentage

$$2 \div 3 = 0.666$$
$$0.666 \times 100 = 66.6\%$$

Changing a Ratio to a Percentage

To change a ratio to a percentage, the ratio is first expressed as a fraction with the first number or term of the ratio becoming the numerator and the second number or term becoming the denominator. For example, the ratio 1:500 when changed to a fraction becomes 1/500. This fraction is then changed to a percentage by the same method shown in the preceding section.

EXAMPLE

Change 1:125 to a percentage

1:125 written as a fraction is 1/125
$$1 \div 125 = 0.008$$
$$0.008 \times 100 = 0.8$$
adding the percent sign = 0.8%

Changing a Percentage to a Ratio

To change a percentage to a ratio, the percentage becomes the numerator and is placed over a denominator of 100.

EXAMPLES

Changing 5% and 10% to ratios

$$5\% \text{ is } \frac{5}{100} = \frac{1}{20} \text{ or } 1:20$$

$$10\% \text{ is } \frac{10}{100} = \frac{1}{10} \text{ or } 1:10$$

Proportions

A proportion is a method of expressing equality between two ratios. An example of two ratios expressed as a proportion is: 3 is to 4 as 9 is to 12. This may also be written as:

$$3:4 \text{ as } 9:12$$

or

$$3:4::9:12$$

or

$$\frac{3}{4} = \frac{9}{12}$$

Proportions may be used to find an unknown quantity. The unknown quantity is assigned a letter, usually X. An example of a proportion with an unknown quantity is 5:10::15:X.

The first and last terms of the proportion are called the *extremes.* In the above expression 5 and X are the extremes. The second and third terms of the proportion are called the *means.* In the above proportion, 10 and 15 are the means.

$$
\begin{array}{c}
\text{means} \\
\swarrow \searrow \\
5:10::15:X \\
\nwarrow \quad \nearrow \\
\text{extremes}
\end{array}
$$

$$
\text{extreme} \; \frac{5}{\text{mean} \; 10} = \frac{15 \; \text{mean}}{X \; \text{extreme}}
$$

To solve for X:

1. Multiply the extremes and place the product (result) to the *left* of the equals sign.

$$5:10::15:X$$
$$5X =$$

2. Multiply the means and place the product to the *right* of the equals sign.

$$5:10::15:X$$
$$5X = 150$$

3. Solve for X by dividing the number to the right of the equal sign by the number to the left of the equals sign (150 ÷ 5).

$$5X = 150$$
$$X = 30$$

4. To prove the answer is correct, substitute the answer (30) for X in the equation.

$$5:10::15:X$$
$$5:10::15:30$$

Then multiply the means and place the product to the left of the equals sign. Then multiply the extremes and place the product to the right of the equals sign.

$$5:10::15:30$$
$$150 = 150$$

If the numbers are the same on both sides of the equals sign, the equation has been solved correctly.

If the proportion has been set up as a fraction, cross-multiply and solve for X.

$$\frac{5}{10} = \frac{15}{X}$$

5 times X = 5X and 10 times 15 = 150
$$5X = 150$$
$$X = 30$$

To set up a proportion, remember that a *sequence must be followed.* If a sequence is not followed, the proportion will be stated incorrectly.

EXAMPLES

If a man can walk 6 *miles* in 2 *hours,* how many *miles* can he walk in 3 *hours?*

miles is to *hours* and *miles* is to *hours*

or

miles:hours::miles:hours

or

$$\frac{miles}{hours} = \frac{miles}{hours}$$

The unknown fact is the number of miles walked in 3 hours:

6 miles:2 hours::X miles:3 hours
$$2X = 18$$
X = 9 miles (he can walk 9 miles in 3 hours)

If there are 15 *grains* in 1 *gram,* 30 *grains* equals how many *grams?*

15 grains:1 gram::30 grains:X grams
$$15X = 30$$
X = 2 grams (30 grains equals 2 grams)

Decimals

Decimals are used in the metric system. A **decimal** is a fraction in which the denominator is 10 or some power of 10. For example, 2/10 (read as two tenths) is a fraction with a denominator of 10; 1/100 (read as one one hundredth) is an example of a fraction with a denominator that is a power of 10 (i.e., 100).

A power (or multiple) of 10 is the *number 1 followed by one or more zeros.* Therefore, 100, 1000, 10,000 and so on are powers of 10 because the number 1 is followed by two, three, and four zeros, respectively. Fractions whose denominators are 10 or a power of 10 are often expressed in decimal form.

Parts of a Decimal

There are three parts to a decimal:

1.25
number(s) **d** number(s)
to the **e** to the
left of **c** right of
the **i** the
decimal **m** decimal
a
l

Types of Decimals

A decimal may consist only of numbers to the right of the decimal point. This is called a **decimal fraction.** Examples of decimal fractions are 0.05, 0.6, and 0.002.

A decimal may also have numbers to the *left* and *right* of the decimal point. This is called a **mixed decimal fraction.** Examples of mixed decimal fractions are 1.25, 2.5, and 7.5.

Both decimal fractions and mixed decimal fractions are commonly referred to as decimals. When there is no number to the left of the decimal, a zero may be written, for example, 0.25. Although in general mathematics the zero may not be required, it should be used in the writing of drug doses in the metric system. *Use of the zero lessens the chance of drug errors,* especially when the dose of a drug is hurriedly written and the decimal point is indistinct. For example, a drug order for dexamethasone is written as dexamethasone .25 mg by one physician and written as dexamethasone 0.25 mg by another. If the decimal point in the first written order is indistinct, the order might be interpreted as 25 mg, which is 100 times the prescribed dose!

Reading Decimals

To read a decimal, the position of the number to the left or right of the decimal point indicates how the decimal is to be expressed.

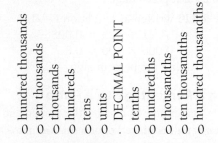

Adding Decimals

When adding decimals, place the numbers in a column so that the whole numbers are aligned to the left of the decimal and the decimal fractions are aligned to the right of the decimal.

EXAMPLE

20.45 + 2.56	2 + 0.25
is written as:	is written as:
20.45	2.00
+2.56	+0.25
23.01	2.25

Subtracting Decimals

When subtracting decimals, the numbers are aligned to the left and right of the decimal in the same manner as for the addition of decimals.

EXAMPLE

20.45 − 2.56	9.74 − 0.45
is written as:	is written as:
20.45	9.74
−2.56	−0.45
17.89	9.29

Multiplying a Whole Number by a Decimal

To multiply a whole number by a decimal, move the decimal point of the product (answer) as many places to the left as there are places to the right of the decimal point.

EXAMPLE

$$\begin{array}{r} 500 \\ \times .05 \\ \hline 2500. \end{array}$$ there is one place to the right ← of the decimal. the decimal point is moved one place to the left

After moving the decimal point, the answer reads 25.

$$\begin{array}{r} 250 \\ \times .3 \\ \hline 750. \end{array}$$ there is one place to the right ← of the decimal. the decimal point is moved one place to the left

After moving the decimal point, the answer reads 75.

Multiplying a Decimal by a Decimal

To multiply a decimal by a decimal, move the decimal point of the product (answer) as many places to the left as there are places to the right in *both* decimals.

EXAMPLE

there are two places to the right
$$\begin{array}{r} 2.75 \\ \times 0.5 \\ \hline 1375. \end{array}$$ ← of the decimal ← plus one place to the right of the decimal move the decimal point three places to the left

After moving the decimal point, the answer reads 1.375.

Dividing Decimals

The **divisor** is a number that is divided into the **dividend**.

EXAMPLE

$$0.69 \div 0.3 \qquad 0.3\overline{)0.69}$$

dividend divisor   divisor dividend

This may be written or spoken as 0.69 divided by 0.3. To divide decimals:

1. The *divisor* is changed to a whole number. In this example, the decimal point is moved one place to the right so that 0.3 now becomes 3, which is a whole number.

$$0.3\overline{)0.69}$$

2. The decimal point in the *dividend* is now moved the *same number of places* to the right. In this example, the decimal point is moved one place to the right, the same number of places the decimal point in the divisor was moved.

$$0.3\overline{)0.69}$$

3. The numbers are now divided.

$$\begin{array}{r} 2.3 \\ 3\overline{)6.9} \end{array}$$

When only the dividend is a decimal, the decimal point is carried to the quotient (answer) in the same position.

EXAMPLES

$$\begin{array}{r} .375 \\ 2\overline{)0.750} \end{array} \qquad \begin{array}{r} 1.736 \\ 2\overline{)3.472} \end{array}$$

To divide when only the divisor is a decimal, for example,

$$.3\overline{)66}$$

1. The divisor is changed to a whole number. In this example the decimal point is moved one place to the right.

$$.3\overline{)66}$$

2. The decimal point in the dividend must also be moved one place to the right.

$$.3\overline{)66.0}$$

3. The numbers are now divided.

$$\begin{array}{r} 220 \\ 3\overline{)660} \end{array}$$

Whenever the decimal point is moved in the dividend *it must also be moved* in the divisor, and whenever the decimal point in the divisor is moved *it must be moved* in the dividend.

Changing a Fraction to a Decimal

To change a fraction to a decimal, divide the numerator by the denominator.

EXAMPLE

$$\frac{1}{5} = 5\overline{)1.0}\;^{.2} \qquad \frac{3}{4} = 4\overline{)3.00}\;^{.75} \qquad \frac{1}{6} = 6\overline{)1.000}\;^{.166}$$

Changing a Decimal to a Fraction

To change a decimal to a fraction:

1. Remove the decimal point and make the resulting whole number the numerator: 0.2 = 2.

2. The denominator is stated as 10 or a power of 10. In this example, 0.2 is read as two *tenths*, and therefore the denominator is 10.

$0.2 = \dfrac{2}{10}$ reduced to the lowest possible number is $\dfrac{1}{5}$

ADDITIONAL EXAMPLES

$$0.75 = \frac{75}{100} = \frac{3}{4} \qquad 0.025 = \frac{25}{1000} = \frac{1}{40}$$

Calculation of Drug Dosages

Although most hospital pharmacies dispense drugs as single doses or in a unit dose system, on occasion the nurse must compute a drug dosage because it differs from the dose of the drug that is available. This is particularly true of small hospitals, nursing homes, physicians' offices, and outpatient clinics that may not have a complete range of all available doses for a particular drug. Because certain situations may require computing the desired amount of drug to be given, nurses must be familiar with the calculation of all forms of drug dosages.

Systems of Measurement

There are three systems of measurement of drug dosages: the **metric system**, the **apothecaries' system**, and **household measurements**. The metric system is the most commonly used system of measurement in medicine. A physician may prescribe a drug dosage in the apothecaries' system, but for the most part this ancient system of measurements is used only occasionally. The household system is rarely used in a hospital setting but may be used to measure drug dosages in the home.

Display 3.1 Metric Measurements

Weight
The unit of weight is the gram.
1 kilogram (kg) = 1000 grams (g)
1 gram (g) = 1000 milligrams (mg)
1 milligram (mg) = 1000 micrograms (mcg)

Volume
The unit of volume is the liter.
1 deciliter (dL) = 10 liters (L)
1 liter (L) = 1000 milliliters (mL)
1 milliliter (mL) = 0.001 liter (L)

Length
The unit of length is the meter.
1 meter (m) = 100 centimeters (cm)
1 centimeter (cm) = 0.01 meter (m)
1 millimeter (mm) = 0.001 meter (m)

The Metric System

The metric system uses decimals (or the decimal system). In the metric system, the **gram** is the unit of weight, the **liter** the unit of volume, and the **meter** the unit of length.

Display 3-1 lists the measurements used in the metric system. The abbreviations for the measurements are given in parentheses.

The Apothecaries' System

The apothecaries' system is an older, less accurate system of measurement than the metric system and may be unfamiliar to some practitioners. Whenever possible, it is preferable to use the metric system. However, because there may be times when the apothecaries' system is used, a review of that system is important.

The apothecaries' system uses whole numbers and fractions. Decimals are *not* used in this system. The whole numbers are written as lowercase Roman numerals, for example, x instead of 10, or v instead of 5.

The units of weight in the apothecaries' system are **grains, drams,** and **ounces.** The units of volume are **minims, fluid drams,** and **fluid ounces.** The units of measurement in this system are not based on exact measurements.

Display 3-2 lists the measurements used in the apothecaries' system.

Household Measurements

When used, household measurements are for volume only. In the hospital, household measurements are rarely used because they are inaccurate when used to measure drug dosages. On occasion, the nurse may use the pint,

Display 3.2 Apothecaries' Measurements

Weight

The units of weight are grains, drams, and ounces.

60 grains = 1 dram

1 ounce = 480 grains

Volume

The units of volume are minims, fluid drams, and fluid ounces.

1 fluid dram = 60 minims

1 fluid ounce = 8 fluid drams

Table 3.1 Approximate Equivalents

Metric	Apothecaries'	Household
Weight		
0.1 mg	gr 1/600	
0.15 mg	gr 1/400	
0.2 mg	gr 1/300	
0.3 mg	gr 1/200	
0.4 mg	gr 1/150	
0.6 mg	gr 1/100	
1 mg	gr 1/60	
2 mg	gr 1/30	
4 mg	gr 1/15	
6 mg	gr 1/10	
8 mg	gr 1/8	
10 mg	gr 1/6	
15 mg	gr 1/4	
20 mg	gr 1/3	
30 mg	gr ss (1/2)	
60 mg	gr 1	
100 mg	gr i ss (1 1/2)	
120 mg	gr ii	
1 g (1000 mg)	gr xv	
Volume		
0.06 mL	min i	
1 mL	min xv or xvi	
4 mL	fluid dram i	1 teaspoon
15 mL	fluid drams iv	1/2 ounce
30 mL	fluid ounce i	1 ounce
500 mL	1 pint	1 pint
1000 mL (1 liter)	1 quart	1 quart

quart, or gallon when ordering, irrigating, or sterilizing solutions or stock solutions. For the ease of a patient taking a drug at home, the physician may order a drug dosage in household measurements.

Display 3-3 lists the more common household measurements.

Conversion Between Systems

To convert between systems, it is necessary to know the equivalents, or what is equal to what in each system. Table 3-1 lists the more common equivalents. These equivalents are only *approximate* because the three systems are different and are not truly equal to each other.

Several methods may be used to convert from one system to another using an equivalent, but most conversions can be done by using proportion.

EXAMPLES

Convert 120 mg (metric) to grains (apothecaries')

Using proportion and the known equivalent 60 mg = gr i (1 grain)

$$1 \text{ gr:60 mg::X gr:120 mg}$$
$$60X = 120$$
$$X = 2 \text{ gr (grains or gr ii)}$$

Note the use of the abbreviations gr and mg when setting up the proportion. This shows that the proportion was stated correctly and helps in identifying the answer as 2 *grains*.

Display 3.3 Household Measurements

3 teaspoons = 1 tablespoon

2 tablespoons = 1 ounce

2 pints = 1 quart

4 quarts = 1 gallon

Convert gr 1/100 (apothecaries') to mg (metric)

Using proportion and the known equivalent 60 mg = 1 gr:

If there are 60 mg in 1 gr, there are X mg in 1/100 gr

$$60 \text{ mg}:1 \text{ gr}::X \text{ mg}:1/100 \text{ gr}$$

$$X = 60 \times \frac{1}{100} = \frac{60}{100} = \frac{3}{5}$$

$$X = \frac{3}{5} \text{ mg}$$

or

$$\frac{60 \text{ mg}}{1 \text{ gr}} = \frac{X \text{ mg}}{1/100} \text{ gr}$$

$$X = 60 \times \frac{1}{100} = \frac{60}{100} = \frac{3}{5}$$

$$X = \frac{3}{5} \text{ mg}$$

Fractions are *not* used in the metric system; therefore, the fraction must be converted to a decimal by dividing the denominator into the numerator, or $3 \div 5 = 0.6$ or

$$5\overline{)3.0}^{.6}$$

Therefore, gr 1/100 is equal to 0.6 mg.

When setting up the proportion, the apothecaries' system was written in Arabic numbers instead of Roman numerals, and their order was reversed (1 gr instead of gr i) so that all numbers and abbreviations are uniform in presentation.

Convert 0.3 milligrams (mg) [metric] to grains (gr) [apothecaries']

Using proportion and the known equivalent 1 mg = g = 1/60

$$1/60 \text{ gr}:1 \text{ mg}::X \text{ gr}:0.3 \text{ mg}$$

$$X = \frac{1}{60} \times 0.3 = \frac{0.3}{60} = \frac{3}{600} = \frac{1}{200}$$

$$X = \frac{1}{200} \text{ grain}$$

or

$$\frac{1/60}{1 \text{ mg}} = \frac{X \text{ gr}}{0.3 \text{ mg}}$$

$$X = \frac{1}{60} \times 0.3 = \frac{0.3}{60} = \frac{3}{600} = \frac{1}{200}$$

$$X = \frac{1}{200} \text{ gr}$$

Therefore, 0.3 mg equals gr 1/200.

There is no rule stating which equivalent must be used. In the above problem, another equivalent (60 mg = 1 gr)

also could have been used. If 60 mg = 1 gr is used, the proportion would be:

$$60 \text{ mg}:1 \text{ gr}::0.3 \text{ mg}:X$$

$$60X = 0.3$$

$$X = 0.005$$

or

$$\frac{60 \text{ mg}}{1 \text{ gr}} = \frac{0.3 \text{ mg}}{X \text{ gr}}$$

$$60X = 0.3$$

$$X = 0.005$$

Therefore, 0.3 mg equals 0.005 gr.

Because decimals are not used in the apothecaries' system, this decimal answer must be converted to a fraction: 0.005 is 5/1000, which, when reduced to its lowest terms, is 1/200. The final answer is now 0.3 mg = gr 1/200.

Converting Within a System

Sometimes it is necessary to convert within the same system, for example, changing grams (g) to milligrams (mg) or milligrams to grams. Proportion and a known equivalent also may be used for this type of conversion.

EXAMPLE

Convert 0.1 gram (g) to milligrams (mg)

Using proportion and the known equivalent 1000 mg = 1g

$$1000 \text{ mg}:1 \text{ g}::X \text{ mg}:0.1 \text{ g}$$

$$X = 1000 \times 0.1$$

$$X = 100 \text{ mg}$$

or

$$\frac{1000 \text{ mg}}{1 \text{ g}} = \frac{X \text{ mg}}{0.1 \text{ g}}$$

$$X = 1000 \times 0.1$$

$$X = 100 \text{ mg}$$

Therefore, 0.1 gram (g) equals 100 milligrams (mg).

Solutions

A **solute** is a substance dissolved in a **solvent**. A solvent may be water or some other liquid. Usually water is used for preparing a solution unless another liquid is specified. Solutions are prepared by using a solid (powder, tablet) and a liquid, or a liquid and a liquid. Today, most solutions are prepared by a pharmacist and not by the nurse.

Examples of how solutions may be labeled include:

- 10 mg/mL—10 mg of the drug in each milliliter

- 1:1000—a solution denoting strength of 1 part of the drug per 1000 parts

- 5 mg/teaspoon—5 mg of the drug in each teaspoon (home use)

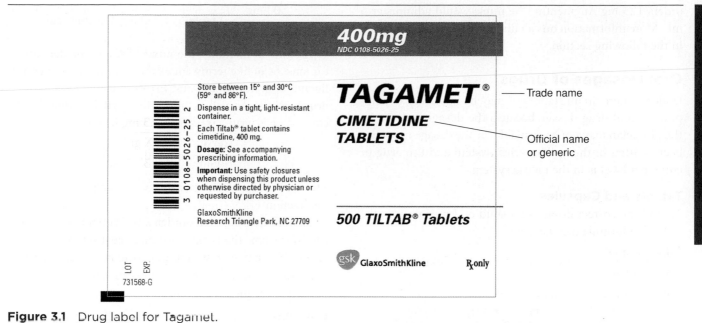

Figure 3.1 Drug label for Tagamet.

Reading Drug Labels

Drug labels give important information the nurse must use to obtain the correct dosage. The unit dose is the most common type of labeling seen in hospitals. The unit dose is a method of dispensing drugs in which each capsule or tablet is packaged separately. At times the drug will come to the nursing unit in a container with a number of capsules or tablets or as a solution. The nurse must then determine the number of capsules/tablets or the amount of solution to administer.

Drug labels usually contain two names: the trade (brand) name and the generic or official name (see Chapter 1). The trade name is capitalized, written first on the label, and identified by the registration symbol. The official or generic name is written in smaller print and usually located under the trade name. Although the drug has only one official name, several companies may manufacture the drug, with each manufacturer using a different trade name. Sometimes

the generic or official name is so widely known that all manufacturers will simply use that name. For example, atropine sulfate is a widely used drug that is so well known that all manufacturers use the official name. In this case only the official name, atropine sulfate, will be found on the label. Drugs may be prescribed by either the trade name or the official or generic name. See Figure 3-1 for an example of a drug label showing the trade and generic names.

The dosage strength is also given on the container. The dosage strength is the average strength given to a patient as one dose. If necessary, the dosage strength is used to calculate the number of tablets or the amount of solution to administer. In liquid drugs there is a specified amount of drug in a given volume of solution, such as 50 mg in 2 mL.

Look at Figure 3-2. In this example, the dosage strength of the Augmentin is 125 mg/5 mL solution. If the physician

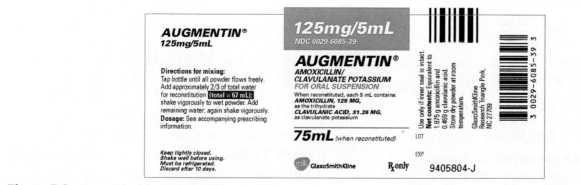

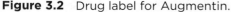

Figure 3.2 Drug label for Augmentin.

orders 125 mg Augmentin, the nurse would administer 5 mL. More information on calculating drug dosages is given in the following section.

Oral Dosages of Drugs

Under certain circumstances, it may be necessary to compute an oral drug dosage because the dosage ordered by the physician may not be available, or the dosage may have been written in the apothecaries' system and the drug or container label is in the metric system.

Tablets and Capsules

To find the correct dosage of a solid oral preparation, the following formula may be used:

$$\frac{\text{dose desired}}{\text{dose on hand}} = \text{dose administered (the unknown or X)}$$

This formula may be abbreviated as

$$\frac{D}{H} = X$$

When the dose ordered by the physician (dose desired) is written in the *same system* as the dose on the drug container (dose on hand), these two figures may be inserted into the formula.

EXAMPLE

The physician orders ascorbic acid 100 mg (metric). The drug is available as ascorbic acid 50 mg (metric).

$$\frac{D}{H} = X$$

$$\frac{100 \text{ mg (dose desired)}}{50 \text{ mg (dose on hand)}} = 2 \text{ tablets of 50-mg ascorbic acid}$$

If the physician had ordered ascorbic acid 0.5 g and the drug container was labeled ascorbic acid 250 mg, a *conversion of grams to milligrams* (because the drug container is labeled in milligrams) would be necessary before this formula can be used. If the 0.5 g were *not* converted to milligrams, the fraction of the formula would look like this:

$$\frac{0.5 \text{ grams}}{250 \text{ milligrams}}$$

A fraction *must* be stated in *like terms*; therefore, proportion may be used to convert grams to milligrams.

$$1000 \text{ mg:1 g::X mg:0.5 g}$$
$$X = 1000 \times 0.5$$
$$X = 500 \text{ mg}$$

After changing 0.5 g to mg, use the formula:

$$\frac{D}{H} = X$$

$$\frac{500 \text{ mg}}{250 \text{ mg}} = 2 \text{ tablets of 250 mg ascorbic acid}$$

As with all fractions, the numerator and the denominator must be of like terms, for example, milligrams over milligrams or grams over grams. Errors in using this and other drug formulas, as well as proportions, will be reduced if the entire dose is written rather than just the numbers.

$$\frac{100 \text{ mg}}{50 \text{ mg}} \text{ rather than } \frac{100}{50}$$

This will eliminate the possibility of using *unlike* terms in the fraction.

Even if the physician's order was written in the apothecaries' system, the drug container most likely would be labeled in the metric system. A conversion of *apothecaries' to metric* will now be necessary because the drug label is written in the metric system.

EXAMPLE

The physician's order reads: codeine sulfate gr 1/4 (apothecaries'). The drug container is labeled: codeine sulfate 15 mg (metric). Grains must be converted to milligrams *or* milligrams converted to grains.

Grains to milligrams:

$$60 \text{ mg:1 gr::X mg:1/4 gr}$$
$$X = 60 \times \frac{1}{4}$$
$$X = 15 \text{ mg}$$

or

$$\frac{60 \text{ mg}}{1 \text{ gr}} = \frac{X \text{ mg}}{1/4 \text{ gr}}$$
$$X = 60 \times \frac{1}{4}$$
$$X = 15 \text{ mg}$$

Therefore, 1/4 grain is approximately equivalent to 15 mg.

Milligrams to grains:

$$60 \text{ mg:1 gr::15 mg:X gr}$$
$$60X = 15$$
$$X = 1/4 \text{ gr}$$

or

$$\frac{60 \text{ mg}}{1 \text{ gr}} = \frac{15 \text{ mg}}{X \text{ gr}}$$
$$60X = 15$$
$$X = \frac{1}{4} \text{ grain}$$

Therefore, 15 mg is approximately equivalent to 1/4 grain.

The formula $\frac{D}{H} = X$ can now be used

$$\frac{D}{H} = X$$

$$\frac{15 \text{ mg}}{15 \text{ mg}} = 1 \text{ tablet}$$

or

$$\frac{1/4 \text{ gr}}{1/4 \text{ gr}} = 1 \text{ tablet}$$

Liquids

In liquid drugs, there is a specific amount of drug in a given volume of solution. For example, if a container is labeled as 10 mg per 5 mL (or 10 mg/5 mL), this means that for every 5 mL of solution there is 10 mg of drug.

As with tablets and capsules, the prescribed dose of the drug may not be the same as what is on hand (or available). For example, the physician may order 20 mg of an oral liquid preparation and the bottle is labeled as 10 mg/5 mL.

The formula for computing the dosage of oral liquids is:

$$\frac{\text{dose desired}}{\text{dose on hand}} \times \text{quantity} = \text{volume administered}$$

This may be abbreviated as

$$\frac{D}{H} \times Q = X$$

The quantity (or Q) in this formula is the amount of liquid in which the available drug is contained. For example, if the label states that there is 15 mg/5 mL, 5 mL is the *quantity* (or *volume*) in which there is 15 mg of this drug.

EXAMPLE

The physician orders oxacillin sodium 125 mg PO oral suspension. The drug is labeled as 250 mg/5 mL. The 5 mL is the amount (quantity or Q) that contains 250 mg of the drug.

$$\frac{D}{H} \times Q = X \text{ (the liquid amount to be given)}$$

$$\frac{125 \text{ mg}}{250 \text{ mg}} \times 5 = X$$

$$\frac{1}{2} \times 5 = 2.5 \text{ ml}$$

Therefore, 2.5 mL contains the desired dose of 125 mg of oxacillin oral suspension.

Liquid drugs may also be ordered in drops (gtt) or minims. With the former, a medicine dropper is usually supplied with the drug and is always used to measure the ordered dosage. Eye droppers are not standardized, and therefore the size of a drop from one eye dropper may be different than one from another eye dropper.

To measure an oral liquid drug in minims, a measuring glass *calibrated in minims* must be used.

Parenteral Drug Dosage Forms

Drugs for parenteral use must be in liquid forms before they are administered. Parenteral drugs may be available in the following forms:

1. As liquids in disposable cartridges or disposable syringes that contain a specific amount of a drug in a specific volume, for example, meperidine 50 mg/mL. After administration, the cartridge or syringe is discarded.

2. In ampules or vials that contain a specific amount of the liquid form of the drug in a specific volume. The vials may be single-dose vials or multidose vials. A multidose vial contains more than one dose of the drug.

3. In ampules or vials that contain powder or crystals, to which a liquid (called a **diluent**) must be added before the drug can be removed from the vial and administered. Vials may be single-dose or multidose vials.

Parenteral Drugs in Disposable Syringes or Cartridges

In some instances a specific dosage strength is not available and it will be necessary to administer less than the amount contained in the syringe.

EXAMPLE

The physician orders diazepam 5 mg IM. The drug is available as a 2-mL disposable syringe labeled 5 mg/mL.

$$\frac{D}{H} \times Q = X$$

$$\frac{5 \text{ mg}}{10 \text{ mg}} \times 2 \text{ mL} = X$$

$$X = \frac{1}{2} \times 2 = 1 \text{ mL}$$

Note that because the syringe contains 2 mL of the drug and that *each* mL contains 5 mg of the drug, there is a total of 10 mg of the drug in the syringe. Because there is 10 mg of the drug in the syringe, half of the liquid in the syringe (1 mL) is discarded and the remaining half (1 mL) is administered to give the prescribed dose of 5 mg.

Parenteral Drugs in Ampules and Vials

If the drug is in liquid form in the ampule or vial, the desired amount is withdrawn from the ampule or vial. In some instances, the entire amount is used; in others, only part of the total amount is withdrawn from the ampule or vial and administered.

Whenever the dose to be administered is different from that listed on the label, the volume to be administered must be calculated. To determine the volume to be administered, the formula for liquid preparations is used. The calculations are the same as those given in the preceding section for parenteral drugs in disposable syringes or cartridges.

EXAMPLES

The physician orders chlorpromazine 12.5 mg IM.

The drug is available as chlorpromazine 25 mg/mL in a 1-mL ampule.

$$\frac{D}{H} \times Q = X$$

$$\frac{12.5 \text{ mg}}{25 \text{ mg}} \times 1 \text{ mL} = X$$

$$\frac{1}{2} \times 1 \text{ mL} = \frac{1}{2} \text{ mL (or 0.5 mL) volume to be administered.}$$

The physician orders hydroxyzine 12.5 mg. The drug is available as hydroxyzine 25 mg/mL in 10-mL vials.

$$\frac{D}{H} \times Q = X$$

$$\frac{12.5 \text{ mg}}{25 \text{ mg}} \times 1 \text{ mL} = \frac{1}{2} \text{ mL (or 0.5 mL)}$$

Therefore, 0.5 mL is withdrawn from the 10-mL multidose vial and administered. In this example, the amount in this or any multidose vial is *not* entered into the equation. What is entered into the equation as quantity (Q) is the amount of the available drug that is contained in a specific volume.

Parenteral Drugs in Dry Form

Some parenteral drugs are available as a crystal or a powder. Because these drugs have a short life in liquid form, they are available in ampules or vials in dry form and must be made a liquid (reconstituted) before they are removed and administered. Some of these products have directions for reconstitution on the label or on the enclosed package insert. The manufacturer may give the following information for reconstitution: (1) the name of the diluent(s) that must be used with the drug, or (2) the amount of diluent that must be added to the drug.

In some instances, the manufacturer supplies a diluent with the drug. If a diluent is supplied, no other stock diluent should be used. Before a drug is reconstituted, the label is carefully checked for instructions.

EXAMPLES

Methicillin sodium: To reconstitute 1-g vial add 1.5 mL of sterile water for injection or sodium chloride injection. Each reconstituted milliliter contains approximately 500 mg of methicillin.

Mechlorethamine: Reconstitute with 10 mL of sterile water for injection or sodium chloride injection. The solution now contains 1 mg/mL of mechlorethamine.

If there is any doubt about the reconstitution of the dry form of a drug and there are no manufacturer's directions, the hospital pharmacist should be consulted.

Once a diluent is added, the volume to be administered is determined. In some cases, the entire amount is given; in others, a part (or fraction) of the total amount contained in the vial or ampule is given.

After reconstitution of any multidose vial, the following information *must* be added to the label:

- Amount of diluent added
- Dose of drug in mL (500 mg/mL, 10 mg/2 mL, etc.)
- The date of reconstitution
- The expiration date (the date after which any unused solution is discarded)

Calculating Intravenous Flow Rates

When the physician orders a drug added to an intravenous (IV) fluid, the amount of fluid to be administered over a specified period, such as 125 mL/h or 1000 mL over 8 hours, must be included in the written order. If no infusion rate has been ordered, 1 L (1000 mL) of IV fluid should infuse over 6 to 8 hours.

To allow the IV fluid to infuse over a specified period, the IV flow rate must be determined. Before using one of the following methods, the drop factor must be known. Drip chambers on the various types of IV fluid administration sets vary. Some deliver 15 drops/mL and others deliver more or less than this number. This is called the *drop factor*. The drop factor (number of drops/mL) is given on the package containing the drip chamber and IV tubing. Three methods for determining the IV infusion rate follow. Methods 1 and 2 can be used when the known factors are the total amount of solution, the drop factor, and the number of hours over which the solution is to be infused.

METHOD 1 *Step 1.* Total amount of solution ÷ number of hours = number of mL/h

Step 2. mL/h ÷ 60 min/h = number of mL/min

Step 3. mL/min × drop factor = number of drops/min

EXAMPLE

1000 mL of an IV solution is to infuse over a period of 8 hours. The drop factor is 14.

Step 1. 1000 mL ÷ 8 hours = 125 mL/h

Step 2. 125 mL ÷ 60 minutes = 2.08 mL/min

Step 3. 2.08 × 14 = 29 drops/min

METHOD 2 *Step 1.* Total amount of solution ÷ number of hours = number of mL/h
Step 2. mL/h × drop factor ÷ 60 = number of drops/min

EXAMPLE

1000 mL of an IV solution is to infuse over a period of 6 hours. The drop factor is 12.

Step 1. 1000 mL ÷ 6 hours = 166.6 mL/h
Step 2. 166.6 × 12 ÷ 60 = 33.33 (33 to 34) drops/min

METHOD 3 This method may be used when the desired amount of solution to be infused in 1 hour is known or written as a physician's order.

$$\frac{\text{drops/mL of given set (drop factor)}}{60 \text{ (minutes in an hour)}} \times \begin{array}{l}\text{total hourly}\\ \text{volume} =\\ \text{drops/min}\end{array}$$

EXAMPLE

If a set delivers 15 drops/min and 240 mL is to be infused in 1 hour:

$$\frac{15}{60} \times 240 = \frac{1}{4} \times 240 = 60 \text{ drops/min}$$

Oral or Parenteral Drug Dosages Based on Weight

The dosage of an oral or parenteral drug may be based on the patient's weight. In many instances, references give the dosage based on the weight in kilograms (kg) rather than pounds (lb). There are 2.2 lb in 1 kg.

When the dosage of a drug is based on weight, the physician, in most instances, computes and orders the dosage to be given. However, errors can occur for any number of reasons. The nurse should be able to calculate a drug dosage based on weight to detect any type of error that may have been made in the prescribing or dispensing of a drug whose dosage is based on weight.

To convert a known weight in kilograms to pounds, multiply the known weight by 2.2.

EXAMPLES

Patient's weight in kilograms is 54
$$54 \times 2.2 = 118.8 \text{ (or 119) lb}$$

Patient's weight in kilograms is 61.5
$$61.5 \times 2.2 = 135.3 \text{ (or 135) lb}$$

To convert a known weight in pounds to kilograms, divide the known weight by 2.2.

EXAMPLES

Patient's weight in pounds is 142
$$142 \div 2.2 = 64.5 \text{ kg}$$

Child's weight in pounds is 43
$$43 \div 2.2 = 19.5 \text{ kg}$$

Once the weight is converted to pounds or kilograms, this information is used to determine drug dosage.

EXAMPLES

A drug dosage is 5 mg/kg/d. The patient weighs 135 lb, which is converted to 61.2 kg.

$$61.2 \text{ kg} \times 5 \text{ mg} = 306.8 \text{ mg}$$

Proportions also can be used:

$$5 \text{ mg:1 kg::X mg:61.2 kg}$$
$$X = 306.8 \text{ mg}$$

A drug dosage is 60 mg/kg/d IV in three equally divided doses.

The patient weighs 143 lb, which is converted to 65 kg.

$$65 \text{ kg} \times 60 \text{ mg} = 3900 \text{ mg/day}$$
$$3900 \text{ mg} \div 3 \text{ (doses per day)} = 1300 \text{ mg each dose}$$

If the drug dosage is based on body surface area (m^2), the same method of calculation may be used.

EXAMPLE

A drug dosage is 60 to 75 mg/m^2 as a single IV injection.
The body surface area (BSA) of a patient is determined by means of a nomogram for estimating BSA (see Appendix D) and is found to be 1.8 m^2. The physician orders 60 mg/m^2.

$$60 \text{ mg} \times 1.8 \text{ m}^2 = 108 \text{ mg}$$

Proportion can also be used:

$$60 \text{ mg: 1 m}^2\text{::X mg:1.8 m}^2$$
$$X = 108 \text{ mg}$$

Dosage Calculation Using Dimensional Analysis

When using **dimensional analysis** (DA) to calculate dosage problems, dosages are written as common fractions. For example:

$$\frac{1 \text{ mL}}{4 \text{ mg}} \quad \frac{5 \text{ mL}}{10 \text{ mg}} \quad \frac{1 \text{ tablet}}{100 \text{ mg}}$$

When written as common fractions, the numerator is the top number. In the example above, 1 mL, 5 mL, and 1 tablet are the numerators.

The numbers on the bottom are called denominators. In the example above, 4 mg, 10 mg, and 100 mg are denominators.

EXAMPLE

The physician orders 10 mg of diazepam. The drug comes in dosage strength of 5 mg/mL. How many milliliters would the nurse administer?

Step 1. To work this problem using DA, always begin by identifying the unit of measure to be calculated. The unit to be calculated will be milliliters or cubic centimeters if the drug is to be administered parenterally. Another drug form is the solid and the unit of measure would be a tablet or capsule. In this problem, the unit of measure to be calculated is milliliters. If the drug is an oral liquid drug, the measurement might be ounces.

Step 2. Write the identified unit of measure to be calculated, followed by an equals sign. In this problem, milliliters is the unit to be calculated, so the nurse writes:

$$mL =$$

Step 3. Next, the dosage strength is written, with the numerator *always expressed in the same unit that was identified before the equals sign.* For example:

$$mL = \frac{1\ mL}{5\ mg}$$

Step 4. Continue by writing the next fraction with the numerator having the same unit of measure as the denominator in the previous fraction. For example, our problem continues:

$$mL = \frac{1\ mL}{5\ mg} \times \frac{10\ mg}{X\ mL}$$

Step 5. The problem is solved by multiplication of the two fractions.

$$mL = \frac{1\ mL}{5\ mg} \times \frac{10\ mg}{X\ mL} = \frac{10\ mg}{5X\ mL} = 2\ mL$$

NOTE: Each alternate denominator and numerator cancel, with only the final unit remaining.

EXAMPLE

Ordered: 200,000 U
On hand: Drug labeled 400,000 U/mL

$$mL = \frac{1\ mL}{400,000\ U} \times \frac{200,000\ U}{X\ mL} = \frac{1}{2}\ mL\ or\ 0.5\ mL$$

Metric Conversions Using Dimensional Analysis

Occasionally, the physician may order a drug in one unit of measure, whereas the drug is available in another unit of measure.

EXAMPLE

The physician orders 0.4 mg of atropine. The drug label reads 400 mcg per 1 mL. This dosage problem is solved by expanding the DA equation by adding one step to the equation.

Step 1. As above, begin by writing the unit of measure to be calculated, followed by an equals sign.

Step 2. Next, express the dosage strength as a fraction with the numerator having the same unit of measure as the number before the equals sign.

Step 3. Continue by writing the next fraction with the numerator having the same unit of measure as the denominator in the previous fraction.

$$mL = \frac{1\ mL}{400\ mcg} \times \frac{mcg}{mg}$$

Step 4. Expand the equation by filling in the missing numbers using the appropriate equivalent. In this problem, the equivalent would be 100 mcg=1 mg. This will convert micrograms to milligrams.

$$mL = \frac{1\ mL}{400\ mcg} \times \frac{1000\ mcg}{1\ mg}$$

Repeat Steps 3 and 4. Continue with the equation by placing the next fraction beginning with the unit of measure of the denominator of the previous fraction.

$$mL = \frac{1\ mL}{400\ mcg} \times \frac{1000\ mcg}{1\ mg} \times \frac{0.4\ mg}{X\ mL}$$

When possible, cancel out the units, leaving only mL.

Step 5. Solve the problem by multiplication. Cancel out the numbers when possible.

$$mL = \frac{1\ mL}{400\ mcg} \times \frac{1000\ mcg}{1\ mg} \times \frac{0.4\ mg}{X\ mL} = \frac{400}{400\ X} = 1\ mL$$

Solve the following problems using DA. Refer to the equivalents table if necessary (see Table 3-1).

EXAMPLE

Ordered: 250 mg.
On hand: Drug labeled 1 g per 1 mL

$$mL = \frac{1\ mL}{1\ g} \times \frac{1\ g}{1000\ mg} \times \frac{250\ mg}{X\ mL} = \frac{1\ mL}{4}\ or\ 0.25\ mL$$

Temperatures

Two scales used in the measuring of temperatures are **Fahrenheit (F)** and **Celsius (C)** (also known as **centigrade**). On the Fahrenheit scale, the freezing point of water is 32° F and the boiling point of water is 212° F. On the Celsius scale, 0° C is the freezing point of water and 100° C is the boiling point of water.

To convert from Celsius to Fahrenheit, the following formula may be used: F = 9/5 C + 32 (9/5 times the temperature in Celsius, then add 32).

EXAMPLE

Convert 38° C to Fahrenheit:

$$F = \frac{9}{5} \times 38° + 32$$
$$F = 68.4° + 32$$
$$F = 100.4°$$

To convert from Fahrenheit to Celsius, the following formula may be used: C = 5/9 (F − 32) (5/9 times the temperature in Fahrenheit minus 32).

EXAMPLE

Convert 100° F to Celsius:

$$C = \frac{5}{9} \times (100 - 32)$$
$$C = \frac{5}{9} \times 68$$
$$C = 37.77 \text{ or } 37.8°$$

Pediatric Dosages

The dosages of drugs given to children are usually less than those given to adults. The dosage may be based on age, weight, or body surface area (BSA).

Body Surface Area

Charts are used to determine the BSA in square meters according to the child's height and weight. Once the BSA is determined, the following formula is used:

$$\frac{\text{surface area of the child in square meters}}{\text{surface area of an adult in square meters*}} \times \text{usual adult dose} = \text{pediatric dose}$$

(See Appendix D for BSA nomograms.)

Weight

Pediatric as well as adult dosages may also be based on the patient's weight in pounds or kilograms. The method of converting pounds to kilograms or kilograms to pounds is explained in a previous section.

EXAMPLE

5 mg/kg
0.5 mg/lb

Today, most pediatric dosages are clearly given by the manufacturer, thus eliminating the need for formulas, except for determining the dosage of some drugs based on the child's weight or BSA.

---

*The figure for the average BSA of an adult in square meters is 1.7.

Review of Arithmetic and Calculation of Drug Dosages

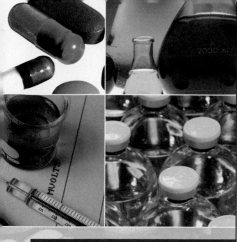

The Nursing Process

Learning Objectives

On completion of this chapter, the student will:

- List the five phases of the nursing process.
- Discuss assessment, analysis, nursing diagnosis, planning, implementation, and evaluation as they apply to the administration of drugs.
- Differentiate between objective and subjective data.
- Discuss how the nursing process may be used in daily life, as well as when administering drugs.
- Identify common nursing diagnoses used in the administration of drugs and nursing interventions related to each diagnosis.

The **nursing process** is a framework for nursing action consisting of problem-solving steps that help members of the health care team provide effective patient care. It is a specific and orderly plan used to gather data, identify patient problems from the data, develop and implement a plan of action, and then evaluate the results of nursing activities, including the administration of drugs.

The five phases of the process are used not only in nursing, but in daily life. For example, when buying a computer one may first think about whether it is really needed, shop in several different stores to find out more about computers (assessment), and then determine what each store has to offer (analysis). At this point, one decides exactly what computer to buy and how to pay for the computer (planning); then the computer is purchased (implementation). After purchase and use, the computer is evaluated (evaluation).

Using the nursing process requires practice, experience, and a constant updating of knowledge. The nursing process is used in this text only as it applies to drug administration. It is not within the scope of this textbook to list all of the assessments, nursing diagnoses, plans, implementations, and evaluations for the medical diagnosis that requires the administration of a specific drug.

The Five Phases of the Nursing Process

Although the nursing process can be described in various ways, it generally consists of five phases: assessment, analysis (or formation of the nursing diagnosis), planning, implementation, and evaluation. Each part is applicable, with modification, to the administration of medications. Figure 4-1 relates the nursing process to administration of medications.

Assessment

Assessment involves collecting objective and subjective data. **Objective data** are facts obtained by means of a physical assessment or physical examination. **Subjective data** are facts supplied by the patient or the patient's family.

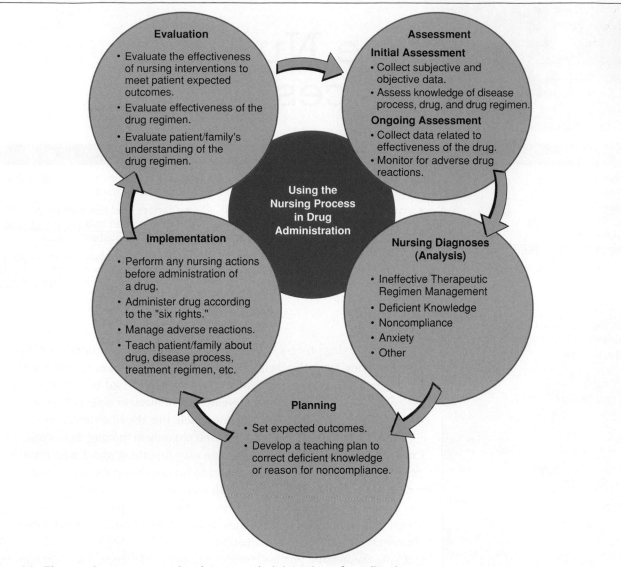

Figure 4.1 The nursing process as it relates to administration of medication.

Assessments are both initial and ongoing. An **initial assessment** is made based on objective and subjective data collected when the patient is first seen in a hospital, outpatient clinic, health care provider's office, or other type of health care facility. The initial assessment usually is more thorough and provides a database (sometimes called a *baseline*) against which later data can be compared and decisions made. The initial assessment provides information that is analyzed to identify problems that can be resolved or alleviated by nursing actions.

Objective data are obtained during an initial assessment through activities, such as examining the skin, obtaining vital signs, palpating a lesion, and auscultating the lungs. A review of the results of any recent laboratory tests and diagnostic studies also is part of the initial physical assessment. Subjective data are acquired during an initial assessment by

obtaining information from the patient, such as a family history of disease, allergy history, occupational history, a description (in the patient's own words) of the current illness or chief complaint, a medical history, and a drug history. In addition to the prescription drugs that the patient may be taking, it is important to know the over-the-counter drugs, vitamins, or herbal therapies that the patient uses. For women of childbearing age, the nurse needs to ask about the woman's pregnancy status and whether or not she is breastfeeding.

An **ongoing assessment** is one that is made at the time of each patient contact and may include the collection of objective data, subjective data, or both. The scope of an ongoing assessment depends on many factors, such as the patient's diagnosis, the severity of illness, the response to treatment, and the prescribed medical or surgical treatment.

The assessment phase (including the initial and ongoing assessment) of the nursing process can be applied to the administration of drugs, with objective and subjective data collected before and after to obtain a thorough baseline or initial assessment. This allows subsequent assessments to be compared with the baseline information. This comparison helps to evaluate the effectiveness of the drug and the presence of any adverse reactions. Ongoing assessments of objective and subjective data are equally important when administering drugs. Important objective data include blood pressure, pulse, respiratory rate, temperature, weight, appearance of the skin, appearance of an intravenous infusion site, and pulmonary status as assessed by auscultation of the lungs. Important subjective data include any statements made by the patient about relief or nonrelief of pain or other symptoms after administration of a drug.

The extent of the assessment and collection of objective and subjective data before and after a drug is administered depends on the type of drug and the reason for its use.

Nursing Diagnosis (Analysis)

After the data collected during assessment are analyzed, the nurse identifies the patient's needs (problems) and formulates one or more nursing diagnoses. A **nursing diagnosis** is not a medical diagnosis; rather, it is a description of the patient's problems and their probable or actual related causes based on the subjective and objective data in the database. A nursing diagnosis identifies problems that can be solved or prevented by **independent nursing actions**—actions that do not require a physician's order and may be legally performed by a nurse. Nursing diagnoses provide the framework for selections of nursing interventions to achieve expected outcomes.

The North American Nursing Diagnosis Association (NANDA) was formed to standardize the terminology used for nursing diagnoses. NANDA continues to define, explain, classify, and research summary statements about health problems related to nursing. NANDA has approved a list of diagnostic categories to be used in formulating a nursing diagnosis. This list of diagnostic categories is periodically revised and updated. In some instances, nursing diagnoses may apply to a specific group or type of drug or a particular patient. One example is Deficient Fluid Volume related to active fluid volume loss (diuresis) secondary to administration of a diuretic. Specific drug-related nursing diagnoses are highlighted in each chapter. However, it is beyond the scope of this book to discuss all possible nursing diagnoses related to a drug or a drug class.

Some of the nursing diagnoses developed by NANDA may be used to identify patient problems associated with drug therapy and are more commonly used when administering drugs. The most frequently used nursing diagnoses related to the administration of drugs include

- Effective Therapeutic Regimen Management
- Ineffective Therapeutic Regimen Management
- Deficient Knowledge
- Noncompliance
- Anxiety

Because these nursing diagnoses are commonly used for the administration of all types of drugs, they will not be repeated for each chapter. The nurse should keep these nursing diagnoses in mind when administering any drug.

Planning

After the nursing diagnoses are formulated, the nurse develops expected outcomes, which are patient oriented. An expected outcome is a direct statement of patient goals to be achieved. The expected outcome describes the maximum level of wellness that is reasonably attainable for the patient. For example, common expected patient outcomes related to drug administration, in general, include

- The patient will effectively manage the therapeutic regimen.
- The patient will understand the drug regimen.
- The patient will comply with the drug regimen.

The expected outcomes define the expected behavior of the patient or family that indicates the problem is being resolved or that progress toward resolution is occurring.

The nurse selects the appropriate interventions on the basis of expected outcomes to develop a plan of action or patient care plan. Planning for nursing actions specific to the drug to be administered can result in greater accuracy in drug administration, enhanced patient understanding of the drug regimen, and improved patient compliance with the prescribed drug therapy after discharge from the hospital. For example, during the initial assessment interview, the patient may report an allergy to penicillin. This information is important, and the nurse must now plan the best methods of informing all members of the health care team of the patient's allergy to penicillin.

The **planning** phase describes the steps for carrying out nursing activities or interventions that are specific and that will meet the expected outcomes. Planning anticipates the implementation phase or the carrying out of nursing actions that are specific to the drug being administered. If, for example, the patient is to receive a drug by the intravenous route, the nurse must plan the materials needed and the patient instruction for administration of the drug by this route. In this instance, the planning phase occurs immediately before the implementation phase and is necessary to carry out the technique of intravenous administration correctly. Failing to plan effectively may result in forgetting to obtain all of the materials necessary for drug administration.

Expected outcomes define the expected behavior of the patient or family that indicates that the problem is being resolved or that progress toward resolution is occurring. Expected outcomes serve as a basis for evaluating the effectiveness of nursing interventions. For example, if the nursing intervention is to "monitor the blood pressure every hour," the expected outcome is that "the patient experiences no further elevation in blood pressure."

Implementation

Implementation is the carrying out of a plan of action and is a natural outgrowth of the assessment and planning phases of the nursing process. When related to the administration of drugs, implementation refers to the preparation and administration of one or more drugs to a specific patient. Before administering a drug, the nurse reviews the subjective and objective data obtained on assessment and considers any additional data, such as blood pressure, pulse, or statements made by the patient. The decision of whether to administer the drug is based on an analysis of all information. For example, a patient is hypertensive and is supposed to receive a drug to lower the blood pressure. Objective data obtained at the time of admission included a blood pressure of 188/110. Additional objective data obtained immediately before the administration of the drug included a blood pressure of 182/110. A decision was made by the nurse to administer the drug because the change in the patient's blood pressure was minimal. However, if the patient's blood pressure was 132/84, and this was only the second dose of the drug, the nurse could decide to withhold the drug and contact the primary health care provider. Giving or withholding a drug or contacting the patient's health care provider are nursing activities related to the implementation phase of the nursing process.

The more common nursing diagnoses used when administering drugs are Effective Therapeutic Regimen Management, Ineffective Therapeutic Regimen Management, Deficient Knowledge, and Noncompliance. Nursing interventions applicable to each of these nursing diagnoses are discussed in the following sections. However, each patient is an individual, and nursing care must be planned on an individual basis after a careful collection and analysis of the data. In addition, each drug is different

and may have various effects in the body. (For drugs discussed in subsequent chapters, some possible nursing diagnoses related to that specific drug are discussed.)

Effective Therapeutic Regimen Management

This nursing diagnosis takes into consideration that the patient is willing to regulate and integrate into daily living the treatment regimen such as the self-administration of medications. For this nursing diagnosis to be used, the patient verbalizes the desire to manage the medication regimen. When the patient is willing and able to manage the treatment regimen, he or she may simply need information concerning the drug, method of administration, what type of reactions to expect, and what to report to the primary health care provider. A patient willing to take responsibility may need the nurse to develop a teaching plan that gives the patient the information needed to manage the therapeutic regimen properly (see Chapter 5 for more information on educating patients).

Ineffective Therapeutic Regimen Management

NANDA defines Ineffective Therapeutic Regimen Management as "a pattern of regulating and integrating into daily living a program for treatment of illness and the sequelae of illness that is unsatisfactory for meeting specific health goals." In the case of medication administration, the patient may not be taking the medication correctly or following the medication regimen prescribed by the health care provider.

The reasons for not following the drug regimen vary (Display 4-1). For example, some people do not fill their

---

Display 4.1 Possible Causes of Ineffective Therapeutic Regimen Management

Extended therapy for chronic illness causes patient to become discouraged

Troublesome adverse reactions

Lack of understanding of the purpose for the drug

Forgetfulness

Misunderstanding of oral or written instructions on how to take the drug

Weak nurse–patient relationships

Lack of funds to obtain drug

Mobility problems

Lack of family support

Cognitive deficits

Visual or hearing defects

From: Carpenito-Moyet L. J. (2006). *Nursing diagnosis: Application to clinical practice* (11th ed., pp. 473–480). Philadelphia: Lippincott Williams & Wilkins.

prescriptions because they do not have enough money to pay for them. Other patients skip doses, take the drug at the wrong times, or take an incorrect dose. Some may simply forget to take the drug; others take a drug for a few days, see no therapeutic effect, and quit.

When working with a patient who is not managing the drug regimen correctly, the nurse must ensure that the patient understands the drug regimen. It is essential to provide written instructions. The nurse must first assess the patient's ability to read English and his or her reading level. Some resources, such as Medline Plus (www.nlm.nih.gov/medlineplus/druginformation.html) offer information in other languages, such as Spanish. If possible, the nurse should allow the patient to administer the drug before he or she is dismissed from the health care facility. The nurse should determine if adequate funds are available to obtain the drug and any necessary supplies. For example, when a bronchodilator is administered by inhalation, a spacer or extender may be required for proper administration. This device is an additional expense. A referral to the social services department of the institution may help the patient when finances are a problem.

For those who forget to take the drug, the nurse may suggest the use of small compartmentalized boxes marked with the day of the week or time the drug is to be taken (Fig. 4-2). These containers can be obtained from the local pharmacy.

It is important to discuss the drug regimen with the patient, including the reason the drug is to be taken, the times, the amount, adverse reactions to expect, and reactions that should be reported. The patient needs a thorough understanding of the desired or expected therapeutic effect

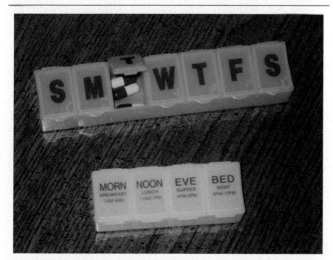

Figure 4.2 Various types of drug containers may be used to help individuals remember to take their medication at the correct time.

and the approximate time expected to attain that effect. For example, a patient may become discouraged after taking an antidepressant for 5 to 7 days and seeing no response. An explanation that 2 to 3 weeks is required before the depression begins to lift will, in many cases, promote compliance.

It is important to provide ways to minimize adverse reactions if possible. For example, many anticholinergic drugs cause dry mouth. The nurse instructs the patient to take frequent sips of water or suck on hard candy to help minimize the discomfort of a dry mouth.

Frequent follow-up sessions are needed to determine compliance with the drug regimen. If a follow-up visit is not feasible, the nurse considers a telephone call or home visit. It is vital that the nurse strive to develop a caring and nurturing relationship with the patient. Compliance is enhanced when a patient trusts the nurse and feels comfortable confiding any problem encountered during drug therapy.

Deficient Knowledge

Deficient Knowledge is the absence or deficiency of cognitive information on a specific subject. In the case of self-administration of drugs, the patient lacks sufficient knowledge to administer the drug regimen correctly. It may also relate to a lack of interest in learning, cognitive limitation, or inability to remember.

Most patients, at least in the initial treatment stages, lack knowledge about the drug, its possible adverse reactions, and the times and method of administration. At times, the patient may lack knowledge about the disease condition. In these situations, the nurse addresses the specific knowledge deficit (e.g., adverse reactions, disease process, method of administration) in words that the patient can understand. It is important for the nurse to determine first what information the patient is lacking and then plan a teaching session that directly pertains to the specific area of need (see Chapter 5 for more information on patient education). If the patient lacks the cognitive ability to understand the information concerning self-administration of drugs, then one or more of the caregivers should be taught to administer the proper treatment regimen.

Noncompliance

Noncompliance is behavior of the patient or caregiver that fails to coincide with the therapeutic plan agreed on by the patient and the health care provider. Patients are noncompliant for various reasons, such as a lack of information about the drug, the reason the drug is prescribed, or the expected or therapeutic results. Some patients find the adverse effects so bothersome that they discontinue taking the drug without notifying the health care provider. Display 4-1 identifies some reasons for this.

Noncompliance also can be the result of anxiety or bothersome side effects. The nurse can relieve anxiety by allowing the patient to express feelings or concerns, by actively listening as the patient verbalizes feelings, and by providing information so that the patient can be fully informed about the drug. Many patients have a tendency to discontinue use of the drug once the symptoms have been relieved. It is important to emphasize the importance of completing the prescribed course of therapy. For example, failure to complete a course of antibiotic therapy may result in recurrence of the infection. To combat noncompliance the nurse finds out the exact reason for the noncompliance, if possible. Factors related to noncompliance are similar to those listed in Display 4-1.

Anxiety

Anxiety is a vague uneasiness or apprehension that manifests itself in varying degrees, from expressions of concern regarding drug regimen to total lack of compliance with the drug regimen. When anxiety is high, the ability to focus on details is reduced. If the patient or caregiver is given information concerning the medication regimen during a high-anxiety state, the patient may not remember the information. This could lead to noncompliance. The anxiety experienced during drug administration depends on the severity of the illness, the occurrence of adverse reactions, and the knowledge level of the patient. Anxiety usually decreases with understanding of the therapeutic regimen. To decrease anxiety before discussing the treatment regimen with the patient, the nurse takes time to talk with and actively listen to the patient. This helps to build a caring relationship and decrease patient anxiety. It is critical for the nurse to allow time for a thorough explanation and to answer all questions and concerns in language the patient can understand.

It is important to identify and address the specific fear and, if possible, reassure the patient that the drug will alleviate the symptoms or, if possible, cure the disorder. The nurse thoroughly explains any procedure. The nurse actively listens and provides encouragement as the patient expresses fears and concerns. Reassurance and understanding on the part of the nurse are required; the amount of reassurance and understanding depends on the individual patient.

Evaluation

Evaluation is a decision-making process that involves determining the effectiveness of the nursing interventions in meeting the expected outcomes. When related to the administration of a drug, this phase of the nursing process is used to evaluate the patient's response to drug therapy. The evaluation is complete if the expected outcomes have been accomplished or if progress has occurred. If the outcomes have not been accomplished, different interventions are needed. During the administration of the drug the expected response is alleviation of specific symptoms or the presence of a therapeutic effect. Evaluation also may be used to determine if the patient or family member understands the drug regimen.

To evaluate the patient's response to therapy, and depending on the drug administered, the nurse may check the patient's blood pressure every hour, inquire whether pain has been relieved, or monitor the patient's pulse every 15 minutes. After evaluation, certain other decisions may need to be made and plans of action implemented. For example, the nurse may need to notify the primary health care provider of a marked change in a patient's pulse and respiratory rate after a drug was administered, or the nurse may need to change the bed linen because sweating occurred after a drug used to lower the patient's elevated temperature was administered.

The nurse can evaluate the patient's or family's understanding of the drug regimen by noting if one or both appear to understand the material that has been presented. Facial expression may indicate that one or both do or do not understand what has been explained. The nurse also may ask questions about the information that has been given to evaluate further the patient's or family's understanding.

Critical Thinking Exercises

1. Mr. Hatfield, aged 69 years, confides to you that he is not taking the drug prescribed by his primary health care provider. He states he took the drug for a while and then quit. Explain some possible reasons Mr. Hatfield could have for not taking his drug. Discuss questions you could ask to assess the reason for Mr. Hatfield's noncompliance.

2. Ms. Heggan is 82 years of age and lives alone. She is prescribed several drugs by the primary health care provider but is worried about taking the drugs and the side effects that might occur. She comes to the outpatient clinic after 1 week, and you learn that she has not filled her prescription and is not taking the drugs. Your nursing diagnosis is Ineffective Therapeutic Regimen Management related to anxiety about taking the prescribed drugs. Determine what information you would seek to obtain from Ms. Heggan. Identify important nursing interventions for this diagnosis.

3. Ms. Taylor is receiving three drugs for the treatment of difficulty breathing and swelling of her legs. You are giving these drugs for the first time. Discuss what questions you would ask Ms. Taylor to obtain subjective data.

Review Questions

1. A patient states that he does not understand why he had to take a specific medication. The most accurate nursing diagnosis for this man would be _____.

   A. Ineffective Therapeutic Regimen Management

   B. Anxiety

   C. Noncompliance

   D. Deficient Knowledge

2. When the nurse enters subjective data in the patient's record, this information is obtained from _____.

   A. the primary care provider

   B. other members of the health care team

   C. the patient or family

   D. laboratory and x-ray reports

3. During the evaluation phase of the nursing process, the nurse makes _____.

   A. decisions regarding the effectiveness of nursing interventions based on the outcome

   B. sure nursing procedures have been performed correctly

   C. notations regarding the patient's response to medical treatment

   D. a list of all adverse reactions the patient has experienced while taking the drug

To check your answers, see Appendix G.

The Nursing Process

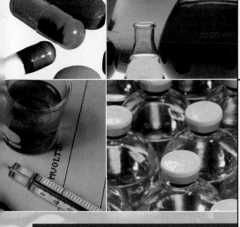

Patient and Family Teaching

Learning Objectives

On completion of this chapter, the student will:

- Identify important aspects of the teaching/learning process.
- Discuss the three domains of learning.
- Discuss important aspects of adult learning.
- Explain how the nursing process can be used to develop a teaching plan.
- Identify basic information to consider when developing a teaching plan.
- Discuss suggestions the nurse can make to the patient to adapt drug administration in the home.

Patient teaching is an integral part of nursing. When a drug is prescribed, the patient and the family must be made aware of all information concerning the drug. The nurse is responsible for supplying the patient with accurate and up-to-date information about the drugs prescribed. The patient must be educated about the drugs being taken while in the hospital as well the drugs to be taken on discharge. Therefore, patient teaching is an ongoing process both while the patient is an inpatient and as the patient prepares for dismissal. The teaching/learning process is the means through which the patient is made aware of the drug regimen.

The Teaching/Learning Process

Teaching is an interactive process that promotes learning. Both the patient and the nurse must be actively involved if teaching is to be effective. **Learning** is acquiring new knowledge or skills. When learning occurs there is a change in the patient's behavior, thinking, or both.

A patient must have **motivation** (having a desire or seeing a need) to learn. Motivation depends on the patient's perception of the need to learn. Education concerning the disease process may be necessary for the patient to become motivated to learn. Encouraging patient participation in planning realistic and attainable goals also promotes motivation. If the patient has no motivation, he or she is likely to be noncompliant.

Creating an accepting and positive atmosphere also enhances learning. Physical discomfort negatively affects the patient's concentration and, thus, the ability to learn. Making sure the patient is not in pain is vital to the teaching/learning process.

The Three Domains of Learning

Learning occurs in three domains: cognitive, affective, and psychomotor. When developing a teaching plan for the patient, the nurse must consider each domain.

Cognitive Domain

The **cognitive domain** refers to intellectual activities such as thought, recall, decision making, and drawing conclusions. In this domain the patient uses previous experiences, prior knowledge, and perceptions to give meaning to new information or to modify previous thinking. The nurse makes use of the patient's cognitive abilities when information is given to the patient or caregivers about the disease process, medication regimen, and adverse reactions. The patient uses the cognitive domain to process the information, ask questions, and make decisions.

Affective Domain

The **affective domain** includes the patient's or caregiver's attitudes, feelings, beliefs, and opinions. Health care providers often ignore these aspects of patient teaching. It is easy to pull a preprinted teaching outline off of the computer or obtain preprinted material. This type of material is often used as a checklist to teach the patient about a drug and the therapeutic regimen. Such checklists are useful in helping the nurse remember important aspects to be covered when teaching the patient about the drug and important information to give to the patient for future reference. However, the use of such checklists fails to take into account the affective domain.

Perhaps the most important prerequisite to learning about the patient's affective behavior is to develop a therapeutic relationship with the patient (a relationship that is based on trust and caring). When the nurse takes the time to develop a therapeutic relationship, the patient/family has confidence in the nurse and more confidence in the information conveyed. The nurse approaches the patient with respect and encourages the expression of thoughts and feelings. Exploring the patient's beliefs about health and illness enhances the nurse's understanding of the patient's affective behavior.

Psychomotor Domain

The **psychomotor domain** involves learning physical skills (such as injection of insulin) or tasks (such as performing a dressing change). The nurse teaches a task or skill using a step-by-step method. The patient is allowed hands-on practice supervised by the nurse. Mastery of the skill is assessed by having the patient or caregiver perform a return demonstration under the watchful eye of the nurse.

Adult Learning

Generally, adults learn only what they feel they need to learn. Adults learn best when they have a strong inner motivation to acquire a new skill or new knowledge. They will learn less if they are passive recipients of "canned" educational content. Adults have a vast array of experiences and knowledge to bring to a new learning experience. Teachers who use this experience will bring about the greatest behavior change. Whereas 83% of adults are visual learners, only 11% learn by listening. Most adults retain the information taught if they are able to "do" something with that new knowledge immediately. For example, in teaching a patient how to administer his or her own insulin, the nurse would demonstrate the technique, allow time for supervised practice, and, as soon as the patient appears ready, allow the patient to prepare and inject the insulin. Most adults prefer an informal learning environment in which mutual exchange and freedom of expression prevail.

The Nursing Process as a Framework for Patient Teaching

The nursing process is a systematic method of identifying patient health needs, devising a plan of care to meet the identified needs, initiating the plan, and evaluating its effectiveness. This process provides the necessary framework to develop an effective teaching plan. However, the teaching plan differs from the nursing process in that the nursing process encompasses all of the patient's health care needs, whereas the teaching plan focuses primarily on the patient's learning needs. Nurses must be actively involved in teaching if they are to educate their patients about the proper way to take their drugs, the possibility of adverse reactions, and the signs and symptoms of toxicity (if applicable).

Assessment

Assessment is the data-gathering phase of the nursing process. Assessment assists the nurse in choosing the best teaching methods and individualizing the teaching plan. To develop an effective teaching plan, the nurse must first determine the patient's needs. Needs stem from three areas: (1) information the patient or family needs to know about a particular drug; (2) the patient's or family member's ability to learn, accept, and use information; and (3) any barriers or obstacles to learning.

Some drugs have simple uses and, therefore, relatively little patient teaching is needed. For example, applying a nonprescription ointment to the skin requires only minimal teaching. Other drugs, such as insulin, require detailed information that may need to be given over several days.

Assessing an individual's ability to learn may be difficult. Not all adults have the same literacy level. The information to be taught should be geared to the patient's educational and reading level. When assessing language and literacy skills, it is important to remember that some patients do not read well. The nurse must carefully assess the patient's ability to communicate. Without accurate communication, learning will not occur. If the patient has a learning impairment, a family member or friend should be included in the teaching process. Most people readily understand what is being taught, but some cannot. For example, a visually impaired patient may be unable to read a label or printed directions supplied by the primary health care provider, pharmacist, or nurse. Another means of teaching will need to be used.

Through assessment, the nurse determines what barriers or obstacles (if any) may prevent the patient or family member from fully understanding the material being presented. Taking into consideration the patient's cultural background is helpful when planning a teaching session. For example, for some patients an interpreter is needed. In other cultures a certain individual (e.g., the mother or the grandmother) is the decision maker in the family. In such cases, it is important for the nurse to include the decision maker and the patient in the teaching session.

Nursing Diagnoses

The nursing diagnosis is formulated after analyzing the information obtained during the assessment phase. Examples of nursing diagnoses related to the administration of drugs are listed in the Nursing Diagnosis Checklist.

Nursing Diagnosis Checklist

✓ **Effective Therapeutic Regimen Management**

✓ **Ineffective Therapeutic Regimen Management** related to lack of knowledge

✓ **Deficient Knowledge** related to the drug regimen, possible adverse reactions, disease process, other factors

The nursing diagnosis Effective Therapeutic Regimen Management generally describes a patient who is successfully managing the medication regimen. The nurse uses this nursing diagnosis to enhance the patient's management by teaching the patient possible adverse reactions that could affect his or her health and how to manage them or reduce the potential harmful effects. This diagnosis does not need related factors because related factors would only indicate the patient's characteristics or ability to manage his or her condition (e.g., motivated or knowledgeable).

The nursing diagnosis Ineffective Therapeutic Regimen Management is useful for discharge teaching, especially when the nurse must teach the client how to manage the medication regimen. Often, chronic illness or a variety of health problems may mean that the patient is taking as many as eight or more medications and may have difficulty managing a complicated medication regimen. This diagnosis describes individuals who are having difficulty achieving positive results. The patient or family must have verbalized the desire to manage the treatment or difficulty with one or more of the prescribed regimens.

Deficient Knowledge is a nursing diagnosis that may be used when the patient has a deficit in cognitive knowledge or psychomotor skills necessary to administer a medication properly. The defining characteristic would be that the patient would report deficient knowledge or request information, or the patient does not correctly perform a prescribed skill necessary to the medication regimen. It is sometimes difficult to know exactly when to use the nursing diagnosis of Deficient Knowledge because all nursing diagnoses have related patient teaching as part of their nursing interventions. If teaching is related directly to a nursing diagnosis, then incorporate the teaching into the plan. Deficient Knowledge should be used cautiously because it is not a human response but a factor relating to or causing the diagnosis. When information (or knowledge) is required to assist the patient with managing the drug in the home setting or after dismissal, the diagnosis Ineffective Therapeutic Regimen Management is indicated.

Planning

Planning is the development of strategies to be used in the teaching plan and the selection of information to be taught. Planning begins with the development of expected outcomes. The nurse then develops a teaching plan based on the expected outcomes using the information gained during the assessment. Display 5-1 identifies important information to include in the teaching plan. Display 5-2 identifies basic information to consider when developing a teaching plan.

Display 5.1 Important Information to Include in the Teaching Plan

1. Therapeutic response expected from the drug
2. Adverse reactions to expect when taking the drug
3. Adverse reactions to report to the nurse or primary health care provider
4. Dosage and route
5. Any special considerations or precautions associated with the particular drug prescribed
6. Additional education regarding special considerations for certain drugs, such as techniques for giving injections, applying topical patches, or instilling eye drops

Display 5.2 Basic Considerations When Developing a Drug Teaching Plan

General material to consider when developing a teaching plan includes information on the dosage regimen and adverse reactions, issues relating to family members, and basic information about drugs, drug containers, and drug storage.

Dosage Regimen

The dosage regimen is an important aspect of the teaching plan. The nurse must consider the following general points when teaching about the dosage regimen:

- Capsules or tablets should be taken with water unless the primary health care provider or pharmacist directs otherwise (e.g., take with food, milk, or an antacid). Some liquids, such as coffee, tea, fruit juice, and carbonated beverages, may interfere with the action of certain drugs.

- It is important not to chew capsules before swallowing; they must be swallowed whole. The patient also should not chew tablets unless they are labeled "chewable." This is because some tablets have special coatings that are required for specific purposes, such as proper absorption of the drug or prevention of irritation of the lining of the stomach.

- The dose (amount) of a drug or the time between doses is never increased or decreased unless directed by the primary health care provider.

- A prescription drug or nonprescription drug course of therapy recommended by a primary health care provider is not stopped or omitted except on the advice of the primary health care provider.

- If the symptoms for which a drug was prescribed do not improve, or become worse, the primary health care provider must be contacted as soon as possible because a change in dosage or a different drug may be necessary.

- If a dose of a drug is omitted or forgotten, the next dose must not be doubled or the drug taken at more frequent intervals unless advised to do so by the primary health care provider.

- All health care workers, including physicians, dentists, nurses, and health personnel, must always be informed of all drugs (prescription and nonprescription) currently being taken on a regular or occasional basis.

- The exact names of all prescription and nonprescription drugs currently being taken should be kept in a wallet or purse for instant reference when seeing a physician, dentist, or other health care provider.

- Check prescriptions carefully when obtaining refills from the pharmacy and report any changes in the prescribed drug (e.g., changes in color, size, shape) to the pharmacist or primary health care provider before taking the drug because an error may have occurred.

- Wear a MedicAlert bracelet or other type of medical identification when taking a drug for a long time. This is especially important for drugs such as anticoagulants, steroids, oral hypoglycemic agents, insulin, or digitalis. In case of an emergency, the bracelet ensures that medical personnel are aware of health problems and current drug therapy.

Adverse Drug Effects

Information about adverse drug effects of the prescribed drug must be included when the nurse develops a teaching plan for the patient. The nurse should teach the patient the following general points about adverse drug effects:

- All drugs cause adverse reactions (side effects). Examples of some of the more common adverse reactions are nausea, vomiting, diarrhea, constipation, skin rash, dizziness, drowsiness, and dry mouth. Some effects may be mild and subside with time or when the primary health care provider adjusts the dosage. In some instances, mild reactions, such as dry mouth, may have to be tolerated. Some adverse reactions, however, are potentially serious and even life-threatening.

- Adverse reactions are always reported to the primary health care provider as soon as possible.

- Medical personnel must be informed of all drug allergies before any treatment or drug is given.

Family Members

The nurse considers the following points concerning family members when developing a teaching plan:

- A drug prescribed for one family member is never given to another family member, relative, or friend unless directed to do so by the primary health care provider.

- The nurse makes sure that all family members or relatives are aware of all drugs, prescription and nonprescription, that are currently being taken by the patient.

Drugs, Drug Containers, and Drug Storage

The following are important facts about drugs, drug containers, and the storage of drugs that the nurse must consider when developing a teaching plan:

Display 5.2 Basic Considerations When Developing a Drug Teaching Plan (continued)

- The term *drug* applies to both nonprescription and prescription drugs.
- A drug must be kept in the container in which it was dispensed or purchased. Some drugs require special containers, such as light-resistant (brown) bottles, to prevent deterioration that may occur on exposure to light.
- The original label on the drug container must not be removed while it is used to hold the drug. All directions on the label (e.g., "shake well before using," "keep refrigerated," "take before meals") must be followed to ensure drug effectiveness.

- Two or more different drugs must never be mixed in one container, even for a brief time, because one drug may chemically affect another. Mixing drugs can also lead to mistaking one drug for another, especially when the size and color are similar.
- All drugs must be kept out of the reach of children and pets.
- Do not expose a drug to excessive sunlight, heat, cold, or moisture because deterioration may occur.
- A prescription must never be saved for later use unless the primary health care provider so advises.

Developing an Individualized Teaching Plan

Teaching plans are individualized because patients' needs are not identical. Areas covered in an individualized teaching plan vary depending on the drug prescribed, the primary health care provider's preference for including or excluding specific facts about the drug, and what the patient needs to know to take the drug correctly. Teaching strategies must reflect individual learning needs and ability. For example, a patient who speaks and reads only Spanish will not benefit from discharge instructions given or written in English. Different strategies must be implemented, such as providing instructions written in Spanish or communicating through another nurse who is fluent in the Spanish language.

Selecting Relevant Information

When developing an individualized teaching plan for patients and their families, the nurse must select information relevant to a specific drug, adapt teaching to the individual's level of understanding, and avoid medical terminology unless terms are explained or defined. Figure 5-1 is a sample form to use when developing a teaching plan. It is important to remember that repetition enhances learning. Several teaching sessions help the nurse to assess better what the patient is actually learning and provide time for clarification. The patient should be encouraged to ask questions and express feelings.

Implementation

Implementation is the actual performance of the interventions identified in the teaching plan—putting the plan into action. Teaching at an appropriate time for each patient fosters learning. For example, patient teaching is not performed when there are visitors (unless they are to be involved in the administration of the patient's drugs), immediately before discharge from the hospital, or if the patient is sedated or in pain.

Teaching should begin a day or more before discharge, at a time when the patient is alone and alert. Teaching continues each day until dismissal. The nurse gears teaching to the patient's level of understanding and, when necessary, provides written as well as oral instructions. If a lot of information is given, it is often best to present the material in two or more sessions. Drug administration modifications may be necessary once the patient is at home. The nurse keeps these modifications in mind when teaching the patient (see Home Care Checklist: Modifying Drug Administration in the Home).

Evaluation

To determine the effectiveness of patient teaching, the nurse evaluates the patient's knowledge of the material presented. Evaluation can occur in several ways, depending on the nature of the information. For example, if the patient is being taught to administer insulin, several demonstrations can be scheduled, followed by a return demonstration by the patient with the nurse observing to evaluate the patient's technique.

Questions such as "Do you understand?" or "Is there anything you don't understand?" should be avoided because the patient may feel uncomfortable admitting a lack of understanding. When factual material is being evaluated, the nurse should periodically ask the patient to list or repeat some of the information presented.

Patient:_____ Medical Diagnosis: _____

Nursing Diagnosis: _____

_____ Effective Therapeutic Regimen Management _____

_____ Ineffective Therapeutic Regimen Management related to _____

_____ Deficient Knowledge related to _____

Expected Outcome: Patient will _____

_____

Identified obstacles to learning: _____

_____

_____

Primary Language: _____

Cultural Considertions: _____

_____

_____

Information to include in teaching session:

Expected therapeutic drug response:

Dosage and route:

Possible adverse reaction:

Adverse reaction to report:

Special considerations:

Teaching session(s)

Date(s)	Present	Evaluation*	Comments
1.			
2.			
3.			

*return demonstration, verbalizes unbderstanding of information, questioned by nurse, other (specify) _____

Figure 5.1   Patient and family medication teaching guide.

Home Care Checklist

Modifying Drug Administration in the Home

Once the patient is at home, some modifications may be necessary to ensure safe drug administration. The nurse provides written instructions, using large print (if necessary), nonglare paper, and words that the patient and caregiver can understand. In addition, it is important to modify your teaching by using the following suggestions:

☑ For patients taking more than one drug, develop a clear, easy-to-read drug schedule or a chart resembling a clock for the patient or caregiver to consult.

☑ Try using a daily calendar as an inexpensive, yet effective, means for scheduling.

☑ If the patient or caregiver has a problem with drug names, refer to the drug by shape or color if appropriate. Another idea is to number bottles and use this number on the drug chart.

☑ If financially feasible, suggest the use of commercially available drug organizers. If the patient cannot afford drug organizers, an egg carton or a muffin tin can be labeled and used as a drug organizer.

☑ If your patient finds it helpful to keep all drugs together, suggest using a bowl, tray, or small box to hold all the containers.

☑ If temporary refrigeration is necessary, suggest the use of a small cooler or insulated bag.

☑ If equipment items such as needles and syringes are used, suggest keeping all the supplies in one area.

☑ If the supplies came in a delivery box, suggest that the patient use it for storage. Other suggestions include using plastic storage containers with snap-on lids or clean, dry glass jars with screw tops.

☑ Advise the patient to use an impervious container with a properly fitting lid, such as a coffee can, for safe disposal of needles and syringes. A plastic milk jug with a lid or a heavy-duty, clean, cardboard milk or juice carton may be used if necessary.

☑ Explain the importance of taking precautions to make sure discarded needles do not puncture the container.

Critical Thinking Exercises

1. Locate the clinical educator in any health care agency in your community whose job it is to educate patients. Discuss with that person his or her thoughts and feelings on patient education, as well as any problems or pitfalls he or she has identified.

2. Interview friends or relatives about their knowledge of the drug(s) prescribed by their primary health care provider. Discuss with them the teaching they received from nurses or other health care providers before they began taking the drugs. Determine what areas could have been included that were not discussed. Analyze how the teaching/learning process was evaluated. Identify any areas that could be improved.

3. Using the form in Figure 5-1, develop a teaching plan for a patient.

Review Questions

1. An interactive process that promotes learning is defined as _____.

   A. motivation

   B. cognitive ability

   C. the psychomotor domain

   D. teaching

2. When developing a teaching plan the nurse assesses the affective learning domain, which means that the nurse considers the patient's _____.

   A. attitudes, feelings, beliefs, and opinions

   B. ability to perform a return demonstration

   C. intellectual ability

   D. home environment

3. Actual development of the strategies to be used in the teaching plan and selection of the information to be taught occur in the _____ phase of the nursing process.

   A. assessment

   B. planning

   C. implementation

   D. evaluation

4. Unless the primary health care provider or pharmacist directs otherwise, the nurse informs the patient to take oral medications with _____.

   A. fruit juice

   B. milk

   C. water

   D. food

5. Mrs. Jones is preparing for dismissal from the hospital tomorrow. She tells you that she has some questions about the medications that she will be taking at home. She explains that the regimen is complicated and she is afraid she will not be able to remember when to take her medications. Which of the following nursing diagnoses would be most appropriate for Mrs. Jones?

   A. Effective Individual Therapeutic Regimen Management

   B. Ineffective Therapeutic Regimen Management

   C. Deficient Knowledge

   D. Risk for Ineffective Home Management

To check your answers, see Appendix G.

Anti-Infectives

The body is equipped with a natural defense system. Infections occur when a **pathogenic** microorganism (which can cause a disease) breaches the defense system. Microbes enter the body in different ways, such as through a break in the skin, or by ingestion, breathing, or contact with the mucous membranes of the body.

This unit discusses drugs used to kill or retard the growth of microorganisms that invade the body. These are classed together as anti-infective drugs. They include drugs used to treat infections from bacteria, viruses, fungi, and protozoans. Those that work to destroy bacteria are categorized according to the chemical classification of the drug and presented in separate chapters. These drugs include the sulfonamides, penicillins, cephalosporins, tetracycline/macrolide/lincosamide group, fluoroquinolone/aminoglycoside group, and miscellaneous anti-infectives.

Drugs that are used against bacteria are either bacteriostatic (they slow or retard the multiplication of bacteria) or bactericidal (they destroy the bacteria). Some drugs are considered *broad spectrum*, meaning they destroy a large number of different types of bacteria from the same strain, such as gram-negative bacteria. Other drugs are specific to particular bacteria and are called *narrow-spectrum* antibiotics.

To determine if a specific type of bacteria is sensitive to an antibiotic drug, culture and sensitivity tests are performed. A culture is performed by placing infectious material obtained from areas such as the skin, respiratory tract, and blood on a culture plate that contains a special growing medium. This growing medium is "food" for the bacteria. After a specified time, the bacteria are examined under a microscope and identified. The sensitivity test involves placing the infectious material on a separate culture plate and then placing small disks impregnated with various antibiotics over the

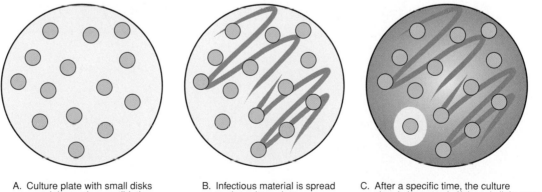

A. Culture plate with small disks containing various antibiotics.

B. Infectious material is spread on the culture plate.

C. After a specific time, the culture plate is inspected. If there is little or no growth around a disk, the bacteria is said to be sensitive to that antibiotic.

In sensitivity testing, small antibiotic disks are placed on a culture plate (**A**). Next, bacterial matter is applied to the plate (**B**). After a specified time, the plate is inspected. An area where few or no bacteria grow indicates that the bacteria are sensitive to the associated antibiotic (**C**, light circle).

area. After a specified time, the culture plate is examined. If there is little or no growth around a disk, the bacteria are considered sensitive to that particular antibiotic. Therefore, the infection will be controlled by this antibiotic. If there is considerable growth around the disk, then the bacteria are considered resistant to that particular antibiotic, and the infection will not be controlled by this antibiotic.

Bacterial resistance is the ability of bacteria to produce substances that inactivate or destroy the antibiotic. Because bacteria have this ability, many more drugs have been developed in addition to the sulfonamides and penicillins to fight bacterial infections. They include cephalosporins, the tetracycline group, and various other drugs.

Antibiotics can disrupt the **normal flora** (nonpathogenic microorganisms in the body), causing a secondary infection or superinfection. This new infection is "superimposed" on the original infection. The destruction of large numbers of nonpathogenic bacteria (normal flora) by the antibiotic alters the chemical environment. This allows uncontrolled growth of bacteria or fungal microorganisms that are not affected by the antibiotic being administered. A superinfection may occur with the use of any antibiotic, especially when these drugs are given for a long time or when repeated courses of therapy are necessary. Therefore, patient teaching is essential to ensure the proper course of therapy to reduce these other infections.

Fungal and protozoal infections have played a more prominent role in recent years because of advances in medical treatments that cause immunosuppression (a reduction in white blood cells). Infections that were minor at one time have become life-threatening in immunosuppressed patients because low numbers of infection-fighting white blood cells leave the body unable to resist the infection.

Viruses are organisms that do not have a typical cell structure and use host cells to grow and divide. Because viruses use the DNA or RNA of other cells, their ability to change has posed a problem in making drugs to treat viral infections. Recent scientific discoveries have led to the production of more effective antiviral drugs.

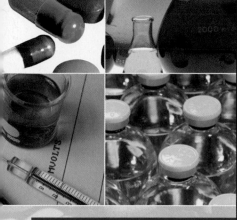

Chapter 6

Sulfonamides

Key Terms

anorexia
antibacterial
aplastic anemia
bacteriostatic
crystalluria
hypersensitivity
leukopenia
pruritus
Stevens-Johnson syndrome
stomatitis
thrombocytopenia
toxic epidermal necrolysis
urticaria

Learning Objectives

On completion of this chapter, the student will:

- Discuss the uses, general drug actions, and general adverse reactions, contraindications, precautions, and interactions for the sulfonamides.
- Discuss important preadministration and ongoing assessment activities the nurse should perform on the patient taking sulfonamides.
- List nursing diagnoses particular to a patient taking sulfonamides.

- Discuss ways to promote an optimal response to therapy, how to manage adverse reactions, and important points to keep in mind when educating patients about the use of the sulfonamides.
- Identify the rationale for increasing fluid intake when taking sulfonamides.
- Describe the objective signs indicating that a severe skin reaction, such as Stevens-Johnson syndrome, is present.

SULFONAMIDES

The sulfonamides (sulfa drugs) were the first antibiotic drugs developed that effectively treated infections. Sulfonamides are **antibacterial** agents, meaning they are active against bacteria. Sulfadiazine, sulfisoxazole, and sulfamethizole are examples of sulfonamide preparations. Although the use of sulfonamides began to decline after the introduction of more effective anti-infectives, such as the penicillins and other antibiotics, these drugs remain important for the treatment of certain types of infections.

Actions

The sulfonamides are primarily **bacteriostatic** because of their ability to inhibit the activity of folic acid in bacterial cell metabolism. Once the rate of bacterial multiplication is slowed, the body's own defense mechanisms (white blood cells) are able to rid the body of the invading microorganisms and therefore control the infection.

Uses

The sulfonamides are often used according to their absorption and excretion rates.

- The sulfonamides are well absorbed by the gastrointestinal system and excreted by the kidneys. They are often used to control urinary tract infections caused by certain bacteria, such as *Escherichia coli*, *Staphylococcus aureus*, and *Klebsiella* and *Enterobacter* species.

- Mafenide (Sulfamylon) and silver sulfadiazine (Silvadene) are topical sulfonamides used in the treatment of infections in second- and third-degree burns.

Additional uses of the sulfonamides are given in the Summary Drug Table: The Sulfonamides.

SUMMARY DRUG TABLE   THE SULFONAMIDES

GENERIC NAME	TRADE NAME	USES	ADVERSE REACTIONS	DOSAGE RANGES
Single Agents				
℞ **sulfadiazine** *sul-fa-dye'-a-zeen*	Microsulfon	Urinary tract infections due to susceptible microorganisms, chancroid, acute otitis media, *Hemophilus influenzae* and meningococcal meningitis, rheumatic fever	Hematologic changes, Stevens-Johnson syndrome, nausea, vomiting, headache, diarrhea, chills, fever, anorexia, crystalluria, stomatitis, urticaria, pruritus	Loading dose: 2–4 g orally; maintenance dose: 2–4 g/d orally in 4–6 divided doses
sulfasalazine *sul-fa-sal'-a-zeen*	Azulfidine, Azulfidine EN-tabs	Ulcerative colitis, rheumatoid arthritis	Same as sulfadiazine; may cause skin and urine to turn orange-yellow	Initial therapy: 1–4 g/d orally in divided doses; maintenance dose: 2 g/d orally in evenly spaced doses (500 mg QID)
℞ **sulfisoxazole** *sul-fi-sox'-a-zole*		Same as sulfadiazine	Same as sulfadiazine	Loading dose: 2–4 g orally; maintenance dose: 4–8 g/d orally in 4–6 divided doses
Multiple Drug Preparations				
trimethoprim (TMP) and sulfamethoxazole (SMZ) *trye-meth'-oh-prim; sul-fa-meth-ox'-a-zole*	Bactrim, Bactrim DS, Septra, Septra DS	Urinary tract infections due to susceptible microorganisms, acute otitis media, traveler's diarrhea due to *Escherichia coli*	Gastrointestinal disturbances, allergic skin reactions, hematologic changes, Stevens-Johnson syndrome, headache	160 mg TMP/800 mg SMZ orally q12h; 8–10 mg/kg/d (based on TMP) IV in 2–4 divided doses
Topical Sulfonamide Preparations				
mafenide *meph'-a-nide*	Sulfamylon	Second- and third-degree burns	Pain or burning sensation, rash, itching, facial edema	Apply to burned area 1–2 times/day
silver sulfadiazine *sil'-ver sul-fa-dye'-a-zeen*	Silvadene, Thermazene, SSD (cream)	Same as mafenide	Leukopenia, skin necrosis, skin discoloration, burning sensation	Same as mafenide

℞ = This drug should be administered at least 1 hour before or 2 hours after a meal.

Adverse Reactions

The sulfonamides are capable of causing a variety of adverse reactions. Some of these are serious or potentially serious; others are mild. **Anorexia** (loss of appetite) is an example of a mild adverse reaction. Other adverse reactions that may occur during therapy include

- Nausea, vomiting
- Diarrhea, abdominal pain
- Chills, fever
- **Stomatitis** (inflammation of the mouth).

In some instances, these may be mild. At other times they may cause serious problems, such as pronounced weight loss, requiring discontinuation of the drug.

Sulfasalazine may cause the urine and skin to take on an orange-yellow color; this is not abnormal. **Crystalluria** (crystals in the urine) may occur during administration of a sulfonamide, although this problem occurs less frequently with some of the newer sulfonamide preparations. Often, this potentially serious problem can be prevented by increasing fluid intake during sulfonamide therapy.

Photosensitivity can be a concern with some of the sulfonamides, and patients should be cautioned to wear protective clothing or sunscreen when outside. In areas where the climate is overcast, solar glare and direct sunshine can cause a sunburn reaction.

Various types of **hypersensitivity** (allergic) reaction may be seen during sulfonamide therapy, including **urticaria** (hives), **pruritus** (itching), generalized skin eruptions, or severe reactions leading to potentially lethal conditions such as toxic epidermal necrolysis or Stevens-Johnson syndrome.

Nursing Alert

Toxic epidermal necrolysis (TEN) and **Stevens-Johnson syndrome** (SJS) are serious and sometimes fatal hypersensitivity reactions. Widespread sloughing of both the skin and mucous membranes can occur. Internal organ involvement can cause death. Patients with SJS may complain of fever, cough, muscular aches and pains, and headache, all of which are signs and symptoms of many other disorders. The nurse must be alert for the additional signs of lesions on the skin and mucous membranes, eyes, and other organs, a diagnostically important indicator of these problems. The lesions appear as red wheals or blisters, often starting on the face, in the mouth, or on the lips, neck, and extremities. These conditions may occur with the administration of other types of drugs. The nurse must notify the primary health care provider and withhold the next dose of the drug. In addition, the nurse must exercise care to prevent injury to the involved areas.

The most frequent adverse reaction seen with the topical application of mafenide is a burning sensation or pain when the drug is applied to the skin. Other possible allergic reactions include rash, itching, edema, and urticaria. Burning, rash, and itching may also be seen with the use of silver sulfadiazine. It may be difficult to distinguish between adverse reactions due to the use of mafenide or silver sulfadiazine and those that occur from a severe burn injury or from other agents used for the management of burns.

The following hematologic changes may occur during prolonged sulfonamide therapy:

- **Thrombocytopenia**—decrease in the number of platelets
- **Aplastic anemia**—anemia due to deficient red blood cell production in the bone marrow
- **Leukopenia**—decrease in the number of white blood cells

These changes are examples of serious adverse reactions. If any of these occur, discontinuation of sulfonamide therapy may be required.

Contraindications

The sulfonamides are contraindicated in patients with hypersensitivity to the sulfonamides, during lactation, and in children younger than 2 years of age. The sulfonamides are not used near the end (at term) of pregnancy (pregnancy category D; see Chapter 1). If the sulfonamides are given near the end of pregnancy, significantly high blood levels of the drug may occur, causing jaundice or hemolytic anemia in the neonate. In addition, the sulfonamides are not used for infections caused by group A beta-hemolytic streptococci because the sulfonamides have *not* been shown to be effective in preventing the complications of rheumatic fever or glomerulonephritis.

Precautions

The sulfonamides are used with caution in patients with renal impairment, hepatic impairment, or bronchial asthma.

These drugs are given with caution to patients with allergies. Safety for use during pregnancy has not been established (pregnancy category C, except at term).

Interactions

The following interactions may occur when a sulfonamide is administered with another agent:

Interacting Drug	Common Use	Effect of Interaction
oral anticoagulants	Blood thinner; prevent clot formation	Increased action of the anticoagulant
methotrexate	Immunosuppression and chemotherapy	Increased bone marrow suppression
hydantoins	Anticonvulsants	Increased serum hydantoin level

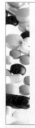

Chronic Care Alert

When diabetic patients are prescribed sulfonamides, assess for a possible hypoglycemic reaction. Sulfonamides may inhibit the (hepatic) metabolism of the oral hypoglycemic drugs tolbutamide (Orinase) and chlorpropamide (Diabinese).

Health Supplement Alert

Cranberries and cranberry juice are commonly used remedies for preventing and relieving symptoms of urinary tract infections (UTIs). The use of cranberries in combination with antibiotics has been recommended by physicians for the long-term suppression of UTIs. Cranberries are thought to prevent bacteria from attaching to the walls of the urinary tract. The suggested amount is 6 ounces of juice twice daily. Extremely large doses can produce gastrointestinal disturbances, such as diarrhea or abdominal cramping. Although cranberries may relieve symptoms or prevent the occurrence of a UTI, their use will not cure a UTI. If an individual suspects a UTI, medical attention is necessary.

NURSING PROCESS

The Patient Receiving a Sulfonamide

ASSESSMENT

PREADMINISTRATION ASSESSMENT

Before the initial administration of the drug, it is important to assess the patient's general appearance and take and record the vital signs. The nurse obtains information regarding the symptoms experienced by the patient and the length of time these symptoms have been present. Depending on the type and location of the infection or disease, the nurse reviews the results of tests, such as a urine culture, urinalysis, complete blood count, intravenous pyelogram, renal function tests, and examination of the stool.

ONGOING ASSESSMENT

During the course of therapy, the nurse evaluates the patient at periodic intervals for response to the drug, that is, a relief of symptoms and a decrease in temperature (if it was elevated before therapy started), as well as the occurrence of any adverse reactions.

The nurse monitors the temperature, pulse, respiratory rate, and blood pressure every 4 hours or as ordered by the primary health care provider. If fever is present and the patient's temperature suddenly increases or if the tempera-

ture was normal and suddenly increases, the nurse contacts the primary health care provider immediately.

The ongoing assessment for patients receiving sulfasalazine for ulcerative colitis includes observation for evidence of the relief or intensification of the symptoms of the disease. The nurse inspects all stool samples and records their number and appearance.

When administering a sulfonamide for a burn, the nurse inspects the burned areas every 1 to 2 hours because some treatment regimens require keeping the affected areas covered with the mafenide or silver sulfadiazine ointment at all times. Any adverse reactions should be reported immediately to the primary health care provider.

Nursing Diagnosis Checklist

✓ **Impaired Urinary Elimination** related to effect on the bladder from sulfonamides

✓ **Impaired Skin Integrity** related to burns

✓ **Impaired Skin Integrity** related to photosensitivity or severe allergic reaction to the sulfonamides

✓ **Risks for (Secondary) Infection** related to lowered white blood cell count resulting from sulfonamide therapy

NURSING DIAGNOSES

Drug-specific nursing diagnoses are highlighted in the Nursing Diagnoses Checklist. Other nursing diagnoses applicable to the drugs are discussed in depth in Chapter 4.

PLANNING

The expected patient outcomes depend on the reason for administration of the sulfonamide but may include an optimal response to drug therapy, meeting patient needs related to the management of adverse drug reactions, and an understanding of and compliance with the prescribed treatment regimen.

IMPLEMENTATION

PROMOTING AN OPTIMAL RESPONSE TO THERAPY

The patient receiving a sulfonamide drug almost always has an active infection. Some patients may be receiving one of these drugs to prevent an infection (prophylaxis) or as part of the management of a disease such as ulcerative colitis.

Unless the primary health care provider orders otherwise, the nurse gives sulfonamides to the patient whose stomach is empty, that is, 1 hour before or 2 hours after meals. If gastrointestinal irritation occurs, the nurse may give sulfasalazine with food or immediately after meals. It is important to instruct the patient to drink a full glass of water (8 ounces) when taking an oral sulfonamide and to drink at least eight large glasses of water each day until therapy is finished.

MONITORING AND MANAGING PATIENT NEEDS

The nurse must observe the patient for adverse reactions, especially an allergic reaction (see Chapter 1). If one or more adverse reactions should occur, the nurse withholds the next dose of the drug and notifies the primary health care provider.

IMPAIRED URINARY ELIMINATION Because one adverse effect of the sulfonamide drugs is altered elimination patterns, it is important that the nurse help the patient maintain adequate fluid intake and output. The nurse can encourage patients to increase fluid intake to 2000 mL or more per day to prevent crystalluria and stone (calculi) formation in the genitourinary tract, as well as to aid in removing microorganisms from the urinary tract. It is important to measure and record the patient's intake and output every 8 hours and notify the primary health care provider if the urinary output decreases or the patient fails to increase his or her oral intake.

Gerontologic Alert

Because renal impairment is common in older adults, the nurse should administer the sulfonamides with great caution. There is an increased danger of the sulfonamides causing additional renal damage when renal impairment is already present. An increase of fluid intake up to 2000 mL (if the older adult can tolerate this amount) decreases the risk of crystals and stones forming in the urinary tract. The older adult may be hesitant to increase oral fluid intake because of fear of incontinence. It is important for the nurse to assess for this fear and teach the patient when to take fluids to maintain continence and reduce the risk of crystal formation.

IMPAIRED SKIN INTEGRITY: BURN INJURY When mafenide or silver sulfadiazine is used in treating burns, the treatment regimen is outlined by the primary health care provider or the personnel in the burn treatment unit. There are various burn treatment regimens, such as debridement (removal of burned or dead tissue from the burned site), special dressings, and cleansing of the burned area. The use of a specific treatment regimen often depends on the extent of the burned area, the degree of the burns, and the physical condition and age of the patient. Other concurrent problems, such as lung damage from smoke or heat or physical injuries that occurred at the time of the burn injury, also may influence the treatment regimen.

When instructed to do so, the nurse cleans and removes debris present on the surface of the skin before each application of mafenide or silver sulfadiazine and applies these drugs with a sterile gloved hand. The drug is applied in a layer approximately 1/16 inch thick; thicker application is not recommended. The patient is kept away from any draft of air because even the slightest movement of air across the burned area can cause pain. It is important to warn the patient that stinging or burning may be felt during, and for a short time after, application of mafenide. Some burning also may be noted with the application of silver sulfadiazine.

IMPAIRED SKIN INTEGRITY: PHOTOSENSITIVITY The skin can become more sensitive to sunlight during sulfonamide therapy. The use of sunscreens is recommended, although they should not be used in place of protective clothing. The skin should be inspected each shift when treatment is started for signs of sores or blisters indicating the possibility of a severe allergic reaction. The skin and mucous membranes should be inspected for up to 14 days after the end of therapy, the period of time during which reactions can still occur.

RISK FOR SECONDARY INFECTION The nurse monitors the patient for leukopenia and thrombocytopenia. Leukopenia may result in signs and symptoms of an infection, such as fever, sore throat, and cough. The nurse protects the patient with leukopenia from individuals who have an infection. With severe leukopenia, the patient may be placed in protective (reverse) isolation.

Thrombocytopenia is manifested by easy bruising and unusual bleeding after moderate to slight trauma to the skin or mucous membranes. The extremities of the patient with thrombocytopenia are handled with care to prevent bruising. Care is taken to prevent trauma when moving the patient. The nurse inspects the skin daily for the extent of bruising and evidence of exacerbation of existing ecchymotic areas. It is important to encourage the patient to use a soft-bristled toothbrush to prevent any trauma to the mucous membranes of the oral cavity. The nurse reports any signs of leukopenia or thrombocytopenia immediately because this is an indication to stop drug therapy.

EDUCATING THE PATIENT AND FAMILY

When a sulfonamide is prescribed for an infection, some outpatients have a tendency to discontinue the drug once symptoms are gone. When teaching the patient and family, the nurse emphasizes the importance of completing the prescribed course of therapy to ensure all microorganisms causing the infection are eradicated. Failure to complete a course of therapy may result in a recurrence of the infection. The nurse should develop a teaching plan to include the following information:

- Take the drug as prescribed.

- Keep all follow-up appointments to ensure the infection is controlled.

- Complete the full course of therapy. Do not discontinue this drug (unless advised to do so by the primary health care provider) even though the symptoms of the infection have disappeared.

- Take the drug on an empty stomach either 1 hour before or 2 hours after a meal (exception: sulfasalazine [Azulfidine] is taken with food or immediately after a meal).

- Take the drug with a full glass of water. Do not increase or decrease the time between doses unless directed to do so by the primary health care provider.

- Drink *at least* eight to ten 8-ounce glasses of fluid every day.

- When taking sulfasalazine, the skin or urine may turn orange-yellow; this is not abnormal. Soft contact lenses may acquire a permanent yellow stain. It is a good idea to seek the advice of an ophthalmologist regarding corrective lenses while taking this drug.

- Prolonged exposure to sunlight may result in skin reactions similar to a severe sunburn (photosensitivity reactions). When going outside, cover exposed areas of the skin or apply a protective sunscreen to exposed areas.

- Notify the primary health care provider immediately if the following should occur: fever, skin rash or other skin problems, nausea, vomiting, unusual bleeding or bruising, sore throat, or extreme fatigue.

EVALUATION

- The therapeutic drug effect is achieved.

- There is no evidence of infection.

- The patient's fluid intake is at least 2000 mL and output is at least 1200 mL daily while taking a sulfonamide.

- The skin is intact and free of inflammation, irritation, or ulcerations.

- Adverse reactions are identified, reported to the primary health care provider, and managed successfully through appropriate nursing interventions.

- The patient verbalizes the importance of complying with the prescribed treatment regimen.

- The patient and family demonstrate an understanding of the drug regimen.

Critical Thinking Exercises

1. Ms. Bartlett, aged 80 years, has been prescribed a sulfonamide for a UTI and is to take the drug for 10 days. You note that Ms. Bartlett seems forgetful and at times confused. Determine what problems might be associated with Ms. Bartlett's mental state and her possible noncompliance with her prescribed treatment regimen.

2. Mr. Garcia is receiving sulfisoxazole for a recurrent bladder infection. When keeping an outpatient clinic appointment, he tells you that he developed a fever and sore throat yesterday. Analyze the steps you would take to investigate his recent problem. Give a reason for your answers.

3. Ms. Watson has diabetes and is taking tolbutamide (Orinase). Her primary care provider prescribes the combination drug trimethoprim and sulfamethoxazole (Septra) for a bladder infection. Discuss any instructions and information you would give to Ms. Watson in the patient education session.

Review Questions

1. A nurse working in the clinic asks how the sulfonamides control an infection. The most accurate answer is that these drugs _____.

   A. encourage the production of antibodies

   B. inhibit folic acid metabolism

   C. reduce urine output

   D. make the urine alkaline, which eliminates bacteria

2. Patients receiving sulfasalazine for ulcerative colitis are told that the drug _____.

   A. is not to be taken with food

   B. rarely causes adverse effects

   C. may cause hair loss

   D. may turn the urine a orange-yellow color

3. When mafenide (Sulfamylon) is applied to a burned area, the nurse _____.

   A. first covers the burned area with a sterile compress

   B. irrigates the area with normal saline solution

C. warns the patient that stinging or burning may be felt

D. instructs the patient to drink two to three extra glasses of water each day

4. The nurse can evaluate the patient's response to therapy by asking him if _____.

   A. he completed the entire course of therapy

   B. his symptoms have been relieved

   C. he has seen any evidence of blood in the urine

   D. has experienced any constipation

Medication Dosage Problems

1. The primary health care provider prescribed sulfasalazine oral suspension 500 mg every 8 hours. The nurse has sulfasalazine oral suspension 250 mg/5 mL on hand. What dosage would the nurse give?

2. The primary health care provider orders sulfamethoxazole 2 g orally initially, followed by 1 g orally two times a day. The nurse has 1000-mg tablets on hand. How many tablets would the nurse give for the initial dose?

To check your answers, see Appendix G.

Sulfonamides

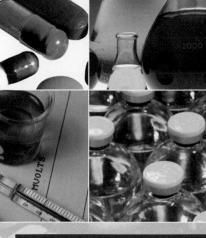

Penicillins

Learning Objectives

On completion of this chapter, the student will:

- Identify the uses, general drug actions, and general adverse reactions, contraindications, precautions, and interactions of the penicillins.

- Identify important preadministration and ongoing assessment activities the nurse should perform on the patient taking penicillin.

- List nursing diagnoses particular to a patient taking penicillin.

- Discuss hypersensitivity reactions and pseudomembranous colitis as they relate to antibiotic therapy.

- Discuss ways to promote optimal response to therapy, nursing actions to minimize adverse effects, and important points to keep in mind when educating patients about the use of penicillins.

The antibacterial properties of natural penicillins were discovered in 1928 by Sir Arthur Fleming while he was performing research on influenza. Ten years later, British scientists studied the effects of natural penicillins on disease-causing microorganisms. However, it was not until 1941 that natural penicillins were used clinically for the treatment of infections. Although used for more than 50 years, the penicillins are still an important and effective group of antibiotics for the treatment of susceptible **pathogens** (disease-causing microorganisms).

Actions

Bacterial cells have select components that differ from human cells, such as specific enzymes and a cell wall. Antibiotics target these differences (Fig. 7-1). The mechanisms of action of the penicillins inhibit the following bacterial cell activities:

- Cell wall synthesis

- DNA or RNA synthesis

- Protein synthesis

There are four groups of penicillins: natural penicillins, penicillinase-resistant penicillins, aminopenicillins, and extended-spectrum penicillins. See the Summary Drug Table: Penicillins for a more complete listing of the penicillins. Display 7-1 also gives examples of the various groups.

Natural Penicillins

Although the sulfonamides were used before the penicillins, the natural penicillins were the first large-scale antibiotics used to combat infection. These drugs worked very well because bacteria have a receptor on the cell wall that attracts the penicillin molecule. When the drug attaches to the cell, a portion of the drug molecule (the **beta-lactam ring**) breaks the cell wall and the cell dies (bactericidal action).

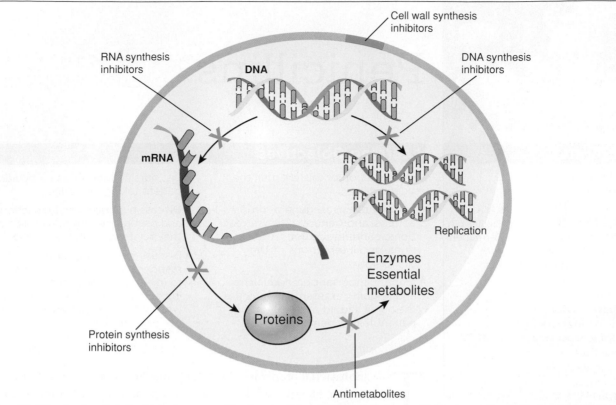

Figure 7.1 Effect of anti-infective drugs on the bacterial cell. (From Adams, M. P., Josephson, D. L., & Holland, L. N. [2005]. *Pharmacology in nursing: A pathophysiologic approach.* ©2005. Adapted by permission of Pearson Education, Inc., Upper Saddle River, NJ.)

Because the natural penicillins have been used for many years, drug-resistant strains of microorganisms have developed, making the natural penicillins less effective than some of the new antibiotics in treating a broad range of infections. Various types of bacterial resistance have developed against the penicillins.

Penicillinase-Resistant Penicillins

One example of **bacterial resistance** is the ability of certain bacteria to produce **penicillinase**, an enzyme that inactivates penicillin. The penicillinase-resistant penicillins were developed to combat this problem.

Display 7.1 Examples of Penicillins

- Natural penicillins—penicillin G and penicillin V
- Penicillinase-resistant penicillins—cloxacillin, dicloxacillin, nafcillin
- Aminopenicillins (broad spectrum)—ampicillin, amoxicillin, bacampicillin
- Extended-spectrum penicillins—mezlocillin, piperacillin, ticarcillin

Aminopenicillins (Broad Spectrum)

The natural penicillins also have a fairly narrow spectrum of activity, which means that they are effective against only a few strains of bacteria. Newer, chemically modified aminopenicillins were developed to combat this problem. These penicillins are a result of chemical treatment of a biological precursor to penicillin. Because of their chemical modifications, they are more slowly excreted by the kidneys and thus have a somewhat wider spectrum of antibacterial activity.

Certain bacteria have developed the ability to produce enzymes called *beta-lactamases*, which are able to destroy the beta-lactam ring. Fortunately, chemicals were discovered that inhibit the activity of these enzymes. Penicillin–beta-lactamase inhibitor combinations are a type of penicillin with a wider spectrum of antibacterial activity. Three examples of these beta-lactamase inhibitors are clavulanic acid, sulbactam, and tazobactam. When these chemicals are used alone, they have little antimicrobial activity. However, when combined with certain penicillins, they extend the spectrum of the penicillin's antibacterial activity. The beta-lactamase inhibitors bind with the penicillin and protect the penicillin from destruction. Examples of combinations of penicillins

SUMMARY DRUG TABLE   PENICILLINS

GENERIC NAME	TRADE NAME	USES	ADVERSE REACTIONS	DOSAGE RANGES
Natural Penicillins (Narrow Spectrum)				
℞ **penicillin G (aqueous)** *pen-i-sill'-in*	Pfizerpen	Infections due to susceptible micro-organisms; syphilis, gonorrhea	Glossitis, stomatitis, gastritis, furry tongue, nausea, vomiting, diarrhea, rash, fever, pain at injection site, hypersensitivity reactions, hematopoietic changes	Up to 20–30 million Units/day IV or IM; dosage may also be based on weight
℞ **penicillin G benzathine**	Bicillin C-R, Bicillin L-A, Permapen	Infections due to susceptible micro-organisms, syphilis; prophylaxis of rheumatic fever or chorea	Same as penicillin G	Up to 2.4 million Units/day IM
℞ **penicillin G procaine**		Infections due to susceptible organisms	Same as penicillin G	600,000–2.4 million Units/day IM
penicillin V	Veetids	Infections due to susceptible organisms	Same as penicillin G	125–500 mg orally q6h or q8h
Semisynthetic Penicillins				
Penicillinase-Resistant Penicillins (Narrow Spectrum)				
℞ **dicloxacillin sodium** *dye-klox-a-sill'-in*		Same as penicillin G	Same as penicillin G	125–250 mg orally q6h
℞ **nafcillin** *naf-sill'-in*		Same as penicillin G	Same as penicillin G	500 mg IV q4
℞ **oxacillin sodium** *ox-a-sill'-in*	Bactocill	Same as penicillin G	Same as penicillin G	500 mg–1 g orally q4–6h; 250 mg–1 g q4–6h IM, IV
Aminopenicillins (Broad Spectrum)				
amoxicillin *a-mox-i-sill'-in*	Amoxil, Trimox	Same as penicillin G	Same as penicillin G	500–875 mg orally q12h or 250 mg orally q8h
℞ **ampicillin, oral** *am-pi-sill'-in*	Principen, Totacillin	Same as penicillin G	Same as penicillin G	250–500 mg orally q6h
℞ **ampicillin sodium, parenteral**		Same as penicillin G	Same as penicillin G	1–12 g/d IM, IV in divided doses q4–6h
Aminopenicillins/Beta–Lactamase Inhibitors				
℞ **amoxicillin and clavulanate potassium** *a-mox-i-sill'-in/ klah-view-lan'-ate*	Augmentin	Same as penicillin G	Same as penicillin G	250 mg orally q8h or 500 mg orally q12h For severe infections: up to 875 mg q12h
℞ **ampicillin/sulbactam** *am-pi-sill'-in/ sull-bak'tam*	Unasyn	Same as penicillin G	Same as penicillin G	1.5 g–3 g q6h IM or IV

SUMMARY DRUG TABLE   (*continued*)

GENERIC NAME	TRADE NAME	USES	ADVERSE REACTIONS	DOSAGE RANGES
Extended-Spectrum Penicillins				
℞ **piperacillin sodium and tazobactam sodium** *pi-per-a-sill'-in/ tay-zoe-back'-tam*	Zosyn	Same as penicillin G	Same as penicillin G	3.375 g–4.5 g q6h IV
℞ **piperacillin sodium** *pi-per-a-sill'-in*		Same as penicillin G	Same as penicillin G	3–4 g q4–6h IV or IM; maximum dosage, 24 g/d
℞ **ticarcillin disodium** *ty-kar-sill'-in*	Ticar	Same as penicillin G	Same as penicillin G	150–300 mg/kg/d IV every 3, 4, or 6 hours; maximum dosage IM, 2–g injection
℞ **ticarcillin and clavulanate potassium** *ty-kar-sill'-in*	Timentin	Same as penicillin G	Same as penicillin G	Up to 3.1 g IV q4–6h or 200–300 mg/kg/d IV in divided doses q4–6h
℞ **carbenicillin indanyl sodium**	Geocillin	UTIs caused by *E. coli, Proteus, Enterobacter*	Same as penicillin G	382–764 mg orally QID

℞ This drug should be administered at least 1 hour before or two hours after a meal.

Display 7.2 Penicillin–Beta-Lactamase Inhibitor Combinations

- Augmentin—combination of amoxicillin and clavulanic acid
- Timentin—combination of ticarcillin and clavulanic acid
- Unasyn—combination of ampicillin and sulbactam
- Zosyn—combination of piperacillin and tazobactam

---

with beta-lactamase inhibitors are given in Display 7-2; also see the Summary Drug Table: Penicillins for more information on these combinations.

Extended-Spectrum Penicillins

Extended-spectrum penicillins are effective against an even wider range of bacteria than the broad-spectrum penicillins. These penicillins are used to destroy bacteria such as *Pseudomonas*.

Identifying the Appropriate Penicillin: Sensitivity and Resistance

After a culture and sensitivity report is received, the strain of microorganisms causing the infection is known

and the antibiotics to which these microorganisms are sensitive and resistant are identified. The primary health care provider then selects the antibiotic to which the microorganism is sensitive because that is the antibiotic that will be effective in the treatment of the infection.

Penicillins are bactericidal against sensitive microorganisms (i.e., those microorganisms that are affected by drug) provided there is an adequate concentration of penicillin in the body. The concentration of any drug in the body is referred to as the *blood level*. An inadequate concentration (or inadequate blood level) of penicillin may produce bacteriostatic activity, which may or may not control the infection.

Uses

Infectious Disease

The natural and semisynthetic penicillins are used in the treatment of bacterial infections caused by susceptible microorganisms. Penicillins may be used to treat infections such as:

- Urinary tract infections (UTIs)
- Septicemia
- Meningitis

- Intra-abdominal infections
- Sexually transmitted diseases (gonorrhea and syphilis)
- Pneumonia and other respiratory infections

Examples of infectious microorganisms (bacteria) that may respond to penicillin therapy include gonococci, staphylococci, streptococci, and pneumococci. A penicillinase-resistant penicillin is used as initial therapy for any suspected staphylococcal infection until culture and sensitivity results are known.

Prophylaxis

Because penicillin targets bacterial cells, it is of no value in treating viral or fungal infections. However, the primary health care provider occasionally prescribes penicillin as **prophylaxis** (prevention) against a potential secondary bacterial infection that can occur in a patient with a viral infection. In these situations the viral infection has weakened the body's defenses and the person is susceptible to other infections, particularly a bacterial infection. Penicillin also may be prescribed as prophylaxis for a potential infection in high-risk individuals, such as those with a history of rheumatic fever. Penicillin is taken several hours or in some instances days before and after an operative procedure, such as dental, oral, or upper respiratory tract procedures, that can result in bacteria entering the bloodstream. Taking penicillin before and after the procedure will usually prevent a bacterial infection in high-risk patients. Penicillin also may be given prophylactically on a continuing basis to those with rheumatic fever or chronic ear infections.

Resistance to Drugs

When antibiotics are used by one person for a while, or by a group of people that live in close proximity, such as a nursing home, drug resistance becomes an issue. Some bacteria may be naturally resistant to an antibiotic or they may acquire a resistance to the drug. When the susceptible bacteria are destroyed, what remains are the resistant bacteria. As a result, strains of drug-resistant bacteria multiply. These can range from the penicillinase enzyme–producing bacteria to **methicillin-resistant *Staphylococcus aureus* (MRSA)**.

MRSA is a type of bacteria that is resistant to certain antibiotics. These antibiotics include methicillin and other, more common antibiotics, such as oxacillin, penicillin, and amoxicillin. According to the Centers for Disease Control and Prevention (2005), staphylococcal infections, including MRSA, occur most frequently among persons who are in hospitals and health care facilities (such as nursing homes and dialysis centers) and who have weakened immune systems. Also emerging is a new resistance associ-

ated with bacteria that have both natural and acquired resistance. An example is vancomycin-resistant enterococci (VRE). This drug resistance is affecting severely ill, immunocompromised patients in intensive care units.

Adverse Reactions

Gastrointestinal Reactions

- **Glossitis** (inflammation of the tongue) when given orally
- **Stomatitis** (inflammation of the mouth), dry mouth
- Gastritis
- Nausea, vomiting
- Diarrhea, abdominal pain

Administration route reactions include pain at the injection site when given intramuscularly (IM) and irritation of the vein and **phlebitis** (inflammation of a vein) when given intravenously (IV).

Hypersensitivity Reactions

A **hypersensitivity** (or allergic) reaction to a drug occurs in some individuals, especially those with a history of allergy to many substances. Signs and symptoms of a hypersensitivity to penicillin are highlighted in Display 7-3.

Anaphylactic shock, which is a severe form of hypersensitivity reaction, also can occur (see Chapter 1). Anaphylactic shock occurs more frequently after parenteral administration but can occur with oral use. This reaction is likely to be immediate and severe in susceptible individuals. Signs of anaphylactic shock include severe hypotension, loss of consciousness, and acute respiratory distress. If not immediately treated, anaphylactic shock can be fatal.

Display 7.3 Signs and Symptoms of Hypersensitivity to Penicillin

Skin rash
Urticaria (hives)
Sneezing
Wheezing
Pruritus (itching)
Bronchospasm (spasm of the bronchi)
Laryngospasm (spasm of the larynx)
Angioedema (also called angioneurotic edema)—swelling of the skin and mucous membranes, especially around and in the mouth and throat
Hypotension—can progress to shock
Signs and symptoms resembling serum sickness—chills, fever, edema, joint and muscle pain, and malaise

Once an individual is allergic to one penicillin, he or she is usually allergic to all of the penicillins. Those allergic to penicillin also have a higher incidence of allergy to the cephalosporins (see Chapter 8). Allergy to drugs in the same or related groups is called **cross-sensitivity** or **cross-allergenicity**.

Superinfections

A **superinfection** can develop rapidly and is potentially serious and even life-threatening. Bacterial superinfections are seen with administration of the oral penicillins and occur in the bowel. Symptoms of bacterial superinfection of the bowel include diarrhea or bloody diarrhea, rectal bleeding, fever, and abdominal cramping. **Pseudomembranous colitis** is a commonly occurring bacterial superinfection.

Nursing Alert

Pseudomembranous colitis may occur after 4 to 9 days of treatment with penicillin or as long as 6 weeks after the drug is discontinued.

Gerontologic Alert

Older adults who are debilitated, chronically ill, or taking penicillin for an extended period are more likely to develop a superinfection. Pseudomembranous colitis is one type of a bacterial superinfection. This potentially life-threatening problem develops because of an overgrowth of the microorganism *Clostridium difficile*. This organism produces a toxin that affects the lining of the colon. Signs and symptoms include severe diarrhea with visible blood and mucus, fever, and abdominal cramps. This adverse reaction usually requires immediate discontinuation of the antibiotic. Mild cases may respond to drug discontinuation. Moderate to severe cases may require treatment with IV fluids and electrolytes, protein supplementation, and oral vancomycin.

Candidiasis or moniliasis is a common type of fungal superinfection. Fungal superinfections commonly occur in the gastrointestinal and reproductive systems. Symptoms include lesions of the mouth or tongue, vaginal discharge, and anal or vaginal itching.

Candidiasis results from yeastlike fungi that usually exist in small numbers in the vagina. The multiplication rate of these microorganisms is normally slowed and kept under control by a strain of bacteria (Döderlein's bacillus)

in the vagina. If penicillin therapy destroys these normal microorganisms of the vagina, the fungi are now uncontrolled, multiply at a rapid rate, and cause symptoms of the fungal infection candidiasis (or moniliasis).

Other Adverse Reactions

Other adverse reactions associated with penicillin include hematopoietic (blood cell) changes:

- Anemia (low red blood cell count)
- Thrombocytopenia (low platelet count)
- Leukopenia (low white blood cell count)
- Bone marrow depression

Contraindications and Precautions

Penicillins are contraindicated in patients with a history of hypersensitivity to penicillin or the cephalosporins.

Penicillins should be used cautiously in patients with renal disease, asthma, bleeding disorders, gastrointestinal disease, pregnancy (Pregnancy Category C) or lactation (may cause diarrhea or candidiasis in the infant), and history of allergies. Any indication of sensitivity is reason for caution.

Interactions

The following interactions may occur when a penicillin is administered with another agent.

Interacting Agent	Common Use	Effect of Interaction
oral contraceptives (with estrogen)	Contraception	Decreased effectiveness of contraceptive agent (with ampicillin, penicillin V).
tetracyclines	Anti-infective	Decreased effectiveness of penicillins
anticoagulants	Prevent blood clots	Increased bleeding risks (with large doses of penicillins)
beta-adrenergic blocking drugs (see Chapter 28)	Blood pressure control and heart problems	May increase the risk for an anaphylactic reaction

Herbal Alert

Goldenseal (*Hydrastis canadensis*) is an herb found growing in the certain areas of the northeastern United States, particularly the Ohio River valley. Goldenseal has long been used alone or in combination with echinacea to treat colds and influenza. However, there is no scientific evidence to support the use of goldenseal for cold and influenza or as a stimulant, as there is for the use of echinacea. Similarly, goldenseal is touted as an "herbal antibiotic," although there is no scientific evidence to support this use either. Another myth surrounding goldenseal's use is that taking the herb masks the presence of illicit drugs in the urine.

There are many traditional uses of the herb, such as an antiseptic for the skin, mouthwash for canker sores, wash for inflamed or infected eyes, and the treatment of sinus infections and digestive problems, such as peptic ulcers and gastritis. Some evidence supports the use of goldenseal to treat diarrhea caused by bacteria or intestinal parasites, such as *Giardia*. The herb is contraindicated during pregnancy and in patients with hypertension. Adverse reactions are rare when the herb is used as directed. However, this herb should not be taken for more than a few days to 1 week. Because of widespread use, destruction of its natural habitats, and renewed interest in its use as an herbal remedy, goldenseal was classified as an "endangered" plant in 1997 by the U.S. government.

NURSING PROCESS

The Patient Receiving Penicillin

ASSESSMENT

PREADMINISTRATION ASSESSMENT

Before administering the first dose of penicillin, the nurse obtains or reviews the patient's general health history. The health history includes an allergy history, a history of all medical and surgical treatments, a drug history, and the current symptoms of the infection. If the patient has a history of allergy, particularly a drug allergy, the nurse must explore this area to ensure the patient is not allergic to penicillin or a cephalosporin.

The nurse should take and record vital signs. When appropriate, it is important to obtain a description of the signs and symptoms of the infection from the patient or family. The nurse assesses the infected area (when possible) and records findings on the patient's chart. It is important to describe accurately any signs and symptoms related to the patient's infection, such as color and type of drainage from a wound, pain, redness and inflammation, color of sputum, or presence of an odor. In addition, the nurse should note the patient's general appearance. A culture and sensitivity test is almost always ordered, and the nurse must obtain the results before giving the first dose of penicillin.

ONGOING ASSESSMENT

The nurse evaluates the patient daily for a response to therapy, such as a decrease in temperature, the relief of symptoms caused by the infection (such as pain or discomfort), an increase in appetite, and a change in the appearance or amount of drainage (when originally present). Once an infection is controlled, patients often look better and even state that they feel better. It is important to record these evaluations on the patient's chart. The nurse notifies the primary health care provider if signs and symptoms of the infection appear to worsen.

Additional **culture and sensitivity tests** may be performed during therapy because microorganisms causing the infection may become resistant to penicillin, or a superinfection may occur. A urinalysis, complete blood count, and renal and hepatic function tests also may be performed at intervals during therapy.

Nursing Alert

The nurse should observe the patient closely for a hypersensitivity reaction, which may occur any time during therapy with the penicillins. If it should occur, it is important to contact the primary health care provider immediately and withhold the drug until the patient is seen by the primary health care provider.

NURSING DIAGNOSES

Drug-specific nursing diagnoses are highlighted in the Nursing Diagnoses Checklist. Other nursing diagnoses applicable to these drugs are discussed in Chapter 4.

Nursing Diagnosis Checklist

✔ **Impaired Skin Integrity** related to hypersensitivity to penicillin

✔ **Risk for Ineffective Respiratory Function** related to an allergic reaction to penicillin

✔ **Diarrhea** related to a bacterial secondary infection or superinfection

✔ **Impaired Oral Mucous Membranes** related to a secondary bacterial or fungal infection

✔ **Impaired Comfort: Increased Fever** related to ineffectiveness of penicillin against the infection

PLANNING

The expected outcomes for the patient depend on the reason for administering penicillin but may include an optimal response to drug therapy, meeting patient needs related to management of common adverse reactions, and an understanding of and compliance with the prescribed drug regimen.

IMPLEMENTATION

PROMOTING OPTIMAL RESPONSE TO THERAPY: PROPER ADMINISTRATION

The results of a culture and sensitivity test take several days because time must be allowed for the bacteria to grow on the culture media. However, infections are treated as soon as possible. In a few instances, the primary health care provider may determine that a penicillin is the treatment of choice until the results of the culture and sensitivity tests are known. In many instances, the primary health care provider selects a broad-spectrum antibiotic for initial treatment because of the many penicillin-resistant strains of microorganisms.

Adequate blood levels of the drug must be maintained for the agent to be effective. Accidental omission or delay of a dose results in decreased blood levels, which will reduce the effectiveness of the antibiotic. It is best to give oral penicillins on an empty stomach, 1 hour before or 2 hours after a meal. Penicillin V, and amoxicillin may be given without regard to meals.

Penicillin is ordered in units or milligrams. The exact equivalency usually is stated on the container or package insert. When preparing a parenteral form of penicillin, the nurse should shake the vial thoroughly before withdrawing the drug to ensure even distribution of the drug in the solution. Some forms of penicillin are in powder or crystalline form and must be made into a liquid (reconstituted) before being withdrawn from the vial. The manufacturer's directions regarding reconstitution are printed on the label or package insert. The manufacturer indicates the type of **diluent** (a solution compatible with the drug) to be used when reconstituting a specific drug. Some powdered or crystalline drugs, when reconstituted with a given amount of diluent, may yield slightly more or less than the amount of the diluent added to the vial. If there is any question regarding the reconstitution of any drug, the nurse consults with a pharmacist. In some health care facilities the drug is prepared in the pharmacy and delivered to the nurse for administration.

When administering penicillin IM, the nurse warns the patient that there may be a stinging or burning sensation at the time the drug is injected into the muscle. Penicillin solutions are often thick or viscous. Discomfort at the time

> **Nursing Alert**
>
> The nurse questions the patient about allergy to penicillin before administering the first dose, even when an accurate drug history has been taken. It is important to tell patients that the drug they are receiving is penicillin because information regarding a drug allergy may have been forgotten at the time the initial drug history was obtained. If a patient states he or she is allergic to penicillin or a cephalosporin, the nurse withholds the drug and contacts the primary health care provider.

of injection occurs because the drug is irritating to the tissues. The nurse inspects previous areas used for injection for continued redness, soreness, or other problems. It is important to inform the primary health care provider if previously used areas for injection appear red or the patient reports pain in the area.

MONITORING AND MANAGING PATIENT NEEDS

IMPAIRED SKIN INTEGRITY. Dermatologic reactions such as hives, rashes, and skin lesions can occur with the administration of penicillin. Treatment of minor hypersensitivity reactions may include administration of an antihistamine such as diphenhydramine (Benadryl) for a rash or itching. In mild cases or where the benefit of the drug outweighs the discomfort of skin lesions, the nurse administers frequent skin care. Emollients, antipyretic creams, or a topical corticosteroid may be prescribed to promote comfort. Harsh soaps and perfumed lotions are avoided. The nurse instructs the patient to avoid rubbing the area and not to wear rough or irritating clothing. It is important to report a rash or hives to the primary health care provider because this may be a precursor to a severe anaphylactic reaction (see section on Hypersensitivity Reactions). In severe cases, the primary health care provider may discontinue the penicillin therapy.

RISK FOR INEFFECTIVE RESPIRATORY FUNCTION. Major hypersensitivity reactions, such as bronchospasm, laryngospasm, hypotension, and angioedema, require immediate treatment with drugs such as epinephrine, cortisone, or an IV antihistamine. When respiratory difficulty occurs, a tracheostomy may need to be performed.

> **Nursing Alert**
>
> After administering penicillin IM in the outpatient setting, the nurse asks the client to wait in the area for at least 30 minutes. Anaphylactic reactions are most likely to occur within 30 minutes after injection.

DIARRHEA. Diarrhea may be an indication of a superinfection of the gastrointestinal tract or pseudomembranous colitis. The nurse inspects all stools and notifies the primary health care provider if diarrhea occurs because it may be necessary to stop the drug. If diarrhea does occur and there appears to be blood and mucus in the stool, it is important to save a sample of the stool and test for occult blood using a test such as Hemoccult. If the stool tests positive for blood, the nurse saves the sample for possible further laboratory analysis.

The nurse observes the patient for other symptoms of a bacterial or fungal superinfection in the vaginal or anal area, such as pain or itching. It is important to report any signs and symptoms of a superinfection to the primary health care provider before administering the next dose of the drug. When symptoms are severe, additional treatment measures may be necessary, such as administration of an antipyretic drug for fever or an antifungal drug.

IMPAIRED ORAL MUCOUS MEMBRANES. The administration of oral penicillin may result in a fungal superinfection in the oral cavity. This condition is characterized by varying degrees of oral mucous membrane inflammation, swollen and red tongue, swollen gums, and pain in the mouth and throat. To detect this problem early, the nurse inspects the patient's mouth daily for evidence of glossitis, sore tongue, ulceration, or a black, furry tongue. The nurse can explain that, if the diet permits, yogurt, buttermilk, or *Acidophilus* capsules may be taken to reduce the risk of fungal superinfection.

The nurse inspects the mouth and gums often and gives frequent mouth care with a nonirritating solution. A soft-bristled toothbrush is used when brushing is needed. A nonirritating soft diet may be required. The nurse monitors the dietary intake to ensure the patient is receiving adequate nutrition. Antifungal agents or local anesthetics are sometimes recommended to soothe the irritated membranes.

IMPAIRED COMFORT: INCREASED FEVER. The nurse takes vital signs every 4 hours, or more often if necessary. It is important to report any increase in temperature to the primary health care provider because additional treatment measures, such as administration of an antipyretic drug or change in the drug or dosage, may be necessary. An increase in body temperature several days after the start of therapy may indicate a secondary bacterial infection or failure of the drug to control the original infection. On occasion the fever may be caused by an adverse reaction to the penicillin. In these cases, the fever can usually be managed by using an antipyretic drug.

EDUCATING THE PATIENT AND FAMILY

Any time a drug is prescribed for a patient, the nurse is responsible for ensuring that the patient has a thorough understanding of the drug, the treatment regimen, and adverse reactions. Some patients do not adhere to the prescribed drug regimen for a variety of reasons, such as failure to comprehend the prescribed regimen or failure to understand the importance of continued and uninterrupted therapy. The nurse describes the drug regimen and stresses the importance of continued and uninterrupted therapy when teaching the patient who is prescribed an antibiotic.

The nurse provides the following information to patients prescribed an antibiotic:

- **Prophylaxis**—Take the drug as prescribed until the primary health care provider discontinues therapy.

- **Infection**—Complete the full course of therapy. Do not stop taking the drug, even if the symptoms have disappeared, unless directed to do so by the primary health care provider. Stopping antibiotic therapy before finishing the prescribed course may allow the infection to return.

- Take the drug at the prescribed times of day because it is important to keep an adequate amount of drug in the body throughout the entire 24 hours of each day.

- **Penicillin (oral)**—Take the drug on an empty stomach either 1 hour before or 2 hours after meals (exceptions: penicillin V and amoxicillin).

- Take each dose with a full 8-oz glass of water.

- **Oral suspensions**—Keep the container refrigerated (if so labeled), shake the drug well before pouring (if so labeled), and return the drug to the refrigerator immediately after pouring the dose. Drugs that are kept refrigerated lose their potency when kept at room temperature. A small amount of the drug may be left after the last dose is taken. Discard any remaining drug because the drug (in suspension form) begins to lose its potency after a few weeks (7 to 14 days).

- To reduce the risk of superinfection during antibiotic therapy, take yogurt, buttermilk, or *Acidophilus* capsules.

- Women who are prescribed ampicillin, and penicillin V and who take birth control pills containing estrogen should use additional contraception measures.

- Never give this drug to other individuals even though their symptoms appear to be the same.

- Notify the primary health care provider immediately if one or more of the following should occur: skin rash; hives (urticaria); severe diarrhea; vaginal or anal itching; black, furry tongue; sores in the mouth; swelling around the mouth or eyes; breathing difficulty; or gastrointestinal disturbances such as nausea, vomiting, and diarrhea. Do not take the next dose of the drug until the problem has been discussed with the primary health care provider.

- Notify the primary health care provider if the symptoms of the infection do not improve or if the condition becomes worse.

- When a penicillin is to be taken for a long time for prophylaxis, you may feel well despite the need for long-term antibiotic therapy. There may be a tendency to omit one or more doses or even neglect to take the drug for an extended time. Never skip doses or stop therapy unless told to do so by the primary health care provider (see Patient and Family Teaching Checklist: Preventing Antibiotic Resistance).

Patient and Family Teaching Checklist

Preventing Antibiotic Resistance

The nurse:

- ✔ Reviews the reason for the drug and the prescribed drug regimen, including drug name, correct dose, and frequency of administration.

- ✔ Stresses the importance of continued and uninterrupted therapy, even if the patient feels better after a few doses.

- ✔ Instructs the patient to continue taking the drug until all the drug is finished or the prescriber discontinues therapy.

- ✔ Urges the patient and family to discard any unused drug once therapy is discontinued or completed.

- ✔ Warns the patient not to use any leftover antibiotic or to take another family member's antibiotic as self-treatment for a suspected infection.

- ✔ Reviews the possible adverse reactions and the signs and symptoms of a new infection or of a worsening infection, both verbally and in writing.

- ✔ Instructs the patient and family to notify the health care provider at once should the patient experience any adverse reactions or signs and symptoms of infection.

EVALUATION

- The therapeutic drug effect is achieved and the infection is controlled.

- Adverse reactions are identified, reported to the primary health care provider, and managed successfully through appropriate nursing interventions.

- The patient and family demonstrate understanding of the drug regimen.

Critical Thinking Exercises

1. Ms. Barker had a bowel resection 4 days ago. After a culture and sensitivity test of her draining surgical wound, the primary health care provider orders penicillin G aqueous IV as a continuous drip. Determine what questions you would ask Ms. Barker before the penicillin is added to the IV solution.

2. After administering penicillin to a patient in an outpatient setting, you request that the patient wait about 30 minutes before leaving. The patient is reluctant to stay, saying that she has a busy schedule. Discuss how you would handle this situation.

3. A 28-year-old married woman with three children is prescribed ampicillin for an upper respiratory infection caused by *Streptococcus pneumoniae*. What information would be important for you to obtain from this woman? What special instructions would you give her because of her sex and age?

Review Questions

1. When reviewing Ms. Robertson's culture and sensitivity test results, the nurse learns that the bacteria causing Ms. Robertson's infection are sensitive to penicillin. The nurse interprets this result to mean that _____.

   A. Ms. Robertson is allergic to penicillin

   B. penicillin will be effective in treating the infection

   C. penicillin will not be effective in treating the infection

   D. the test must be repeated to obtain accurate results

2. Mr. Thomas, who is receiving oral penicillin, reports he has a sore mouth. On inspection, the nurse notes a black, furry tongue and bright red oral mucous membranes. The primary care provider is notified immediately because these symptoms may be caused by _____.

A. a vitamin C deficiency

B. a superinfection

C. dehydration

D. poor oral hygiene

3. The nurse correctly administers penicillin V _____.

A. 1 hour before or 2 hours after meals

B. without regard to meals

C. with meals to prevent gastrointestinal upset

D. every 3 hours around the clock

4. After administering penicillin in an outpatient setting, the nurse _____.

A. asks the patient to wait 10 to 15 minutes before leaving the clinic

B. instructs the patient to report any numbness or tingling of the extremities

C. keeps pressure on the injection site for 10 minutes

D. asks the patient to wait in the area for at least 30 minutes

Medication Dosage Problems

1. A patient is prescribed amoxicillin for oral suspension. The drug is reconstituted to a solution of 250 mg/5 mL. Answer the following questions:

How much amoxicillin will 1 teaspoon contain? _____ The primary care provider prescribes 500 mg. How many milliliters (mL) will the nurse administer? _____

2. The primary care provider orders 500 mg of Augmentin oral suspension. Read the label below to answer the following questions:

250

AUGMENTIN®
125mg/5mL

125mg/5mL
NDC 0029-6085-23

Directions for mixing:
Tap bottle until all powder flows freely. Add approximately 2/3 of total water for reconstitution (total = 90 mL); shake vigorously to wet powder. Add remaining water; again shake vigorously.
Dosage: See accompanying prescribing information.

AUGMENTIN®
AMOXICILLIN/
CLAVULANATE
POTASSIUM
FOR ORAL SUSPENSION
When reconstituted, each 5 mL contains:
AMOXICILLIN, 125 MG, as the trihydrate
CLAVULANIC ACID, 31.25 MG, as clavulanate potassium

100mL
(when reconstituted)

Keep tightly closed.
Shake well before using.
Must be refrigerated.
Discard after 10 days.

gsk GlaxoSmithKline   Ronly   9405705-E

Use only if inner seal is intact.
Net contents: Equivalent to 2.5 g amoxicillin and 0.625 g clavulanic acid.
Store dry powder at room temperature.
GlaxoSmithKline
Research Triangle Park, NC 27709

3 0029-6085-23 2

LOT

EXP.

A. How much water will be required for reconstitution? _____

B. Describe the process you would go through to reconstitute this drug. _____

C. When reconstituted, what will be the strength of the solution? _____

To check your answers, see Appendix G.

Penicillins

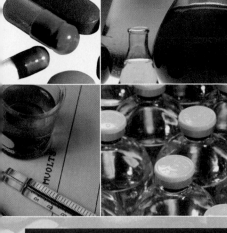

Cephalosporins

Learning Objectives

On completion of this chapter, the student will:

- Explain the difference between the first-, second-, third-, and fourth-generation cephalosporins.
- Discuss uses, general drug action, adverse reactions, contraindications, precautions, and interactions associated with the cephalosporins.
- Discuss important preadministration and ongoing assessment activities

- the nurse should perform on the patient taking cephalosporins.
- List nursing diagnoses particular to a patient taking cephalosporins.
- Discuss ways to promote an optimal response to therapy, how to manage common adverse reactions, special considerations related to administration, and important points to keep in mind when educating patients about the use of the cephalosporins.

The cephalosporins are a valuable group of drugs that are effective in the treatment of infection with almost all of the strains of bacteria affected by the penicillins, as well as some strains of bacteria that have become resistant to penicillin. The cephalosporins are structurally and chemically related to penicillin.

The cephalosporins are divided into first-, second-, third-, and fourth-generation drugs. Particular cephalosporins also may be differentiated within each group according to the microorganisms that are sensitive to the drug. In general, progression from the first-generation to the fourth-generation drugs shows an increase in the sensitivity of gram-negative microorganisms and a decrease in the sensitivity of gram-positive microorganisms. For example, a first-generation cephalosporin would be more useful against gram-positive microorganisms than would a third-generation cephalosporin. This scheme of classification is becoming less clearly defined as newer drugs are introduced. The fourth generation of cephalosporins has a broader spectrum and longer duration of resistance to beta-lactamase (see Chapter 7). These drugs are used to treat urinary tract and skin infections and hospital-acquired pneumonias. Examples of first-, second-, third-, and fourth-generation cephalosporins are listed in Display 8-1. For a more complete listing, see the Summary Drug Table: Cephalosporins.

Display 8.1 Examples of First-, Second-, Third-, and Fourth-Generation Cephalosporins

- First generation—cephalexin (Keflex), cefazolin (Ancef)
- Second generation—cefaclor (Ceclor), cefoxitin (Mefoxin), cefuroxime (Zinacef)
- Third generation—cefoperazone (Cefobid), cefotaxime (Claforan), ceftriaxone (Rocephin)
- Fourth generation—cefepime (Maxipime)

SUMMARY DRUG TABLE　CEPHALOSPORINS

GENERIC NAME	TRADE NAME	USES	ADVERSE REACTIONS	DOSAGE RANGES
First-Generation Cephalosporins				
cefadroxil *saf-a-drox'-ill*	Duricef	Infections due to susceptible microorganisms	Nausea, vomiting, diarrhea, hypersensitivity reactions, superinfection, nephrotoxicity, headache, Stevens-Johnson syndrome, pseudomembranous colitis	1–2 g/d orally in divided doses
cefazolin sodium *sef-a'-zoe-lin*	Ancef, Kefzol	Same as cefadroxil; perioperative prophylaxis	Same as cefadroxil	250 mg–1 g IM, IV q6–12h Perioperative: 0.5–1 g IM, IV
cephalexin *sef'-a-lex-in*	Keflex, Biocef, Keftab	Same as cefadroxil	Same as cefadroxil	1–4 g/d orally in divided doses
cephradine *sef'-rah-deen*	Velosef	Same as cefadroxil	Same as cefadroxil	250 mg–1g q6–12h
Second-Generation Cephalosporins				
cefaclor *sef'-a-klor*	Ceclor	Infections due to susceptible microorganisms	Nausea, vomiting, diarrhea, hypersensitivity reactions, nephrotoxicity, headache, hematologic reactions	250 mg orally q8h
cefotetan *sef-oh-tee'-tan*	Cefotan	Same as cefaclor; perioperative prophylaxis	Same as cefaclor	1–2 g IM, IV q12h for 5–10 d; perioperative; 1–2 g in a single dose IV
cefoxitin *sef-ox'-i -tin*	Mefoxin	Same as cefaclor; perioperative prophylaxis	Same as cefaclor	1–2 g IM q6–8h
cefpodoxime *sef-poed-ox'-eem*	Vantin	Same as cefaclor; STD treatment	Same as cefaclor	100–400 mg/d orally in equally divided doses
cefprozil *saf-proe'-zil*	Cefzil	Same as cefaclor	Same as cefaclor	250–500 mg orally q12h
cefuroxime *sef-yoor-ox'-eem*	Ceftin, Zinacef	Same as cefaclor; preoperative prophylaxis	Same as cefaclor	250 mg orally BID; 750 mg–1.5 g IM or IV q8h
Ⓡ **loracarbef** *lor-ah-kar'-bef*	Lorabid	Same as cefaclor	Same as cefaclor	200–400 mg orally q12h
Third-Generation Cephalosporins				
cefdinir *sef'-din-er*	Omnicef	Same as cefaclor	Same as cefaclor	300 mg orally q12h or 600 mg orally q24h orally
cefditoren *sef'-di-tore-en*	Spectracef	Same as cefaclor	Same as cefaclor	200–400 mg orally BID
cefoperazone *sef-oh-per'-a zone*	Cefobid	Same as cefaclor	Same as cefaclor	2–4 g/d IM, IV in equally divided doses
cefotaxime *sef-oh-taks'-eem*	Claforan	Same as cefaclor; perioperative prophylaxis	Same as cefaclor	2–8 g/d IM, IV in equally divided doses q6–8h; maximum 12 g/d

GENERIC NAME	TRADE NAME	USES	ADVERSE REACTIONS	DOSAGE RANGES
ceftazidime *sef-taz'-i-deem*	Ceptaz	Same as cefaclor	Same as cefaclor	250 mg–2g IV, IM q8–12h
Ⓡ **ceftibuten hydrochloride** *sef-ta-byoo'-ten*	Cedax	Same as cefaclor	Same as cefaclor	400 mg/d for 10 d
ceftizoxime *sef-tih-zox'-eem*	Cefizox	Same as cefaclor	Same as cefaclor	500 mg IM IV q8–12h; maximum 12 g/d
ceftriaxone *sef-try-ax'-on*	Rocephin	Same as cefaclor; perioperative prophylaxis; gonorrhea	Same as cefaclor	1–2 g/d IM, IV q12h maximum 4 g/d; perioperative, 1 g IV; gonorrhea, 1 g IM as a single dose
Fourth-Generation Cephalosporins				
cefepime hydrochloride *sef'-ah-pime*	Maxipime	Same as cefaclor	Same as cefaclor	0.5–2 g IV, IM q12h

Ⓡ This drug should be administered at least 1 hour before or 2 hours after a meal.

Actions

Cephalosporins have a beta-lactam ring and target the bacterial cell wall, making it defective and unstable. This action is similar to the action of penicillin. The cephalosporins are usually bactericidal.

Uses

The cephalosporins are used in the treatment of infections caused by bacteria, including:

- Respiratory infections
- **Otitis media** (ear infection)
- Bone/joint infections
- Genitourinary tract and other infections caused by bacteria.

Culture and sensitivity tests (see Chapter 7) are performed whenever possible to determine which antibiotic, including a cephalosporin, will best control an infection caused by a specific strain of bacteria.

The cephalosporins also may be used throughout the **perioperative period**, that is, during the preoperative, intraoperative, and postoperative periods, to prevent infection in patients having surgery on a contaminated or potentially contaminated area, such as the gastrointestinal (GI) tract or vagina. In some instances, a specific drug may be recommended for postoperative prophylactic use only.

Adverse Reactions

Gastrointestinal Reactions

- Nausea
- Vomiting
- Diarrhea

Other Body System Reactions

- Headache
- Dizziness
- **Malaise**
- Heartburn
- Fever
- **Nephrotoxicity** (damage to the kidneys by a toxic substance)
- Hypersensitivity (allergic) reactions—may occur with administration of the cephalosporins and may range from mild to life-threatening. Mild hypersensitivity reactions include pruritus, urticaria, and skin rashes; the more serious reactions include Stevens-Johnson syndrome and hepatic and renal dysfunction.
- **Aplastic anemia** (anemia due to deficient red blood cell production)
- Toxic epidermal necrolysis (death of the epidermal layer of the skin)

Cephalosporins

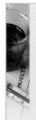

Nursing Alert

Because of the close relationship of the cephalosporins to penicillin, a patient who is allergic to penicillin also may be allergic to the cephalosporins. Approximately 10% of the people allergic to a penicillin drug are also allergic to a cephalosporin drug.

Administration route reactions include pain, tenderness, and inflammation at the injection site when given intramuscularly (IM), and phlebitis or **thrombophlebitis** (inflammation of a vein with formation of a clot in the vein) along the vein when given intravenously (IV). Therapy with cephalosporins may result in a bacterial or fungal superinfection. Diarrhea may be an indication of pseudomembranous colitis, which is one type of bacterial superinfection (see Chapter 7).

Contraindications and Precautions

The nurse should not administer cephalosporins if the patient has a history of allergies to cephalosporins or penicillins.

Cephalosporins should be used cautiously in patients with renal disease, hepatic impairment, bleeding disorder, pregnancy (pregnancy category B), and known penicillin allergy.

Interactions

The following interactions may occur when a cephalosporin is administered with another agent:

Interacting Drug	Common Use	Effect of Interaction
aminoglycosides	Anti-infective	Increased risk for nephrotoxicity
oral anticoagulants	Blood thinner	Increased risk for bleeding

The blood level of certain cephalosporins may increase when administered with other drugs, such as the diuretic furosemide (Lasix) and cefuroxime. Probenecid (Benemid, used for gout pain) will increase the levels of most cephalosporins (*except* cefoperazone, ceftazidime, and ceftriaxone).

Nursing Alert

A **disulfiram-like reaction** may occur if alcohol is consumed within 72 hours after administration of certain cephalosporins (i.e., cefamandole, cefoperazone, and cefotetan). Symptoms of a disulfiram-like reaction (associated with the use of disulfiram [Antabuse], a drug used to treat alcoholism) include flushing, throbbing in the head and neck, respiratory difficulty, vomiting, sweating, chest pain, and hypotension. Severe reactions may cause arrhythmias and unconsciousness.

NURSING PROCESS

The Patient Receiving a Cephalosporin
ASSESSMENT
PREADMINISTRATION ASSESSMENT

Before the administration of the first dose of a cephalosporin, it is important to obtain a general health history. The health history includes an allergy history, a history of all medical and surgical treatments, a drug history, and the current symptoms of the infection. If the patient has a history of allergy, particularly a drug allergy, the nurse explores this area to ensure that the patient is not allergic to a cephalosporin. Patients with a history of an allergy to penicillin may also be allergic to a cephalosporin. If an allergy to either of these drug groups is suspected, the nurse informs the primary health care provider of this before the first dose of the drug is given. The nurse should check to be sure any culture and sensitivity tests are done before the first dose of the drug is administered. Liver and kidney function tests may be ordered by the primary health care provider.

ONGOING ASSESSMENT

An ongoing assessment is important in evaluating the patient's response to therapy, such as a decrease in temperature, the relief of symptoms caused by the infection (e.g., pain or discomfort), an increase in appetite, and a change in the appearance or amount of drainage (when originally present). The nurse notifies the primary health care provider if signs of the infection appear to worsen. The nurse checks the patient's skin regularly for rash and is alert for any loose stools or diarrhea.

NURSING DIAGNOSES

Drug-specific nursing diagnoses are highlighted in the Nursing Diagnoses Checklist. Other, more general nursing diagnoses are discussed in Chapter 4.

Nursing Diagnoses Checklist

✔ **Risk for Impaired Skin Integrity** related to hypersensitivity to cephalosporin therapy

✔ **Risk for Impaired Comfort: Increased Fever** related to ineffectiveness of cephalosporin against the infection

✔ **Impaired Urinary Elimination** related to nephrotoxic effects

✔ **Diarrhea** related to superinfection

PLANNING

The expected outcomes for the patient depend on the reason for administration but may include an optimal response to therapy (infectious process controlled), meeting patient needs related to the management of adverse drug reactions, and an understanding of and compliance with the prescribed treatment regimen.

IMPLEMENTATION

PROMOTING AN OPTIMAL RESPONSE TO THERAPY

ORAL ADMINISTRATION The nurse must question the patient about allergy to cephalosporins or the penicillins before administering the first dose, even when an accurate drug history has been taken. Information regarding a drug allergy may have been forgotten or not documented at the time the initial drug history was obtained. If a patient gives a history of possible cephalosporin or penicillin allergy, the nurse withholds the drug and contacts the primary health care provider.

The nurse administers cephalosporins around the clock to the patient to provide adequate blood levels. Most cephalosporins may be taken with food to prevent gastric upset. Loracarbef (Lorabid) and ceftibuten (Cedax) should not be taken with food. The nurse should administer these oral medications at least 1 hour before or 2 hours after meals. However, if the patient experiences GI upset, the nurse can administer the drug with food. The absorption of oral cefuroxime and cefpodoxime is increased when given with food.

Some cephalosporins are available as powder for a suspension and are reconstituted by a pharmacist or a nurse. The nurse should shake oral suspensions well before administering them. It is important to keep this form of the drug refrigerated until it is used.

PARENTERAL ADMINISTRATION The nurse should read the manufacturer's package insert for each drug for instructions regarding reconstitution of powder for injection, storage of unused portions, life of the drug after it is reconstituted, methods of IV administration, and precautions to be taken when the drug is administered.

Some cephalosporins are given by direct IV infusion, intermittent infusion, or continuous infusion. When the direct IV method is used, the nurse gives the dose directly into a vein. Intermittent IV infusion is given using "Y" tubing while another solution is being given on a continuous basis. When this method is used, the nurse clamps off the IV fluid given on a continuous basis while the drug is allowed to infuse. Continuous IV infusion requires that the nurse add the drug to a specified amount of an IV solution at a drip rate or volume per hour prescribed by the primary health care provider.

Nursing Alert

When the drug is given IV, the nurse inspects the needle insertion site for signs of extravasation or infiltration (see Chapter 2). In addition, the needle insertion site and the area above the site are inspected several times a day for signs of redness, which may indicate phlebitis or thrombophlebitis. If either problem occurs, the nurse contacts the primary health care provider and the IV infusion must be discontinued and restarted in another vein, preferably in another extremity.

Gerontologic Alert

When a cephalosporin is given IM, the nurse injects the drug into a large muscle mass, such as the gluteus muscle or lateral aspect of the thigh. If the patient has been nonambulatory for any length of time or has paralysis, the nurse assesses the muscle carefully because the large muscle may be atrophied. It is important to rotate injection sites. The nurse warns the patient that at the time the drug is injected into the muscle, there may be a stinging or burning sensation and the area may be sore for a short time. The nurse informs the primary health care provider if previously used areas for injection appear red or if the patient reports continued pain in the area.

Chronic Care Alert

People with phenylketonuria (PKU) need to be aware that the oral suspension cefprozil (Cefzil) contains phenylalanine, a substance that people with PKU cannot process. In addition, diabetic patients who use urine testing for determining diabetic medicine dosing and who are prescribed cephalosporins need to be aware that this drug may interfere with accurate test results. The primary care provider should be consulted before diet and drug changes are made.

Cephalosporins

MONITORING AND MANAGING PATIENT NEEDS

The nurse observes the patient closely for any adverse drug reactions, particularly signs and symptoms of a hypersensitivity reaction.

IMPAIRED SKIN INTEGRITY The nurse inspects the skin every 4 hours for redness, rash, or lesions that appear as red wheals or blisters. It is important to report a rash or hives to the primary health care provider because this may be a precursor to a severe, possibly fatal syndrome (Stevens-Johnson) or anaphylactic reaction (see Chapters 6 and 7). When a rash or irritation is present, the nurse administers frequent skin care. Emollients, antipyretic creams, or a topical corticosteroid may be prescribed. An antihistamine may be prescribed. Harsh soaps and perfumed lotions are avoided. The nurse instructs the patient to avoid rubbing the area and not to wear rough or irritating clothing. In severe cases of skin impairment, the primary health care provider may discontinue the cephalosporin therapy. The nurse closely observes the patient for signs and symptoms of a bacterial or fungal superinfection (see Chapter 7). If a superinfection occurs, the nurse contacts the primary health care provider before the next dose of the drug is due.

IMPAIRED COMFORT: INCREASED FEVER The nurse takes vital signs every 4 hours or as ordered by the primary health care provider. It is important to report any increase in temperature to the primary health care provider because additional treatment measures, such as administration of an antipyretic drug or change in the drug or dosage, may be necessary.

IMPAIRED URINARY ELIMINATION Nephrotoxicity may occur with the administration of cephalosporins. An early sign of this adverse reaction may be a decrease in urine output. The nurse should measure and record the fluid intake and output and notify the primary health care provider if the output is less than 500 mL daily. Any changes in the fluid intake-and-output ratio or in the appearance of the urine also may indicate nephrotoxicity. It is important that the nurse report these findings to the primary health care provider promptly.

Gerontologic Alert

The older adult is more susceptible to the nephrotoxic effects of the cephalosporins, particularly if renal function is already diminished because of aging or disease. If renal impairment is present, a lower dosage and monitoring of blood creatinine levels are indicated. Blood creatinine levels greater than 4 mg/dL indicate serious renal impairment. In elderly patients with decreased renal function, a dosage adjustment may be necessary.

DIARRHEA Frequent liquid stools may be an indication of a superinfection or pseudomembranous colitis. If pseudomembranous colitis occurs, it is usually seen 4 to 10 days after treatment is started.

The nurse inspects each bowel movement and immediately reports to the primary health care provider the occurrence of diarrhea or loose stools containing blood and mucus because it may be necessary to discontinue drug therapy and institute treatment for diarrhea, a superinfection, or pseudomembranous colitis.

If blood and mucus appear to be in the stool, the nurse saves a sample of the stool and tests for occult blood using a test such as Hemoccult. If the stool tests positive for blood, the sample is saved for possible additional laboratory testing for blood.

EDUCATING THE PATIENT AND FAMILY

The nurse carefully reviews the dosage regimen with the patient and family and provides the following information:

- Complete the full course of therapy. Do not stop the drug even if the symptoms have disappeared unless directed to do so by the primary health care provider.

- Take the drug at the prescribed times of day because it is important to keep an adequate amount of drug in the body throughout the entire 24 hours of each day.

- Consider taking each dose with food or milk if GI upset occurs after administration.

- Oral suspensions—keep the container refrigerated (if so labeled), shake the drug well before pouring (if so labeled), and return the drug to the refrigerator immediately after pouring the dose. Drugs that require refrigeration lose their potency when kept at room temperature. If a small amount of the drug is left after the last dose is taken, discard it because the drug (in suspension form) begins to lose potency after a few weeks.

- Avoid drinking alcoholic beverages when taking the cephalosporins and for 3 days after completing the course of therapy because severe reactions may occur.

- Notify the primary health care provider immediately if any one or more of the following occurs: vomiting, skin rash, hives (urticaria), severe diarrhea, vaginal or anal itching, sores in the mouth, swelling around the mouth or eyes, breathing difficulty, or GI disturbances, such as nausea, vomiting, and diarrhea. Do not take the next dose of the drug until the problem is discussed with the primary health care provider (see Home Care Checklist: Teaching About Superinfection).

Home Care Checklist

Teaching About Superinfection

Antibiotics are one of the most commonly administered types of drug therapy in the home. Any patient taking antibiotics, especially cephalosporins, is susceptible to superinfection. The nurse makes sure the patient knows the signs and symptoms of superinfection.

A bacterial superinfection commonly occurs in the bowel. The nurse teaches the patient to report any of the following:

☑ Fever

☑ Burning sensation in the mouth or throat

☑ Localized redness, inflammation, and excoriation, particularly inside the mouth, in the groin, or in skin folds of the anogenital area

☑ Abdominal cramps

☑ Scaly, reddened, papular rash commonly in the breast folds, axillae, groin, or umbilicus

☑ Diarrhea, possibly severe with visible blood and mucus

A fungal superinfection commonly occurs in the mouth, vagina, and anogenital areas. The nurse teaches the patient to report any of the following:

☑ Creamy white, lacelike patches on the tongue, mouth, or throat

☑ White or yellow vaginal discharge

☑ Anal or vaginal itching

Cephalosporins

- Never give this drug to another individual even though his or her symptoms appear to be the same as yours.

- Notify the primary health care provider if the symptoms of the infection do not improve or if the condition becomes worse.

EVALUATION

- Therapeutic effect is achieved.

- No evidence of infection.

- Adverse reactions are identified, reported to the primary health care provider, and managed successfully with nursing interventions.

- The skin is intact and free of inflammation, irritation or ulcerations.

- Urine output is at least 500 mL/d.

- The patient does not experience diarrhea.

- Patient and family demonstrate understanding of the drug regimen.

- Patient verbalizes importance of complying with the prescribed therapeutic regimen.

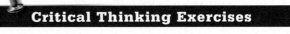

Critical Thinking Exercises

1. Mr. Jonas is receiving a cephalosporin IM. He tells you that he has had to get out of bed several times this morning because he has diarrhea. Determine what questions you would ask Mr. Jonas. Analyze what steps you would take to resolve this problem.

2. A patient who is a recent immigrant to the United States is seen in the outpatient clinic for a severe upper respiratory infection. The primary health care provider prescribes a cephalosporin and asks you to give the patient instructions for taking the drug. You note that the patient appears to understand very little English. Discuss how you would solve this problem. Determine what information you would include in a teaching plan and how you would evaluate the effectiveness of the teaching plan for this patient.

3. Describe what assessments you would make if you suspect that a patient receiving a cephalosporin is experiencing Stevens-Johnson syndrome.

Review Questions

1. The nurse observes a patient taking a cephalosporin for common adverse reactions, which include _____.

A. hypotension, dizziness, urticaria

B. nausea, vomiting, diarrhea

C. skin rash, constipation, headache

D. bradycardia, pruritus, insomnia

2. When giving a cephalosporin by the IM route, the nurse tells the patient that _____.

   A. a stinging or burning sensation and soreness at the site may be experienced

   B. the injection site will be red for several days

   C. all injections will be given in the same area

   D. the injection will not cause any discomfort

3. A nurse asks why it is so important to determine if the patient is allergic to penicillin before the first dose of the cephalosporin is given. The most correct answer is that persons allergic to penicillin _____.

   A. are usually allergic to most antibiotics

   B. respond poorly to antibiotic therapy

   C. require higher doses of other antibiotics

   D. have a higher incidence of allergy to the cephalosporins

4. The nurse observes a patient receiving a cephalosporin for Stevens-Johnson syndrome. The signs and symptoms that might indicate this syndrome include _____.

   A. swelling of the extremities

   B. increased blood pressure and pulse rate

   C. lesions on the skin or mucous membranes

   D. pain in the joints

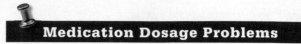

Medication Dosage Problems

1. Ceclor 500 mg is prescribed for a patient. Use the drug label below to determine the dosage:

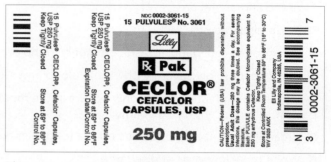

The nurse would administer _____.

2. The physician prescribes 1 g of Mefoxin (cefoxitin) for parenteral administration. Mefoxin is available in a solution of 250 mg/1 mL. What amount of Mefoxin would the nurse prepare? _____

To check your answers, see Appendix G.

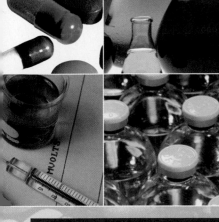

Chapter 9

Tetracyclines, Macrolides, and Lincosamides

Learning Objectives

On completion of this chapter, the student will:

- Discuss the uses, general drug action, adverse reactions, contraindications, precautions, and interactions of the tetracyclines, macrolides, and lincosamides.
- Discuss important preadministration and ongoing assessment activities the nurse should perform on the patient taking a tetracycline, macrolide, or lincosamide.

- List nursing diagnoses particular to a patient taking a tetracycline, macrolide, or lincosamide.
- Discuss ways to promote an optimal response to therapy, how to manage adverse reactions, and important points to keep in mind when educating patients about the use of a tetracycline, macrolide, or lincosamide.

This chapter discusses three groups of broad-spectrum antibiotics: the tetracyclines, the macrolides, and the lincosamides. Examples of the tetracyclines include doxycycline (Vibramycin), minocycline (Minocin), and tetracycline (Sumycin). Examples of the macrolides include azithromycin (Zithromax), clarithromycin (Biaxin), and erythromycin (E-Mycin). The lincosamides include clindamycin (Cleocin) and lincomycin (Lincocin). The Summary Drug Table: Tetracyclines, Macrolides, and Lincosamides describes the types of broad-spectrum antibiotics discussed in this chapter.

TETRACYCLINES

The tetracyclines are a group of anti-infectives composed of natural and semisynthetic compounds. They are useful in select infections when the organism shows sensitivity (see Chapter 7) to the tetracyclines, such as cholera, Rocky Mountain spotted fever, and typhus.

Actions

The tetracyclines exert their effect by inhibiting bacterial protein synthesis, which is a process necessary for reproduction of the microorganism.

Uses

These antibiotics are effective in the treatment of infections caused by a wide range of gram-negative and gram-positive microorganisms. Tetracyclines are used as

SUMMARY DRUG TABLE   TETRACYCLINES, MACROLIDES, AND LINCOSAMIDES

GENERIC NAME	TRADE NAME	USES	ADVERSE REACTIONS	DOSAGE RANGES
Tetracyclines				
℞ **demeclocycline** *deh-meh-kloe-sye'-kleen*	Declomycin	Treatment of infections due to susceptible microorganisms	Nausea, vomiting, diarrhea, dizziness, headache, hypersensitivity reactions, photosensitivity reactions, pseudomembranous colitis, hematologic changes, discoloration of teeth in fetus and young children	150 mg orally QID or 300 mg orally BID; gonorrhea: 600 mg orally initially then 300 mg orally q12h for 4 days
℞ **doxycycline** *dox-i-sye'-kleen*	Vibra-Tabs, Vibramycin	Same as demeclocycline	Same as demeclocycline	100 mg orally q12h first day then 100 mg/d orally Severe infections: 100 mg q12h
minocycline *min-oh-sye'-kleen*	Minocin, Minocin IV	Same as demeclocycline	Same as demeclocycline	200 mg orally initially then 100 mg orally q12h
oxytetracycline *ox-i-tet-ra-sye'-kleen*	Terramycin	Same as demeclocycline	Same as demeclocycline	250 mg IM daily
℞ **tetracycline** *tet-ra-sye'-kleen*	Sumycin	Same as demeclocycline	Same as demeclocycline	1–2 g/d orally in 2–4 divided doses
tigecycline (glycylcycline similar to tetracycline)	Tygacil	Complicated skin structures and complicated intra-abdominal infections	Nausea, vomiting, diarrhea	100 mg IV initially then 50 mg IV q12h
Macrolides				
℞ **azithromycin** *ay-zi-thro-my'-cin*	Zithromax	Same as demeclocycline	Nausea, vomiting, diarrhea, abdominal pains, hypersensitivity reactions, pseudomembranous colitis	500 mg orally first day then 250 mg/d orally for 4 days
clarithromycin *klar-ith-ro-my'-cin*	Biaxin	Same as demeclocycline	Same as azithromycin	250–500 mg orally q12h
dirithromycin *dir-ith-ro-my'-cin*		Same as demeclocycline	Anorexia, constipation, dry mouth, hypersensitivity reactions, photosensitivity reactions, pseudomembranous colitis, electrolyte imbalance	500 mg orally for 7–14 days
℞ **erythromycin base** *er-ith-roe-my'-sin*	E-Mycin, Eryc	Same as demeclocycline	Same as azithromycin	250 mg orally q6h or 333 mg q8h
erythromycin ethylsuccinate	EryPed, E.E.S.	Same as demeclocycline	Same as azithromycin	400 mg orally q6h
telithromycin *tell-ith-roe-my'-sin*	Ketek	Same as demeclocycline	Visual disturbance, nausea, diarrhea, vomiting, headache, dizziness	800 mg orally q24h

GENERIC NAME	TRADE NAME	USES	ADVERSE REACTIONS	DOSAGE RANGES
troleandomycin	Tao	Same as demeclocycline	Same as clindamycin	250–500 mg orally QID
Lincosamides				
clindamycin *klin-da-my'-sin*	Cleocin	Same as demeclocycline	Abdominal pain, esophagitis, nausea, vomiting, diarrhea, skin rash, pseudomembranous colitis, hypersensitivity reactions	Serious infection: 150–450 mg orally q6h; severe infecton: 600–2700 mg/d in 2–4 equal doses; life-threatening infection: up to 4.8 g/d IV, IM
℞ **lincomycin** *lin-koe-my'-sin*	Lincocin	Same as demeclocycline	Same as clindamycin	500 mg orally q6–8h; 600 mg IM q12–24h; up to 8 g/d IV in life-threatening situations

℞ This drug should be administered at least 1 hour before or 2 hours after a meal.

broad-spectrum antibiotics when penicillin is contraindicated, and also to treat the following infections:

- Rickettsial diseases (Rocky Mountain spotted fever, typhus fever, and tick fevers)

- Intestinal amebiasis

- Some skin and soft tissue infections

- Uncomplicated urethral, endocervical, or rectal infections caused by *Chlamydia trachomatis*

- Severe acne as an **adjunctive treatment** (therapy used in addition to a primary treatment)

- Infection with *Helicobacter pylora* (a bacterium in the stomach that can cause peptic ulcer) in combination with metronidazole and bismuth subsalicylate.

Growing resistance to the drugs is a problem with the tetracyclines.

Adverse Reactions

Gastrointestinal Reactions

- Nausea or vomiting

- Diarrhea

- Epigastric distress

- Stomatitis

- Sore throat

Other Body System Reactions

- Skin rashes

- Photosensitivity reaction (demeclocycline seems to cause the most serious photosensitivity reaction,

whereas minocycline is least likely to cause this type of reaction).

Contraindications

The tetracyclines are contraindicated in the patient known to be hypersensitive to any of the tetracyclines; during pregnancy because of the possibility of toxic effects to the developing fetus (pregnancy category D); and during lactation and in children younger than 9 years.

Nursing Alert

The tetracyclines are not given to children younger than 9 years of age unless their use is absolutely necessary because these drugs may cause permanent yellow-gray-brown discoloration of the teeth. The use of the tetracyclines, especially prolonged or repeated therapy, may result in overgrowth of nonsusceptible bacterial or fungal organisms.

Precautions

Tetracyclines should be used cautiously in patients with impaired renal function (when degradation of the tetracyclines occurs, the agents are highly toxic to the kidneys) and those with liver impairment (doses greater that 2 g/day can be extremely damaging to the liver).

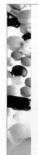

Chronic Care Alert

Tetracyclines may increase the risk of toxicity in patients who take digitalis drugs for heart disease. The effects of toxicity could last for months after tetracycline administration discontinues. Caution the patient and family to inform the primary care provider about the tetracycline drug therapy should digitalis toxicity symptoms appear.

Interactions

The following interactions may occur when a tetracycline is administered with another agent:

Interacting Drug or Agent	Common Use	Effect of Interaction
antacids containing aluminum, zinc, magnesium, or bismuth salts	Relief of heartburn and gastrointestinal (GI) upset	Decreased effectiveness of tetracycline
oral anticoagulants	Blood thinner	Increased risk for bleeding
oral contraceptives	Birth control	Decreased effectiveness of contraceptive agent (breakthrough bleeding or pregnancy)
digoxin	Management of heart disease	Increased risk for digitalis toxicity (see Chapter 38)

Chronic Care Alert

Tetracyclines may reduce insulin requirements in patients with diabetes. Blood glucose levels should be monitored frequently during tetracycline therapy.

MACROLIDES

The macrolides are effective against a wide variety of pathogenic organisms, particularly infections of the respiratory and genitourinary tract.

Actions

The macrolides are bacteriostatic or bactericidal in susceptible bacteria. The drugs act by causing changes in protein function and synthesis.

Uses

These antibiotics are effective as prophylaxis before dental or other procedures in patients allergic to penicillin and in the treatment of

- A wide range of gram-negative and gram-positive infections
- Acne vulgaris and skin infections
- Upper respiratory infections caused by *Hemophilus influenzae* (with sulfonamides)

Adverse Reactions

Gastrointestinal reactions include the following:

- Nausea
- Vomiting
- Diarrhea
- Abdominal pain or cramping

As with almost all antibacterial drugs, pseudomembranous colitis may occur, ranging in severity from mild to life-threatening. Visual disturbances (associated with telithromycin) may also occur.

Contraindications

These drugs are contraindicated in patients with a hypersensitivity to the macrolides and in patients with preexisting liver disease. Telithromycin (Ketek) should not be ordered if a patient is taking cisapride (Propulsid) or pimozide (Orap).

Precautions

Macrolides should be used cautiously in patients who have liver dysfunction or **myasthenia gravis** (a disease that affects the myoneural junction in nerves and is manifested by extreme weakness and exhaustion of the muscles), or who are pregnant or lactating (azithromycin and erythromycin are in pregnancy category B; clarithromycin, dirithromycin, troleandomycin, and telithromycin are in pregnancy category C).

Interactions

The following interactions may occur when a macrolide is administered with another agent:

Interacting Drug	Common Use	Effect of Interaction
antacids (kaolin, aluminum salts, or magaldrate)	Relief of GI upset such as diarrhea	Decreased absorption and effectiveness of macrolide
digoxin	Management of cardiac and respiratory disorders	Increased serum levels
anticoagulants	Blood thinner	Increased risk of bleeding
clindamycin, lincomycin, or chloramphenicol	Anti-infective agent	Decreased therapeutic activity of the macrolide
theophylline	Management of respiratory problems, such as asthma	Increased serum theophylline level

LINCOSAMIDES

The lincosamides, another group of anti-infectives with a high potential for toxicity, are usually used only for treating serious infections in which penicillin or erythromycin (a macrolide) is not effective.

Actions

The lincosamides act by inhibiting protein synthesis in susceptible bacteria, causing cell death.

Uses

These antibiotics are effective in the treatment of infections caused by a wide range of gram-negative and gram-positive microorganisms. The lincosamides are used for the more serious infections and may be used in conjunction with other antibiotics.

Adverse Reactions

Gastrointestinal Reactions

- Abdominal pain
- Esophagitis
- Nausea
- Vomiting
- Diarrhea

Other Body System Reactions

- Skin rash
- **Blood dyscrasias** (an abnormality of the blood cell structure or function)

These drugs also can cause pseudomembranous colitis, which may range from mild to very severe. Discontinuing the drug may relieve mild symptoms of pseudomembranous colitis.

Contraindications

The lincosamides are contraindicated in infants younger than 1 month of age and in patients

- Hypersensitive to the lincosamides
- Taking cisapride (Propulsid) or the antipsychotic drug pimozide (Orap)
- With minor bacterial or viral infections

Precautions

These drugs should be used cautiously in patients with a history of GI disorders, renal disease, liver impairment, or myasthenia gravis (lincosamides have neuromuscular blocking action).

Interactions

The following interactions may occur when a lincosamide is administered with another agent:

Interacting Drug	Common Use	Effect of Interaction
kaolin- or aluminum-based antacids	Relief of stomach upset	Decreased absorption of the lincosamide
neuromuscular blocking drugs (see Chapter 21)	Anesthesia	Increased action of neuromuscular blocking drug, possibly leading to severe and profound respiratory depression

NURSING PROCESS

The Patient Receiving a Tetracycline, Macrolide, or Lincosamide

ASSESSMENT

PREADMINISTRATION ASSESSMENT

It is important to establish an accurate database before the administration of any antibiotic. The nurse should identify and record signs and symptoms of the infection. Signs and symptoms may vary and often depend on the organ or system involved and whether the infection is external or internal. Examples of some of the signs and symptoms of an infection in various areas of the body are pain, drainage, redness, changes in the appearance of sputum, general malaise, chills and fever, cough, and swelling.

The nurse obtains a thorough allergy history, especially a history of drug allergies. Some antibiotics have a higher incidence of hypersensitivity reactions in those with a history of allergy to drugs or other substances. If the patient has a history of allergies and has not told the primary health care provider, the nurse should not administer the first dose of the drug until the problem is discussed with the primary health care provider.

It also is important to take and record vital signs before the first dose of the antibiotic is given. The primary health care provider may order culture and sensitivity tests, and these should also be performed before the first dose of the drug is given. Other laboratory tests such as renal and hepatic function tests, complete blood count, and urinalysis may also be ordered by the primary health care provider.

ONGOING ASSESSMENT

An ongoing assessment is important during therapy with the tetracyclines, macrolides, and lincosamides. The nurse should take vital signs every 4 hours or as ordered by the primary health care provider. The nurse must notify the primary health care provider if there are changes in the vital signs, such as a significant drop in blood pressure, an increase in the pulse or respiratory rate, or a sudden increase in temperature. Each day, the nurse compares current signs and symptoms of the infection against the initial signs and symptoms and records any specific findings in the patient's chart.

When an antibiotic is ordered for prevention of a secondary infection (prophylaxis), the nurse observes the patient for signs and symptoms that may indicate the beginning of an infection despite the prophylactic use of the antibiotic. If signs and symptoms of an infection occur, the nurse must report them to the primary health care provider.

NURSING DIAGNOSES

Drug-specific nursing diagnoses are highlighted in the Nursing Diagnoses Checklist. Other nursing diagnoses applicable to these drugs are discussed in Chapter 4.

Nursing Diagnosis Checklist

✓ **Impaired Comfort: Increased Fever** related to ineffectiveness of anti-infective therapy

✓ **Risk for Injury** related to visual disturbances from telithromycin treatment

✓ **Diarrhea** related to superinfection secondary to anti-infective therapy, adverse drug reaction

---

PLANNING

The expected outcomes for the patient may include an optimal response to therapy, which includes control of the infectious process or prophylaxis of bacterial infection, meeting of patient needs related to the management of adverse drug effects, and an understanding of and compliance with the prescribed treatment regimen.

IMPLEMENTATION

PROMOTING AN OPTIMAL RESPONSE TO THERAPY

These drugs are of no value in the treatment of infections caused by a virus or fungus. There may be times when a secondary bacterial infection has occurred or may occur when the patient has a fungal or viral infection. The primary health care provider may then order one of the broad-spectrum antibiotics, but its purpose is for preventing (prophylaxis) or treating a secondary bacterial infection that could potentially develop after the primary fungal or viral infection.

ORAL ADMINISTRATION Adverse reactions to most anti-infective drugs include nausea, vomiting, or abdominal pain. Patients may want to eat foods when these drugs are administered to reduce the GI problems. It is important for the nurse to know how medications will be affected if taken with foods.

Tetracyclines It is important to give the tetracyclines on an empty stomach. The exceptions are minocycline (Minocin) and oxytetracycline (Terramycin), which may be taken with food. All tetracyclines should be given with a full glass of water (240 mL).

> ### Nursing Alert
>
> The nurse should not give tetracyclines along with dairy products (milk or cheese), antacids, laxatives, or products containing iron. When the aforementioned drugs are prescribed, the nurse makes sure they are given 2 hours before or after the administration of a tetracycline. Food or drugs containing calcium, magnesium, aluminum, or iron prevent the absorption of the tetracyclines if ingested concurrently.

Macrolides The nurse gives clarithromycin, troleandomycin, and telithromycin without regard to meals, and clarithromycin may be taken with milk, if desired. Azithromycin is given 1 hour or more before a meal or 2 hours or more after a meal. Dirithromycin is given with food or within 1 hour of eating. Erythromycin is given on an empty stomach (1 hour before or 2 hours after meals) and with 180 to 240 mL of water.

Lincosamides Food impairs the absorption of lincomycin. The patient should take nothing by mouth (except water) for 1 to 2 hours before and after taking lincomycin. The nurse should give clindamycin with food or a full glass of water.

PARENTERAL ADMINISTRATION When these drugs are given intramuscularly, the nurse inspects previous injection sites for signs of pain or tenderness, redness, and swelling. Some antibiotics may cause temporary local reactions, but persistence of a localized reaction should be reported to the primary health care provider. It is important to rotate injection sites and record the site used for injection in the patient's chart.

When these drugs are given intravenously (IV), the nurse should inspect the needle site and area around the needle for signs of extravasation of the IV fluid or signs of tenderness, pain, and redness (which may indicate phlebitis or thrombophlebitis). If these symptoms are apparent, the nurse should restart the IV in another vein and bring the problem to the attention of the primary health care provider.

MONITORING AND MANAGING PATIENT NEEDS

The nurse observes the patient at frequent intervals, especially during the first 48 hours of therapy. It is important to report to the primary health care provider the occurrence of any adverse reaction before the next dose of the drug is due. The nurse should report serious adverse reactions, such as a severe hypersensitivity reaction, respiratory difficulty, severe diarrhea, or a decided drop in blood pressure, to the primary health care provider immediately because a serious adverse reaction may require emergency intervention.

IMPAIRED COMFORT: INCREASED FEVER The nurse monitors the temperature at frequent intervals, usually every 4 hours unless the patient has an elevated temperature. When the patient has an elevated temperature the nurse checks the temperature, pulse, and respirations every hour until the temperature returns to normal, and administers an antipyretic medication if prescribed by the primary care provider.

RISK FOR INJURY Telithromycin (Ketek) is a drug related to the macrolides. It can cause the patient's eyes to have difficulty focusing and accommodating to light. Patients should be cautioned regarding the potential for accidents and injury when driving, operating machinery, or engaging in other hazardous activities.

DIARRHEA Diarrhea may be an indication of a superinfection or pseudomembranous colitis, both of which can be serious. The nurse should inspect all stools for blood or mucus. If diarrhea does occur and blood and mucus appear to be in the stool, the nurse saves a sample of the stool and tests for occult blood using a test such as Hemoccult. If the stool tests positive for blood, the nurse saves the stool for possible further laboratory analysis.

The nurse should encourage the patient with diarrhea to drink fluids to replace those lost with the diarrhea. It is also important to maintain an accurate intake and output record to help determine fluid balance.

The nurse observes the patient for other signs and symptoms of a bacterial or fungal superinfection, such as vaginal or anal itching, sores in the mouth, diarrhea, fever, chills, and sore throat. It is important to report any new signs and symptoms occurring during antibiotic therapy to the primary health care provider, who must then decide if these problems are part of the original infection or if a superinfection has occurred.

EDUCATING THE PATIENT AND FAMILY

The patient and family must understand the prescribed therapeutic regimen. It is not uncommon for patients to stop taking a prescribed drug because they feel better. A detailed plan of teaching helps to reduce the incidence of this problem.

The nurse should explain, in easy-to-understand terms, the adverse reactions associated with the specific prescribed antibiotic. The nurse advises the patient to contact the primary health care provider if any potentially serious adverse reactions, such as hypersensitivity reactions, moderate to severe diarrhea, sudden onset of chills and fever, sore throat, or sores in the mouth, occur.

The nurse develops a teaching plan that includes the following information:

- Take the drug at the prescribed time intervals. These intervals are important because a certain amount of the drug must be in the body at all times for the infection to be controlled.

- Do not increase or omit the dose unless advised to do so by the primary health care provider.

- Complete the entire course of treatment. Never stop the drug, except on the advice of a primary health care provider, before the course of treatment is completed even if symptoms improve or disappear. Failure to complete the prescribed course of treatment may result in a return of the infection.

- Take each dose with a full glass of water. Follow the directions given by the pharmacist regarding taking the drug on an empty stomach or with food (see Home Care Checklist: Avoiding Drug–Food Interactions).

- Notify the primary health care provider if symptoms of the infection become worse or there is no improvement in the original symptoms after about 5 days.

- Avoid the use of alcoholic beverages during therapy unless use has been approved by the primary health care provider.

- When a tetracycline has been prescribed, avoid exposure to the sun or any type of tanning lamp or bed. When exposure to direct sunlight is unavoidable, completely cover the arms and legs and wear a wide-brimmed hat to protect the face and neck. Application of a sunscreen may or may not be effective. Therefore, consult the primary health care provider before using a sunscreen to prevent a photosensitivity reaction.

EVALUATION

The therapeutic effect is achieved: the patient has no evidence of infection; the patient's normal vision is unaffected; and the patient does not experience diarrhea.

Home Care Checklist

Avoiding Drug–Food Interactions

☑ In some instances, drugs may be taken with food or milk to minimize the risk for GI upset. However, most tetracyclines, when given with foods containing calcium, such as dairy products, are not absorbed as well as when they are taken on an empty stomach. So, if the patient is to receive tetracycline at home, it is important to be sure he or she knows to take the drug on an empty stomach, 1 hour before or 2 hours after a meal.

☑ Be sure to teach the patient to read labels in the grocery store and beware of items (e.g., cereals) that may be fortified with calcium.

☑ In addition, the nurse teaches the patient to avoid the following dairy products before or after taking tetracycline:

- Milk (whole, low-fat, skim, condensed, or evaporated) and milkshakes
- Cream (half-and-half, heavy, light), sour cream, coffee creamers, and creamy salad dressings
- Eggnog
- Cheese (natural and processed) and cottage cheese
- Yogurt and frozen yogurt
- Ice cream, ice milk, and frozen custard

- Adverse reactions are identified, reported to the primary health care provider, and managed successfully through appropriate nursing interventions.

- The patient and family demonstrate understanding of the drug regimen.

- The patient verbalizes the importance of complying with the prescribed therapeutic regimen.

Critical Thinking Exercises

1. Ms. Jones has been prescribed tetracycline. She works nights and is home sleeping during the day. To decrease the possibility of noncompliance with the treatment regimen, discuss how and what you would teach Ms. Jones about her drug regimen.

2. Mr. Park, a patient in a nursing home, has been receiving clarithromycin (Biaxin) for an upper respiratory infection for 9 days. The nurse assistant reports that he has had fecal incontinence for the past 2 days. Analyze whether this matter should be investigated.

3. When taking the drug history of Mr. Woods, a patient in the outpatient clinic, you note that he has been taking 0.25 mg digoxin, one baby aspirin, and the tetracycline minocycline (Minocin). Based on your knowledge of the tetracyclines, determine whether there is any reason to be concerned about the drug regimen that Mr. Woods is on. Explain your answer.

4. Ms. Evans, aged 75 years, is to be dismissed on a regimen of doxycycline (Vibramycin). You note that she is alert and has good communication skills. Because she lives alone, she will be responsible for administering her own drug. Devise a teaching plan for Ms. Evans. You may want to use the teaching plan form in Chapter 5.

Review Questions

1. A patient asks the nurse why the primary health care provider prescribed an anti-infective when she was told that she has a viral infection. The correct response by the nurse is that the antibiotic may be used to prevent a _____.

   A. primary fungal infection

   B. repeat viral infection

   C. secondary bacterial infection

   D. breakdown of the immune system

2. A patient is receiving erythromycin for an infection. The patient's response to therapy is best evaluated by _____.

   A. monitoring vital signs every 4 hours

   B. comparing initial and current signs and symptoms

   C. monitoring fluid intake and output

   D. asking the patient if he is feeling better

3. When asked to describe a photosensitivity reaction, the nurse correctly states that this reaction may be described as a(n) _____.

   A. tearing of the eyes on exposure to bright light

   B. aversion to bright lights and sunlight

   C. sensitivity to products in the environment

   D. exaggerated sunburn reaction when the skin is exposed to sunlight

4. When giving one of the macrolide antibiotics, the nurse assesses the patient for the most common adverse reactions, which are _____.

   A. related to the GI tract

   B. skin rash and urinary retention

   C. sores in the mouth and hypertension

   D. related to the nervous system

Medication Dosage Problems

1. Mr. Baker is prescribed azithromycin for a lower respiratory tract infection. The nurse tells Mr. Baker to take the drug on an empty stomach. Azithromycin is available in 250-mg tablets. The primary health care provider has ordered 500 mg on the first day, followed by 250 mg on days 2 to 5. How many tablets would Mr. Baker take on the first day? _____ On the last day of therapy? _____

2. A patient is prescribed 600 mg of lincomycin every 12 hours IM. The drug is available as 300 mg/mL. How many milliliters would the nurse administer?

3. A patient is prescribed 200 mg of minocycline oral suspension initially, followed by 100 mg orally every 12 hours. The minocycline is available as an oral suspension of 50 mg/5 mL. How many milliliters would the nurse administer as the initial dose? _____

To check your answers, see Appendix G.

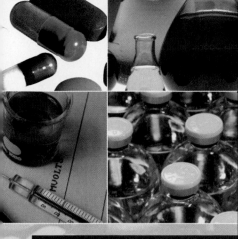

Chapter 10

Fluoroquinolones and Aminoglycosides

Key Terms

bactericidal
bowel preparation
broad spectrum
enteric-coated
extended-release
hematuria
hepatic coma
nephrotoxicity
neuromuscular blockade
neurotoxicity
ototoxicity
photosensitivity
proteinuria

Learning Objectives

On completion of this chapter, the student will:

- Discuss the uses, general drug action, contraindications, precautions, interactions, and adverse reactions of the fluoroquinolones and aminoglycosides.

- Discuss preadministration and ongoing assessment activities the nurse should perform on the patient taking the fluoroquinolones and aminoglycosides.

- List nursing diagnoses particular to a patient receiving a fluoroquinolone or aminoglycoside.

- Discuss ways to promote an optimal response to therapy, how to manage adverse reactions, and important points to keep in mind when educating patients about the use of a fluoroquinolone or aminoglycoside.

A s antibiotics became resistant to various microorganisms, researchers sought to develop more powerful drugs that would be effective against these resistant pathogens. The fluoroquinolones and aminoglycosides are two groups of **broad-spectrum** antibiotics that resulted from this research. The Summary Drug Table: Fluoroquinolones and Aminoglycosides lists the drugs discussed in this chapter.

FLUOROQUINOLONES

The fluoroquinolones include ciprofloxacin (Cipro), gatifloxacin (Tequin), lomefloxacin (Maxaquin), moxifloxacin (Avelox), and ofloxacin (Floxin).

Actions

The fluoroquinolones exert their **bactericidal** effect by interfering with the synthesis of bacterial DNA. This interference prevents cell reproduction, leading to death of the bacteria.

Uses

The fluoroquinolones are effective in treating infections caused by gram-positive and gram-negative microorganisms. They are primarily used in the treatment of

- Lower respiratory infections

- Bone and joint infections

- Urinary tract infections

SUMMARY DRUG TABLE   FLUOROQUINOLONES AND AMINOGLYCOSIDES

GENERIC NAME	TRADE NAME	USES	ADVERSE REACTIONS	DOSAGE RANGES
Fluoroquinolones				
ciprofloxacin *si-proe'-flox-a sin*	Cipro, Cipro IV	Treatment of infections due to susceptible microorganisms	Nausea, diarrhea, headache, abdominal discomfort, photosensitivity, superinfections, hypersensitivity reactions	250–750 mg orally q12h; 200–400 mg IV q12h
gatifloxacin *ga-tah-flox'-a-sin*	Tequin	Same as ciprofloxacin	Same as ciprofloxacin	200–400 mg once daily orally, IV
gemifloxacin *jem-ah-flox'-a-sin*	Factive	Bronchitis and pneumonia	Vomiting, diarrhea, stomach pain, restlessness, dizziness, confusion, taste changes, sleep disturbances	320 mg/d orally
levofloxacin *lee-voe-flox'-a-sin*	Levaquin	Same as ciprofloxacin	Same as ciprofloxacin	250–750 mg/d orally, IV
lomefloxacin *loh-meh-flox'-a-sin*	Maxaquin	Same as ciprofloxacin	Same as ciprofloxacin	400 mg orally once daily
moxifloxacin *mocks-ah-flox'-a-sin*	Avelox	Same as ciprofloxacin	Same as ciprofloxacin	400 mg/d orally
℞ **norfloxacin** *nor-flox'-a-sin*	Noroxin	Same as ciprofloxacin, urinary tract infections, uncomplicated gonorrhea, prostatitis	Same as ciprofloxacin	400 mg orally q12h; 800 mg as single dose for gonorrhea
ofloxacin *oe-flox'-a-sin*	Floxin	Same as ciprofloxacin	Same as ciprofloxacin	200–400 mg orally, IV q12h
Aminoglycosides				
amikacin *am-i-kay'-sin*	Amikin	Treatment of serious infections caused by susceptible strains of microorganisms	Nausea, vomiting, diarrhea, rash, ototoxicity, nephrotoxicity, hypersensitivity reactions, neurotoxicity, superinfections, neuromuscular blockade	15 mg/kg IM, IV, in divided doses, not to exceed 1.5 g/d
gentamicin *jen-ta-mye'-sin*		Same as amikacin	Same as amikacin	3 mg/kg/d in 3 divided doses IM or IV For life-threatening infection: 5 mg/kg/d in divided doses
kanamycin *kan-a-mye'-sin*	Kantrex	Same as amikacin; for hepatic coma and for suppression of intestinal bacteria	Same as amikacin	7.5–15 mg/kg/d in divided doses IM, not to exceed 15 mg/kg/d in divided doses IV; not to exceed 1.5 g/d
neomycin *nee-o-mye'-sin*		Same as amikacin, same as kanamycin	Same as amikacin	Preoperative prophylaxis: 1 g/d orally for 3 days Hepatic coma: 4–12 g/d in divided doses

GENERIC NAME	TRADE NAME	USES	ADVERSE REACTIONS	DOSAGE RANGES
paramycin sulfate *para-mye'-sin*	Humetin	Hepatic coma, intestinal amebiasis	Same as amikacin	25–35 mg/kg/d
streptomycin *strep-toe-mye'-sin*		Same as amikacin, treatment of tuberculosis	Same as amikacin	15 mg/kg/d IM or 25–30 mg/kg IM 2–3 times per week
tobramycin *toe-bra-mye'-sin*		Same as amikacin	Same as amikacin	3–5 mg/kg/d IM, IV in 3 equal doses

Ⓡ This drug should be administered at least 1 hour before or 2 hours after a meal.

- Infections of the skin
- Sexually transmitted diseases

Ciprofloxacin, norfloxacin, and ofloxacin are available in ophthalmic forms for infections in the eyes.

Adverse Reactions

Common adverse effects include
- Nausea
- Diarrhea
- Headache
- Abdominal pain or discomfort
- Dizziness
- **Photosensitivity**, which is a more serious adverse reaction seen with the administration of the fluoroquinolones, especially lomefloxacin and sparfloxacin.

The administration of any drug may result in a hypersensitivity reaction, which can range from mild to severe and, in some cases, be life-threatening. Mild hypersensitivity reactions may require only discontinuing the drug, whereas the more serious reactions require immediate treatment (see Chapters 1 and 7). Bacterial or fungal superinfections and pseudomembranous colitis (see Chapter 7) may occur with the use of both of these drugs. See the Summary Drug Table: Fluoroquinolones and Aminoglycosides for more information.

Contraindications and Precautions

The fluoroquinolones are contraindicated in patients with a history of hypersensitivity to the fluoroquinolones, in children younger than 18 years of age, and in pregnancy (category C). These drugs also are contraindicated in patients whose lifestyles do not allow for adherence to the precautions regarding photosensitivity.

The fluoroquinolones are used cautiously in patients with renal impairment, patients with a history of seizures, older patients, and patients on dialysis.

Interactions

The following interactions may occur when a fluoroquinolone is administered with another agent:

Interacting Drug	Common Use	Effect of Interaction
theophylline	Management of respiratory problems, such as asthma	Increased serum theophylline level
cimetidine	Management of gastrointestinal (GI) upset	Interferes with elimination of the antibiotic
oral anticoagulants	Blood thinner	Increased risk of bleeding
antacids, iron salts, or zinc	Relief of heartburn and GI upset	Decreased absorption of the antibiotic
nonsteroidal anti-inflammatory drugs (NSAIDs)	Relief of pain and inflammation	Risk of seizure activity

There is also a risk of severe cardiac arrhythmias when the fluoroquinolones gatifloxacin and moxifloxacin are administered with drugs that increase the QT interval (e.g., quinidine, procainamide, amiodarone, sotalol).

AMINOGLYCOSIDES

The aminoglycosides include amikacin (Amikin), gentamicin, kanamycin (Kantrex), neomycin, streptomycin, and tobramycin.

Actions

The aminoglycosides exert their bactericidal effect by blocking a step in protein synthesis necessary for bacterial multiplication. They disrupt the functional ability of the bacterial cell wall, causing cell death.

Uses

The aminoglycosides are used primarily in the treatment of infections caused by gram-negative microorganisms. In addition, the drugs may be used to reduce bacteria (normal flora) in the bowel when patients are having abdominal surgery or when a patient is in a hepatic coma. Because the oral aminoglycosides are poorly absorbed, they are useful in suppressing GI bacteria. For example, kanamycin (Kantrex) and neomycin are used before surgery to reduce intestinal bacteria. It is thought this reduces the possibility of abdominal infection that may occur after surgery on the bowel. This drug treatment protocol is called a **bowel preparation** (bowel prep).

Kanamycin, neomycin, and paromomycin are used orally in the management of **hepatic coma**. In this disorder, liver failure results in an elevation of blood ammonia levels. By reducing the number of ammonia-forming bacteria in the intestines, blood ammonia levels may be lowered, thereby temporarily reducing some of the symptoms associated with this disorder.

Adverse Reactions

General system reactions include the following:
- Nausea
- Vomiting
- Anorexia
- Rash
- Urticaria

More serious adverse reactions may lead to discontinuation of the drug. These reactions include:

- **Nephrotoxicity** (damage to the kidneys by a toxic substance)
- **Ototoxicity** (damage to the hearing organs by a toxic substance)
- **Neurotoxicity** (damage to the nervous system by a toxic substance)

Signs and symptoms of nephrotoxicity may include **proteinuria** (protein in the urine), **hematuria** (blood in the urine), increase in the blood urea nitrogen (BUN) level, decrease in urine output, and an increase in the serum creatinine concentration. Nephrotoxicity is usually reversible once the drug is discontinued.

Signs and symptoms of ototoxicity include tinnitus (ringing in the ears), dizziness, roaring in the ears, vertigo, and a mild to severe loss of hearing. If hearing loss occurs, it is usually permanent. Ototoxicity may occur during drug therapy or even after therapy is discontinued. The short-term administration of kanamycin and neomycin as a preparation for bowel surgery rarely causes these two adverse reactions.

Signs and symptoms of neurotoxicity include numbness, skin tingling, circumoral (around the mouth) paresthesia, peripheral paresthesia, tremors, muscle twitching, convulsions, muscle weakness, and **neuromuscular blockade** (acute muscular paralysis and apnea).

The administration of the aminoglycosides may result in a hypersensitivity reaction, which can range from mild to severe and, in some cases, be life threatening. Mild hypersensitivity reactions may require only discontinuing the drug, whereas the more serious reactions require immediate treatment. When aminoglycosides are given, individual drug references, such as the package insert, should be consulted for more specific adverse reactions. As with other anti-infectives, bacterial or fungal superinfections and pseudomembranous colitis (see Chapter 7) may occur with the use of these drugs.

Contraindications

The aminoglycosides are contraindicated in patients with hypersensitivity to aminoglycosides, preexisting hearing loss, myasthenia gravis, and parkinsonism. They are also contraindicated during lactation or pregnancy (pregnancy category C, except for neomycin, amikacin, gentamicin, kanamycin, netilmicin, and tobramycin, which are in pregnancy category D). Aminoglycosides are also contraindicated for long-term therapy because of the potential for ototoxicity and nephrotoxicity.

Precautions

The aminoglycosides are used cautiously in elderly patients and patients with renal failure (dosage adjustments may be necessary) and neuromuscular disorders.

Interactions

The following interactions may occur when an aminoglycoside is administered with another agent:

Interacting Drug	Common Use	Effect of Interaction
cephalosporins	Anti-infective agent	Increased risk of nephrotoxicity
loop diuretics (water pills)	Management of edema and water retention	Increased risk of ototoxicity
Pavulon or Anectine (general anesthetics)	Anesthesia (e.g., for surgery)	Increased risk of neuromuscular blockade

NURSING PROCESS

The Patient Receiving a Fluoroquinolone or Aminoglycoside

ASSESSMENT

PREADMINISTRATION ASSESSMENT

Before administering a fluoroquinolone or aminoglycoside, the nurse identifies and records the signs and symptoms of the infection. It is particularly important for the nurse to obtain a thorough allergy history, especially a history of drug allergies. The nurse should take and record vital signs as well.

The primary health care provider may order culture and sensitivity tests, and the culture is obtained before the first dose of the drug is given. When an aminoglycoside is to be given, laboratory tests such as renal and hepatic function tests, complete blood count, and urinalysis also may be ordered. In persons with impaired hearing or at risk for hearing loss, a hearing test may be recommended.

When kanamycin or neomycin is given for hepatic coma, the nurse must evaluate the patient's level of consciousness and ability to swallow.

ONGOING ASSESSMENT

During drug therapy with the aminoglycosides or fluoroquinolones, it is important for the nurse to perform an ongoing assessment. In general, the nurse compares the initial signs and symptoms of the infection, which were recorded during the initial assessment, with the current signs and symptoms. The nurse then records these findings in the patient's chart. When kanamycin or neomycin is given for hepatic coma, the nurse evaluates and records the patient's general condition and changes in mentation daily.

The nurse monitors the patient's vital signs every 4 hours or as ordered by the primary health care provider. The nurse should notify the primary health care provider if there are changes in the vital signs, such as a significant drop in blood pressure, an increase in the pulse or respiratory rate, or a sudden increase in temperature.

When an aminoglycoside is being administered, it is important to monitor the patient's respiratory rate because neuromuscular blockade has been reported with the administration of these drugs. The nurse reports any changes in the respiratory rate or rhythm to the primary health care provider because immediate treatment may be necessary.

NURSING DIAGNOSES

Drug-specific nursing diagnoses are highlighted in the Nursing Diagnoses Checklist. Other nursing diagnoses applicable to these drugs are discussed in Chapter 4.

Nursing Diagnoses Checklist

✔ **Risk for Impaired Comfort** related to fever

✔ **Altered Thought Process** related to increased ammonia blood levels

✔ **Risk for Impaired Skin Integrity** related to photosensitivity

✔ **Acute Pain** related to tissue injury during drug therapy

✔ **Risk for Injury** related to paresthesia secondary to neurotoxicity

✔ **Ineffective Tissue Perfusion: Renal** related to adverse drug reactions to aminoglycosides

✔ **Disturbed Sensory Perception: Auditory** related to adverse drug reactions to aminoglycosides

✔ **Diarrhea** related to superinfection secondary to antibiotic therapy adverse drug reaction

PLANNING

The expected outcomes for the patient may include an optimal response to therapy, which includes control of the infectious process, meeting of patient needs related to the management of adverse drug reactions, and an understanding of and compliance with the prescribed treatment regimen.

IMPLEMENTATION

PROMOTING AN OPTIMAL RESPONSE TO THERAPY

A variety of adverse reactions can be seen with the administration of the fluoroquinolones or aminoglycosides. The nurse observes the patient, especially during the first 48 hours of therapy. It is important to report the occurrence of any adverse reaction to the primary health care provider before the next dose of the drug is due. If a serious adverse reaction, such as a hypersensitivity reaction, respiratory difficulty, severe diarrhea, or a decided drop in blood pressure, occurs the nurse contacts the primary health care provider immediately.

The nurse always listens to, evaluates, and reports any complaints the patient may have; certain complaints may be an early sign of an adverse drug reaction. The nurse should report all changes in the patient's condition and any new problems that occur (e.g., nausea or diarrhea) as soon as possible. It is then up to the primary health care provider to decide if these changes or problems are a part of the patient's infectious process or the result of an adverse drug reaction.

The nurse encourages patients who receive the fluoroquinolones to increase their fluid intake. Norfloxacin is given on an empty stomach (e.g., 1 hour before or 2 hours after meals). Some drugs are made so that they release the drug over time in the body; these formulations are known as **extended-release** (XR) drugs, sustained-release (SR), or controlled-release (CR) drugs. Because the amount of drug would be too great if released in the body at once, it is important to swallow these medications whole. Patients should not crush, chew, or break extended-release medications. If the patient is taking an antacid, ciprofloxacin and moxifloxacin should be administered 2 to 4 hours before or 6 to 8 hours after the antacid.

When kanamycin or neomycin is given to suppress intestinal bacteria before surgery, the primary health care provider's orders regarding the timing of the administration of the drug are extremely important. Omission of a dose or failure to give the drug at the specified time may result in inadequate suppression of intestinal bacteria. When neomycin is given, enteric-coated erythromycin (see Chapter 9) may be given at the same time as part of bowel preparation. **Enteric-coated** tablets have a special coating that prevents the drug from being absorbed in the stomach. Absorption takes place lower in the GI tract when the coating has dissolved.

MONITORING AND MANAGING PATIENT NEEDS

IMPAIRED COMFORT: INCREASED FEVER The infectious process is accompanied by an elevation in temperature. When the patient is being treated for the infection, the nurse must monitor the vital signs, particularly the body temperature. As the anti-infective works to rid the body of the infectious organism, the body temperature should return to normal. The nurse monitors the vital signs (temperature, pulse, and respiration) frequently to assess the drug's effectiveness in eradicating the infection. The nurse checks the vital signs every 4 hours, or more frequently if the temperature is elevated. The primary health care provider is notified if a temperature rises over 101° F.

ALTERED THOUGHT PROCESS: HEPATIC COMA When the aminoglycosides kanamycin and neomycin are administered orally as treatment for hepatic coma, the nurse exercises care. During the early stages of this disorder, various changes in the level of consciousness may be seen. At times, the patient may appear lethargic and respond poorly to commands. Because of these changes in the level of consciousness, the patient may have difficulty swallowing, and a danger of aspiration is present. If the patient appears to have difficulty taking an oral drug, the nurse withholds the drug and contacts the primary health care provider.

IMPAIRED SKIN INTEGRITY The fluoroquinolone drugs, particularly lomefloxacin, cause dangerous photosensitivity reactions. Patients have experienced severe reactions even when they used sunscreen or sunblock products. Patients should be cautioned to wear cover-up clothing with long sleeves and wide-brimmed hats when outside in addition to sunblock preparations. Patients should be aware that glare during hazy or cloudy days can cause skin reactions as readily as direct sunlight on a clear day.

ACUTE PAIN: TISSUE INJURY For intravenously administered fluoroquinolones or aminoglycosides, as with other caustic drugs, the nurse inspects the needle site and the area around the needle every hour for signs of extravasation of the IV fluid. The nurse performs these assessments more frequently if the patient is restless or uncooperative. It is important to check the rate of infusion every 15 minutes and adjust it as needed. The nurse should inspect the vein used for the IV infusion every 4 hours for signs of tenderness, pain, and redness (which may indicate phlebitis or thrombophlebitis). If these are apparent, the nurse must restart the IV in another vein and bring the problem to the attention of the primary health care provider.

All fluoroquinolone drugs can cause pain, inflammation, or rupture of a tendon. The Achilles tendon is particularly vulnerable. This problem can be so severe that prolonged disability results, and, at times, surgical intervention may be necessary to correct the problem.

RISK FOR INJURY The nurse should be alert for symptoms such as numbness or tingling of the skin, circumoral paresthesia, peripheral paresthesia (numbness or tingling in the extremities), tremors, and muscle twitching or weakness. The nurse reports any symptom of neurotoxicity immediately to the primary health care provider. Convulsions can occur if the drug is not discontinued.

Nursing Alert

Neuromuscular blockade or respiratory paralysis may occur after administration of the aminoglycosides. Therefore, it is extremely important that any symptoms of respiratory difficulty be reported immediately. If neuromuscular blockade occurs, it may be reversed by the administration of calcium salts, but mechanical ventilation may be required.

INEFFECTIVE TISSUE PERFUSION: RENAL The patient taking an aminoglycoside is at risk for nephrotoxicity. The nurse measures and records the intake and output and notifies the primary health care provider if the output is less than 750 mL/d. It is important to keep a record of the fluid intake and output as well as the patient's daily weight to assess hydration and renal function. The nurse encourages fluid intake to 2000 mL/d (if the patient's condition permits). Any changes in the intake-and-output ratio or in the appearance of the urine may indicate nephrotoxicity. The nurse reports these types of changes to the primary health care provider promptly. In turn, the primary health care provider may order daily laboratory tests (e.g., serum creatinine and BUN) to monitor renal function. The nurse reports elevations in the creatinine or BUN level to the primary health care provider because elevation may indicate renal dysfunction.

DISTURBED SENSORY PERCEPTION: AUDITORY The patient taking aminoglycosides is at risk for ototoxicity. Auditory changes are irreversible, usually bilateral, and may be partial or total. The risk is greater in patients with renal impairment or those with preexisting hearing loss. It is important for the nurse to detect any problems with hearing and report them to the primary health care provider because continued drug administration could lead to permanent hearing loss.

Nursing Alert

To detect ototoxicity, the nurse carefully evaluates the patient's complaints or comments related to hearing, such as a ringing or buzzing in the ears or difficulty hearing. If hearing problems do occur, the nurse reports this problem to the primary health care provider immediately. To monitor for damage to the eighth cranial nerve, an evaluation of hearing may be done by audiometry before and throughout the course of therapy.

DIARRHEA Because superinfections and pseudomembranous colitis can occur during therapy with these drugs, the nurse checks the patient's stools and reports any incidence of diarrhea immediately because this may indicate a superinfection or pseudomembranous colitis. If diarrhea does occur and blood and mucus appear in the stool, the nurse should save a sample of the stool and test it for occult blood using a test such as Hemoccult. If the stool tests positive for blood, it is important to save the sample for possible additional laboratory tests.

EDUCATING THE PATIENT AND FAMILY

Carefully planned patient and family education is important to foster compliance, relieve anxiety, and promote therapeutic effect. The nurse explains all adverse reactions associated with the specific prescribed antibiotic to the patient. The nurse advises the patient of the signs and symptoms of potentially serious adverse reactions, such as hypersensitivity reactions, moderate to severe diarrhea, and sudden onset of chills and fever. The nurse should explain to the patient the necessity of contacting the primary health care provider immediately if such symptoms occur. To reduce the incidence of noncompliance with the treatment regimen, a teaching plan is developed to include the information that appears in the Home Care Checklist.

EVALUATION

- The therapeutic effect is achieved, the infection is controlled, and the bowel is cleansed sufficiently if surgery is to occur.
- The patient reports no pain or injury.

Home Care Checklist

Taking Fluoroquinolone or Aminoglycoside Antibiotics

☑ Take the drug at the prescribed time intervals. These time intervals are important because a certain amount of the drug must be in the body at all times for the infection to be controlled.

☑ Drink six to eight 8-ounce glasses of fluid while taking these drugs and take each dose with a full glass of water.

☑ Do not increase or omit the dose unless advised to do so by the primary health care provider.

☑ Complete the entire course of treatment. Do not stop the drug, except on the advice of a primary health care provider, before the course of treatment is completed even if symptoms improve or disappear. Failure to complete the prescribed course of treatment may result in a return of the infection.

☑ Follow the directions supplied with the prescription regarding taking the drugs with meals or on an empty stomach. Take drugs that must be taken on an empty stomach, 1 hour before or 2 hours after a meal.

☑ Distinguish between immediate- and extended-release medications. Do not break, chew, or crush extended-release medications.

☑ Notify the primary health care provider if symptoms of the infection become worse or if original symptoms do not improve after 5 to 7 days of drug therapy.

☑ Avoid any exposure to sunlight or ultraviolet light (tanning beds, sunlamps) while taking these drugs and for several weeks after completing the course of therapy. Wear sunblock, sunglasses, and protective clothing when exposed to sunlight.

☑ Avoid tasks requiring mental alertness until response to the drug is known.

Specific Instructions Regarding Fluoroquinolone Therapy

☑ When taking the fluoroquinolones, report any signs of tendinitis, such as pain or soreness in the leg, shoulder, or back of the heel. Periodic applications of ice may help relieve the pain. Until tendinitis or tendon rupture can be excluded, rest the involved area and avoid exercise.

☑ Do not take antacids or drugs containing iron or zinc because these drugs will decrease absorption of the fluoroquinolone.

Specific Instructions Regarding Aminoglycoside Therapy

☑ Notify the primary health care provider of any ringing in the ears or difficulty hearing, numbness or tingling around the mouth or in the extremities, and of any change in urinary patterns.

Specific Instructions for Preoperative Bowel Preparation

☑ When taking an aminoglycoside for preparation of the bowel before surgery, take the prescribed drug at the exact times indicated on the prescription container. Some bowel prep regimens are complex. For example, when kanamycin is prescribed for suppression of intestinal bacteria in preparation for bowel surgery, the drug is given orally every hour for 4 hours followed by 1 gram every 6 hours for 36 to 72 hours.

• The patient's hearing is intact.

• The patient's fluid intake is at least 2000 mL and output is at least 1200 mL daily while taking these drugs.

• Adverse reactions are identified, reported to the primary health care provider, and managed successfully through nursing interventions.

• The patient and family demonstrate understanding of the drug regimen.

• The patient verbalizes the importance of complying with the prescribed therapeutic regimen.

Critical Thinking Exercises

1. Mr. Baker is receiving amikacin (Amikin) IV as treatment for a bacterial septicemia. When checking a drug reference you note that this drug is an aminoglycoside. Considering the most serious toxic

effects associated with this group of drugs, determine what daily assessments you would perform to detect early signs and symptoms of these adverse drug effects.

2. Ms. Carson is seen in the outpatient clinic for a severe respiratory infection and is prescribed ciprofloxacin. Discuss what you would include in the teaching plan for this patient.

3. A patient is prescribed ciprofloxacin for a severe respiratory infection. For what serious adverse reaction(s) should the nurse warn the patient to be especially observant? What common adverse reactions should the patient be aware of? What important information should the nurse include in the teaching plan concerning adverse reactions?

Review Questions

1. Mr. Allison is taking gentamicin for a severe gram-negative infection. The nurse observes him for signs of neurotoxicity, which include _____.

    A. anorexia and abdominal pain

    B. decreased urinary output and dark, concentrated urine

    C. muscle twitching and numbness

    D. headache and agitation

2. Patients taking a fluoroquinolone are encouraged to _____.

    A. nap 1 to 2 hours daily while taking the drug

    B. eat a high-protein diet

    C. increase their fluid intake

    D. avoid foods high in carbohydrate

3. Which of the following complaints by a man taking tobramycin would be most indicative that he is experiencing ototoxicity?

    A. tingling of the extremities

    B. complaints that he is unable to hear the television

    C. changes in mental status

    D. short periods of dizziness

4. A patient is prescribed moxifloxacin. The nurse notes that the patient is also taking an antacid. The nurse correctly administers moxifloxacin _____.

    A. once daily orally, 4 hours before the antacid

    B. twice daily orally, immediately after the antacid

    C. once daily IM without regard to the administration of the antacid

    D. every 12 hours IV without regard to the administration of the antacid

5. The nurse is asked why kanamycin is given as a "bowel prep" before GI surgery. The nurse correctly replies that _____.

    A. abdominal surgery requires starting antibiotic therapy 4 days before surgery

    B. the bacteria found in the bowel cannot be destroyed after surgery

    C. a reduction of intestinal bacteria lessens the possibility of postoperative infection

    D. anesthesia makes the bowel resistant to an antibiotic after surgery

Medication Dosage Problems

1. A patient is prescribed 40 mg of tobramycin IM. Use the drug label shown below to determine the amount of drug to administer:

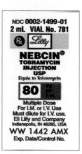

The nurse would administer _____.

2. The primary health care provider prescribed 400 mg gatifloxacin orally daily for 7 days. The drug is available in 200-mg tablets. How many tablets would the nurse administer each day?

To check your answers, see Appendix G.

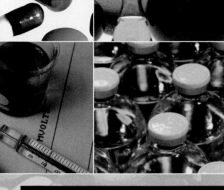

Chapter 11

Miscellaneous Anti-Infectives

Key Terms

phenylketonuria
red-man syndrome
vancomycin-resistant
Enterococcus faecium (VREF)

Learning Objectives

On completion of this chapter, the student will:

- Discuss the uses, general drug actions, adverse reactions, contraindications, precautions, and interactions of the drugs presented in this chapter.
- Discuss preadministration and ongoing assessments necessary with the administration of the drugs presented in this chapter.
- Identify nursing assessments that are performed when a drug is

potentially nephrotoxic or ototoxic.

- List nursing diagnoses particular to a patient taking the anti-infective drugs presented in this chapter.
- Discuss ways to promote optimal response to therapy and important points to keep in mind when educating patients about the use of the anti-infectives presented in this chapter.

The anti-infectives discussed in this chapter are singular drugs, that is, they are not related to each other and do not belong to any one of the drug groups discussed in Chapters 6 through 10. Some of these drugs are used only for the treatment of one type of infection, whereas others may be limited to the treatment of serious infections not treatable by other anti-infectives.

LINEZOLID

Actions and Uses

Linezolid (Zyvox) is the first drug in a new drug class. It is an oxazolidinone that acts by binding to a site on a specific ribosomal RNA and preventing the formation of a component necessary for the bacteria to replicate. It is both bacteriostatic (i.e., to enterococci and staphylococci) and bactericidal (i.e., against streptococci). The drug is used in the treatment of **vancomycin-resistant *Enterococcus faecium* (VREF)**, health care– and community-acquired pneumonias, and skin and skin structure infections, including those caused by methicillin-resistant *Staphylococcus aureus* (MRSA).

Adverse Reactions

The most common adverse reactions include

- Nausea
- Vomiting
- Diarrhea
- Headache and dizziness

- Insomnia
- Rash

Less common adverse reactions include

- Fatigue
- Depression
- Nervousness
- Photosensitivity

Pseudomembranous colitis and thrombocytopenia are the most serious adverse reactions caused by linezolid.

Contraindications and Precautions

Linezolid is contraindicated in patients who are allergic to the drug or are pregnant (category C) or lactating, and in patients with **phenylketonuria**.

Linezolid is used cautiously in patients with bone marrow depression, hepatic dysfunction, renal impairment, hypertension, and hyperthyroidism.

Interactions

The following interactions may occur when linezolid is administered with another agent:

- Antiplatelet drugs (aspirin or the nonsteroidal anti-inflammatory drugs [NSAIDs])—increased risk of bleeding and thrombocytopenia
- Monamine oxidase inhibitor (MAOI) antidepressants—decreased effectiveness
- Large amounts of food containing tyramine (e.g., aged cheese, caffeinated beverages, yogurt, chocolate, red wine, beer, pepperoni)—risk of severe hypertension.

CARBAPENEMS

Action and Uses

The carbapenems inhibit synthesis of the bacterial cell wall and cause the death of susceptible cells. Meropenem (Merrem IV) is used for intra-abdominal infections and bacterial meningitis. Imipenem-cilastatin (Primaxin) is used to treat serious infections, endocarditis, and septicemia. Ertapenem (Invanz) is used to treat serious infections and community-acquired pneumonia caused by bacteria.

Adverse Reactions

The most common adverse reactions with the carbapenems include nausea, vomiting, diarrhea, and rash. These drugs also can cause an abscess or phlebitis at the injection site. An abscess is suspected if the injection site appears red or is tender and warm to the touch. Tissue sloughing at the injection site also may occur. For more information, see Summary Drug Table: Miscellaneous Anti-infectives.

Contraindications, Precautions, and Interactions

Carbapenems are contraindicated in patients who are allergic to cephalosporins and penicillins and in patients with renal failure. This drug is not recommended in children younger than 3 months or for women during pregnancy (category B) or lactation. Carbapenems are used cautiously in patients with central nervous system (CNS) disorders, seizure disorders, or renal or hepatic failure. The excretion of carbapenems is inhibited when the drug is administered to a patient also taking probenecid (Benemid).

SPECTINOMYCIN

Actions and Uses

Spectinomycin (Trobicin) is chemically related to but different from the aminoglycosides (see Chapter 10). This drug exerts its action by interfering with bacterial protein synthesis. Spectinomycin is used for treating gonorrhea in patients who are allergic to penicillins, cephalosporins, or probenecid (Benemid).

Adverse Reactions

Soreness at the injection site, urticaria, dizziness, rash, chills, fever, and hypersensitivity reactions may occur as side effects of this drug.

Contraindications, Precautions, and Interactions

Spectinomycin is contraindicated in patients with known hypersensitivity to the drug. In addition, the drug should

SUMMARY DRUG TABLE   MISCELLANEOUS ANTI-INFECTIVES

GENERIC NAME	TRADE NAME	USES	ADVERSE REACTIONS	DOSAGE RANGES
aztreonam *az'-tree-oh-nam*	Azactam	Gram-negative bacterial infections	Nausea, diarrhea, hypotension, rash and headache	500 mg–1 g q8–12h
daptomycin *dap-toe-mye'-sin*	Cubicin	Complicated skin and skin structure infections	Nausea, diarrhea, constipation, rash, vein irritation	4 mg/kg IV daily for 7–14 d
ertapenem *er-tah-pen'-em*	Invanz	Serious infections and community acquired pneumonia	Nausea, diarrhea, headache, altered mental status, vein irritation	1 g IV daily
fosfomycin tromethamine *foss-foe-mye'-sin*	Monurol	Urinary tract infections	Nausea, diarrhea, headache, vaginal itch, runny nose	3-g packet mixed with water, orally daily
imipenem-cilastatin	Primaxin	Serious infections caused by *Staphylococcus* sp, *Streptococcus* sp, and *Escherichia coli*	Nausea, diarrhea	125–500 mg q6h, not to exceed 4 g/d
linezolid *lih-nez'-oh-lid*	Zyvox	Infections with vancomycin-resistant *Enterococcus faecium*; pneumonia from *Staphylococcus aureus* and penicillin-susceptible *Streptococcus pneumoniae*; skin and skin structure infections	Nausea, diarrhea, headache, insomnia, pseudomembranous colitis	600 mg orally or IV q12h
meropenem *meh-row-pen'-em*	Merrem IV	Intra-abdominal and soft tissue infections caused by multiresistant gram-negative organisms	Headache, diarrhea, abdominal pain, nausea, pain and inflammation at injection site, pseudo-membranous colitis	1 g IV q8h
quinupristin-dalfopristin	Synercid	Vancomycin-resistant *E. faecium*	Vein inflammation, nausea, vomiting, diarrhea	7.5 mg/kg IV q8h
spectinomycin *spek-tin-oe-mye'-cin*	Trobincin	Gonorrhea	Soreness at injection site, urticaria, dizziness, rash, chills, fever, hypersensitivity reactions	2 g IM as single dose; up to 4 g IM
vancomycin *van-koe-mye'-cin*	Vancocin, Vancoled	Serious susceptible gram-positive infections not responding to treatment with other antibiotics	Nephrotoxicity, ototoxicity, nausea, chills, fever, urticaria, sudden fall in blood pressure, redness on face, neck, arms, and back	500 mg–2 g/d orally in divided doses; 500 mg IV q6h or 1 g IV q12h

Miscellaneous Anti-Infectives

not be given to infants. If another sexually transmitted disease (STD) is present with gonorrhea, additional anti-infectives may be needed to eradicate the infectious processes. Safe use during pregnancy (category B) or lactation or in children has not been established. No significant drug or food interactions for spectinomycin are known.

VANCOMYCIN

Actions and Uses

Vancomycin (Vancocin) acts against susceptible gram-positive bacteria by inhibiting bacterial cell wall synthesis and increasing cell wall permeability. This drug is used in the treatment of serious gram-positive infections that do not respond to treatment with other anti-infectives. It also may be used in treating anti-infective–associated pseudomembranous colitis caused by *Clostridium difficile*.

Adverse Reactions

Nephrotoxicity (damage to the kidneys) and ototoxicity (damage to the organs of hearing) may be seen with the administration of this drug. Additional adverse reactions include nausea, chills, fever, urticaria, sudden fall in blood pressure with parenteral administration, and skin rashes.

Contraindications, Precautions, and Interactions

This drug is contraindicated in patients with known hypersensitivity to vancomycin. Vancomycin is used cautiously in patients with renal or hearing impairment and during pregnancy (category C) and lactation. When administered with other ototoxic and nephrotoxic drugs, additive effects may occur. In other words, one drug alone may not cause the hearing or kidney problem, but when another drug with similar adverse effects is given with vancomycin, the patient is more likely to experience a problem.

AZTREONAM

Actions and Uses

Aztreonam has a beta-lactam nucleus, and therefore it is called a *monobactam*. The monobactams have bactericidal action and are used to treat gram-negative microorganisms.

Adverse Reactions

Nausea, vomiting and diarrhea, hypotension, rash, and headache are common adverse reactions. As with many other anti-infectives, there is a risk of pseudomembranous colitis. The nurse needs to assess stools for blood when the patient has diarrhea.

Contraindications, Precautions, and Interactions

This drug is contraindicated in patients with a known hypersensitivity to aztreonam. Aztreonam should not be used during pregnancy (pregnancy category B) or lactation. This drug should be used cautiously in patients with renal or hepatic impairment. Patients sensitive to penicillins, cephalosporins, or carbapenems should be monitored carefully for cross-sensitivity.

QUINUPRISTIN/DALFOPRISTIN

Actions and Uses

Quinupristin/dalfopristin is a bacteriostatic agent used in the treatment of VREF. It has bactericidal action against both methicillin-susceptible and methicillin-resistant staphylococci.

Adverse Reactions

This drug is irritating to the vein. After peripheral infusion of quinupristin/dalfopristin, the vein should be flushed with 5% dextrose in water (D_5W) because the drug is incompatible with saline or heparin flush solutions. Other adverse reactions include nausea, vomiting, and diarrhea.

Contraindications, Precautions, and Interactions

This drug is contraindicated in patients with a known hypersensitivity to quinupristin/dalfopristin. Because prolonged use of anti-infectives can disrupt normal flora, the patient should be monitored for secondary bacterial or fungal infections. This drug should not be used during pregnancy (category B) and lactation. When taking quinupristin/dalfopristin the serum levels of the following drugs may increase: antiretrovirals, antineoplastic and immunosuppressant agents, calcium channel blockers, benzodiazepines, and cisapride.

DAPTOMYCIN

Actions and Uses

Daptomycin is a member of a new category of antibacterial agents called *cyclic lipopeptides*. This drug binds to the cell membrane, depolarizing the wall and inhibiting protein DNA and RNA synthesis, which causes the bacterial cell to die. Daptomycin is used to treat complicated skin and skin structure bacterial infections.

Adverse Reactions

The most common adverse reactions are gastrointestinal. They include nausea, diarrhea, and constipation. In addition, the vein can become irritated from intravenous administration.

Contraindications, Precautions, and Interactions

This drug is contraindicated in patients with a known hypersensitivity to daptomycin, and it should not be used during pregnancy (category B) or lactation. Daptomycin should be used cautiously in patients taking warfarin (Coumadin).

FOSFOMYCIN TROMETHAMINE

Actions and Uses

Fosfomycin tromethamine (Monurol) is an anti-infective used to treat urinary tract infections.

Adverse Reactions

Headache, nausea and diarrhea, rhinitis, and vaginitis are the most common adverse reactions to fosfomycin tromethamine treatment.

Contraindications, Precautions, and Interactions

This drug is contraindicated in patients with a known hypersensitivity to fosfomycin tromethamine. This drug should not be used during pregnancy (category B) or lactation. This drug should be used cautiously in patients taking metoclopramide (Reglan).

NURSING PROCESS

The Patient Receiving a Miscellaneous Anti-Infective

ASSESSMENT
PREADMINISTRATION ASSESSMENT

Before administering these drugs, the nurse takes and records the patient's vital signs and identifies and records the symptoms of the infection. It is very important to take a thorough allergy history, especially a history of drug allergies. When culture and sensitivity tests are ordered, they must be performed before the first dose of the drug is given. Other laboratory tests, such as renal and hepatic function tests, complete blood count, and urinalysis, also may be ordered before and during drug therapy for early detection of toxic reactions.

ONGOING ASSESSMENT

The nurse should monitor the patient's vital signs every 4 hours or as ordered by the primary health care provider. It is important to notify the primary health care provider if there are changes in the vital signs, such as a significant drop in blood pressure, an increase in the pulse or respiratory rate, or a sudden increase in temperature.

The nurse observes the patient at frequent intervals, especially during the first 48 hours of therapy. It is important to report any adverse reaction to the primary health care provider before the next dose of the drug is due.

NURSING DIAGNOSES

Drug-specific nursing diagnoses are highlighted in the Nursing Diagnoses Checklist. Other nursing diagnoses applicable to these drugs are discussed in Chapter 4.

PLANNING

The expected outcomes for the patient depend on the reason for administration of the anti-infective, but may include an optimal response to drug therapy, meet patient needs

☑ Nursing Diagnoses Checklist

✓ **Anxiety** related to feelings about seriousness of illness, route of administration, other factors (specify)

✓ **Diarrhea** related to adverse drug reaction, super-infection

✓ **Acute Pain** related to intramuscular injection or vein irritation

✓ **Risk for Impaired Urinary Elimination** related to adverse drug effects (nephrotoxicity)

✓ **Risk for Disturbed Sensory Perception: Auditory** related to adverse drug effects (ototoxicity)

in relation to the management of adverse drug reactions, a decrease in anxiety, and an understanding of and compliance with the prescribed drug regimen.

IMPLEMENTATION

PROMOTING AN OPTIMAL RESPONSE TO THERAPY

Monitoring each patient for the response to drug therapy and for the appearance of adverse reactions is an integral part of promoting an optimal response to therapy. The nurse immediately reports serious adverse reactions, such as signs and symptoms of a hypersensitivity reaction or superinfection, respiratory difficulty, or a marked drop in blood pressure.

INTRAMUSCULAR ADMINISTRATION To promote an optimal response to therapy when giving these drugs intramuscularly (IM), the nurse inspects previous injection sites for signs of pain or tenderness, redness, and swelling. In addition, the nurse reports any persistent local reaction to the primary health care provider. It also is important to develop a plan for rotating injection sites and recording the site used after each injection.

INTRAVENOUS ADMINISTRATION When these drugs are administered intravenously (IV), the nurse inspects the needle site and area around the needle at frequent intervals for signs of extravasation of the IV fluid. More frequent assessments are performed if the patient is restless or uncooperative. Many of the miscellaneous anti-infectives irritate the vein when administered by the IV route.

The rate of infusion is checked every 15 minutes and adjusted as needed. This is especially important when administering vancomycin because rapid infusion of the drug can result in severe hypotension and shock. The nurse inspects the vein used for the IV infusion every 4 to 8 hours for signs of tenderness, pain, and redness (which

may indicate phlebitis or thrombophlebitis). If these symptoms are apparent, the IV infusion is restarted in another vein and the problem brought to the attention of the primary health care provider.

⚠ Nursing Alert

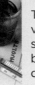

The nurse should administer each IV dose of vancomycin over 60 minutes. Too rapid an infusion may result in a sudden and profound fall in blood pressure and shock. When giving the drug IV, the nurse closely monitors the infusion rate and the patient's blood pressure. The nurse reports any decrease in blood pressure or occurrence of throbbing neck or back pain. These symptoms could indicate a severe adverse reaction referred to as red-neck or **red-man syndrome**. Symptoms of this syndrome include a sudden and profound fall in blood pressure, fever, chills, paresthesias, and erythema (redness) of the neck and back.

The nurse reports patient complaints of difficulty hearing or tinnitus (ringing in the ears) to the primary health care provider before the next dose is due. In addition, the nurse monitors the fluid intake and output and brings any decrease in the urinary output to the attention of the primary health care provider.

MONITORING AND MANAGING PATIENT NEEDS

ANXIETY Patients may exhibit varying degrees of anxiety related to their illness and infection and the necessary drug therapy. When these drugs are given by the parenteral route, patients may experience anxiety because of the discomfort or pain that accompanies an IM injection or IV administration. The nurse reassures the patient that every effort will be made to reduce pain and discomfort, although complete pain relief may not always be possible.

DIARRHEA Diarrhea may be a sign of a superinfection or pseudomembranous colitis, both of which are adverse reactions that may be seen with the administration of any anti-infective. The nurse checks each stool and reports any changes in color or consistency. When these drugs are given as part of the treatment for pseudomembranous colitis, it is important to record the color and consistency of each stool to determine the effectiveness of therapy.

ACUTE PAIN Pain at the injection site may occur when these drugs are given IM. The nurse warns the patient that discomfort may be felt when it is injected and that additional discomfort may be experienced for a brief time afterward. The nurse places a warm, moist compress over the injection site to help alleviate the discomfort. Many of these anti-infectives are irritating to the vein when administered IV. The nurse should read instructions carefully for infusion rates. The proper flush solution is used after the infusion to keep the vein open and minimize irritation.

IMPAIRED URINARY ELIMINATION It is important for the nurse to monitor for nephrotoxicity. The nurse measures and records intake and output while the patient is receiving these drugs. Any changes in the intake–output ratio or in the appearance of the urine must be reported immediately because these may indicate nephrotoxicity.

DISTURBED SENSORY PERCEPTION: AUDITORY The nurse also closely monitors for ototoxicity in all patients receiving an anti-infective. It is important to report any ringing in the ears, difficulty hearing, or dizziness to the primary health care provider. Changes in hearing may not be noticed initially by the patient, but when changes occur they usually progress from difficulty in hearing high-pitched sounds to problems hearing low-pitched sounds.

EDUCATING THE PATIENT AND FAMILY

Whenever a drug is prescribed for a patient, the nurse is responsible for ensuring that the patient has a thorough understanding of the drug, the treatment regimen, and the potential adverse reactions.

To decrease the chance of noncompliance, the nurse emphasizes the following points when any of these drugs are prescribed on an outpatient basis:

- Take the drug at the prescribed time intervals. These time intervals are important because a certain amount of the drug must be in the body at all times for the infection to be controlled.

- Take the drug with food or on an empty stomach as directed on the prescription container.

- Do not increase or omit the dose unless advised to do so by the primary health care provider.

- Complete the entire course of treatment. Do not stop the drug, except on the advice of a primary health care provider, before the course of treatment is completed even if symptoms have improved or have disappeared. Failure to complete the prescribed course of treatment may result in a return of the infection.

- Notify the primary health care provider if symptoms of the infection become worse or there is no improvement in the original symptoms after about 5 to 7 days.

- Contact the primary health care provider as soon as possible if a rash, fever, sore throat, diarrhea, chills, extreme fatigue, easy bruising, ringing in the ears, difficulty hearing, or other problems occur.

- Avoid drinking alcoholic beverages unless use has been approved by the primary health care provider.

EVALUATION

- The therapeutic drug effect is achieved and the infection is controlled.

- Adverse reactions are identified, reported to the primary health care provider, and managed successfully.

- Pain or discomfort after IM or IV administration is relieved or eliminated.

- Anxiety is reduced.

- The patient and family demonstrate understanding of the drug regimen.

Critical Thinking Exercises

1. The charge nurse asks you to discuss the drug quinupristin/dalfopristin (Synercid) and VREF at a team conference. Determine what specific points about preventing transmission of this condition you would discuss at the conference.

2. Mr. Stone is receiving vancomycin. One adverse reaction that may be seen with the administration of this drug is ototoxicity. Rather than ask Mr. Stone directly whether he is having any problem with his hearing, discuss how you might determine if ototoxicity might be occurring.

3. Mr. Reeves has a severe infection and is receiving Synercid. What specific action should the nurse take when terminating the IV infusion? Give a rationale for your answer.

Review Questions

1. When educating a patient about the drug linezolid, the nurse instructs the patient _____.

   A. to take the drug without food to enhance absorption

   B. to avoid foods high in tyramine such as chocolate, coffee, tea, and red wine

   C. to avoid alcohol for at least 10 days after taking the drug

   D. that frequent liver function tests will be necessary while taking the drug

2. When giving a drug that is potentially neurotoxic, the nurse reports which of the patient's complaints related to neurotoxicity?

   A. light-headedness and abdominal pain

   B. severe headache and feeling chilly

   C. numbness of the extremities and dizziness

   D. blurred vision and tinnitus

3. When giving spectinomycin to Mr. Jackson for gonorrhea, the nurse advises him to _____.

   A. return for a follow-up examination

   B. limit his fluid intake to 1200 mL/d while taking the drug

   C. return the next day for a second injection

   D. avoid drinking alcohol for the next 10 days

4. When monitoring the IV infusion of vancomycin, the nurse makes sure the drug infuses over a period of 60 minutes because rapid infusion can result in _____.

   A. fluid overload and respiratory distress

   B. a sudden and profound fall in blood pressure

   C. fluid deficit and dehydration

   D. a sudden and severe rise in blood pressure

Medication Dosage Problems

1. A patient is prescribed 500 mg of vancomycin orally every 6 hours. The drug is available in 500-mg tablets. The nurse administers _____.

2. Aztreonam 500 mg IV is ordered. The drug is available in a vial with 500 mg/15 mL. The nurse administers _____.

3. The primary health care provider prescribes linezolid 400 mg orally. The drug is available as an oral suspension in a strength of 100 mg/5 mL. The nurse administers _____.

To check your answers, see Appendix G.

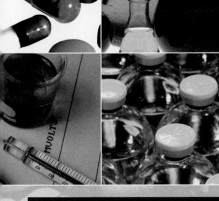

Antitubercular Drugs

Learning Objectives

On completion of this chapter, the student will:

- Discuss the drugs used in the treatment of tuberculosis.
- Discuss the uses, general drug actions, contraindications, precautions, interactions, and general adverse reactions associated with the administration of the antitubercular drugs.
- Discuss important preadministration and ongoing assessment activities the nurse should perform on the

patient taking an antitubercular drug.
- List nursing diagnoses particular to a patient taking an antitubercular drug.
- Describe directly observed therapy (DOT).
- Discuss ways to promote an optimal response to therapy, how to manage adverse reactions, and important points to keep in mind when educating patients about the use of the antitubercular drugs.

Tuberculosis (TB) is a major health problem throughout the world; almost 2 million deaths each year are caused by TB. The World Health Organization (WHO) predicts that 8 million people worldwide will contract this disease each year. Individuals living in crowded conditions, those with compromised immune systems, and individuals with debilitative conditions are especially susceptible to TB.

Tuberculosis is an infectious disease caused by the *Mycobacterium tuberculosis* bacterium. The pathogen is also referred to as the *tubercle bacillus*. The disease is transmitted from one person to another by droplets dispersed in the air when an infected person coughs or sneezes. These droplet nuclei are then inhaled by noninfected persons. Although TB primarily affects the lungs, other organs may be affected also. For example, if the immune system is inadequate, the infection can spread from the lungs to other organs of the body. **Extrapulmonary** (outside of the lungs) tuberculosis is the term used to distinguish TB affecting the lungs from infection with the *M. tuberculosis* bacillus in other organs of the body. Organs that can be affected include the liver, kidneys, spleen, and uterus. People with human immunodeficiency virus (HIV) infection are at risk for TB because of their compromised immune systems.

Tuberculosis responds well to long-term treatment with a combination of three or more antitubercular drugs. Antitubercular drugs are used to treat active cases of TB. They are also used as **prophylactic** (preventative) therapy to prevent the spreading of TB. The drugs used to treat TB do not "cure" the disease, but they do render the patient noninfectious to others. Antitubercular drugs are classified as primary (first-line) and secondary (second-line) drugs. Primary drugs provide the foundation for treatment. Secondary drugs are less effective and more toxic than primary drugs. These drugs are used in various combinations to treat TB. Sensitivity testing may be done to determine the most effective combination treatment, especially in areas of the country where patients may become resistant to therapy.

Nursing Alert

Active TB in patients infected with HIV can be difficult to diagnose. Because the patients' immune systems are deficient, TB skin tests may not show a reaction even when the disease is present. X-ray studies, sputum analyses, or physical examinations may be needed to diagnose *M. tuberculosis* infection accurately in patients with HIV infection.

Secondary drugs are used to treat extrapulmonary TB or drug-resistant organisms. The primary antitubercular drugs are discussed in this chapter. Both primary and secondary antitubercular drugs are listed in the Summary Drug Table: Antitubercular Drugs. Certain fluoroquinolones such as ciprofloxacin, ofloxacin, and levofloxacin have proven effective against TB and are considered secondary drugs (see Chapter 10).

Actions

Most antitubercular drugs are bacteriostatic against the *M. tuberculosis* bacillus. These drugs usually act to inhibit bacterial cell wall synthesis, which slows the multiplication rate of the bacteria. Only isoniazid is bactericidal, with rifampin and streptomycin having some bactericidal activity.

Uses

Antitubercular drugs are used with other drugs to treat active TB. Isoniazid (INH), however, may be used alone in preventive therapy (prophylaxis). For example, when a person is diagnosed with TB, family members of the infected individual must be given prophylactic treatment with isoniazid for 6 months to 1 year. Display 12-1 identifies prophylactic uses for isoniazid.

Standard Treatment

Standard treatment for TB is divided into two phases: the initial phase followed by a continuing phase. During the initial phase, drugs are used to kill the rapidly multiplying *M. tuberculosis* and to prevent drug resistance. The initial phase lasts approximately 2 months and the continuing phase approximately 4 months, with the total treatment regimen lasting for 6 to 9 months, depending on the patient's response to therapy.

Display 12.1 Prophylactic Uses for Isoniazid (INH)

Isoniazid may be used in the following situations:
- Household members and other close associates of those recently diagnosed as having tuberculosis
- Those whose tuberculin skin test has become positive in the last 2 years
- Those with positive skin tests whose radiographic (x-ray) findings indicate nonprogressive, healed, or **quiescent** (causing no symptoms) tubercular lesions
- Those at risk of developing tuberculosis (e.g., those with Hodgkin's disease, severe diabetes mellitus, leukemia, and other serious illnesses and those receiving corticosteroids or drug therapy for a malignancy)
- All patients younger than 35 years (primarily children to age 7) who have a positive skin test
- Persons with acquired immunodeficiency syndrome (AIDS) or those who are positive for the human immunodeficiency virus (HIV) and have a positive tuberculosis skin test or a negative tuberculosis skin test but a history of a prior significant reaction to purified protein derivative (a skin test for tuberculosis)

The initial phase involves using the following drugs: isoniazid (INH), rifampin (Rifadin), and pyrazinamide, along with ethambutol (Myambutol). The Centers for Disease Control and Prevention (CDC) recommends that treatment begin as soon as possible after the diagnosis of TB. The recommended treatment regimen is for the administration of rifampin, isoniazid, pyrazinamide, and ethambutol for a minimum of 2 months. The second or continuation phase includes only the drugs rifampin and isoniazid. The CDC recommends this phase for 4 months or up to 7 months in special populations. These special circumstances include

- Positive sputum culture after completion of initial treatment
- Cavitary (hole or pocket of) disease and positive sputum culture after initial treatment
- Noninclusion of pyrazinamide in the initial treatment
- A positive sputum culture after initial treatment in a patient with previously diagnosed HIV infection

Retreatment

At times treatment fails because of inadequate initial drug treatment or noncompliance with the therapeutic regimen.

When treatment fails, retreatment is necessary. Retreatment generally includes the use of four or more antitubercular drugs. Retreatment drug regimens most often consist of the secondary drugs ethionamide (Trecator), aminosalicylic acid (Paser), cycloserine (Seromycin), and capreomycin (Capastat). Ofloxacin (Floxin) and ciprofloxacin (Cipro) may also be used in retreatment. Sometimes during retreatment, seven or more drugs may be used, with the ineffective drugs discontinued when susceptibility test results are available. Treatment is individualized based on the susceptibility of the microorganism. Up to 24 months of continued treatment after sputum cultures are no longer positive for TB can be part of the plan.

Resistance to the Antitubercular Drugs

Of increasing concern is the development of mutant strains of TB that are resistant to many of the antitubercular drugs currently in use. Bacterial resistance develops, sometimes rapidly, with the use of antitubercular drugs. Treatment is individualized and based on laboratory studies identifying the drugs to which the organism is susceptible. The CDC recommends using three or more drugs with initial therapy, as well as in retreatment, because using a combination of drugs slows the development of bacterial resistance. Tuberculosis caused by drug-resistant organisms should be considered in patients who have no response to therapy and in patients who have been treated in the past.

This chapter discusses the following primary antitubercular drugs: ethambutol, isoniazid, pyrazinamide, and rifampin. Other primary and secondary drugs are listed in the Summary Drug Table: Antitubercular Drugs.

ETHAMBUTOL

Adverse Reactions

Generalized Reactions

- Dermatitis and pruritus
- Joint pain
- Anorexia
- Nausea and vomiting

More Severe Reactions

- **Anaphylactoid reactions** (unusual or exaggerated allergic reactions)

- **Optic neuritis** (a decrease in visual acuity and changes in color perception); optic neuritis is dose related

Contraindications, Precautions, and Interactions

Ethambutol is not recommended for patients with a history of hypersensitivity to the drug or children younger than 13 years. The drug is used with caution during pregnancy (category B), in patients with hepatic or renal impairment, and in patients with diabetic retinopathy or cataracts.

ISONIAZID

Adverse Reactions

The incidence of adverse reactions appears to be higher when larger doses of isoniazid are prescribed.

Generalized Reactions

- Nausea and vomiting
- Epigastric distress
- Fever
- Skin eruptions
- Hematologic changes
- Jaundice
- Hypersensitivity

Toxicity

- **Peripheral neuropathy** (numbness and tingling of the extremities) is the most common symptom of toxicity.
- Severe, and sometimes fatal, hepatitis has been associated with isoniazid therapy and may appear after many months of treatment.

Contraindications and Precautions

Isoniazid is contraindicated in patients with a history of hypersensitivity to the drug. The drug is used with caution during pregnancy (category C) or lactation and in patients with hepatic and renal impairment.

SUMMARY DRUG TABLE   ANTITUBERCULAR DRUGS

GENERIC NAME	TRADE NAME	USES	ADVERSE REACTIONS	DOSAGE RANGES
Primary (First-Line) Drugs				
ethambutol *eth-am'-byoo-tole*	Myambutol	Pulmonary tuberculosis (TB)	Optic neuritis, fever, pruritus, headache, nausea, anorexia, dermatitis, hypersensitivity, psychic disturbances	15–25 mg/kg/d orally
℞ **isoniazid (INH)** *eye-soe-nye'-a-zid*	Laniazid, Nydrazid	Active TB; prophylaxis for TB	Peripheral neuropathy, nausea, vomiting, epigastric distress, jaundice, hepatitis, pyridoxine deficiency, skin eruptions, hypersensitivity	*Active TB*: up to 300 mg/d orally or 15 mg/kg 2–3 times weekly *TB prophylaxis*: 300 mg/d orally
pyrazinamide *peer-a-zin'-a-mide*		Active TB	Hepatotoxicity, nausea, vomiting, diarrhea, myalgia, rashes	15–30 mg/kg/d orally maximum 3 g/d orally; 50–70 mg/kg twice weekly orally
rifabutin *rif-ah-byou'-tin*	Mycobutin	*Mycobacterium avium*	Nausea, vomiting, diarrhea, rash, discolored urine	300 mg/d orally or 150 mg orally BID
℞ **rifampin** *rif-am'-pin*	Rifadin, Rimactane	Active TB	Heartburn, drowsiness, fatigue, dizziness, epigastric distress, hematologic changes, renal insufficiency, rash, body fluid discoloration	600 mg/d orally, IV
Combination Drugs				
isoniazid 150 mg and rifampin 300 mg	Rifamate	TB	See individual drugs	1–2 tablets daily orally
isoniazid 50 mg, rifampin 120 mg, and pyrazinamide 300 mg	Rifater	TB	See individual drugs	1–2 tablets daily orally
Secondary (Second-Line) Drugs				
aminosalicylate *a-meen-oh-sal'-sa-late* (*p*-aminosalicylic acid; 4-aminosalicylic acid)	Paser	TB	Nausea, vomiting, diarrhea, abdominal pain, hypersensitivity reactions	4 g (1 packet) orally TID
capreomycin sulfate *kap-ree-oh-mye'-sin*	Capastat Sulfate	TB	Hypersensitivity reactions, nephrotoxicity, hepatic impairment, pain and induration at injection site, ototoxicity	1 g/d (maximum 20 mg/kg/d) IM
cycloserine *sye-kloe-ser'-een*	Seromycin	TB	Convulsions, somnolence, confusion, renal impairment, sudden development of congestive heart failure, psychoses	500 mg–1 g orally in divided doses

GENERIC NAME	TRADE NAME	USES	ADVERSE REACTIONS	DOSAGE RANGES
ethionamide *e-thye-on-am'-ide*	Trecator	TB	Nausea, vomiting, diarrhea, headache	15–20 mg/kg/d orally
streptomycin *strep-toe-mye'-sin* (although still available, this drug is seldom used)		TB; infections due to susceptible microorganisms	Nephrotoxicity, ototoxicity, numbness, tingling, paresthesia of the face, nausea, dizziness	15 mg/kg but no more than 1 g IM daily (120 g therapeutic maximum)

Ⓡ This drug should be administered at least 1 hour before or 2 hours after a meal.

Interactions

The following interactions may occur when isoniazid is administered with another agent:

Interacting Drug	Common Use	Effect of Interaction
antacids containing aluminum salts	Relief of heartburn and gastrointestinal upset	Reduced absorption of isoniazid
anticoagulants	Blood thinner	Increased risk for bleeding
phenytoin	Antiseizure drug	Increased serum levels of phenytoin
alcohol (in beverages)	Calming effect	Higher incidence of drug-related hepatitis

When isoniazid is taken with foods containing tyramine, such as aged cheese and meats, bananas, yeast products, and alcohol, an exaggerated sympathetic-type response can occur (i.e., hypertension, increased heart rate, and palpitations).

PYRAZINAMIDE

Adverse Reactions

Generalized Reactions

- Nausea and vomiting
- Diarrhea
- Myalgia (aches)
- Rashes

Hepatotoxicity

Hepatotoxicity is the principal adverse reaction seen with pyrazinamide use. Symptoms of hepatotoxicity may range from none (except for slightly abnormal hepatic function test results) to a more severe reaction such as jaundice.

Contraindications and Precautions

Pyrazinamide is contraindicated in patients with a history of hypersensitivity to the drug, acute **gout** (a metabolic disorder resulting in increased levels of uric acid and causing severe joint pain), or severe hepatic damage.

Pyrazinamide should be used cautiously in patients during pregnancy (category C) and lactation and in patients with hepatic and renal impairment, HIV infection, and diabetes mellitus.

Interactions

When pyrazinamide is administered with allopurinol (Zyloprim), colchicine, or probenecid (Benemid), all antigout medications, its effectiveness decreases.

RIFAMPIN

Adverse Reactions

Generalized reactions include the following:
- Nausea and vomiting
- Epigastric distress, heartburn, fatigue
- **Vertigo** (dizziness)
- Rash
- Reddish-orange discoloration of body fluids (urine, tears, saliva, sweat, and sputum)
- Hematologic changes, renal insufficiency

Antitubercular Drugs

Contraindications and Precautions

Rifampin is contraindicated in patients with a history of hypersensitivity to the drug. The drug is used with caution during pregnancy (category C) and lactation and in patients with hepatic or renal impairment.

Interactions

The following interactions may occur when rifampin is administered with another agent:

Interacting Drug	Common Use	Effect of Interaction
digoxin	Management of cardiac problems	Decreased serum levels of digoxin
oral contraceptives	Birth control	Decreased contraceptive effectiveness
isoniazid	Antitubercular agent	Higher risk of hepatotoxicity
oral anticoagulants	Blood thinner	Increased risk for bleeding
oral hypoglycemics	Antidiabetic agent	Decreased effectiveness of oral hypoglycemic agent
chloramphenicol	Anti-infective agent	Increased risk for seizures
phenytoin	Antiseizure agent	Decreased effectiveness of phenytoin
verapamil	Management of cardiac problems and blood pressure	Decreased effectiveness of verapamil

NURSING PROCESS

The Patient Receiving an Antitubercular Drug

ASSESSMENT

PREADMINISTRATION ASSESSMENT

Once the diagnosis of TB is confirmed, the primary health care provider selects the drug that will best con-trol the spread of the disease and make the patient non-infectious to others. Many laboratory and diagnostic tests may be necessary before starting antitubercular therapy, including radiographic studies, culture and sensitivity tests, and various types of laboratory tests, such as a complete blood count. It also is important to assess the family history and a history of contacts if the patient has active TB.

Depending on the severity of the disease, patients may be treated initially in the hospital and then discharged for supervised follow-up care, or they may have all treatment instituted on an outpatient basis.

ONGOING ASSESSMENT

When performing the ongoing assessment, the nurse observes the patient daily for the appearance of adverse reactions. These observations are especially important when a drug is known to be nephrotoxic or ototoxic. It is important to report any adverse reactions to the primary health care provider. In addition, the nurse carefully monitors vital signs daily or as frequently as every 4 hours when the patient is hospitalized.

NURSING DIAGNOSES

Drug-specific nursing diagnoses are highlighted in the Nursing Diagnoses Checklist. The nursing diagnosis of Ineffective Therapeutic Regimen Management may be especially important with patients considering the long-term therapy required to treat TB. Refer to interventions discussed in Chapter 4 to deal with those patient needs.

Nursing Diagnoses Checklist

✔ **Acute Pain** related to frequent injection of anti-tubercular drug

✔ **Imbalanced Nutrition: Less than Body Requirements** related to gastric upset and general poor health status

✔ **Risk of Ineffective Therapeutic Regimen Management** related to indifference, lack of knowledge, long-term treatment regimen, other factors

PLANNING

The expected outcomes for the patient may include an optimal response to antitubercular therapy, meeting patient needs related to the management of common adverse reactions, and an understanding of and compliance with the prescribed treatment regimen.

IMPLEMENTATION

PROMOTING AN OPTIMAL RESPONSE TO THERAPY

The diagnosis, along with the necessity of long-term treatment and follow-up, is often distressing to the patient. Patients with a diagnosis of TB may have many questions about the disease and its treatment. As such, the nurse allows time for the patient and family members to ask questions. In some instances, it may be necessary to refer the patient to other health care workers, such as a social service worker or a dietitian.

MONITORING AND MANAGING PATIENT NEEDS

Managing adverse reactions in patients taking antitubercular drugs is an important responsibility of the nurse. The nurse must continuously observe for signs of adverse reactions and immediately report them to the primary health care provider

ACUTE PAIN: FREQUENT PARENTERAL INJECTIONS

When administering the antitubercular drug by the parenteral route, the nurse is careful to rotate the injection sites. At the time of each injection, the nurse inspects previous injection sites for signs of swelling, redness, and tenderness. If a localized reaction persists or if the area appears to be infected, it is important to notify the primary health care provider.

IMBALANCED NUTRITION: LESS THAN BODY REQUIREMENTS

When TB affects patients who live in crowded and impoverished conditions, malnutrition may be prevalent. In some cases alcoholism may compound the patient's difficulties. This complicates the administration of drugs and compromises the general condition of the patient's gastrointestinal tract. Ethambutol (Myambutol) should be given at the same time daily and may be given without regard to food. Pyrazinamide may also be given with food. The nurse should give other antitubercular drugs by the oral route and on an empty stomach, unless gastric upset occurs. If gastric upset occurs, it is important to notify the primary health care provider before the next dose is given. If a dose is missed, the nurse should tell the patient not to double the dose the next day. An alternative, twice-weekly dosing regimen has been developed to promote compliance on an outpatient basis. This may improve patient nutrition by decreasing the gastric upset of frequent dosing. Combination drugs (e.g., Rifater, which contains isoniazid, rifampin, and pyrazinamide) are being manufactured to promote compliance and reduce the need to take multiple drugs that produce gastric upset.

The nurse teaches the patient to minimize alcohol consumption because of the increased risk of hepatitis. Frequently, the inclusion of pyridoxine (vitamin B_6) is recommended to promote nutrition and prevent neuropathy.

It is helpful to explain to patients that their bodily fluids (urine, feces, saliva, sputum, sweat, and tears) may be colored reddish-orange from the different drugs and that this is normal. It is even more important to teach the patient that this is different from the skin and eye color changes that could indicate hepatic dysfunction (jaundice). The nurse must carefully monitor all patients at least monthly for any evidence of liver dysfunction. It is important to instruct patients to report any of the following symptoms: anorexia, nausea, vomiting, fatigue, weakness, yellowing of the skin or eyes, darkening of the urine, or numbness in the hands and feet

Gerontologic Alert

Older adults are particularly susceptible to a potentially fatal hepatitis when taking isoniazid, especially if they consume alcohol on a regular basis. Two other antitubercular drugs, rifampin and pyrazinamide, can cause liver dysfunction in the older adult as well. Careful observation and monitoring for signs of liver impairment are necessary (e.g., increased serum aspartate aminotransferase [AST], alanine aminotransferase [ALT], and bilirubin levels, and jaundice).

INEFFECTIVE THERAPEUTIC REGIMEN MANAGEMENT

Because the antitubercular drugs must be taken for prolonged periods, compliance with the treatment regimen becomes a problem and increases the risk of development of resistant strains of TB. To help prevent the problem of noncompliance, **directly observed therapy** (DOT) is used to administer these drugs. With DOT, the patient makes periodic visits to the office of the primary care provider or the health clinic, where the drug is taken in the presence of the nurse. The nurse watches the patient swallow each dose of the medication regimen. In some cases, the nurse uses DOT to administer the antitubercular drug in the patient's home, place of employment, or school. DOT may occur daily or two to three times weekly, depending on the patient's health care regimen. Studies indicate that taking the drugs intermittently does not cause a drop in the therapeutic blood levels of antitubercular drugs, even if the drugs are given only two or three times a week.

EDUCATING THE PATIENT AND FAMILY

Antitubercular drugs are given for a long time, and careful patient and family education and close medical supervision are necessary. Noncompliance can be a problem whenever a disease or disorder requires long-term treatment. For this reason, the DOT method of administration is preferred. The patient and family must understand that short-term therapy is of no value in treating this disease. The nurse remains alert for statements made by the patient or family that may indicate future noncompliance with the drug regimen necessary in controlling the disease. See Patient and Family Teaching Checklist: Increasing Compliance in Tubercular Drug Treatment Program for more information.

Patient and Family Teaching Checklist

Increasing Compliance in Tubercular Drug Treatment Program

The nurse:

✔ Discusses tuberculosis, its causes and communicability, and the need for long-term therapy for disease control.

✔ Reinforces that short-term treatment is ineffective.

✔ Reviews the drug therapy regimen, including the prescribed drugs, doses, and frequency of administration.

✔ Reassures the patient that various combinations of drugs are effective in treating tuberculosis.

✔ Urges the patient to take the drugs exactly as prescribed and not to omit, increase, or decrease the dosage unless directed to do so by the health care provider.

✔ Instructs the patient about possible adverse reactions and the need to notify prescriber should any occur.

✔ Arranges for direct observation therapy with the patient and family.

✔ Instructs the patient in measures to minimize gastrointestinal upset.

✔ Advises the patient to avoid alcohol and the use of nonprescription drugs, especially those containing aspirin, unless use is approved by the health care provider.

✔ Reassures the patient and family that the results of therapy will be monitored by periodic laboratory and diagnostic tests and follow-up visits with the health care provider.

EVALUATION

- The therapeutic effect is achieved.

- Adverse reactions are identified, reported to the primary health care provider, and managed successfully.

- The patient verbalizes an understanding of treatment methods and the importance of continued follow-up care.

- The patient and family demonstrate understanding of the drug regimen.

- The patient complies with the prescribed drug regimen.

Critical Thinking Exercises

1. Ms. Burns has been diagnosed with TB. She is concerned because her primary health care provider has informed her that the treatment regimen consists of three drugs, isoniazid, rifampin, and pyrazinamide, taken for the next 2 months, followed by a 4-month treatment regimen with two of the drugs. Determine what rationales the nurse can give Ms. Burns for the use of multiple drugs and the need for long-term therapy.

2. While Mr. Johnson is taking isoniazid, explain what instructions the nurse should give him concerning side effects.

Review Questions

1. The nurse explains to the patient that to slow bacterial resistance to an antitubercular drug, the primary health care provider may prescribe _____.

   A. at least three antitubercular drugs

   B. an antibiotic to be given with the drug

   C. vitamin B_6

   D. that the drug be given only once a week

2. Which of the following drugs is the only antitubercular drug to be prescribed alone?

   A. rifampin

   B. pyrazinamide

   C. streptomycin

   D. isoniazid

3. The nurse monitors the patient taking isoniazid for toxicity. The most common symptom of toxicity is _____.

    A. peripheral edema

    B. circumoral edema

    C. peripheral neuropathy

    D. jaundice

4. Which of the following is a dose-related adverse reaction to ethambutol?

    A. peripheral neuropathy

    B. optic neuritis

    C. hyperglycemia

    D. fatal hepatitis

5. Which of the following antitubercular drugs is contraindicated in patients with gout?

    A. rifampin

    B. streptomycin

    C. isoniazid

    D. pyrazinamide

Medication Dosage Problems

1. A patient is prescribed isoniazid syrup 300 mg. The isoniazid is available as 50 mg/mL. The nurse should administer _____.

2. Oral rifampin 600 mg is prescribed. The drug is available in 150-mg tablets. The nurse should administer _____.

To check your answers, see Appendix G.

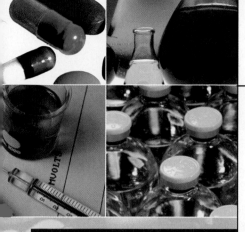

Chapter 13

Leprostatic Drugs

Key Terms

hemolysis
leprosy
Mycobacterium leprae

Learning Objectives

On completion of this chapter, the student will:

- Discuss the drugs used in the treatment of leprosy.
- Discuss the uses, general drug action, contraindications, precautions, interactions, and general adverse reactions associated with the administration of the leprostatic drugs.
- Discuss important preadministration and ongoing assessment

activities the nurse should perform on the patient taking a leprostatic drug.

- List nursing diagnoses particular to a patient taking a leprostatic drug.
- Discuss the ways to promote an optimal response to therapy, how to manage adverse reactions, and important points to keep in mind when educating patients about the use of the leprostatic drugs.

Leprosy is a chronic, communicable disease that is difficult to spread and has a long incubation period. Since 1985, the prevalence of leprosy has dropped by 90%. Less than 0.8 per 10,000 people suffered from the disease in 2004. Leprosy can be considered a public health success story because of drug therapy. Today leprosy remains a major public health problem in only nine countries around the world. About 100 new cases are diagnosed yearly in the United States (primarily the southern states, Hawaii, and U.S. possessions).

Leprosy, also referred to as *Hansen's disease*, is caused by the bacterium *Mycobacterium leprae*. Peripheral nerves are affected, causing sensory loss and muscle weakness. The traditional fear of leprosy relates to skin involvement, which may present with lesions confined to a few isolated areas or may be fairly widespread over the entire body. Dapsone, clofazimine (Lamprene), rifampin (Rifadin; see Chapter 12), and ethionamide (Trecator; see Chapter 12) are drugs currently used to treat leprosy. The inflammation associated with the disease is treated with drugs covered in Unit III, Drugs Used to Manage Pain. Treatment with the leprostatic drugs provides a good prospect for controlling the disease and preventing complications; to date, drug resistance has not occurred. The leprostatic drugs are listed in the Summary Drug Table: Leprostatic Drugs.

CLOFAZIMINE

Actions and Uses

Clofazimine (Clomid) has anti-inflammatory action and is bactericidal against *M. leprae*. The action of this drug is to bind with the DNA of the mycobacterium, causing cell death. Clofazimine is used for primary combined leprosy therapy and the inflammation of nodular disease (erythema nodosum leprosum).

SUMMARY DRUG TABLE   LEPROSTATIC DRUGS

GENERIC NAME	TRADE NAME	USES	ADVERSE REACTIONS	DOSAGE RANGES
clofazimine *kloe-fazz'-ih-meen*	Lamprene	Leprosy	Skin pigmentation (pink to brown), skin dryness, rash, abdominal/epigastric pain, nausea, vomiting, burning or itching of the eyes, dizziness, headache	100 mg/d orally
dapsone *dap'-sone*		Leprosy; dermatitis herpetiformis; *Pneumocystis carinii* pneumonia; pneumonia prophylaxis	Hemolytic anemia, headache, insomnia, phototoxicity, nausea, vomiting, anorexia, rash, fever, jaundice, toxic epidermal necrolysis	50–300 mg/d orally
rifampin *see Chapter 12*				
ethionamide *see Chapter 12*				

Adverse Reactions

Generalized adverse reactions include

- Dry skin and eyes
- Pink-red to brown pigmentation of the skin, body fluids, and conjunctiva
- Abdominal/epigastric pain
- Diarrhea, nausea, vomiting
- Dizziness and headache

Contraindications, Precautions, and Interactions

Clofazimine is used cautiously in patients with gastrointestinal disorders and diarrhea as well as during pregnancy and lactation (pregnancy category C). Infants born while the mother receives therapy can be discolored, as can those breast-feeding from a treated mother. No significant drug–drug interactions are associated with the use of clofazimine.

DAPSONE

Actions and Uses

Dapsone is used to treat leprosy because it is bactericidal and bacteriostatic against *M. leprae*. Dapsone may also be used for treating dermatitis herpetiformis, a chronic, inflammatory skin disease. This drug has also been effective in prophylactic treatment of *Pneumocystis carinii* pneumonia (PCP).

Adverse Reactions

Generalized Reactions

- Nausea, vomiting, anorexia
- Skin rash
- Headache

More Severe Reactions

- **Hemolysis** (destruction of red blood cells) and jaundice
- Toxic epidermal necrolysis (TEN)

Contraindications, Precautions, and Interactions

Dapsone is used with caution during pregnancy (category C) and in patients with anemia, severe cardiopulmonary disease, and hepatic dysfunction. The drug is contraindicated during lactation. Substantial amounts of dapsone are excreted in breast milk and can cause hemolytic reactions in neonates. When dapsone is administered with pyrimethamine (an antimalarial drug), the interaction involves a greater risk for hemolysis.

NURSING PROCESS

The Patient Receiving a Leprostatic Drug

ASSESSMENT

PREADMINISTRATION ASSESSMENT

It is important to perform a complete physical examination and history before the initiation of therapy. The nurse examines the involved areas and describes them in detail on the patient's record to provide a database, or baseline, for comparison during therapy.

ONGOING ASSESSMENT

These drugs are often given on an outpatient basis. Each time the patient is seen in the clinic or primary health care provider's office, the nurse performs a general physical examination, with particular attention given to the affected areas.

NURSING DIAGNOSES

A drug-specific nursing diagnosis for the patient receiving a leprostatic drug is Disturbed Body Image related to skin and tissue deformities or discoloration. More general nursing diagnoses applicable to these drugs are discussed in depth in Chapter 4.

PLANNING

The expected outcomes for the patient may include an optimal response to drug therapy, meeting patient needs related to the management of adverse drug reactions, and an understanding of and compliance with the prescribed treatment regimen.

IMPLEMENTATION

PROMOTING AN OPTIMAL RESPONSE TO THERAPY

It is important to give the leprostatic drugs orally and with food to minimize gastric upset. The primary health care provider may order antitubercular drugs, such as rifampin or ethionamide, concurrently during initial therapy to minimize bacterial resistance to the leprostatic drugs.

MONITORING AND MANAGING PATIENT NEEDS

DISTURBED BODY IMAGE The word *leprosy* has struck fear into people for ages. Older people may still talk of leprosy, or a popular movie, such as *Motorcycle Diaries*, may show leper colonies where patients were secluded from the rest of the population because of fear of contagion (catching or spreading the deforming disease). Treatment to prevent deformity with a leprostatic drug is successful, yet may require many years. These patients are faced with long-term medical drug therapy and possibly severe disfigurement.

In addition to the disease, patients can experience changes in skin pigmentation from treatment. This leads to patients feeling self-conscious about their appearance. Some patients may become depressed or despondent. The drug clofazimine (Lamprene) has been associated with patients committing suicide while being treated, but this is extremely rare. The nurse must spend time with these patients, allowing them to verbalize their anxieties, anger, and fears. It is also important for the nurse to acknowledge these feelings as being both valid and important to the patient. Referring patients to a support group or other patients to talk may be helpful.

EDUCATING THE PATIENT AND FAMILY

The nurse is alert to patient statements regarding compliance with the long-term treatment regimen. It is important to note factors, such as depression or indifference, that suggest treatment noncompliance and to take a positive approach to patient and family teaching. The nurse informs the patient that changes in skin pigmentation may occur, ranging from red to brownish-black. Skin discoloration may take months to years to reverse after drug therapy is discontinued. The nurse should educate the patient and family regarding supportive services to deal with this body change.

To ensure compliance with the treatment regimen, the nurse explains the dosage schedule, possible adverse effects, and the importance of scheduled follow-up visits. In particular, the nurse emphasizes the importance of adhering to the prescribed dosage schedule.

EVALUATION

- The therapeutic drug effect is achieved.
- The patient has resources to deal with anticipated body image changes

- The patient verbalizes an understanding of treatment modalities and the importance of continued follow-up care.

- The patient and family demonstrate understanding of the drug regimen.

- The patient complies with the prescribed drug regimen.

Critical Thinking Exercises

1. Mr. Winters is very anxious about his newly diagnosed leprosy and his treatment regimen with dapsone. Discuss what you could do to decrease his anxiety. Determine what information you would include when educating Mr. Winters about the treatment regimen.

2. Ms. York, a young single woman, has been prescribed clofazimine daily to manage her leprosy. Discuss how you would address her fears of being out in public and dating should she experience pigment changes to her skin.

Review Questions

1. Before administration of the initial dose of a leprostatic drug, it is most important for the nurse to assess _____.

   A. range of motion

   B. mental ability

   C. vital signs

   D. peripheral sensation

2. Which of the following adverse reactions would the nurse expect with the administration of clofazimine?

   A. Hypotension

   B. Blurred vision

   C. Pigmentation of the skin

   D. Jaundice

3. Which of the following hematologic changes may result from the administration of dapsone?

   A. Hemolysis

   B. Leukopenia

   C. Decreased platelets

   D. Increase in the hematocrit

4. When educating the patient about taking a leprostatic drug, the nurse would include which of the following information?

   A. This drug regimen will require that you take the drug faithfully for at least 3 months.

   B. Take the drug with food to minimize gastric upset.

   C. Skin lesions should clear within 3 days.

   D. The drug should be taken on an empty stomach at bedtime to minimize gastric upset.

Medication Dosage Problems

1. The patient is prescribed 150 mg of dapsone. On hand are 25-mg tablets. The nurse administers _____.

2. A patient with leprosy is prescribed clofazimine 100 mg/d orally. The drug is available in 50-mg tablets. The nurse administers _____.

To check your answers, see Appendix G.

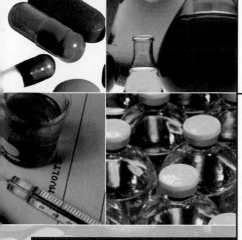

Antiviral Drugs

Learning Objectives

On completion of this chapter, the student will:

- Discuss the uses, general drug actions, adverse reactions, contraindications, precautions, and interactions of antiviral drugs.
- Discuss important preadministration and ongoing assessment activities the nurse should perform on the patient receiving an antiviral/antiretroviral drug.

- List nursing diagnoses particular to a patient taking an antiviral drug.
- List possible goals for a patient taking an antiviral/antiretroviral drug.
- Discuss ways to promote an optimal response to therapy and manage adverse reactions, and special considerations to keep in mind when educating the patient and the family about the antiviral/antiretroviral drugs.

Compared with a fungus or bacterium, a virus is a very tiny, infectious organism. A virus enters the body through various routes. It can be swallowed, inhaled, injected with a contaminated needle, or transmitted through the bite of an insect. To reproduce, the virus needs the cellular material of another living cell (the host cell). The virus attaches to a cell, enters it, and releases its DNA or RNA inside the cell. The viral material takes control of the cell and forces it to replicate the virus. The cell releases new viruses, which go on to infect other cells. The infected cell usually dies because the virus keeps it from performing its normal functions (Fig. 14-1).

More than 200 viruses have been identified as capable of producing disease. Common viral infections are those of the nose, throat, and respiratory system. An example is the common cold or influenza. A wart comes from a common virus that infects the skin. Other common viral infections are caused by the herpes viruses. Eight different herpes viruses infect people. Systemic viral infections occur when a virus attacks the nervous system (West Nile), liver (hepatitis C), or white blood cells (immunodeficiency diseases). The drugs used to treat viral infection can be split into two categories: antiviral and antiretroviral agents. For a more complete listing, see the Summary Drug Table: Antiviral Drugs.

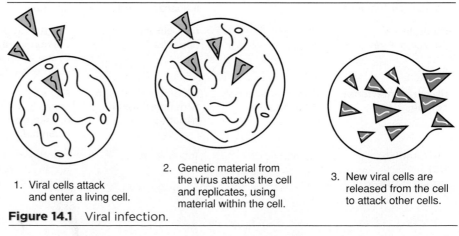

1. Viral cells attack and enter a living cell.

2. Genetic material from the virus attacks the cell and replicates, using material within the cell.

3. New viral cells are released from the cell to attack other cells.

Figure 14.1 Viral infection.

SUMMARY DRUG TABLE ANTIVIRAL DRUGS

GENERIC NAME	TRADE NAME	USES	ADVERSE REACTIONS	DOSAGE RANGES
Antivirals				
acyclovir *ay-sye'-kloe-ver*	Zovirax	HSV herpes zoster, varicella zoster	Nausea, vomiting, diarhea, fever, headache, dizziness, confusion, rashes, myalgia	Oral: 200–800 mg q4h for 5 doses per day, treat for 5–10 d; IV: 5–10 mg/kg q8h; Topical: apply to lesions q3h
adefovir dipivoxil *ah-def'-oh-veer*	Hepsera	Chronic hepatitis B	Asthenia, headache, abdominal pain	10 mg/d orally
amantadine *a-man'-ta-deen*	Symmetrel	Prevention and treatment of influenza A; Parkinson's disease	Nausea, diarrhea, dizziness, hypotension, insomnia	200 mg/d orally or 100 mg daily for patient over age 65; begin before flu exposure and continue 10 d postexposure
cidofovir *si-doh'-foh-vir*	Vistide	Retinitis in patients with AIDS	Headache, nausea, vomiting, diarrhea, anorexia, dyspnea, alopecia, rash, neutropenia, fever, chills	5 mg/kg IV once a week for 2 wk, then once every 2 wk for maintenance
entecavir *en-te'-ka-veer*	Baraclude	Chronic hepatitis B	Dizziness, fatigue, headache	0.5–1 mg/d orally
famciclovir *fam-sye'-kloe-vir*	Famvir	Acute herpes zoster, HSV-2	Fatigue, fever, nausea, vomiting, diarrhea, sinusitis, constipation, headache	Herpes zoster: 500 mg orally q8h for 7 d; HSV-2: 125 mg orally BID for 5d
foscarnet *foss-kar'-net*	*Foscavir*	CMV retinitis; acyclovir-resistant HSV-1 and 2	Headache, seizures, nausea, vomiting, diarrhea, anemia, abnormal renal function test results	CMV retinitis: 90–120 mg/kg/d IV; HSV: 40 mg/kg IV q8–12h
ganciclovir *gan-sye'-kloe-vir*	Cytovene	CMV prevention in transplant recipients	Anorexia, vomiting, diarrhea, fever, sweats, anemia, leukopenia	5 mg/kg IV q12h for 14–21 d, then daily
oseltamivir *oh-sell-tam'-ih-veer*	Tamiflu	Treatment of influenza A and B	Nausea, vomiting, diarrhea	75 mg orally BID for 5d
ribavirin *rye-ba-vye'-rin*	Virazole	RSV, chronic hepatitis C	Worsening of pulmonary status, bacterial pneumonia, hypotension	Administered by aerosol with special aerosol generator
ribavirin/interferon combination	Copegus, Rebetol, Ribaspheres	In combination with with interferon for hepatitis C	Fatigue, headache, myalgia, anorexia, nausea, vomiting, insomnia, nervousness	800–1200 mg orally BID
rimantadine HCl *ri-man'-ta-deen*	Flumadine	Influenza A	Lightheadedness, dizziness, insomnia, nausea, anorexia	100 mg/d orally BID

GENERIC NAME	TRADE NAME	USES	ADVERSE REACTIONS	DOSAGE RANGES
valacyclovir *val-ah-sye'-kloe-ver*	Valtrex	Genital herpes; herpes zoster	Nausea, headache	Genital herpes initial: 1 g BID for 10 d Recurrent infection: 500 mg orally BID for 5 d Herpes zoster: 1 g orally TID for 7d
valganciclovir *val-gan-si'-klo-veer*	Valcyte	CMV retinitis, CMV prevention in transplant recipients	Headache, insomnia, diarrhea, nausea, vomiting, pancytopenia, fever	900 mg orally BID; Transplant recipient start 10 d before transplantation and continue 100 d after transplantation
zanamivir *zan-am'-ah-ver*	Relenza	Influenza A, B	Nausea, headache, rhinitis	5 mg inhalation q12h
Topical Antivirals				
docosanol *doe-koe-nah'-zole*	Abreva	HSV-1 and 2	Headache, skin irritation	Apply to lesions 5 times daily
imiquimod *im-ee'-kwee-mod*	Aldara	External genitalia and perianal warts	Local skin irritation, itching, excoriation, flaking	Apply externally 3 times weekly
penciclovir *pen-sye'-kloe-ver*	Denavir	HSV-1 and 2	Headache, taste perversion	Apply q2h for 4 d during waking hours
vidarabine *vy-darc'-ah-been*	Ara-A, Vira-A	Keratitis, keratoconjunctivitis caused by HSV-1 and 2	Burning, itching, irritation, tearing, sensitivity to light	Ophthalmic ointment: 0.5 inch into lower conjunctival sac 2–5 times daily
Antiretrovirals				
abacavir sulfate *ab-ah-kav'-ear*	Ziagen	HIV infection	Nausea, vomiting, diarrhea, anorexia, liver dysfunction	300 mg orally BID
amprenavir *am-prenn'-ah-veer*	Agenerase	HIV infection	Peripheral and circumoral paresthesias, nausea, vomiting, diarrhea, abdominal pain, rash, pruritus	1200 mg orally BID
atazanavir sulfate *ah-taz'-ah-nah-veer*	Reyataz	HIV infection	Nausea, rash	300-400 mg/d
delavirdine *dell-ah-vur'-den*	Rescriptor	HIV infection	Headache, nausea, diarrhea	400 mg orally TID
ⓡ didanosine (ddI) *dye-dan'-oh-sin*	Videx	HIV infection	Headache, nausea, rash, vomiting, peripheral neuropathy, abdominal pain, diarrhea	Oral: 400 mg/d or 200 mg BID; for patients weighing less than 60 kg, 250 mg/d or 125 mg BID
efavirenz *ef-ah-vi'-renz*	Sustiva	HIV infection	Rash, pruritus, dizziness, insomnia, fatigue, nausea, vomiting	600 mg/d orally
emtricitabine *em-tra-cye'-tah-ben*	Emtriva	HIV infection	Headache, nausea, vomiting, diarrhea, rash	200 mg/d orally

Antiviral Drugs

⬤ SUMMARY DRUG TABLE   *(continued)*

GENERIC NAME	TRADE NAME	USES	ADVERSE REACTIONS	DOSAGE RANGES
enfuvirtide *en-foo-veer'-tide*	Fuzeon	HIV infection	Injection site discomfort, induration, erythema	90 mg subcutaneous injection BID
fosamprenavir *foss-am-pren'-ah-veer*	Lexiva	HIV infection	Headache, nausea, vomiting, diarrhea, rash	1400 mg/d orally
indinavir *in-din'-ah-veer*	Crixivan	HIV infection	Headache, nausea, vomiting, diarrhea, kidney/bladder stones	800 mg orally q8h
lamivudine (3TC) *lam-ah-vew'-deen*	Epivir, Epivir-HB	HIV infection, chronic hepatitis B infection	Headache, nausea, diarrhea, nasal congestion, cough, fatigue	HIV: 150 mg orally BID HBV: 100 mg/d orally daily
nelfinavir *nell-fin'-a-veer*	Viracept	HIV infection	Diarrhea	750 mg orally TID or 1250 mg orally BID
nevirapine *neh-veer'-ah-peen*	Viramune	HIV infection	Rash, fever, headache, nausea, stomatitis, liver dysfunction	200 mg orally BID
ritonavir *ri-ton'-ah-veer*	Norvir	HIV infection	Peripheral and circumoral paresthesias, nausea, vomiting, diarrhea, anorexia	600 mg orally BID
saquinavir, saquinavir mesylate *sa-kwen'-a-veer*	Fortovase, Invirase	HIV infection	Headache, nausea, diarrhea, heartburn, flatulence	Fortovase: Six 200-mg capsules orally TID Invirase: Three 200-mg capsules orally TID
stavudine *stay-vew'-den*	Zerit	HIV infection	Headache, nausea, diarrhea, fever, rash, peripheral neuropathy	40 mg orally q12h
tenofovir disoproxil fumarate *te-no'-fo-veer*	Viread	HIV infection	Nausea, vomiting, diarrhea, flatulence	300 mg/d orally
tipranavir *tih-pran'-ah-veer*	Aptivus	HIV infection	Nausea, diarrhea	500 mg orally BID
zalcitabine *zal-cye'-tay-been*	Hivid	HIV infection	Peripheral neuropathy, abnormal liver function	0.75 mg orally q8h
zidovudine (AZT) *zid-o-vew'-den*	Retrovir	HIV infection	Asthenia, malaise, weakness, headache, anorexia, diarrhea, nausea, abdominal pain, dizziness, insomnia, anemia, agranulocytosis	600 mg/d orally in divided doses; 1 mg/kg IV q4h
Antiretroviral Combinations				
abacavir/lamivudine	Epzicom	See individual drugs above	See individual drugs above	One tablet daily (600 mg/300 mg dose)
abacavir/lamivudine/ zidovudine	Trizivir	See individual drugs above	See individual drugs above	One tablet orally twice daily (300 mg/150 mg/300 mg dose)
emtricitabine/ tenofovir disoproxil fumarate	Truvada	See individual drugs above	See individual drugs above	One tablet orally BID (200 mg/300 mg dose)

GENERIC NAME	TRADE NAME	USES	ADVERSE REACTIONS	DOSAGE RANGES
lamivudine/ zidovudine	Combivir	See individual drugs above	See individual durgs above	One tablet orally BID (150 mg/300 mg dose)
lopinavir/ritonavir *low-pin'-ah-veer/ ri-ton'-ah-veer*	Kaletra	See individual drugs above	See individual drugs above	One tablet orally BID (400 mg/100 mg dose)

Ⓡ This drug should be administered at least 1 hour before or 2 hours after a meal.

ANTIVIRALS

Actions

Drugs that combat viral infections are called *antiviral drugs*. Antiviral drugs work by interfering with the virus's ability to reproduce in a cell. Antiviral medications are limited in their ability to treat viral infections because viruses are tiny and replicate inside cells, changing how the cell works depending on the type of cell they invade. In comparison, a bacterial organism is relatively large and commonly reproduces outside of cells (e.g., in the bloodstream). This makes antiviral drugs more difficult to develop. Antiviral drugs can be toxic to human cells, and viruses can develop resistance to antiviral drugs. Antibiotics are not effective against viral infections, but if a person has a bacterial infection in addition to a viral infection, an antibiotic is often necessary.

Herbal Alert

Lemon balm is a perennial herb with heart-shaped leaves that has been used for hundreds of years. Its scientific name is *Melissa officinalis*. Traditionally the herb has been used for Graves' disease, as a sedative, an antispasmodic, and an antiviral agent. When used topically, lemon balm has antiviral activity against herpes simplex virus (HSV). No adverse reactions have been reported when lemon balm is used topically.

Uses

Labeled Uses

Although infections caused by viruses are common, antiviral drugs have limited use because they are effective against only a small number of specific viral infections (Display 14-1). Antiviral drugs are used in the treatment or prevention of infections caused by:

- Cytomegalovirus (CMV) in transplant recipients
- Herpes simplex virus (HSV) 1 and 2 (genital) and herpes zoster
- Human immunodeficiency virus (HIV)
- Influenza A and B (respiratory tract illness)
- Respiratory syncytial virus (RSV; severe lower respiratory tract infection primarily affecting children)
- Hepatitis B and C

Unlabeled Uses

Because there are a limited number of antiviral drugs and more than 200 viral diseases, the primary health care provider may decide to prescribe an antiviral drug for an unlabeled use even though its effectiveness for that use is not documented. Approval by the U.S. Food and Drug Administration (FDA) is necessary for a drug to be prescribed. On occasion, the use of a drug for a specific disorder or condition may be under investigation, or it may be approved for use in another country. In this instance, the drug may be prescribed by the primary health care provider for the condition under investigation. The use of the drug for a specific disorder or condition that is not officially approved by the FDA is called an **unlabeled use**. Examples of unlabeled uses of the antiviral drugs include treatment of CMV and HSV infections after transplantation procedures and varicella pneumonia; the treatment of CMV retinitis in immunocompromised patients; and the use of ribavirin (in aerosol form) for influenza A and B, acute and chronic hepatitis, herpes genitalis, and measles (in oral form).

Adverse Reactions

Gastrointestinal Reactions

- Nausea, vomiting
- Diarrhea

Display 14.1 Description of Viral Infections

Cytomegalovirus (CMV)

CMV, a virus of the herpes family, is a common viral infection. Healthy individuals may become infected yet have no symptoms. However, immunocompromised patients (such as those with HIV or cancer) may have the infection. Symptoms include malaise, fever, pneumonia, and superinfection. Infants may acquire the virus from the mother while in the uterus, resulting in learning disabilities and mental retardation. CMV can infect the eye, causing retinitis. Symptoms of CMV retinitis are blurred vision and decreased visual acuity. Visual impairment is irreversible and can lead to blindness if untreated.

Herpes simplex virus (HSV)

HSV is divided into HSV-1, which causes oral, ocular, or facial infections, and HSV-2, which causes genital infection. However, either type can cause disease at either body site. HSV-1 causes painful vesicular lesions in the oral mucosa, face, or around the eyes. HSV-2 or genital herpes is usually transmitted by sexual contact and causes painful vesicular lesions on the mucous membranes of the genitalia. Vaginal lesions may appear as mucous patches with grayish ulcerations. The patient may appear irritable, lethargic, and jaundiced, and may have difficulty breathing or experience seizures. The lesions usually heal within 2 weeks. Immunosuppressed patients may develop a severe systemic disease.

Herpes zoster

Herpes zoster (shingles) is caused by the varicella (chickenpox) virus. It is highly contagious. The virus causes chickenpox in the child and is easily spread via the respiratory system. Recovery from childhood chickenpox results in the infection lying dormant in the nerve cells. The virus may become reactivated later in life as the older adult's immune system weakens or the individual becomes ill with other disorders. The lesions of herpes zoster appear as pustules along a sensory nerve route. Pain often continues for several months after the lesions have healed.

Human immunodeficiency virus (HIV)

HIV or AIDS is a type of viral infection transmitted through an infected person's bodily secretions, such as blood or semen. HIV destroys the immune system, causing the body to develop opportunistic infections such as Kaposi's sarcoma, *Pneumocystis carinii* pneumonia, or tuberculosis. Symptoms include chills and fever, night sweats, dry productive cough, dyspnea, lethargy, malaise, fatigue, weight loss, and diarrhea.

Influenza

Influenza, commonly called the "flu," is an acute respiratory illness caused by influenza viruses A and B. Symptoms include fever, cough, sore throat, runny or stuffy nose, headache, muscle aches, and extreme fatigue. Most people recover within 1 to 2 weeks. Influenza may cause severe complications such as pneumonia in children, the elderly, and other vulnerable groups. The viruses causing influenza continually change over time, which enables them to evade the immune system of the host. These rapid changes in the most commonly circulating types of influenza virus necessitate annual changes in the composition of the "flu" vaccine.

Respiratory syncytial virus (RSV)

RSV infection is highly contagious and affects mostly children, causing bronchiolitis and pneumonia. Infants younger than 6 months are the most severely affected. In adults, RSV causes colds and bronchitis, with fever, cough, and nasal congestion. When RSV affects immunocompromised patients, the consequences can be severe and sometimes fatal.

Other Reactions

- Headache
- Rash
- Fever
- Insomnia

Contraindications

The nurse should not administer antivirals if the patient has a history of allergies to the drug or other antivirals. Cidofovir (Vistide) should not be given to patients who have renal impairment or in combination with medications that are nephrotoxic, such as aminoglycosides. Ribavirin should not be used in patients with unstable cardiac disease. These drugs should be used during pregnancy (pregnancy categories B and C) and lactation only when the benefit outweighs the risk to the fetus or child (ribavirin is in pregnancy category X).

Precautions

Antivirals should be used cautiously in patients with renal impairment, low blood cell counts, history of epilepsy (rimantadine), and history of respiratory disease (zanamivir).

Interactions

The following interactions may occur when an antiviral is administered with another agent:

Interacting Drug	Common Use	Effect of Interaction
probenecid	Gout treatment	Increased serum levels of the antivirals
cimetidine	Gastric upset, heartburn	Increased serum level of the antiviral valacyclovir
ibuprofen	Pain relief	Increased serum level of the antiviral adefovir
imipenem-cilastatin	Anti-infective agent	With ganciclovir only, increased risk of seizures
anticholinergic agents	Management of bladder spasms	With amantadine only, increased adverse reactions of anticholinergic agent
theophylline	Management of respiratory problems	With acyclovir only, increased serum level of theophylline

ANTIRETROVIRALS

Actions

The human immunodeficiency virus (HIV) that causes acquired immunodeficiency syndrome (AIDS) is a **retrovirus**. Retroviruses attack the host cell just like a virus; the difference is that RNA is the primary component of the virus instead of DNA. Retroviruses also contain an enzyme called *reverse transcriptase* that is used to turn the RNA of the virus into DNA, helping to reproduce more of the virus. To control the disease effectively, a number of drugs are used that work at different portions of the life cycle of the virus. This multidrug therapy is called **highly active antiretroviral therapy (HAART)**. The following types of drugs are used in HAART (for more information see the Summary Drug Table: Antiviral Drugs):

- Protease inhibitors, which block the protease enzyme so the new viral particles cannot mature

- Reverse transcriptase inhibitors, which block the reverse transcriptase enzyme so the HIV material can not change into DNA in the new cell
- Attachment and fusion inhibitors, which prevent the attachment or fusion of HIV to a cell

Uses

Antiretroviral drugs are used in the treatment of HIV infection and AIDS.

Adverse Reactions

Gastrointestinal Reactions

- Nausea, vomiting
- Diarrhea
- Altered taste

Other Reactions

- Headache, fever, and chills
- Rash
- Numbness and tingling in the **circumoral** area (around the mouth) or peripherally, or both

Contraindications

The nurse should not administer antiretrovirals if the patient has a history of allergies to the drug or other antiretrovirals. Women who are lactating should not use antiretroviral drugs. Antiretrovirals should not be prescribed to the patient who is using cisapride, pimozide, triazolam, midazolam, or an ergot derivative. Ritonavir is contraindicated if the patient is taking bupropion (Wellbutrin), zolpidem (Ambien), or an antiarrhythmic drug.

Precautions

Antiretrovirals should be used cautiously in patients with diabetes mellitus, impaired hepatic function, pregnancy (pregnancy categories B and C), or hemophilia. Caution should be used for the patient taking indinavir who has a history of kidney or bladder stone formation. If a patient has a sulfonamide allergy, the drugs fosamprenavir and amprenavir should be used cautiously.

Interactions

The following interactions may occur when an antiretroviral is administered with another agent:

Interacting Drug	Common Use	Effect of Interaction
antifungals	Eliminate or manage fungal infections	Increased serum level of the antiretroviral
clarithromycin	Treat bacterial infection	Increased serum level of both drugs
sildenafil	Treat erectile dysfunction	Increased adverse reactions of sildenafil
opioid analgesics	Pain relief	Risk of toxicity with ritonavir
anticoagulant, anticonvulsant, antiparasitic agents	Prevent blood clots, seizures, parasitic infections, respectively	Decreased effectiveness when taking ritonavir
interleukins	Prevent severely low platelet counts usually related to chemotherapy	Risk of antiretroviral toxicity
fentanyl	Analgesia, used typically with procedures requiring anesthesia	Increased serum level of fentanyl
oral contraceptives	Birth control	Decreased effectiveness of the birth control agent

NURSING PROCESS

The Patient Receiving an Antiviral/Antiretroviral Drug

ASSESSMENT

PREADMINISTRATION ASSESSMENT

Preadministration assessment of the patient receiving an antiviral drug depends on the patient's symptoms or diagnosis. These patients may have a serious infection that weakens their natural defenses against disease. Before administering the antiviral drug, the nurse determines the patient's general state of health and resistance to infection. The nurse then records the patient's symptoms and complaints. In addition, the nurse takes and records the patient's vital signs. Additional assessments may be necessary in certain types of viral infections or in patients who are acutely ill. For example, before treatment of patients with HSV-1 or HSV-2 infection, the nurse inspects the areas of the body affected with the lesions (e.g., the mouth, face, eyes, or genitalia) as a baseline for comparison during therapy.

ONGOING ASSESSMENT

The ongoing assessment depends on the reason for giving the antiviral drug. It is important to make a daily assessment for improvement of the signs and symptoms identified in the initial assessment. The nurse monitors for and reports any adverse reactions from the antiviral drug. In addition, the nurse inspects the intravenous (IV) infusion site several times a day for redness, inflammation, or pain and reports any signs of phlebitis.

NURSING DIAGNOSES

Drug-specific nursing diagnoses are highlighted in the Nursing Diagnoses Checklist. Other, more general nursing diagnoses applicable to the antiviral drugs are discussed in Chapter 4.

Nursing Diagnoses Checklist

✓ **Risk for Imbalanced Nutrition: Less Than Body Requirements** related to adverse reaction of antiviral drugs

✓ **Risk for Impaired Skin Integrity** related to initial infection, adverse drug reactions, administration of the antiviral drug

✓ **Risk for Injury** related to patient's mental status, peripheral neuropathy, and generalized weakness

✓ **Body Image Disturbance** related to body fat redistribution

✓ **Acute Pain** related to kidney or bladder stones or inflammation caused by antiviral drugs

---

PLANNING

The expected outcomes for the patient depend on the reason for administration of the antiviral drug, but may include an optimal response to therapy, meeting of patient needs related to the management of adverse reactions, and an understanding of and compliance with the prescribed treatment regimen.

IMPLEMENTATION

PROMOTING AN OPTIMAL RESPONSE TO THERAPY

Because these drugs may be used in the treatment of certain types of severe and sometimes life-threatening viral infections, the patient may be concerned about the diagnosis and prognosis. The nurse should allow the patient and family members time to talk and ask questions about treatment methods, especially when the drug is given IV. It is important to prepare the antiviral drugs according to the manufacturer's directions. The administration rate is ordered by the primary health care provider.

AMANTADINE The nurse administers this drug for the prevention or treatment of respiratory tract illness caused by influenza A virus. Some patients are prescribed this drug to manage extrapyramidal effects caused by drugs used to treat parkinsonism. The nurse should observe the patient for adverse effects similar to those associated with anticholinergic drugs (see Chapter 30).

RIBAVIRIN The nurse gives ribavirin by inhalation using a small particle aerosol generator (SPAG-2 aerosol generator). It is important to discard and replace the solution every 24 hours. This drug can worsen respiratory status. Sudden deterioration of respiratory status can occur in infants receiving ribavirin, and it is important to monitor respiratory function closely throughout therapy. The nurse should immediately report any worsening of respiratory function to the primary health care provider. Female caregivers should know that the drug is a pregnancy category X drug and women of childbearing age should take care not to inhale the drug. In patients requiring mechanical ventilation, treatment should be provided only by health care providers familiar with the specific ventilator.

MONITORING AND MANAGING PATIENT NEEDS

RISK FOR IMBALANCED NUTRITION: LESS THAN BODY REQUIREMENTS The metabolic needs of patients with HIV infection are demanding. Because the antiviral drugs may cause anorexia, nausea, or vomiting, providing adequate nutrition becomes a real challenge. The gastrointestinal (GI) effects range from mild to severe. Many of the drugs can be given without regard to food. One exception is didanosine (Videx). This drug is provided in a buffered or enteric-coated form. The nurse mixes the buffered powder with 4 oz of water (not juice), stirs until dissolved, and gives it to the patient to drink immediately. The nurse avoids generating dust when preparing the medication.

The patient may be able to tolerate small, frequent meals with soft, nonirritating foods if nausea is mild. Frequent sips of carbonated beverages or hot tea may be helpful for others. It is important to keep the atmosphere clean and free of odors. The nurse provides good oral care before and after meals. Sometimes daily-dose drugs can be given at bedtime to reduce the nausea. If nausea is severe or the patient is vomiting, the nurse notifies the primary health care provider.

RISK FOR IMPAIRED SKIN INTEGRITY The nurse monitors any skin lesions carefully for worsening or improvement. Should the lesions not improve, the nurse informs the primary health care provider. Accurate observation and documentation are essential. If an antiviral drug is administered topically, the nurse uses gloves when applying to avoid spreading the infection. These drugs may also cause a rash as an adverse reaction. The nurse notes and reports any rash to the primary health care provider.

When administering the drug by the IV route, the nurse must closely observe the injection site for signs of phlebitis. The nurse takes care to prevent trauma because even slight trauma can result in bruising if the platelet count is low. If injections are given, pressure is applied at the injection site to prevent bleeding. Occasionally, headache or a slight fever may occur in patients taking antiviral drugs. An analgesic may be prescribed to manage these effects. Depending on the patient's symptoms, the nurse monitors vital signs every 4 hours or as ordered by the primary health care provider.

RISK FOR INJURY Some patients with a viral infection are acutely ill. Others may experience fatigue, lethargy, dizziness, or weakness as an adverse reaction to the antiviral/antiretroviral agent. The nurse monitors these patients carefully. Call lights are placed in a convenient place for the patient and are answered promptly by the nurse. If fatigue, dizziness, confusion, or weakness is present, the patient may require assistance with ambulation or activities of daily living. The nurse plans activities so as to provide adequate rest periods. Other drugs can damage the peripheral nerves, especially when used with other neurotoxic agents. The nurse watches for signs of peripheral neuropathy (numbness, tingling, or pain in the feet or hands). It is important to report these signs immediately to the primary health care provider.

Antiviral Drugs

DISTURBED BODY IMAGE Patients taking the protease inhibitors (saquinavir, ritonavir, indinavir, nelfinavir, fos-amprenavir, amprenavir, and atazanavir) have experienced redistribution of body fat. Movement is to the center of the body, so patients appear to have thinner arms and legs with a rounder abdomen or enlarged breasts. Sometimes body fat relocates to the area behind the neck (sometimes called a *buffalo hump*). The nurse should spend time with these patients, encouraging them to verbalize their feelings regarding this change in appearance. It is also important for the nurse to acknowledge these feelings as being both valid and important to the patient.

ACUTE PAIN The drug indinavir (Crixivan) has been known to cause kidney or bladder stones in patients. Antiretroviral drugs have been known to cause acute pancreatitis. Patients should be assessed for pain when the nurse performs a routine vital signs check. Any pain should be explored for location and intensity. When assessing the patient for GI problems such as nausea, vomiting, abdominal pain, and jaundice, the nurse should be alert because these are symptoms of pancreatitis, and particular care should be taken in assessment of pain. Acute, sudden-onset pain should be reported to the primary health care provider for both treatment and further assessment for more involved disease.

> ### Nursing Alert
>
> Patients receiving antiretroviral drugs for HIV infection may continue to contract opportunistic infections and other complications of HIV disease. The nurse monitors all patients closely for signs of infection such as fever (even low-grade fever), malaise, sore throat, or lethargy. All caregivers are reminded to use good hand-washing technique.

> ### Herbal Alert
>
> Individuals have tried *St. John's wort* for both the antidepressive and antiviral effects of the supplement. Researchers have found that in patients with HIV infection who receive prescribed protease inhibitors, the effectiveness of drug therapy is reduced if the patient also takes St. John's wort. Patients need to be instructed to disclose the use of all over-the-counter medications and supplements to their primary health care provider to prevent potentially harmful interactions.

EDUCATING THE PATIENT AND FAMILY

When an antiviral drug is given orally, the nurse explains the dosage regimen to the patient and family and instructs the patient to take the drug exactly as directed for the full course of therapy. If a dose is missed, the patient should take it as soon as remembered but should not double the dose at the next dosage time. Any adverse reactions should be reported to the primary health care provider or the nurse. The patient must understand that these drugs do not cure viral infections, but they can decrease symptoms and increase feelings of well-being.

The nurse instructs patients to report any symptoms of infection, such as an elevated temperature (even a slight elevation), sore throat, difficulty breathing, weakness, or lethargy. Again, the nurse reviews possible signs of pancreatitis (nausea, vomiting, abdominal pain, jaundice) and peripheral neuropathy (tingling, burning, numbness, or pain in the hands or feet). Any indication of pancreatitis or peripheral neuropathy must be reported at once.

The nurse includes the following information in the teaching plan for antiviral drugs:

- Antiviral drugs are not a cure for viral infections, but they will shorten the course of disease outbreaks and promote healing of the lesions. The drugs will not prevent the spread of the disease to others. Topical drugs should not be applied more frequently than prescribed but should be applied with a finger cot or gloves. All lesions should be covered. There should be no sexual contact while lesions are present. Notify the primary health care provider if burning, stinging, itching, or rash worsens or becomes pronounced.

- Some drugs cause photosensitivity, so precautions should be taken when going outdoors, such as wearing sunscreen, head coverings, and protective clothing. Patients should also refrain from using tanning beds.

- Some patients have experienced an acute exacerbation of the disease when medications used to treat hepatitis B are stopped. Hepatic function should be closely monitored in these patients.

- Those taking antiretrovirals should be cautioned that there is an increased risk of adverse reactions (hypotension, visual disturbances, prolonged penile erection) when the drug sildenafil (Viagra) is used. Symptoms should be reported promptly to the primary health care provider.

- Some drugs affect mental status. Activities requiring mental alertness, such as driving a car, should be delayed until the effect of the drug is apparent because vision and coordination can be affected. Patients should rise slowly from a prone to a sitting position to decrease the possibility of lightheadedness caused by orthostatic hypotension. Changes, such as nervousness, tremors, slurred speech, or depression, should be reported.

- Some patients are on an alternate dosage schedule. In this case, it is important to mark the calendar to designate the days the drug is to be taken.

- Patients taking saquinavir need to know that the two brand name drugs (Invirase and Fortovase) are not interchangeable.

- Zanamivir (Relenza) is taken every 12 hours for 5 days using a "Diskhaler" delivery system. If a bronchodilator is also prescribed for use at the same time, the bronchodilator is used before the zanamivir. The drug may cause dizziness. The patient should use caution when driving an automobile or operating dangerous machinery. Treatment with this drug does not decrease the risk of transmission of influenza to others.

EVALUATION

- The therapeutic effect is achieved and symptoms of the disease process subside or diminish.

- Adverse reactions are identified, reported to the primary health care provider, and managed successfully through nursing interventions.

- The patient and family demonstrate an understanding of the drug regimen.

- The patient verbalizes the importance of complying with the prescribed treatment regimen.

Critical Thinking Exercises

1. A young mother is concerned because her 2-month-old daughter was diagnosed with RSV. The infant is receiving inhalation treatments with ribavirin. The mother questions this treatment. Describe how the nurse could explain treatment with ribavirin to the mother. Discuss what possible effects the drug could have on the infant and on the mother.

2. Ms. Jenkins, aged 77 years, has herpes zoster. The primary health care provider prescribes acyclovir 200 mg every 4 hours during Ms. Jenkins' waking hours. Discuss what information you would give Ms. Jenkins concerning herpes zoster, the drug regimen, and the possible adverse reactions.

3. Jim, age 25 years, has recently received a diagnosis of HIV infection and is prescribed a treatment regimen of zidovudine and lamivudine. Determine what information you would give him concerning the drugs he will be taking. What adverse reactions would you discuss with him?

Review Questions

1. Which of the following adverse reactions would the nurse expect in a patient receiving acyclovir by the oral route?

   A. Nausea and vomiting

   B. Constipation and urinary frequency

   C. Conjunctivitis and blurred vision

   D. Nephrotoxicity

2. Which of the following would the nurse report immediately in a 3-month-old patient receiving ribavirin?

   A. Any worsening of the respiratory status

   B. Refusal to take foods or fluids

   C. Drowsiness

   D. Constipation

3. The nurse is administering didanosine properly when _____.

   A. tablets are crushed and mixed thoroughly with 1 oz of water

   B. the drug is prepared for subcutaneous injection

   C. the drug is given with meals

   D. the drug is given mixed with orange juice or apple juice

4. Administration of antiretrovirals can result in _____.

   A. abnormal hair growth

   B. body fat redistribution

   C. cardiac arrest

   D. discoloration of the skin

Antiviral Drugs

Medication Dosage Problems

1. The patient is prescribed amantadine 200 mg. The drug is available in 100-mg tablets. The nurse administers _____.

2. A patient is prescribed 2 inhalations of zanamivir. The drug is available as one 5-mg blister per inhalation and is to be given with a "Diskhaler" device. How many milligrams will the nurse administer with 2 inhalations?

3. The nurse is to administer 100 mg of zidovudine orally. The drug is available as syrup 50 mg/5 mL. The nurse administers _____.

To check your answers, see Appendix G.

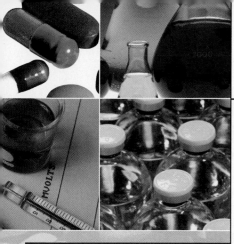

Chapter 15

Antifungal Drugs

Key Terms

candidiasis
fungicidal
fungistatic
fungus
mycotic infections
onychomycosis
thrush
tinea corporis
tinea cruris
tinea pedis

Learning Objectives

On completion of this chapter, the student will:

- Distinguish between superficial and systemic fungal infections.

- Discuss the uses, general drug action, adverse reactions, contraindications, precautions, and interactions of antifungal drugs.

- Discuss important preadministration and ongoing assessment activities the nurse should perform on the patient receiving an antifungal drug.

- List nursing diagnoses particular to a patient taking an antifungal drug.

- List possible goals for a patient taking an antifungal drug.

- Discuss ways to promote an optimal response to therapy, how to manage adverse reactions, and important points to keep in mind when educating the patient and the family about the antifungal drugs.

A fungus is a single-celled, colorless plant that lacks chlorophyll. Fungi that cause disease in humans may be yeastlike or moldlike; the resulting infections are called **mycotic infections** or fungal infections.

Fungal infections range from superficial skin infections to life-threatening systemic infections. Systemic fungal infections are serious infections that occur when fungi gain entrance into the interior of the body.

The superficial mycotic infections occur on the surface of, or just below, the skin or nails. Superficial infections include **tinea pedis** (athlete's foot), **tinea cruris** (jock itch), **tinea corporis** (ringworm), **onychomycosis** (nail fungus), and yeast infections, such as those caused by *Candida albicans*, known as **candidiasis**. Candidiasis affects women in the vulvovaginal area and immunocompromised patients with chronic conditions in both the perineal and oral cavity. Infection of the mouth by the microorganism *C. albicans* is commonly called **thrush**. Patients who are at increased risk for candidal infections are those who have diabetes, are pregnant, or are taking oral contraceptives, antibiotics, or corticosteroids.

Deep mycotic infections develop inside the body, such as in the lungs, brain, or gastrointestinal tract. Treatment for deep mycotic infections is often difficult and prolonged. The Summary Drug Table: Antifungal Drugs identifies drugs that are used to combat fungal infections.

Actions

Antifungal drugs may be **fungicidal** (able to destroy fungi) or **fungistatic** (able to slow or retard the multiplication of fungi). Amphotericin B (Fungizone IV), miconazole (Monistat), nystatin (Mycostatin), voriconazole (Vfend), micafungin (Mycamine), and ketoconazole (Nizoral) are thought to have an effect on the cell membrane of the fungus. The fungicidal or fungistatic effect of these drugs appears to

SUMMARY DRUG TABLE   ANTIFUNGAL DRUGS

GENERIC NAME	TRADE NAME	USES	ADVERSE REACTIONS	DOSAGE RANGES
amphotericin B desoxycholate *am-foe-ter'-i-sin*	Fungizone IV	Systemic fungal infections	Headache, hypotension, fever, shaking, chills, malaise, nausea, vomiting, diarrhea, abnormal renal function, joint and muscle pain	Desoxycholate: 1–1.5 mg/kg/d IV
amphotericin B, lipid-based	Abelcet, AmBisome, Amphotec	Systemic fungal infection, cryptococcal meningitis in patients with human immunodeficiency virus infection	Headache, hypotension, fever, shaking, chills, malaise, nausea, vomiting, diarrhea, abnormal renal function, joint and muscle pain	Lipid-based: 3–6 mg/kg/d IV
caspofungin acetate *kass-poe-fun'-jin*	Cancidas	Invasive aspergillosis, hepatic insufficiency	Headache, rash, nausea, vomiting, abdominal pain, hematologic changes, fever	70 mg loading dose IV, followed by 50 mg/d IV for at least 14 d
fluconazole *floo-kon'-a-zole*	Diflucan	Oropharyngeal and esophageal candidiasis, vaginal candidiasis, cryptococcal meningitis	Headache, nausea, vomiting, diarrhea, skin rash	50–400 mg/d orally, IV
flucytosine (5-FC) *floo-sye'-toe-seen*	Ancobon	Systemic fungal infections	Nausea, diarrhea, rash, anemia, leukopenia, thrombocytopenia, renal insufficiency	50–150 mg/kg/d orally q6h
griseofulvin *griz-ee-oh-full'-vin*	Fulvicin U/F, Grifulvin V, Gris-PEG	Ringworm infections of the skin, hair, nails	Nausea, vomiting, diarrhea, oral thrush, headache, rash, urticaria	For ringworm and jock itch: 330–375 mg orally in a single or divided dose. For athlete's foot: 660–750 mg/d orally in divided doses; take for 2–6 wk until the infection is completely gone
itraconazole *eye-truh-kon'-uh-zole*	Sporanox	Systemic fungal infections, may be used for nail infections	Nausea, vomiting, diarrhea, rash, abdominal pain, edema, hypokalemia in dosages over 600 mg/d	200–400 mg/d orally; IV as a single or divided dose Nail infections: 200 mg BID for 1 wk, then repeat in 3 wk
ketoconazole *kee-toe-kon'-uh-zole*	Nizoral	Treatment of systemic fungal infections	Nausea, vomiting, abdominal pain, headache, pruritus	200 mg/d orally; may increase to 400 mg/d orally

GENERIC NAME	TRADE NAME	USES	ADVERSE REACTIONS	DOSAGE RANGES
micafungin sodium *mye-ka-fun'-jin*	Mycamine	Esophageal candidiasis, candidal infection prevention in stem cell transplantation	Rash, pruritus, facial swelling, vasodilation, flushing, headache, dizziness, anorexia, nausea, vomiting	150 mg/d IV
nystatin, oral *nye-stat'-in*	Mycostatin	Non-esophageal gastrointestinal membrane candidiasis	Rash, diarrhea, nausea, vomiting	500,000–1 million units TID
terbinafine *ter-bin'-a-feen*	Lamisil	Nail fungal infections	Headache, nausea, flatulence, diarrhea, rash	250 mg/d for 6–12 wk
voriconazole *vor-ih-kon'-ah-zole*	Vfend	Aspergillus systemic fungal infections	Visual disturbances, fever, rash, headache, anorexia, nausea, vomiting, diarrhea, peripheral edema, photosensitivity	Loading dose: 6 mg/kg q12h for the first day Maintenance: If tolerated orally: 200 mg q12h; if unable to take orally: 4 mg/kg q 12h IV until able to switch to oral drug

be related to their concentration in body tissues. Fluconazole (Diflucan) has fungistatic activity that appears to result from the depletion of sterols (a group of substances related to fats) in the fungus cells.

Griseofulvin (Grisactin) exerts its effect by being deposited in keratin precursor cells, which are then gradually lost (because of the constant shedding of top skin cells), and replaced by new, noninfected cells. The mode of action of flucytosine (Ancobon) is to inhibit DNA and RNA synthesis in the fungi. Clotrimazole (Lotrimin, Mycelex) binds with phospholipids in the fungal cell membrane, increasing permeability of the cell and resulting in loss of intracellular components (Tables 15-1 and 15-2).

Uses

Antifungal drugs are used prophylactically to prevent fungal infection in immunocompromised patients. They are also used to treat

- Superficial and deep fungal infections
- Systemic infections such as aspergillosis, candidiasis, and cryptococcal meningitis
- Superficial infections of nailbeds and oral, anal, and vaginal areas

The specific uses of antifungal drugs appear in the Summary Drug Table: Antifungal Drugs. Miconazole is an antifungal drug used to treat vulvovaginal "yeast" infections and is representative of all the vaginal antifungal agents. Fungal infections of the skin or mucous membranes may be treated with topical or vaginal preparations. A listing of the topical antifungal drugs appears in Table 15-1, and the vulvovaginal antifungal agents are listed in Table 15-2.

Herbal Alert

Researchers have identified several *antifungal herbs* that are effective against tinea pedis, such as tea tree oil (*Melaleuca alternifolia*) and garlic (*Allium sativum*). Tea tree oil comes from an evergreen tree native to Australia. The herb has been used as a nonirritating, antimicrobial for cuts, stings, wounds, burns, and acne. It can be found in shampoos, soaps, and lotions.

Tea tree oil should not be ingested orally but is effective when used topically for minor cuts and stings. Topical application is most effective when used in a cream with at least 10% tea tree oil. Several commercially prepared ointments are available. The cream is applied to affected areas twice daily for several weeks.

Garlic is also used as an antifungal. A cream of 0.4% ajoene (the antifungal component of garlic) was found to relieve symptoms of athlete's foot and, like tea tree oil, is applied twice daily.

Antifungal Drugs

Table 15.1 Topical Antifungal Drugs

Generic Name (Form)	Trade names	Uses
amphotericin B (cream or lotion)	Fungizone	Mycotic infections
butenafine HCl (cream)	Mentax	Mycotic infections
ciclopirox (cream, lotion)	Loprox, Penlac Nail Lacquer	Tinea pedis, tinea cruris, tinea corporis, mild to moderate onychomycosis of fingernails and toenails
clioquinol (cream)		Tinea pedis, tinea cruris, and other ringworm infections
clotrimazole (cream, solution, lotion)	Lotrimin	Tinea pedis, tinea cruris, tinea corporis
econazole (cream)	Spectazole	Tinea pedis, tinea cruris, tinea corporis
gentian violet (solution)		Abrasions, minor cuts, surface injuries, and superficial fungus infections
haloprogin	Halotex	Tinea pedis, tinea cruris, tinea corporis
miconazole nitrate (cream, solution, spray)	Fungoid Tincture, Lotrimin, Micatin, Monistat	Tinea pedis, tinea cruris, tinea corporis
naftifine (cream, gel)	Naftin	Cutaneous or mucocutaneous mycotic infections
oxiconazole nitrate (cream, lotion)	Oxistat	Tinea pedis, tinea cruris, tinea corporis
sulconazole nitrate (cream, solution)	Exelderm	Tinea pedis, tinea cruris, tinea corporis
tolnaftate (cream, solution, gel, spray)	Aftate, Genaspor, Tinactin, Ting	Tinea pedis, tinea cruris, tinea corporis
triacetin (solution, cream, spray)	Fungoid, Ony-Clear Nail	Tinea pedis, tinea cruris, tinea corporis
undecylenic acid (ointment, cream, powder)	Cruex, Desenex	Tinea pedis; relief and prevention of diaper rash, itching, burning and chafing, prickly heat; tinea cruris; excessive perspiration, irritation of the groin area

Adverse Reactions

Topical Administration: Integumentary Reactions

- Irritation and burning sensation
- Redness, stinging
- Abdominal pain (vaginal preparations)

Systemic Administration

- Headache
- Rash
- Anorexia and malaise
- Abdominal, joint, or muscle pain
- Nausea, vomiting, diarrhea

Table 15.2 Vaginal Antifungal Drugs

Generic Name	Select Trade Name(s)
butoconazole nitrate *byoo-toe-koe'-nuh-zole*	Femstat 3, Gynazole-1, Mycelex-3
clotrimazole *kloe-trye'-ma-zole*	Lotrimin 3, Mycelex-7,
miconazole nitrate *mi-kon'-a-zole*	Monistat 3, Monistat 7, Monistat Dual Pak, M-Zole 3 Combination Pack
nystatin *nye-stat'-in*	
terconazole *ter-kon'-a-zole*	Terazol 7, Terazol 3
tioconazole *tee-o-kon'-a-zole*	Monistat 1, Vagistat-1

Contraindications

Antifungal drugs are contraindicated in patients with a history of allergy to the drug. Most of the systemic antifungal medications are contraindicated during pregnancy and lactation, and are used only when the situation is life-threatening and outweighs the risk to the fetus.

Griseofulvin is not recommended for those with severe liver disease, and voriconazole is contraindicated when patients are taking the following medications: terfenadine, astemizole, sirolimus, rifampin, rifabutin, carbamazepine, ritonavir, ergot alkaloids, or long-acting barbiturates.

Both voriconazole and itraconazole are contraindicated in patients taking cisapride, pimozide, or quinidine. The systemic agent itraconazole should not be used to treat fungal nail infections in patients with a history of heart failure.

Precautions

Antifungals should be used cautiously in patients with renal dysfunction or hepatic impairment. Specific precautions include

- Use amphotericin B cautiously in patients who have electrolyte imbalances or who currently use antineoplastic drugs (because severe bone marrow suppression can result).

- Administer griseofulvin cautiously with penicillin because of possible cross-sensitivity.

- Itraconazole should be used with caution in patients with human immunodeficiency virus (HIV) infection or hypochlorhydria (low levels of stomach acid).

Interactions

Possible interactions depend on the individual drugs, and many interactions can occur. See Table 15-3 for more information.

NURSING PROCESS

The Patient Receiving an Antifungal Drug

ASSESSMENT

PREADMINISTRATION ASSESSMENT

The nurse assesses the patient for signs of the infection before giving the first dose of an antifungal drug. Superficial fungal infections of the skin or skin structures (e.g., hair, nails) are inspected and their description entered on the patient's record to provide baseline data. The nurse carefully documents any skin lesions, such as rough, itchy patches, cracks between the toes, and sore and reddened areas, to obtain an accurate database. It also is important to ask about pain and to describe white plaques or sore areas on mucous membranes of the oral or perineal areas, as well as any vaginal discharge. The nurse takes and records vital signs. The nurse weighs the patient scheduled to receive amphotericin or flucytosine because the dosage of the drug is determined according to the patient's weight.

ONGOING ASSESSMENT

The ongoing assessment involves careful observation of the patient every 2 to 4 hours for adverse drug reactions when the antifungal drug is given by the oral or parenteral route. When these drugs are administered topically or on an outpatient basis, the nurse must instruct the patient what to look for when gathering ongoing assessment data. This should include signs of improvement and adverse reactions, both minor and severe (requiring immediate notification of the primary health care provider).

NURSING DIAGNOSES

Drug-specific nursing diagnoses are highlighted in the Nursing Diagnoses Checklist. More general nursing diagnoses applicable to these drugs are discussed in depth in Chapter 4.

Table 15.3 Possible Interactions Between Antifungal and Other Drugs

Interacting Drug	Common Use	Effect of Interaction
Amphotericin B		
corticosteroids	Reduce Inflammation	Risk for severe hypokelemia
digoxin	Management of cardiac problems	Increased risk of digitalis toxicity
aminoglycosides	Anti-infective agent	Increased risk of nephrotoxicity
cyclosporine	Immunosuppressant (particularly for transplant recipients)	Increased risk of nephrotoxicity
flucytosine	Antifungal	Drug toxicity
miconazole	Antifungal for vaginal infections	Decreased effectiveness of amphotericin B
Fluconazole		
oral hypoglycemics	Diabetes control	Increased effect of oral hypoglycemic
phenytoin	Seizure control	Decreased effectiveness of phenytoin
Griseofulvin		
barbiturates	Sedation	Decreased effectiveness of sedative
oral contraceptives	Birth control	Decreased effectiveness of birth control (breakthrough bleeding, pregnancy, or amenorrhea)
salicylates	Analgesia, pain relief	Decreased serum level of pain reliever
Itraconazole		
digoxin and cyclosporine	See above	Elevated blood levels of itraconazole
phenytoin, histamine antagonists	Antiseizure drug and gastrointestinal acid suppressant, respectively	Decreased blood levels of itraconazole
isoniazid and rifampin	Antitubercular drugs	Decreased blood levels of itraconazole
Ketoconazole		
histamine antagonists and antacids	Control of gastrointestinal upset	Decreased absorption of Ketoconazole
rifampin or isoniazid	Antitubercular drugs	May decrease the blood levels of ketoconazole
Voriconazole		
methadone, tacrolimus, the statins, benzodiazepines, calcium channel blockers	Addiction control and pain relief, immunosuppressant, lipid-lowering agents, sedative hypnotics, and blood pressure or angina control, respectively	Increased effectiveness of voriconazole
sulfonylureas	Diabetes control	Hypoglycemia
vinca alkaloids	Antineoplastic (chemotherapy) agents	Increased risk of neurotoxicity

Interacting Drug	Common Use	Effect of Interaction
Micafungin		
sirolimus	Immunosuppression	Risk of greater immunosuppression
nifedipine	Management of angina (chest pain)	Risk of nifedipine toxicity
Terbinafine		
beta blockers and antidepressants	Cardiac problems and depression, respectively	Increased effectiveness of the beta blocker and antidepressant
Fluconazole, ketoconazole, itraconazole, vorixonazole, or griseofulvin		
warfarin	Blood thinner	Increased risk of bleeding

Nursing Diagnoses Checklist

✔ **Disturbed Body Image** related to changes in skin and mucous membranes

✔ **Impaired Comfort** related to IV administration of amphotericin B

✔ **Risk for Ineffective Tissue Perfusion: Renal** related to adverse reactions of the antifungal drug

PLANNING

The expected outcomes for the patient depend on the reason for administering the antifungal drug, but may include a therapeutic response to the antifungal drug, patient needs related to the management of adverse reactions, and an understanding of and compliance with the prescribed treatment regimen.

IMPLEMENTATION

PROMOTING AN OPTIMAL RESPONSE TO THERAPY: ADMINISTERING SPECIFIC ANTIFUNGAL DRUGS

AMPHOTERICIN B Amphotericin B is given only under close supervision in the hospital setting. Its use is reserved for serious and potentially life-threatening fungal infections. The nurse administers this drug daily or every other day over several days or months.

The intravenous (IV) solution of amphotericin B is light sensitive and should be protected from exposure to light. If the solution is used within 8 hours, there is negligible loss of drug activity. Therefore, once the drug is reconstituted, the nurse should administer the medication immediately because the typical IV infusion is for a period of 6 hours or more. The nurse should consult the primary health care provider or hospital pharmacist regarding whether to use a protective covering for the infusion container.

Nursing Alert

Renal damage is the most serious adverse reaction to the use of amphotericin B. Renal impairment usually improves with a modification of the dosage regimen (reduced dosage or increased time between doses). Serum creatinine levels and blood urea nitrogen (BUN) levels are checked frequently during the course of therapy to monitor kidney function. If the BUN exceeds 40 mg/dL or the serum creatinine level exceeds 3 mg/dL, the primary health care provider may discontinue the drug or reduce the dosage until renal function improves.

TOPICAL ANTIFUNGAL INFECTION PREPARATIONS

When these drugs are applied topically to the skin, the nurse inspects the area at the time of each application for localized skin reactions. When these drugs are administered vaginally, the nurse questions the patient regarding any discomfort or other sensations experienced after insertion of the antifungal preparation. The nurse notes improvement or deterioration of lesions of the skin, mucous membranes, or vaginal secretions in the chart. It is important for the nurse to evaluate and chart the patient's response to therapy daily.

When a vaginal fungal infection is treated with miconazole during pregnancy, a vaginal applicator may be contraindicated. Manual insertion of the vaginal tablets may be preferred. Because small amounts of these drugs may be absorbed from the vagina, they are used during the first trimester only when essential.

Oral thrush infections (candidiasis) may be treated with oral solutions. The patient is instructed to swish and hold the solution in the mouth for several seconds (or as long as possible), gargle, then swallow the solution. Oral infections also may be treated with medication lozenges. Sometimes the vaginal troche preparation of an antifungal medication is prescribed for oral use. The patient needs specific instructions on how to use the medication to prevent confusion and improper use.

MONITORING AND MANAGING PATIENT NEEDS

DISTURBED BODY IMAGE Superficial and deep fungal infections respond slowly to antifungal therapy. The lesions caused by the fungal infections may cause the patient to feel negatively about the body or a body part. In addition, many patients experience anxiety and depression over the fact that therapy must continue for a prolonged period and that results are slow to appear. Depending on the method of treatment, patients may be faced with many problems during therapy and therefore need time to talk about problems as they arise. Examples of these problems may be the cost of treatment, hospitalization (when required), the failure of treatment adequately to control the infection, and loss of income. It is important for the nurse to develop a therapeutic nurse–patient relationship that conveys an attitude of caring and fosters a sense of trust. The nurse listens to the patient's concerns and assists the patient in accepting the situation as temporary. The nurse encourages the patient to verbalize any feelings or anxiety about the effect of the disorder on body image. The nurse explains the disorder and the treatment regimen in terms the patient can understand and discusses the need at times for long-term treatment to eradicate the infection. The nurse must help the patient and the family to understand that therapy must be continued until the infection is under control. In some cases, therapy may take weeks or months.

IMPAIRED COMFORT: MEDICATION ADMINISTRATION
When the nurse administers amphotericin B by IV infusion, immediate adverse reactions can occur. Nausea, vomiting, hypotension, tachypnea, fever, and chills (sometimes called *rigors*) may occur within 15 to 20 minutes of beginning the IV infusion. To prevent these adverse reactions, patients may be premedicated with antipyretics, antihistamines, or antiemetics. It is important to monitor the patient's temperature, pulse, respirations, and blood pres-

sure carefully during the first 30 minutes to 1 hour of treatment. The nurse should monitor vital signs every 2 to 4 hours during therapy, depending on the patient's condition. The nurse also checks the IV infusion rate and the infusion site frequently during administration of the drug. This is especially important if the patient is restless or confused.

Patients should be taught before the drug is given that the side effects can be uncomfortable. Warm blankets should be provided for patient comfort. Reassurance is given to the patient that the medications administered before the antifungal are to help ease the adverse reactions. Instruction should include that the reactions decrease with ongoing therapy.

RISK FOR INEFFECTIVE TISSUE PERFUSION: RENAL
When the patient is taking a drug that is potentially toxic to the kidneys, the nurse must carefully monitor fluid intake and output. In some instances, the nurse may need to perform hourly measurements of urine output. Periodic laboratory tests are usually ordered to monitor the patient's response to therapy and detect toxic reactions. Serum creatinine and BUN levels are checked frequently during the course of therapy to monitor kidney function. If the BUN exceeds 40 mg/dL or if the serum creatinine level exceeds 3 mg/dL, the primary health care provider may discontinue the drug therapy or reduce the dosage until renal function improves.

> ### Gerontologic Alert
>
> Before administering fluconazole to an elderly patient or a patient with renal impairment, the primary health care provider may order a creatinine clearance test. The nurse reports the laboratory results to the primary health care provider because the dosage may be adjusted based on the test results.

EDUCATING THE PATIENT AND FAMILY

If the patient is being treated with topical antifungal drugs, the nurse includes the following points in the teaching plan (also see Home Care Checklist: Using Topical Antifungal Drugs):

- Clean the involved area and apply the ointment or cream to the skin as directed by the primary health care provider.

- Do not increase or decrease the amount used or the number of times the ointment or cream should be applied unless directed to do so by the primary health care provider.

Home Care Checklist

Using Topical Antifungal Drugs

Often patients are required to apply topical drugs for fungal infections of the skin. Most of the adverse effects that occur with topical drugs are a result of applying the drug improperly. Typically, if applied correctly, the drug usually is not systemically absorbed. However, many times, patients think that if a little or some is good, then "more is better." Applying more than the amount necessary increases the patient's risk for systemic absorption. To ensure that the patient applies the topical antifungal drug properly, the nurse includes the following points in the teaching plan:

☑ Gather all necessary supplies and wash hands before starting.

☑ Wash the area first to remove any debris and old drug.

☑ Pat the area dry with a clean cloth.

☑ Open the container (or tube) and place the lid or cap upside down on the counter or surface.

☑ Use a tongue blade, gloved finger (either with a nonsterile gloved hand or finger cot), cotton swab, or gauze pad to remove the drug, then apply it to the skin.

☑ Wipe the drug onto the affected area using long smooth strokes in the direction of hair growth.

☑ Apply a thin layer of drug to the area (more is *not* better).

☑ Use a new tongue blade, applicator, or clean gloved finger to remove additional drug from the container (if necessary).

☑ Apply a clean, dry dressing (if appropriate) over the area.

Antifungal Drugs

- During treatment for a ringworm infection, keep towels and facecloths for bathing separate from those of other family members to avoid the spread of the infection. It is important to keep the affected area clean and dry.

Drug-specific teaching points include:

- *Flucytosine*: Nausea and vomiting may occur with this drug. Reduce or eliminate these effects by taking a few capsules at a time during a 15-minute period. If nausea, vomiting, or diarrhea persists, notify the primary health care provider as soon as possible.

- *Griseofulvin*: Beneficial effects may not be noticed for some time; therefore, take the drug for the full course of therapy. Avoid exposure to sunlight and sunlamps because an exaggerated skin reaction (which is similar to a severe sunburn) may occur even after a brief exposure to ultraviolet light. Notify the primary health care provider if fever, sore throat, or skin rash occurs.

- *Ketoconazole*: Complete the full course of therapy as prescribed by the primary health care provider. Do not take this drug with an antacid. In addition, avoid the use of nonprescription drugs unless use of a specific drug is approved by the primary health care provider. This drug may produce headache, dizziness, and drowsiness. If drowsiness or dizziness occur, use caution while driving or performing other hazardous tasks. Notify the primary health care provider if pronounced abdominal pain, fever, or diarrhea occurs.

- *Itraconazole*: The drug is taken with food. Therapy continues for at least 3 months until infection is controlled. Report unusual fatigue, yellow skin, darkened urine, anorexia, nausea, and vomiting.

- *Miconazole*: If the drug (cream or tablet) is administered vaginally, insert the drug high in the vagina using the applicator provided with the product. Wear a sanitary napkin after insertion of the drug to prevent staining of the clothing and bed linen. Continue taking the drug during the menstrual period if vaginal route is being used. Do not have intercourse while taking this drug, or advise the partner to use a condom to avoid reinfection. To prevent recurrent infections, avoid nylon and tight-fitting garments. If there is no improvement in 5 to 7 days, stop using the drug and consult a primary care provider because a more serious infection may be present. If abdominal pain, pelvic pain, rash, fever, or offensive-smelling vaginal discharge is present, do not use the drug, but notify the primary health care provider.

EVALUATION

- The therapeutic effect occurs and signs and symptoms of infection improve.

- Optimal skin integrity is maintained.

- Adverse reactions are identified, reported to the primary health care provider, and managed through appropriate nursing interventions.

- The patient and family demonstrate an understanding of the drug regimen.

- The patient verbalizes the importance of complying with the prescribed treatment regimen.

Critical Thinking Exercises

1. A nurse is preparing to administer amphotericin B to a patient with a systemic mycotic infection. This is the first time the nurse has administered amphotericin B. Determine what information the nurse should be aware of concerning the administration of this drug. Explain your answer.

2. Mr. Harding, aged 35 years, has received a diagnosis of fungal infection. The primary health care provider has prescribed a topical antifungal drug. Develop a teaching plan for the application of a topical antifungal drug.

Review Questions

1. Mr. Carr is receiving amphotericin B for a systemic fungal infection. Which of the following would most likely indicate to the nurse that Mr. Carr is experiencing an adverse reaction to amphotericin B?

   A. Fever and chills

   B. Abdominal pain

   C. Drowsiness

   D. Flushing of the skin

2. Which of the following laboratory tests would the nurse monitor in patients receiving flucytosine?

   A. Liver function tests

   B. Complete blood count

   C. Renal functions tests

   D. Prothrombin levels

3. The nurse monitors a patient taking itraconazole for the most common adverse reaction, which is _____.

   A. nausea

   B. hypokalemia

   C. irregular pulse

   D. confusion

4. The nurse would withhold griseofulvin if the patient has _____.

   A. anemia

   B. respiratory disease

   C. had a recent myocardial infarction

   D. severe liver disease

Medication Dosage Problems

1. A patient weighs 140 pounds. If amphotericin B 1.5 mg/kg/d is prescribed, what is the total daily dosage of amphotericin B for this patient?

2. The primary care provider has prescribed fluconazole 200 mg orally initially, followed by 100 mg orally daily. On hand are fluconazole 100-mg tablets. What would the nurse administer as the initial dose?

To check your answers, see Appendix G.

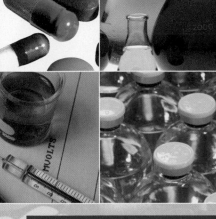

Chapter 16

Antiparasitic Drugs

Key Terms

amebiasis
anthelmintic
cinchonism
helminthiasis
merozoites
over the counter
parasite
sporozoites

Learning Objectives

On completion of this chapter, the student will:

- Discuss the uses, general drug action, adverse effects, contraindications, precautions, and interactions of the drugs used in the treatment of helminthic infections, protozoal infections, and amebiasis.
- Discuss important preadministration and ongoing assessment activities the nurse should perform with the patient taking an anthelmintic, anti-malarial, antiprotozoal, or amebicidal drug.
- List nursing diagnoses particular to a patient taking an anthelmintic, antimalarial, antiprotozoal, or amebicidal drug.
- Discuss ways to promote an optimal response to therapy, how to manage adverse reactions, and important points to keep in mind when educating patients about the use of the anthelmintics, antimalarials, antiprotozoals, and amebicides.

A parasite is an organism that lives in or on another organism (the host) without contributing to the survival or well-being of the host. **Helminthiasis** (invasion of the body by parasitic worms), protozoan infections (such as malaria), and **amebiasis** (invasion of the body by single-celled parasites) are worldwide health problems. What makes these diseases even more concerning is the frequency of global air travel in our society. Conditions once confined to specific parts of the world can now be spread in hours or days by air travel.

ANTHELMINTIC DRUGS

Roundworms, pinworms, whipworms, hookworms, and tapeworms are examples of helminths. The most common parasitic worm across the world is the roundworm. In the United States, the most common worm seen is the pinworm. **Anthelmintic** (against helminths) drugs are used to treat helminthiasis. Table 16-1 lists the organisms that cause helminth infections.

Actions and Uses

Although the actions of anthelmintic drugs vary, their primary purpose is to kill parasites. *Albendazole* (Albenza) interferes with the synthesis of the parasite's microtubules, resulting in death of susceptible larva. This drug is used to treat larval forms of pork tapeworm and to treat liver, lung, and peritoneum disease caused by the dog tapeworm.

Mebendazole (Vermox) blocks the uptake of glucose by the helminth, resulting in depletion of the helminth's own glycogen. This drug is used to treat whipworm, pinworm, roundworm, American hookworm, and the common hookworm.

163

SUMMARY DRUG TABLE   ANTHELMINTIC DRUGS

GENERIC NAME	TRADE NAME	USES	ADVERSE REACTIONS	DOSAGE RANGES
albendazole *al-ben'-dah-zohl*	Albenza	Parenchymal neurocysticercosis due to pork tapeworms, hydatid disease (caused by the larval form of the dog tapeworm)	Abnormal liver function test results, abdominal pain, nausea, vomiting, headache, dizziness	Weight greater than or equal to 60 kg: 400 mg Weight less than 60 kg: 15 mg/kg/d
mebendazole *me-ben'-dah-zole*	Vermox	Treatment of whipworm, pinworm, roundworm, common and American hookworm	Transient abdominal pain, diarrhea	100 mg orally morning and evening for 3 consecutive days; Pinworm: 100 mg orally as a single dose
pyrantel* *pi-ran'-tel*	Antiminth, Reese's Pinworm	Treatment of pinworm and roundworm	Anorexia, nausea, vomiting, abdominal cramps, diarrhea, rash (serious)	11 mg/kg orally as a single dose; maximum dose, 1000 mg
thiabendazole *thye-a-ben'-da-zole*	Mintezol	Treatment of threadworm	Hypersensitivity reactions, drowsiness, dizziness, rash (serious)	Weight less than 150 lb: 10 mg/lb per dose orally Weight greater than 150 lb: 1.5 g/dose orally Maximum daily dose, 3 g

*This product is sold over the counter without prescription in drugstores.

The activity of *pyrantel* (Antiminth) is due probably to its ability to paralyze the helminth. Paralysis causes the helminth to release its grip on the intestinal wall, after which it can be excreted in the feces. Pyrantel is used to treat roundworm and pinworm.

The exact mechanism of action of *thiabendazole* (Mintezol) is unknown. This drug appears to suppress egg or larval production, and therefore may interrupt the life cycle of the helminth. Thiabendazole is used to treat threadworm.

Table 16.1 Common Names and Causative Organisms of Parasitic Infections

Common Name	Causative Organism
Roundworm	*Ascaris lumbricoides*
Pinworm	*Enterobius vermicularis*
Whipworm	*Trichuris trichiura*
Threadworm	*Strongyloides stercoralis*
Hookworm	*Ancylostoma duodenale, Necator americanus*
Beef tapeworm	*Taenia saginata*
Pork tapeworm	*Taenia solium*
Fish tapeworm	*Diphyllobothrium latum*

Adverse Reactions

Generalized adverse reactions include

- Drowsiness, dizziness
- Nausea, vomiting
- Abdominal pain and cramps, diarrhea

Adverse reactions associated with the anthelmintic drugs, if they do occur, are usually mild when the drug is used in the recommended dosage. Rash is a serious adverse reaction to pyrantel, which is sold **over the counter** (without a prescription). As such, patients may begin self-treatment before notifying their primary health provider. Therefore, it is important for the nurse to instruct the patient to notify the primary health care provider if this skin reaction occurs. For more information, see the Summary Drug Table: Anthelmintic Drugs.

Contraindications and Precautions

The anthelmintic drugs are contraindicated in patients with known hypersensitivity to the drugs and during pregnancy (category C). They should be used cautiously in lactating patients and patients with hepatic or renal impairment, and malnutrition or anemia.

Interactions

The following interactions may occur when an anthelmintic is administered with another agent:

Interacting Drug	Common Use	Effect of Interaction
albendazole (Albenza)		
dexamethasone	Inflammation or immunosuppression	Increased effectiveness of albendazole
cimetidine (Tagamet)	Relief of gastrointestinal (GI) problems, such as heartburn	Increased effectiveness of albendazole
mebendazole (Vermox)		
hydantoins and carbamazepine (Tegretol)	Seizure control	Lower levels of mebendazole
thiabendazole (Mintezol)		
xanthine derivatives	Management of respiratory problems	Increased serum level, possible toxic effects of the xanthines

NURSING PROCESS

The Patient Receiving an Anthelmintic Drug

ASSESSMENT

PREADMINISTRATION ASSESSMENT

Patients with massive helminth infections may or may not be acutely ill. The acutely ill patient requires hospitalization, but many individuals with helminth infections can be treated on an outpatient basis. The diagnosis of a helminth infection is made by examination of the stool for ova and all or part of the helminth. Several stool specimens may be necessary before the helminth is seen and identified. The patient history also may lead to a suspicion of a helminth infection, but some patients have no symptoms.

When a pinworm infection is suspected, the nurse will frequently instruct the parent how to take a specimen from the anal area, preferably early in the morning before the patient gets out of bed. Specimens are taken by swabbing the perianal area with a cellophane tape–covered swab. The nurse also may need to weigh the patient if the drug's dosage is determined by weight or if the patient is acutely ill.

ONGOING ASSESSMENT

Unless ordered otherwise, the nurse should save all stools that are passed after the drug is given. It is important to inspect each stool visually for passage of the helminth. If stool specimens are to be saved for laboratory examination, the nurse follows hospital procedure for saving the stool and transporting it to the laboratory. If the patient is acutely ill or has a massive infection, it is important to monitor vital signs every 4 hours and measure and record fluid intake and output. The nurse observes the patient for adverse drug reactions, as well as severe episodes of diarrhea. It is important to notify the primary health care provider if these occur.

NURSING DIAGNOSES

The nursing diagnoses depend on the patient and the type of helminth infection. Drug-specific nursing diagnoses are highlighted in the Nursing Diagnoses Checklist. Other nursing diagnoses are discussed in depth in Chapter 4.

Nursing Diagnoses Checklist

- ✓ **Imbalanced Nutrition: Less Than Body Requirements** related to infestation with helminthes
- ✓ **Ineffective Therapeutic Regimen: Family**

PLANNING

The expected outcomes for the patient may include a reduction in anxiety, an optimal response to therapy, meeting of patient needs related to the management of adverse reactions, and an understanding of and compliance with the prescribed therapeutic regimen.

IMPLEMENTATION

PROMOTING AN OPTIMAL RESPONSE TO THERAPY

The diagnosis of a helminth infection is often distressing to patients and their family. The nurse should allow time to explain the treatment and future preventive measures, as well as to allow the patient or family members to discuss their concerns and ask questions.

Depending on hospital policy, as well as the type of helminth, linen precautions may be necessary. The nurse wears gloves when changing bed linens, emptying bedpans, or obtaining or handling stool specimens. It is important to wash hands thoroughly after removing the gloves. The nurse instructs the patient to wash his or her hands thoroughly after personal care and use of the bedpan.

MONITORING AND MANAGING PATIENT NEEDS

RISK FOR IMBALANCED NUTRITION: LESS THAN BODY REQUIREMENTS Gastrointestinal upset may occur, causing nausea, vomiting, abdominal pain, and diarrhea. Taking the drug with food often helps to alleviate the nausea. The patient may require frequent, small meals of easily digested food. The nurse considers the patient's food preferences and encourages the patient to eat nutritious, balanced meals. If vomiting is present, the primary health care provider may prescribe an antiemetic or a different anthelmintic agent. If the patient has diarrhea, the nurse notifies the primary health care provider because a change in the drug regimen may be needed. The nurse keeps a record of the number, consistency, color, and frequency of stools. The nurse also monitors fluid intake and output and makes sure patient is clean and the room free of odor.

INEFFECTIVE THERAPEUTIC REGIMEN MANAGEMENT: FAMILY Pinworm infections may present in children as fussiness or crankiness. They may pull at their clothing in attempts to scratch at an anal itch. As children play with each other, they may pass the disease to another child. When the infection is diagnosed, multiple members of the family may be infected, and all household members may need to be treated. It is important to wash all bedding and bed clothes once treatment has started. Families need to be taught the importance of handwashing before meals and after using the bathroom.

EDUCATING THE PATIENT AND FAMILY

When an anthelmintic is prescribed on an outpatient basis, the nurse gives the patient or a family member complete instructions about taking the drug, as well as household precautions that should be followed until the helminth is eliminated from the intestine. The nurse develops a patient education plan to include the following:

- Follow the dosage schedule exactly as printed on the prescription container. It is absolutely necessary to follow the directions for taking the drug to eradicate the helminth.
- Follow-up stool specimens will be necessary because this is the only way to determine the success of drug therapy.
- To prevent reinfection and the infection of others in the household, change and launder bed linens and undergarments daily, separately from those of other members of the family.
- Daily bathing (showering is best) is recommended. Disinfect toilet facilities daily, and disinfect the bathtub or

shower stall immediately after bathing. Use the disinfectant recommended by the primary health care provider or use chlorine bleach. Scrub the surfaces thoroughly and allow the disinfectant to remain in contact with the surfaces for several minutes.
- Wash the hands thoroughly after urinating or defecating and before preparing and eating food. Clean under the fingernails daily and avoid putting fingers in the mouth or biting the nails.
- Report any symptoms of infection (low-grade fever or sore throat) or thrombocytopenia (easy bruising or bleeding).
- Albendazole can cause serious harm to a developing fetus. Inform women of childbearing age of this. Explain that a barrier contraceptive is recommended during the course of therapy and for 1 month after discontinuing the therapy.

EVALUATION

- The therapeutic effect is achieved.
- Adverse reactions are identified, reported to the primary health care provider, and managed successfully using appropriate nursing interventions.
- The infection is resolved.
- Stool specimens or perineal swabs are negative for parasites.
- The patient verbalizes an understanding of the therapeutic regimen modalities and the importance of continued follow-up testing.
- The patient describes or lists measures used to prevent the spread of infection to others.
- The patient verbalizes the importance of complying with the prescribed treatment regimen and preventive measures.

ANTIPROTOZOAL DRUGS

Protozoa are single-celled animals. Drugs used to treat or prevent malaria are called *antimalarial drugs*. Three antimalarial drugs are discussed in the chapter: chloroquine, doxycycline, and quinine sulfate. Although rare in the United States, with global travel more people may be at risk depending on where they go. The protozoal infections seen in America include giardiasis (contracted from contaminated food or water) and toxoplasmosis (seen in immunocompromised patients). Examples of antiprotozoal drugs in use today are listed in the Summary Drug Table: Antimalarial and Antiprotozoal Drugs.

SUMMARY DRUG TABLE ANTIMALARIAL AND ANTIPROTOZOAL DRUGS

GENERIC NAME	TRADE NAME	USES	ADVERSE REACTIONS	DOSAGE RANGES
Primary Antimalarial Drugs				
chloroquine *klor'-oh-kwin*	Aralen	Treatment and prevention of malaria	Hypotension, electrocardiographic changes, headache, nausea, vomiting, anorexia, diarrhea, abdominal cramps, visual disturbances	Treatment: 160–200 mg IM and repeat in 6 h if necessary Prevention: 300 mg orally weekly; begin 1–2 wk before travel and continue for 4 wk after return from endemic area
doxycycline *dox-i-sye'-kleen*	Monodox, Vibramycin, Vibra-Tabs	Short-term prevention of malaria	Photosensitivity, anorexia, nausea, vomiting, diarrhea, superinfection, rash	100 mg orally daily, 1–2 d before travel and for 4 wk after return from endemic area
quinine sulfate *kwi'-nine*		Treatment of malaria	Nausea, vomiting, cinchonism, skin rash, visual disturbances	260–650 mg TID for 6–12 d
Other Antimalarial Drugs				
atovaquone and proguanil hydrochloride *ah-toe'-vuh-kwone and pro-gwa'-nill*	Malarone	Prevention and treatment of malaria	Headache, fever, myalgia, abdominal pain, diarrhea	Prevention: 1–2 d before travel, 1 tablet orally per day during period of exposure and for 7 d after exposure Treatment: 4 tablets orally daily for 3 d
mefloquine hydrochloride *me'-flow-kwin*	Lariam	Prevention and treatment of malaria	Vomiting, dizziness, disturbed sense of balance, nausea, fever, headache, visual disturbances	Prevention: begin 1 wk before travel, 250 mg/wk mg/wk orally, continue for 4 wk after return from endemic area Treatment: 5 tablets orally as a single dose
primaquine phosphate *prim'-a-kween*		Treatment of malaria	Nausea, vomiting, epigastric distress, abdominal cramps	26.3. mg/d orally for 14 d
pyrimethamine *peer-i-meth'-a-meen*	Daraprim	Prevention and treatment of malaria	Nausea, vomiting, hematologic changes, anorexia	Prevention: 25 mg orally once weekly Treatment: 50 mg/d for 2 d
sulfadoxine and pyrimethamine *sul-fa-dox'-een and peer-i-meth'-a-meen*	Fansidar	Prevention and treatment of malaria	Hematolotic changes, nausea, emesis, headache, hypersensitivity reactions, Stevens-Johnson syndrome	Prevention: 1 tablet orally weekly Treatment: 2–3 tablets orally as a single dose
Antiprotozoal Drugs				
atovaquone *nita-zocks'-a-nide*	Mepron	Prevention of *Pneumocystis carinii pneumonia* (PCP)	Nausea, vomiting, diarrhea, headache, rash	750 mg orally BID for 21 d
nitazoxanide *nita-zocks'-a-nide*	Alinia	Diarrhea caused by *Giardia lamblia*	Abdominal pain, nausea, vomiting, diarrhea, headache	500 mg orally q 12h with food

Antiparasitic Drugs

SUMMARY DRUG TABLE *(continued)*

GENERIC NAME	TRADE NAME	USES	ADVERSE REACTIONS	DOSAGE RANGES
pentamidine isethionate *pen-ta'-mih-deen*	Pentam 300, Nebupent	*P. carinii pneumonia* (PCP)	IM: pain at injection site Fatigue, metallic taste, anorexia, shortness of breath, dizziness, rash, cough	Injection: 4 mg/kg IM or IV daily, for 14d Aerosol (preventative): 300 mg/wk for 4 wk by nebulizer
tinidazole *teh-nye'-da-zoll*	Tindamax	*Giardia lamblia,* trichomoniasis	Nausea, vomiting, metallic taste	Single dose of 2 g orally

Actions

Malaria is transmitted from person to person by certain species of the *Anopheles* mosquito. The four different protozoans causing malaria are *Plasmodium falciparum*, *P. malariae*, *P. ovale*, and *P. vivax*. The plasmodium causing malaria must enter the mosquito to develop, reproduce, and be transmitted. When the mosquito bites a person infected with malaria, it ingests the plasmodium. In the mosquito's stomach, **sporozoites** (an animal reproductive cell) form; these make their way to the salivary glands of the mosquito. When the mosquito bites a noninfected person, the sporozoites enter the person's bloodstream and lodge in the liver and other tissues. The sporozoites then reproduce and form **merozoites** (cells formed as a result of asexual reproduction). The merozoites then divide and enter the red blood cells of the person, where they form the plasmodium. The symptoms of malaria (shaking, chills, and fever) appear when the merozoites enter the individual's red blood cells.

Antimalarial drugs interfere with, or are active against, the life cycle of the plasmodium, primarily when it is present in the red blood cells. Destruction at this stage of the plasmodium life cycle prevents the development of the plasmodium. This in turn keeps the mosquito (when the mosquito bites an infected individual) from ingesting the plasmodium, thus effectively ending the plasmodium life cycle (Fig. 16-1).

Uses

Antimalarial drugs are used for suppressing (the prevention of malaria) or treating (the management of an attack) malaria. Not all antimalarial drugs are effective in sup-

pressing or treating all four of the *Plasmodium* species that cause malaria. In addition, resistant strains have developed, and some antimalarial drugs are no longer effective against some of these strains. The primary health care provider must select the antimalarial drug that reportedly is effective, at present, for treating the type of malaria the individual has or for preventing the type of malaria that the individual may be exposed to in a specific area of the world.

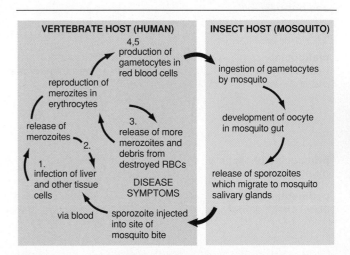

Figure 16.1 Life cycle of the malarial parasite. Points numbered on the illustration indicate the location in the malarial life cycle where specific drugs might be effective. **(1)** Chlorguanide, pyrimethamine, and primaquine used for causal prophylaxis. **(2)** Primaquine used to prevent relapses. **(3)** Drugs against the erythrocytic phase: potent action—chloroquine, amodiaquine, quinine; limited action—primaquine and chlorguanide. **(4)** Gametocidal drugs: primaquine. **(5)** Gametocyte-sterilizing drugs: chlorguanide, pyrimethamine. (RBCs, red blood cells).

Adverse Reactions

Gastrointestinal reactions include

- Anorexia
- Nausea, vomiting
- Abdominal cramping and diarrhea

Other body system reactions may include

- Headache and dizziness
- Visual disturbances or tinnitus
- Hypotension or changes detected on an electrocardiogram (ECG; associated with chloroquine)
- Photosensitivity (associated with doxycycline)
- **Cinchonism**—a group of symptoms associated with quinine administration, including tinnitus, dizziness, headache, GI disturbances, and visual disturbances. These symptoms usually disappear when the dosage is reduced.

Contraindications and Precautions

Antimalarial drugs are contraindicated in patients with known hypersensitivity. All the drugs are contraindicated during pregnancy (chloroquine, pregnancy category C; doxycycline, pregnancy category D; quinine, pregnancy category X). Quinine should not be prescribed for patients with myasthenia gravis because it may cause respiratory distress and dysphagia. Antimalarial drugs should be used cautiously in children, lactating patients, and those who have hepatic or renal disease or bone marrow depression.

Interactions

Foods that acidify the urine (cranberries, plums, prunes, meats, cheeses, eggs, fish, and grains) may interact with chloroquine and increase its excretion, thereby decreasing the effectiveness of the antimalarial drug. The following interactions may also occur when an antimalarial is administered with another agent:

Interacting Drug	Common Use	Effect of Interaction
antacids	GI upset	Decreased absorption of the antimalarial
iron	Treat anemia	Decreased absorption of the antimalarial
digoxin	Treat cardiac disease	Increased risk of digoxin toxicity
doxycycline (Vibramycin)		
barbiturates, phenytoin, and carbamazepine	Anticonvulsant agents	Decreased effectiveness of doxycycline
Quinine		
warfarin	Blood thinner, prevents blood clots	Increased risk of bleeding

NURSING PROCESS

The Patient Receiving an Antimalarial Drug

ASSESSMENT

PREADMINISTRATION ASSESSMENT

When an antimalarial drug is given to a hospitalized patient, the preadministration assessment includes vital signs and a summary of the nature and duration of the symptoms. Laboratory tests may be ordered for the diagnosis of malaria. Additional laboratory tests, such as a complete blood count, may be ordered to determine the patient's general health status.

ONGOING ASSESSMENT

If the patient is hospitalized with malaria, the nurse takes the vital signs every 4 hours or as ordered by the primary health care provider. The nurse observes the patient every 1 to 2 hours for malaria symptoms (headache, nausea, muscle aching, and high fever). Improvement or exacerbation of signs and symptoms of malaria is documented and reported to the primary health care provider. Antipyretics may be ordered for fever. If the patient is acutely ill, the nurse carefully measures and records the fluid intake and output. In some instances, intravenous (IV) fluids may be required.

NURSING DIAGNOSES

The specific nursing diagnoses for a patient receiving an antimalarial depend on the reason for administration (prevention or treatment) of the antimalarial drug. Drug-specific nursing diagnoses are highlighted in the Nursing Diagnoses Checklist.

> ### Nursing Diagnoses Checklist
>
> ✓ **Risk for Imbalanced Nutrition: Less Than Body Requirements** related to adverse drug reactions or disease process (malaria)
>
> ✓ **Risk for Injury** related to adverse reactions
>
> ✓ **Disturbed Sensory Perception: Visual** related to adverse drug reactions

PLANNING

The expected outcomes for the patient may include an optimal response to therapy, maintenance of adequate nutrition, meeting patient needs related to the management of common adverse reactions, and an understanding of and compliance with the prescribed therapeutic or prevention regimen.

IMPLEMENTATION

PROMOTING AN OPTIMAL THERAPEUTIC RESPONSE

When administering an antimalarial drug, such as chloroquine, for prophylaxis (prevention), therapy should begin 2 weeks before exposure and continue for 6 to 8 weeks after the client leaves the area where malaria is prevalent. Initial treatment with quinine may be given parenterally. When administered IV, quinine should be well diluted and administered slowly. The nurse must frequently examine the injection site and areas along the vein because quinine is irritating to the vein. Parenteral injection of chloroquine is avoided because the drug can cause respiratory distress, shock, and cardiovascular collapse when given intramuscularly (IM) or IV. If chloroquine must be given parenterally, the route should be changed to oral as soon as possible.

MONITORING AND MANAGING PATIENT NEEDS

RISK FOR IMBALANCED NUTRITION: LESS THAN BODY REQUIREMENTS Patients receiving an antimalarial drug may experience nausea. Good nutrition is essential in the healing process. The nurse assists patients to identify food preferences and aversions and helps them in planning a nutritious diet. The nurse can consult a registered dietitian

if necessary. If the patient is hospitalized with an active case of malaria, the nurse keeps the room clean and pleasant during mealtime. Meals should be nutritious and attractively served. Several small meals may be preferable to three large meals.

RISK FOR INJURY Some patients experience dizziness and hypotensive episodes when taking antimalarial drugs. The nurse should frequently monitor blood pressure if the patient is hospitalized. If dizziness occurs, the nurse may need to assist the patient with ambulation. The nurse instructs the patient to rise slowly from a reclining position, sit a few minutes before standing, and stand a few minutes before beginning to walk. When the patient is taking these drugs on an outpatient basis, the nurse instructs the patient to avoid driving or performing hazardous tasks if dizziness occurs.

DISTURBED SENSORY PERCEPTION VISUAL The patient taking chloroquine may experience a number of visual disturbances, such as disturbed color vision, blurred vision, night blindness, diminished visual fields, or optic atrophy. The nurse should therefore ask the patient to describe any visual disturbances.

> ### Nursing Alert
>
> The nurse reports any visual disturbance in patients taking chloroquine to the primary health care provider. Irreversible retinal damage has occurred in patients on long-term therapy with this drug.

Frequent ophthalmic examinations are necessary for patients receiving long-term or high-dose regimens of chloroquine. When vision is affected, the patient is assessed for the extent of visual impairment. If treatment is taking place outside the hospital, it is important to instruct the patient not to drive until examined by an ophthalmologist. Environmental safety is accomplished by measures such as positioning doors and furniture so they are out of walkways, removing scatter rugs, placing items frequently used in convenient places, and strategically placing grab bars to aid the patient in maintaining balance. Assistance with ambulation may be necessary.

EDUCATING THE PATIENT AND FAMILY

When an antimalarial drug is prescribed for preventing malaria (suppression), the nurse thoroughly reviews the drug regimen with the patient. When the drug is to be taken once a week, the nurse advises the patient to select a day of the week that will best remind him or her to take the drug. The nurse emphasizes the importance of taking the drug exactly as prescribed because failure to take the drug on an exact schedule will not give protection against malaria.

When an antimalarial drug is used for preventing malaria and taken once a week, the patient also must take the drug on the same day each week. The prevention program is usually started 1 week before the individual departs to an area where malaria is prevalent.

Because the patient must have a complete understanding of the therapeutic regimen, the nurse and patient review the drug dosage schedule, stressing the importance of adhering to the prescribed schedule. The following additional information is relevant to specific antimalarial drugs:

- *Chloroquine:* Take chloroquine with food or milk. Avoid foods that acidify the urine (cranberries, plums, prunes, meats, cheeses, eggs, fish, and grains). This drug may cause diarrhea, loss of appetite, nausea, stomach pain, or vomiting; the primary health care provider should be notified if these symptoms become pronounced. Chloroquine may cause the urine to take on a yellow or brownish discoloration; this is normal and will go away when the drug therapy is discontinued. Notify the primary health care provider if any of the following occur:

  - Visual changes

  - Ringing in the ears, difficulty in hearing

  - Fever, sore throat

  - Unusual bleeding or bruising, unusual skin coloration (blue-black)

  - Skin rash

  - Unusual muscle weakness

- *Doxycycline:* This drug can cause photosensitivity. Even relatively brief exposure to sunlight may cause sunburn. Avoid exposure to the sun by wearing protective clothing (e.g., long-sleeved shirts and wide-brimmed hats) and by using a sunscreen.

- *Quinine:* Take this drug with food or immediately after a meal. Do not drive or perform other hazardous tasks requiring alertness if blurred vision or dizziness occurs. Do not chew the tablet or open the capsule because the drug is irritating to the stomach. If itching, rash, fever, difficult breathing, or vision problems

occur, stop taking the drug and notify the primary health care provider.

EVALUATION

- The therapeutic effect is achieved.

- Adverse reactions are identified, reported to the health care provider, and managed using appropriate nursing interventions.

- The patient verbalizes the importance of complying with the prescribed therapeutic or prophylactic regimen.

- The patient verbalizes an understanding of the prophylaxis or treatment schedule.

AMEBICIDES

Amebicides (drugs that kill amebas) are used to treat amebiasis caused by the parasite *Entamoeba histolytica*. An ameba is a one-celled organism found in soil and water. Examples of amebicides are listed in the Summary Drug Table: Amebicides.

Actions and Uses

There are two types of amebiasis: intestinal and extraintestinal. In the intestinal form, the ameba is confined to the intestine. Metronidazole (Flagyl) is used to treat intestinal amebiasis. Metronidazole is also used to treat infections caused by susceptible microorganisms, such as is discussed in Chapter 9. Paromomycin is an aminoglycoside with amebicidal activity that also is used to treat intestinal amebiasis.

In the extraintestinal form, the ameba is found outside of the intestine, such as in the liver. The extraintestinal form of amebiasis is more difficult to treat. Chloroquine hydrochloride (Aralen) is used to treat extraintestinal amebiasis.

Adverse Reactions

Gastrointestinal adverse reactions include
- Nausea, vomiting, anorexia
- Abdominal cramps and diarrhea

Other body system adverse reactions include
- Skin eruptions
- Fever, chills, headache

SUMMARY DRUG TABLE   AMEBICIDES

GENERIC NAME	TRADE NAME	USES	ADVERSE REACTIONS	DOSAGE RANGES
chloroquine hydrochloride *klor'-oh-kwin*	Aralen	Extraintestinal amebiasis when oral therapy not feasible	Hypotension, electrocardiographic changes, headache, nausea, vomiting, anorexia, diarrhea, abdominal cramps, visual disturbances	200–250 mg IM for 10–12 d
chloroquine phosphate	Aralen Phosphate	Extraintestinal amebiasis	See above	1 g/d for 2 d, then 500 mg/d for 2–3 wk
metronidazole *me-troe-ni'-da-zole*	Flagyl	Treatment of intestinal amebiasis, trichomoniasis, anaerobic microorganisms	Headache, nausea, peripheral neuropathy, disulfiram-like interaction with alcohol	750 mg orally TID for 5–10 d
paromomycin *par-oh-moe-mye'-sin*	Humatin	Treatment of intestinal amebiasis	Nausea, vomiting, diarrhea	25–35 mg/kg/d in 3 divided doses with meals for 5–10 d

- Vertigo, hypotension, and ECG changes with chloroquine
- Peripheral neuropathy (numbness and tingling of the extremities) with metronidazole
- Nephrotoxicity and ototoxicity with paromomycin

Contraindications and Precautions

Amebicides are contraindicated in patients with known hypersensitivity. Metronidazole is contraindicated during the first trimester of pregnancy (pregnancy category B).

Amebicides should be used cautiously in patients during pregnancy and lactation (metronidazole can be given during the second and third trimesters) and in patients with thyroid disease (iodoquinol interferes with the results of thyroid function tests up to 6 months after therapy), blood dyscrasias, seizure disorders, severe hepatic impairment (metronidazole), bowel disease (paromomycin use interferes with absorption causing ototoxicity and renal impairment), or history of alcohol dependency.

Interactions

The following interactions may occur when metronidazole is administered with another agent:

Interacting Drug	Common Use	Effect of Interaction
cimetidine	Management of GI upset or heartburn	Decreased metabolism of metronidazole
phenobarbital	Sedative	Increased metabolism of metronidazole
warfarin	Blood thinner, prevent blood clots	Increased risk of bleeding

NURSING PROCESS

The Patient Receiving an Amebicide

ASSESSMENT

PREADMINISTRATION ASSESSMENT

Diagnosis of amebiasis is made by examining the stool, as well as by considering the patient's symptoms. Once the patient has received a diagnosis of amebiasis, local health department regulations often require investigation into the source of infection. A thorough history of foreign travel is necessary. If the patient has not traveled to a foreign country, further investigation of the patient's lifestyle, such as local travel, use of restaurants, and the local water supply (especially well water) may be necessary to identify the source of the infection. In addition, it is common practice to test immediate family members for amebiasis.

Before the first dose of an amebicide is given, the nurse records the patient's vital signs and weight, evaluates the general physical status of the patient, and looks for evidence of dehydration, especially if severe vomiting and diarrhea have occurred.

ONGOING ASSESSMENT

If the patient is acutely ill or has vomiting and diarrhea, the nurse measures the fluid intake and output and observes the patient closely for signs of dehydration. The nurse takes vital signs every 4 hours or as ordered by the primary health care provider.

NURSING DIAGNOSES

The specific nursing diagnoses used depend on the type of amebiasis and the condition of the patient. Drug-specific nursing diagnoses are highlighted in the Nursing Diagnoses Checklist. More general nursing diagnoses are discussed in greater depth in Chapter 4.

Nursing Diagnoses Checklist

✓ **Diarrhea** related to amebiasis

✓ **Risk for Deficient Fluid Volume** related to amebiasis

✓ **Imbalanced Nutrition: Less Than Body Requirements** related to adverse effects of drug therapy

---

PLANNING

The expected outcomes for the patient may include an optimal response to therapy, management of common adverse reactions, an absence of diarrhea, meeting of patient needs related to the maintenance of an adequate intake of fluids, maintenance of adequate nutrition, an understanding of the therapeutic regimen (hospitalized patients), and an understanding of and compliance with the prescribed therapeutic regimen (outpatients).

IMPLEMENTATION

PROMOTING AN OPTIMAL RESPONSE TO THERAPY

The patient with amebiasis may or may not be acutely ill. Nursing management depends on the condition of the patient and the information obtained during the initial assessment.

Isolation is usually not necessary, but hospital policy may require isolation procedures. Stool precautions are usually necessary. The nurse washes his or her hands thoroughly after all patient care and the handling of stool specimens.

MONITORING AND MANAGING PATIENT NEEDS

DIARRHEA AND RISK FOR FLUID VOLUME DEFICIT The nurse records the number, character, and color of stools passed. Daily stool specimens may be ordered to be sent to the laboratory for examination. The nurse immediately delivers all stool specimens saved for examination to the laboratory because the organisms die (and therefore cannot be seen microscopically) when the specimen cools. The nurse should inform laboratory personnel that the patient has amebiasis because the specimen must be kept at or near body temperature until examined under a microscope.

The nurse observes the patient with severe or frequent episodes of diarrhea for symptoms of a fluid volume deficit. If dehydration is apparent, the nurse notifies the primary health care provider. If the patient is or becomes dehydrated, oral or IV fluid and electrolyte replacement may be necessary.

IMBALANCED NUTRITION: LESS THAN BODY REQUIREMENTS Because most amebicides cause GI upset, particularly nausea, the maintenance of adequate nutrition is important. A discussion of eating habits, food preferences, and food aversions assists in meal planning. The nurse monitors body weight daily to identify any changes (increase or decrease). The nurse should make sure that meals are well balanced nutritionally, appetizing, and attractively served. Small, frequent meals (five to six daily) may be more appealing than three large meals. The nurse may consult the dietitian if necessary.

EDUCATING THE PATIENT AND FAMILY

The nurse stresses the importance of completing the full course of treatment (see the Home Care Checklist: Administering Pentamidine at Home). The nurse should provide the following information to patients receiving an amebicide on an outpatient basis:

- *Follow directions*: Take the drug exactly as prescribed. Complete the full course of therapy to eradicate the ameba. Failure to complete treatment may result in a recurrence of the infection.

- *Prevention*: Follow measures to control the spread of infection. Wash hands immediately before eating or preparing food and after defecation.

- *Food service—chefs and wait staff*: Food handlers should not resume work until a full course of treatment is completed and stools do not contain the ameba.

- *Chloroquine*: Notify the primary health care provider if any of the following occurs: ringing in the ears, difficulty

Home Care Checklist

Administering Pentamidine at Home

The patient may be required to receive aerosol pentamidine at home. Before discharge, the nurse checks to make sure that arrangements have been made to deliver the specialized equipment and supplies, such as a Respirgard II nebulizer and diluent, to the home. The nurse also instructs the patient and caregiver on how to administer the drug, for example:

☑ Prepare the solution immediately before its use.

☑ Dissolve the contents of one vial in 6 mL sterile water and protect the solution from light.

☑ Place the entire solution in the prebulizer's reservoir. Do not put any other drugs into the reservoir.

☑ Attach the tubing to the nebulizer and reservoir.

☑ Place the mouthpiece in your mouth and turn on the nebulizer.

☑ Breathe in and out deeply and slowly. The entire treatment should last 30 to 45 minutes.

☑ Tap the reservoir periodically to ensure that all of the drug is aerosolized.

☑ When the treatment is finished, turn off the nebulizer.

☑ Clean the equipment according to the manufacturer's instructions.

☑ Allow tubing, reservoir, and mouthpiece to air dry.

☑ Store the equipment in a clean plastic bag and put it away for the next dose.

☑ Use a calendar to mark the days you are to receive the drug and check off each time you've done the treatment.

---

hearing, visual changes, fever, sore throat, or unusual bleeding or bruising.

- *Iodoquinol*: Notify the primary health care provider if nausea, vomiting, or other GI distress becomes severe.

- *Metronidazole*: This drug may cause gastric upset. Take this drug with food or meals. Avoid the use of alcohol, in any form, until the course of treatment is completed. The ingestion of alcohol may cause a mild to severe reaction, with symptoms of severe vomiting, headache, nausea, abdominal cramps, flushing, and sweating. These symptoms may be so severe that hospitalization is required.

- *Paromomycin*: Take this drug three times a day with meals. Report any ringing in the ears, dizziness, severe GI upset, decrease in urinary output, or other urinary difficulties.

EVALUATION

- The therapeutic effect is achieved.

- Adverse reactions are identified, reported to the primary health care provider, and managed successfully through nursing interventions.

- Bowel elimination is normal.

- The patient verbalizes an understanding of the therapeutic modalities and importance of continued follow-up care.

- The patient verbalizes the importance of complying with the prescribed therapeutic regimen.

Critical Thinking Exercises

1. While he was living outside the country for 3 years, Mr. Evans became infected with a helminth. The parasite has been identified and the appropriate drug prescribed. Discuss the points you would include in a teaching plan for this patient.

2. A child in a family of four children is found to have pinworms. Determine what you would include in a teaching plan to prevent the spread of pinworms to other family members.

3. Explain what precautions should be taken when administering paromomycin.

4. Mr. Adkins, aged 68 years, is being treated with metronidazole for intestinal amebiasis. He tells you that he lives alone, eats out for most of his meals,

and likes to have a glass of wine before retiring. Analyze what information would be most important for you to give Mr. Adkins before he begins taking metronidazole.

Review Questions

1. When discussing the adverse reactions of an anthelmintic, the nurse correctly states that _____.

   A. patients must be closely observed for 2 hours after the drug is given

   B. adverse reactions are usually mild when recommended doses are used

   C. most patients experience severe adverse reaction and must be monitored closely

   D. there are no adverse reactions associated with these drugs

2. A patient asks how antimalarial drugs prevent or treat malaria. The nurse correctly responds that this group of drugs _____.

   A. kills the mosquito that carries the protozoa

   B. interferes with the life cycle of the protozoa causing malaria

   C. ruptures the red blood cells that contain merozoites

   D. increases the body's natural immune response to the protozoa

3. When explaining the drug regimen to a patient who will be taking chloroquine for the prevention of malaria, the nurse instructs the patient _____.

   A. to take the drug on an empty stomach

   B. to protect the skin from the sun because the drug can cause severe sunburn

   C. therapy should begin 2 weeks before exposure

   D. to take the drug with a citrus drink to enhance absorption

4. While administering paromomycin, the nurse monitors the patient for which of the following adverse reactions?

   A. Ototoxicity

   B. Cinchonism

   C. Convulsions

   D. Hypertension

Medication Dosage Problems

1. Pyrantel 360 mg is prescribed. The drug is available in 180-mg capsules. The nurse administers _____.

2. Hydroxychloroquine 0.4 g is ordered. The drug is available in 200-mg tablets. The nurse administers _____.

To check your answers, see Appendix G.

Antiparasitic Drugs

Drugs Used to Manage Pain

How do people protect their bodies from harm? Typically they sense danger and pull away or remove themselves from the harmful object or situation. The body uses pain to warn about potential or actual danger to body tissues. The danger can be something outside the body, such as heat, or inside the body, such as a blood clot. **Pain** is the unpleasant sensory and emotional perceptions associated with actual or potential tissue damage.

The nervous system is the agent involved in the recognition and perception of pain. Essentially, nerve fibers in the tissue are stimulated by stretching (an example would be the swelling of a blood clot that would force the nerve to stretch) or a noxious substance, such as a flame or a pin prick. In the **peripheral** (outside or distal) tissues, the nerve endings (or receptors) are activated and send a message to the spinal cord. Here the nerve impulses are transferred across different nerve pathways in the central nervous system and sent to the brainstem. From this area the message goes to the brain cortex, where the perception of pain occurs.

Kinds of Pain

The two basic types of pain are acute pain and chronic pain. **Acute pain** is brief and lasts less than 3 to 6 months. Causes can range from a sunburn to postoperative, procedural, or traumatic pain. Acute pain usually subsides when the injury heals. **Chronic pain** lasts more than 6 months and is associated with specific diseases, such as cancer, sickle cell disease, and end-stage organ or system failure. Various neuropathic and musculoskeletal disorders, such as headaches, fibromyalgia, rheumatoid arthritis, and osteoarthritis, are also causes of chronic pain.

Pain is treated with medications that correct or help to heal the site of tissue and nerve damage or stimulation (peripherally) or that change the brain's perception of the pain signal (centrally). When patients recover more slowly than expected from injury and illness, pain may be the key factor.

Pain management in acute and chronic illness is an important responsibility of the nurse. In managing pain, the nurse needs to overcome the three main barriers to proper pain management, which have to do with assessment, intervention, and evaluation:

- Primary health care providers do not prescribe proper pain medicine doses.
- Nurses do not administer adequate medication for relief of pain.
- Patients to not report accurate levels of pain.

The factors associated with these barriers to successful pain management are too numerous to be examined in detail in this unit, but nurses should be sensitive to patient needs and to their role in providing adequate pain control.

Analgesics and Pain Assessment

Analgesics are drugs used to relieve pain. To prescribe effective analgesics for pain management, the primary health care provider needs two key assessments about pain from the nurse: location and

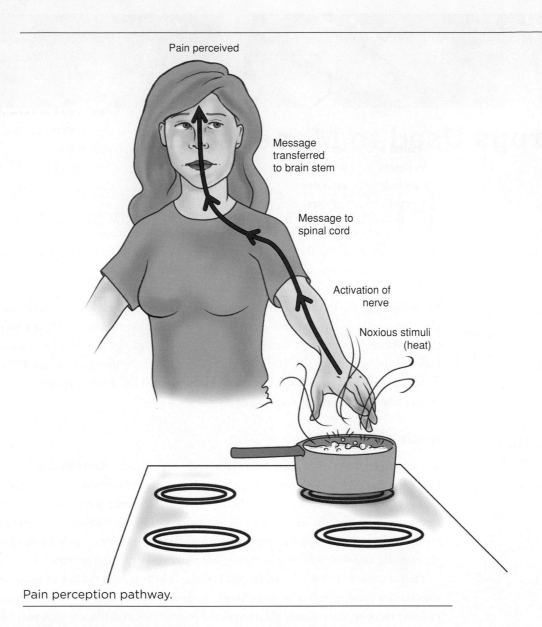

Pain perceived

Message
transferred
to brain stem

Message to
spinal cord

Activation of
nerve

Noxious stimuli
(heat)

Pain perception pathway.

intensity. Assessment of location helps the primary health care provider prescribe drugs that target the pain peripherally or centrally. The strength of the analgesic is determined by the patient's report of the pain's intensity. The World Health Organization (WHO) uses a three-step analgesic ladder based on intensity as a guideline for treating pain (see Chapter 19 for detailed information).

Pain Management

The four chapters in this unit deal with drugs used in managing pain. These drugs are classified into two broad categories:

- Nonopioid analgesics, which include salicylates, nonsalicylates, and the nonsteroidal anti-inflammatory drugs (NSAIDs)

- Opioid analgesics

Opioid is the general term used for the opium-derived or synthetic analgesics used in pain control. **Narcotic** is a term referring to the properties of a drug to produce numbness or a stupor-like state. Although the terms *opioid* and *narcotic* were once interchangeable, law enforcement agencies have generalized the term *narcotic* to mean a drug that is addictive and abused or used illegally.

The nonopioid analgesics are a group of drugs used to relieve mild to moderate pain. They can be divided into three categories: salicylates, nonsalicylates (acetaminophen), and NSAIDs. A number of combination nonopioid analgesics are available over the counter and by prescription as well. The NSAIDs have emerged as important drugs in the treatment of the chronic pain and inflammation associated with disorders such as rheumatoid arthritis and osteoarthritis.

As described by the WHO pain ladder (see Chapter 19), treatment of moderate to severe pain may include both an opioid and a nonopioid analgesic. Manufacturers make drug products containing a combination of these drugs for ease of administration and standard selection of dosage combinations so the primary health care provider can prescribe the most effective pain relief. These are listed in Chapter 19.

The major uses of the opioid analgesics are relief or management of moderate to severe acute and chronic pain. The ability of an opioid analgesic to relieve pain depends on several factors, such as the drug, the dose, the route of administration, the type of pain, the patient, and the length of time the drug has been administered.

The key nursing role in administering nonopioid and opioid drug therapy is careful assessment of pain and monitoring of the patient's response to the medications.

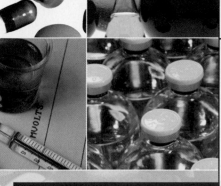

Chapter 17

Nonopioid Analgesics: Salicylates and Nonsalicylates

Key Terms

aggregation
analgesic
antipyretic
jaundice
opioid
pain
pancytopenia
prostaglandins
Reye's syndrome
salicylates
salicylism
tinnitus

Learning Objectives

On completion of this chapter, the student will:

- Discuss the types, uses, general drug actions, common adverse reactions, contraindications, precautions, and interactions of the salicylates and acetaminophen.

- Discuss important preadministration and ongoing assessment activities the nurse should perform for the patient taking salicylates or acetaminophen.

- List nursing diagnoses particular to a patient taking the salicylates or acetaminophen.

- Discuss the ways to promote an optimal response to therapy, how to manage common adverse reactions, and important points to keep in mind when educating patients about the use of the salicylates or acetaminophen.

This chapter deals with the nonopioid analgesics: the salicylates and acetaminophen. Subsequent chapters cover the nonsteroidal anti-inflammatory drugs (NSAIDs) and the **opioid** analgesics. Both opioid and nonopioid analgesics are used to treat pain. **Pain** can be described as "the unpleasant sensory and emotional perception associated with actual or potential tissue damage" (International Association for the Study of Pain, 1979).* Important tasks for the nurse caring for a patient with pain include early and ongoing assessment and intervention to promote healing.

Understanding Pain

To treat pain effectively, the nurse needs a good understanding of the patient's pain experience. This is challenging because sometimes patients feel the provider is too busy to worry about the pain, or a previous bad pain management situation will make the patient think providers do not want or know how to treat the pain. In addition, patients sometimes offer only a vague or poor description of their pain experience. Therefore, it is essential that the nurse conduct a through pain assessment. The nurse needs to know what the pain is like initially and how the pain changes after medications are administered. Guidelines for the initial pain assessment are listed in Display 17-1.

---

* International Association for the Study of Pain. (1979). Subcommittee on Taxonomy: Pain terms: A list with definitions and notes on usage. *Pain, 6*, 249.

Many nurses think of pain as the fifth vital sign, with assessment of pain just as important as the assessment of pulse, respiration, blood pressure, and temperature. The following subject areas may help to guide the pain assessment.

Assessment Guidelines

- Patient's subjective description of the pain (What does the pain feel like?)
- Location(s) of the pain
- Intensity, severity, and duration
- Any factors that influence the pain
- Quality of the pain
- Patterns of coping
- Effects of previous therapy (if applicable)
- Nurses' observations of patient's behavior

Sample Assessment Questions

Questions to include in the assessment of pain may include the following:

- Does the pain keep you awake at night? Prevent you from falling asleep or staying asleep?
- What makes your pain worse? What makes it better?
- Can you describe what your pain feels like? Sharp, stabbing, burning, or throbbing?
- Does the pain affect your mood? Are you depressed? Irritable? Anxious?
- What over-the-counter or herbal remedies have you used for the pain?
- Does the pain affect your activity level? Are you able to walk? Perform self-care activities?

Pain Assessment

The intensity of pain is subjective because the sensation of pain is a complex phenomenon that is uniquely experienced by each individual. Nurses may find it difficult to find signs of pain to measure objectively that match the level of distress reported by the patient. Therefore, the patient's report of pain should always be taken seriously.

Failure to assess pain adequately is a major factor in the undertreatment of pain.

To understand the patient's pain level, the nurse asks the patient to describe the pain using a standardized pain scale measurement tool. The patient is taught to rate the pain on a scale of 0 to 10, with 0 being "no pain" and 10 being the "most severe pain imagined" by the patient. Sometimes it is hard for patients to think about their pain experience in a quantitative manner, like assigning a number to it. For those who find it difficult to quantify pain numerically, other methods to describe pain have been developed. Many of these are visual and may be useful, such as scales of colors or facial expressions. The Wong-Baker FACES Pain Rating Scale (Fig. 17-1) is an example of a visual tool to measure pain. This is especially helpful with children or populations that have trouble understanding or cannot tell the nurse about their pain using numbers.

Many nurses consider pain as the fifth vital sign and assessment of pain just as important as the assessment of temperature, pulse, respirations, and blood pressure. Accurate assessment of pain is necessary if pain management is to be effective. Patients with pain are often undertreated because of an inadequate nursing assessment.

SALICYLATES

The **salicylates** are drugs derived from salicylic acid. Salicylates are useful in pain management because of their **analgesic** (pain-relieving), **antipyretic** (fever-reducing), and anti-inflammatory effects. Examples include aspirin (acetylsalicylic acid) and magnesium salicylate. Specific salicylates are listed in the Summary Drug Table: Nonopioid Analgesics: Salicylates and Nonsalicylates.

Herbal Alert

Willow bark has a long history of use as an analgesic. Willows are trees or shrubs that grow in moist places, often along river banks in temperate or cold climates. When used as a medicinal herb, willow bark is collected in early spring

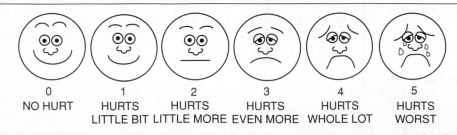

0	1	2	3	4	5
NO HURT	HURTS LITTLE BIT	HURTS LITTLE MORE	HURTS EVEN MORE	HURTS WHOLE LOT	HURTS WORST

Figure 17.1 Wong-Baker FACES Pain Rating Scale. (From Hockenberry, M. J., Wilson, D., & Winkelstein, M. L. [2005]. *Wong's essentials of pediatric nursing* [7th ed., p. 1259]. St. Louis: Mosby.)

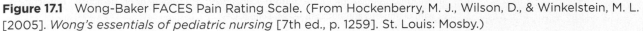

SUMMARY DRUG TABLE NONOPIOID ANALGESICS: SALICYLATES AND NONSALICYLATES

GENERIC NAME	TRADE NAME	USES	ADVERSE REACTIONS	DOSAGE RANGES
Salicylates				
aspirin (acetylsalicylic acid) *ass'-purr-in*	Bayer, Ecotrin, Ecotrin (enteric coated), Empirin	Analgesic, antipyretic, anti-inflammatory	Nausea, vomiting, epigastric distress, gastrointestinal bleeding, tinnitus, allergic and anaphylactic reactions; salicylism with overuse	325–650 mg orally or rectally q4h, up to 8 g/d
buffered aspirin	Ascriptin, Asprimox, Bufferin, Alka-Seltzer with Aspirin	Same as aspirin	Same as aspirin	Same as aspirin
diflunisal *dye-floo-'ni-sal*	Dolobid	Same as aspirin	Same as aspirin	250–500 mg q8–12h (maximum dose, 1.5 g/d)
magnesium salicylate *mag-nee'-see-um sal-ih'-sah-late*	Bufferin, Ecotrin	Same as aspirin	Same as aspirin	650 mg orally q4h or 1090 mg TID
salsalate *sal-sa'-late*	Amigesic, Disalcid	Anti-inflammatory	Same as aspirin	3000 mg/d orally in divided doses
Nonsalicylate				
acetaminophen (APAP) *a-sea-tah-min'-oh-fen*	Tempra, Tylenol	Analgesic, antipyretic	Rare when used as directed; skin eruptions, urticaria, hemolytic anemia, pancytopenia, jaundice, hepatotoxicity	325–650 mg/d orally q4–6h; maximum dose, 4 g/d

Nonopioid Analgesics

Herbal Alert *(continued)*

from young branches. In addition to its use as a pain reliever, the bark and leaves of various willow species have been used to lower fever and reduce inflammation. The salicylates were isolated from willow bark and identified as the most likely source of the bark's anti-inflammatory effects. The chemical structure was replicated in the laboratory and mass produced as synthetic salicylic acid. Years later, a modified version (acetylsalicylic acid) was first sold as aspirin. Aspirin became the most widely used pain reliever, fever reducer, and anti-inflammatory agent, leaving willow bark to be cast aside. The synthetic anti-inflammatory drugs work quickly and have a higher potency than willow bark. Willow bark takes longer to work and fairly high doses may be needed to achieve a noticeable effect. However, fewer adverse reactions are associated with willow bark than with the salicylates. Although adverse reactions are rare with willow bark, it should be used with caution in patients with peptic ulcers and medical conditions in which aspirin is contraindicated.

Actions

Salicylates lower body temperature by dilating peripheral blood vessels. The blood flows out to the extremities, resulting in the dissipation of the heat of fever, which in turn cools the body. The analgesic action of the salicylates is due to the inhibition of prostaglandins. **Prostaglandins** are fatty acid derivatives found in almost every tissue of the body and body fluid. When prostaglandins are released, the sensitivity of pain receptors in the tissue increases, making the patient more likely to feel pain. Salicylates inhibit the production of prostaglandins, making pain receptors less likely to send the pain message to the brain. The reduction in prostaglandins is also thought to account for the anti-inflammatory activity of salicylates.

Aspirin more potently inhibits prostaglandin synthesis and has greater anti-inflammatory effects than other salicylates. In addition, aspirin also prolongs the bleeding time by inhibiting the **aggregation** (clumping) of platelets. When bleeding time is prolonged, it takes a longer time for the blood to clot after a cut, surgery, or other injury to the skin or mucous membranes. Other salicylates do not have as great an effect on platelets as aspirin. This effect of aspirin on platelets is irreversible and lasts for the life of the platelet (7 to10 days).

Uses

The salicylate nonopioid analgesics are used for

- Relieving mild to moderate pain.

- Reducing elevated body temperature (exception: diflunisal, which is not used as an antipyretic).

- Treating inflammatory conditions, such as rheumatoid arthritis, osteoarthritis, and rheumatic fever.

- Decreasing the risk of myocardial infarction in those with unstable angina or previous myocardial infarction (aspirin only).

- Reducing the risk of transient ischemic attacks or strokes in men who have had transient ischemia of the brain due to fibrin platelet emboli (aspirin only). This use has been found to be effective only in men (not women).

- Helping maintain pregnancy in special at-risk populations (low-dose aspirin therapy). For example, it may be used to prevent or treat inadequate uterine–placental blood flow.

Adverse Reactions

Gastrointestinal (GI) reactions include

- Gastric upset, heartburn, nausea, vomiting

- Anorexia

- GI bleeding

Although salicylates are relatively safe when taken as recommended on the label or by the primary health care provider, their use can occasionally result in more serious reactions. Loss of blood through the GI tract may occur with salicylate use. The amount of blood lost is insignificant when one normal dose is taken. However, use of these drugs over a long period, even in normal doses, can result in significant blood loss. Some individuals are allergic to aspirin and the other salicylates. Allergy to the salicylates may be manifested by hives, rash, angioedema, bronchospasm with asthma-like symptoms, and anaphylactoid reactions.

Contraindications

The salicylates are contraindicated in patients with known hypersensitivity to the salicylates or the NSAIDs. Because the salicylates prolong bleeding time, they are contraindicated in those with bleeding disorders or tendencies. These include patients with GI bleeding (from any cause), blood dyscrasias (abnormalities), and those receiving anticoagulant or antineoplastic drugs. Salicylates are classified as pregnancy category D (aspirin) and C drugs and are used cautiously during pregnancy and lactation. Children or teenagers with influenza or chickenpox should not take the salicylates, particularly aspirin, because their use appears to be associated with **Reye's syndrome** (a life-threatening condition characterized by vomiting and lethargy progressing to coma).

Precautions

Salicylates should be used cautiously in patients during lactation and in those with hepatic or renal disease, preexisting hypoprothrombinemia, and vitamin K deficiency. The drugs are also used with caution in patients with GI irritation, such as peptic ulcers, and in patients with mild diabetes or gout.

Chronic Care Alert

Aspirin is an over-the-counter medication that patients may use to self-treat for pain. Some may take more aspirin than the recommended dosage, and toxicity can then result in a condition called **salicylism**. Signs and symptoms of salicylism include dizziness, **tinnitus** (a ringing sound in the ear), impaired hearing, nausea, vomiting, flushing, sweating, rapid, deep breathing, tachycardia, diarrhea, mental confusion, lassitude, drowsiness, respiratory depression, and coma (from large doses). Mild salicylism usually occurs with repeated administration of large doses of a salicylate. This condition is reversible with reduction of the drug dosage.

Interactions

Foods containing salicylates (e.g., curry powder, paprika, licorice, prunes, raisins, and tea) may increase the risk of adverse reactions. The following interactions may occur when a salicylate is administered with another agent:

Interacting Drug	Common Use	Effect of Interaction
anticoagulant	Blood thinner	Increased risk for bleeding
NSAIDs	Pain relief	Increased serum levels of the NSAID
activated charcoal	Antidote (usually to poisons)	Decreased absorption of the salicylates
antacids	Relief of gastric upset, heartburn	Decreased effects of the salicylates
carbonic anhydrase inhibitors	Reduction of intraocular pressure; also used as diuretic	Increased risk for salicylism

NONSALICYLATES

The major drug classified as a nonsalicylate analgesic is acetaminophen (APAP). It is the most widely used aspirin substitute for patients who are allergic to aspirin or who experience extreme gastric upset when taking aspirin. Acetaminophen is also the drug of choice for treating children with fever and flulike symptoms.

Actions

Acetaminophen is a nonsalicylate, nonopioid analgesic whose mechanism of action is unknown. The analgesic and antipyretic activity of acetaminophen is the same as the salicylates. However, acetaminophen does not possess anti-inflammatory action and is of no value in the treatment of inflammation or inflammatory disorders. Acetaminophen does not inhibit platelet aggregation; therefore, it is the analgesic of choice when bleeding tendencies are an issue.

Uses

Acetaminophen is used for
- Treating mild to moderate pain.
- Reducing elevated body temperature (fever).
- Managing pain and discomfort associated with arthritic disorders.

The drug is particularly useful for those with aspirin allergy and bleeding disorders, such as bleeding ulcer or hemophilia, those receiving anticoagulant therapy, and those who have recently had minor surgical procedures.

Adverse Reactions

Adverse reactions to acetaminophen are rare when the drug is used as directed. Adverse reactions associated with acetaminophen usually occur with chronic use or when the recommended dosage is exceeded. They include
- Skin eruptions, urticaria (hives)
- Hemolytic anemia
- **Pancytopenia** (a reduction in all cellular components of the blood)
- Hypoglycemia
- **Jaundice** (yellow discoloration of the skin), hepatotoxicity (damage to the liver), and hepatic failure

Acute acetaminophen poisoning or toxicity can occur after a single 10- to 15-g dose of acetaminophen. Doses of 20 to 25 g may be fatal. With excessive doses, the liver cells undergo necrosis (die), and death can result from liver failure. The risk of liver failure increases in patients who drink alcohol habitually. Signs of acute acetaminophen toxicity include nausea, vomiting, confusion, liver tenderness, hypotension, cardiac arrhythmias, jaundice, and acute hepatic and renal failure.

Contraindications and Precautions

Hypersensitivity to acetaminophen is a contraindication to its use. Hepatotoxicity has occurred in habitual alcohol users after therapeutic dosages. The individual taking acetaminophen should avoid alcohol if taking more than an occasional dose of acetaminophen and avoid taking acetaminophen concurrently with the salicylates or the NSAIDs. Acetaminophen is classified as a pregnancy category B drug and is used cautiously during pregnancy and lactation. If an analgesic is necessary, it appears safe for short-term use. The drug is used cautiously in patients with severe or recurrent pain or high or continued fever because this may indicate a serious untreated illness. If pain persists for more than 5 days or if redness or swelling is present, the primary health care provider should be consulted.

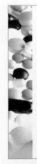

Gerontologic Alert

If liver damage is present in an older adult, acetaminophen should be used with caution.

Interactions

The following interactions may occur when acetaminophen is administered with another agent:

Interacting Drug	Common Use	Effect of Interaction
barbiturates	Sedation, central nervous system depressants	Increased possibility of toxicity and decreased effect of acetaminophen
hydantoins	Anticonvulsants	Increased possibility of toxicity and decreased effect of acetaminophen
isoniazid and rifampin	Tuberculosis medications	Increased possibility of toxicity and decreased effect of acetaminophen
loop diuretics	Control of fluid imbalance	Decreased effectiveness of the diuretic

Chronic Care Alert

Polypharmacy interactions: When administering acetaminophen to diabetic patients, care needs to be taken when blood glucose testing is done. Acetaminophen may alter blood glucose test results, resulting in falsely lower blood glucose values. As a result, inaccurate and lower doses of antidiabetic medications may be given to the patient taking acetaminophen.

NURSING PROCESS

The Patient Receiving a Salicylate or a Nonsalicylate

ASSESSMENT

PREADMINISTRATION ASSESSMENT

The patient's pain scale rating and location of the pain are the two key data items of every pain assessment (see Fig. 17-1). Before giving a nonopioid analgesic to a patient, the nurse assesses the type, onset, intensity, and location of the pain (see Display 17-1). It is important to determine if this problem is different in any way from previous episodes of pain or discomfort. If the patient is receiving a nonopioid analgesic for an arthritic, musculoskeletal disorder or soft tissue inflammation, the nurse should examine the joints or areas involved. The appearance of the skin over the joint or affected area or any limitation of motion is documented. The nurse evaluates the patient's ability to carry out activities of daily living. This important information is used to develop a care plan, as well as to evaluate the response to drug therapy.

Nursing Alert

Before administering acetaminophen, the nurse assesses the overall health and alcohol usage of the patient. Patients who are malnourished or who consume alcohol habitually are at greater risk for developing hepatotoxicity (damage to the liver) with the use of acetaminophen.

ONGOING ASSESSMENT

During the ongoing assessment, the nurse monitors the patient for relief of pain and reassesses the patient's pain rating 30 to 60 minutes after administration of the drug. If pain persists, it is important to assess and document its severity, location, and intensity. (Examples of questions to ask the patient appear in Display 17-1.) The nurse monitors the vital signs every 4 hours or more frequently if necessary. Hot, dry, flushed skin and a decrease in urinary output may develop. If temperature elevation is prolonged, dehydration can occur. The nurse also assesses the joints for decreased inflammation and greater mobility. Any adverse reactions, such as unusual or prolonged bleeding or dark stools, are reported to the primary care provider.

NURSING DIAGNOSES

Drug-specific nursing diagnoses are highlighted in the Nursing Diagnoses Checklist. Other nursing diagnoses applicable to these drugs are discussed in depth in Chapter 4.

PLANNING

The expected outcomes of the patient depend on the reason for administering a nonopioid analgesic, but may include an optimal response to drug therapy, which includes relief of pain and fever, supporting patient needs related to the management of adverse drug reactions, and an understanding of and compliance with the prescribed treatment regimen.

Nursing Diagnoses Checklist

✓ **Impaired Comfort** related to fever of the disease process (e.g., infection or surgery)

✓ **Chronic** or **Acute Pain** related to peripheral nerve damage and/or tissue inflammation due to the aspirin therapy

✓ **Impaired Physical Mobility** related to muscle and joint stiffness

✓ **Disturbed Sensory Perception**: **Auditory** related to adverse drug reactions

IMPLEMENTATION

PROMOTING AN OPTIMAL RESPONSE TO THERAPY

SALICYLATES The patient should avoid salicylates for at least 1 week before any type of major or minor surgery, including dental surgery, because of the possibility of postoperative bleeding. In addition, the patient should not use salicylates after any type of surgery until complete healing has occurred because of the effects of salicylates on platelets. The patient may use acetaminophen or an NSAID after surgery or a dental procedure, when relief of mild pain is necessary.

The nurse observes the patient for adverse drug reactions. When high doses of salicylates are administered (e.g., to those with severe arthritic disorders), the nurse observes the patient for signs of salicylism. Should signs of salicylism occur, the nurse should notify the primary health care provider before the next dose is given because a reduction in dose or determination of the plasma salicylate level may be necessary. Therapeutic salicylate levels are between 100 and 300 mcg/mL. The following are the symptoms associated with increasing levels of salicylates:

- Levels greater than 150 mcg/mL may result in symptoms of mild salicylism, namely tinnitus (ringing sound in the ear), difficulty hearing, dizziness, nausea, vomiting, diarrhea, mental confusion, central nervous system depression, headache, sweating, and hyperventilation (rapid, deep breathing).

- Levels greater than 250 mcg/mL may result in symptoms of mild salicylism plus headache, diarrhea, thirst, and flushing.

- Levels greater than 400 mcg/mL may result in respiratory alkalosis, hemorrhage, excitement, confusion, asterixis (involuntary jerking movements especially of the hands), pulmonary edema, convulsions, tetany (muscle spasms), fever, coma, shock, and renal and respiratory failure.

Nursing Alert

Serious GI toxicity can cause bleeding, ulceration, and perforation and can occur at any time during therapy, with or without symptoms. Although minor GI problems are common, the nurse should remain alert for ulceration and bleeding in patients receiving long-term therapy, even if no previous gastric symptoms have been experienced.

The nurse monitors the patient for signs and symptoms of acute salicylate toxicity or salicylism. Initial treatment includes induction of emesis or gastric lavage to remove any unabsorbed drug from the stomach. Activated charcoal diminishes salicylate absorption if given within 2 hours of ingestion. Further therapy is supportive (reduce hyperthermia and treat severe convulsions with diazepam). Hemodialysis is effective in removing the salicylate but is used only in patients with severe salicylism.

ACETAMINOPHEN The nurse administers acetaminophen with a full glass of water. The patient may take this drug with meals or on an empty stomach. Symptoms of overdosage include nausea, vomiting, diaphoresis, and generalized malaise. Acute overdosage may be treated with administration of the drug acetylcysteine (Mucomyst) to prevent liver damage.

Nursing Alert

The nurse immediately reports any signs of acetaminophen toxicity, such as nausea, vomiting, anorexia, malaise, diaphoresis, abdominal pain, confusion, liver tenderness, hypotension, arrhythmias, jaundice, and any other indication of acute hepatic or renal failure. Early diagnosis is important because liver failure may be reversible. Toxicity is treated with gastric lavage, preferably within 4 hours of ingestion of the acetaminophen. Liver function studies are performed frequently. Acetylcysteine (Mucomyst) is an antidote to acetaminophen toxicity and acts by protecting liver cells and destroying acetaminophen metabolites. It is administered by nebulizer within 24 hours after ingestion of the drug and after the gastric lavage.

MONITORING AND MANAGING PATIENT NEEDS

IMPAIRED COMFORT If the patient is receiving the analgesic for reduction of elevated body temperature, the nurse checks the temperature immediately before and 45 to 60 minutes after administration of the drug. If a suppository form of the drug is used, it is important to check the patient after 30 minutes for retention of the suppository. If the drug fails to lower an elevated temperature, the nurse notifies the primary health care provider because other means of temperature control, such as a cooling blanket, may be necessary. Patients can be made more comfortable by changing the clothing and bedding when it becomes damp because of the fluid loss during fever.

However, some health care providers may not prescribe an antipyretic for the patient with an elevated temperature because evidence suggests that fever is the result of the immune system's production of disease-fighting antibodies. The decision to treat an elevated temperature with an antipyretic is an individual one, based on the cause of the fever, the amount of discomfort to the patient, and the patient's physical condition.

PAIN The nurse notifies the primary health care provider if the salicylate or acetaminophen fails to relieve the patient's pain or discomfort. The nurse gives the salicylate with food, milk, or a full glass of water to prevent gastric upset. The nurse checks to see if a new pain experience may be caused by gastric bleeding or inflammation. If gastric distress occurs, the nurse notifies the primary health care provider because other drug therapy may be necessary. An antacid may be prescribed to minimize GI distress. The nurse also checks the color of the stools. Black or dark stools or bright red blood in the stool may indicate GI bleeding. The nurse reports to the primary care provider any change in the color of the stool.

IMPAIRED PHYSICAL MOBILITY The patient may have an acute or chronic disorder with varying degrees of mobility. The patient may be in acute pain or have long-standing mild to moderate pain. Along with the pain there may be skeletal deformities, such as the joint deformities seen with advanced rheumatoid arthritis. Considering the nature of the patient's condition, the nurse's assistance with ambulation may be required. The nurse determines the degree of immobility of the patient and assists the patient as needed.

> ### Gerontologic Alert
>
> The salicylates are prescribed for the pain and inflammation associated with arthritis. Because older adults have a higher incidence of both rheumatoid arthritis and osteoarthritis and may use the nonopioid analgesics on a long-term basis, they are particularly vulnerable to GI bleeding. The nurse should encourage the patient to take the drug with a full glass of water or with food because this may decrease the GI effects.

DISTURBED SENSORY PERCEPTION: AUDITORY The nurse also should assess the patient for tinnitus or impaired hearing. Tinnitus or impaired hearing probably indicates high blood salicylate levels. If this is suspected, the nurse should withhold the drug and report any sensory alterations immediately. It is a good idea to explain to the patient that hearing loss disappears gradually after the drug therapy is discontinued.

> ### Nursing Alert
>
> Studies suggest that the use of salicylates (especially aspirin) may be involved in the development of Reye's syndrome in children with chickenpox or influenza. This rare but life-threatening disorder is characterized by vomiting and lethargy, progressing to coma. Therefore, use of salicylates in children with chickenpox, fever, or flulike symptoms is not recommended. Acetaminophen is recommended for managing symptoms associated with these disorders.

EDUCATING THE PATIENT AND FAMILY

In some instances, a nonopioid analgesic may be prescribed for a prolonged period, such as when the patient has arthritis. Some patients may discontinue use of the drug, fail to take the drug at the prescribed or recommended intervals, increase the dose, or decrease the time interval between doses, especially if there is an increase or decrease in their symptoms. The patient and family must understand that the drug is to be taken even though symptoms have been relieved. The nurse develops a teaching plan to include the following general points:

- Take the drug exactly as prescribed by the primary health care provider. Do not increase or decrease the dosage, and do not take any over-the-counter (OTC) drugs without first consulting the primary health care provider. Notify the primary health care provider or dentist if the pain is not relieved.

- Take the drug with food or a full glass of water unless indicated otherwise by the primary health care provider. If gastric upset occurs, take the drug with food or milk. If the problem persists, contact the primary health care provider.

- Inform all health care providers, including dentists, when these drugs are taken on a regular or occasional basis.

- If the drug is used to reduce fever, contact the primary health care provider if the temperature continues to remain elevated for more than 24 hours.

- Do not consistently use an OTC nonopioid analgesic to treat chronic pain without first consulting the primary health care provider.

- Severe or recurrent pain or high or continued fever may indicate serious illness. If pain persists more than 10 days in adults, or if fever persists more than 3 days, consult the primary health care provider.

SALICYLATES Advise patients taking a salicylate to notify the primary health care provider if any of the following symptoms occur: ringing in the ears, GI pain, nausea, vomiting, flushing, sweating, thirst, headache, diarrhea, episodes of unusual bleeding or bruising, or dark stools (see Home Care Checklist: Detecting Gastrointestinal Bleeding). When teaching about salicylates, also include the following information:

- All drugs deteriorate with age. Salicylates often deteriorate more rapidly than many other drugs. If there is a vinegar odor to the salicylate, discard the entire contents of the container. Purchase salicylates in small amounts when used on an occasional basis. Keep the container tightly closed at all times because salicylates deteriorate rapidly when exposed to air, moisture, and heat.

- The ingredients of some OTC drugs include aspirin. The name of the salicylate may not appear in the name of the drug, but it is listed on the label. Do not use these products while taking a salicylate, especially during high-dose or long-term salicylate therapy. Consult the pharmacist about the product's ingredients if in doubt.

- If surgery or a dental procedure, such as tooth extraction or gum surgery, is anticipated, notify the primary health care provider or dentist. Salicylates may be discontinued 1 week before the procedure because of the possibility of postoperative bleeding.

Home Care Checklist

Detecting Gastrointestinal Bleeding

The patient with pain and inflammation from a musculoskeletal disorder commonly receives salicylates or NSAIDs (see Chapter 18). These drugs are readily available over the counter (OTC). So a patient who is prescribed one drug, such as an NSAID, may also take an OTC salicylate, such as aspirin, for headaches or additional pain relief. When taken alone, these drugs may cause gastrointestinal (GI) irritation, possibly leading to GI bleeding. If taken in combination or with high doses, or for long periods of time, the patient's risk for GI bleeding increases dramatically. Be sure to teach your patient how to look for signs and symptoms of GI bleeding. Instruct the patient to report any of the following:

☑ Abdominal pain or distention, especially any sudden increases

☑ Vomiting that appears
  - bright red or blood streaked (indicates fresh or recent bleeding)
  - dark red, brown, or black, similar to the consistency of coffee grounds (indicates partial digestion of retained blood)

☑ Stools that appear
  - black, loose, and tarry
  - bright red, red streaked, maroon, or dark mahogany colored

Also instruct your patient how to check the stools for occult blood (guaiac) by doing the following:

1. Gather necessary supplies, including chemical testing solution, testing card, and applicator.

2. After passing stool and opening the flap of the testing card, obtain a sample of stool and place a thin smear on the first window or slot marked as "1" or "A."

3. Then, obtain a second sample from another area of the same stool and place a thin smear on the second window or slot marked as "2" or "B."

4. Close the flap of the test card and place the card in the proper packaging material for transfer to the health care provider for analysis.

Nonopioid Analgesics

ACETAMINOPHEN When teaching patients and families about acetaminophen, include the following information:

- If taking medication for arthritis, do not change from aspirin to acetaminophen without consulting the primary health care provider. Acetaminophen lacks the anti-inflammatory properties of aspirin.

- Notify the primary health care provider if any of the following adverse reactions occur: dyspnea, weakness, dizziness, bluish discoloration of the nailbeds, unexplained bleeding, bruising, or sore throat.

- Avoid the use of alcoholic beverages.

EVALUATION

- Pain is relieved, and discomfort is reduced or eliminated.

- Body temperature is normal.

- Adverse reactions are identified, reported to the primary health care provider, and managed through nursing interventions.

- The patient verbalizes the importance of complying with the prescribed treatment regimen.

- The patient demonstrates an understanding of the treatment regimen and adverse effects of the drug.

Critical Thinking Exercises

1. On a visit to the outpatient clinic, Ms. Cain tells you that she takes aspirin daily for the minor aches and pains she experiences. Determine what you might want to discuss with Ms. Cain to explore her use of this drug. Discuss what you might incorporate into the teaching plan to increase her knowledge of the drug and prevent any complications.

2. Jim, aged 49, is at the outpatient clinic with complaints of muscular aches and pain. He is currently taking a nonprescription aspirin product. He states he is experiencing some gastric upset. He tells you that he plans to begin taking Tylenol because he has heard that it does not cause an upset stomach. What assessments would be important for the nurse to make? What information would you give Jim concerning the Tylenol?

Review Questions

1. At a team conference, the nurse explains that the anti-inflammatory actions of the salicylates are most likely due to _____.

   A. a decrease in the prothrombin time

   B. a decrease in the productions of endorphins

   C. the inhibition of prostaglandins

   D. vasodilation of the blood vessels

2. Which of the following symptoms would the nurse expect in a patient experiencing salicylism?

   A. Dizziness, tinnitus, mental confusion

   B. Diarrhea, nausea, weight loss

   C. Constipation, anorexia, rash

   D. Weight gain, hyperglycemia, urinary frequency

3. When administering a salicylate, the nurse correctly administers the drug _____.

   A. between meals

   B. with a carbonated beverage

   C. with food or milk

   D. dissolved in juice

4. A nurse instructs the patient taking aspirin to avoid foods containing salicylates because this increases the risk of adverse reactions. Which foods should the patient avoid?

   A. Salt, soft drinks

   B. Broccoli, milk

   C. Prunes, tea

   D. Liver, pepper

5. While taking acetaminophen, patients who consume alcohol habitually are monitored by the nurse for symptoms of toxicity, which include _____.

   A. hypertension

   B. visual disturbances

   C. liver tenderness

   D. skin lesions

6. Which of the following drugs would the nurse most likely administer to a child with an elevated temperature?

   A. Baby aspirin

   B. Acetaminophen

   C. Fenoprofen

   D. Diflunisal

Medication Dosage Problems

1. The physician orders acetaminophen elixir 180 mg orally. Acetaminophen elixir is available in a 120-mg/mL solution. The nurse administers _____.

2. Aspirin 650 mg orally is prescribed. On hand is aspirin in 325-mg tablets. The nurse administers _____.

To check your answers, see Appendix G.

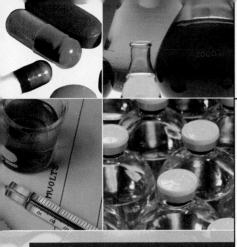

Chapter 18

Nonopioid Analgesics: Nonsteroidal Anti-Inflammatory Drugs (NSAIDs)

Key Terms

cyclooxygenase
cyclooxygenase-1 (COX-1)
cyclooxygenase-2 (COX-2)

Learning Objectives

On completion of this chapter, the student will:

- Discuss the types, uses, general drug actions, common adverse reactions, contraindications, precautions, and interactions of the NSAIDs.

- Discuss important preadministration and ongoing assessment activities the nurse should perform on the patient taking the NSAIDs.

- List nursing diagnoses particular to a patient taking an NSAID.

- Discuss the ways to promote an optimal response to therapy, how to manage common adverse reactions, and important points to keep in mind when educating patients about the use of NSAIDs.

B ecause of the action of nonsteroidal anti-inflammatory drugs (NSAIDs), some texts include the salicylates in the NSAID group, whereas others do not. Although the chemical and physiologic effects are similar, this text discusses the salicylates in a separate chapter (see Chapter 17). The NSAIDs are nonopioid analgesics. This chapter covers general information on the NSAIDs, which are listed in the Summary Drug Table: Nonsteroidal Anti-inflammatory Drugs. Like the salicylates, the NSAIDs have anti-inflammatory, antipyretic, and analgesic effects.

Actions

The NSAIDs are so named because they have anti-inflammatory effects, but do not belong to the steroidal group of substances and thus do not possess the adverse reactions associated with the steroids (see Chapter 50). In addition, NSAIDs have analgesic and antipyretic properties. Although their exact mechanisms of actions are not known, the NSAIDs are thought to act by inhibiting prostaglandin synthesis by inhibiting the action of the enzyme **cyclooxygenase**. This enzyme is responsible for prostaglandin synthesis. The NSAIDs act to inhibit the activity of two related enzymes:

SUMMARY DRUG TABLE   NONSTEROIDAL ANTI-INFLAMMATORY DRUGS

GENERIC NAME	TRADE NAME	USES	ADVERSE REACTIONS	DOSAGE RANGES
diclofenac potassium *dye-kloe'-fen-ak*	Cataflam	Acute or chronic pain of rheumatoid arthritis, osteoarthritis, ankylosing spondylitis, and dysmenorrhea	Nausea, gastric or duodenal ulcer formation, GI bleeding	50–200 mg orally divided into 2 or 3 doses
etodolac *ee-toe-doe'-lak*	Lodine	Osteoarthritis, rheumatoid arthritis, and acute pain	Dizziness, nausea, dyspepsia, rash, constipation, bleeding, diarrhea, tinnitus	300–500 mg BID; maximum daily dose 1200 mg
fenoprofen calcium *fen-oh-proe'-fen*	Nalfon	Same as etodolac	Same as etodolac	300–600 mg orally 3 or 4 times daily; maximum daily dose 3.2 g
flurbiprofen *flure-bih'-proe-fen*	Ansaid	Same as etodolac	Same as etodolac	Up to 300 mg/d orally in divided doses
ibuprofen *eye-byoo'-proe-fen*	Advil, Motrin, Nuprin	Mild to moderate pain, rheumatoid disorders, painful dysmenorrhea, fever	Nausea, dizziness, dyspepsia, gastric or duodenal ulcer, GI bleeding, headache	400 mg orally q4–6h; maximum daily dose 3.2 g
indomethacin *in-doe-meth'-a-sin*	Indocin	Rheumatoid disorders	Nausea, constipation, gastric or duodenal ulcer, GI bleeding, hematologic changes	25–50 mg orally, 3 to 4 times daily
ketoprofen *kee-toe-proe'-fen*	Orudis KT, Oruvail	Mild to moderate pain, rheumatoid disorders, aches and fever	Dizziness, visual disturbances, nausea, constipation, vomiting, diarrhea, gastric or duodenal ulcer formation, GI bleeding	12.5–75 mg orally, TID
ketorolac *kee'-toe-role-ak*	Toradol	Moderate to severe acute pain	Dyspepsia, nausea, GI pain and bleeding	Single dose: 60 mg IM or 30 mg IV Multiple dosing: 10 mg q4–6h; maximum daily dose 40 mg
meclofenamate sodium *me-kloe-fen-am'-ate*		Rheumatoid arthritis, mild to moderate pain, dysmenorrhea	Headache, dizziness, tiredness, insomnia, nausea, dyspepsia, constipation, rash, bleeding	50–400 mg orally q4–6h, maximum dose 400 mg/d
mefenamic acid *me-fe-nam'-ick*	Ponstel	Episodic acute mild to moderate pain (less than 1 wk duration)	Dizziness, tiredness, nausea, dyspepsis, rash, constipation, bleeding, diarrhea	250–500 mg q6h
meloxicam *mel-ox'-i-kam*	Mobic	Osteoarthritis	Nausea, dyspepsia, GI pain, headache, dizziness, somnolence, insomnia, rash	7.5–15 mg/d orally
nabumetone *nah-byew'-meh-tone*	Relafen	Rheumatoid arthritis and osteoarthritis	Dizziness, tiredness, nausea, dyspepsia, rash, constipation, bleeding, diarrhea	1000–2000 mg/d orally
naproxen *na-prox'-en*	Aleve, Anaprox, Naprosyn, Naprelan	Rheumatoid arthritis and osteoarthritis, mild to moderate pain, dysmenorrhea, general aches and fever	Dizziness, headache, nausea, vomiting, gastric or duodenal ulcer, GI bleeding	250–500 mg q6–8h orally; maximum daily dose 1.25 g

GENERIC NAME	TRADE NAME	USES	ADVERSE REACTIONS	DOSAGE RANGES
oxaprozin *ocks-a-pro'-zin*	Daypro	Rheumatoid arthritis and osteoarthritis	Dizziness, nausea, dyspepsia, rash, constipation, GI bleeding, diarrhea	1200 mg/d orally
piroxicam *peer-ox'-I-kam*	Feldene	Mild to moderate pain, rheumatoid arthritis and osteoarthritis	Nausea, vomiting, diarrhea, gastric or duodenal ulcer, GI bleeding	20 mg/d orally as a single dose or 10 mg orally BID
sulindac *sul-in'-dak*	Clinoril	Mild to moderate pain, rheumatoid arthritis, ankylosing spondylitis, osteoarthritis, gouty arthritis	Nausea, vomiting, diarrhea, constipation, gastric or duodenal ulcer, GI bleeding	150–200 mg orally BID
tolmetin sodium *tole'-met-in*	Tolectin	Rheumatoid arthritis and osteoarthritis	Nausea, vomiting, diarrhea, constipation, gastric or duodenal ulcer, GI bleeding	400 mg orally TID or BID; maximum daily dose 1800 mg
COX-2 Inhibitor				
celecoxib *sell-ah-cocks'-ib*	Celebrex	Acute pain, rheumatoid arthritis, ankylosing spondylitis, primary dysmenorrhea, and osteoarthritis; reduction of colorectal polyps in familial adenomatous polyposis	Headache, dyspepsia, rash See cardiovascular precautions	100–200 mg orally BID

- **cyclooxygenase-1 (COX-1)**, the enzyme that helps to maintain the stomach lining, and
- **cyclooxygenase-2 (COX-2)**, the enzyme that triggers pain and inflammation.

The traditional NSAIDs, such as ibuprofen and naproxen, are thought to regulate pain and inflammation by blocking COX-2. However, these drugs also inhibit COX-1, the enzyme that helps maintain the lining of the stomach. Therefore, blocking the effects of COX-2 produces the pain relief and blocking the effects of COX-1 produces the adverse reactions. This inhibition of COX-1 causes unwanted gastrointestinal (GI) reactions, such as stomach irritation and ulcers. The newer NSAID celecoxib (Celebrex) appears to work by specifically inhibiting the COX-2 enzyme, without inhibiting the COX-1 enzyme. Celecoxib relieves pain and inflammation with less potential for GI adverse reactions.

Uses

The NSAIDs are used for the treatment of
- Pain associated with osteoarthritis, rheumatoid arthritis, and other musculoskeletal disorders

- Mild to moderate pain
- Primary dysmenorrhea (menstrual cramps)
- Fever (reduction)

Adverse Reactions

Gastrointestinal System Reactions

- Nausea, vomiting, dyspepsia
- Anorexia, dry mouth
- Diarrhea, constipation
- Epigastric pain, indigestion, abdominal distress or discomfort, bloating
- Intestinal ulceration, stomatitis
- Jaundice

Central Nervous System Reactions

- Dizziness, anxiety, lightheadedness, vertigo
- Headache
- Drowsiness, somnolence (sleepiness), insomnia
- Confusion, depression
- Stroke, psychic disturbances

Nonopioid Analgesics

Cardiovascular Reactions

- Decrease or increase in blood pressure
- Congestive heart failure, cardiac arrhythmias
- Myocardial infarction

Renal Reactions

- Polyuria (excessive urination), dysuria (painful urination), oliguria (reduced urine output)
- Hematuria (blood in the urine), cystitis
- Elevated blood urea nitrogen (BUN)
- Acute renal failure in those with impaired renal function

Sensory Reactions

- Taste change
- Rhinitis (runny nose)
- Tinnitus (ringing in the ears)
- Visual disturbances, blurred or diminished vision, diplopia (double vision), swollen or irritated eyes, photophobia (sensitivity to light), reversible loss of color vision

Hematologic Reactions

- Pancytopenia (reduction in blood cell components), thrombocytopenia (reduced platelet count)
- Neutropenia (abnormally few neutrophils), eosinophilia (low eosinophil count), leukopenia (reduced white blood cell count), agranulocytosis (reduced granulocyte count)
- Aplastic anemia

Skin Reactions

- Rash, erythema (redness), irritation, skin eruptions
- Ecchymosis (subcutaneous hemorrhage), purpura (excessive skin hemorrhage causing red-purple patches under the skin)
- Exfoliative dermatitis, Stevens-Johnson syndrome

Metabolic/Endocrine Reactions

- Decreased appetite, weight increase or decrease
- Flushing, sweating
- Menstrual disorders, vaginal bleeding
- Hyperglycemia or hypoglycemia (high or low blood sugar)

Other

- Thirst, fever, chills
- Vaginitis

Contraindications

The NSAIDs are contraindicated in patients with known hypersensitivity. There is a cross-sensitivity to other NSAIDs. Therefore, if a patient is allergic to one NSAID, there is an increased risk of an allergic reaction with any other NSAID. Hypersensitivity to aspirin is a contraindication for all NSAIDs. In general, the NSAIDs are contraindicated during the third trimester of pregnancy and during lactation. Celecoxib is contraindicated in patients who are allergic to the sulfonamides or have a history of cardiac disease or stroke. Ibuprofen is contraindicated in those who have hypertension, peptic ulceration, or GI bleeding.

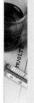

Nursing Alert

Celecoxib is associated with an increased risk of serious cardiovascular thrombosis, myocardial infarction, and stroke, all of which can be fatal. All NSAIDs may carry a similar risk. The nurse should always question the patient regarding a history of risk for or actual cardiovascular disease before administering NSAIDs. Because of this risk, celecoxib should not be used to relieve postoperative pain from coronary artery bypass graft (CABG).

Precautions

The NSAIDs should be used cautiously during pregnancy (category B), by elderly patients (increased risk of ulcer formation in patients older than 65 years), and by patients with bleeding disorders, renal disease, cardiovascular disease, or hepatic impairment.

Interactions

The following interactions may occur when an NSAID is administered with another agent:

Interacting Drug	Common Use	Effect of Interaction
anticoagulants	Blood thinner	Increased risk of bleeding
lithium	Antipsychotic drug used for bipolar disorder	Increased effectiveness and possible toxicity of lithium
cyclosporine	Antirejection agent (immuno-suppressant)	Increased effectiveness of cyclosporine
hydantoins	Anticonvulsant	Increased effectiveness of anticonvulsant
diuretics	Excretion of extra body fluid	Decreased effectiveness of diuretic
antihypertensive drugs	Blood pressure control	Decreased effectiveness of antihypertensive drug
acetaminophen in long-term use	Pain relief	Increased risk of renal impairment

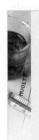

Nursing Alert

Ibuprofen is available to individuals as an over-the-counter (OTC) drug that may be purchased without a prescription. When assessing patients with pain, the nurse should ask what medications the patient is currently taking or has tried for pain relief already. Because of the risk of Reye's syndrome from aspirin, ibuprofen is used in treatment of children with juvenile arthritis and for fever reduction in children 6 months to 12 years of age.

NURSING PROCESS

The Patient Receiving a Nonsteroidal Anti-inflammatory Drug

ASSESSMENT

PREADMINISTRATION ASSESSMENT

Before administering an NSAID, the nurse needs to determine if the patient has any history of allergy to aspirin or any other NSAID. The nurse determines if the patient has a history of GI bleeding, cardiovascular disease, stroke, hypertension, peptic ulceration, or impaired hepatic or renal function. If so, the nurse notifies the primary health care provider before administering an NSAID.

In addition, before giving an NSAID to a patient, the nurse assesses and documents the type, onset, intensity, and location of the pain. It is important to determine if this problem is different in any way from previous episodes of pain or discomfort. If the patient is receiving an NSAID for arthritis, a musculoskeletal disorder, or soft tissue inflammation, the nurse should examine the joints or areas involved. The appearance of the skin over the joint or affected area or any limitation of motion is documented. The nurse evaluates the patient's ability to carry out activities of daily living. This important information is used to develop a care plan, as well as to evaluate the response to drug therapy.

ONGOING ASSESSMENT

During the ongoing assessment, the nurse monitors the patient for relief of pain. The nurse reassesses the patient's pain rating 30 to 60 minutes after administration of the drug. If pain persists, it is important to assess its severity, location, and intensity. Then, every 4 hours, or more frequently if necessary, the nurse monitors the vital signs. Hot, dry, flushed skin and a decrease in urinary output may develop if temperature elevation is prolonged; consequently, dehydration can occur. The nurse assesses the joints for a decrease in inflammation and greater mobility. The nurse reports adverse reactions, such as unusual or prolonged bleeding or dark-colored stools, to the primary health care provider.

NURSING DIAGNOSES

Drug-specific nursing diagnoses are highlighted in the Nursing Diagnoses Checklist. Other nursing diagnoses applicable to these drugs are discussed in depth in Chapter 4.

Nursing Diagnoses Checklist

✓ **Acute or Chronic Pain** related to peripheral tissue damage caused by the disease process or GI bleeding or inflammation from NSAID therapy

✓ **Impaired Physical Mobility** related to muscle and joint stiffness

✓ **Disturbed Sensory Perception: Visual** related to adverse drug reactions

PLANNING

The expected outcomes for the patient depend on the reason for administration of the NSAID, but may include an optimal response to drug therapy, which includes relief of pain and fever, supporting the patient's needs related to the management of adverse reactions, and an understanding of and compliance with the prescribed treatment regimen.

IMPLEMENTATION

PROMOTING AN OPTIMAL RESPONSE TO THERAPY

The nurse should give the NSAID with food, milk, or antacids. Patients who do not experience adequate pain relief using one NSAID may have success using another NSAID. However, several weeks of treatment may be necessary to achieve full therapeutic response.

MONITORING AND MANAGING PATIENT NEEDS

PAIN The NSAIDs are prescribed for the pain and inflammation associated with arthritis. Because older adults have a higher incidence of both rheumatoid arthritis and osteoarthritis and may use the NSAID on a long-term basis, they are particularly vulnerable to GI bleeding. The nurse should encourage the patient to take the drug with a full glass of water or with food because this may decrease the GI effects. The nurse checks whether a new pain experience may be caused by gastric bleeding or inflammation.

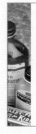

Gerontologic Alert

Age appears to increase the possibility of adverse reactions to the NSAIDs. The risk of serious ulcer disease in adults older than 65 years is increased with higher doses of the NSAIDs. Use greater care and begin with reduced dosages in the elderly, increasing the dosage slowly.

IMPAIRED PHYSICAL MOBILITY The nurse provides comfort measures to the patient with pain from the limbs or joints affected by the various musculoskeletal disorders. Limbs are supported by proper positioning; applications of heat or cold, joint rest, and avoidance of joint overuse are additional comfort measures. Various orthopedic devices, such as splints and braces, may be used to support inflamed joints. The use of assistive mobility devices, such as canes, crutches, and walkers, eases pain by limiting movement or stress from weight bearing on painful joints. The nurse may need to assist the patient while ambulating or using assistive devices to walk. Patients with osteoarthritis should exhibit an increased range of motion and a reduction in tenderness, pain, stiffness, and swelling.

It is important to observe the patient receiving an NSAID for adverse drug reactions throughout therapy. GI reactions are the most common and can be severe, especially in those prone to upper GI tract disease. Cardiovascular reactions can be very severe and even lead to death.

Because of the severity of some of these adverse drug reactions, the nurse notifies the primary health care provider of any complaints the patient may have.

Nursing Alert

The nurse withholds the next dose and notifies the primary health care provider immediately if any gastric or cardiac symptoms occur.

DISTURBED SENSORY PERCEPTION: VISUAL The NSAIDs may cause visual disturbances. The nurse reports any complaints of blurred or diminished vision or changes in color vision to the primary health care provider. Corneal deposits and retinal disturbances may also occur. The primary health care provider may discontinue therapy if ocular changes are noted. Blurred vision may be significant and warrants thorough examination. Because visual changes may be asymptomatic, patients on long-term therapy require periodic eye examinations.

EDUCATING THE PATIENT AND FAMILY

In many instances, an NSAID may be prescribed for a prolonged period, such as when the patient has arthritis. Some patients may discontinue their drug use, fail to take the drug at the prescribed or recommended intervals, increase the dose, or decrease the time interval between doses, especially if there is an increase or decrease in their symptoms. The patient and family must understand that the drug is to be taken even though symptoms have been relieved. The nurse develops a teaching plan to include the following information:

- Take the drug exactly as prescribed by the primary health care provider. Do not increase or decrease the dosage, and do not take any OTC drugs without first consulting the primary health care provider. Notify the primary health care provider or dentist if pain is not relieved.

- Take the drug with food or a full glass of water unless indicated otherwise by the primary health care provider. If gastric upset occurs, take the drug with food or milk. If the problem persists, contact the primary health care provider.

- Whether taking an NSAID on a regular or occasional basis, inform all health care providers, including dentists, that you are taking it.

- If the drug is used to reduce fever, contact the primary health care provider if the temperature remains elevated for more than 24 hours after beginning therapy.

Home Care Checklist

Using Over-the-Counter Nonsteroidal Anti-inflammatory Drugs

Quite a few NSAIDs are available as OTC products. OTC formulations such as ibuprofen (Advil, Motrin, and Nuprin), ketoprofen (Orudis), and naproxen sodium (Aleve) are available to any consumer. The potential for misuse and abuse is high, especially when one is confronted by the large number of advertisements on television and in print heralding the wonderful benefits of these products.

Now, more than ever, patients need to be educated about these products. A thorough drug history and knowledge of the consumer's underlying disorder are essential to setting up an effective teaching program. In addition to the topics that are normally addressed with any drug teaching plan, the nurse stresses the following:

☑ Indications for using the drug (the reason the patient might take it)

☑ Dosage information, including frequency and maximum daily amounts

☑ Possible drug–drug and drug–food interactions

☑ Possible adverse effects, including life-threatening ones such as bleeding, cardiovascular, and stroke risk

☑ Need to read and heed all manufacturer's instructions, including the number of days that the patient should use the drug and when to notify the physician (e.g., if fever is not resolved within 3 days or pain persists)

Although this is not a foolproof remedy for eliminating possible misuse and abuse, thorough patient education can help minimize the risk of problems associated with OTC NSAIDs.

- Do not consistently use an OTC nonopioid analgesic to treat chronic pain without first consulting the primary health care provider.

- Severe or recurrent pain or high or continued fever may indicate serious illness. If pain persists more than 10 days in adults, or if fever persists more than 3 days, consult the primary health care provider.

- Avoid using aspirin or other salicylates when taking an NSAID.

- The drug may take several days to produce an effect (relief of pain and tenderness). If some or all of the symptoms are not relieved after 2 weeks of therapy, continue taking the drug, but notify the primary health care provider.

- These drugs may cause drowsiness, dizziness, or blurred vision. Use caution while driving or performing tasks that require alertness.

- Notify the primary health care provider if any of the following adverse reactions occur: skin rash, itching, visual disturbances, weight gain, edema, diarrhea, black stools, nausea, vomiting, chest/leg pain, numbness or persistent headache. See the Home Care Checklist: Using Over-the-Counter Nonsteroidal Anti-inflammatory Drugs.

EVALUATION

- Pain is relieved, and discomfort is reduced or eliminated.

- Body temperature is normal.

- Patients with joint disease report better mobility.

- Adverse reactions are identified, reported to the primary health care provider, and managed.

- The patient verbalizes the importance of complying with the prescribed treatment regimen.

- The patient demonstrates an understanding of the treatment regimen and adverse effects of the drug.

Critical Thinking Exercises

1. Mr. Nunn, aged 68 years, has been prescribed an NSAID for the treatment of arthritis and has been taking the drug for 2 weeks. During an outpatient appointment, Mr. Nunn tells you that he has noticed very little, if any, improvement in his arthritis and complains of nausea, difficulty hearing, constipation, and bloating. Analyze what steps you might take to investigate this problem. Give a reason for your answers.

Nonopioid Analgesics

2. Ms. Parker, aged 72 years, is prescribed celecoxib for osteoarthritis. She is confused at times and has difficulty hearing. In developing a teaching plan for Ms. Parker, discuss what assessments would be important. Identify points to include in her teaching plan.

Review Questions

1. The nurse observes a patient for which of the common adverse reactions when administering naproxen?

   A. Headache, dyspepsia

   B. Blurred vision, constipation

   C. Anorexia, tinnitus

   D. Stomatitis, confusion

2. An elderly patient is receiving sulindac. The nurse is aware that older adults taking NSAIDs are at increased risk for _____.

   A. ulcer disease

   B. stroke

   C. myocardial infarction

   D. gout

3. When a patient is receiving an NSAID, the nurse must monitor the patient for _____.

   A. agitation, which indicates nervous system involvement

   B. urinary retention, which indicates renal insufficiency

   C. decrease in white blood cell count, which increases the risk for infection

   D. gastrointestinal symptoms, which can be serious and sometimes fatal

4. Which of the following statements would the nurse be certain to include in a teaching plan for the patient taking an NSAID?

   A. If GI upset occurs, take this drug on an empty stomach.

   B. Avoid the use of aspirin or other salicylates when taking these drugs.

   C. These drugs can cause extreme confusion and should be used with caution.

   D. Relief from pain and inflammation should occur within 30 minutes after the first dose.

Medication Dosage Problems

1. Naproxen (Naprosyn) oral suspension 250 mg is prescribed. The dosage on hand is oral suspension 125 mg/5 mL. The nurse administers _____.

2. The physician orders celecoxib (Celebrex) 200 mg orally. The nurse has celecoxib 100-mg tablets on hand. The nurse administers _____.

To check your answers, see Appendix G.

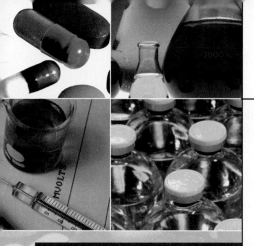

Opioid Analgesics

Learning Objectives

On completion of this chapter, the student will:

- Discuss the uses, general drug action, general adverse reactions, contraindications, precautions, and interactions of the opioid analgesics.

- Discuss important preadministration and ongoing assessment activities the nurse should perform on the patient taking the opioid analgesics.

- List nursing diagnoses particular to a patient taking an opioid analgesic.

- Discuss ways to promote optimal response to therapy, how to manage adverse reactions, and important points to keep in mind when educating patients about the use of opioid analgesics.

O pioid analgesics are the analgesics obtained from the opium plant. More than 20 different alkaloids are obtained from the unripe seed of the opium poppy. The analgesic properties of opium have been known for hundreds of years. The opioid analgesics are controlled substances (see Chapter 1) used to treat moderate to severe pain centrally in the brain. These drugs do not change the tissues where the pain sensation originates; instead, they change how the patient perceives the pain sensation.

Pain is universal. The World Health Organization (WHO) has addressed the problem of pain by developing a "pain ladder" that directs treatment for pain in three steps (Fig. 19-1). For mild pain, a Step 1 nonopioid analgesic may be prescribed. If necessary, an adjuvant (extra helping) agent may be used to promote the pain-relieving effect. If pain persists or worsens even with appropriate dosage increases, a Step 2 or Step 3 analgesic is indicated. Step 2 and Step 3 analgesics contain opioid substances. Most patients with severe pain require a Step 2 or Step 3 analgesic.

OPIOID ANALGESICS

The opiates are natural substances obtained from raw opium. They include morphine sulfate, codeine, hydrochlorides of opium alkaloids, and camphorated tincture of opium. Morphine sulfate, when extracted from raw opium and treated chemically, yields the semisynthetic opioids hydromorphone, oxymorphone, oxycodone, and heroin. Heroin is an illegal narcotic substance in the United States and is not used in medicine. Synthetic opioids are those manufactured analgesics with properties and actions similar to the natural opioids. Examples of synthetic opioid analgesics are methadone, levorphanol, remifentanil, and meperidine. Additional analgesics are listed in the Summary Drug Table: Opioid Analgesics.

SUMMARY DRUG TABLE   OPIOID ANALGESICS

GENERIC NAME	TRADE NAME	USES	ADVERSE REACTIONS*	DOSAGE RANGES
Agonists				
alfentanil HCl *al-fen'-ta-nil*	Alfentha	Anesthetic adjunct	Respiratory depression, skeletal muscle rigidity, constipation, nausea, vomiting	Individualize dosage and titrate to obtain desired effect
Codeine *koe'-deen*		Moderate to severe pain, antitussive, anesthetic adjunct	Sedation, sweating, headache, dizziness, lethargy, confusion, lightheadedness	Analgesic: 15–60 mg q4–6h orally, SC, IM
fentanyl *fen'-ta-nil*	Sublimaze	Severe pain, anesthetic adjunct	Sweating, headache, vertigo, lethargy, confusion, nausea, vomiting, respiratory depression	Same as alfentanil
fentanyl transdermal systems	Duragesic	Chronic pain unmanaged by other opioids	Sedation, sweating, headache, vertigo, lethargy, confusion, lightheadedness, nausea, vomiting	Individualized dosage: 25–175-mcg transdermal patch (dose is amount absorbed per hour)
fentanyl transmucosal system	Actiq	Management of breakthrough cancer pain	Sedation, sweating, headache, vertigo, lethargy, confusion, lightheadedness, nausea, vomiting	200–1600 mcg/dose , depending on pain severity
hydromorphone *hy-droe-mor'-fone*	Dilaudid	Moderate to severe pain	Sedation, vertigo, lethargy, confusion, lightheadedness, nausea, vomiting	2–4 mg orally, q4–6h; 3 mg q6–8h rectally; 1–2 mg IM or SC q4–6h
levorphanol tartrate *lee-vor'-fa-nole*	Levo-Dromoran	Moderate to severe pain, preoperative sedation	Dizziness, nausea, vomiting, dry mouth, sweating, respiratory depression	2 mg orally, q3–6h; 1 mg IV q3–8h
meperidine *me-per'-i-deen*	Demerol	Acute moderate to severe pain, preoperative sedation, anesthetic adjunct	Lightheadedness, constipation, dizziness, nausea, vomiting, respiratory depression	50–150 mg orally, IM, SC, q3–4h
methadone *meth'-a-doan*	Dolophine	Severe pain; treatment of opioid dependence	Lightheadedness, dizziness, sedation, nausea, vomiting, constipation	Analgesic: 2.5–10 mg orally, IM, SC q4h; detoxification: 10–40 mg orally, IV
morphine sulfate *mor'-feen*	Roxanol, Avinza, Kadian; timed release: MS Contin, Oramorph SR	Acute/chronic pain, preoperative sedation, anesthetic adjunct, dyspnea	Sedation, hypotension, increased sweating, constipation, dizziness, drowsiness, nausea, vomiting, dry mouth, somnolence, respiratory depression	Acute pain relief: 10–30 mg q4h; chronic pain relief: individualized
oxycodone *ox-ee-koe'-doan*	Roxicodone; timed release: OxyContin	Moderate to severe pain	Lightheadedness, sedation, constipation, dizziness, nausea, vomiting, sweating, respiratory depression	10–30 mg orally q4h
oxymorphone *ox-ee-mor'-fone*	Numorphan	Moderate to severe pain, preoperative sedation, obstetric analgesia	Lightheadedness, sedation, constipation, dizziness, nausea, vomiting, respiratory depression	1–1.5 mg SC or IM q4–6h

GENERIC NAME	TRADE NAME	USES	ADVERSE REACTIONS*	DOSAGE RANGES
propoxyphene *proe-pox'-i-feen*	Darvon, Darvon-N	Moderate to severe pain	Lightheadedness, sedation, constipation, dizziness, nausea, vomiting, respiratory depression	65–100 mg orally q4h; maximum dose 600 mg/d
remifentanil HCl *reh-mih-fen'-tah-nill*	Ultiva	Anesthetic adjunct	Lightheadedness, skeletal muscle rigidity, nausea, vomiting, respiratory depression, sweating	Same as alfentanil
sufentanil *suh-fen'-tah-nill*	Sufenta	Anesthetic adjunct	Same as alfentanil	Same as alfentanil
tramadol *tram'-a-doll*	Ultram	Moderate to severe chronic pain	Same as morphine sulfate	Titrate individual dose starting at 25 mg up to 100 mg/d
Agonists-Antagonists				
buprenorphine *byoo-pre-nor'-feen*	Buprenex, Suboxone, Subutex	Moderate to severe chronic pain, treatment of opioid dependence	Lightheadedness, sedation, dizziness, nausea, vomiting, respiratory depression	Parenteral: 0.03 mg q6h IV or IM Sublingual: 12–16 mg/d
butorphanol *byoo-tor'-fa-nole*	Stadol, Stadol NS	Acute pain, anesthetic adjunct	Lightheadedness, sedation, constipation, dizziness, nausea, vomiting, respiratory depression	1–4 mg IM, 0.5–2 mg IV; Nasal spray (NS): 1 mg (spray), repeat in 60–90 min; may repeat q3–4h
nalbuphine *nal'-byoo-feen*	Nubain	Moderate to severe chronic pain, anesthetic adjunct	Lightheadedness, sedation, constipation, dizziness, nausea, vomiting, respiratory depression	10 mg/70 kg SC, IM, or IV q3–6h
pentazocine *pen-taz'-oh-seen*	Talwin, Talwin Nx	Same as nalbuphine	Same as nalbuphine	30–60 mg IM, SC, IV q3–4h; maximum daily dose 360 mg

*The adverse reactions of the narcotic analgesics are discussed extensively in the chapter. Some of the reactions may be less severe or intense than others.

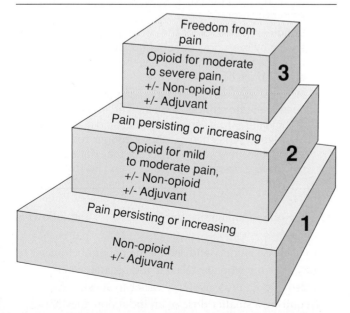

Figure 19.1 World Health Organization pain relief ladder (© World Health Organization 2005. Redrawn with permission.)

Actions

Cells in the central nervous system (CNS) have receptor sites called *opiate receptors*. Although opiates are attracted to many different receptor sites, the mu and kappa receptors are the ones that produce the analgesic, sedative, and euphoric effects associated with analgesic drugs.

Drugs that bind well to a receptor are called *agonist* agents. An opioid analgesic may be classified as an agonist, partial agonist, and mixed agonist-antagonist. The **agonist** binds to a receptor and causes a response. A **partial agonist** binds to a receptor, but the response is limited (i.e., is not as great as with the agonist). An **agonist-antagonist** has properties of both the agonist and antagonist. These drugs have some agonist activity at the receptor sites and some antagonist activity at the receptor sites. Antagonists bind to a receptor and cause no response. An antagonist can reverse the effects of the agonist. This reversal is possi-

Table 19.1 Bodily Responses Associated With Opioid Receptor Sites

Receptor	Bodily Response
Mu	Morphine-like supraspinal analgesia, respiratory and physical depression, miosis, reduced GI motility
Delta	Dysphoria, psychotomimetic effects (e.g., hallucinations), respiratory and vasomotor stimulations caused by drugs with antagonist activity
Kappa	Sedation and miosis

ble because the antagonist competes with the agonist for a receptor site. Drugs that act as opioid antagonists are discussed in Chapter 20.

In addition to the pain-relieving effects, other, nonintended responses occur when the opiate receptor sites are stimulated. These include respiratory depression, decreased gastrointestinal (GI) motility, and **miosis** (pinpoint pupils). Table 19-1 identifies the responses in the body associated with three of the opiate receptors. The actions of the opioid analgesics on the various organs and structures of the body (also called *secondary pharmacologic effects*) are shown in Display 19-1. With long-term use, the patient's body adapts to these secondary effects. The one body system that does not adapt and compensate is the GI system. Slow GI motility and the resulting constipation are always a problem in opioid therapy.

The most widely used opioid, morphine sulfate is an effective drug for moderately severe to severe pain. Morphine sulfate is considered the prototype (model) opioid. Morphine sulfate is considered the gold standard in pain management. Morphine sulfate's actions, uses, and ability to relieve pain are the standards against which other opioid analgesics are often compared. Charts called *equal-analgesic conversions* compare other opioid doses with the doses of morphine sulfate that would be used for the same level of pain control.

Other opioids, such as meperidine and levorphanol, are effective for the treatment of moderate to severe pain. For mild to moderate pain, the primary health care provider may order an opioid such as codeine or pentazocine.

Uses

The opioid analgesics are used primarily for the treatment of moderate to severe acute and chronic pain and in the treatment and management of opiate dependence. In addi-

Display 19.1 Secondary Pharmacologic Effects of the Opioid Analgesics

- **Cardiovascular**—peripheral vasodilation, decreased peripheral resistance, inhibition of baroreceptors (pressure receptors located in the aortic arch and carotid sinus that regulate blood pressure), orthostatic hypotension and fainting
- **Central nervous system**—euphoria, drowsiness, apathy, mental confusion, alterations in mood, reduction in body temperature, feelings of relaxation, dysphoria (depression accompanied by anxiety); nausea and vomiting are caused by direct stimulation of the emetic chemoreceptors located in the medulla. The degree to which these occur usually depends on the drug and the dose.
- **Dermatologic**—histamine release, pruritus, flushing, and red eyes
- **Gastrointestinal**—decrease in gastric motility (prolonged emptying time); decrease in biliary, pancreatic, and intestinal secretions; delay in digestion of food in the small intestine; increase in resting tone, with the potential for spasms, epigastric distress, or biliary colic (caused by constriction of the sphincter of Oddi). These drugs can cause constipation and anorexia.
- **Genitourinary**—urinary urgency and difficulty with urination, caused by spasms of the ureter. Urinary urgency also may occur because of the action of the drugs on the detrusor muscle of the bladder. Some patients may experience difficulty voiding because of contraction of the bladder sphincter.
- **Respiratory**—depressant effects on respiratory rate (caused by a reduced sensitivity of the respiratory center to carbon dioxide)
- **Cough**—suppression of the cough reflex (antitussive effect) by exerting a direct effect on the cough center in the medulla. Codeine has the most noticeable effect on the cough reflex.
- **Medulla**—Nausea and vomiting can occur when the chemoreceptor trigger zone located in the medulla is stimulated. To a varying degree, opioid analgesics also depress the chemoreceptor trigger zone. Therefore, nausea and vomiting may or may not occur when these drugs are given.

tion, the opioid analgesics may be used for the following reasons:

- To decrease anxiety and sedate the patient before surgery. Patients who are relaxed and sedated when an anesthetic agent is given are easier to anesthetize (requiring a smaller dose of an induction anesthetic), as well as easier to maintain under anesthesia.

- To support anesthesia (i.e., as an adjunct during anesthesia)

- To promote obstetric analgesia

- To relieve anxiety in patients with dyspnea (breathing difficulty) associated with pulmonary edema

- Administered intrathecally or epidurally, to control pain for extended periods without apparent loss of motor, sensory, or sympathetic nerve function

- To relieve pain associated with a myocardial infarction (morphine sulfate is the agent of choice)

- To manage opiate dependence

- To induce conscious sedation before a diagnostic or therapeutic procedure in the hospital setting

- To treat severe diarrhea and intestinal cramping (camphorated tincture of opium may be used)

- To relieve severe, persistent cough (codeine may be helpful, although the drug's use has declined)

Adverse Reactions

Central Nervous System Reactions

- Euphoria, weakness, headache

- Lightheadedness, dizziness, sedation

- Miosis, insomnia, agitation, tremor

- Increased intercranial pressure, impairment of mental and physical tasks

Respiratory System Reactions

- Depression of rate and depth of breathing

Gastrointestinal Reactions

- Nausea, vomiting

- Dry mouth, biliary tract spasms

- Constipation, anorexia

Cardiovascular System Reactions

- Facial flushing

- Tachycardia, bradycardia, palpitations

- Peripheral circulatory collapse

Genitourinary System Reactions

- Urinary retention or hesitancy

- Spasms of the ureters and bladder sphincter

Allergic Reactions

- Pruritus, rash, and urticaria

Other

- Sweating, pain at injection site, and local tissue irritation

Contraindications

All opioid analgesics are contraindicated in patients with known hypersensitivity to the drugs. These drugs are contraindicated in patients with acute bronchial asthma, emphysema, or upper airway obstruction and in patients with head injury or increased intracranial pressure. The drugs are also contraindicated in patients with convulsive disorders, severe renal or hepatic dysfunction, and acute ulcerative colitis. The opioid analgesics are pregnancy category C drugs (oxycodone is in pregnancy category B) and are not recommended for use during pregnancy or labor because they may prolong labor or cause respiratory depression in the neonate. The use of opioid analgesics is recommended during pregnancy only if the benefit to the mother outweighs the potential harm to the fetus.

Precautions

Opioid analgesics should be used cautiously in elderly patients and in patients considered "opioid naive," that is, patients who have not been medicated with opioid drugs before and who are consequently at greatest risk for respiratory depression. The drugs should be administered cautiously in patients undergoing biliary surgery (because of the risk for spasm of the sphincter of Oddi; in these patients meperidine is the drug of choice). Patients who are lactating should wait at least 4 to 6 hours after taking the drug to breast-feed the infant. Additional precautions apply to patients with undiagnosed abdominal pain, hypoxia, supraventricular tachycardia, prostatic hypertrophy, and renal or hepatic impairment.

Interactions

The following interactions may occur when an opioid analgesic is administered with another agent:

Interacting Drug	Common Use	Effect of Interaction
alcohol	Social occasions	Increased risk for CNS depression
antihistamines	Prevent or relieve allergic reactions	Increased risk for CNS depression
antidepressants	Alleviate depression	Increased risk for CNS depression
sedatives	Sedation	Increased risk for CNS depression
phenothiazines	Relief of agitation, anxiety, vomiting	Increased risk for CNS depression
opioid agonist-antagonist (Nubain, Talwin)	Gynecologic or obstetric pain relief	Opioid withdrawal symptoms (if long-term opioid use)
barbiturates	Used in general anesthesia	Respiratory depression, hypotension, or sedation

Herbal Alert

The term *passion flower* is used to denote many of the approximately 400 species of herb in the genus *Passiflora*. Passion flower has been used in medicine to treat pain, anxiety, and insomnia. Some herbalists use it to treat symptoms of parkinsonism. Passion flower is often used in combination with other natural substances, such valerian, chamomile, and hops, for promoting relaxation, rest, and sleep. Although no adverse reactions have been reported, large doses may cause CNS depression. The use of passion flower is contraindicated in pregnancy and in patients taking the monoamine oxidase inhibitors (MAOIs). Passion flower contains coumarin, and the risk of bleeding may be increased in patients taking warfarin (Coumadin) and passion flower. The following are recommended dosages for passion flower:

- Tea: 1-4 cups per day (made with 1 tablespoon of the crude herb per cup)
- Tincture (2 g/5 mL): 2 teaspoons (10 mL) 3-4 times daily
- Dried herb: 2 g 3-4 times daily.

NURSING PROCESS

The Patient Receiving an Opioid Analgesic for Pain

ASSESSMENT

PREADMINISTRATION ASSESSMENT

As part of the preadministration assessment, the nurse assesses and documents the type, onset, intensity, and location of the pain. The nurse documents a description of the pain (e.g., sharp, dull, stabbing, throbbing) and an estimate of when the pain began. Further questioning and more detailed information about the pain are necessary if the pain is of a different type than the patient had been experiencing previously or if it is in a different area.

The nurse reviews the patient's health history, allergy history, and past and current drug therapies. This is especially important when an opioid is given for the first time because data may be obtained during the initial history and physical assessment that require the nurse to contact the primary health care provider. For example, the patient may state that nausea and vomiting occurred when he or she was given a drug for pain several years ago. Further questioning of the patient is necessary because this information may influence the primary health care provider's decision to administer a specific opioid drug.

ONGOING ASSESSMENT

The nurse obtains the blood pressure, pulse and respiratory rate, and pain rating in 5 to 10 minutes if the drug is given intravenously (IV), 20 to 30 minutes if the drug is administered intramuscularly or subcutaneously, and 30 or more minutes if the drug is given orally. It is important to notify the primary health care provider if the analgesic is ineffective because a higher dose or a different opioid analgesic may be required.

During the ongoing assessment, it is important for the nurse to ask about the pain regularly and believe the patient and family in their reports of pain. Nursing judgment must be exercised because not all instances of a change in pain type, location, or intensity require notifying the primary health care provider. For example, if a patient recovering from recent abdominal surgery experiences pain in the calf of the leg (suggesting venous thrombosis), the nurse should immediately notify the primary health care provider. However, it is not important to contact the primary health care provider for pain that is slightly worse because the patient has been moving in bed.

The *opioid-naive* patient who does not use opioids routinely and is being given an opioid drug for acute pain relief or a surgical procedure is at greatest risk for respiratory depression after opioid administration. Respiratory depression may occur in patients receiving a normal dose if the patient is vulnerable (e.g., in a weakened or debilitated state). Elderly, **cachectic** (malnourished/general poor health), or debilitated patients may have a reduced initial dose until their response to the drug is known. If the patient's respiratory rate is 10 breaths/min or less, the nurse monitors the patient at more frequent intervals and notifies the primary health care provider immediately. Patients involved in long-term opioid therapy for pain relief build tolerance to the physical adverse effects of the drugs; respiratory depression is typically not seen in these patients.

When an opiate is used as an antidiarrheal drug, the nurse records each bowel movement, as well as its appearance, color, and consistency. The nurse should notify the primary health care provider immediately if diarrhea is not relieved or becomes worse, if the patient has severe abdominal pain, or if blood in the stool is noted.

NURSING DIAGNOSES

Drug-specific nursing diagnoses are highlighted in the Nursing Diagnoses Checklist. Other nursing diagnoses applicable to these drugs are discussed in depth in Chapter 4.

Nursing Diagnoses Checklist

✔ **Ineffective Breathing Pattern** related to pain and effects on breathing center by opioids

✔ **Risk for Injury** related to dizziness or lightheadedness from opioid administration

✔ **Constipation** related to the decreased gastrointestinal motility caused by opioids

✔ **Imbalanced Nutrition: Less Than Body Requirements** related to anorexia caused by opioids

PLANNING

The expected outcomes of the patient may include relief of pain, supporting the patient needs related to the management of adverse reactions, an understanding of **patient-controlled analgesia** (when applicable), absence of injury, adequate nutrition intake, and understanding of and compliance with the prescribed treatment regimen.

IMPLEMENTATION
RELIEVING ACUTE PAIN

Patient-controlled analgesia (PCA) allows patients to administer their own analgesic by means of an IV pump system (Fig. 19-2). The patient does not have to wait for the nurse to administer the medicine. Pumps are preset with small amounts of the opioid medication that the patient can administer by pushing a button on the pump. The medication can be delivered, for example, when the patient begins to feel pain or when the patient wishes to ambulate but wants some medication to prevent pain on getting out of bed. Many postoperative patients require less opioid when they can self-administer the medicine for pain. When patients take less opioid, they also experience fewer unpleasant adverse reactions, such as nausea and constipation. Because the self-administration system is under the control of the nurse, who adds the drug to the infusion pump and sets the time interval (or lockout interval) between doses, the patient cannot receive an overdose of the drug.

RELIEVING CHRONIC SEVERE PAIN

Morphine sulfate is the most widely used drug in the management of chronic severe pain. The fact that this drug can

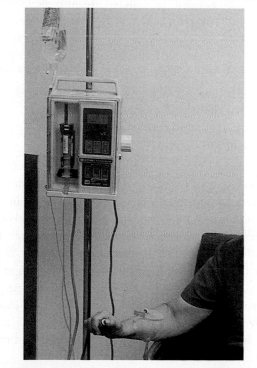

Figure 19.2 Patient-controlled analgesia allows the client to self-administer medication, as necessary, to control pain.

Opioid Analgesics

Table 19.2 Opioid/Nonopioid Combination Oral Analgesics

Brand Name	Opioid	Nonopioid
Tylenol #3	codeine 30 mg	acetaminophen 300 mg
Loratab	hydrocodone 2.5 mg	acetaminophen 167 mg
Vicodin	hydrocodone 5 mg	acetaminophen 500 mg
Vicodin ES	hydrocodone 7.5 mg	acetaminophen 750 mg
Percodan	oxycodone 5 mg	aspirin 325 mg
Percocet	oxycodone 5 mg	acetaminophen 325 mg
Roxicet	oxycodone 5 mg	acetaminophen 325 mg
Darvon-Compound 65	propoxyphene 65 mg	aspirin 389 mg; caffeine 32.4 mg
Darvocet-N 50	propoxyphene 50 mg	acetaminophen 325 mg
Darvocet-N 100	propoxyphene 100 mg	acetaminophen 650 mg

be given orally, subcutaneously, intramuscularly, IV, and rectally in the form of a suppository makes it tremendously versatile. Medication for chronic pain should be scheduled around the clock and not given on a PRN (as-needed) basis. With any chronic pain medication, the oral route is preferred as long as the patient can swallow or can tolerate sublingual administration.

Using the concept of the WHO pain ladder for chronic pain, medications that work to relieve pain both peripherally and centrally will be ordered. To provide good pain relief based on the pain ladder, drugs that combine a nonopioid and an opioid analgesic are available. These drugs work well at dealing with the inflammation at the peripheral site, as well as modifying the pain perception centrally in the brain. Table 19-2 lists many of these drugs and their combination ingredients.

Controlled-released forms of opioids are indicated for the management of moderate to severe pain when a continuous, around-the-clock analgesic is needed for an extended time. Examples of these drugs include oxycodone (Oxy-Contin) and morphine sulfate (Oramorph SR). The medication is given once every 8 to 12 hours; the actual drug is slowly released over time so the patient does not get all the medication at once. Controlled-released drugs are not intended for use as a PRN analgesic. The patient may experience fewer adverse reactions with oxycodone products than with morphine sulfate, and the drug is effective and safe for elderly patients. Controlled-release tablets should be swallowed whole and are not to be broken, chewed, or crushed.

When long-acting forms of the opioids are used, a fast-acting form may be given for breakthrough pain. These are typically ordered on a PRN basis to be used between the

long-acting doses for acute pain episodes. Morphine sulfate in oral or sublingual tablets is commonly used. Oral transmucosal fentanyl (Actiq) is also used to treat breakthrough pain.

Fentanyl transdermal is a transdermal system that is effective in the management of severe pain associated with diseases like cancer. The transdermal system allows for a timed-release patch containing the drug fentanyl to be activated over a 72-hour period. A small number of patients may require systems applied every 48 hours. The nurse monitors for adverse effects in the same manner as for other opioid analgesics.

Gerontologic Alert

The transdermal route should be used with caution in the elderly because the amount of subcutaneous tissue is reduced in the aging process. The transdermal route of drug administration is used because it treats severe pain most effectively, and should not be used simply for the convenience of administration.

When pain is best relieved by a combination of drugs and not just the opioid analgesics alone, a mixture of an oral opioid and other drugs may be used to obtain relief. Brompton's mixture is one of the most commonly used solutions. In addition to the opioid, such as morphine sulfate or methadone, other drugs may be used in the solution, including antidepressants, stimulants, aspirin, acetaminophen, and tranquilizers. The pharmacist prepares the solution according to the primary health care provider's instructions. It is necessary to monitor for the adverse reactions of each drug contained in the solution. The time interval for administration varies. Some primary health care providers may order the mixture on a PRN basis; others may order it given at regular intervals.

Over time, the patient taking an opioid analgesic develops tolerance to it. The rate at which tolerance develops varies according to the dosage, the route of administration, and the individual. Patients taking oral medications develop tolerance more slowly than those taking the drugs parenterally. Some patients develop tolerance quickly and need larger doses every few weeks, whereas others are maintained on the same dosage schedule throughout the course of the illness.

The fear of respiratory depression is a concern for many nurses administering an opioid, and some nurses may hesitate to administer the drug. However, respiratory depression rarely occurs in patients using an opioid for chronic pain. In fact, these patients usually develop tolerance to the respiratory depressant effects of the drug very quickly. Nurses should be more concerned about adverse effects on the GI system. The decrease in GI motility causes constipation, nausea, acute abdominal pain, and anorexia. It is important to provide a thorough, aggressive bowel program to patients when they are taking opioid medications.

Nursing Alert

When patients experience a drop in respiratory rate, the nurse should attempt to increase the rate by coaching the patient to breathe. Should an antidote be needed, naloxone (Narcan) should be administered with great caution and only when necessary in patients receiving an opioid for severe pain. Naloxone removes all of the pain-relieving effects of the opioid and may lead to withdrawal symptoms or the return of intense pain.

USING EPIDURAL PAIN MANAGEMENT

Administration of morphine sulfate and fentanyl by the epidural route has provided an alternative to the intramuscular or oral route. **Epidural** administration consists of a catheter placed into the epidural space, which is the space outside the dura mater of the brain and spinal cord. Analgesia is produced by the drug's direct effect on the opiate receptors in the dorsal horn of the spinal cord. This approach was introduced with the idea that very small doses of opioid would provide long-lasting pain relief with significantly fewer systemic adverse reactions. Epidural

administration offers several advantages over other routes, including lower total dosages of the drug used, fewer adverse reactions, and greater patient comfort.

Access to the epidural route is made through the use of a percutaneous epidural catheter. The placement of the catheter requires strict aseptic technique by a skilled physician. The epidural catheter is placed into the space between the dura mater and the vertebral column (Fig. 19-3). Drug injected through the catheter spreads freely throughout the tissues in the space, interrupting pain conduction at the points where sensory nerve fibers exit from the spinal cord.

The administration of the opioid is either by bolus or by continuous infusion pump.

This type of pain management is used for postoperative pain, labor pain, and intractable chronic pain. Patients experience pain relief with fewer adverse reactions; the adverse reactions experienced are those related to processes under direct CNS control. The most serious adverse reaction associated with the epidurally administered opioids is respiratory depression. Patients using epidural analgesics for chronic pain are monitored for respiratory problems with an apnea monitor. The patient may also experience sedation, confusion, nausea, pruritus, or urinary retention. Fentanyl is increasingly used as an alternative to morphine sulfate because patients experience fewer adverse reactions.

Nursing Alert

Epidural analgesia should be administered only by those specifically trained in the use of IV and epidural anesthetics. Oxygen, resuscitative, and intubation equipment should be readily available.

Nursing care includes close monitoring of the patient for respiratory depression immediately after insertion of the epidural catheter and throughout therapy. Vital signs are taken every 30 minutes, apnea monitors are used, and an opioid antagonist, such as naloxone, is readily available.

Policies and procedures for administering, monitoring, and documenting drugs given through the epidural route must be specific to the nurse practice act in each state and in accordance with federal and state regulations. This type of analgesia is most often managed by registered nurses with special training in the care and management of epidural catheters.

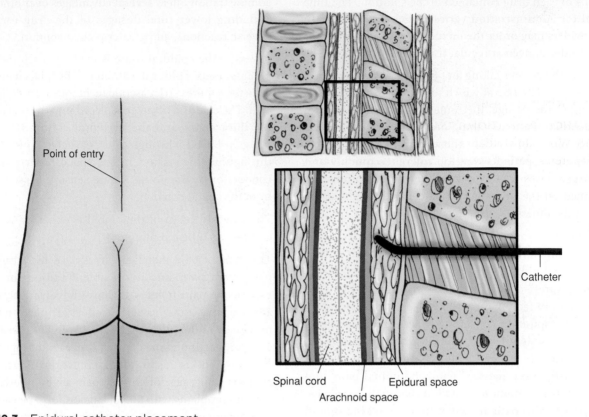

Figure 19.3 Epidural catheter placement.

MONITORING AND MANAGING PATIENT NEEDS

The nurse should contact the primary health care provider immediately if any of the following are present:

- A significant decrease in the respiratory rate or a respiratory rate of 10 breaths/min or below.

- A significant increase or decrease in the pulse rate or a change in the pulse quality.

- A significant decrease in blood pressure (systolic or diastolic) or a systolic pressure below 100 mm Hg.

INEFFECTIVE BREATHING PATTERN Opioids may depress the cough reflex. The nurse should encourage patients receiving an opioid, even for a few days, to cough and breathe deeply every 2 hours. This task prevents the pooling of secretions in the lungs, which can lead to hypostatic pneumonia and other lung problems. The patient may be fearful that exercise will cause even greater pain. The nurse should perform tasks, such as getting the patient out of bed, and encourage therapeutic activities, such as deep breathing, coughing, and leg exercises (when ordered), when the drug is producing its greatest analgesic effect, usually 1 to 2 hours after the nurse administers the opioid. If the patient experiences nausea

and vomiting, the nurse should notify the primary health care provider. A different analgesic or an antiemetic may be necessary.

RISK FOR INJURY Opioids may produce orthostatic hypotension, which in turn results in dizziness. The nurse immediately reports to the primary health care provider any significant change in the patient's vital signs. Particularly vulnerable are postoperative patients and individuals whose ability to maintain blood pressure has been compromised. The nurse should assist the patient with ambulatory activities and with rising slowly from a sitting or lying position. Miosis (pinpoint pupils) may occur with the administration of some opioids and is most pronounced with morphine sulfate, hydromorphone, and hydrochlorides of opium alkaloids. Miosis decreases the ability to see in dim light. The nurse keeps the room well lit during daytime hours and advises the patient to seek assistance when getting out of bed at night.

CONSTIPATION Most patients should begin taking a stool softener or laxative with the initial dose of an opioid analgesic. Decreased GI motility due to the opioids, in addition to lower food and water intake and decreased mobility, cause the constipation. The nurse keeps a daily record of bowel movements and informs the primary health care provider if constipation appears to be a problem. Many patients need to continue taking a laxative for as long as they take an opioid analgesic. If the patient is constipated despite the use of a stool softener or laxative, the primary health care provider may prescribe an enema or other means of relieving constipation.

IMBALANCED NUTRITION: LESS THAN BODY REQUIREMENTS When an opioid is prescribed for a prolonged time, anorexia (loss of appetite) may occur. Those receiving an opioid for pain relief caused by a terminal illness often have severe anorexia from the disease and the opioid. The nurse assesses food intake after each meal. When anorexia is prolonged, the nurse weighs the patient as ordered by the primary health care provider. It is important for the nurse to notify the primary health care provider of continued weight loss and anorexia. Supplements may be ordered and administered orally, enterally, or parenterally.

OPIOID DRUG DEPENDENCE Patients receiving the opioid analgesics for acute pain do not develop physical dependence. Delays in medication administration cause patients to ask repeatedly for pain medication. This behavior is sometimes interpreted as drug-seeking behavior or it may be associated with the fear of making a patient drug dependent. Nurses are also fearful that patients with a history of psychologic dependence might become dependent again when given pain medication. These individuals experience pain, too. They need to be provided adequate pain relief to *prevent* returning to dependency behaviors. Typically it is the behavior of the nurses and primary health care providers in delaying administration of opioids for good pain control that causes the problems associated with appearances of dependence.

Drug dependence can, however, occur in a newborn whose mother was dependent on opiates during pregnancy. Withdrawal symptoms in the newborn usually appear during the first few days of life. Symptoms include irritability, excessive crying, yawning, sneezing, increased respiratory rate, tremors, fever, vomiting, and diarrhea.

MANAGEMENT OF OPIOID DEPENDENCE Two opioids are used in the treatment and management of opiate dependence: levomethadyl and methadone. Levomethadyl is given in an opiate dependency clinic to maintain control over the delivery of the drug. Because of its potential for serious and life-threatening prearrhythmic effects, levomethadyl is reserved for treating addicted patients who have had no response to other treatments. Levomethadyl is not taken daily; the drug is administered three times a week (Monday/Wednesday/Friday or Tuesday/Thursday/Saturday). Daily use of the usual dose will cause serious overdose.

> **Nursing Alert**
>
> If transferring from levomethadyl to methadone, the nurse should wait 48 hours after the last dose of levomethadyl before administering the first dose of methadone or other opioid.

Methadone, a synthetic opioid, may be used for the relief of pain, but it also is used in the detoxification and maintenance treatment of those dependent on opioids. Detoxification involves withdrawing the patient from the opioid while preventing withdrawal symptoms. Maintenance therapy is designed to reduce the patient's desire to return to the drug that caused dependence, as well as to prevent withdrawal symptoms. Dosages vary with the patient, the length of time the individual has been dependent, and the average amount of drug used each day. Patients enrolled in an outpatient methadone program for detoxification or maintenance therapy on methadone must continue to receive methadone when hospitalized. In adults, withdrawal symptoms are known as the *abstinence syndrome* (see Display 19-2 for more information).

Display 19.2 Symptoms of the Abstinence Syndrome

Early Symptoms
Yawning, lacrimation, rhinorrhea, sweating

Intermediate Symptoms
Mydriasis, tachycardia, twitching, tremor, restlessness, irritability, anxiety, anorexia

Late Symptoms
Muscle spasm, fever, nausea, vomiting, kicking movements, weakness, depression, body aches, weight loss, severe backache, abdominal and leg pains, hot and cold flashes, insomnia, repetitive sneezing, increased blood pressure, respiratory rate, and heart rate

---

EDUCATING THE PATIENT AND FAMILY

The nurse informs the patient that the drug he or she is receiving is for pain. It also is a good idea to include additional information, such as how often the drug can be given and the name of the drug being given. If a patient is receiving drugs through a PCA infusion pump, the nurse discusses the following points:

- The location of the control button that activates the administration of the drug

- The difference between the control button and the button to call the nurse (when both are similar in appearance and feel)

- The machine regulates the dose of the drug as well as the time interval between doses

- If the control button is used too soon after the last dose, the machine will not deliver the drug until the correct time

- Pain relief should occur shortly after pushing the button

- Call the nurse if pain relief does not occur after two successive doses

Opioids for outpatient use may be prescribed in the oral form or as a timed-release transdermal patch. In certain cases, such as when terminally ill patients are being cared for at home, the nurse may give the family instruction in the parenteral administration of the drug or use of an IV pump (see Home Care Checklist: Using an Analgesia IV Pump in the Home).

When an opioid has been prescribed, the nurse includes the following points in the teaching plan:

- This drug may cause drowsiness, dizziness, and blurring of vision. Use caution when driving or performing tasks requiring alertness.

Home Care Checklist

Using an Analgesic IV Pump in the Home

In some situations, opioid analgesics may be ordered for pain relief using IV equipment at home. If the patient will be receiving IV analgesics at home, the nurse makes sure to review the following steps with the patient and the caregiver:

☑ How the pump works

☑ What drug is being given

☑ When to administer a dose

☑ What the power source is (battery or electricity)

☑ What to do if the battery fails or a power failure occurs

☑ How to check the insertion site

☑ How to change the cartridge or syringe

If the patient or caregiver will be responsible for changing the drug cartridge or syringe, the nurse teaches the following steps:

☑ Gather new syringe with drug (if refrigerated, remove it at least 30 minutes before using).

☑ Attach pump-specific tubing to the drug.

☑ Prime the tubing.

☑ Turn off the pump and clamp the infusion tubing.

☑ Remove the tubing from the infusion site.

☑ Flush the site (if ordered).

☑ Remove used cartridge or syringe from the pump.

☑ Insert the new cartridge or syringe into the pump.

☑ Connect the new infusion tubing to the infusion site.

☑ Turn on the pump and have the patient provide a drug dose when needed.

- Avoid the use of alcoholic beverages unless use has been approved by the primary health care provider. Alcohol may intensify the action of the drug and cause extreme drowsiness or dizziness. In some instances, the use of alcohol and an opioid can have extremely serious and even life-threatening consequences that may require emergency medical treatment.

- Take the drug as directed on the container label and do not exceed the prescribed dose. Contact the primary health care provider if the drug is not effective.

- If GI upset occurs, take the drug with food.

- Notify the primary health care provider if nausea, vomiting, and constipation become severe.

- To administer the transdermal system, remove the system from the package and immediately apply it to the skin of the upper torso. To ensure complete contact with the skin surface, press for 10 to 20 seconds with the palm of the hand. After 72 hours, remove the system and, if continuous therapy is prescribed, apply a new system. Use only water to cleanse the site before application because soaps, oils, and other substances may irritate the skin. Rotate site of application. The used patch should be folded carefully so the system adheres to itself.

EVALUATION

- The therapeutic effect occurs and pain is relieved.

- The patient demonstrates the ability to use PCA effectively.

- Adverse reactions are identified, reported to the primary health care provider, and managed through appropriate nursing interventions.

- No evidence of injury is seen.

- Body weight is maintained.

- Diet is adequate.

- The patient and family demonstrate understanding of the drug regimen.

Critical Thinking Exercises

1. Ms. Taylor is receiving meperidine for postoperative pain management. In assessing Ms. Taylor approximately 20 minutes after receiving an injection of meperidine, the nurse discovers Ms. Taylor's vital signs are blood pressure 80/50 mm Hg, pulse rate 120 bpm, and respiratory rate 8/min. Determine what action, if any, the nurse should take.

2. Mr. Talley, a 64-year-old retired schoolteacher, has cancer and is to receive morphine through an IV infusion pump into a central line Hickman catheter. His wife is eager to help, yet her arthritis makes tasks requiring fine motor skills difficult. Formulate a teaching plan for this family that includes the use of the IV pump, adverse reactions to expect, and what adverse reactions to report.

3. Roger Baccus, aged 23 years, is prescribed meperidine (Demerol) for postoperative pain. You discover in his health history on the chart that he has a history of alcohol and drug use. Determine how to ensure that all the nursing staff will provide him with adequate pain management during his hospital stay.

4. Discuss the important preadministration assessments that must be made on the patient receiving an opioid analgesic.

5. Joe Thompson, aged 48 years, is taking morphine sulfate to manage severe pain occurring as the result of heart failure. The primary health care provider has prescribed an around-the-clock dosage regimen. Joe is asking for the pain drug 1 to 2 hours before the next dose is due. What strategies would you use to determine if this is the correct dosing of opioid analgesic?

Review Questions

1. The nurse explains to the patient that some opioids may be used as part of the preoperative medication regimen to _____.

    A. increase intestinal motility

    B. facilitate passage of an endotracheal tube

    C. enhance the effects of the skeletal muscle relaxant

    D. lessen anxiety and sedate the patient

2. Each time the patient requests an opioid analgesic, the nurse must_____.

    A. check the patient's diagnosis

    B. talk to the patient to see if he is awake

    C. determine the exact location and intensity of the pain

    D. administer the drug with food to prevent gastric upset

Opioid Analgesics

3. Which of the following findings requires that the nurse immediately contact the health care provider?

A. A pulse rate of 80 bpm

B. Complaint of breakthrough pain

C. A respiratory rate of 20/min

D. A systolic blood pressure of 140 mm Hg

4. When administering opioid analgesics to an elderly patient, the nurse monitors the patient closely for _____.

A. an increased heart rate

B. euphoria

C. confusion

D. a synergistic reaction

5. When administering a timed-release medication to a patient, the nurse must be aware that _____.

A. it should not be crushed

B. the medication is stronger

C. serious cardiac arrhythmias may develop

D. CNS stimulation is possible

Medication Dosage Problems

1. A patient is prescribed oral morphine sulfate 12 mg. The dosage available is 10 mg/mL. The nurse administers _____.

2. A patient is prescribed fentanyl (Sublimaze) 50 mcg IM 30 minutes before surgery. The nurse has available a vial with a dosage strength of 0.05 mg/1 mL. The nurse calculates the dosage and administers _____.

To check your answers, see Appendix G.

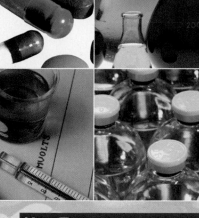

Opioid Antagonists

Learning Objectives

On completion of this chapter, the student will:

- Discuss the uses, general drug action, general adverse reactions, contraindications, precautions, and interactions of the opioid antagonists.
- Discuss important preadministration and ongoing assessment activities the nurse should perform on the patient receiving the opioid antagonists.
- List nursing diagnoses particular to a patient taking an opioid antagonist.
- Discuss ways to promote optimal response to therapy, how to manage adverse reactions, and important points to keep in mind when educating patients about the use of opioid antagonists.

An **antagonist** is a substance that counteracts the action of something else. A drug that is an opioid antagonist has a greater affinity for a cell receptor than an opioid drug (agonist), and by binding to the cell it prevents a response to the opioid. Thus, an opioid antagonist reverses the actions of an opioid. One of the most severe adverse reactions to opioid treatment is respiratory depression. Specific antagonists have been developed to reverse the respiratory depression associated with the opioids. The two opioid antagonists in use today are naloxone (Narcan) and nalmefene (Revex). Naloxone is capable of restoring respiratory function within 1 to 2 minutes after administration. Naltrexone (another antagonist) is used primarily to treat alcohol dependence and to block the effects of suspected opioids if they are being used by the person undergoing treatment for alcohol dependence.

OPIOID (NARCOTIC) ANTAGONISTS

Actions

Administration of an antagonist prevents or reverses the effects of opioid drugs. The antagonist reverses the opioid effects by competing for the opiate receptor sites and displacing the opioid drug (see Chapter 19). If the individual has taken or received an opioid, the effects of the opioid are reversed. An antagonist drug is not selective for specific adverse reactions. When an antagonist is given to reverse a specific adverse reaction, such as respiratory depression, it is important to remember the antagonist reverses *all* effects. Therefore, a patient who receives an antagonist to reverse respiratory effects will also experience a reversal of pain relief—that is, the pain will return. If the individual has not taken or received an opioid, an antagonist has no drug effect.

Uses

The opioid antagonists are used for the treatment of

- Postoperative acute respiratory depression
- Opioid adverse effects (reversal)
- Suspected acute opioid overdosage

Adverse Reactions

Generalized reactions include
- Nausea and vomiting
- Sweating
- Tachycardia
- Increased blood pressure
- Tremors

See the Summary Drug Table: Opioid Antagonists for more information.

Contraindications, Precautions, and Interactions

Antagonists are contraindicated in those with a hypersensitivity to the opioid antagonists. Antagonists are used cautiously in those who are pregnant (pregnancy category B), in infants of opioid-dependent mothers, and in patients with an opioid dependency or cardiovascular disease. These drugs also are used cautiously during lactation.

These drugs may produce withdrawal symptoms in individuals who are physically dependent on the opioid. Antagonists may prevent the action or intended use of opioid antidiarrheals, antitussives, and analgesics.

NURSING PROCESS

The Patient Receiving an Opioid Antagonist for Respiratory Depression

ASSESSMENT

PREADMINISTRATION ASSESSMENT

Patients involved in long-term opioid therapy for pain relief build tolerance to the physical adverse effects of the drugs. It is the patient who does not use opioids routinely and who is being given an opioid drug for acute pain relief or a surgical procedure who is at most risk for respiratory depression after opioid administration. These patients are described as **opioid naive**.

Sometimes the somnolence and pain relief produced by the opioid drug will slow the patient's breathing pattern. This can be alarming to the nurse if the respiratory rate has been rapid because of anxiety and pain. The nurse should make efforts to arouse the patient and coach his or her breathing pattern if possible. Before administration of the antagonist, the nurse obtains the blood pressure, pulse, and respiratory rate and reviews the record for the drug suspected of causing the symptoms of respiratory depression. If there is sufficient time, the nurse also should review the initial health history, allergy history, and current treatment modalities.

SUMMARY DRUG TABLE   OPIOID ANTAGONISTS

GENERIC NAME	TRADE NAME	USES	ADVERSE REACTIONS	DOSAGE RANGES
nalmefene nal'-me-feen	Revex	Complete or partial reversal of opioid effects after surgery or overdose	Nausea, vomiting, tachycardia, hypertension, return of postoperative pain, fever, dizziness	Postoperative opioid reversal: 0.25 mcg/kg; may be repeated in 2–5-min increments
naloxone HCl nal-ox'-own	Narcan	Same as nalmefene	Same as nalmefene	Postoperative opioid reversal: 0.1–0.2 mg IV at 2–3 min intervals Suspected opioid overdose: 0.4–2 mg IV at 2–3-min intervals

ONGOING ASSESSMENT

As part of the ongoing assessment during the administration of the antagonist, the nurse monitors the blood pressure, pulse, and respiratory rate at frequent intervals, usually every 5 minutes, until the patient responds. This monitoring is more frequent if respiratory depression occurs in the immediate postoperative setting. After the patient has shown a response to the drug, the nurse monitors vital signs every 5 to 15 minutes. The nurse should notify the primary health care provider if any adverse drug reactions occur because additional medical treatment may be needed. The nurse monitors the respiratory rate, rhythm, and depth; pulse; blood pressure; and level of consciousness until the effects of the opioid wear off.

Nursing Alert

The effects of some opioids may last longer than the effects of naloxone (Narcan). A repeat dose of naloxone may be ordered by the primary health care provider if results obtained from the initial dose are unsatisfactory. The duration of close patient observation depends on the patient's response to the administration of the opioid antagonist.

NURSING DIAGNOSES

Drug-specific nursing diagnoses are highlighted in the Nursing Diagnoses Checklist. Other nursing diagnoses applicable to these drugs are discussed in depth in Chapter 4.

Nursing Diagnoses Checklist

✔ **Impaired Spontaneous Ventilation** related to brain response to slow breathing induced by the opioid drug

✔ **Acute Pain** related to antagonist drug displacing opioid drug at cell receptor sites

PLANNING

The expected outcome for the patient with respiratory depression is an optimal response to therapy and support of patient needs related to the management of adverse drug effects. This is essentially a return to normal respiratory rate, rhythm, and depth. The nurse meets the patient's needs by providing adequate ventilation of the body as well as continued pain relief.

IMPLEMENTATION
PROMOTING AN OPTIMAL RESPONSE TO THERAPY

Frequently the use of naloxone (Narcan) is in the controlled setting of the postanesthesia recovery unit (postanesthesia care unit [PACU] or surgical recovery room). As the patient awakens from the deep operative sleep, the nurse balances the need for continued pain relief against the person's ability to breathe independently after the procedure.

MONITORING AND MANAGING PATIENT NEEDS

IMPAIRED SPONTANEOUS VENTILATION. Depending on the patient's condition, the nurse may use cardiac monitoring, artificial ventilation (respirator), and other drugs during and after the administration of naloxone. It is important to keep suction equipment readily available because abrupt reversal of opioid-induced respiratory depression may cause vomiting. The nurse must maintain a patent airway and should turn and suction the patient as needed.

If naloxone is given by intravenous (IV) infusion, the primary health care provider orders the IV fluid and amount, the drug dosage, and the infusion rate. Giving the drug by IV infusion requires use of a secondary line, an IV piggyback or an IV push.

Nursing Alert

When naloxone (Narcan) is used to reverse respiratory depression and the resulting somnolence, the drug is given by slow IV push until the respiratory rate begins to increase and somnolence abates. Keep in mind that giving a rapid bolus will cause withdrawal and return of intense pain.

ACUTE PAIN. When the antagonist drug is given to patients, they experience pain abruptly because the opioid no longer works in the body. The nurse assesses the pain level and begins to treat the pain again. The nurse needs to review the circumstances that led to the use of the antagonist as an opioid reversal drug. Steps can then be taken to resume pain relief without the adverse reaction.

If the patient is in a setting where family members may be present, it is the nurse's responsibility to educate the family about the action of the drug and what they will see happen. It can be distressing for others to see a person experience intense pain when the antagonist begins to work if they do not understand the reason for the intervention.

The nurse monitors fluid intake and output and notifies the primary health care provider of any change in the fluid intake–output ratio. Of course, the nurse should notify the primary health care provider if there is any sudden change in the patient's condition.

EVALUATION

- The therapeutic effect is achieved.
- The patient's respiratory rate, rhythm, and depth are normal.
- Pain relief is resumed.

Critical Thinking Exercises

1. Explain the term *opiate naive* and describe which patients are more likely to experience respiratory depression and which patients are not as likely to experience this adverse reaction to opioid therapy.

2. Discuss important preadministration and ongoing nursing assessments you would make when giving a patient naloxone for severe respiratory depression caused by morphine sulfate.

Review Questions

1. Which opioid antagonist would most likely be prescribed for treatment of a patient who is experiencing an opioid overdose?

   A. naltrexone

   B. naloxone

   C. naproxen

   D. nifedipine

2. Which patient, given an opioid analgesic for acute pain, should the nurse monitor most closely for respiratory distress?

   A. The patient with cancer taking morphine sulfate regularly

   B. The athlete who is taking Percocet for a leg injury

   C. The man who has never used an opioid pain medication

   D. The methadone client with a broken arm

Medication Dosage Problems

1. A patient is prescribed 0.8 mg naloxone IV for postoperative respiratory depression caused by morphine. Available is a vial with 1 mg/mL. The nurse administers _____.

2. In the recovery room, the physician prescribes naloxone 0.4 mg by injection as the initial dose for opioid-induced respiratory depression; it may be followed in 5 minutes with 0.2 mg. Orders read that the nurse should contact the primary health care provider when a total of 1 mg is given. How many times can the nurse give the drug before contacting the primary health care provider?

To check your answers, see Appendix G.

Drugs That Affect the Neuromuscular System

The nervous system is a complex part of the human body concerned with the regulation and coordination of body activities such as movement, digestion, sleep, and elimination of waste products. The musculoskeletal system comprises the bones, joints, and muscles that provide the body with movement. Although separate body systems, they work together as the neuromuscular system to provide our bodies with the ability to live, work, and play. Drugs discussed in Unit IV affect both these body systems.

The nervous system has two main divisions: the central nervous system (CNS) and the peripheral nervous system (PNS). The CNS consists of the brain and the spinal cord. The CNS receives, integrates, and interprets nerve impulses. The PNS connects all parts of the body with the CNS.

CENTRAL NERVOUS SYSTEM

The CNS processes information to and from the PNS and is the center of coordination and control for the entire body. Drugs that affect the CNS alter mood, sensation, and the interpretation of information in the brain. The body is quick to respond to some of these drugs, and they are used for a short duration. Chapter 21 discusses anesthetics—drugs used to eliminate sensation and the perception of pain. Drugs that depress the CNS are used to treat anxiety (Chapter 22) and insomnia (Chapter 23).

Other drugs that act on the CNS are used to change mood or behavior. These drugs may take many days or even weeks to produce a therapeutic response. Chapter 24 discusses drugs used to treat depression, which is one of the most common mental health disorders. Depression is characterized by impaired functioning and feelings of intense sadness, helplessness, and worthlessness. People experiencing major depressive episodes exhibit physical and psychological symptoms, such as appetite disturbances, sleep disturbances, and loss of interest in job, family, and other activities usually enjoyed.

Many drugs stimulate the CNS, but only a few are used therapeutically; these are known as CNS stimulants (Chapter 25). These drugs may be used to reverse respiratory depression or to treat children with attention deficit hyperactivity disorder (ADHD).

A psychotic disorder is characterized by extreme personality disorganization and the loss of contact with reality. Drugs given to patients with a psychotic disorder, such as schizophrenia, are called *antipsychotic drugs* or *neuroleptics*. The antipsychotic drugs are discussed in Chapter 26.

PERIPHERAL NERVOUS SYSTEM

Chapters 27 through 30 focus on drugs that affect the peripheral nerves in the body. The PNS comprises all nerves outside of the brain and spinal cord. The PNS is divided into the somatic nervous system and the autonomic nervous system. The somatic branch of the PNS is concerned with sensation

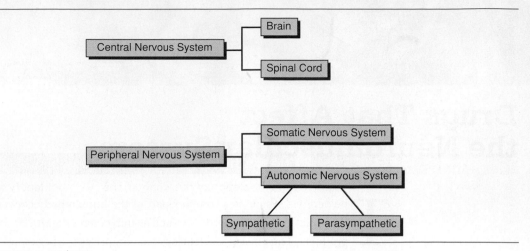

The nervous system.

and voluntary movement. The sensory part of the somatic nervous system sends messages to the brain concerning the internal and external environment, such as sensations of heat, pain, cold, and pressure. The movement part of the somatic nervous system is concerned with the voluntary movement of skeletal muscles, such as those used in walking, talking, or writing a letter.

The autonomic branch of the PNS is concerned with functions essential to the survival of the organism. Functional activity of the autonomic nervous system is not controlled consciously (i.e., the activity is automatic). This system controls blood pressure, heart rate, gastrointestinal activity, and glandular secretions.

The autonomic branch is further divided into the sympathetic and the parasympathetic nervous systems. The sympathetic nervous system tends to regulate the expenditure of energy and is operative when the organism is confronted with stressful situations. The sympathetic system is also called the *adrenergic branch*. Chapter 27 discusses drugs that mimic the effects of the sympathetic system— the adrenergic drugs. Drugs that block or inhibit the system are called *antiadrenergic drugs* or *adrenergic blocking drugs*; they are covered in Chapter 28.

The parasympathetic nervous system helps conserve body energy and is partly responsible for such activities as slowing the heart rate, digesting food, and eliminating bodily wastes. The parasympathetic nervous system is known as the *cholinergic branch*. Drugs that enhance neuro-transmission are discussed in Chapter 29; those that block transmission are covered in Chapter 30.

The remaining chapters of this unit (Chapters 31 through 34) discuss drugs that not only affect the nervous system but exert influence over the musculoskeletal system. Drugs that control seizure activity are presented in Chapter 31. Degenerative diseases (Parkinson's disease, Alzheimer's disease, and gout) that affect both the musculoskeletal and neurologic systems are covered in Chapters 32 through 34.

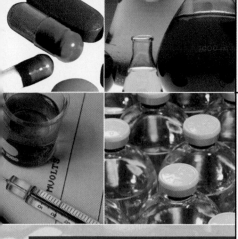

Anesthetic Drugs

Learning Objectives

On completion of this chapter, the student will:

- State the uses of local anesthesia, methods of administration, and nursing responsibilities when administering a local anesthetic.

- Describe the purpose of a preanesthetic drug and the nursing responsibilities associated with the administration of a preanesthetic drug.

- Identify several drugs used for local and general anesthesia.

- List and briefly describe the four stages of general anesthesia.

- Discuss important nursing responsibilities associated with caring for a patient receiving a preanesthesic drug and during the postanesthesia care (recovery room) period.

nesthesia is a loss of feeling or sensation. Anesthesia may be induced by various drugs that can bring about partial or complete loss of sensation. There are two types of anesthesia: local anesthesia and general anesthesia. **Local anesthesia**, as the term implies, is the provision of a sensation-free state in a specific area (or region). With a local anesthetic, the patient is fully awake but does not feel pain in the area that has been anesthetized. However, some procedures performed under local anesthesia may require the patient to be sedated. Although not fully awake, sedated patients may still hear what is going on around them. **General anesthesia** is the provision of a sensation-free state for the entire body. When a general anesthetic is given, the patient loses consciousness and feels no pain. Reflexes, such as the swallowing and gag reflexes, are lost during deep general anesthesia (Fig. 21-1). Both physicians and nurses administer anesthesia. An **anesthesiologist** is a physician with special training in administering anesthesia. A nurse **anesthetist** is a nurse with a master's degree and special training who is qualified to administer anesthetics.

LOCAL ANESTHESIA

The various methods of administering a local anesthetic include topical application, local infiltration, and regional anesthesia.

Topical Anesthesia

Topical anesthesia involves the application of the anesthetic to the surface of the skin, open area, or mucous membrane. The anesthetic may be applied with a cotton swab or sprayed on the area. This type of anesthesia may be used to desensitize the skin or mucous membrane to the injection of a deeper local anesthetic. In some instances, topical anesthetics may be applied by the nurse.

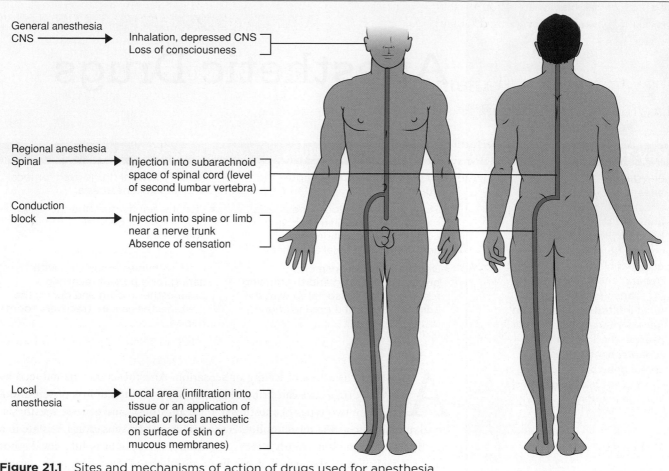

Figure 21.1   Sites and mechanisms of action of drugs used for anesthesia.

Local Infiltration Anesthesia

Local infiltration anesthesia is the injection of a local anesthetic drug into tissues. This type of anesthesia may be used for dental procedures, the suturing of small wounds, or making an incision into a small area, such as that required for removing a superficial piece of tissue for biopsy.

Regional Anesthesia

Regional anesthesia is the injection of a local anesthetic around nerves so that the area supplied by these nerves will not send pain signals to the brain. The anesthetized area is usually larger than the area affected by local infiltration anesthesia. Spinal anesthesia and conduction blocks are two types of regional anesthesia.

Spinal Anesthesia

Spinal anesthesia is a type of regional anesthesia that involves the injection of a local anesthetic drug into the subarachnoid space of the spinal cord, usually at the level of the second lumbar vertebra. There is a loss of feeling (anesthesia) and movement in the lower extremities, lower abdomen, and perineum.

Conduction Blocks

A **conduction block** is a type of regional anesthesia produced by injection of a local anesthetic drug into or near a nerve trunk. Examples of a conduction block include an **epidural block** (injection of a local anesthetic into the space surrounding the dura of the spinal cord); a **transsacral** (caudal) **block** (injection of a local anesthetic into the epidural space at the level of the sacrococcygeal notch); and **brachial plexus block** (injection of a local anesthetic into the brachial plexus). Epidural, especially, and transsacral blocks are often used in obstetrics. A brachial plexus block may be used for surgery of the arm or hand.

Preparing the Patient for Local Anesthesia

Depending on the procedure performed, preparing the patient for local anesthesia may or may not be similar to preparing the patient for general anesthesia. For example, administering a local anesthetic for dental surgery or for suturing a small wound may require that the nurse explain to the patient how the anesthetic will be administered, take the patient's allergy history, and, when applicable, prepare the area to be anesthetized, which may involve cleaning the area with an antiseptic or shaving the area. Other local anesthetic procedures may require the patient to be fasting (taking in nothing by mouth) because a sedative may also be administered. The nurse may administer an intravenous (IV) sedative such as the central nervous system (CNS) depressant drug midazolam (Versed) during some local anesthetic procedures, such as cataract surgery or surgery performed under spinal anesthesia.

Administering Local Anesthesia

The physician or dentist administers a local injectable anesthetic. These drugs may be mixed with epinephrine to cause local vasoconstriction. The drug stays in the tissue longer when epinephrine is used. This is contraindicated, however, when the local anesthetic is used on an extremity. When preparing these medications, the nurse should proceed cautiously and be aware of when epinephrine is to be used and when it should not be used. Table 21-1 lists the more commonly used local anesthetics.

Nursing Responsibilities When Caring for a Patient Receiving Local Anesthesia

When caring for a patient receiving local anesthesia, the nurse may be responsible for applying a dressing to the surgical area if appropriate. Depending on the reason for using local anesthesia, the nurse also may be responsible

Table 21.1 Example of Local Anesthetics

Generic Name	Trade Name
articaine HCl	Septocaine
bupivacaine HCl	Marcaine HCl
chloroprocaine HCl	Nesacaine, Nesacaine-MPF
lidocaine HCl	Xylocaine
mepivacaine HCl	Carbocaine, Isocaine HCl
prilocaine HCl	Citanest HCl
procaine HCl	Novocain
ropivacaine HCl	Naropin

for observing the area for bleeding, oozing, or other problems after the administration of the anesthetic.

PREANESTHETIC DRUGS

A **preanesthetic drug** is one given before the administration of anesthesia. The nurse usually gives a preanesthetic drug before the administration of general anesthesia, but occasionally may give it before injection of the local anesthetic to sedate the patient. The preanesthetic agent may consist of one drug or a combination of drugs.

Uses of Preanesthetic Drugs

The general purpose, or use, of the preanesthetic drug is to prepare the patient for anesthesia. The more specific purposes of these drugs include the following:

- Opioid or antianxiety drug—to decrease anxiety and apprehension immediately before surgery. The patient who is calm and relaxed can be anesthetized more quickly, usually requires a smaller dose of an induction drug, may require less anesthesia during surgery, and may have a smoother recovery from the anesthesia period (awakening from anesthesia).

- Cholinergic blocking drug—to decrease secretions of the upper respiratory tract. Some anesthetic gases and volatile liquids are irritating to the lining of the respiratory tract and thereby increase mucous secretions. The cough and swallowing reflexes are lost during general anesthesia, and excessive secretions can pool in the lungs, resulting in pneumonia or atelectasis (lung collapse) during the postoperative period. The administration of a cholinergic blocking drug, such as glycopyrrolate (Robinul), dries up secretions of the upper respiratory tract and decreases the possibility of excessive mucus production.

- Antiemetic—to decrease the incidence of nausea and vomiting during the immediate postoperative recovery period.

Gerontologic Alert

Preanesthetic drugs may be omitted in patients aged 60 years or older because many of the medical disorders for which these drugs are contraindicated are seen in older individuals. For example, atropine and glycopyrrolate, drugs that can be used to decrease secretions of the upper respiratory tract, are contraindicated in certain medical disorders, such as prostatic hypertrophy, glaucoma, and myocardial ischemia. Other preanesthetic drugs that depress the CNS, such as opioids, barbiturates, and antianxiety drugs, with or without antiemetic properties, may be contraindicated in the older individual.

Selection of Preanesthetic Drugs

The preanesthetic drug is usually selected by the anesthesiologist and may consist of one or more drugs (Table 21-2). An opioid (see Chapter 19), antianxiety drug (see Chapter 22), or barbiturate (see Chapter 23) may be given to relax or sedate the patient. Barbiturates are used only occasionally; opioids are usually preferred for sedation. A cholinergic blocking drug (see Chapter 30) is given to dry secretions in the upper respiratory tract. Scopolamine and glycopyrrolate also have mild sedative properties, and atropine may or may not produce some sedation. Antianxiety drugs have sedative action; when combined with an opioid, they allow for a lowering of the opioid dosage because they also have the ability to potentiate (increase the effect of) the sedative action of the opioid. Diazepam (Valium), an antianxiety drug, is one of the more commonly used drugs for preoperative sedation.

Nursing Responsibilities

When caring for a patient receiving a preanesthetic drug, the nurse assesses the patient's physical status and gives an explanation of the anesthesia. In some hospitals, the anesthesiologist examines the patient the day or evening before

Table 21.2 Examples of Preanesthetic Drugs

Generic Name	Trade Name
Opioids	
fentanyl	Sublimaze
meperidine hydrochloride	Demerol
morphine sulfate	
Barbiturates	
pentobarbital	Nembutal Sodium
secobarbital	Seconal
Cholinergic Blocking Drugs	
atropine sulfate	
glycopyrrolate	Robinul
scopolamine	
Antianxiety Drugs With Antiemetic Properties	
hydroxyzine	Atarax, Vistaril
Antianxiety Drugs	
chlordiazepoxide	Librium
diazepam	Valium
lorazepam	Ativan
midazolam	Versed
Sedative Drugs	
droperidol	Inapsine

surgery, although this may not be possible in emergency situations. Some hospitals use operating room or postanesthesia care unit (PACU) staff members to visit the patient before surgery to explain certain facts, such as the time of surgery, the effects of the preanesthetic drug, preparations for surgery, and the PACU. Proper explanation of anesthesia, the surgery itself, and the events that may occur in preparation for surgery, as well as care after surgery, requires a team approach. The nurse's responsibilities include the following:

- Describes or explains the preparations for surgery ordered by the physician. Examples of preoperative preparations include fasting from midnight (or the time specified by the physician), enema, shaving of the operative site, use of a hypnotic for sleep the night before, and the preoperative injection about 30 minutes before surgery.

- Describes or explains immediate postoperative care, such as that given in the PACU (also called the *recovery room*) or a special postoperative surgical unit, and the activities of the health care team during this period. The nurse explains that the patient's vital signs will be monitored frequently and that other equipment, such as IV lines and fluids and hemodynamic (cardiac) monitors, may be used.

- Demonstrates, describes, and explains postoperative patient activities, such as deep breathing, coughing, and leg exercises.

- Emphasizes the importance of pain control, and makes sure the patient understands that relieving pain early on is better than trying to hold out, not take the medicine, and later attempt to relieve the pain. The nurse teaches the patient how to use the patient-controlled analgesia (PCA) pump.

- Tailors the preoperative explanations to fit the type of surgery scheduled. Not all of these teaching points may be included in every explanation.

GENERAL ANESTHESIA

The administration of general anesthesia requires the use of one or more drugs. The choice of anesthetic drug depends on many factors, including:
- The general physical condition of the patient
- The area, organ, or system being operated on
- The anticipated length of the surgical procedure

The anesthesiologist selects the anesthetic drugs that will produce safe anesthesia, **analgesia** (absence of pain), and, in some surgeries, effective skeletal muscle relaxation. General anesthesia is most commonly achieved when the anesthetic vapors are inhaled or administered IV. Volatile liquid anesthetics produce anesthesia when their vapors are inhaled. **Volatile liquids** are liquids that evaporate on exposure to air. Examples of volatile liquids include halothane, desflurane, and enflurane. Gas anesthetics are combined with oxygen and administered by inhalation. Examples of gas anesthetics are nitrous oxide and cyclopropane.

Drugs Used for General Anesthesia

Barbiturates and Similar Agents

Methohexital (Brevital), which is an ultrashort-acting barbiturate, is used
- For induction of anesthesia
- For short surgical procedures with minimal painful stimuli

- In conjunction with or as a supplement to other anesthetics

These types of drugs have a rapid onset and a short duration of action. They depress the CNS to produce hypnosis and anesthesia but do not produce analgesia. Recovery after a small dose is rapid.

Etomidate (Amidate), a nonbarbiturate, is used for induction of anesthesia. Etomidate also may be used to supplement other anesthetics, such as nitrous oxide, for short surgical procedures. It is a hypnotic without analgesic activity.

Propofol (Diprivan) is used for induction and maintenance of anesthesia. It also may be used for sedation during diagnostic procedures and procedures that use a local anesthetic. This drug also is used for continuous sedation of intubated or respiratory-controlled patients in intensive care units.

Benzodiazepines

Midazolam (Versed), a short-acting benzodiazepine CNS depressant, is used as a preanesthetic drug to relieve anxiety; for induction of anesthesia; for conscious sedation before minor procedures, such as endoscopy; and to supplement nitrous oxide and oxygen for short surgical procedures. When the drug is used for induction anesthesia, the patient gradually loses consciousness over a period of 1 to 2 minutes.

Ketamine

Ketamine (Ketalar) is a rapid-acting general anesthetic. It produces an anesthetic state characterized by profound analgesia, cardiovascular and respiratory stimulation, normal or enhanced skeletal muscle tone, and occasionally mild respiratory depression. Ketamine is used for diagnostic and surgical procedures that do not require relaxation of skeletal muscles, for induction of anesthesia before the administration of other anesthetic drugs, and as a supplement to other anesthetic drugs.

Gases and Volatile Liquids

Nitrous oxide is the most commonly used anesthetic gas. It is a weak anesthetic and is usually used in combination with other anesthetic drugs. It does not cause skeletal muscle relaxation. The chief danger in the use of nitrous oxide is hypoxemia. Nitrous oxide is nonexplosive and is supplied in blue cylinders.

Enflurane (Ethrane) is a volatile liquid anesthetic that is delivered by inhalation. Induction and recovery from anesthesia are rapid. Muscle relaxation for abdominal surgery is adequate, but greater relaxation may be necessary and may require the use of a skeletal muscle relaxant.

Enflurane may produce mild stimulation of respiratory and bronchial secretions when used alone. Hypotension may occur when anesthesia deepens.

Halothane (Fluothane) is a volatile liquid given by inhalation for induction and maintenance of anesthesia. Induction and recovery from anesthesia are rapid, and the depth of anesthesia can be rapidly altered. Halothane does not irritate the respiratory tract, and an increase in tracheobronchial secretions usually does not occur. Halothane produces moderate muscle relaxation, but skeletal muscle relaxants may be used in certain types of surgeries. This anesthetic may be given with a mixture of nitrous oxide and oxygen.

Isoflurane (Forane) is a volatile liquid given by inhalation. It is used for induction and maintenance of anesthesia.

Methoxyflurane (Penthrane), a volatile liquid, provides analgesia and anesthesia. It is usually used with nitrous oxide but may also be used alone. Methoxyflurane does not produce good muscle relaxation, and a skeletal muscle relaxant may be required.

Desflurane (Suprane), a volatile liquid, is used for induction and maintenance of anesthesia. A special vaporizer is used to deliver this anesthetic because delivery by mask results in irritation of the respiratory tract.

Sevoflurane (Ultane) is an inhalational analgesic. It is used for induction and maintenance of general anesthesia in adult and pediatric patients for inpatient and outpatient surgical procedures.

Opioids

The opioid analgesic fentanyl (Sublimaze) and the neuroleptic drug (major tranquilizer) droperidol (Inapsine) may be used together as a single drug called Innovar. The combination of these two drugs results in **neuroleptanalgesia**, which is characterized by general quietness, reduced motor activity, and profound analgesia. Complete loss of consciousness may not occur unless other anesthetic drugs are used. A combination of fentanyl and droperidol may be used for the tranquilizing effect and analgesia for surgical and diagnostic procedures. It may also be used as a preanesthetic for the induction of anesthesia and in the maintenance of general anesthesia.

The use of droperidol as a tranquilizer, an antiemetic to reduce nausea and vomiting during the immediate postanesthesia period, as an induction drug, and as an adjunct to general anesthesia has decreased because of its association with fatal cardiac arrhythmias. Fentanyl may be used alone as a supplement to general or regional anesthesia. It may also be administered alone or with other drugs as a preoperative drug and as an analgesic during the immediate postoperative period.

Table 21.3 Examples of Muscle Relaxants Used During General Anesthesia

Generic Name	Trade Name
atracurium besylate	Tracrium
cisatracurium besylate	Nimbex
doxacurium chloride	Nuromax
mivacurium chloride	Mivacorn
pancuronium bromide	Pavulon
succinylcholine chloride	Anectine

Remifentanil (Ultiva) is used for induction and maintenance of general anesthesia and for continued analgesia during the immediate postoperative period. This drug is used cautiously in patients with a history of hypersensitivity to fentanyl.

Skeletal Muscle Relaxants

The various skeletal muscle relaxants that may be used during general anesthesia are listed in Table 21-3. These drugs are administered to produce relaxation of the skeletal muscles during certain types of surgeries, such as those involving the chest or abdomen. They may also be used to facilitate the insertion of an endotracheal tube. Their onset of action is usually rapid (45 seconds to a few minutes), and their duration of action is 30 minutes or more.

Stages of General Anesthesia

General surgical anesthesia is divided into the following stages:

- Stage I—analgesia
- Stage II—delirium
- Stage III—surgical analgesia
- Stage IV—respiratory paralysis

Display 21-1 describes the stages of general anesthesia more completely. With newer drugs and techniques, the stages of anesthesia may not be as prominent as those described in Display 21-1. In addition, movement through the first two stages is usually very rapid.

Anesthesia begins with a loss of consciousness. This is part of the induction phase (stage I). The patient is now relaxed and can no longer comprehend what is happening. After consciousness is lost, additional anesthetic drugs are

Display 21.1 Stages of General Anesthesia

Stage I

Induction is a part of stage I anesthesia. It begins with the administration of an anesthetic drug and lasts until consciousness is lost. With some induction drugs, such as the short-acting barbiturates, this stage may last only 5 to 10 seconds.

Stage II

Stage II is the stage of delirium and excitement. This stage is also brief. During this stage, the patient may move about and mumble incoherently. The muscles are somewhat rigid, and the patient is unconscious and cannot feel pain. During this stage, noises are exaggerated and even quiet sounds may seem extremely loud to the patient. If surgery were attempted at this stage, there would be a physical reaction to painful stimuli, yet the patient would not remember sensing pain. During these first two stages of anesthesia, the nurse and other health care professionals avoid any unnecessary noise or motion.

Stage III

Stage III is the stage of surgical analgesia and is divided into four parts, planes, or substages. The anesthesiologist differentiates these planes by the character of the respirations, eye movements, certain reflexes, pupil size, and other factors. The levels of the planes range from plane 1 (light) to plane 4 (deep). At plane 2 or 3, the patient is usually ready for the surgical procedure.

Stage IV

Stage IV is the stage of respiratory paralysis and is a rare and dangerous stage of anesthesia. At this stage, respiratory arrest and cessation of all vital signs may occur.

administered. Some of these drugs are also used as part of the induction phase, as well as for deepening anesthesia. Depending on the type of surgery, an endotracheal tube also may be inserted to provide an adequate airway and to assist in administering oxygen and other anesthetic drugs. The endotracheal tube is removed during the postanesthesia period once the gag and swallowing reflexes have resumed. If an IV line was not inserted before the patient's arrival in surgery, it is inserted by the anesthesiologist before the administration of an induction drug.

Nursing Responsibilities

Preanesthesia

Before surgery, and during the administration of general anesthesia, the nurse has the following responsibilities:

- Performing the required tasks and procedures as prescribed by the physician and hospital policy before surgery and recording these tasks on the patient's chart. Examples of these tasks include administering a hypnotic agent before surgery, shaving the operative area, taking vital signs, seeing that the operative consent form is signed, checking that all jewelry or metal objects are removed from the patient, administering enemas, inserting a catheter, inserting a nasogastric tube, and teaching.

- Checking the chart for any recent abnormal laboratory test results. If a recent abnormal laboratory test finding was included in the patient's chart shortly before surgery, the nurse must make sure that the surgeon and the anesthesiologist are aware of the abnormality. The nurse attaches a note to the front of the chart and may also contact the surgeon or anesthesiologist by telephone.

- Placing a list of known or suspected drug allergies or idiosyncrasies on the front of the chart.

- Administering the preanesthetic (preoperative) drug.

- Instructing the patient to remain in bed and placing the bed's side rails up once the preanesthetic drug has been given.

Nursing Alert

Preanesthetic drugs must be administered on time to produce their intended effects. Failure to give the preanesthetic drug on time may result in such events as increased respiratory secretions caused by the irritating effect of anesthetic gases and the need for an increased dose of the induction drug because the preanesthetic drug has not had time to sedate the patient.

Postanesthesia: PACU

After surgery, the nurse has the following responsibilities, which vary according to where the nurse first sees the postoperative patient:

- Admitting the patient to the unit according to hospital procedure or policy.

- Checking the airway for patency, assessing the respiratory status, and giving oxygen as needed.

- Positioning the patient to prevent aspiration of vomitus and secretions.

- Checking blood pressure and pulse, IV lines, catheters, drainage tubes, surgical dressings, and casts.

- Reviewing the patient's surgical and anesthesia records.

- Monitoring the blood pressure, pulse, and respiratory rate every 5 to 15 minutes until the patient is discharged from the area.

- Checking the patient every 5 to 15 minutes for emergence from anesthesia. Suctioning is provided as needed.

- Exercising caution in administering opioids. The nurse must check the patient's respiratory rate, blood pressure, and pulse before these drugs are given and 20 to 30 minutes after administration (see Chapter 20). The physician is contacted if the respiratory rate is below 10 before the drug is given or if the respiratory rate falls below 10 after the drug is given.

- Discharging the patient from the area to his or her room or other specified area. The nurse must record all drugs administered and nursing tasks performed before the patient leaves the PACU.

Critical Thinking Exercises

1. Mr. Cantu's family asks you why a drug is being given before he goes to surgery for a bowel resection. When checking the chart, you note that Mr. Cantu has an order for meperidine HCl (Demerol) 50 mg IM and glycopyrrolate (Robinul) 0.35 mg IM 30 minutes before surgery. Describe how you would explain to the family the purpose of the preanesthetic drugs that are to be given to Mr. Cantu.

2. A nurse you are working with complains she was reprimanded and asked to fill out an incident report for not giving a preanesthetic drug on time. She states that she feels she is being unfairly accused of an error because the drug was given 10 minutes before the patient was taken to surgery. Explain why this is a potentially serious error.

3. Discuss the most important responsibilities of the nurse in the postanesthesia care unit after a patient has undergone general anesthesia.

Review Questions

1. When planning preoperative care, the nurse expects that a preanesthetic medication usually is given _____ before the patient is transported to surgery.

   A. 20 minutes

   B. 30 minutes

   C. 40 minutes

   D. 60 minutes

2. Which of the following drugs is the most commonly used gas for general anesthesia?

   A. Ethylene

   B. Enflurane

   C. Nitrous oxide

   D. Sevoflurane

3. Neuroleptanalgesia is used to promote general quietness, reduce motor activity, and induce profound analgesia. Which of the following two drugs are used in combination to accomplish neuroleptanalgesia?

   A. Fentanyl and droperidol

   B. Morphine and glycopyrrolate

   C. Atropine and meperidine

   D. Fentanyl and midazolam

4. One use of skeletal muscle relaxants as part of general anesthesia is to _____.

   A. prevent movement during surgery

   B. facilitate insertion of the endotracheal tube

   C. allow for deeper anesthesia

   D. produce additional anesthesia

Medication Dosage Problems

1. As a preoperative medication for a patient going to surgery, the anesthesiologist prescribes meperidine HCl (Demerol) 50 mg IM. Meperidine is available in solution of 50 mg/mL. The nurse prepares to administer _____.

2. Glycopyrrolate (Robinul) is prescribed for a patient as part of the preoperative preparation for surgery. The drug dose recommendation is 0.002 mg/lb. The patient weighs 150 lb. The nurse expects the primary care provider to prescribe _____.

To check your answers, see Appendix G.

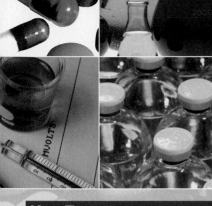

Chapter 22

Antianxiety Drugs

Key Terms

antianxiety drugs
anxiety
anxiolytics

Learning Objectives

On completion of this chapter, the student will:

- Discuss the uses, general drug actions, general adverse reactions, contraindications, precautions, and interactions associated with the administration of the antianxiety drugs.
- Discuss important preadministration and ongoing assessment activities

the nurse should perform on the patient taking antianxiety drugs.

- List nursing diagnoses particular to a patient taking antianxiety drugs.
- Discuss ways to promote an optimal response to therapy, how to manage common adverse reactions, and important points to keep in mind when educating patients about the use of antianxiety drugs.

Anxiety is a feeling of apprehension, worry, or uneasiness that may or may not be based on reality. Anxiety may be seen in many types of situations, ranging from the "jitters" and excitement of a new job to the acute panic that may be seen during withdrawal from alcohol. Although a certain amount of anxiety is normal, excess anxiety interferes with day-to-day functioning and can cause undue stress in the lives of certain individuals. Drugs used to treat anxiety are called *antianxiety drugs*. Another term that refers to the antianxiety drugs is **anxiolytics**.

Antianxiety drugs include the benzodiazepines and the nonbenzodiazepines. Examples of the benzodiazepines include alprazolam (Xanax), chlordiazepoxide (Librium), diazepam (Valium), and lorazepam (Ativan). Long-term use of benzodiazepines can result in physical or psychological dependence. Therefore, these drugs are classified as schedule IV in the Controlled Substances Act by the Drug Enforcement Agency (DEA) regulations (see Chapter 1). Nonbenzodiazepines useful as antianxiety drugs include buspirone (BuSpar), doxepin (Sinequan), and hydroxyzine (Atarax).

Actions

Anxiolytic drugs exert their tranquilizing effect by blocking certain neurotransmitter receptor sites. In turn, this prevents the neurotransmission of the anxious perception and the body's physical reaction to the anxiety. Benzodiazepines exert their tranquilizing effect by potentiating the effects of gamma-aminobutyric acid (GABA), an inhibitory transmitter. Nonbenzodiazepines exert their action in various ways. For example, buspirone is thought to act on the brain's serotonin receptors. Hydroxyzine (Atarax or Vistaril) produces its antianxiety effect by acting on the hypothalamus and brainstem reticular formation.

Uses

Antianxiety drugs are used in the management of

- Anxiety disorders and panic attacks
- Preanesthetic sedation and muscle relaxation
- Convulsions or seizures
- Alcohol withdrawal

Adverse Reactions

Frequent, early reactions include

- Mild drowsiness or sedation
- Lightheadedness or dizziness
- Headache

Other adverse body system reactions include

- Lethargy, apathy, fatigue
- Disorientation
- Anger
- Restlessness
- Nausea, constipation or diarrhea, dry mouth
- Visual disturbances

See the Summary Drug Table: Antianxiety Drugs for more information.

Dependence

Long-term use of antianxiety drugs may result in physical drug dependence and tolerance (increasingly larger dosages required to obtain the desired effect). Withdrawal symptoms have occurred when the drug is stopped after as few as 4 to 6 weeks of therapy with a benzodiazepine.

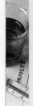

Nursing Alert

Symptoms of benzodiazepine withdrawal include increased anxiety, concentration difficulties, tremor, and sensory disturbances, such as paresthesias, photophobia, hypersomnia, and metallic taste.

Typically, withdrawal symptoms are more likely to occur when the benzodiazepine is taken for 3 months or more and is abruptly discontinued. Therefore, antianxiety

Display 22.1 Symptoms of Withdrawal

- Increased anxiety
- Fatigue
- Hypersomnia
- Metallic taste
- Concentration difficulties
- Headache
- Tremors
- Numbness in the extremities
- Nausea
- Sweating
- Muscle tension and cramps
- Psychoses
- Hallucinations
- Memory impairment
- Convulsions (possible)

drugs must never be discontinued abruptly. Instead, a gradually decreasing dosage schedule (known as *tapering*) should be used when the drug is to be stopped. The onset of withdrawal symptoms usually occurs within 1 to 10 days after discontinuing the drug, with the duration of withdrawal symptoms from 5 days to 1 month. Symptoms of withdrawal are identified in Display 22-1.

Some antianxiety drugs, such as buspirone (BuSpar), are associated with less physical dependence potential and less effect on motor ability and cognition than others.

Contraindications

The nurse should not administer antianxiety drugs to patients with known hypersensitivity, psychoses, and acute narrow-angle glaucoma. The benzodiazepines are contraindicated during pregnancy (category D drugs) and labor because of reports of floppy infant syndrome manifested by sucking difficulties, lethargy, and hypotonia seen in the newborn. Lactating women should also avoid the benzodiazepines because of the effect on the infant, who becomes lethargic and loses weight.

Buspirone (BuSpar) is a pregnancy category B drug and hydroxyzine is a pregnancy category C drug. Their safety is still questionable because adequate studies have not been performed in pregnant women. All of these drugs are also contraindicated when patients are in a coma or shock, and if the vital signs of the patient in acute alcoholic intoxication are low.

SUMMARY DRUG TABLE ANTIANXIETY DRUGS

GENERIC NAME	TRADE NAME	USES	ADVERSE REACTIONS	DOSAGE RANGES
Benzodiazepines				
alprazolam *al-prah'-zoe-lam*	Niravam, Xanax	Anxiety disorders, short-term relief of anxiety, panic attacks	Transient mild drowsiness, lightheadedness, headache, depression, constipation, diarrhea, dry mouth	0.25–0.5 mg orally TID, may be increased to 4 mg/d in divided doses
chlordiazepoxide *klor-dye-az-e-pox'-ide*	Librium	Anxiety disorders, short-term relief of anxiety, acute alcohol withdrawal	Same as alprazolam	Anxiety: 5–25 mg orally 3 or 4 times daily Acute alcohol withdrawal: 50–100 mg IM, then 25–50 mg IM
clonazepam *klon-az'-eh-pam*	Klonopin	Panic disorder, anticonvulsant	Same as alprazolam	0.25 mg orally BID
clorazepate *klor-az'-eh-pate*	Tranxene, Tranxene SD	Anxiety disorders, short-term relief of anxiety, acute alcohol withdrawal, anticonvulsant	Same as alprazolam	Anxiety: 15–60 mg/d orally in divided doses Acute alcohol withdrawal: Up to 90 mg/d with taper-off schedule
diazepam *dye-az'-eh-pam*	Valium	Anxiety disorders, short-term relief of anxiety, acute alcohol withdrawal, anticonvulsant, preoperative muscle relaxant	Same as alprazolam	Individualize dosage: 2–10 mg IM, IV, or orally 2–4 times daily
lorazepam *lor-az'-eh-pam*	Ativan	Anxiety disorders, short-term relief of anxiety, preanesthetic	Same as alprazolam	1–10 mg/d orally in divided doses; when used as preanesthetic: up to 4 mg IM, IV
oxazepam *ox-az'-eh-pam*		Anxiety disorders, short-term relief of anxiety	Same as alprazolam	10–30 mg orally 3–4 times daily
Nonbenzodiazepines				
buspirone HCl *byoo-spye'-rone*	BuSpar	Anxiety disorders, short-term relief of anxiety	Dizziness, drowsiness	15–60 mg/d orally in divided doses
doxepin HCl *docks'-e-pin*	Sinequan	Anxiety and depression	Same as buspirone	75–150 mg/d, up to 300 mg/d for those severely ill

SUMMARY DRUG TABLE *(continued)*

GENERIC NAME	TRADE NAME	USES	ADVERSE REACTIONS	DOSAGE RANGES
hydroxyzine *high-drox'-ih-zeen*	Atarax, Vistaril	Anxiety and tension associated with psychoneurosis, pruritus, preanesthetic sedative	Dry mouth, transitory drowsiness, involuntary motor activity	25–100 mg orally QID Preanesthetic: 50–100 mg orally or 25–100 mg IM
meprobamate *me-proe-ba'-mate*	Miltown	Anxiety disorders, short-term relief of anxiety	Drowsiness, ataxia, nausea, dizziness, slurred speech, headache, weakness, vomiting, diarrhea	1.2–1.6 g/d orally in 3–4 doses, not to exceed 2.4 g/d

Precautions

Antianxiety drugs are used cautiously in elderly patients and in patients with impaired liver function, impaired kidney function, or debilitation.

Interactions

The following interactions may occur when an anxiolytic is administered with another agent:

Interacting Drug	Common Use	Effect of Interaction
alcohol	Relaxation and enjoyment in social situations	Increased risk for central nervous system (CNS) depression or convulsions
analgesics	Pain relief	Increased risk for CNS depression
tricyclic antidepressants	Management of depression	Increased risk for sedation and respiratory depression
antipsychotics	Control of psychotic symptoms	Increased risk for sedation and respiratory depression
digoxin	Management of cardiac problems	Increased risk for digitalis toxicity

Herbal Alert

Kava is a popular herbal remedy thought to relieve stress, anxiety, and tension; promote sleep; and provide relief from menstrual discomfort. Kava's benefits are not supported by science, and the U.S. Food and Drug Administration (FDA) has issued an alert indicating that the use of kava may cause liver damage. Because kava-containing products have been associated with liver-related injuries (e.g., hepatitis, cirrhosis, and liver failure), the safest way to use kava is to take the herb occasionally for episodes of anxiety, rather than on a daily basis. It is important that individuals who use a kava-containing dietary supplement and experience signs of liver disease immediately consult their primary health care provider. Symptoms of liver disease include jaundice, urine with a brownish discoloration, nausea, vomiting, light-colored stools, weakness, and loss of appetite. Adverse effects experienced with the use of dietary supplements should be reported to the FDA's Med-Watch program (see Appendix B). Identifying kava-containing products can be difficult. Careful reading of the "Supplement Facts" information on the label may identify kava by any of the following names: kava, ava, ava pepper, awa, kava root, kava-kava, kew, *Piper methysticum* G. Forst, *Piper methysticum*, sakau, tonga, yangona.

NURSING PROCESS

The Patient Receiving an Antianxiety Drug
ASSESSMENT
PREADMINISTRATION ASSESSMENT

A patient receiving an antianxiety drug may be treated in the hospital or in an outpatient setting. Before starting therapy for the hospitalized patient, the nurse obtains a complete medical history, including mental status and anxiety level. In the case of mild anxiety, patients may (but sometimes may not) give a reliable history of their illness.

When severe anxiety is present, the patient may be unable to communicate effectively. Therefore, it is important to obtain portions of the history from a family member or friend. During the intake history, the nurse observes the patient for behavioral signs indicating anxiety (e.g., inability to focus, extreme restlessness, facial grimaces, tense posture).

Physical assessment should include the blood pressure, pulse, respiratory rate, and weight. Physiologic manifestations of anxiety can include increased blood pressure and pulse rate, increased rate and depth of respiration, and increased muscle tension. An anxious patient may have cool and pale skin.

The nurse makes sure to obtain a history of any past drug or alcohol use. This information can help establish what the patient has used in the past as coping mechanisms. Individuals with mild anxiety or depression do not necessarily require inpatient care. These patients are usually seen at periodic intervals in the primary health care provider's office or in a mental health outpatient setting. The preadministration assessments of the outpatient are the same as those for the hospitalized patient.

ONGOING ASSESSMENT

An ongoing assessment is important for the patient taking an antianxiety drug. The nurse checks the patient's blood pressure before drug administration. If systolic pressure has dropped 20 mm Hg, the nurse withholds the drug and notifies the primary health care provider. The nurse periodically monitors the patient's mental status and anxiety level during therapy and assesses for improvement or worsening of behavioral and physical signs identified in the preadministration assessment.

The nurse can ask the patient or a family member about adverse drug reactions or any other problems occurring during therapy. The nurse then brings these reactions or problems to the attention of the primary health care provider. The nurse documents a general summary of the patient's outward behavior and any complaints or problems in the patient's record. The nurse then compares new information with previous notations and observations.

NURSING DIAGNOSES

Drug-specific nursing diagnoses are highlighted in the Nursing Diagnoses Checklist. Other nursing diagnoses applicable to these drugs are discussed in depth in Chapter 4.

Nursing Diagnoses Checklist

- ✓ **Risk for Injury** related to dizziness or hypotension and gait problems
- ✓ **Impaired Comfort** related to dryness in gastrointestinal tract from medications
- ✓ **Ineffective Individual Coping** related to situation causing anxiety

---

PLANNING

The expected patient outcomes may include an optimal response to drug therapy, support of patient needs in relation to managing adverse drug reactions, and a knowledge of and compliance with the prescribed therapeutic regimen.

IMPLEMENTATION

PROMOTING AN OPTIMAL RESPONSE TO THERAPY

During initial therapy, the nurse observes the patient closely for adverse drug reactions. Some adverse reactions, such as episodes of postural hypotension and drowsiness or dry mouth, may need to be tolerated because drug therapy must continue. The antianxiety drugs are not recommended for long-term use. When the antianxiety drugs are used for short periods (1 to 2 weeks), tolerance, dependence, or withdrawal symptoms usually do not develop. The nurse reports any signs of tolerance or dependence, such as the patient needing larger doses of drug or complaint of increased anxiety and agitation (see Display 22-1).

MONITORING AND MANAGING PATIENT NEEDS

RISK FOR INJURY When these drugs are given in the outpatient setting, the nurse should instruct both the patient and family about the adverse reactions (dizziness, lightheadedness or ataxia) that can cause a patient to fall and become injured. This is very important when the drugs are administered to elderly patients in an outpatient setting.

Gerontologic Alert

Benzodiazepines are excreted more slowly in older adults, causing a prolonged drug effect. The drugs may accumulate in the blood, resulting in an increase in adverse reactions or toxicity. For this reason, the initial dose should be small, and the dose increased gradually until a therapeutic response is obtained.

However, lorazepam and oxazepam are relatively safe for older adults when given in normal dosages. Buspirone (BuSpar) also is a safe choice for older adults with anxiety because it does not cause excessive sedation, and the risk of falling is not as great.

When the patient is hospitalized, the nurse develops a nursing care plan to meet the patient's individual needs. Vital signs can be monitored at frequent intervals, usually three or four times daily. Patients can be monitored for symptoms such as dizziness or lightheadedness. Patients can be instructed to stay in bed and call for assistance to get up out of the bed or chair, and may need to be supervised for all ambulatory activities. The nurse should provide total assistance with activities of daily living to the patient experiencing extreme sedation. This includes help with eating, dressing, and ambulating. In some instances, such as when a hypotensive episode occurs, the vital signs are taken more often. Then the nurse reports any significant change in the vital signs to the primary health care provider. The sedation and drowsiness that sometimes occur with the use of an antianxiety drug may decrease as therapy continues.

Parenteral administration is indicated primarily in acute states when it is difficult for the patient to take the medication by mouth. When these drugs are given intramuscularly (IM), the nurse gives them in a large muscle mass, such as the gluteus muscle. The nurse observes the patient closely for at least 3 hours after parenteral administration. The patient is kept lying down (when possible) for 30 minutes to 3 hours after the drug is given.

Gerontologic Alert

Parenteral (intravenous [IV] or IM) administration to older adults, the debilitated, and those with limited pulmonary reserve requires that the nurse exert extreme care because the patient may experience apnea and cardiac arrest. Resuscitative equipment should be readily available during parenteral (particularly IV) administration.

IMPAIRED COMFORT Antianxiety drugs can cause both dryness of the mucous membranes and slower transit in the intestines, leading to constipation. Nursing interventions to relieve some of these reactions may include offering frequent sips of water to relieve dry mouth and provide adequate hydration. The patient may also chew sugarless gum or suck on hard candy to reduce discomfort from dry mouth. The nurse may administer oral antianxiety drugs with food or meals to decrease the possibility of gastrointestinal upset. Meals should include fiber, fruits, and vegetables to aid in preventing constipation. However, the nurse should use great care when administering these drugs orally because some patients have difficulty swallowing (because of a dry mouth or other causes).

INEFFECTIVE INDIVIDUAL COPING When the patient is an outpatient, the nurse observes the patient for a response to therapy at the time of each clinic visit. In some instances, the nurse may question the patient or a family member about the response to therapy. The type of questions asked depends on the patient and the diagnosis, and may include open-ended questions such as "How are you feeling?" "Do you seem to feel less nervous?" or "Would you like to tell me how everything is going?" Many times the nurse may need to rephrase questions or direct the conversation toward other subjects until these patients feel comfortable enough to discuss their therapy.

Once the patient has reduced the anxious behavior, the nurse may be able to help the patient identify what is precipitating the panic attacks or causing anxiety. It is important for the nurse to help patients understand that there are health care providers who can help them gain skills to cope with situations before the anxious behavior returns.

Although rare, benzodiazepine toxicity may occur from an overdose of the drug. Benzodiazepine toxicity causes sedation, respiratory depression, and coma. Flumazenil (Romazicon) is an antidote (antagonist) for benzodiazepine toxicity and acts to reverse the sedation, respiratory depression, and coma within 6 to 10 minutes after IV administration. Adverse reactions to flumazenil include agitation, confusion, seizures, and, in some cases, symptoms of benzodiazepine withdrawal. Adverse reactions to flumazenil, related to the symptoms of benzodiazepine withdrawal, are relieved by the administration of the benzodiazepine.

EDUCATING THE PATIENT AND FAMILY

The nurse evaluates the patient's ability to assume responsibility for taking drugs at home. The nurse explains any adverse reactions that may occur with a specific antianxiety drug and encourages the patient or family members to contact the primary health care provider immediately if a serious adverse reaction occurs. The nurse should include the following points in a teaching plan for the patient or family member:

• Take the drug exactly as directed. Do not increase, decrease, or omit a dose or discontinue use of this drug unless directed to do so by the primary health care provider.

• Do not discontinue use of the drug abruptly because withdrawal symptoms may occur.

• Avoid driving or performing other hazardous tasks if drowsiness occurs.

- Do not take any nonprescription drug unless the specific drug has been approved by the primary health care provider.

- Inform physicians, dentists, and other health care providers of therapy with this drug.

- Do not drink alcoholic beverages unless approval is obtained from the primary health care provider.

- If dizziness occurs when changing position, rise slowly when getting out of bed or a chair. If dizziness is severe, always have help when changing positions.

- If dryness of the mouth occurs, relieve it by taking frequent sips of water, sucking on hard candy, or chewing gum (preferably sugarless).

- Prevent constipation by eating foods high in fiber, increasing fluid intake, and exercising if condition permits.

- Keep all appointments with the primary health care provider because close monitoring of therapy is essential.

- Report any unusual changes or physical effects to the primary health care provider.

EVALUATION

- The therapeutic effect is achieved.

- The patient reports a decrease in feelings of anxiety.

- Adverse reactions are identified, reported to the primary health care provider, and managed successfully through appropriate nursing interventions.

- The patient verbalizes the importance of complying with the prescribed therapeutic regimen.

- The patient and family demonstrate an understanding of the drug regimen.

Critical Thinking Exercises

1. Ms. Stovall, aged 66 years, is hospitalized for congestive heart failure. She is improving, but has been complaining of feelings of anxiety. Her respirations are 32 breaths/min, heart rate 88 beats/min, and blood pressure 118/60 mm Hg. The primary health care provider prescribes alprazolam (Xanax) 0.25 mg orally three times a day. What precautions would the nurse expect to be taken because of Ms. Stovall's age? Discuss what assessment findings would indicate increased anxiety.

2. The primary health care provider prescribes lorazepam (Ativan) for short-term management of

anxiety. What information would be included in a teaching plan for this patient?

3. A patient is prescribed buspirone (BuSpar) 5 mg orally three times a day to be taken on an outpatient basis. What assessments would be important for the nurse to make when the patient comes to the clinic for a visit?

Review Questions

1. Alprazolam (Xanax) is contraindicated in patients with _____.

   A. a psychotic disorder
   B. congestive heart failure
   C. diabetes
   D. hypertension

2. Which of the following drugs is a schedule IV controlled substance?

   A. hydroxyzine (Vistaril)
   B. doxepin HCl (Sinequan)
   C. buspirone HCl (BuSpar)
   D. chlordiazepoxide (Librium)

3. Which of the following is a sign of drug withdrawal and not an adverse reaction?

   A. Dizziness
   B. Metallic taste
   C. Constipation
   D. Sedation

4. The benzodiazepines are pregnancy category D drugs that should not be taken while lactating because the newborn may become _____.

   A. depressed
   B. excited and irritable
   C. lethargic and lose weight
   D. hypoglycemic

Medication Dosage Problems

1. Hydroxyzine (Vistaril) 100 mg IM is prescribed. Available is a vial with 100 mg hydroxyzine per milliliter. The nurse administers _____.

2. The patient is prescribed 30 mg oxazepam three times a day orally. The drug is available in 15-mg tablets. The nurse administers _____.

To check your answers, see Appendix G.

Antianxiety Drugs

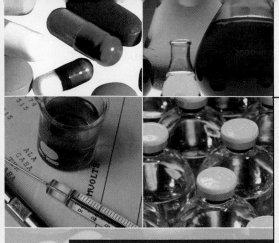

Chapter 23

Sedatives and Hypnotics

Key Terms

ataxia
hypnotic
sedative

Learning Objectives

On completion of this chapter, the student will:

- Differentiate between a sedative and a hypnotic.
- Discuss the uses, general drug actions, adverse reactions, contraindications, precautions, and interactions of the sedatives and hypnotics.
- Discuss important preadministration and ongoing assessment activities

the nurse should perform with the patient taking a sedative or hypnotic.

- List nursing diagnoses particular to a patient taking a sedative or hypnotic.
- Discuss ways to promote an optimal response to therapy, how to manage common adverse reactions, and important points to keep in mind when educating patients about the use of a sedative or hypnotic.

The sedatives and hypnotics are primarily used to treat insomnia. According to the National Sleep Foundation, insomnia affects nearly 70 million people in the United States. It may be caused by lifestyle changes, such as a new job or moving to a new town, returning to school, jet lag, chronic pain, headaches, stress, or anxiety.

In many cases, insomnia occurs during hospitalization. Patients are in unfamiliar surroundings that are unlike the home situation. There are noises and lights at night, which often interfere with or interrupt sleep. An important part of meeting patient needs during illness is to help the patient gain rest and sleep. Sleep deprivation may interfere with the healing process; therefore, a hypnotic may be given. These drugs also may be prescribed for short-term use to promote sleep after discharge from the hospital.

A **hypnotic** is a drug that induces drowsiness or sleep, that is, it allows the patient to fall asleep and stay asleep. Hypnotics are given at night or at the hour of sleep (HS). A **sedative** is a drug that produces a relaxing, calming effect. Sedatives are usually given during daytime hours, and although they may make the patient drowsy, they usually do not produce sleep.

Sedatives and hypnotics may be divided into two classes: barbiturates and nonbarbiturates. The nonbarbiturates are classified into two groups: benzodiazepines and miscellaneous sedatives and hypnotics. Barbiturates were once the drugs of choice to treat insomnia and anxiety. The nonbarbiturates are now used as sedatives more frequently than the barbiturates because the benzodiazepines are more effective in treating insomnia and the adverse reactions of barbiturates are more severe. The benzodiazepines are also used as antianxiety drugs (see Chapter 22). Examples of the benzodiazepines discussed in this chapter include estazolam (ProSom), flurazepam (Dalmane), and quazepam (Doral).

The miscellaneous sedatives and hypnotics consist of a group of nonrelated drugs. Examples of the nonrelated group of drugs include eszopiclone (Lunesta),

SUMMARY DRUG TABLE — SEDATIVES AND HYPNOTICS

GENERIC NAME	TRADE NAME	USES	ADVERSE REACTIONS	DOSAGE RANGES
Benzodiazepines				
estazolam *es-taz'-e-lam*	ProSom	Hypnotic	Headache, heartburn, nausea, palpitations, rash, somnolence, vomiting, weakness, body and joint pain	1–2 mg orally
flurazepam *flur-az'-e-pam*	Dalmane	Hypnotic	Same as estazolam	15–30 mg orally
quazepam *kwa'-ze-pam*	Doral	Hypnotic	Same as estazolam	7.5–15 mg orally
temazepam *te-maz'-e-pam*	Restoril	Hypnotic	Same as estazolam	15–30 mg orally
triazolam *trye-ay'-zoe-lam*	Halcion	Sedative, hypnotic	Same as estazolam	0.125–0.5 mg orally at bedtime
Nonbenzodiazepines				
eszopiclone	Lunesta	Chronic insomnia	Headache, somnolence, taste changes, chest pain, migraine, edema	1–3 mg orally at bedtime
ramelteon	Rozerem	Insomnia	Dizziness, headache	8 mg orally at bedtime
zaleplon *zal'-ah-plahn*	Sonata	Transient insomnia	Dizziness, headache, rebound insomnia, nausea, myalgia	10 mg orally at bedtime
℞ zolpidem tartrate *zol'-pih-dem*	Ambien, Ambien CR (*controlled release*)	Transient insomnia	Drowsiness, headache, myalgia, nausea	10 mg orally at bedtime
Barbiturates				
pentobarbital sodium *pen-toe-bar'-bi-tall*	Nembutal Sodium	Sedative, hypnotic, preoperative sedation	Respiratory and CNS depression, nausea, vomiting, constipation, diarrhea, bradycardia, hypotension, syncope, hypersensitivity reactions, headache	Available only in parenteral form: 100 mg deep IM or IV, may titrate up to 200–500 mg
secobarbital sodium *see-koe-bar'-bi-tall*	Seconal	Hypnotic, preoperative sedation	Same as pentobarbital sodium	Hypnotic: 100 mg orally at bedtime Sedation: 200–300 mg orally 1–2 h before procedure

℞ This drug should not be administered with food (especially high-fat meals).

zaleplon (Sonata), and zolpidem (Ambien). Barbiturates, benzodiazepines, and the miscellaneous sedatives and hypnotics are listed in the Summary Drug Table: Sedatives and Hypnotics.

Actions

Barbiturates

All barbiturates have essentially the same mode of action. Depending on the dose given, these drugs are capable of producing central nervous system (CNS) depression and mood alteration ranging from mild excitation to mild sedation, hypnosis (sleep), and deep coma. These drugs also are respiratory depressants; the degree of depression usually depends on the dose given. When these drugs are used as hypnotics, their respiratory depressant effect is usually similar to that occurring during sleep.

Benzodiazepines and the Miscellaneous Sedatives and Hypnotics

The nonbarbiturate sedatives and hypnotics have essentially the same mode of action as the barbiturates, that is, they depress the CNS. The benzodiazepine effect on GABA (gamma-aminobutyric acid) to potentiate neural inhibition is discussed in Chapter 22. However, these drugs have a lesser effect on the respiratory rate—another reason why they are chosen over barbiturates for insomnia.

Like the barbiturates, the miscellaneous drugs' sedative or hypnotic effects diminish after approximately 2 weeks. Persons taking these drugs for longer than 2 weeks may have a tendency to increase the dose to produce the desired effects (e.g., sleep, sedation). Physical tolerance and psychological dependence may occur, especially after prolonged use of high doses. However, their addictive potential appears to be less than that of the barbiturates. Discontinuing use of a sedative or hypnotic after prolonged use may result in mild to severe withdrawal symptoms.

Uses

The sedative and hypnotic drugs are used in the treatment of
- Insomnia
- Convulsions or seizures

They are also used as adjuncts for anesthesia and for
- Preoperative sedation
- Conscious sedation

Gerontologic Alert

Elderly patients may require a smaller hypnotic dose, and in some instances, a sedative dose produces sleep.

Adverse Reactions

- Nervous system reactions include dizziness, drowsiness, and headache.
- A common gastrointestinal reaction is nausea.

Contraindications

These drugs are contraindicated in patients with known hypersensitivity to the sedatives or hypnotics. The nurse should not administer these drugs to comatose patients, those with severe respiratory problems, those with a history of drug and alcohol habitual use, or to pregnant or lactating women. The barbiturates are classified as pregnancy category D drugs.

Benzodiazepines (e.g., estazolam, quazepam, temazepam, triazolam) used for sedation are classified as pregnancy category X drugs. Most miscellaneous sedatives and hypnotics are pregnancy category B or C drugs.

Nursing Alert

Women taking the barbiturates or the benzodiazepines should be warned of the potential risk to the fetus so that contraceptive methods may be instituted, if necessary. A child born to a mother taking benzodiazepines may experience withdrawal symptoms during the postnatal period.

Precautions

Sedatives and hypnotics should be used cautiously in lactating patients and in patients with hepatic or renal impairment, habitual alcohol use, and mental health problems.

Gerontologic Alert

The nurse uses these drugs cautiously in older adults or in those who are debilitated because these patients are more sensitive to the effects of the sedatives or hypnotics.

Interactions

The following interactions may occur when a sedative or hypnotic is administered with another agent:

Interacting Drug	Common Use	Effect of Interaction
antidepressants	Management of depression	Increased sedative effect
opioid analgesics	Pain relief	Increased sedative effect
antihistamines	Relief of allergy symptoms (runny nose and itching)	Increased sedative effect
phenothiazines (e.g., Thorazine)	Management of agitation and psychotic symptoms	Increased sedative effect
cimetidine (Tagamet)	Management of gastric upset	Increased sedative effect
Alcohol	Relaxation and enjoyment in social situations	Increased sedative effect

Health Supplement Alert

Melatonin is a hormone produced by the pineal gland in the brain. Melatonin has been used in treating insomnia, overcoming jet lag, and improving the effectiveness of the immune system, and as an antioxidant. The most significant use—at low doses—is the short-term treatment of insomnia. Melatonin obtained from animal pineal tissue is not recommended for use because of the risk of contamination. The synthetic form of melatonin does not carry this risk. However, melatonin is an over-the-counter (OTC) dietary supplement and has not been evaluated for safety, effectiveness, and purity by the U.S. Food and Drug Administration. All of the potential risks and benefits may not be known. Supplements should be purchased from a reliable source to minimize the risk of contamination. Individuals should consult with their primary health care provider or a pharmacist before using the supplement. Possible adverse reactions include headache and depression. Drowsiness may occur within 30 minutes after taking the supplement. The drowsiness may persist for an hour or more, affecting any activity that requires mental alertness, such as

Health Supplement Alert *(continued)*

driving. Although uncommon, allergic reactions (difficulty breathing, hives, or swelling of lips, tongue, or face) to melatonin have been reported. The supplement should be stopped and emergency care sought.

NURSING PROCESS

The Patient Receiving a Sedative or Hypnotic

ASSESSMENT

PREADMINISTRATION ASSESSMENT

Before administering a sedative or hypnotic, the nurse takes and records the patient's blood pressure, pulse, and respiratory rate. In addition to the vital signs, the nurse assesses the patient's needs by asking the following questions:

- Is the patient uncomfortable? If the reason for discomfort is pain, an analgesic, rather than a hypnotic, may be required.

- Is it too early for the patient to receive the drug? Is a later hour preferred?

- Does the patient receive an opioid analgesic every 4 to 6 hours? A hypnotic may not be necessary because an opioid analgesic can also induce drowsiness and sleep.

- Are there disturbances in the environment that may keep the patient awake and decrease the effectiveness of the drug?

- Is the sedative for a surgical procedure, and is its administration correctly timed?

- Has a consent form for the procedure been signed before the medication is given? Informed consent cannot be established if the patient has medication in his or her system.

Barbiturates have little or no analgesic action, so the nurse does not give these drugs if the patient has pain and cannot sleep. Barbiturates, when given in the presence of pain, may cause restlessness, excitement, and delirium.

If the patient is receiving one of these drugs for daytime sedation, the nurse assesses the patient's general mental state and level of consciousness. If the patient appears sedated and difficult to awaken, the nurse withholds the drug and contacts the primary health care provider as soon as possible.

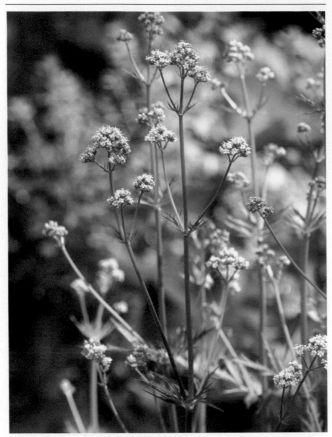

Figure 23.1 The root of the herb valerian is used medicinally. (From Facts and Comparisons. [2003]. *Guide to popular natural products* [3rd ed., p. I–16]. St. Louis: Facts and Comparisons.)

Herbal Alert

Valerian was originally used in Europe and was brought to North America on the *Mayflower* (Fig. 23-1). The herb is widely used for its sedative effects in conditions of mild anxiety or restlessness. It is particularly useful in individuals with insomnia. Valerian improves overall sleep quality by shortening the length of time it takes to fall asleep and decreasing the number of nighttime awakenings.

Formulated as a tea, tablet, capsule, or tincture, valerian is classified as "generally recognized as safe" (GRAS) for use in the United States. When used as an aid to sleep, valerian is taken approximately 1 hour before bedtime; less is used for anxiety. Valerian can be used in combination with other calming herbs, such as lemon balm or chamomile. It may take 2 to 4 weeks before the full therapeutic effect (i.e., improvement of mood and sleep patterns) occurs. Individuals have been known to experience withdrawal symptoms when they stop taking valerian abruptly.

ONGOING ASSESSMENT

Before administering the drug each time, the nurse should perform an assessment that includes the patient's vital signs (temperature, pulse, respiration, and blood pressure) and level of consciousness (e.g., alert, confused, or lethargic). This is especially important when the drug is to be given as needed (PRN). After assessing the patient, the nurse makes a decision regarding administration of the drug.

The nurse checks to see if the drug helped the patient sleep on previous nights. If not, a different drug or dose may be needed, and the nurse should consult the primary health care provider regarding the drug's ineffectiveness.

If the patient has a PRN order for an opioid analgesic or other CNS depressant and a hypnotic, the nurse should consult the primary health care provider regarding the time interval between administration of these drugs. Usually, at least 2 hours should elapse between administration of a hypnotic and any other CNS depressant, but this interval may vary, depending on factors such as the patient's age and diagnosis.

Nursing Alert

The nurse withholds the drug and notifies the primary health care provider if one or more vital signs significantly vary from the database, if the respiratory rate is 10 breaths/min or below, or if the patient appears lethargic. In addition, it is important to determine if there are any factors (e.g., noise, lights, pain, discomfort) that would interfere with sleep and whether these may be controlled or eliminated.

NURSING DIAGNOSES

Drug-specific nursing diagnoses are highlighted in the Nursing Diagnoses Checklist. Other nursing diagnoses applicable to these drugs are discussed in depth in Chapter 4.

Nursing Diagnoses Checklist

✔ **Risk for Injury** related to drowsiness or impaired memory

✔ **Ineffective Breathing Pattern** related to respiratory depression

✔ **Ineffective Individual Coping** related to excessive use of medication

PLANNING

The expected outcomes for the patient depend on the reason for administration of a sedative or hypnotic but may include an optimal response to drug therapy (e.g., sedation or sleep), support of patient needs related to management of adverse drug reactions, and an understanding of and compliance with the postdischarge drug regimen.

IMPLEMENTATION

PROMOTING AN OPTIMAL RESPONSE TO THERAPY

To promote the effects of the sedative or hypnotic drug, the nurse provides supportive care, such as back rubs, night lights or a darkened room, and a quiet atmosphere. The patient is discouraged from drinking beverages containing caffeine, such as coffee, tea, or cola drinks, which can contribute to wakefulness.

The nurse never leaves hypnotics and sedatives at the patient's bedside to be taken at a later hour; hypnotics and sedatives are controlled substances (see Chapter 1). In addition, the nurse never leaves these drugs unattended in the nurses' station, hallway, or other areas to which patients, visitors, or hospital personnel have direct access.

Nursing Alert

Some sleep medicines (zolpidem) may cause memory loss or amnesia. A person may not remember getting up out of bed, driving, or eating. These drugs should be taken when a person plans for 7 to 8 hours of sleep.

MONITORING AND MANAGING PATIENT NEEDS

RISK FOR INJURY It is important that the nurse observe the patient for adverse drug reactions. During periods when the patient is excited or confused, the nurse protects the patient from harm and provides supportive care and a safe environment. The nurse assesses the patient receiving a sedative dose and determines what safety measures must be taken. After administration of a hypnotic, the nurse may raise the side rails of the bed and advise the patient to remain in bed and to call for assistance if it is necessary to get out of bed. Patients receiving sedative doses may or may not require this safety measure, depending on the patient's response to the drug. The nurse assesses the patient receiving a hypnotic 1 to 2 hours after the drug is given to evaluate the effect of the drug. The nurse notifies the primary health care provider if the patient fails to sleep, awakens one or more times during the night, or experiences an adverse drug reaction. In some instances, supplemental doses of a hypnotic may be ordered if the patient awakens during the night.

Excessive drowsiness and headache the morning after a hypnotic has been given (drug hangover) may occur in some patients. The nurse reports this problem to the primary health care provider because a smaller dose or a different drug may be necessary. The nurse assists the patient with ambulation, if necessary. When getting out of bed the patient is encouraged to rise to a sitting position first, wait a few minutes, and then rise to a standing position.

Patients using these drugs in an outpatient setting are taught about the hazards of operating machinery or involvement in other potentially hazardous tasks until they are sure that concentration and focus are not affected.

Gerontologic Alert

The older adult is at greater risk for oversedation, dizziness, confusion, or **ataxia** (unsteady gait) when taking a sedative or hypnotic. The nurse checks elderly and debilitated patients for marked excitement, CNS depression, and confusion. If excitement or confusion occurs, the nurse observes the patient at frequent intervals (as often as every 5 to 10 minutes may be necessary) for the duration of this occurrence and institutes safety measures to prevent injury. If oversedation, extreme dizziness, or ataxia occurs, the nurse notifies the primary health care provider.

INEFFECTIVE BREATHING PATTERN Sedatives and hypnotics depress the CNS and can cause respiratory depression. The nurse carefully assesses respiratory function (rate, depth, and quality) before administering a sedative, 30 minutes to 1 hour after administering the drug, and frequently thereafter. When administering barbiturates, the nurse needs to be aware that the possibility of adverse reactions is greater than that from other sedatives and hypnotics.

Nursing Alert

The onset of symptoms of barbiturate toxicity may not occur until several hours after the drug is administered. Symptoms of acute toxicity include CNS and respiratory depression, constriction or paralytic dilation of the pupils, tachycardia, hypotension, lowered body temperature, oliguria, circulatory collapse, and coma. The nurse should report any symptoms of toxicity to the primary health care provider immediately.

Treatment of barbiturate toxicity is mainly supportive (i.e., maintaining a patent airway, oxygen administration, and monitoring vital signs and fluid balance). The patient may require treatment for shock, respiratory assistance, administration of activated charcoal, and, in severe cases of toxicity, hemodialysis.

The nurse should instruct the patient not to drink alcohol when taking sedatives or hypnotics. Alcohol is a CNS depressant, as are the sedatives and hypnotics. When alcohol and a sedative or hypnotic are taken together, there is an additive effect and an increase in CNS depression, which has, on occasion, resulted in death. The nurse must emphasize the importance of abstaining from alcohol use while taking this drug and stress that the use of alcohol and any one of these drugs can result in serious effects.

INEFFECTIVE INDIVIDUAL COPING Sedatives and hypnotics are best given for no more than 2 weeks and preferably for a shorter time. Sedatives and hypnotics can become less effective after they are taken for a prolonged period. Thus, there may be a tendency to increase the dose without consulting the primary health care provider. To ensure compliance with the treatment regimen, the nurse emphasizes the importance of not increasing or decreasing the dose unless a change in dosage is recommended by the primary health care provider. In addition, the nurse stresses the importance of not repeating the dose during the night if sleep is interrupted or sleep lasts only a few hours, unless the primary health care provider has approved taking the drug more than once per night.

Although the practice is not recommended, a patient with sleep disturbances may be taking one of these drugs for an extended period of time. A barbiturate or miscellaneous sedative and hypnotic can cause drug dependency. The nurse must never suddenly discontinue use of these drugs when there is a question of possible dependency. Patients who have been taking a sedative or hypnotic for several weeks should gradually withdraw from taking the drug to prevent withdrawal symptoms (see Chapter 22). Symptoms of withdrawal include restlessness, excitement, euphoria, and confusion. Withdrawal can result in serious consequences, especially in those with existing diseases or disorders.

EDUCATING THE PATIENT AND FAMILY

In educating the patient and family about sedatives and hypnotics, several general points must be considered. The nurse gives the patient and family an explanation of the prescribed drug and dosage regimen, as well as situations that should be avoided. The nurse develops a teaching plan to include one or more of the following items of information:

- The primary health care provider usually prescribes these drugs for short-term use only.

- If the drug appears to be ineffective, contact the primary health care provider. Do not increase the dose unless advised to do so by the primary health care provider.

- Notify the primary health care provider if any adverse drug reactions occur.

- Do not drink any alcoholic beverage 2 hours before, with, or 8 hours after taking the drug.

- When taking the drug as a sedative, be aware that the drug can impair the mental and physical abilities required for performing potentially dangerous tasks, such as driving a car or operating machinery.

- Observe caution when getting out of bed at night after taking a drug for sleep. Keep the room dimly lit and remove any obstacles that may result in injury when getting out of bed. Never attempt to drive or perform any hazardous task after taking a drug intended to produce sleep.

- Do not use these drugs if you are pregnant, considering becoming pregnant, or breast-feeding.

- Do not use OTC cold, cough, or allergy drugs while taking this drug unless their use has been approved by the primary health care provider. Some of these products contain antihistamines or other drugs that also may cause mild to extreme drowsiness. Others may contain an adrenergic drug, which is a mild stimulant, and therefore will defeat the purpose of the sedative or hypnotic.

- Do not take zolpidem with a high-fat meal or snack because fat interferes with absorption of the drug.

EVALUATION

- The therapeutic effect is achieved.

- The sleep pattern is improved.

- Adverse drug reactions are identified, reported to the primary health care provider, and managed successfully through appropriate nursing interventions.

- The patient and family demonstrate an understanding of and comply with the prescribed therapeutic regimen.

- The patient verbalizes an understanding of what to avoid while taking the drug.

Critical Thinking Exercises

1. Ms. Parker's husband was killed in an automobile accident, and she has had trouble coping with her loss. She complains of being unable to sleep for

more than an hour before she wakes. The primary health care provider prescribes a hypnotic, 1 capsule per night for use during the next 3 weeks. In 2 weeks, she calls the primary health care provider's office and asks for a refill of her prescription. Determine what questions you would you ask Ms. Parker. Explain why you would ask them.

2. Mr. Davidson, who is 57 years old, is to be discharged after major bowel surgery. The primary health care provider gives him a prescription for 24 tablets of zolpidem (Ambien). When reading Mr. Davidson's chart you note that he works part time on weekends as a bartender. Discuss what you would emphasize when explaining the prescription to Mr. Davidson.

3. Mr. Allen, who is hospitalized in the coronary care unit with a myocardial infarction, is restless and tells you that although he has been able to sleep other nights while in the hospital, he is unable to sleep tonight. Although he has an order for flurazepam (Dalmane) 30 mg at bedtime (HS), analyze what you would investigate before making a decision regarding administration of the hypnotic.

4. Discuss and give a rationale for situations or conditions in which sedatives would be contraindicated.

5. Explain why sedatives or hypnotics must be given cautiously to older adults.

Review Questions

1. Ms. Brown has arthritis in her lower back, and the pain keeps her awake at night. She asks if she can have a "sleeping pill." In considering her request, the nurse must take into account that _____.

   A. hypnotics might not be the drug of choice when pain causes insomnia

   B. a hypnotic may be given instead of an analgesic to relieve her pain

   C. hypnotics often increase the pain threshold

   D. a hypnotic plus an analgesic is best given in this situation

2. Which of these of these assessments should the nurse report immediately to the primary health provider?

   A. Dizziness when arising from the chair

   B. Heart rate of 80 beats/min

   C. Respiration rate of 8/min

   D. Joint pain

3. When giving a hypnotic to Ms. Green, aged 82 years, the nurse is aware that _____.

   A. smaller doses of the drug are usually given to older patients

   B. elderly patients usually require larger doses of a hypnotic

   C. older adults excrete the drug faster than younger adults

   D. dosages of the hypnotic may be increased each night until the desired effect is achieved

4. Which of the following points should be included in a teaching plan for a patient taking a sedative or hypnotic?

   A. An alcoholic beverage may be served 1 to 2 hours before a sedative is taken without any ill effects.

   B. Dosage of the sedative may be increased if sleep is not restful.

   C. These drugs may safely be used for 6 months to 1 year when given for insomnia.

   D. Do not use any over-the-counter cold, cough, or allergy medications while taking a sedative or hypnotic.

5. Which of the following sedatives/hypnotics is a pregnancy category X drug?

   A. zolpidem (Ambien)

   B. amobarbital (Amytal)

   C. temazepam (Restoril)

   D. eszopiclone (Lunesta)

Medication Dosage Problems

1. Triazolam (Halcion) 0.125 mg is prescribed. The drug is available in 0.125-mg tablets. The nurse administers _____.

2. Eszopiclone (Lunesta) 2 mg is prescribed for insomnia. The drug is available in 1-mg tablets. The nurse administers _____.

To check your answers, see Appendix G.

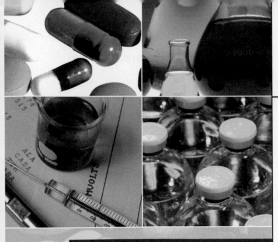

Chapter 24

Antidepressant Drugs

Key Terms

depression
dysphoric
endogenous
neurohormones
orthostatic hypotension
priapism
tardive dyskinesia
tyramine

Learning Objectives

On completion of this chapter, the student will:

- Define depression and identify symptoms of a major depressive episode.
- Name the different types of antidepressant drugs.
- Discuss the uses, general drug actions, general adverse reactions, contraindications, precautions, and interactions of the antidepressant drugs.

- Discuss important preadministration and ongoing assessment activities that the nurse should perform on the patient taking antidepressant drugs.
- List nursing diagnoses particular to a patient taking antidepressant drugs.
- Discuss ways to promote an optimal response to therapy, how to manage common adverse reactions, and important points to keep in mind when educating patients about the use of antidepressant drugs.

Depression may be described as feeling sad, unhappy, or "down in the dumps." Most of us feel this way at one time or another for short periods. A major depressive episode is a depressed or **dysphoric** (extreme or exaggerated sadness, anxiety, or unhappiness) mood that interferes with daily functioning. To be classified as clinical depression, five or more of the symptoms listed in Display 24-1 need to occur daily or nearly every day for a period of 2 weeks or more. It should be noted that the symptoms of clinical depression are not the result of normal bereavement, such as the loss of a loved one, or another disease, such as hypothyroidism.

Clinical depression is treated with antidepressant drugs, and psychotherapy is used with the antidepressants in treating major depressive episodes. The four types of antidepressants are

- Tricyclic antidepressants (TCAs)
- Monoamine oxidase inhibitors (MAOIs)

Display 24.1 Symptoms of Depression

- Feelings of hopeless or helplessness
- Diminished interest in activities of life
- Significant weight loss or gain (without dieting)
- Insomnia (inability to sleep) or hypersomnia (excessive sleeping)
- Agitation, restlessness, or irritability
- Fatigue or loss of energy
- Feelings of worthlessness
- Excessive or inappropriate guilt
- Diminished ability to think or concentrate, or indecisiveness
- Recurrent thoughts of death or suicide (or suicide attempt)

- Selective serotonin reuptake inhibitors (SSRIs)
- Miscellaneous, unrelated drugs

TRICYCLIC ANTIDEPRESSANTS
Actions

For several years it was thought that the antidepressants blocked the reuptake of the **endogenous** (produced by the body) neurotransmitters norepinephrine and serotonin. This action resulted in stimulation of the central nervous system (CNS) and alleviation of the depressed mood. This theory is now being questioned. New research indicates that the effects of the antidepressants are related to slow adaptive changes in norepinephrine and serotonin receptor systems. Treatment with the antidepressants is thought to produce complex changes in the sensitivities of both presynaptic and postsynaptic receptor sites. The antidepressants increase the sensitivity of postsynaptic alpha-adrenergic and serotonin receptors and decrease the sensitivity of the presynaptic receptor sites. This enhances recovery from the depressive episode by making neurotransmission activity more effective, as visualized in Figure 24-1. The TCAs, such as amitriptyline and doxepin (Sinequan), inhibit reuptake of norepinephrine or serotonin in the brain.

Uses

Tricyclic antidepressant drugs are used in the treatment of
- Depressive episodes
- Bipolar disorder
- Obsessive-compulsive disorders
- Chronic neuropathic pain
- Depression accompanied by anxiety disorders
- Enuresis

Unlabeled uses include peptic ulcer disease, sleep apnea, panic disorder, bulimia nervosa, premenstrual symptoms, and some dermatologic problems. These drugs may be used with psychotherapy in severe cases.

Adverse Reactions

Generalized body system reactions include
- Anticholinergic effects (e.g., sedation, dry mouth, visual disturbances, urinary retention)
- Constipation and photosensitivity

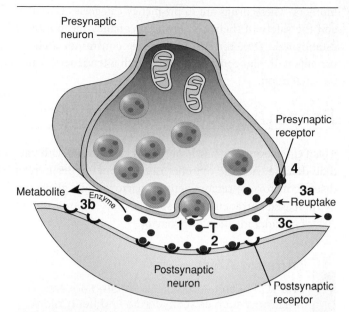

Figure 24.1 Schematic illustration of (1) neurotransmitter (T) release; (2) binding of transmitter to postsynaptic receptor; termination of transmitter action by (3a) reuptake of transmitter into the presynaptic terminal, (3b) enzymatic degradation, or (3c) diffusion away from the synapse; and (4) binding of transmitter to presynaptic receptors for feedback regulation of transmitter release. (From Porth, C. M. [2005]. *Pathophysiology: Concepts of altered health states* [7th ed., p. 1121]. Philadelphia: Lippincott Williams & Wilkins.)

Nursing Alert

Although the TCAs are not considered antipsychotic agents, the drug amoxapine has been associated with tardive dyskinesia and neuroleptic malignant syndrome (NMS). **Tardive dyskinesia** is a syndrome of involuntary movement that may be irreversible. Symptoms of NMS are similar and include muscle rigidity, altered mental status, and autonomic system problems, such as tachycardia or sweating. These syndromes tend to occur more readily in elderly women, and the drug should be discontinued, the primary health care provider notified immediately, and treatment of adverse effects begun quickly.

Contraindications

The TCAs are contraindicated in patients with known hypersensitivity to the drugs. The TCAs are not given within 14 days of the MAOI antidepressants, to patients with a recent myocardial infarction, or to children or lactating

Antidepressant Drugs

mothers. These drugs are in pregnancy categories C and D, and the safety of their use during pregnancy has not been established. Doxepin (Sinequan) is contraindicated in patients with glaucoma or in those with a tendency for urinary retention.

Precautions

The TCAs should be used cautiously in patients with cardiac disease, hepatic or renal impairment, hyperthyroid disease, history of seizure activity, narrow-angle glaucoma or increased intraocular pressure, urinary retention, and risk of suicidal ideation or behavior.

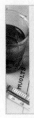

Nursing Alert

The TCAs can cause cardiac-related adverse reactions, such as tachycardia and heart block. The nurse therefore gives these drugs with caution to the person with preexisting cardiac disease, and to the elderly.

Interactions

The following interactions may occur when a TCA is administered with another agent:

Interacting Drugs	Common Use	Effect of Interaction
sedatives and hypnotics, and analgesics	Sedation and pain relief, respectively	Increased risk of respiratory and nervous system depression
dicumarol	Blood thinner	Increased risk for bleeding
cimetidine (Tagamet)	Treatment of gastric upset	Increased anticholinergic symptoms (dry mouth, urinary retention, blurred vision).
MAOIs	Antidepressant agents	Increased risk for hypertensive episodes, severe convulsions, and hyperpyretic episodes
adrenergic agents	Neuromuscular agents	Increased risk for arrhythmias and hypertension

MONOAMINE OXIDASE INHIBITORS

Actions

Drugs classified as MAOIs inhibit the activity of monoamine oxidase, a complex enzyme system responsible for inactivating certain neurotransmitters. Blocking monoamine oxidase results in an increase in endogenous epinephrine, norepinephrine, dopamine, and serotonin in the nervous system. An increase in these **neurohormones** (secreted rather than transmitted neurosubstances) stimulates the CNS. New drugs have been developed and MAOIs are typically not the first drugs chosen for treating depression. Tranylcypromine (Parnate) is an example of an MAOI.

Uses

The MAOI antidepressants are used in the treatment of depressive episodes, and may be used in conjunction with psychotherapy in severe cases. Unlabeled uses include bulimia, night terrors, migraine headaches, seasonal affective disorder, and multiple sclerosis.

Adverse Reactions

- Neuromuscular reactions include orthostatic hypotension, dizziness, vertigo, headache, and blurred vision.

- Gastrointestinal (GI) and genitourinary system reactions include constipation, dry mouth, nausea, diarrhea, and impotence.

- A serious adverse reaction associated with MAOIs is hypertensive crisis (extremely high blood pressure), which may occur when foods containing **tyramine** (an amino acid) are eaten (see Home Care Checklist: Avoiding Drug–Food Interactions With MAOIs).

Nursing Alert

One of the earliest symptoms of hypertensive crisis is headache (usually occipital), followed by a stiff or sore neck, nausea, vomiting, sweating, fever, chest pain, dilated pupils, and bradycardia or tachycardia. If a hypertensive crisis occurs, immediate medical intervention is necessary to reduce the blood pressure. Strokes (cerebrovascular accidents) and death have been reported.

Home Care Checklist

Avoiding Drug–Food Interactions With MAOIs

If your patients are taking monoamine oxidase inhibitors (MAOIs), they need to avoid foods containing tyramine. Otherwise they may experience a life-threatening reaction, hypertensive crisis. Be sure to instruct your patients to avoid the following foods:

☑ Aged cheese (e.g., blue, Camembert, cheddar, Emmenthaler, mozzarella, parmesan, romano, Stilton, Swiss)

☑ Sour cream

☑ Yogurt

☑ Beef or chicken livers

☑ Pickled herring

☑ Fermented meats (e.g., bologna, pepperoni, salami, dried fish)

☑ Undistilled alcoholic beverages (e.g., imported beer, ale, red wine, especially Chianti and sherry)

☑ Caffeinated beverages (e.g., coffee, tea, colas)

☑ Chocolate

☑ Certain fruits and vegetables (e.g., avocado, bananas, fava beans, figs, raisins, sauerkraut)

☑ Yeast extracts

☑ Soy sauce

Contraindications and Precautions

The MAOI antidepressants are contraindicated in the elderly and in patients with known hypersensitivity to the drugs, pheochromocytoma, liver and kidney disease, cerebrovascular disease, hypertension, history of headaches, or congestive heart failure. Safety has not been established for use in patients younger than 16 years or during pregnancy (category C) or lactation.

The MAOIs should be used cautiously in patients with impaired liver function, history of seizures, parkinsonian symptoms, diabetes, hyperthyroidism, or risk of suicidal ideation or behavior.

Interactions

The following interactions may occur when an MAOI antidepressant is administered with another agent (see Home Care Checklist: Avoiding Drug–Food Interactions With MAOIs):

Interacting Drugs or Agent	Common Use	Effect of Interaction
sedatives and hypnotics, and analgesics	Sedation and pain relief, respectively	Increased risk for adverse reactions during surgery
thiazide diuretic	Relief of fluid retention	Increased hypotensive effects of the MAOI
meperidine	Pain relief	Increased risk for hypertensive episodes, severe convulsions, and hyperpyretic episodes
adrenergic agents	Neuromuscular agent	Increased risk for cardiac arrhythmias and hypertension
tyramine or tryptophan	Amino acids found in some foods	Hypertensive crisis, which may occur up to 2 weeks after the MAOI is discontinued

SELECTIVE SEROTONIN REUPTAKE INHIBITORS

Actions

The SSRIs inhibit CNS uptake of serotonin (a CNS neurotransmitter). The increase in serotonin levels is thought to act as a stimulant to reverse depression.

Uses

The SSRIs are used in the treatment of

- Depressive episodes
- Obsessive-compulsive disorders
- Bulimia nervosa

  Unlabeled uses include panic; premenstrual syndrome and post-traumatic stress disorders; generalized anxiety and social phobias; Raynaud's disease; migraine headaches; diabetic neuropathy; and hot flashes. These drugs may be used with psychotherapy in severe cases.

Adverse Reactions

Neuromuscular Reactions

- Somnolence, dizziness
- Headache, insomnia
- Tremor, weakness

Gastrointestinal and Genitourinary System Reactions

- Constipation, dry mouth, nausea
- Pharyngitis, runny nose, and abnormal ejaculation

Contraindications

The SSRIs are contraindicated in patients with a hypersensitivity to the drugs and during pregnancy (category C). Patients taking cisapride (Propulsid), pimozide (Orap), or carbamazepine (Tegretol) should not take fluoxetine (Prozac).

Precautions

The SSRI antidepressants should be used cautiously in patients with diabetes mellitus, cardiac disease, impaired liver or kidney function, and risk for suicidal ideation or behavior. Patients should not be switched to an SSRI antidepressant drug within 2 weeks of stopping an MAOI antidepressant.

Interactions

The following interactions may occur when an SSRI is administered with another agent:

Interacting Drugs	Common Use	Effect of Interaction
other antidepressants	Treatment of depression	Increased risk of toxic effects
cimetidine	Relief of gastric upset	Increased anticholinergic symptoms (dry mouth, urinary retention, blurred vision)
aspirin or nonsteroidal anti-inflammatory drugs (NSAIDs)	Relief of inflammation and pain	Increased risk for GI bleeding
lithium (interaction with fluoxetine)	Treatment of bipolar disorder	Increased risk of lithium toxicity

  Note that the effectiveness of fluoxetine (Prozac) is decreased in patients who smoke cigarettes during administration of the drug.

Herbal Alert

The SSRIs should not be administered with preparations containing *St. John's wort* because there is an increased risk for a severe sedative effect.

MISCELLANEOUS ANTIDEPRESSANTS

Actions

The mechanism of action of most of the miscellaneous antidepressants is not clearly understood. It is thought that they affect neurotransmission of serotonin, norepinephrine, and dopamine. Examples of this group of drugs include venlafaxine (Effexor) and bupropion (Wellbutrin).

Uses

Miscellaneous antidepressant drugs may be used in conjunction with psychotherapy in severe cases or alone in the treatment of

- Depressive episodes
- Depression accompanied by anxiety disorders
- Diabetic peripheral neuropathic pain

Unlabeled uses include enhancing weight loss and treating aggressive behaviors, neuropathic pain, menstrual disorders, cocaine withdrawal and alcohol cravings, fibromyalgia, and stress incontinence.

Adverse Reactions

Neuromuscular Reactions

- Somnolence, migraine headache
- Hypotension, dizziness, lightheadedness, and vertigo
- Blurred vision, photosensitivity, insomnia, nervousness or agitation, and tremor

Gastrointestinal Reactions

- Nausea, dry mouth, anorexia, thirst
- Diarrhea, constipation, bitter taste

Generalized Body System Reactions

- Fatigue, tachycardia, and palpitations
- Change in libido, impotence
- Skin rash, itching, vasodilation resulting in flushing and excessive sweating

Additional adverse reactions and adverse reactions associated with the use of all the antidepressant drugs are listed in the Summary Drug Table: Antidepressants.

Contraindications

The miscellaneous antidepressant drugs are contraindicated in patients with known hypersensitivity to the drugs. Among the miscellaneous antidepressants, bupropion (Wellbutrin) and maprotiline are pregnancy category B drugs. Other miscellaneous antidepressants discussed in this chapter are in pregnancy category C. Safe use of the antidepressants during pregnancy has not been established. They should be used during pregnancy only when the potential benefits outweigh the potential hazards to the developing fetus. Maprotiline should not be used with patients who have a seizure disorder or during the acute phase of a myocardial infarction. Patients taking cisapride, pimozide, or carbamazepine

should not take nefazodone HCl because of risk for hepatic failure.

> ### Nursing Alert
>
> The smoking cessation product Zyban is a form of the antidepressant drug bupropion. Smokers should not use Zyban if they are currently taking the drug bupropion (Wellbutrin) for management of depression because of the possibility of bupropion overdose.

Precautions

Miscellaneous antidepressants should be used cautiously in patients with cardiac disease, renal or hepatic impairment, hyperthyroid disease, or risk of suicidal ideation or behavior.

Interactions

The following interactions may occur when a miscellaneous antidepressant is administered with another agent:

Interacting Drug	Common Use	Effect of Interaction
sedatives and hypnotics; analgesics	Sedation and pain relief, respectively	Increased risk of respiratory and nervous system depression
warfarin	Anticoagulation (blood thinner)	Increased risk for bleeding
cimetidine	GI upset	Increased anticholinergic symptoms (dry mouth, urinary retention, blurred vision)
antihypertensive agents	Treatment of high blood pressure	Increased risk for hypotension
MAOIs	Antidepressant	Increased risk for hypertensive episodes, severe convulsions, and hyperpyretic episodes

SUMMARY DRUG TABLE ANTIDEPRESSANTS

GENERIC NAME	TRADE NAME	USES	ADVERSE REACTIONS	DOSAGE RANGES
Tricyclic Antidepressants				
amitriptyline *am-ee-trip'-ti-leen*		Depression, neuropathic pain, eating disorders	Sedation, anticholinergic effects (dry mouth, dry eyes, urinary retention), constipation	Up to 150 mg/d orally in divided doses; 20–30 mg IM QID; severely depressed hospitalized patient up to 300 mg/d orally Do not administer IV
amoxapine *a-mox'-a-peen*		Depression accompanied by anxiety	Same as amitriptyline	50 mg orally 2–3 times daily up to 300 mg/d, if poor response may go up to 600 mg/d
clomipramine *kloe-mi'-pra-meen*	Anafranil	Obsessive-compulsive disorder	Same as amitriptyline, sexual dysfunction	25–250 mg/d orally in divided doses
desipramine *dess-ip'-ra-meen*	Norpramin	Depression, eating disorders	Same as amitriptyline	100–200 mg/d orally, not to exceed 300 mg/d
doxepin *dox'-e-pin*	Sinequan	Anxiety or depression, emotional symptoms accompanying organic disease	Same as amitriptyline	25–150 mg/d orally in divided doses
imipramine *im-ip'-ra-meen*	Tofranil, Tofranil PM	Depression, enuresis, eating disorders	Same as amitriptyline	100–200 mg/d orally in divided doses Childhood enuresis (older than 6y): 25 mg/d 1 h before bedtime, not to exceed 2.5 mg/kg/d
nortriptyline *not-trip'-ti-leen*	Aventyl, Pamelor	Depression, premenstrual symptoms	Same as amitriptyline	25 mg orally 3–4 times/d; not to exceed 150 mg/d
protriptyline *proe-trip'-ti-leen*	Vivactil	Depression, sleep apnea	Same as amitriptyline	15–40 mg/d orally in 3–4 doses, not to exceed 60 mg/d
trimipramine *trye-mi'-pra-meen*	Surmontil	Depression, peptic ulcer disease	Same as amitriptyline	75–150 mg/d orally in divided doses, not to exceed 300 mg/d
Monoamine Oxidase Inhibitors				
phenelzine *fen'-el-zeen*	Nardil	Atypical depression	Orthostatic hypotension, vertigo, dizziness, nausea, constipation, dry mouth, diarrhea, headache, restlessness, blurred vision, hypertensive crisis	45–90 mg/d orally in divided doses
tranylcypromine *tran-ill-sip'-roe-meen*	Parnate	Atypical depression	Same as phenelzine	30–60 mg/d orally in divided doses
isocarboxazid *eye-so-car-box'-a-zid*	Marplan	Depression	Same as phenelzine	10–40 mg/d orally

GENERIC NAME	TRADE NAME	USES	ADVERSE REACTIONS	DOSAGE RANGES
Selective Serotonin Reuptake Inhibitors				
citalopram *si-tal'-oh-pram*	Celexa	Depression, panic disorder, post-traumatic stress disorder (PTSD), premenstrual disorder	Nausea, dry mouth, sweating, somnolence, insomnia, anorexia, diarrhea	20–40 mg/d orally
escitalopram oxalate	Lexapro	Depression, generalized anxiety disorder, panic disorder	Headache, insomnia, somnolence, nausea	10–20 mg/d orally
fluoxetine *floo-ox'-e-teen*	Prozac, Prozac Weekly, Sarafem	Depression, bulimia, OCD, panic disorder, premenstrual dysphoric disorder (Sarafem only)	Anxiety, nervousness, somnolence, insomnia, drowsiness, asthenia, tremor, headache, nausea, diarrhea, constipation, dry mouth, anorexia	20 mg/d orally in the morning or up to 80 mg/d (dose split between morning and at noon)
fluvoxamine *floo-voks'-a-meen*		OCD, depression	Headache, nervousness, somnolence, insomnia, nausea, diarrhea, dry mouth, constipation, dyspepsia, ejaculatory disturbances	50–300 mg/d orally in divided doses
paroxetine *par-ox'-e-teen*	Paxil	Depression, OCD, panic disorder, general anxiety disorder, social anxiety disorder, post-traumatic stress syndrome	Headache, tremors, somnolence, nervousness, dizziness, insomnia, nausea, diarrhea, constipation, dry mouth, sweating, weakness, sexual dysfunction	20–50 mg/d orally
sertraline *sir'-trah-leen*	Zoloft	Depression, OCD, panic disorders, post-traumatic stress disorder	Headache, drowsiness, anxiety, dizziness, insomnia, fatigue, nausea, diarrhea, dry mouth, ejaculatory disturbances, sweating	50–200 mg/d orally
Miscellaneous Drugs				
bupropion HCl *byoo-proe'-pee-on*	Wellbutrin, Wellbutrin SR, Zyban (smoking cessation)	Depression, neuropathic pain, attention deficit hyperactivity disorder (ADHD), smoking cessation (Zyban)	Agitation, dizziness, dry mouth, insomnia, sedation, headache, nausea, vomiting, tremor, constipation, weight loss, anorexia, excess sweating	100–300 mg/d orally in divided doses; sustained release, 1 tablet BID orally
duloxetine HCl *doo-locks'-eh-teen*	Cymbalta	Depression, diabetic peripheral neuropathy, fibromyalgia, stress incontinence	Insomnia, dry mouth, nausea, constipation	40–60 mg/d orally
maprotiline *ma-proe'-ti-leen*		Depression, anxiety associated with depression	Sedation, dry mouth, constipation, orthostatic hypotension	75–150 mg/d orally; for severe depression, dosage may increase to 225 mg/d orally

Antidepressant Drugs

SUMMARY DRUG TABLE   (*continued*)

GENERIC NAME	TRADE NAME	USES	ADVERSE REACTIONS	DOSAGE RANGES
mirtazapine *mer-tah'-zah-peen*	Remeron	Depression	Sedation, dry mouth, constipation, orthostatic hypotension	15–45 mg/d orally
nefazodone *ne-faz'-oh-done*		Depression	Somnolence, insomnia, dizziness, nausea, dry mouth, constipation, headache, weakness	200–600 mg/d orally in divided doses
trazodone *traz'-oh-done*	Desyrel	Depression, alcohol craving	Drowsiness, dizziness, priapism, dry mouth, nausea, vomiting, constipation, fatigue, nervousness	150–400 mg/d orally in divided doses, not to exceed 600 mg/d
venlafaxine *ven-la-fax'-een*	Effexor, Effexor XR	Depression, anxiety disorders, premenstrual disorder	Headache, insomnia, dizziness, nervousness, weakness, anorexia, nausea, constipation, dry mouth, somnolence, sweating	75–225 mg/d orally in divided doses

Herbal Alert

Patients should be assessed for use of herbal preparations containing *St. John's wort* because of the potential for adverse reactions when taken with antidepressants.

NURSING PROCESS

The Patient Receiving an Antidepressant Drug

ASSESSMENT

PREADMINISTRATION ASSESSMENT

A patient receiving an antidepressant drug may be treated in the hospital or in an outpatient setting. Before starting therapy for the hospitalized patient, the nurse obtains a complete medical history. The nurse assesses the patient's mental status to determine the degree of depression and obtain a baseline for comparison with future assessments. The patient may report feelings of anxiety, worthlessness, guilt, helplessness, and hopelessness. The nurse documents any subjective feelings as well as slowness to answer questions, a monotone speech pattern, and any sadness or crying.

The preadministration assessments of the outpatient are basically the same as those for the hospitalized patient. The nurse obtains a complete medical history and a history of the symptoms of the depression from the patient, a family member, or the patient's hospital records. The nurse performs a physical assessment, which includes obtaining blood pressure measurements on both arms with the patient in a sitting position, pulse and respiratory rate, and weight.

During the initial interview, the nurse observes the patient for symptoms of depression and the potential for suicide. It is important for the nurse to note the presence of suicidal thoughts. The nurse accurately documents in the patient's record and reports to the primary health care provider any statements concerning suicide and the ability of the patient to carry out any suicidal intentions. If the patient does make statements about suicide, the nurse must ask about intent using simple, straightforward questions.

ONGOING ASSESSMENT

The nurse monitors vital signs at least daily as part of the ongoing assessment. The vital signs are monitored more frequently if the drug used is one that carries the risk for a hypertensive or hypotensive adverse reaction. The nurse reports any significant change in the vital signs to the primary health care provider.

OUTPATIENT ASSESSMENT Ultimately, the hospitalized patient may be discharged from the acute care setting. Some patients, such as those with mild depression, do not require inpatient care. These patients are usually seen at periodic intervals in the primary health care provider's office or in a mental health outpatient setting.

At the time of each visit to the primary health care provider or clinic, the nurse observes the patient for a response to therapy. In some instances, the nurse may question the patient or a family member about the response to therapy. The type of questions asked depends on the patient and the diagnosis and may include questions such as

- How are you feeling?
- How would you describe your depressed feelings?
- How would you rate your depression?
- Would you like to tell me how everything is going?

Many times the nurse may need to rephrase questions or direct conversation toward other subjects until the patient feels comfortable and can discuss therapy. The nurse should ask the patient or a family member about adverse drug reactions or any other problems occurring during therapy because it is important to bring these reactions or problems to the attention of the primary health care provider. The nurse documents in the patient's record a general summary of the patient's outward behavior and any complaints or problems and compares these notations with previous notations and observations.

NURSING DIAGNOSES

Drug specific nursing diagnoses are highlighted in the Nursing Diagnoses Checklist. Other nursing diagnoses applicable to these drugs are discussed in depth in Chapter 4.

Nursing Diagnoses Checklist

✔ **Self-Care Deficit Syndrome** related to inability to participate in activities of daily living secondary to somnolence, drowsiness, and depressive state

✔ **Disturbed Sleep Pattern** related to depression, adverse drug reactions (e.g., excessive drowsiness)

✔ **Imbalanced Nutrition: Less Than Body Requirements** related to anorexia, constipation, and depression

✔ **Risk for Suicide** related to suicidal ideation and adverse reaction to antidepressive drug

✔ **Acute Pain** related to priapism

PLANNING

The expected outcomes of the patient depend on the reason for administration of an antidepressant, but may include an optimal response to drug therapy, support of patient needs related to the management of adverse drug reactions, and an understanding of and compliance with the prescribed therapeutic regimen.

IMPLEMENTATION
PROMOTING AN OPTIMAL RESPONSE TO THERAPY

Response to antidepressant medications is not rapid. It can take a number of weeks for the drugs to take effect. Fluoxetine (Prozac) is an example of a drug that may take as long as 4 weeks to attain a full therapeutic effect. Some adverse reactions, such as dry mouth, episodes of **orthostatic hypotension**, and drowsiness, appear long before the intended effect of the antidepressant. The inability to deal with the unpleasantness of these adverse reactions is one of the greatest reasons patients stop taking the antidepressants. The two adverse reactions patients have the most trouble tolerating are somnolence and dry mouth. During initial therapy or whenever the dosage is increased or decreased, the nurse observes the patient closely for adverse drug reactions and any behavioral changes. The nurse reports to the primary health care provider any change in behavior or the appearance of adverse reactions because a further increase or decrease in dosage may be necessary or use of the drug may need to be discontinued.

When caring for hospitalized patients with depression, the nurse must develop a nursing care plan to meet the patient's individual needs. When the antidepressants are given parenterally, the nurse gives these drugs intramuscularly (IM) in a large muscle mass, such as the gluteus muscle. The nurse keeps the patient lying down (when possible) for about 30 minutes after administering the drug.

MONITORING AND MANAGING PATIENT NEEDS

SELF-CARE DEFICIT SYNDROME Initially, the patient may need assistance with self-care because patients with depression often do not have the physical or emotional energy to perform self-care activities. This is complicated by the fact that many antidepressants cause excessive drowsiness during the initial stages of treatment, and patients may need assistance with ambulation and self-care activities. These problems usually subside as the depression lifts and tolerance to the adverse reactions builds with continued use of the antidepressant. To minimize the risk for injury, the nurse assists the patient when necessary and makes the environment as safe as possible. When orthostatic hypotension is an effect of drug therapy, the nurse instructs the patient to rise from a lying position to a sitting position. The patient remains in a sitting position for a few minutes before rising to a standing position. Position changes are made slowly, with the nurse at the bedside to offer assistance if necessary.

If the patient has a difficult time with self-care because of the depression or sedative effects of the antidepressants, the nurse provides total assistance with activities of daily living, including help with eating, dressing, and ambulating. However, the nurse encourages self-care, whenever possible, allowing sufficient time for the patient to accomplish tasks to the fullest extent of his or her ability. It is important for the nurse to provide positive feedback when appropriate. As a therapeutic effect of the drug is attained, the patient will be able to resume self-care (if no other physical conditions interfere).

The nurse writes behavioral records at periodic intervals, the frequency of which depends on hospital or unit guidelines. An accurate assessment of the patient's behavior aids the primary health care provider in planning therapy and thus becomes an important part of nursing management. Patients with a poor response to drug therapy may require dosage changes, a change to another antidepressant drug, or the addition of other therapies to the treatment regimen.

DISTURBED SLEEP PATTERN Many of the antidepressant drugs cause somnolence. This adverse reaction is one of the greatest reasons patients stop taking the medication. When the nurse administers the drug at night, the sedative effects promote sleep, and the adverse reactions appear less troublesome. An exception to this is the SSRIs; it is best to administer those medications in the morning.

The nurse should assess the environment to help promote sleep at night and wakefulness during the day. Drapes should be shut at night and opened in the day to let in light, and clocks should be available for the patient to see the time of day. These activities will help the patient to reorient to daytime and nighttime, thereby promoting an effective sleep pattern.

IMBALANCED NUTRITION: LESS THAN BODY REQUIREMENTS Depressed patients may not feel like eating; therefore, they lose weight. This can be potentiated by the adverse reactions of anorexia and constipation. The nurse monitors dietary intake and helps the dietitian in providing nutritious meals, taking into consideration foods that the patient likes and dislikes. Fluid intake and foods high in fiber are important for the patient to prevent constipation. Weighing the patient weekly is important for monitoring weight loss or gain. To minimize the dry mouth that frequently accompanies administration of the antidepressants, the nurse provides good oral hygiene, frequent sips of fluids, and sugarless gum or hard candy.

Patients receiving MAOIs require strict dietary control because foods containing tyramine should not be eaten.

The nurse asks family members and visitors not to bring food to the patient and explains why this is important. When an MAOI is prescribed, it is critical that the nurse give the patient a list of foods containing tyramine and to emphasize the importance of not eating foods on the list. If the patient has trouble understanding this dietary restriction, it may be necessary to observe the patient closely when eating in a community setting to be sure food is not taken or accepted from other patients.

RISK FOR SUICIDE Patients with a high suicide potential require protection from suicidal acts and a well-supervised environment. For patients with severe depression, suicide precautions are important until a therapeutic effect is achieved. When the patient is hospitalized, policies of observation must be strictly followed for the patient's protection.

Of greatest concern to the nurse is the depressed patient who has suicidal ideation, but has not been identified as such. Patients in a depressive state may lack the energy to carry out plans for ending their own life. Because the full therapeutic effect of the antidepressant may not be attained for 10 days to 4 weeks, patients have time to gain enough energy to carry out an injurious act upon themselves. Patients with suicidal tendencies must be monitored closely. Report any expressions of guilt, hopelessness, or helplessness, insomnia, weight loss, and direct or indirect threats of suicide.

Oral administration requires great care because some patients have difficulty swallowing (e.g., because of a dry mouth). After administration of an oral drug, the nurse inspects the patient's oral cavity to be sure the drug has been swallowed. If the patient resists having his or her oral cavity checked, the nurse reports this refusal to the primary health care provider. Patients planning suicide may try to keep the drug on the side of the mouth or under the tongue and not swallow in an effort to hoard or save enough of the drug to commit suicide at a later time. Other patients may refuse to take the drug. If the patient refuses to take the drug, the nurse contacts the primary health care provider regarding this problem because parenteral administration of the drug may be necessary.

Gerontologic Alert

Older men with prostatic enlargement are at increased risk for urinary retention when they take the tricyclic antidepressants.

ACUTE PAIN An uncommon but potentially serious adverse reaction of trazodone (Desyrel) is **priapism** (a persistent erection of the penis). This can be very painful and if not treated within a few hours, priapism can result in impotence. Because this can be an embarrassing adverse reaction, the nurse needs to instruct the patient to report any prolonged or inappropriate penile erection. The drug is discontinued immediately and the primary care provider notified. Injection of alpha-adrenergic stimulants (e.g., norepinephrine) may be helpful in treating priapism. In some cases, surgical intervention may be required.

EDUCATING THE PATIENT AND FAMILY

Once some patients are discharged to the home setting, noncompliance with drug therapy is a problem because of unpleasant adverse drug effects. This is why it is very important for the nurse to educate the patient or family members thoroughly about the importance of managing the reactions so that the patient will continue the proper drug regimen. The nurse evaluates the patient's ability to assume responsibility for taking drugs at home (see Patient and Family Teaching Checklist: Promoting Patient Responsibility for Antidepressant Drug Therapy). The administration of antidepressant drugs becomes a family responsibility if the outpatient appears to be unable to manage his or her own drug therapy.

The nurse explains any adverse reactions that may occur with a specific antidepressant drug and encourages the patient or family member to contact the primary health care provider immediately if a serious drug reaction occurs. The nurse includes the following points in a teaching plan for the patient or family member:

- Inform the primary health care provider, dentist, and other medical personnel of therapy with this drug.

- If dizziness occurs when changing position, rise slowly when getting out of bed or a chair. If dizziness is severe, always have help when changing positions.

- Relieve dry mouth by taking frequent sips of water, sucking on hard candy, or chewing gum (preferably sugarless gum).

- Keep all clinic appointments or appointments with the primary health care provider because close monitoring of therapy is essential.

- Do not take the antidepressants during pregnancy. Notify the primary health care provider if you are pregnant or wish to become pregnant.

- Report any unusual changes or physical effects to the primary health care provider.

Patient and Family Teaching Checklist

Promoting Patient Responsibility for Antidepressant Drug Therapy

The nurse:

✔ Explains the reason for drug therapy, including the type of antidepressant prescribed, drug name, dosage, and frequency of administration.

✔ Enlists the aid of family members to ensure compliance with therapy, including checking patient's oral cavity to be sure drug has been swallowed.

✔ Urges the patient to take the drug exactly as prescribed and not to increase or decrease dosage, omit doses, or discontinue use of the drug unless directed to do so by health care provider.

✔ Advises that full therapeutic effect may not occur for several weeks.

✔ Instructs in signs and symptoms of behavioral changes indicative of therapeutic effectiveness or increasing depression and suicidal tendencies.

✔ Reviews measures to reduce the risk for suicide.

✔ Instructs about possible adverse reactions with instructions to notify health care provider should any occur.

✔ Reinforces safety measures such as changing positions slowly and avoiding driving or hazardous tasks.

✔ Advises avoidance of alcohol and use of nonprescription drugs unless use is approved by health care provider.

✔ Encourages patient to inform other health care providers and medical personnel about drug therapy regimen.

✔ Instructs in measures to minimize dry mouth.

✔ Emphasizes importance of avoiding foods containing tyramine (if MAOIs are prescribed) and provides written list of foods to avoid.

✔ Reassures results of therapy will be monitored by periodic laboratory tests and follow-up visits with the health care provider.

✔ Assists with arrangements for follow-up visits.

- Avoid prolonged exposure to sunlight or sunlamps because an exaggerated reaction to the ultraviolet light may occur (photosensitivity), resulting in a burn.

- For male patients who take trazodone (Desyrel) and who experience prolonged, inappropriate, and painful erections, stop taking the drug and notify the primary care provider.

EVALUATION

- The therapeutic effect is achieved.

- No evidence of injury is apparent.

- The patient is able to perform self-care.

- Adverse reactions are identified, reported to the primary health care provider, and managed successfully through appropriate nursing interventions.

- The patient verbalizes an understanding of treatment modalities and importance of continued follow-up care.

- The patient verbalizes the importance of complying with the prescribed therapeutic regimen.

- The patient and family demonstrate understanding of the drug regimen.

Critical Thinking Exercises

1. Mr. Hopkins has been severely depressed for several months. Two weeks ago the primary care provider prescribed amitriptyline 30 mg orally four times a day. His family is concerned because he is still depressed. They are requesting that the dosage be increased. Discuss what information you will give Mr. Hopkins and his family and what assessments you can make.

2. Ms. Jefferson has been taking phenelzine (Nardil) for depression. She reports having a "bad headache" at the back of her head. Determine what assessment would be most important to make. Explain what action, if any, you would take.

3. Mr. Jones is prescribed trazodone (Desyrel), and the nurse is preparing discharge instructions. What are the most important points to cover at the teaching session?

Review Questions

1. When administering an antidepressant to a patient contemplating suicide, it is most important for the nurse to _____.

A. have the patient remain upright for at least 30 minutes after taking the antidepressant

B. assess the patient in 30 minutes for a therapeutic response to the drug

C. monitor the patient for an occipital headache

D. inspect the patient's oral cavity to be sure the drug was swallowed

2. Which of the following adverse reactions would the nurse expect to find in a patient taking amitriptyline?

A. Constipation and abdominal cramps

B. Bradycardia and double vision

C. Sedation and dry mouth

D. Polyuria and hypotension

3. The nurse instructs the patient taking a monoamine oxidase inhibitor (MAOI) not to eat foods containing _____.

A. glutamine

B. sugar

C. tyramine

D. large amounts of iron

4. Which of the following antidepressants would be most likely to cause the patient to have a seizure?

A. amitriptyline

B. bupropion

C. sertraline

D. venlafaxine

Medication Dosage Problems

1. The primary care provider prescribes trazodone (Desyrel) 150 mg orally. Available are 50-mg tablets. The nurse administers _____.

2. The primary care provider prescribes oral paroxetine (Paxil) 50 mg/d. The drug is available as oral suspension with a strength of 10 mg/5 mL. The nurse administers _____.

To check your answers, see Appendix G.

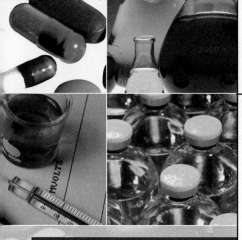

Chapter 25

Central Nervous System Stimulants

Key Terms

analeptics
anorexiants
attention deficit hyperactivity
  disorder
narcolepsy

Learning Objectives

On completion of this chapter, the student will:

- List the three types of central nervous system (CNS) stimulants.

- Discuss the uses, general drug actions, general adverse reactions, contraindications, precautions, and interactions of the CNS stimulants.

- Discuss important preadministration and ongoing assessment activities

the nurse should perform on the patient taking a CNS stimulant.

- List nursing diagnoses particular to a patient taking a CNS stimulant.

- Discuss ways to promote an optimal response to drug therapy, how to manage common adverse drug reactions, and important points to keep in mind when educating patients about the use of CNS stimulants.

This chapter discusses the drugs that stimulate the central nervous system (CNS) and the nursing implications related to their administration. The CNS stimulants include the **analeptics**, drugs that stimulate the respiratory center of the brain and cardiovascular system; the **anorexiants**, drugs used to suppress the appetite; and the amphetamines, used to treat children with attention deficit hyperactivity disorder. Other drugs being developed for the treatment of children will include fewer amphetamines because of their high abuse potential and their ability to produce euphoria and wakefulness.

Actions

Analeptics increase the depth of respirations by stimulating special receptors located in the carotid arteries and upper aorta. These special receptors (called *chemoreceptors*) are sensitive to the amount of oxygen in arterial blood. Stimulation of these receptors results in an increase in the depth of respirations. In larger doses, drugs like doxapram (Dopram) increase the respiratory rate by stimulating the medulla.

One of the most widely used CNS stimulants is caffeine. It is a mild-to-potent analeptic CNS stimulant. The degree of its stimulating effect depends on the dose administered. Caffeine stimulates the CNS at all levels, including the cerebral cortex, the medulla, and the spinal cord. Caffeine has mild analeptic (respiratory-stimulating) activity. Other actions include cardiac stimulation (which may produce tachycardia), dilation of coronary and peripheral blood vessels, constriction of cerebral blood vessels, and skeletal muscle stimulation. Caffeine also has mild diuretic activity. People take caffeine on their own in the form of coffee, tea, or even chocolate, yet caffeine's use as a therapeutic drug for stimulation in the neonatal setting is growing.

Modafinil (Provigil), another analeptic, is used to treat **narcolepsy** (a disorder that causes an uncontrollable desire to sleep during normal waking hours even though the individual has a normal nighttime sleeping pattern). The exact mechanism of action is not known, but the drug is thought to bind to dopamine, thereby reducing the number of episodes. It does not cause cardiac and other systemic stimulatory effects like the other CNS stimulants.

The amphetamines are sympathomimetic (i.e., adrenergic) drugs that stimulate the CNS (see Chapter 27). Their drug action results in an elevation of blood pressure, wakefulness, and an increase or decrease in pulse rate. Amphetamines also produce a euphoric state that increases their dependency potential, making their use less frequent.

One condition successfully treated by amphetamines is **attention deficit hyperactivity disorder** (ADHD) in children. ADHD is a condition of both children and adults and is characterized by inattention, hyperactivity, and impulsivity. Symptoms appear early in a child's life. Because these behaviors alone can be normal in any individual, it is important that the child receive a thorough examination and appropriate diagnosis by a well-qualified professional before drug therapy is initiated. How amphetamines, which are CNS stimulants, work in ADHD is unknown.

The anorexiants are nonamphetamine drugs pharmacologically similar to the amphetamines. Like the amphetamines, their ability to suppress the appetite is thought to be due to their action on the appetite center in the hypothalamus.

Uses

The CNS stimulants are used in the treatment of

- ADHD

- Drug-induced respiratory depression

- Postanesthesia respiratory depression, without reduction of analgesia

- Narcolepsy

- Sleep apnea

- Exogenous obesity

- Fatigue (caffeine)

Adverse Reactions

Neuromuscular Reactions

- Excessive CNS stimulation, headache, dizziness

- Apprehension, disorientation, and hyperactivity

Other

- Nausea, vomiting, cough, dyspnea

- Urinary retention, tachycardia, and palpitations

For more information on adverse reactions, see the Summary Drug Table: Central Nervous System Stimulants.

Contraindications

The CNS stimulants are contraindicated in patients with known hypersensitivity or convulsive disorders, and in those with ventilation disorders (e.g., chronic obstructive pulmonary disease [COPD]). The nurse should not administer CNS stimulants to patients with cardiac problems, severe hypertension, or hyperthyroidism. CNS stimulants are not recommended as treatment for depression. Amphetamines and anorexiants should not be taken concurrently or within 14 days of antidepressant medications. In addition, the amphetamines are contraindicated in patients with glaucoma. Most anorexiants are classified as pregnancy category X and should not be used during pregnancy. Although sibutramine (Meridia) is a pregnancy category C drug, its safety has not been proven.

> **Nursing Alert**
>
> The amphetamines and anorexiants have abuse and addiction potential. These drugs are recommended only for short-term use in selected patients for the treatment of obesity. Long-term use of amphetamines for obesity may result in tolerance to the drug and a tendency to increase the dose. Extreme psychological dependency may also occur.

Precautions

The CNS stimulants should be used cautiously in patients with respiratory illness, renal or hepatic impairment, and history of substance abuse. The CNS stimulants should be used cautiously in pregnant or lactating women.

SUMMARY DRUG TABLE CENTRAL NERVOUS SYSTEM STIMULANTS

GENERIC NAME	TRADE NAME	USES	ADVERSE REACTIONS	DOSAGE RANGES
Analeptics				
caffeine *kaf-een'*	Cafcit, Stay Awake, No Doz, Vivarin	Fatigue, drowsiness, as adjunct in analgesic formulation, respiratory depression	Palpitations, nausea, vomiting, insomnia, tachycardia, restlessness	100–200 mg orally q3–4h Respiratory depression: 500 mg/1g IM, IV
doxapram HCl *docks'-a-pram*	Dopram	Respiratory depression: postanesthesia, drug-induced, acute respiratory insufficiency superimposed on COPD	Dizziness, headache, apprehension, disorientation, nausea, cough, dyspnea, urinary retention	0.5–1 mg/kg IV
modafinil *moe-daf'-in-ill*	Provigil	Narcolepsy, obstructive sleep apnea	Headache, nausea	200–400 mg/d orally
Amphetamines				
amphetamine sulfate *am-fet'-a-meen*		Narcolepsy, ADHD, exogenous obesity	Insomnia, nervousness, headache, tachycardia, anorexia, dizziness, excitement	Narcolepsy: 5–60 mg/d orally in divided doses ADHD: 5 mg BID, increase by 10 mg/wk until desired effect Obesity. 5–30 mg/d orally in divided doses
amphetamine/ dextroamphetamine *decks-troe-am-fet'-a meen*	Adderall	Narcolepsy, ADHD	Same as amphetamine	Same as amphetamine
dexmethylphenidate *dex-meth-thyl-fen'-i-date*	Focalin	ADHD	Nervousness, insomnia, loss of appetite, abdominal pain, weight loss, tachycardia, skin rash	2.5 mg orally BID; maximum dosage, 20 mg/d
dextroamphetamine sulfate	Dexedrine, Dextrostat	Narcolepsy, ADHD	Same as amphetamine	Narcolepsy: 5–60 mg/d orally in divided doses ADHD: up to 40 mg/d orally
methamphetamine *meth-am-fet'-a-meen*	Desoxyn	ADHD, exogenous obesity	Same as amphetamine	ADHD: Up to 25 mg/d orally Obesity: 5 mg orally 30 min before meals
methylphenidate HCl *meh-thill-fen'-ih-date*	Concerta, Metadate CD & ER, Ritalin, Methylin	ADHD, narcolepsy	Insomnia, anorexia, dizziness, headache, abdominal pain	5–60 mg/d orally

Central Nervous System Stimulants

● SUMMARY DRUG TABLE *(continued)*

GENERIC NAME	TRADE NAME	USES	ADVERSE REACTIONS	DOSAGE RANGES
Anorexiants				
benzphetamine HCl *benz-fet'-a-meen*	Didrex	Obesity	Insomnia, nervousness, headache, dry mouth, palpitations, tachycardia, dizziness, excitement	25–50 mg orally 1–3 times/d
diethylpropion HCl *die-eth'-uhl-pro'-pee-ahn*	Tenuate, Tenuate Dospan	Obesity	Same as benzphetamine	Immediate release: 25 mg orally TID Sustained release: 75 mg once daily
phendimetrazine tartrate	Bontril, Bontril PDM	Obesity	Same as benzphetamine	35 mg orally 2–3 times/d
phentermine HCl *fen-ter'-meen*	Ionamin, Adipex-P	Obesity	Same as benzphetamine	8 mg orally TID or 15–37.5 mg orally as a single daily dose
sibutramine HCl *si-byoo'-tra-meen*	Meridia	Obesity	Insomnia, headache, dry mouth, constipation, rhinitis, pharyngitis	5–15 mg orally once daily
Miscellaneous Drugs				
atomoxetine	Strattera	ADHD (acts like antidepressant rather than stimulant)	Headache, decreased appetite, abdominal pain, vomiting, cough	Initial dose: 40 mg/d orally, may increase up to 100 mg/d orally

ADHD, attention deficit hyperactivity disorder; COPD, chronic obstructive pulmonary disease.

Interactions

The following interactions may occur when a CNS stimulant is administered with another agent:

Interacting Drug	Common Use	Effect of Interaction
anesthetics	Anesthesia during surgical procedures	Increased risk of cardiac arrhythmias
theophylline	Respiratory problems, such as asthma	Increased risk of hyperactive behaviors
oral contraceptives	Birth control	Decreased effectiveness of the oral contraceptive when taken with modafinil (Provigil; used for treatment of narcolepsy)

NURSING PROCESS

The Patient Receiving a Central Nervous System Stimulant

ASSESSMENT

Assessment of the patient receiving a CNS stimulant depends on the drug, the patient, and the reason for administration.

PREADMINISTRATION ASSESSMENT

RESPIRATORY DEPRESSION When a CNS stimulant is prescribed for respiratory depression, initial patient assessments include the blood pressure, pulse, and respiratory rate. It is important to note the depth of the respirations and any pattern to the respiratory rate, such as shallow respirations or alternating deep and shallow respirations. The nurse reviews recent laboratory test results (if any), such as arterial blood gas studies. It is important to review the chart to identify the drugs given that caused the respiratory depression.

ATTENTION DEFICIT HYPERACTIVITY DISORDER When an amphetamine is prescribed for any reason, the nurse weighs the patient and takes the blood pressure, pulse, and respiratory rate before starting drug therapy. The nurse should initially observe the child with ADHD for the various patterns of abnormal behavior. The nurse records a summary of the behavior pattern in the patient's chart to provide a comparison with future changes that may occur during therapy. If the child is hospitalized, the nurse enters a daily summary of the child's behavior in the patient's record. This provides a record of the results of therapy.

OBESITY When an anorexiant or amphetamine is used as part of obesity treatment, the drug is usually prescribed for outpatient use. The nurse obtains and records the blood pressure, pulse, respiratory rate, and weight before therapy is started and at each outpatient visit.

ONGOING ASSESSMENT

RESPIRATORY DEPRESSION After administering an analeptic, the nurse carefully monitors the patient's respiratory rate and pattern until the respirations return to normal. The nurse also monitors the level of consciousness, the blood pressure, and pulse rate at 5- to 15-minute intervals or as ordered by the primary health care provider. The nurse may draw blood for arterial blood gas analysis at intervals to determine the effectiveness of the analeptic, as well as the need for additional drug therapy. It is important to observe the patient for adverse drug reactions and to report their occurrence immediately to the primary health care provider.

NURSING DIAGNOSES

Drug-specific nursing diagnoses are highlighted in the Nursing Diagnoses Checklist. Other nursing diagnoses applicable to these drugs are discussed in depth in Chapter 4.

Nursing Diagnoses Checklist

✔ **Disturbed Sleep Pattern** related to CNS stimulation and hyperactivity, nervousness, insomnia, other (specify)

✔ **Ineffective Breathing Pattern** related to respiratory depression

✔ **Imbalanced Nutrition: Less Than Body Requirements** related to diminished appetite

---

PLANNING

The expected outcomes for the patient depend on the reason for administration of a CNS stimulant, but may include an optimal response to therapy, support of patient needs related to management of adverse drug reactions, and an understanding of the drug regimen.

IMPLEMENTATION
PROMOTING AN OPTIMAL RESPONSE TO THERAPY

Amphetamines may be used in the short-term treatment of exogenous obesity (obesity caused by a persistent calorie intake that is greater than needed by the body). However, their use in treating exogenous obesity has declined because the long-term use of the amphetamines for obesity carries the potential for dependence and abuse.

MONITORING AND MANAGING PATIENT NEEDS

DISTURBED SLEEP PATTERN When CNS stimulant therapy causes insomnia, the nurse administers the drug early in the day (when possible) to diminish sleep disturbances. The patient is provided with distracting activities and encouraged not to nap during the day.

Other stimulants, such as coffee, tea, or cola drinks, are avoided. In some patients, nervousness, restlessness, and palpitations may occur. The vital signs are checked every 6 to 8 hours or more often if tachycardia, hypertension, or palpitations occur. The adverse drug reactions that may occur with amphetamine use may be serious enough to require discontinuation of the drug. In some instances, the adverse drug effects are mild and may even disappear during therapy. In many cases, these adverse reactions diminish with continued use as physical tolerance develops. The nurse informs the primary care provider of all adverse reactions. If tolerance does develop, the dosage is not increased.

Gerontologic Alert

Older adults are especially sensitive to the effects of the CNS stimulants and may exhibit excessive anxiety, nervousness, insomnia, and mental confusion. Cardiovascular disorders, common in the older adult, may be worsened by the CNS stimulants. Careful monitoring is important because these reactions may result in the need to discontinue use of the drug.

These drugs may also be helpful in managing narcolepsy, a disorder manifested by an uncontrollable desire to sleep during normal waking hours even though the individual has a normal nighttime sleeping pattern. The individual with narcolepsy may fall asleep from a few minutes to a few hours many times in one day. The disorder begins in adolescence or young adulthood and persists throughout life.

INEFFECTIVE BREATHING PATTERN Respiratory depression can be a serious event requiring administration of a respiratory stimulant. When an analeptic drug is administered, the nurse notes and records the rate, depth, and character of the respirations before the drug is given. This provides a baseline for evaluating the effectiveness of drug therapy. Also before administering the drug, the nurse ensures that the patient has a patent airway. Oxygen is usually administered before, during, and after drug administration. After administration, the nurse monitors respirations closely and records the effects of therapy.

When respiratory depression occurs in the postsurgical setting, the nurse should assess carefully the patient's level of pain. Respiratory depression can occur after a surgical procedure from the combination of drugs used to produce anesthesia. Opioid reversal drugs, such as naloxone (Narcan), that reverse the effects of opioid agents replace the pain relief drug at the receptor site of the cell. This means that the patient can experience a sudden and severe return of pain because the pain relief effect of the drug is eliminated along with the reversal of respiratory depression. Use of analeptic drugs for respiratory stimulation can enhance the breathing pattern without changing the effect of the opioid drug. Therefore, breathing improves and pain relief continues for the patient.

Nausea and vomiting may occur with the administration of an analeptic; therefore, the nurse should keep a suction machine nearby in case the patient vomits. Urinary retention may result from doxapram administration; therefore, the nurse measures intake and output and notifies the primary health care provider if the patient cannot void or the bladder appears to be distended on palpation.

IMBALANCED NUTRITION: LESS THAN BODY REQUIREMENTS One of the adverse reactions to the use of CNS stimulants for the child with ADHD is decreased appetite. Although decreased appetite is a desired effect when treating a patient with weight problems, it is not desirable when treating ADHD. Long-term treatment with the CNS stimulants is also thought possibly to retard growth in children. Therefore it is important to monitor weight and growth patterns of children on long-term treatment with the CNS stimulant drugs.

The nurse instructs parents to monitor the eating patterns of the child while he or she is taking CNS stimulants. Parents should be taught to prepare nutritious meals and snacks. A good breakfast is important to provide because the child in school may not feel hungry at lunch time. The child should be checked frequently with height and weight measurements to monitor growth. When a CNS stimulant, such as dextroamphetamine, is administered to treat a child with ADHD, the drug regimen may be interrupted periodically under direction of the primary health provider to evaluate the effectiveness of drug management.

EDUCATING THE PATIENT AND FAMILY

The nurse explains the therapeutic regimen and adverse drug reactions to the patient and family. The type of information included in the teaching plan depends on the drug and the reason for its use. It is important to emphasize the need to follow the recommended dosage schedule. The nurse may include the following additional teaching points:

- *ADHD*: Give the drug in the morning 30 to 45 minutes before breakfast and before lunch. Do not give the drug in the late afternoon. Keep a journal of the child's behavior, including the general pattern of behavior, socialization with others, and attention span. Bring this record to each primary health care provider or clinic visit because this record may help the primary health care provider determine future drug dosages or additional treatment modalities. The primary health care provider may prescribe drug therapy only on school days, when high levels of attention and performance are necessary.

- *Narcolepsy*: Keep a record of the number of times per day that periods of sleepiness occur, and bring this record to each visit to the primary health care provider or clinic.

- *Amphetamines and anorexiants*: These drugs are taken early in the day to avoid insomnia. Do not increase the dose or take the drug more frequently, except on the advice of the primary health care provider. These drugs may impair the ability to drive or perform hazardous tasks and may mask extreme fatigue. If dizziness, lightheadedness, anxiety, nervousness, or tremors occur, contact the primary care provider. Avoid or decrease the use of coffee, tea, and carbonated beverages containing caffeine (see Patient and Family Teaching Checklist: Using Anorexiants for Weight Loss).

- *Caffeine (oral, nonprescription)*: Over-the-counter caffeine preparations should be avoided if the individual has a history of heart disease, high blood pressure, or stomach ulcers. These products are intended for occasional use and should not be used if heart palpitations, dizziness, or lightheadedness occurs.

Patient and Family Teaching Checklist

Using Anorexiants for Weight Loss

The nurse:

☑ Reviews reasons for the drug and prescribed drug regimen, including drug name, dosage, and frequency of administration.

☑ Stresses the importance of taking the drug exactly as prescribed, including not to increase the dose or take more frequently unless instructed to do so by the prescriber.

☑ Reinforces use of drug for short-term therapy only.

☑ Warns about possible abuse, drug tolerance, and psychological dependency.

☑ Reviews possible adverse reactions, especially CNS overstimulation, with instructions to notify the health care provider immediately should any occur.

☑ Instructs to take drug early in day to minimize insomnia.

☑ Cautions about safety measures because of possible impairment in ability to drive or perform hazardous tasks.

☑ Advises to avoid other stimulants, including those containing caffeine such as coffee, tea, and cola drinks; provides a written list of foods to avoid.

☑ Urges to read labels of foods and nonprescription drugs for possible stimulant content.

☑ Reinforces prescribed dietary and exercise program for weight reduction, both verbally and in writing.

☑ Reassures that results of therapy will be monitored by continued follow-up visits with health care provider.

☑ Arranges for follow-up visits as necessary.

EVALUATION

• The parent or child reports that the child's behavior and school performance are improved.

• Desired weight loss is achieved.

• Respiratory depression is reversed.

• The patient reports fewer episodes of inappropriate sleep patterns.

• Adverse reactions are identified and managed through appropriate nursing interventions.

• The patient complies with the prescribed drug regimen.

• The patient and family demonstrate an understanding of the drug regimen.

• The patient verbalizes the importance of complying with the prescribed therapeutic regimen.

Critical Thinking Exercises

1. Ms. Stone is given a special diet and prescribed an anorexiant to help her lose 20 lb before she has reconstructive knee surgery. Determine what instructions you would include in a teaching plan for this patient.

2. Mr. Trent has narcolepsy and is prescribed amphetamine 10 mg/d. Develop questions you would ask Mr. Trent when he returns to the clinic for evaluation after 1 month of therapy.

3. Ms. Allison is admitted to the postsurgical recovery area and prescribed an analeptic for respiratory depression. Discuss what preadministration and ongoing assessments you would make when caring for Ms. Allison.

4. Discuss precautions that should be taken when administering the CNS stimulants.

Review Questions

1. Initial assessment of the child with attention deficit hyperactivity disorder includes _____.
   A. assessing to which stimuli the child responds the most
   B. determining the child's intelligence
   C. obtaining a summary of the child's behavior pattern
   D. obtaining vital signs

2. When assessing the patient receiving doxapram for chronic pulmonary disease, the nurse observes the patient for adverse drug reactions, which may include _____.
   A. headache, dizziness, variations in heart rate
   B. diarrhea, drowsiness, hypotension
   C. decreased respiratory rate, weight gain, bradycardia
   D. fever, dysuria, constipation

3. When teaching a patient with narcolepsy who is receiving an amphetamine, the nurse instructs the patient to _____.

   A. record the times of the day the medication is taken

   B. take the medication at bedtime as well as in the morning

   C. take the drug with meals

   D. keep a record of how often periods of sleepiness occur

4. When administering an amphetamine, the nurse first checks to see if the patient is taking or has taken a monoamine oxidase inhibitor (MAOI) because _____.

   A. a lower dosage of the amphetamine may be needed

   B. a higher dosage of the amphetamine may be needed

   C. the amphetamine can be substituted as the anti-depressant drug

   D. the amphetamine is not given within 14 days of the MAOI

Medication Dosage Problems

1. Phentermine hydrochloride 8 mg three times a day orally is prescribed as an adjunct for weight loss. The total amount of drug the patient will receive daily is _____. Is this an appropriate dose for this drug?

2. Modafinil 400 mg is prescribed. The drug is available in 200-mg tablets. The nurse administers _____.

To check your answers, see Appendix G.

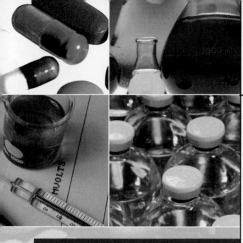

Chapter 26

Antipsychotic Drugs

Key Terms

- agranulocytosis
- akathisia
- anhedonia
- bipolar disorder
- delusions
- dystonia
- extrapyramidal syndrome
- flattened affect
- hallucinations
- neuroleptic malignant syndrome
- photophobia
- photosensitivity
- tardive dyskinesia

Learning Objectives

On completion of this chapter, the student will:

- List the uses, general drug actions, general adverse reactions, contraindications, precautions, and interactions associated with the administration of the antipsychotic drugs.
- Discuss important preadministration and ongoing assessment activities

the nurse should perform on the patient taking an antipsychotic drug.

- List nursing diagnoses particular to a patient taking an antipsychotic drug.
- Discuss ways to promote an optimal response to therapy, how to manage common adverse reactions, and important points to keep in mind when educating patients about the use of the antipsychotic drugs.

A ntipsychotic drugs are administered to patients experiencing a psychotic disorder. The term *psychosis* refers to a group of symptoms that affect mood and behavior. **Hallucinations** (false perceptions having no basis in reality) or **delusions** (false beliefs that cannot be changed with reason) are usually present. Other symptoms include disorganized speech, behavior disturbance, social withdrawal, **flattened affect** (absence of an emotional response to any situation or condition), and **anhedonia** (finding no pleasure in activities that are normally pleasurable).

Although lithium is not a true antipsychotic drug, it is considered with the antipsychotics because of its use in regulating the severe fluctuations of the manic phase of **bipolar disorder** (a psychiatric disorder characterized by severe mood swings from extreme hyperactivity to depression). During the manic phase, the person experiences altered thought processes, which can lead to bizarre delusions. The drug diminishes the frequency and intensity of hyperactive (manic) episodes.

Actions

Antipsychotic drugs are thought to act by inhibiting or blocking the release of the neurotransmitter dopamine in the brain and possibly increasing the firing of nerve cells in certain areas of the brain. These effects may be responsible for the ability of these drugs to suppress the symptoms of certain psychotic disorders. Because these drugs block dopamine transmission, they also produce unpleasant extrapyramidal effects (see Adverse Reactions). Examples of antipsychotic drugs include chlorpromazine (Thorazine), haloperidol (Haldol), and lithium.

Another group of antipsychotic drugs is classified as atypical antipsychotics. It is believed they act on serotonin receptors as well as on the dopamine receptors in the brain. They are termed *atypical* because the typical extrapyramidal side effects are lessened. Examples of the atypical antipsychotic drugs include clozapine (Clozaril) and aripiprazole (Abilify). The Summary Drug Table: Antipsychotic Drugs gives a more complete listing of the antipsychotic drugs.

SUMMARY DRUG TABLE   ANTIPSYCHOTIC DRUGS

GENERIC NAME	TRADE NAME	USES	ADVERSE REACTIONS	DOSAGE RANGES
Typical Antipsychotics				
Chlorpromazine HCl *klor-proe'-ma-zeen*	Thorazine	Psychotic disorders, nausea, vomiting, intractable hiccups	Hypotension, drowsiness, tardive dyskinesia, nasal congestion, dry mouth, dystonia, extra-pyramidal symptoms (EPS), behavioral changes, photosensitivity	Psychiatric disorders: up to 400 mg/d orally in divided doses Nausea and vomiting: 10–25 mg orally, 25–50 mg IM, 50–100 mg rectally
fluphenazine HCl *floo-fen'-a-zeen*	Prolixin	Psychotic disorders	Drowsiness, tachycardia, EPS, dystonia, akathisia, hypotension	0.5–10 mg/d orally in divided doses, up to 20mg/d; 1.25–10 mg/d IM in divided doses
haloperidol *ha-loe-per'-i-dole*	Haldol	Psychotic disorders; Tourette's syndrome, hyperactivity, behavior problems in children	EPS, akathisia, dystonia, TD, drowsiness, headache, dry mouth, orthostatic hypotension	0.5–5 mg orally BID or TID with dosage up to 100 mg/d in divided doses; 2–5 mg IM Children 0.05–0.075 mg/kg/d orally
lithium *lith'-ee-um*	Eskalith, Lithobid	Manic episodes of bipolar disorder	Headache, drowsiness, tremors, nausea, polyuria (see Table 26–1)	Based on lithium serum levels; average dose range is 900–1800 mg/d orally in divided doses
loxapine *lox'-a-peen*	Loxitane	Psychotic disorders	EPS, akathisia, dystonia, TD, drowsiness, headache, dry mouth, orthostatic hypotension	10–100 mg/d orally, not to exceed 250 mg/d
molindone HCl *moe-lyn'-dun*	Moban	Schizophrenia	EPS, drowsiness, increased libido, TD, rash, nausea, dry mouth, constipation	50–100 mg/d orally in divided doses
perphenazine *per-fen'-a- zeen*		Psychotic disorders	Hypotension, postural hypotension, TD, photophobia, urticaria, nasal congestion, dry mouth, akathisia, dystonia, pseudoparkinsonism, behavioral changes, headache, photosensitivity	Psychotic disorders; 4–16 mg orally 2–4 times/d
pimozide *pi'-moe-zide*	Orap	Tourette's syndrome	Parkinson-like symptoms, motor restlessness, dystonia, oculogyric crisis, TD, dry mouth, diarrhea, headache, rash, drowsiness	Initial dose: 1–2 mg/d orally Maintenance dose: up to 10mg/d orally
prochlorperazine *proe-klor-per'-a-zeen*	Compazine	Psychotic disorders, nausea, vomiting, anxiety	EPS, sedation, TD, dry eyes, blurred vision, constipation, dry mouth, photosensitivity	Psychotic disorders: up to 150 mg orally, 10–20 mg IM Nausea, vomiting: 15–40 mg/d orally in divided doses Anxiety: 5 mg orally TID

GENERIC NAME	TRADE NAME	USES	ADVERSE REACTIONS	DOSAGE RANGES
promazine HCl *proe'-ma-zeen*	Sparine	Psychotic disorders	Drowsiness, EPS, dystonia, akathisia, hypotension	10–200 mg orally, IM q4–6h
thioridazine *thee-o-rid'-a-zeen*		Schizophrenia	Cardiac arrhythmias, drowsiness, TD, nausea, dry mouth, constipation, diarrhea	50–100 mg orally TID, not to exceed 800 mg/d
thiothixene *thigh-o-thicks'-een*	Navane	Schizophrenia	EPS, drowsiness, nausea, diarrhea, TD	6–30 mg/d orally, not to exceed 60 mg/d
trifluoperazine HCl *try-floo-oh-per'-a-zeen*	Stelazine	Psychotic disorders, anxiety	Drowsiness, pseudoparkinsonism, dystonia, akathisia, TD, photophobia, blurred vision, dry mouth, salivation, nasal congestion, nausea, discolored urine (pink to red-brown	Psychosis: 4–20 mg/d orally in divided doses Anxiety: 1–2 mg orally BID

Atypical Antipsychotics

GENERIC NAME	TRADE NAME	USES	ADVERSE REACTIONS	DOSAGE RANGES
aripiprazole	Abilify	Psychotic disorders	Agitation, akathisia, anxiety, drowsiness, headache, constipation, dry mouth, nausea	10–30 mg/d orally
clozapine *kloe'-za-peen*	Clozaril, Fazaclo	Severely ill schizophrenic patients with no response to other therapies	Drowsiness, sedation, akathisia, tachycardia, nausea, agranulocytosis	Initial dose:25–50 mg/d, titrate up to 300–400 mg/d orally, not to exceed 900 mg/d
olanzapine *oh-lan'-za-peen*	Zyprexa	Schizophrenia, short-term treatment of manic episodes of bipolar disorder	Agitation, dizziness, nervousness, akathisia, constipation, fever, weight gain	5–20 mg/d orally
olanzapine/fluoxetine *oh-lan'-za-peen* *floo-ox'-e-teen*	Symbyax	Bipolar depressive episodes	Same as olanzapine	6-mg/25-mg combination tablet taken in the evening orally
quetiapine fumarate *kwe-tie'-ah-pine*	Seroquel	Psychotic disorders	Orthostatic hypotension, dizziness, vertigo, nausea, constipation, dry mouth diarrhea, headache, restlessness, blurred vision	150–750 mg/d orally in divided doses
risperidone *ris-per'-i-done*	Risperdal	Psychotic disorders	Agitation, dizziness, nervousness, akathisia, constipation, fever, weight gain	1–3 mg orally BID
ziprasidone HCl *zih-pray'-sih-dohn*	Geodon	Schizophrenia, bipolar mania, acute agitation	Somnolence, drowsiness, sedation, headache, arrhythmias, dyspepsia, fever, constipation, EPS	80 mg orally BID

TD, tardive dyskinesia; EPS, extrapyramidal syndrome.

Antipsychotic Drugs

Uses

The antipsychotic drugs are used in the treatment of

- Acute and chronic psychoses
- Bipolar (manic-depressive) illness
- Agitated behaviors associated with dementia

Selected drugs may be used for their adverse effects to treat minor conditions; for example, chlorpromazine (Thorazine) may be used to treat uncontrollable hiccoughs, and chlorpromazine and prochlorperazine (Compazine) are used as antiemetics.

Special Considerations: Lithium

Lithium carbonate is rapidly absorbed after oral administration. The most common adverse reactions include tremors, nausea, vomiting, thirst, and polyuria. Toxic reactions may occur when serum lithium levels are greater than 1.5 mEq/L (Table 26-1). Because some of these toxic reactions are potentially serious, lithium blood level measurements are usually obtained during therapy, and the dosage of lithium is adjusted accordingly.

Adverse Reactions

Generalized System Reactions

- Sedation, headache, hypotension
- Dry mouth, nasal congestion
- Urticaria, **photophobia** (intolerance to light), **photosensitivity** (abnormal sensitivity when exposed to light). Photosensitivity can result in severe sunburn when patients taking antipsychotic drugs are exposed to the sun or ultraviolet light, such as a tanning bed.

Behavioral Changes

- Possible increase in the intensity of the psychotic symptoms
- Lethargy, hyperactivity, paranoid reactions, agitation, and confusion

A decrease in dosage may eliminate some of these symptoms, but it also may be necessary to try another drug. Changes in psychotic behaviors may not be seen for days or weeks, although adverse reactions affecting the patient's ability to feel or move may occur before then. Patients may independently stop using the drug because of the unpleasantness of the reactions, thus causing the psychotic symptoms to return. It is important for the nurse to monitor for these conditions and notify the primary health care provider immediately. Three of the more serious motor syndromes are described in the following sections.

Table 26.1 Lithium Toxicity

Serum Lithium Level	Signs of Toxicity
1.5–2 mEq/L	Diarrhea, vomiting, nausea, drowsiness, muscular weakness, lack of coordination (early signs of toxicity)
2–3 mEq/L	Giddiness, ataxia, blurred vision, tinnitus, vertigo, increasing confusion, slurred speech, blackouts, myoclonic twitching or movement of entire limbs, choreoathetoid movements, urinary or fecal incontinence, agitation or manic-like behavior, hyperreflexia, hypertonia, dysarthria
More than 3 mEq/L	May produce a complex clinical picture involving multiple organs and organ systems, including seizures (generalized and focal), arrhythmias, hypotension, peripheral vascular collapse, stupor, muscle group twitching, spasticity, coma

Extrapyramidal Syndrome

Among the most significant adverse reactions associated with the antipsychotic drugs are the extrapyramidal effects. The term **extrapyramidal syndrome** (EPS) refers to a group of adverse reactions affecting the extrapyramidal portion of the nervous system as a result of antipsychotic drugs. This part of the nervous system affects body posture and promotes smooth and uninterrupted movement of various muscle groups. Antipsychotics disturb the function of the extrapyramidal portion of the nervous system, causing abnormal muscle movement. Extrapyramidal effects include Parkinson-like symptoms, akathisia, and dystonia (Display 26-1). Extrapyramidal effects usually diminish with a reduction in the dosage of the antipsychotic drug. Typically, the primary health care provider prescribes an antiparkinsonism drug, such as benztropine (see Chapter 32), to reduce the incidence of Parkinson-like symptoms.

> **Display 26.1 Extrapyramidal Syndrome (EPS)**
>
> - Parkinson-like symptoms—fine tremors, muscle rigidity, masklike appearance of the face, slowness of movement, slurred speech, and unsteady gait
> - **Akathisia**—extreme restlessness and increased motor activity
> - **Dystonia**—facial grimacing and twisting of the neck into unnatural positions

Tardive Dyskinesia

Tardive dyskinesia (TD) is a syndrome consisting of irreversible, involuntary dyskinetic movements. Tardive dyskinesia is characterized by rhythmic, involuntary movements of the tongue, face, mouth, or jaw and sometimes the extremities. The tongue may protrude, and there may be chewing movements, puckering of the mouth, and facial grimacing. TD is a late-appearing reaction and may be observed in patients receiving an antipsychotic drug or after discontinuation of antipsychotic drug therapy. Because TD is non-reversible, drug therapy must be discontinued when symptoms occur during the course of therapy. Because of the risk of TD, it is best to use the smallest dose and the shortest duration of treatment that produces a satisfactory clinical response. The use of atypical antipsychotic drugs has increased because they are less likely to cause TD effects.

Neuroleptic Malignant Syndrome

Neuroleptic malignant syndrome (NMS) is a rare reaction characterized by a combination of extrapyramidal effects, hyperthermia, and autonomic disturbance. It typically occurs within 1 month after the antipsychotic drug regimen is begun. NMS is potentially fatal and requires intensive symptomatic treatment and immediate discontinuation of the drug causing the syndrome. Once the antipsychotic drug is discontinued, recovery occurs within 7 to 10 days.

Contraindications

The antipsychotics are contraindicated in patients with known hypersensitivity to the drugs, in comatose patients, and in those who are severely depressed, have bone marrow depression, blood dyscrasias, Parkinson's disease (haloperidol), liver impairment, coronary artery disease, or severe hypotension or hypertension.

Antipsychotic drugs are classified as pregnancy category C drugs (except for clozapine, which is pregnancy category B). Safe use of these drugs during pregnancy and lactation has not been clearly established. Antipsychotics should be used only when clearly needed and when the potential benefit outweighs any potential harm to the fetus.

Lithium is contraindicated in patients with hypersensitivity to tartrazine, renal or cardiovascular disease, sodium depletion, and dehydration, and in patients receiving diuretics. Lithium is a pregnancy category D drug and is contraindicated during pregnancy and lactation. For women of childbearing age, contraceptives may be prescribed while they are taking lithium.

Precautions

The antipsychotic drugs are used cautiously in patients with respiratory disorders, glaucoma, prostatic hypertrophy, epilepsy, decreased renal function, and peptic ulcer disease.

Gerontologic Alert

Because drug metabolism and excretion are altered in elderly or debilitated patients, doses may be instituted at one-half to one-third the recommended dose for younger adults and increased more gradually than in younger adults.

Lithium is monitored carefully in patients who sweat profusely, experience diarrhea or vomiting, or who have an infection or fever causing fluid loss.

Interactions

The following interactions may occur when an antipsychotic is administered with another agent:

Interacting Drug	Common Use	Effect of Interaction
anticholinergic drugs	Management of gastrointestinal (GI) problems such as peptic ulcer disease	Increased risk for TD and psychotic symptoms
immunologic drugs	Treatment of chronic illness such as cancer, arthritis, human immunodeficiency virus (HIV) infection	Increased severity of bone marrow suppression
antacids	Relief of GI upset, heartburn	Decreased effectiveness of lithium
loop diuretics	Management of cardiac problems	Increased risk for lithium toxicity
lithium combined with other antipsychotics	Management of psychotic symptoms	Increased risk for lithium toxicity
alcohol	Relaxation and enjoyment in social situations	Increased risk for central nervous system depression

The Patient Receiving an Antipsychotic Drug

ASSESSMENT

PREADMINISTRATION ASSESSMENT

A patient receiving an antipsychotic drug may be treated in the hospital or in an outpatient setting. The nurse assesses the patient's mental status before and periodically throughout therapy. The nurse must note the presence of hallucinations or delusions and document them accurately in the patient's record.

Before starting therapy for the hospitalized patient, the nurse obtains a complete mental health, social, and medical history. In the case of psychosis, patients often are unable to give a reliable history of their illness. When available, the nurse obtains the mental health history from a family member or friend. As the history is taken, the nurse observes the patient for any behavior patterns that appear to be deviations from normal. Examples of deviations include poor eye contact, failure to answer questions completely, inappropriate answers to questions, a monotone speech pattern, and inappropriate laughter, sadness, or crying.

During the initial assessment, the nurse may need to rely more on observation of the patient than actual physical assessment. Ideally, assessment should include obtaining blood pressure, pulse, respiratory rate, and weight. The patient may react violently because of the psychosis; therefore, touching the patient may be contraindicated.

Some patients, such as those with mild schizophrenia, do not require inpatient care. The nurse usually sees these patients at periodic intervals in the mental health outpatient setting. The initial assessments of the outpatient are basically the same as those for the hospitalized patient. The nurse obtains a complete medical history and a history of the symptoms of the mental disorder from the patient, a family member, or the patient's hospital records. During the initial interview, the nurse observes the patient for what appear to be deviations from a normal behavior pattern. The nurse also should assess the patient's vital signs and body weight.

ONGOING ASSESSMENT

Many antipsychotic drugs are administered for a long time, which makes the ongoing assessment an important part of determining therapeutic drug effects and monitoring for adverse reactions, particularly EPS (see Display 26-1) and TD. The role of the nurse is important in the administration of these drugs both in the inpatient and clinic settings for the following reasons:

- The patient's response to drug therapy on an inpatient basis requires around-the-clock assessments because frequent dosage adjustments may be necessary during therapy.

- Accurate assessments for the appearance of adverse drug effects assume a greater importance when the patient may be unable to verbalize physical changes to the primary health care provider or nurse.

NURSING DIAGNOSES

Drug-specific nursing diagnoses are highlighted in the Nursing Diagnoses Checklist. Other nursing diagnoses applicable to these drugs are discussed in depth in Chapter 4.

✔ Nursing Diagnoses Checklist

✔ **Risk for Injury** related to hypotension or sedation

✔ **Impaired Physical Mobility** related to impaired motor ability

✔ **Risk for Infection** related to agranulocytosis

✔ **Imbalanced Fluid Volume** related to lithium toxicity

PLANNING

The expected outcomes for the patient depend on the reason for drug administration, but may include an optimal response to drug therapy, meeting of patient needs related to management of adverse drug reactions, an absence of injury, and compliance with the prescribed therapeutic regimen.

IMPLEMENTATION

PROMOTING AN OPTIMAL RESPONSE TO THERAPY

The nurse develops a nursing care plan to meet the patient's individual needs.

MANAGING CARE OF THE INPATIENT Behavioral records should be written at periodic intervals (frequency depends on hospital or unit guidelines). An accurate description of the patient's behavior aids the primary health care provider in planning therapy and thus becomes an important part of nursing management. Patients with a poor response to drug therapy may require dosage changes, a change to another psychotherapeutic drug, or the addition of other therapies to the treatment regimen. However, it is important for the nurse to know that full response to antipsychotic drugs takes several weeks.

If the patient's behavior is violent or aggressive, antipsychotic drugs may have to be given parenterally. The nurse may require assistance in securing the patient and should give the drugs intramuscularly (IM) in a large muscle mass, such as the gluteus muscle. The nurse keeps the patient lying down (when possible) for about 30 minutes after administering the drug.

Nursing Alert

In combative patients or those who have serious manifestations of acute psychosis (e.g., hallucinations or loss of contact with reality), parenteral administration may be repeated every 1 to 4 hours until the desired effects are obtained. The nurse monitors the patient closely for cardiac arrhythmias or rhythm changes, or hypotension.

The nurse may give antipsychotic drugs orally as a single daily dose or in divided doses several times a day. Oral administration, especially in the long-term care setting, requires great care because some patients have difficulty swallowing (because of a dry mouth or other causes). After administration of an oral drug, the nurse inspects the patient's oral cavity to be sure the drug has been swallowed. If the patient resists having his or her oral cavity checked, the nurse reports this refusal to the primary health care provider.

Other patients may refuse to take the drug altogether. The nurse should never force a patient to take an oral drug. If the patient refuses the drug, the nurse contacts the primary health care provider regarding this problem because parenteral administration of the medication may be necessary.

Oral liquid concentrates are available for patients who can more easily swallow a liquid. To aid in administration to debilitated or elderly patients, oral drugs can be mixed in liquids such as fruit juices, tomato juice, milk, or carbonated beverages. Semisolid foods, such as soups or puddings, may also be used.

MANAGING CARE OF THE OUTPATIENT At the time of each visit of the patient to the primary health care provider's office or clinic, the nurse observes the patient for a response to therapy. In some instances, the nurse may question the patient or a family member about the response to therapy. The questions asked depend on the patient and the diagnosis, and may include questions such as

- How are you feeling?
- How do your nerves feel compared to before the medicine?
- Would you like to tell me how everything is going?

Many times the nurse may need to rephrase questions or direct conversation toward other subjects until these patients feel comfortable and are able to discuss their therapy.

The nurse asks the patient or a family member about adverse drug reactions or any other problems occurring during therapy. The nurse brings these reactions or problems to the attention of the primary health care provider. The nurse should document in the patient's record a general summary of the patient's outward behavior and any complaints or problems. The nurse then compares these notations with previous notations and observations.

MONITORING AND MANAGING PATIENT NEEDS

The patient may need to tolerate some adverse reactions, such as dry mouth, episodes of orthostatic hypotension, and drowsiness during drug therapy. Nursing interventions to relieve some of these reactions may include offering frequent sips of water, assisting the patient out of the bed or chair, and supervising all ambulatory activities.

RISK FOR INJURY The antipsychotic drugs may cause extreme drowsiness and sedation, especially during the first or second weeks of therapy. This reaction may impair mental or physical abilities. The nurse provides total assistance with activities of daily living to the patient experiencing extreme sedation, including help with eating, dressing, and ambulating. If hypotension or sedation occurs with these drugs, administration at bedtime helps to minimize the risk of injury. During hypotensive episodes it is important to monitor vital signs at least daily; depending on the patient's behavior, the nurse may monitor vital signs more frequently. The nurse should report any significant change in vital signs to the primary health care provider.

Drowsiness usually diminishes after 2 or 3 weeks of therapy. However, if the patient continues to be troubled by drowsiness and sedation, the primary health care provider may decide to prescribe a lower dosage.

IMPAIRED PHYSICAL MOBILITY During initial therapy or whenever the dosage is increased or decreased, the nurse observes the patient closely for adverse drug reactions, including TD. The nurse may use the Abnormal Involuntary Movement Scale (AIMS) to screen the patient for symptoms (Display 26-2) and any behavioral changes. Because these adverse effects are considered "late stage," the nurse needs to be alert to their presence. The nurse reports to the primary health care provider any change in behavior or the appearance of adverse reactions. An immediate decrease in dosage will not change the condition, but may prevent further deterioration of the patient.

Display 26.2 Abnormal Involuntary Movement Scale (AIMS) Screening Tool

Client identification: _____   Date: _____
Rated by: _____

Either before or after completing the examination procedure, observe the client unobtrusively at rest (e.g., in waiting room). The chair to be used in this examination should be a hard, firm one without arms.

After observing the client, he or she may be rated on a scale of 0 (none), 1 (minimal), 2 (mild), 3 (moderate), and 4 (severe) according to the severity of symptoms.

Ask the client whether there is anything in his/her teeth (i.e., gum, candy, etc.) and, if there is, to remove it.

Ask client about the current condition of his/her teeth. Ask client if he/she wears dentures. Do teeth or dentures bother client now?

Ask client whether he/she notices any movement in mouth, face, hands, or feet. If yes, ask to describe and to what extent the movements currently bother patient or interfere with his/her activities.

0 1 2 3 4	Ask client to tap thumb with each finger as rapidly as possible for 10–15 seconds; separately with right hand, then with left hand. (Observe facial and leg movements.)
0 1 2 3 4	Flex and extend client's left and right arms (one at a time).
0 1 2 3 4	*Ask client to stand up. (Observe in profile. Observe all body areas again, hips included.)
0 1 2 3 4	Have client sit in chair with hands on knees, legs slightly apart, and feet flat on floor (look at entire body for movements while in this position)
0 1 2 3 4	Ask client to sit with hands hanging unsupported. If male, hands between legs; if female and wearing a dress, hands hanging over knees. (Observe hands and other body areas.)
0 1 2 3 4	Ask client to open mouth. (Observe tongue at rest within mouth.) Do this twice.
0 1 2 3 4	Ask client to protrude tongue. (Observe abnormalities of tongue movement.) Do this twice.
0 1 2 3 4	Ask client to extend both arms outstretched in front with palms down. (Observe trunk, legs, and mouth.)
0 1 2 3 4	*Have client walk a few paces, turn, and walk back to chair. (Observe hands and gait.) Do this twice.

_____
* Activated movements.

From Videbeck, S. L. (2006). *Psychiatric mental health nursing* (3rd ed., p. 284) Philadelphia: LWW.

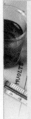

Nursing Alert

Because there is no known treatment for tardive dyskinesia (TD) and because it is irreversible in patients, the nurse must immediately report symptoms. These include rhythmic, involuntary movements of the tongue, face, mouth, jaw, or the extremities.

Patients can experience mobility problems if EPS occurs while taking the antipsychotic drugs. The nurse observes the patient for extrapyramidal effects, which include muscular spasms of the face and neck, the inability to sleep or sit still, tremors, rigidity, or involuntary rhythmic movements.

The nurse also assists with ambulation and reassures the patient that symptoms will decline when the dosage of the antipsychotic is decreased. In addition, the nurse notifies the primary health care provider of the occurrence of these symptoms because they may indicate a need for dosage adjustment.

RISK FOR INFECTION The use of the drug clozapine has been associated with severe **agranulocytosis**, or decreased white blood cell (WBC) count. This bone marrow suppression can make the patient more susceptible to illness and infection. To ensure close monitoring of this adverse reaction, clozapine is available only through a patient management system (a program that combines WBC testing, patient monitoring, and pharmacy and drug distribution services). Only a 1-week supply of this drug is dispensed at a time. A weekly WBC count is done throughout therapy and for 4 weeks after therapy is discontinued. In addition, the nurse monitors the patient for adverse reactions that indicate bone marrow suppression: lethargy, weakness, fever, sore throat, malaise, mucous membrane ulceration, or "flulike" complaints.

IMBALANCED FLUID VOLUME Fluid volume determines the concentration of lithium in the blood. The dosage of lithium is individualized according to serum levels and clinical response to the drug. The desirable serum lithium level is between 0.6 and 1.2 mEq/L. Blood samples are drawn immediately before the next dose of lithium (8 to 12 hours after the last dose) when lithium levels are relatively stable. During the acute phase, the nurse monitors serum lithium levels twice weekly or until the patient's manic phase is under control. During maintenance therapy, the serum lithium levels are monitored every 2 to 4 months.

Lithium toxicity is closely related to serum lithium levels and can occur even when the drug is administered at therapeutic doses. Adverse reactions are seldom observed at serum lithium levels of less than 1.5 mEq/L, except in the patient who is especially sensitive to lithium. Toxic symptoms may occur with serum lithium levels of 1.5 mEq/L or greater. Levels should not exceed 2 mEq/L (see Table 26-1). Therefore, the nurse must continually monitor patients taking lithium for signs of toxicity, such as diarrhea, vomiting, nausea, drowsiness, muscular weakness, and lack of coordination. For early symptoms, the primary health care provider may order a dosage reduction or discontinue the drug for 24 to 48 hours and then gradually restart the drug therapy at a lower dosage.

Gerontologic Alert

Older adults are at increased risk for lithium toxicity because of a decreased rate of excretion. Lower dosages may be necessary to decrease the risk of toxicity.

For patients receiving lithium therapy, the nurse increases the oral fluid intake to about 3000 mL/d. It is important to keep fluids readily available and to offer extra fluids throughout waking hours. If there is any question regarding the oral fluid intake, the nurse monitors intake and output.

EDUCATING THE PATIENT AND FAMILY

Noncompliance is a problem with some patients once they are discharged to the home setting. It is important for the nurse to evaluate accurately the patient's ability to assume responsibility for taking drugs at home. The administration of antipsychotic drugs becomes a family responsibility if the outpatient appears to be unable to manage his or her own drug therapy.

The nurse explains any adverse reactions that may occur with a specific antipsychotic drug and encourages the patient or family members to contact the primary health care provider immediately if a serious drug reaction occurs. The nurse includes the following points in a teaching plan for the patient or family member:

- Keep all primary care provider and clinic appointments because close monitoring of therapy is essential.
- Report any unusual changes or physical effects to the primary health care provider.
- Take the drug exactly as directed. Do not increase, decrease, or omit a dose or discontinue use of this drug unless directed to do so by the primary health care provider.
- Do not drive or perform other hazardous tasks if drowsiness occurs.
- Do not take any nonprescription drug unless use of a specific drug has been approved by the primary health care provider.
- Inform physicians, dentists, and other medical personnel of therapy with this drug.
- Do not drink alcoholic beverages unless approval is obtained from the primary health care provider.
- If dizziness occurs when changing position, rise slowly when getting out of bed or a chair. If dizziness is severe, always have help when changing positions.
- To relieve dry mouth, take frequent sips of water, suck on hard candy, or chew gum (preferably sugarless).
- Notify your primary care provider if you become pregnant or intend to become pregnant during therapy.
- Immediately report the occurrence of the following adverse reactions: restlessness, inability to sit still, muscle spasms, masklike expression, rigidity, tremors, drooling, or involuntary rhythmic movements of the mouth, face, or extremities.
- Avoid exposure to the sun. If exposure is unavoidable, wear sunblock, keep arms and legs covered, and wear a sun hat.

Antipsychotic Drugs

- Note that only a 1-week supply of clozapine is dispensed at a time. The drug is obtained through a special program designed to ensure the required blood monitoring. Weekly WBC laboratory tests are required. Immediately report any signs of weakness, fever, sore throat, malaise, or flulike symptoms to the primary health care provider.

- Note that olanzapine is available as a tablet to swallow or as an orally disintegrating tablet. When using the orally disintegrating tablet, peel back the foil on the blister packaging. Using dry hands, remove the tablet, and place the entire tablet in the mouth. The tablet will disintegrate immediately with or without liquid.

- Remember to take lithium with food or immediately after meals to avoid stomach upset. Drink at least 10 large glasses of fluid each day and add extra salt to food. Prolonged exposure to the sun may lead to dehydration. If any of the following occurs, do not take the next dose and immediately notify the primary health care provider: diarrhea, vomiting, fever, tremors, drowsiness, lack of muscle coordination, or muscle weakness.

EVALUATION

- The therapeutic effect is achieved and psychotic behavior is decreased.

- Adverse reactions are identified, reported to the primary health care provider, and managed successfully through appropriate nursing interventions.

- No evidence of injury is seen.

- The patient verbalizes an understanding of treatment modalities and the importance of continued follow-up care.

- The patient verbalizes the importance of complying with the prescribed therapeutic regimen.

- The patient and family demonstrate understanding of the drug regimen.

Critical Thinking Exercises

1. Ms. Brown comes to the mental health clinic for a follow-up visit. She is taking lithium to control a bipolar disorder. Ms. Brown tells you that she is concerned because her "hands are always shaking" and "sometimes I walk like I have been drinking alcohol." Explain how you would explore this problem with Ms. Brown.

2. As a nurse on the mental health unit, you are assigned to discuss extrapyramidal effects at a team conference. Discuss how you would present and explain this topic. Describe the points you would stress.

3. Your patient is prescribed clozapine for schizophrenia that has not responded to other drugs. You must explain this new therapy to the family. Discuss what points to include in this family teaching session.

Review Questions

1. A patient taking chlorpromazine for schizophrenia is also prescribed the antiparkinsonism drug benztropine. What is the best explanation for adding an antiparkinsonism drug to the drug regimen?

   A. Antiparkinsonism drugs prevent symptoms of tardive dyskinesia, such as involuntary movements of the face and tongue.

   B. Antiparkinsonism drugs promote the effects of chlorpromazine.

   C. Antiparkinsonism drugs are given to reduce the possibility of symptoms such as fine tremors, muscle rigidity, and slow movement.

   D. Antiparkinsonism drugs help to decrease hallucinations and delusions in patients with schizophrenia.

2. Which of the following reactions would the nurse expect to see in a patient experiencing tardive dyskinesia?

   A. Muscle rigidity, dry mouth, insomnia

   B. Rhythmic, involuntary movements of the tongue, face, mouth, or jaw

   C. Muscle weakness, paralysis of the eyelids, diarrhea

   D. Dyspnea, somnolence, muscle spasms

3. Which of the following symptoms would indicate to the nurse that a patient taking lithium is experiencing toxicity?

   A. Constipation, abdominal cramps, rash

   B. Stupor, oliguria, hypertension

   C. Nausea, vomiting, diarrhea

   D. Dry mouth, blurred vision, difficulty swallowing

4. In giving discharge instructions to a patient taking lithium, the nurse stresses that the patient should _____.

  A. eat a diet high in carbohydrates and low in proteins

  B. increase oral fluid intake to approximately 3000 mL/d

  C. have blood drawn before each dose of lithium is administered

  D. avoid eating foods high in amines

Medication Dosage Problems

1. A patient is prescribed haloperidol 3 mg IM. The drug is available in solution of 2 mg/mL. The nurse would administer _____.

2. Oral Thorazine 50 mg is prescribed. Use the drug label below to determine the correct dosage. The nurse administers _____.

Store between 15° and 30°C (59° and 86°F). Dispense in a tight, light resistant container. Each tablet contains chlorpromazine hydrochloride, 25 mg. **Dosage:** See accompanying prescribing information. **Important:** Use safety closures when dispensing this product unless otherwise directed by physician or requested by purchaser.

GlaxoSmithKline
Research Triangle Park, NC 27709
731562-AN

NDC 0007-5074-20
25mg
THORAZINE®
CHLORPROMAZINE HCl TABLETS
100 Tablets   R only
gsk GlaxoSmithKline

3. Lithium 600 mg is prescribed. Use the drug label below to determine the correct dosage. The nurse administers _____.

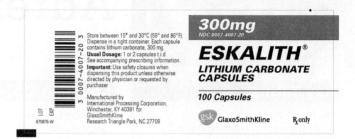

Store between 15° and 30°C (59° and 86°F). Dispense in a tight container. Each capsule contains lithium carbonate, 300 mg. **Usual Dosage:** 1 or 2 capsules t.i.d. See accompanying prescribing information. **Important:** Use safety closures when dispensing this product unless otherwise directed by physician or requested by purchaser.

Manufactured by International Processing Corporation, Winchester, KY 40391 for GlaxoSmithKline Research Triangle Park, NC 27709
670876-W

NDC 0007-4007-20
300mg
ESKALITH®
LITHIUM CARBONATE CAPSULES
100 Capsules
gsk GlaxoSmithKline   R only

To check your answers, see Appendix G.

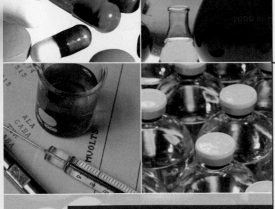

Adrenergic Drugs

Learning Objectives

On completion of this chapter, the student will:

- Discuss the activity of the autonomic nervous system, specifically the sympathetic branch.
- Discuss the types of shock, physiologic responses of shock, and the use of adrenergic drugs in the treatment of shock.
- Discuss the uses, general drug actions, contraindications, precautions, interactions, and adverse reactions associated with the administration of adrenergic vasopressor drugs.

- Discuss important preadministration and ongoing assessment activities the nurse should perform on the patient taking adrenergic drugs.
- List nursing diagnoses particular to a patient taking the adrenergic drugs.
- Discuss ways to promote an optimal response to therapy, how to manage common adverse reactions, and important points to keep in mind when educating patients about the use of adrenergic drugs.

One component of the **peripheral nervous system** (see unit introduction) is a system of nerves that automatically regulates bodily functions—the **autonomic nervous system**. This system is further divided into the **sympathetic** and the **parasympathetic** nervous system branches. The sympathetic branch is regulated by involuntary control. In other words, a person does not have control over what this system does. These nerves are activated when the body is confronted with stressful situations, such as danger, intense emotion, or severe illness. The sympathetic branch has control over a person's heart rate, breathing rate, and ability to divert blood to the skeletal muscles—to enable a person to run, for example. Activation of this branch is often called the *fight-or-flight response*. Another term for the sympathetic branch is the **adrenergic** branch because the system is based on the neurohormone adrenalin (epinephrine).

Norepinephrine is a **neurotransmitter** produced naturally by the body. It is the primary neurotransmitter in the sympathetic branch of the autonomic nervous system.

In the sympathetic branch of the autonomic nervous system, adrenergic drugs produce activity similar to the neurotransmitter norepinephrine. Another name for these drugs is **sympathomimetic** (mimic the actions of the sympathetic nervous system) drugs. The adrenergic drugs produce pharmacologic effects similar to the effects that occur in the body when the sympathetic nerves (norepinephrine) and the medulla (epinephrine) are stimulated. The primary effects of these drugs occur on the heart, the blood vessels, and the smooth muscles, such as the bronchi of the lung (Table 27-1). Metaraminol (Aramine) and isoproterenol (Isuprel) are examples of adrenergic drugs.

Table 27.1 Action of the Autonomic Nervous System on Body Organs and Structures

Organs or Structures	Sympathetic (Adrenergic) Effects	Types of Sympathetic (Adrenergic) Receptor	Parasympathetic (Cholinergic) Effects
Heart	Increase in heart rate, heart muscle contractility, increase in speed of atrioventricular conduction	β	Decrease in heart rate, decrease in heart muscle contractility
Blood vessels 1. Skin, mucous membranes 2. Skeletal muscle	Constriction Usually dilation	α Cholinergic,* β	
Bronchial muscles	Relaxation	β	Contraction
Gastrointestinal 1. Muscle motility, tone 2. Sphincters 3. Gallbladder	Decrease Usually contraction Relaxation	β α	Increase Usually relaxation Contraction
Urinary bladder 1. Detrusor muscle 2. Trigone, sphincter muscles	Relaxation Contraction	β α	Contraction Relaxation
Eye 1. Radial muscle of iris 2. Sphincter muscle of iris 3. Ciliary muscle	Contraction (pupil dilates)	α	 Contraction (pupil constricts) Contraction
Skin 1. Sweat glands 2. Pilomotor muscles	Increased activity in localized areas Contraction (gooseflesh)	Cholinergic* α	
Uterus	Relaxation	β	
Salivary glands	Thickened secretions	α	Copious, watery secretions
Liver	Glycogenolysis	β	
Lacrimal and nasopharyngeal glands			Increased secretion
Male sex organs	Emission	α	Erection

α, alpha; β, beta.
*Cholinergic transmission, but nerve cell chain originates in the thoracolumbar part of the spinal cord and is therefore sympathetic.

Actions

The purpose of stimulating the sympathetic (adrenergic) nerves is to divert blood flow to the vital organs so that the body can deal with a stressful situation. In general, adrenergic drugs produce one or more of the following responses in varying degrees:

- Central nervous system—wakefulness, quick reaction to stimuli, quickened reflexes
- Autonomic nervous system—relaxation of the smooth muscles of the bronchi; constriction of blood vessels, sphincters of the stomach; dilation of coronary blood vessels; decrease in gastric motility
- Heart—increase in the heart rate
- Metabolism—increased use of glucose (sugar) and liberation of fatty acids from adipose tissue

Adrenergic Nerve Receptors

The degree to which any organ is affected by the sympathetic nervous system depends on which postsynaptic nerve receptor sites are activated (Fig. 27-1). Adrenergic

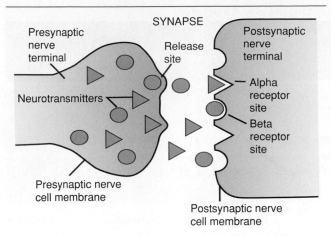

Figure 27.1 Neurotransmission in the peripheral nervous system. Neurotransmitter molecules (e.g., norepinephrine), released by the presynaptic nerve, cross the synapse and bind with alpha and beta receptors in the cell membrane of the postsynaptic nerve, resulting in the transmission of the nerve impulse.

nerves have either alpha (α) or beta (β) receptors. Drugs that act on the receptors are called *selective* or *nonselective*. Adrenergic drugs may be selective (act on α receptors or β receptors only) or nonselective (act on both α and β receptors). For example, isoproterenol acts chiefly on β receptors; it is considered a selective drug. Epinephrine is a nonselective drug and acts on both α and β receptors.

Whether an adrenergic drug acts on α, β, or α and β receptors accounts for the variation of responses to this group of drugs. Table 27-2 lists the type of adrenergic nerve receptor that corresponds with each action of the autonomic nervous system on the body. The α and β receptors can be further grouped as α_1- and α_2-adrenergic receptors and β_1- and β_2-adrenergic receptors.

Uses

Adrenergic drugs have a wide variety of uses and may be given for the treatment of

- Hypovolemic and septic shock
- Moderately severe to severe episodes of hypotension
- Control of superficial bleeding during surgical and dental procedures of the mouth, nose, throat, and skin
- Cardiac decompensation and arrest
- Allergic reactions (anaphylactic shock, angioneurotic edema)
- Temporary treatment of heart block
- Ventricular arrhythmias (under certain conditions)
- Respiratory distress (as bronchodilators)
- Nasal congestion and glaucoma (topical formulation)

Adrenergic drugs may also be used as a vasoconstricting adjunct to local anesthetics to prolong anesthetic action in the tissues. The adrenergic drugs used primarily as **vasopressors** (drugs that raise the blood pressure because of their ability to constrict blood vessels) are listed in the Summary Drug Table: Adrenergic Drugs. Sympathomimetics are also used as bronchodilators in the treatment of respiratory problems (see Chapter 37) or topically in the treatment of glaucoma (see Chapter 57).

Shock

The adrenergic drugs are important in the care and treatment of patients in shock. **Shock** is a state of inadequate tissue perfusion. In shock, the supply of arterial blood and oxygen flowing to the cells and tissues is inadequate. To counteract the symptoms of shock, the body initiates physiologic mechanisms (e.g., the release of epinephrine and norepinephrine). In some situations, the body is able to compensate and blood pressure is maintained. However, if

Table 27.2 Effects of the Adrenergic Receptors

Receptor	Site	Effect
α_1	Peripheral blood vessels	Vasoconstriction of peripheral blood vessels
α_2	Presynaptic neuron	Regulates release of neurotransmitters; decreases tone, motility, and secretions of gastrointestinal tract
β_1	Myocardium	Increased heart rate, increased force of myocardial contraction
β_2	Peripheral blood vessels Bronchial smooth muscles	Vasodilation of peripheral vessels Bronchodilation

α, alpha; β, beta.

SUMMARY DRUG TABLE ADRENERGIC DRUGS

GENERIC NAME	TRADE NAME	USES	ADVERSE REACTIONS	DOSAGE RANGES
dobutamine HCl *doe-byoo'-ta-meen*		Cardiac decompensation due to depressed contractility caused by organic heart disease or cardiac surgical procedures	Headache, nausea, increased heart rate, increase in systolic blood pressure, palpitations, anginal and nonspecific chest pain	2.5–10 mcg/kg/min IV (up to 40 mcg/kg/min); titrate to patient's hemodynamic and renal status
dopamine *doe'-pa-meen*		Shock due to myocardial infarction, trauma, open heart surgery, renal failure, and chronic cardiac decompensation in congestive heart failure	Nausea, vomiting, ectopic beats, tachycardia, anginal pain, palpitations, hypotension, dyspnea	2–50 mcg/kg/min IV (infusion rate determined by patient's response)
epinephrine *ep-i-nef'-rin*	EpiPen	Ventricular standstill; treatment and prophylaxis of cardiac arrest, heart block; mucosal congestion of hay fever, rhinitis, and acute sinusitis; prolong regional/local anesthetics; anaphylactic reactions	Anxiety, restlessness, headache, lightheadedness, dizziness, nausea, dysuria, pallor	Cardiac arrest: 0.5–1.0 mg IV Respiratory distress (e.g., anaphylaxis): 0.1–0.25 mg
isoproterenol *eye-sew-proe-tare'-e-nall*	Isuprel	Injection: shock, bronchospasm during anesthesia, cardiac standstill and arrhythmias Inhalation: acute bronchial asthma, emphysema, bronchitis, bronchiectasis	Anxiety, sweating, flushing, headache, lightheadedness, dizziness, nausea, vomiting, tachycardia	Shock: 4 mcg/mL diluted solution IV Cardiac arrhythmias, cardiac standstill: 0.02–0.06 mg of diluted solution IV, or 1:5000 solution intracardiac injection
metaraminol *met-a-ram'-i-nole*	Aramine	Hypotension with spinal anesthesia, hypotension due to hemorrhage, drug reactions, surgical complication, shock associated with brain damage	Headache, apprehension, palpitations, nausea, projectile vomiting, urinary urgency	2–10 mg IM, SC; 15–100 mg in 250- or 500-mL solution IV

Adrenergic Drugs

SUMMARY DRUG TABLE *(continued)*

GENERIC NAME	TRADE NAME	USES	ADVERSE REACTIONS	DOSAGE RANGES
midodrine *mid'-oh-dryn*	ProAmatine	Orthostatic hypotension, only when patient is considerably impaired	Paresthesias, headache, pain, dizziness, supine hypertension, bradycardia, piloerection, pruritus, dysuria, chills	10 mg orally TID during daylight hours when patient is upright
norepinephrine (levarterenol) *nor-ep-i-nef'-rin*	Levophed	Shock, hypotension, cardiac arrest	Restlessness, headache, dizziness, bradycardia, hypertension	2–4 mcg/min, rate adjusted to maintain desired blood pressure

shock is untreated and compensatory mechanisms of the body fail, irreversible shock occurs and death follows. There are three types of shock: hypovolemic shock, cardiogenic shock, and distributive shock. Table 27-3 describes the various types of shock.

Various clinical manifestations may be present in a patient in shock. For example, in the early stages of shock the extremities may be warm because vasodilation is initiated and the blood flow to the skin and extremities is maintained. If the condition is untreated, blood flow to vital organs, skin, and extremities is compromised. The patient becomes cool and clammy, which is referred to as "cool" or "cold" shock. Regardless of the type, shock results in a decrease in cardiac output, decrease in arterial blood pressure (hypotension), reabsorption of water

by the kidneys (causing a decrease in urinary output), decrease in the exchange of oxygen and carbon dioxide in the lungs, increase in carbon dioxide and decrease in oxygen in the blood, hypoxia (decreased oxygen reaching the cells), and increased concentration of intravascular fluid. This scenario compromises the functioning of vital organs such as the heart, brain, and kidneys. The various physiologic responses caused by shock are listed in Table 27-4.

The adrenergic drugs are useful in improving hemodynamic status by improving myocardial contractility and increasing heart rate, which results in increased cardiac output. Peripheral resistance is increased by vasoconstriction. In cardiogenic shock or advanced shock associated with low cardiac output, the adrenergic drug may be used

Table 27.3 Types of Shock

Type*	Description
Hypovolemic	Occurs when the blood volume is significantly diminished. *Examples*: hemorrhage; fluid loss caused by burns, dehydration, or excess diuresis.
Cardiogenic-obstructive shock	Occurs when cardiac output is insufficient and perfusion to the vital organs cannot be maintained. *Examples*: a result of acute myocardial infarction, ventricular arrhythmias, congestive heart failure, or severe cardiomyopathy. Obstructive shock is categorized with cardiogenic shock. It occurs when obstruction of blood flow results in inadequate tissue perfusion. *Examples*: pericardial tamponade, restrictive pericarditis, and severe cardiac valve dysfunction.
Distributive (vasogenic) shock	Occurs when there are changes to the blood vessels causing dilation, but no additional blood volume. The blood is redistributed within the body. This category is further differentiated: • Septic shock—circulatory insufficiency resulting from overwhelming infection (e.g., central line infection) • Anaphylactic shock—hypersensitivity resulting in massive systemic vasodilation (e.g., drug allergic reaction) • Neurogenic shock—interference with peripheral nervous system control of blood vessels (e.g., spinal cord injury)

*Other causes of shock include hypoglycemia, hypothyroidism, and Addison's disease.

Table 27.4 Physiologic Manifestations of Shock

Body System	Possible Signs and Symptoms
Integumentary (skin)	Pallor, cyanosis, cold and clammy, sweating
Central nervous system	Agitation, confusion, disorientation, coma
Cardiovascular	Hypotension, tachycardia, arrhythmias, wide pulse pressure, gallop rhythm
Respiratory	Tachypnea, pulmonary edema
Renal	Urinary output less than 20 mL/h
Metabolic (endocrine)	Acidosis

with a vasodilating drug. A vasodilator, such as nitroprusside (see Chapter 41) or nitroglycerin (see Chapter 40), improves myocardial performance because the adrenergic drug maintains blood pressure.

Adverse Reactions

The adverse reactions associated with the administration of adrenergic drugs depend on the drug used, the dose administered, and individualized patient response. Some of the more common adverse reactions include

- Cardiac arrhythmias (bradycardia and tachycardia)
- Headache
- Nausea and vomiting
- Increased blood pressure (which may reach dangerously high levels)

Additional adverse reactions for specific adrenergic drugs are listed in the Summary Drug Table: Adrenergic Drugs.

Gerontologic Alert

The older adult is especially vulnerable to adverse reactions of the adrenergic drugs, particularly epinephrine. In addition, older adults are more likely to have preexisting cardiovascular disease that predisposes them to potentially serious cardiac arrhythmias. The nurse closely monitors all elderly patients taking an adrenergic drug. It is important to report any changes in the pulse rate or rhythm immediately. In addition, epinephrine may temporarily increase tremor and rigidity in older adults with Parkinson's disease.

Contraindications

Adrenergic drugs are contraindicated in patients with known hypersensitivity. Isoproterenol is contraindicated in patients with tachyarrhythmias, tachycardia, or heart block caused by digitalis toxicity, ventricular arrhythmias, and angina pectoris. Dopamine is contraindicated in those with pheochromocytoma (adrenal gland tumor), unmanaged arrhythmias, and ventricular fibrillation. Epinephrine is contraindicated in patients with narrow-angle glaucoma, and as a local anesthetic adjunct in fingers and toes. Norepinephrine is contraindicated in patients who are hypotensive from blood volume deficits. Midodrine causes severe hypertension in the patient who is lying down (supine); therefore, it is used for orthostatic hypotension only when the patient is considerably impaired.

Nursing Alert

Supine hypertension is a potentially dangerous adverse reaction in the patient taking midodrine. The drug should be given only to patients whose lives are impaired despite standard treatment offered. The nurse can minimize this reaction by administering midodrine during the day while the patient is in an upright position. The following is a suggested dosing schedule for the administration of midodrine: shortly before arising in the morning, midday, and late afternoon (not after 6:00 PM). Drug therapy should continue only in the patient whose orthostatic hypotension improves during the initial treatment.

Precautions

These drugs are used cautiously in patients with coronary insufficiency, cardiac arrhythmias, angina pectoris, diabetes, hyperthyroidism, occlusive vascular disease, or prostatic hypertrophy. Patients with diabetes may require an increased dosage of insulin. Adrenergic drugs are classified as pregnancy category C and are used with extreme caution during pregnancy.

Interactions

The following interactions may occur when an adrenergic drug is administered with another agent:

Interacting Drug	Common Use	Effect of Interaction
antidepressants	Treatment of depression	Increased sympathomimetic effect
oxytocin	Induction of uterine contractions	Increased risk of hypertension
bretylium	Treatment of severe cardiac problems	Increased risk of arrhythmias

There is an increased risk of seizures, hypotension, and bradycardia when dopamine is administered with phenytoin (Dilantin). Metaraminol (Aramine) is used cautiously in patients taking digoxin because of an increased risk for cardiac arrhythmias. There is an increased risk of hypertension when dobutamine is administered with the β-adrenergic blocking drugs.

NURSING PROCESS

The Patient Receiving an Adrenergic Drug

ASSESSMENT

Assessment of the patient receiving an adrenergic drug differs depending on the drug, the patient, and the reason for administration. For example, assessment of the patient in shock who is to be treated with norepinephrine is different from that for the patient receiving epinephrine with a local anesthetic while having a tooth cavity repaired. Both are receiving adrenergic drugs, but the circumstances are much different.

Herbal Alert

Ephedra (Ma Huang) and the many substances of the *Ephedra* genus have been used medicinally (e.g., *E. sinica* and *E. intermedia*). Ephedra (ephedrine) preparations have traditionally been used to relieve cold symptoms and improve respiratory function, and as an adjunct in weight loss. Large doses may cause a variety of adverse reactions, such as hypertension and irregular heart rate. The use of ephedra has shifted from relief of respiratory problems to an aid to weight loss and enhanced athletic performance. Before taking this herb, the patient should consult the primary health care provider. Ephedra should not be used with the cardiac glycosides,

Herbal Alert (continued)

halothane, guanethidine, monoamine oxidase inhibitors (MAOIs), or oxytocin, or by patients taking St. John's wort. The U.S. Food and Drug Administration (FDA) warns the public not to take ephedrine-containing dietary supplements. Stroke and heart attack have resulted from taking these products. Many producers of weight loss supplements are removing the ephedra component because of potential legal liability.

PREADMINISTRATION ASSESSMENT

When a patient is to receive an adrenergic agent for shock, the nurse obtains the blood pressure, pulse rate and quality, and respiratory rate and rhythm. The nurse assesses the patient's symptoms, problems, or needs before administering the drug and records any subjective or objective data on the patient's chart. In emergencies, the nurse must make assessments quickly and accurately. This information provides an important database that is used during treatment.

A general survey of the patient also is necessary. It is important to look for additional symptoms of shock, such as cool skin, cyanosis, diaphoresis, and a change in the level of consciousness. Other assessments may be necessary if the hypotensive episode is due to trauma, severe infection, or blood loss.

ONGOING ASSESSMENT

During the ongoing assessment, the nurse observes the patient for the effect of the drug, such as improved breathing of the patient with asthma, or response of blood pressure to the administration of the vasopressor. During therapy, the nurse evaluates and documents the drug effect. The nurse also takes and documents the vital signs. Comparison of assessments made before and after administration may help the primary health care provider determine future use of the drug for this patient. It is important to report adverse drug reactions to the primary health care provider as soon as possible.

NURSING DIAGNOSES

Drug-specific nursing diagnoses are highlighted in the Nursing Diagnoses Checklist. Other nursing diagnoses applicable to these drugs are discussed in depth in Chapter 4.

PLANNING

The expected outcomes of the patient depend on the reason for administering an adrenergic agent, but may include an optimal response to drug therapy, support of patient needs related to management of adverse drug reactions, and an understanding of the reason the drug is being given.

✓ **Ineffective Tissue Perfusion** related to hypovolemia, blood loss, impaired distribution of fluid,
impaired circulation, impaired transport of oxygen
across alveolar and capillary bed, other (specify)

✓ **Decreased Cardiac Output** related to altered
heart rate and/or rhythm

✓ **Disturbed Sleep Pattern** related to adverse
reactions (nervousness) to the drug and the
environment

IMPLEMENTATION

PROMOTING AN OPTIMAL RESPONSE TO THERAPY

Management of the patient receiving an adrenergic agent
varies and depends on the drug used, the reason for
administration, and the patient's response to the drug. In
most instances, adrenergic drugs are potent and potentially dangerous. The nurse must exercise great care in the
calculation and preparation of these drugs for administration. Although adrenergic drugs are potentially dangerous,
proper supervision and management before, during, and
after administration will minimize the occurrence of any
serious problems. The nurse reports and documents any
complaint the patient may have while taking the adrenergic drugs. However, nursing judgment is necessary when
reporting adverse reactions. The nurse must report some
adverse effects, such as the development of cardiac
arrhythmias, immediately, regardless of the time of day or
night. The nurse also should report other adverse effects,
such as anorexia, but this is usually not an emergency.

Management of shock is aimed at providing basic life support (airway, breathing, and circulation) while attempting
to correct the underlying cause. Antibiotics, inotropes,
hormones (e.g., insulin, thyroid), and other drugs may be
used to treat the underlying disease. However, the initial
pharmacologic intervention is aimed at supporting the circulation with vasopressors.

MONITORING AND MANAGING PATIENT NEEDS

INEFFECTIVE TISSUE PERFUSION If the patient is being
given the adrenergic drug for hypotension, there is already
a problem with tissue perfusion. Administration of the
adrenergic drug may correct the problem or, if the blood
pressure becomes too high, tissue perfusion may again be a
problem. By maintaining the blood pressure at the systolic
rate prescribed by the primary health care provider tissue
perfusion will be maintained.

When a patient is in shock and experiencing ineffective
tissue perfusion there is a decrease in oxygen, resulting in
an inability of the body to nourish its cells at the capillary
level. If the patient has marked hypotension, the administration of a vasopressor is required. The primary health
care provider determines the cause of the hypotension and
then selects the best method of treatment. Some hypotensive episodes require the use of a less potent vasopressor,
such as metaraminol, whereas at other times a more potent
vasopressor, such as dobutamine, dopamine, or norepinephrine (Levophed), is necessary.

The nurse considers the following points when administering the potent vasopressors dopamine and norepinephrine:

• Use an electronic infusion pump to administer these
drugs.

• Do not mix dopamine with other drugs, especially
sodium bicarbonate or other alkaline intravenous (IV)
solutions. Check with the hospital pharmacist before
adding a second drug to an IV solution containing this
drug.

• Administer norepinephrine and dopamine only by the
IV route. Do not dilute these drugs in an IV solution
before administration. The primary health care provider
orders the IV solution, the amount of drug added to the
solution, and the initial rate of infusion.

• Monitor blood pressure every 2 minutes from the
beginning of therapy until the desired blood pressure is
achieved, then monitor the blood pressure and pulse
rate at frequent intervals, usually every 5 to 15 minutes,
during the administration of these drugs.

• Adjust the rate of administration according to the
patient's blood pressure. The rate of administration of
the IV solution is increased or decreased to maintain
the patient's blood pressure at the systolic pressure
ordered by the primary health care provider.

• Readjustment of the rate of flow of the IV solution is
often necessary. The frequency of adjustment depends
on the patient's response to the vasopressor.

• Inspect the needle site and surrounding tissues at frequent intervals for leakage (extravasation, infiltration)
of the solution into the subcutaneous tissues surrounding the needle site. If leakage occurs, establish another
IV line immediately, discontinue the IV containing the
vasopressor, and notify the primary health care provider.
These drugs are particularly damaging when they leak
into surrounding tissues. The nurse should know the
extravasation protocol and have orders signed by the
primary health provider to implement the protocol.

• Never leave the patient receiving these drugs unattended.

Monitoring the patient in shock requires vigilance on the part of the nurse. The patient's heart rate, blood pressure, and electrocardiogram are monitored continuously. Urine output is measured often (usually hourly), and accurate intake and output measurements are taken. Monitoring of central venous pressure by a central venous catheter provides an estimate of the patient's fluid status. Sometimes additional hemodynamic monitoring is necessary with a pulmonary artery catheter. The use of a pulmonary artery catheter allows the nurse to monitor a number of parameters, such as cardiac output and peripheral vascular resistance. The nurse adjusts therapy according to the primary health care provider's instructions.

The less potent vasopressors, such as metaraminol, also require close patient supervision during administration. The nurse follows the same procedure as for norepinephrine and dopamine, but may take blood pressure and pulse determinations at less frequent intervals, usually every 15 to 30 minutes. The nurse needs sound clinical judgment to determine the frequency because there is no absolute minimum or maximum time limit between determinations.

DECREASED CARDIAC OUTPUT The heart rate and stroke volume determine cardiac output. The stroke volume is determined in part by the contractile state of the heart and the amount of blood in the ventricle available to be pumped out. The interventions listed to support tissue perfusion also help to support the cardiac output of the patient in shock.

When the patient is in shock, it is important for the nurse to monitor vital signs (heart rate and rhythm, respiratory rate, and blood pressure) carefully and often (every 15 to 30 minutes) to determine the severity of shock. For example, as cardiac output decreases, compensatory tachycardia develops to increase cardiac output. As shock deepens, the pulse volume becomes progressively weaker and assumes a "thready" feel. The heart rate increases and the heart rhythm may become irregular. Initially the respiratory rate is rapid as the patient experiences air hunger, but in profound shock the respiratory rate decreases. Blood pressure decreases as shock progresses.

Nursing Alert

Regardless of the actual numeric reading of the blood pressure, a progressive fall of the blood pressure is serious. The nurse reports to the primary health care provider any progressive fall of the blood pressure, a fall in systolic blood pressure below 100 mm Hg, or any fall of 20 mm Hg or more of the patient's normal blood pressure.

DISTURBED SLEEP PATTERN Often adrenergic drugs are used in the critical care setting where the typical daily pattern of activities is usually disrupted. These units can be as busy in the middle of the night as they are in the middle of the day. Patients can easily get confused regarding the time of day. This can cause a great deal of stress in the patient. It is helpful to identify circumstances that disturb sleep, such as the nurse taking vital signs during the night or turning the overhead light on during the night. The nurse plans care with as few interruptions as possible or makes modifications. For example, to filter light, curtains can be drawn over windows and between patients in the critical care units. The nurse has to weigh the importance of monitoring patient status and vital signs or providing comfort interventions when administering the adrenergic drugs. A thorough explanation of the reason for close monitoring of the vital signs by the nurse is necessary. In addition, caffeinated beverages are avoided, especially after 5:00 PM. Other sleep aids may be used (e.g., warm milk, back rub, progressive relaxation, or bedtime snack).

EDUCATING THE PATIENT AND FAMILY

Only medical personnel give some adrenergic drugs, such as the vasopressors. The nurse's responsibility for teaching involves explaining the drug to the patient or family. Depending on the situation, the nurse may include facts such as how the drug will be given (e.g., the route of administration) and what results are expected. The nurse must use judgment regarding some of the information given to the patient or family regarding administration of an adrenergic drug in life-threatening situations because certain facts, such as the seriousness of the patient's condition, are usually best explained by the primary health care provider.

EDUCATING THE PATIENT RECEIVING MIDODRINE When midodrine is given to patients with severe orthostatic hypotension, the nurse explains the importance of taking the drug during daytime hours when the patient is upright. The patient can take doses in 3-hour intervals if needed to control symptoms. The drug should not be taken within 4 hours of bedtime. In addition, to control supine hypertension, a potentially fatal adverse reaction, the patient should not become fully supine. The nurse explains that it may be necessary to sleep with the head of the bed elevated. If urinary retention is a problem, the patient is instructed to urinate before taking the drug. The nurse stresses the importance of returning for regular medical evaluation. The patient is instructed to report any changes in vision, pounding in the head when lying down, slow heart rate, or difficulty urinating.

EVALUATION

- The therapeutic effect is achieved.

- Adverse reactions are identified, reported to the primary health care provider, and managed successfully.

- The patient verbalizes an understanding of treatment modalities and the importance of continued follow-up care.

Critical Thinking Exercises

1. Mr. Cole is receiving dopamine for the treatment of severe hypotension. In planning the care for Mr. Cole, determine what would be the most important aspects of nursing management. Explain your answers.

2. Plan a teaching program to explain the autonomic nervous system to a group of nurses at a staff education meeting.

3. Discuss the preadministration assessment for a patient requiring an adrenergic drug for hypotension.

4. Describe the different types of shock and causes of each.

Review Questions

1. The physician prescribes norepinephrine, a potent vasopressor, to be administered to a patient in shock. The rate of the administration of the IV fluid containing the norepinephrine is _____.

   A. maintained at a set rate of infusion

   B. adjusted per protocol to maintain the patient's blood pressure

   C. given at a rate not to exceed 5 mg/min

   D. discontinued when the blood pressure is 100 mm Hg systolic

2. At what intervals would the nurse monitor the blood pressure of a patient administered norepinephrine?

   A. Every 5 to 15 minutes

   B. Every 30 minutes

   C. Every hour

   D. Every 4 hours

3. Which of the following are the common adverse reactions the nurse would expect with the administration of the adrenergic drugs?

   A. Bradycardia, lethargy, bronchial constriction

   B. Increase in appetite, nervousness, drowsiness

   C. Anorexia, vomiting, hypotension

   D. Headache, nervousness, nausea

4. When dobutamine is administered with the β-adrenergic blocking drugs, the nurse is aware of an increased risk for _____.

   A. seizures

   B. arrhythmias

   C. hypotension

   D. hypertension

Medication Dosage Problems

1. An adult with a honey bee allergy was stung and calls the nurse at the clinic. The patient has two EpiPens at home. The solution is 1 mg/mL and each EpiPen contains 0.3 mL. What drug dose has the patient taken if two injections were already given? _____

2. The physician orders 0.5 mg of 1:1000 epinephrine solution IV. The drug is available in 1:1000 solution 1 mg/mL. The nurse administers _____.

To check your answers, see Appendix G.

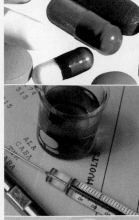
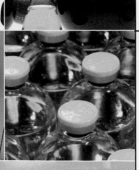

Chapter 28

Adrenergic Blocking Drugs

Key Terms

- alpha-adrenergic blocking drugs
- alpha/beta-adrenergic blocking drugs
- antiadrenergic drugs
- beta-adrenergic blocking drugs
- cardiac arrhythmia
- first-dose effect
- glaucoma
- orthostatic hypotension
- pheochromocytoma
- postural hypotension
- sympatholytic

Learning Objectives

On completion of this chapter, the student will:

- List the four types of adrenergic blocking drugs.
- Discuss the uses, general drug actions, general adverse reactions, contraindications, precautions, and interactions of the adrenergic blocking drugs.
- Discuss important preadministration and ongoing assessment activities the nurse should perform on the patient taking adrenergic blocking drugs.

- List nursing diagnoses particular to a patient taking adrenergic blocking drugs.
- Discuss ways to promote an optimal response to therapy, how to manage common adverse reactions, nursing actions that may be taken to minimize orthostatic or postural hypotension, and important points to keep in mind when educating patients about the use of adrenergic blocking drugs.

N orepinephrine is a substance that transmits nerve impulses across the sympathetic branch of the autonomic nervous system (see figure in the unit introduction). Activation of these nerves is sometimes called our *fight-or-flight response.* Drugs that facilitate transmission are called *adrenergic* drugs. Drugs that reverse the response are called *adrenergic blocking* drugs. Also called **sympatholytic** drugs, these agents block the transmission of norepinephrine in the sympathetic system. Drugs blocking neurotransmission in the sympathetic nervous system work *directly* by blocking the receptor, or *indirectly* by preventing release of norepinephrine. They may be divided into four groups:

- **Alpha (α)-adrenergic blocking drugs**—drugs that block α-adrenergic receptors. These drugs produce their greatest effect on the α receptors of the adrenergic nerves that control the vascular system.

- **Beta (β)-adrenergic blocking drugs**—drugs that block β-adrenergic receptors. These drugs produce their greatest effect on the β receptors of adrenergic nerves, primarily the β receptors of the heart.

- **Alpha/beta (α/β)-adrenergic blocking drugs**—drugs that block both α- and β-adrenergic receptors. These drugs act on both α and β nerve fibers.

- **Antiadrenergic drugs**—drugs that prevent the release of the neurotransmitter. These drugs can block the adrenergic nerve impulse in both the central and peripheral nervous systems.

Each of these groups is discussed individually, followed by an example of the Nursing Process for the group as a whole. See the Summary Drug Table: Adrenergic Blocking Drugs for a more complete listing of these drugs.

SUMMARY DRUG TABLE ADRENERGIC BLOCKING DRUGS

GENERIC NAME	TRADE NAME	USES	ADVERSE REACTIONS	DOSAGE RANGES
Alpha-Adrenergic Blocking Drugs				
phentolamine *fen-tole'-a-meen*	Regitine	Diagnosis of pheochromocytoma, hypertensive episodes before and during surgery, prevention/ treatment of dermal necrosis after IV administration of norepinephrine or dopamine	Weakness, dizziness, flushing, nausea, vomiting, orthostatic hypotension	5 mg IV, IM Tissue necrosis: 5-10 mg in 10 mL saline solution infiltrated into affected area
Beta-Adrenergic Blocking Drugs				
acebutolol HCl *a-se-byoo'-toe-lol*	Sectral	Hypertension, ventricular arrhythmias	Bradycardia, dizziness, weakness, hypotension, nausea, vomiting, diarrhea,nervousness	Hypertension: 400 mg orally in 1-2 doses Arrhythmias: 400-1200 mg/d orally in divided doses
atenolol *a-ten'-oh-lol*	Tenormin, Tenoretic	Hypertension, angina, acute MI	Bradycardia, dizziness, fatigue, weakness, hypotension, nausea, vomiting, diarrhea, nervousness	50-200 mg/d orally Acute MI: 5 mg IV over 5 min, may be repeated
betaxolol HCl *beh-tax'-oh-lol*	Kerlone	Hypertension	Bradycardia, dizziness, hypotension, bronchospasm, nausea, vomiting, diarrhea, nervousness	10-20 mg/d orally
bisoprolol *bye-sew'-proe-lol*	Zebeta	Hypertension	Same as acebutolol	2.5-10 mg orally daily; maximum dose, 20 mg orally daily
carteolol *kar'-tee-oh-lol*		Hypertension	Same as acebutolol	2.5-10 mg/d orally
esmolol HCl *ess'-moe-lol*	Brevibloc	Supraventricular tachycardia, noncompensatory tachycardia	Hypotension, weakness, lightheadedness, urinary retention	50-250 mcg/kg/min IV
metoprolol *me-toe'-proe-lol*	Lopressor, Toprol-XL	Hypertension, angina, MI, CHF	Dizziness, hypotension, CHF, cardiac arrhythmia, nausea, vomiting, diarrhea	100-450 mg/d orally; 5 mg IV Extended release; 50-100 mg/d orally
nadolol *nay-doe'-lol*	Corgard	Angina, hypertension	Dizziness, hypotension nausea, vomiting, diarrhea, CHF, cardiac arrhythmia	40-240 mg/d orally
penbutolol *pen-byoo'-toe-lol*	Levatol	Hypertension	Bradycardia, dizziness, hypotension, nausea, vomiting, diarrhea	20 mg orally daily
pindolol *pen'-doe-loe*	Visken	Hypertension	Bradycardia, dizziness, hypotension, nausea, vomiting, diarrhea	10-60 mg/d orally BID

Adrenergic Blocking Drugs

SUMMARY DRUG TABLE *(continued)*

GENERIC NAME	TRADE NAME	USES	ADVERSE REACTIONS	DOSAGE RANGES
propranolol *pro-pran'-oh-lol*	Inderal	Cardiac arrhythmias, MI, angina, hypertension, migraine prophylaxis, pheochromocytoma, essential tremor	Bradycardia, dizziness, hypotension, nausea, vomiting, diarrhea, bronchospasm, hyperglycemia, pulmonary edema	Arrhythmias: 10–30 mg orally TID, QID Hypertension: 120–240 mg/d orally in divided doses Angina: 80–320 mg/d orally in divided doses Migraine: 160–240 mg/d orally in divided doses
Ⓡ **sotalol HCl** *soh'-ta-lole*	Betapace, Betapace AF	Ventricular arrhythmias (maintain normal sinus rhythm— Betapace AF only)	Dizziness, hypotension, nausea, vomiting, diarrhea, respiratory distress	160–320 mg/d orally in divided doses
timolol maleate *tih'-mo-lol*	Blocadren	Hypertension, MI, migraine prophylaxis	Dizziness, hypotension, nausea, vomiting, diarrhea, pulmonary edema	Hypertension: 10–40 mg/d orally in divided doses MI: 10 mg orally BID Migraine: 20 mg/d orally
Topical Preparations				
betaxolol HCl (ophthalmic) *beh-tax'-oh-lol*	Betoptic	Glaucoma	Brief ocular discomfort, tearing	1 gtt BID
timolol maleate (ophthalmic)	Timoptic	Glaucoma	Ocular irritation, tearing	1 gtt BID
Alpha/Beta-Adrenergic Blocking Drugs				
carvedilol *car-veh'-dih-lol*	Coreg	Hypertension, CHF, left ventricular dysfunction	Bradycardia, hypotension, cardiac insufficiency, fatigue, dizziness, diarrhea	6.25–25 mg orally BID
labetalol *lah-bet'-ah-lol*	Trandate	Hypertension	Fatigue, drowsiness, insomnia, hypotension, impotence, diarrhea	200–400 mg/d orally in divided doses IV: 20 mg over 2 min with blood pressure monitoring, may repeat
Antiadrenergic Drugs: Centrally Acting				
clonidine HCl *kloe'-ni'-deen*	Catapres, Catapres-TTS (transdermal)	Severe pain in patients with cancer, hypertension	Drowsiness, dizziness, sedation, dry mouth, constipation, syncope, dreams, rash	100–600 mcg/d orally Transdermal: release rate 0.1–0.3 mg/24 h
guanabenz acetate *gwan'-ah-benz*		Hypertension	Dry mouth, sedation, dizziness, headache, weakness, arrhythmias	4–32 mg orally BID
guanfacine HCl *gwan'-fa-sine*	Tenex	Hypertension	Dry mouth, somnolence, asthenia, dizziness, headache, constipation, fatigue	1–3 mg/d orally at bedtime
methyldopa or methyldopate HCl *meth'-ill-done-pa, meth'-ill-doe-pate*		Hypertension, hypertensive crisis	Bradycardia, aggravation of angina pectoris, heart failure, sedation, headache, rash, nausea, vomiting, nasal congestion	250 mg orally BID or TID; maintenance dose, 2 g/d; 250–500 mg q6h IV

GENERIC NAME	TRADE NAME	USES	ADVERSE REACTIONS	DOSAGE RANGES
Antiadrenergic Drugs: Peripherally Acting				
alfuzosin *al-foo-zow'-sin*	Uroxatral	Hypertension, BPH	Headache, dizziness	10 mg orally daily
doxazosin mesylate	Cardura	BPH	Headache, dizziness, fatigue	1-16 mg orally daily
mecamylamine *mek-a-mill'-a-meen*	Inversine	Hypertension	Dizziness, syncope, dry mouth, nausea, constipation, urinary retention	2.5 mg orally BID
prazosin *pray-zoe'-sin*	Minipress	Hypertension	Dizziness, postural hypotension, drowsiness, headache, loss of strength, palpitation, nausea	1-20 mg orally daily in divided doses
reserpine *reh-sir'-pine*	Serpalan	Hypertension, psychosis	Bradycardia, dizziness, nausea, vomiting, diarrhea, nasal congestion	0.1-0.5 mg orally daily
tamsulosin *tam-soo-low' sin*	Flomax	BPH	Headache, ejaculatory dysfunction, dizziness, rhinitis	0.4 mg orally daily
terazosin *tare-ah'-zoe-sin*	Hytrin	Hypertension, BPH	Dizziness, postural hypotension, headache, dyspnea, nasal congestion	1-20 mg orally daily

BPH, benign prostatic hyperplasia; CHF, congestive heart failure; MI, myocardial infarction.
Ⓡ This drug should be administered at least 1 hour before or 2 hours after a meal.

ALPHA-ADRENERGIC BLOCKING DRUGS

Actions

Stimulation of α-adrenergic nerves results in vasoconstriction (see Table 27-1 in Chapter 27). If stimulation of α-adrenergic nerves is interrupted or blocked, the result is vasodilation. This is the direct opposite of the effect of an adrenergic drug with α activity. The primary drugs used in this category cause vasodilation by relaxing the smooth muscle of blood vessels. These drugs are discussed in Chapter 40. Phentolamine (Regitine) is an example of an α-adrenergic blocking drug.

Uses

α-Adrenergic blocking drugs are used in the treatment of
- Hypertension caused by **pheochromocytoma** (a tumor of the adrenal gland that produces excessive amounts of epinephrine and norepinephrine)
- Hypertension during preoperative preparation

They are also used to prevent or treat tissue damage caused by extravasation of dopamine.

Adverse Reactions

Administration of an α-adrenergic blocking drug may result in weakness, orthostatic hypotension, cardiac arrhythmias, hypotension, and tachycardia. See the Summary Drug Table: Adrenergic Blocking Drugs for more information

Contraindications, Precautions, and Interactions

α-Adrenergic blocking drugs are contraindicated in patients who are hypersensitive to the drugs and in patients with coronary artery disease. These drugs are used cautiously during pregnancy (category C) and lactation, after a recent myocardial infarction (MI), and in patients with renal failure or Raynaud's disease. When phentolamine (Regitine) is administered with epinephrine, there is decreased vasoconstrictor and hypertensive action.

Adrenergic Blocking Drugs

BETA-ADRENERGIC BLOCKING DRUGS

Actions

β-Adrenergic blocking drugs are also called *β blockers*. These drugs decrease the stimulation of the sympathetic nervous system on certain tissues. β-Adrenergic receptors are found mainly in the heart. Stimulation of β receptors of the heart results in an increase in the heart rate. Blocking the nerve impulse of β-adrenergic nerves decreases the heart rate and dilates the blood vessels (Fig. 28-1). These drugs decrease the heart's excitability, decrease cardiac workload and oxygen consumption, and provide membrane-stabilizing effects that contribute to the antiarrhythmic activity of the β-adrenergic blocking drugs. Examples of β-adrenergic blocking drugs used for cardiac purposes are esmolol (Brevibloc) and propranolol (Inderal).

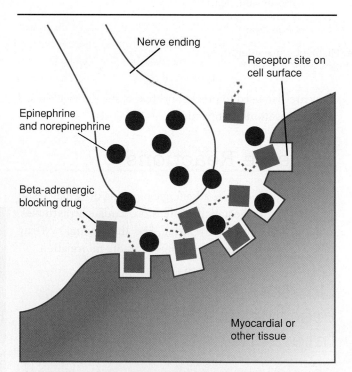

Figure 28.1 Beta-adrenergic blocking drugs prevent epinephrine and norepinephrine from occupying receptor sites on cell membranes. This action alters cell functions normally stimulated by epinephrine and norepinephrine, according to the number of receptor sites occupied by the beta-blocking drugs. (Adapted by J. Harley from *Encyclopedia Britannica Medical and Health Annual*. Chicago: Encyclopedia Britannica, 1983.)

β-Adrenergic blocking drugs such as betaxolol (Betoptic) and timolol (Timoptic) are used to treat glaucoma. **Glaucoma** is a narrowing or blockage of the drainage channels (canals of Schlemm) between the anterior and posterior chambers of the eye. This results in a buildup of pressure (increased intraocular pressure) in the eye. Blindness may occur if glaucoma is left untreated. When the above drugs are used topically as ophthalmic drops, they appear to reduce the production of aqueous humor in the anterior chamber of the eye, lessening the effects of glaucoma.

Uses

β-Adrenergic blocking drugs are used in the treatment of
- Hypertension
- **Cardiac arrhythmia** (abnormal rhythm of the heart), such as ventricular or supraventricular tachycardia
- Migraine headaches
- Angina pectoris
- Glaucoma (topical ophthalmic eye drops)

β-Adrenergic blockers are also used to prevent reinfarction in patients with a recent MI (1 to 4 weeks after the MI).

Adverse Reactions

- Cardiac reactions that affect the body in a generalized manner include orthostatic hypotension, bradycardia, dizziness, vertigo, and headache.
- Gastrointestinal (GI) reactions include hyperglycemia, nausea, vomiting, and diarrhea.
- Another body system reaction is bronchospasm (especially in those with a history of asthma).

Many of these reactions are mild and may disappear with therapy. More serious adverse reactions include symptoms of congestive heart failure (i.e., dyspnea, weight gain, peripheral edema).

Gerontologic Alert

Older adults are at increased risk for adverse reactions when taking the β-adrenergic blocking drugs. The nurse should monitor the older adult closely for confusion, heart failure, worsening of angina, shortness of breath, and peripheral vascular insufficiency (e.g., cold extremities, paresthesia of the hands, weak peripheral pulses).

Contraindications, Precautions, and Interactions

These drugs are contraindicated in patients with an allergy to the β blockers, in patients with sinus bradycardia, second- or third-degree heart block, or heart failure, and in those with asthma, emphysema, or hypotension. The drugs are used cautiously in patients with diabetes, thyrotoxicosis, or peptic ulcer.

The following interactions may occur when a β-adrenergic blocker is administered with another agent:

Interacting Drug	Common Use	Effect of Interaction
antidepressants (monoamine oxidase inhibitors [MAOIs], selective serotonin reuptake inhibitors [SSRIs])	Management of depression	Increased effect of the β blocker, bradycardia
nonsteroidal anti-inflammatory drugs (NSAIDs), salicylates	Pain relief	Decreased effect of the β blocker
loop diuretics	Management of cardiovascular problems	Increased risk of hypotension
clonidine	Management of cardiovascular problems	Increased risk of paradoxical hypertensive effect
cimetidine	Management of GI problems	Increased serum level of the β blocker and higher risk of β blocker toxicity
lidocaine	Management of cardiac problems	Increased serum level of the β blocker and higher risk of β blocker toxicity

ALPHA/BETA-ADRENERGIC BLOCKING DRUGS

Actions

α/β-Adrenergic blocking drugs block the stimulation of both the α- and β-adrenergic receptors, resulting in peripheral vasodilation. The two drugs in this category are carvedilol (Coreg) and labetalol (Trandate).

Uses

Carvedilol is used to treat essential hypertension and in congestive heart failure to reduce progression of the disease. Labetalol is used in the treatment of hypertension, either alone or in combination with another drug such as a diuretic.

Adverse Reactions

Most adverse effects of α/β-adrenergic blocking drugs are mild and do not require discontinuation of therapy. General body system adverse reactions include fatigue, dizziness, hypotension, drowsiness, insomnia, weakness, diarrhea, dyspnea, chest pain, bradycardia, and skin rash.

Contraindications, Precautions, and Interactions

α/β Blockers are contraindicated in patients with hypersensitivity to the drugs, bronchial asthma, decompensated heart failure, and severe bradycardia. The drugs are used cautiously in patients with drug-controlled congestive heart failure, chronic bronchitis, or impaired hepatic or cardiac function, in those with diabetes, and during pregnancy (category C) and lactation.

The following interactions may occur when an α/β-adrenergic blocker is administered with another agent:

Interacting Drug	Common Use	Effect of Interaction
antidepressants (tricyclics and SSRIs)	Management of depression	Increased risk of tremors
cimetidine	Management of GI problems	Increased effect of the adrenergic blocker
halothane	Anesthetic for surgery	Increased effect of the adrenergic blocker
clonidine	Management of cardiovascular problems	Increased effect of the clonidine
digoxin	Management of cardiac problems	Increased serum level of the digoxin and higher risk of digoxin toxicity

Adrenergic Blocking Drugs

ANTIADRENERGIC DRUGS

Actions

One group of antiadrenergic drugs inhibits the release of norepinephrine from certain adrenergic nerve endings in the peripheral nervous system. This group is composed of peripherally acting (i.e., acting on peripheral structures) antiadrenergic drugs. An example of a peripherally acting antiadrenergic drug is prazosin (Minipress). The other antiadrenergic drugs are called *centrally acting* antiadrenergic drugs because they act on the central nervous system (CNS) rather than on the peripheral nervous system. This group affects specific CNS centers, thereby decreasing some of the activity of the sympathetic nervous system. Although the action of both types of antiadrenergic drugs is somewhat different, the results are basically the same. An example of a centrally acting antiadrenergic drug is clonidine (Catapres).

Uses

Antiadrenergic drugs are used mainly for the treatment of certain cardiac arrhythmias and hypertension (see the Summary Drug Table: Adrenergic Blocking Drugs).

Adverse Reactions

- Dry mouth, drowsiness, sedation, anorexia, rash, malaise, and weakness are generalized reactions to antiadrenergic drugs that work on the CNS.

- Hypotension, weakness, lightheadedness, and bradycardia are adverse reactions associated with the administration of the peripherally acting antiadrenergic drugs.

Contraindications, Precautions, and Interactions

The centrally acting antiadrenergic drugs are contraindicated in active hepatic disease, antidepressant therapy using MAOIs, and in patients with a history of hypersensitivity to these drugs. The centrally acting antiadrenergic drugs are used cautiously in patients with a history of liver disease or renal impairment, and during pregnancy and lactation.

The peripherally acting antiadrenergic drugs are contraindicated in patients with a hypersensitivity to any of the drugs. Reserpine (Serpasil) is contraindicated in patients who have an active peptic ulcer or ulcerative colitis and in patients who are mentally depressed. Reserpine is used cautiously in patients with a history of depression, in those with renal impairment or cardiovascular disease, and during pregnancy and lactation.

The following interactions may occur when an antiadrenergic drug is administered with another agent:

Interacting Drug	Common Use	Effect of Interaction
adrenergic drugs	Management of cardiovascular problems	Increased risk of hypertension
levodopa	Management of Parkinson's disease	Decreased effect of the levodopa, hypotension
anesthetic agents	Surgical anesthesia	Increased effect of the anesthetic
β blockers	Management of cardiovascular problems	Increased risk of hypertension
lithium	Treatment of psychosis	Increased risk of lithium toxicity
haloperidol	Treatment of psychosis	Increased risk of psychotic behavior

NURSING PROCESS

The Patient Receiving an Adrenergic Blocking Drug

ASSESSMENT

Assessment depends on the drug, the patient, and the reason for administration.

PREADMINISTRATION ASSESSMENT

The nurse establishes an accurate database before any adrenergic blocking drug is administered for the first time. If, for example, the patient has a peripheral vascular disease, the nurse notes the subjective and objective symptoms of the disorder during the initial assessment. If the drug is given for anginal pain, the nurse records the onset, type (e.g., sharp, dull, squeezing), radiation, location, intensity, and duration of anginal pain. The nurse also questions the patient regarding any precipitating factors of the anginal pain, such as exertion or emotional stress.

Once drug therapy is started, evaluation of the effects of therapy can be made by comparing the patient's current symptoms with the symptoms experienced before therapy was initiated.

Patients with hypertension must have their blood pressure and pulse taken on both arms in sitting, standing, and supine positions before therapy is begun. If the patient has a cardiac arrhythmia, the initial assessment includes taking the pulse rate, determining the pulse rhythm, and noting the patient's general appearance.

Subjective data (i.e., the patient's complaints or description of symptoms) also are obtained at this time, and the primary health care provider usually orders an electrocardiogram. Additional diagnostic studies and laboratory tests also may be ordered.

If the drug is given to treat congestive heart failure (e.g., carvedilol), the patient is assessed for evidence of the disease, such as dyspnea (especially on exertion), peripheral edema, distended neck veins, and cough.

ONGOING ASSESSMENT

It is important for the nurse to perform ongoing assessment of the patient receiving adrenergic blocking drug therapy. This assessment often depends on the reason the drug is administered. For all adrenergic blocking drugs, it is important for the nurse to observe these patients continually for the appearance of adverse reactions. Some adverse reactions are mild, whereas others, such as diarrhea, may cause a problem, especially if the patient is elderly or debilitated.

Ongoing assessment of patients receiving adrenergic blocking drugs for cardiac arrhythmias depends on the type of arrhythmia and the method of treatment. Some cardiac arrhythmias, such as ventricular fibrillation, are life-threatening and require immediate attention. Other arrhythmias are serious and require treatment but are not life-threatening. If propranolol is given for angina, the nurse should ask the patient about the relief of symptoms and should record responses on the patient's chart.

NURSING DIAGNOSES

Drug-specific nursing diagnoses are highlighted in the Nursing Diagnoses Checklist. Other nursing diagnoses applicable to these drugs are discussed in depth in Chapter 4.

PLANNING

The expected outcomes for the patient depend on the reason for administration of an adrenergic blocking drug, but

> ### Nursing Diagnosis Checklist
>
> ✔ **Impaired Comfort** related to adverse effects of medication
>
> ✔ **Ineffective Tissue Perfusion: Peripheral** related to adverse drug response (hypotension)
>
> ✔ **Risk for Injury** related to vertigo, dizziness, weakness, and syncope secondary to hypotension

may include an optimal response to drug therapy, meeting of patient needs related to the management of adverse reactions, and an understanding of and compliance with the prescribed drug regimen.

IMPLEMENTATION

PROMOTING AN OPTIMAL RESPONSE TO THERAPY

Most adrenergic blocking drugs may be given without regard to food. However, the nurse should administer drugs preventing release of neurotransmitters (antiadrenergics) at the same time each day because the fluctuation in blood level can affect blood pressure. Sotalol (Betapace) is given on an empty stomach because food may reduce absorption of the drug.

When adrenergic blocking drugs are given to patients to control hypertension, angina, or cardiac arrhythmias, it is important to communicate with the primary health care provider about the patient's response to therapy. When given for a cardiac arrhythmia, these drugs can provoke new or worsen existing ventricular arrhythmias. If angina worsens or does not appear to be controlled by the drug, the nurse should contact the primary health care provider immediately. When the drug is administered for hypertension, the nurse monitors the patient for a decrease in blood pressure. If there is a significant rise in blood pressure, the nurse administers the dose and notifies the primary health care provider immediately because additional drug therapy may be necessary.

When a β-adrenergic blocking ophthalmic preparation, such as timolol, is administered to patients with glaucoma, it is important to insist that they have periodic follow-up examinations by an ophthalmologist. At these examinations, the intraocular pressure should be measured to determine the effectiveness of drug therapy.

MONITORING AND MANAGING PATIENT NEEDS

IMPAIRED COMFORT Some patients may experience one or more adverse drug reactions during treatment with adrenergic blocking drugs. As with any drug, the nurse must report adverse reactions to the primary health care provider and record the reactions on the patient's chart. Nursing judgment in this matter is necessary because some adverse reactions are serious or potentially serious. In these cases, the nurse should withhold the next dose of the drug and contact the primary health care provider immediately. The nurse also reports to the primary health care provider any adverse reactions that pose no serious threat. Adverse reactions that pose no serious threat to the patient's well-being, such as dry mouth or mild constipation, may have to be tolerated by the patient. It is important to assure the patient that, in some instances, these less serious reactions disappear or lessen in intensity over time.

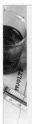

Nursing Alert

When administering a sympatholytic drug, such as propranolol (Inderal), the nurse should take an apical pulse rate and blood pressure before giving the drug. If pulse is below 60 beats/min, if there is any irregularity in the patient's heart rate or rhythm, or if systolic blood pressure is less than 90 mm Hg, the nurse should withhold the drug and contact the primary health care provider.

However, even minor adverse drug reactions can be distressing to the patient, especially when they persist for a long time. Therefore, when possible, the nurse should relieve minor adverse reactions with simple nursing measures. For example, the nurse can assist the patient with dry mouth by giving frequent sips of water or by allowing the patient to suck on a piece of hard candy (provided that the patient does not have diabetes or is not on a special diet that limits sugar intake) to relieve a dry mouth. The nurse can help relieve a patient's constipation by encouraging increased fluid intake, unless extra fluids are contraindicated. The primary health care provider also may order a laxative or stool softener. It is important for the nurse to maintain a daily record of bowel elimination. The nurse can help the patient minimize certain GI side effects, such as anorexia, diarrhea, and constipation, by administering drugs at a specific time in relation to meals, with food, or with antacids.

INEFFECTIVE TISSUE PERFUSION: PERIPHERAL During therapy with an adrenergic blocking drug for hypertension, the nurse should take the patient's blood pressure before each dose is given. Some patients have an unusual response to the drugs. In addition, some drugs may, in some individuals, decrease the blood pressure at a more rapid rate than other drugs. It is important to

monitor the patient's blood pressure on both arms and in the sitting, standing, and supine positions for the first week or more of therapy. Once the patient's blood pressure has stabilized, the nurse should take the blood pressure before each drug administration using the same arm and position for each reading. It is a good idea to make a notation on the medication administration record or care plan about the position and arm used for blood pressure determinations. Measuring the blood pressure near the end of the dosing interval or near the end of the day after the last dose of the day helps to determine if the blood pressure is controlled throughout the day.

The patient with a life-threatening arrhythmia may receive an adrenergic blocking drug, such as propranolol, by the intravenous (IV) route. When these drugs are administered IV, cardiac monitoring is necessary. Patients not in a specialized unit, such as a coronary care unit, are usually transferred to one as soon as possible. When administering these drugs for a life-threatening arrhythmia, it is important for the nurse to supervise the patient continually, monitor the blood pressure and respiratory rate frequently, and perform cardiac monitoring.

When propranolol is administered orally for a less serious cardiac arrhythmia, cardiac monitoring is usually not necessary. The nurse should monitor the patient's blood pressure and pulse rate and rhythm at varying intervals, depending on the length of treatment and the patient's response to the drug.

RISK FOR INJURY Administration of the adrenergic blocking drugs may cause hypotension. If the drug is administered for hypertension, then a decrease in blood pressure is expected.

Nursing Alert

If a significant decrease in blood pressure (a drop of 20 mm Hg systolic or a systolic pressure below 90 mm Hg) occurs after a dose of an adrenergic blocking drug, the nurse should withhold the drug and notify the primary health care provider immediately. A dosage reduction or discontinuation of the drug may be necessary. Some adrenergic blocking drugs (e.g., prazosin or terazosin) may cause a first-dose effect. A **first-dose effect** occurs when the patient experiences marked hypotension (or postural hypotension) and syncope with sudden loss of consciousness with the first few doses of the drug.

Display 28.1 Minimizing the Effects of Adrenergic Blocking Drugs

Assisting patients to minimize the uncomfortable effects of adrenergic blocking drugs can be challenging. The following measures may be useful:

- Instruct patients to rise slowly from a sitting or lying position.
- Provide assistance for the patient getting out of bed or a chair if symptoms of postural hypotension are severe. Place the call light nearby and instruct patients to ask for assistance each time they get in and out of bed or a chair.
- Assist the patient in bed to a sitting position and have the patient sit on the edge of the bed for about 1 minute before ambulating.
- Help seated patients to a standing position and instruct them to stand in one place for about 1 minute before ambulating.
- Remain with the patient while he or she is standing in one place, as well as during ambulation.
- Instruct the patient to avoid standing in one place for prolonged periods. This is rarely a problem in the hospital but should be included in the patient and family discharge teaching plan.
- Teach the patient to avoid taking hot showers or baths, which tend to increase vasodilation.

The first-dose effect may be minimized by decreasing the initial dose and administering the dose at bedtime. The dosage can then be slowly increased every 2 weeks until a full therapeutic effect is achieved. If the patient experiences syncope, the nurse places the patient in a recumbent position and treats supportively. This effect is self-limiting and in most cases does not recur after the initial period of therapy. Lightheadedness and dizziness are more common than loss of consciousness. The following paragraphs discuss these effects and provide interventions for management.

On occasion, patients receiving an adrenergic blocking drug may experience postural or orthostatic hypotension. **Postural hypotension** is characterized by a feeling of lightheadedness and dizziness when the patient suddenly changes from a lying to a sitting or standing position, or from a sitting to a standing position. **Orthostatic hypotension** is characterized by similar symptoms and occurs when the patient changes or shifts position after standing in one place for a long period. See Display 28-1 for tips on how to minimize these adverse reactions.

Symptoms of postural or orthostatic hypotension often lessen with time, and the patient may be allowed to get out of bed or a chair slowly without assistance. The nurse must exercise good judgment in this matter. Allowing the patient to rise from a lying or sitting position without help is done only when the determination has been made that the symptoms have lessened and ambulation poses no danger of falling.

EDUCATING THE PATIENT AND FAMILY

Some patients do not adhere to the prescribed drug regimen for a variety of reasons, such as failure to comprehend the prescribed regimen, the cost of drug therapy, and failure to understand the importance of continued and uninterrupted therapy. If the nurse detects failure to adhere to the prescribed drug regimen, he or she should investigate the possible cause of the problem. In some instances, financial assistance may be necessary; in other instances, patients need to know why they are taking a drug and why therapy must be continuous to attain and maintain an optimal state of health and well-being.

The nurse should describe the drug regimen and stress the importance of continued and uninterrupted therapy when teaching the patient who is prescribed an adrenergic blocking drug. Patient education will differ according to the reason the adrenergic blocking drug is prescribed.

EDUCATING THE PATIENT WITH HYPERTENSION, CARDIAC ARRHYTHMIA, OR ANGINA If a β-adrenergic blocking drug has been prescribed for hypertension, cardiac arrhythmia, angina, or other cardiac disorders, the patient must have a full understanding of the treatment regimen. In some instances, the primary health care provider may advise the hypertensive patient to lose weight or eat a special diet, such as a low-salt diet. A special diet also may be recommended for the patient with angina or a cardiac arrhythmia. When appropriate, the nurse should stress the importance of diet and weight loss in the therapy of hypertension.

It is important to include the following additional points in the teaching plan for the patient with hypertension, angina, or a cardiac arrhythmia:

- Do not stop taking the drug abruptly, except on the advice of the primary health care provider. Most of these drugs require that the dosage be gradually decreased to prevent precipitation or worsening of adverse effects.
- Notify the primary health care provider promptly if adverse drug reactions occur.
- Observe caution while driving or performing other hazardous tasks because these drugs (β-adrenergic blockers) may cause drowsiness, dizziness, or lightheadedness.

Patient and Family Teaching Checklist

Monitoring Blood Pressure

The nurse:

✔ Teaches the patient and a family member how to take an accurate blood pressure reading. This involves choosing the correct instrument and teaching the patient the steps in taking a blood pressure reading.

✔ Supervises the patient and a family member during several trial blood pressure readings to ensure accuracy of the measurements.

✔ Suggests to the patient that the same arm and body position be used each time the blood pressure is taken.

✔ Explains that the blood pressure can vary slightly with emotion, the time of day, and the position of the body.

✔ Explains that a slight change in readings is normal, but if a drastic change in either or both the systolic or diastolic readings occurs, the patient should contact the primary health care provider as soon as possible.

• Immediately report any signs of congestive heart failure (weight gain, difficulty breathing, or edema of the extremities).

• Do not use any nonprescription drug (e.g., cold or flu preparations or nasal decongestants) unless use of a specific drug has been approved by the primary health care provider.

• Inform dentists and other primary health care providers of therapy with this drug.

• Keep all primary health care provider appointments because close monitoring of therapy is essential.

• Check with a primary health care provider or pharmacist to determine if the drug is to be taken with food or on an empty stomach.

In addition, when an adrenergic blocking drug is prescribed for hypertension, the primary health care provider may want the patient to monitor his or her own blood pressure between office visits. This may enable the number of visits to the primary health care provider's office to be reduced and will help the patient learn to manage his or her own health (see Patient and Family Teaching Checklist: Monitoring Blood Pressure).

EDUCATING THE PATIENT WITH GLAUCOMA When an adrenergic blocking drug has been prescribed for glaucoma, the nurse demonstrates the technique of eye drop instillation and explains the prescribed treatment regimen to the patient. Adherence to the instillation schedule is stressed because omitting or discontinuing the drug without approval of the primary care provider may result in a marked increase in intraocular pressure, which can lead to blindness. The nurse should tell patients with glaucoma who are using adrenergic blocking eye drops to contact their primary health care provider if eye pain, excessive tearing, or any change in vision occurs.

EVALUATION

• The therapeutic effect is achieved and hypertension, cardiac arrhythmia, or glaucoma is controlled.

• Adverse reactions are identified, reported to the primary health care provider, and managed successfully through appropriate nursing interventions.

• No evidence of injury related to orthostatic or postural hypotension is seen.

• The patient and family demonstrate an understanding of the drug regimen.

Critical Thinking Exercises

1. Ms. Martin has been prescribed propranolol (Inderal) for hypertension. She arrives at the outpatient clinic and tells you that she is having episodes of dizziness and at times feels as if she is going to faint. Discuss how you would investigate this problem and what information you could give Ms. Martin that might help her.

2. Mr. Garcia was prescribed labetalol (Trandate) 100 mg orally twice daily for hypertension. The primary health care provider wants him to monitor his blood pressure once daily. Determine what assessments you would make. Develop a teaching plan for Mr. Garcia that would help him in monitoring his blood pressure and taking labetalol.

3. A new nurse says that she is unsure about how the adrenergic blocking drugs work. Discuss the four types of adrenergic blocking drugs and how each one works in the body.

Review Questions

1. A patient is to receive a β-adrenergic drug for hypertension. Before the drug is administered, the most important assessment the nurse performs is _____.

   A. weighing the patient

   B. obtaining blood for laboratory tests

   C. taking a past medical history

   D. taking the blood pressure on both arms

2. When an adrenergic blocking drug is given for a life-threatening cardiac arrhythmia, which of the following activities would the nurse expect to be a part of patient care?

   A. Daily electrocardiograms

   B. Fluid restriction to 1000 mL/d

   C. Daily weights

   D. Cardiac monitoring

3. To prevent complications when administering a β-adrenergic blocking drug to an elderly patient, the nurse would be particularly alert for _____.

   A. vascular insufficiency (e.g., weak peripheral pulses and cold extremities)

   B. complaints of an occipital headache

   C. insomnia

   D. hypoglycemia

4. The patient with glaucoma will likely receive a(n) _____.

   A. α/β-adrenergic blocking drug

   B. α-adrenergic blocking drug

   C. β-adrenergic blocking drug

   D. antiadrenergic drug

Medication Dosage Problems

1. The primary health care provider prescribes 60 mg propranolol oral solution. The drug is available in an oral solution with a strength of 4 mg/mL. The nurse administers _____.

2. A patient has just had a dose increase to 12.5 mg of carvedilol. The patient has a bottle with 3.125-mg tablets and insists on finishing the bottle before buying a different strength. The nurse tells the patient to administer _____.

To check your answers, see Appendix G.

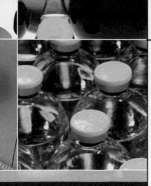

Chapter 29

Cholinergic Drugs

Key Terms

- acetylcholine
- acetylcholinesterase
- cholinergic crisis
- miosis
- micturition
- muscarinic receptors
- myasthenia gravis
- nicotinic receptors
- parasympathomimetic drugs

Learning Objectives

On completion of this chapter, the student will:

- Discuss important aspects of the parasympathetic nervous system.
- Discuss the uses, drug actions, general adverse reactions, contraindications, precautions, and interactions of the cholinergic drugs.
- Identify important preadministration and ongoing assessment activities

- the nurse should perform on the patient taking cholinergic drugs.
- List nursing diagnoses particular to a patient taking cholinergic drugs.
- Discuss ways to promote an optimal response to therapy, how to manage common adverse reactions, and important points to keep in mind when educating the patient about the use of cholinergic drugs.

Acetylcholine (ACh) is the substance that transmits nerve impulses across the parasympathetic branch of the autonomic nervous system. There are two types of receptors in the parasympathetic nervous branch: **muscarinic receptors** (which stimulate smooth muscle) and **nicotinic receptors** (which stimulate skeletal muscle). Stimulation of this pathway results in the opposite reactions to those triggered by the adrenergic system. Blood vessels dilate, sending blood to the gastrointestinal (GI) tract. Secretions and peristalsis are activated and salivary glands increase production. The heart slows and pulmonary bronchioles constrict. The smooth muscle of the bladder contracts and the pupils of the eyes constrict. Activation of these nerves is sometimes called the *rest-and-digest* response.

What makes the parasympathetic system function differently is the enzyme acetylcholinesterase. **Acetylcholinesterase** (AChE) is an enzyme that can inactivate the neurotransmitter ACh, thereby preventing the nerve synapse from continuing the nerve impulse. Cholinergic drugs mimic the activity of the parasympathetic nervous system. They also are called **parasympathomimetic drugs**. Drugs that inhibit the enzyme AChE are called *anticholinesterases* or *acetylcholinesterase inhibitors*. See the Summary Drug Table: Cholinergic Drugs for a more complete listing of these drugs.

Actions

Cholinergic drugs may act like the neurotransmitter acetylcholine (ACh) or they may inhibit the release of the enzyme acetylcholinesterase (AChE).

Myasthenia gravis is a disease that involves rapid fatigue of skeletal muscles because of the lack of ACh released at the nerve endings of parasympathetic nerves. Cholinergic drugs that prolong the activity of ACh by inhibiting the release of AChE are called *indirect-acting cholinergics* or *anticholinesterase muscle stimulants*. Drugs used to treat this disorder act indirectly to inhibit the activity of AChE and promote muscle contraction.

SUMMARY DRUG TABLE CHOLINERGIC DRUGS

GENERIC NAME	TRADE NAME	USES	ADVERSE REACTIONS	DOSAGE RANGES
Anticholinesterase Muscle Stimulants				
ambenonium *am-be-noe'-nee-um*	Mytelase	Myasthenia gravis	Increased bronchial secretions, cardiac arrhythmias, muscle weakness, urinary frequency	5–75 mg orally TID, QID
edrophonium *ed-roe-fone'-ee-yum*	Enlon, Tensilon	Diagnosis of myasthenia gravis	Increased bronchial secretions, cardiac arrhythmias, muscle weakness, urinary frequency	2–10 mg IV, look for cholinergic reaction (muscle weakness)
guanidine *goo-wan'-eh-deen*		Myasthenic syndrome (Eaton-Lambert disease)	Palpitations, numbness in lips/ extremities, dry mouth, nausea, abdominal cramping	10–30 mg/kg/d, titrate until adverse reaction occurs
pyridostigmine bromide *peer-id-oh-stig'-meen*	Mestinon, Regonol	Myasthenia gravis	Increased bronchial secretions, cardiac arrhythmias, muscle weakness	Average dose is 600 mg/d orally at spaced intervals
Urinary Cholinergics				
bethanechol chloride *be-than'-e-kole*	Duvoid, Urecholine	Acute nonobstructive urinary retention, neurogenic atony of urinary bladder with urinary retention	Abdominal discomfort, headache, diarrhea, nausea, salivation, urgency	10–50 mg orally BID to QID; 2.5–5 mg SC TID to QID
Topical Ophthalmics				
carbachol, topical *kar'-ba-kole*	Miostat	Glaucoma	Temporary reduction of visual acuity, headache	1–2 gtt in eye up to 3 times daily
pilocarpine HCl *pye-loe-kar'-peen*	Pilopine	Glaucoma	Temporary reduction in visual acuity, headache	1–2 gtt in eye 1–6 times daily

The parasympathetic branch of the autonomic nervous system partly controls the process of **micturition** (voiding of urine) by constricting the detrusor muscle and relaxing the bladder sphincter (see Table 27-1). Micturition is both a voluntary and involuntary act. Urinary retention (not caused by a mechanical obstruction, such as a stone in the bladder) results when micturition is impaired. Treatment of urinary retention with cholinergic drugs causes contraction of the bladder smooth muscles and passage of urine. Cholinergic drugs that act like ACh are called *direct-acting cholinergics.*

Glaucoma is a disorder of increased pressure within the eye caused by an obstruction of the outflow of aqueous humor through the canal of Schlemm. In the normal eye, the aqueous humor flows from the ciliary body to the posterior chamber of the eye, through the pupil, and out the canal of Schlemm into the venous circulation (Fig. 29-1).

This flow of aqueous humor keeps the pressure in the eye within normal limits. Glaucoma may be treated by topical application (e.g., eye drops) of a cholinergic drug, such as carbachol or pilocarpine. Treatment of glaucoma with a cholinergic drug produces **miosis** (constriction of the iris). This opens the blocked channels and allows the normal passage of aqueous humor, thereby reducing intraocular pressure.

Uses

The major uses of the cholinergic drugs are in the treatment of

- Urinary retention
- Myasthenia gravis
- Glaucoma

Cholinergic Drugs

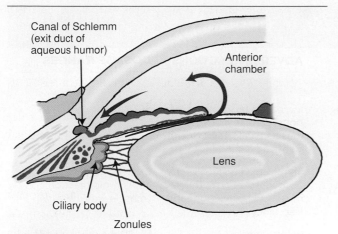

Figure 29.1 In the normal eye, aqueous humor flows through the ciliary body into the posterior chamber, through the pupil into the anterior chamber, and out through the trabecular meshwork to the canal of Schlemm and into the venous circulation.

Adverse Reactions

Topical administration usually produces few adverse effects, but a temporary reduction of visual acuity (sharpness) and headache may occur. With the exception of those applied topically, cholinergic drugs are not selective in action. General adverse reactions include

- Nausea, diarrhea, abdominal cramping
- Salivation
- Flushing of the skin
- Cardiac arrhythmias and muscle weakness

Contraindications

These drugs are contraindicated in patients with known hypersensitivity to the drugs, asthma, peptic ulcer disease, coronary artery disease, and hyperthyroidism. Bethanecol is contraindicated in those with mechanical obstruction of the GI or genitourinary tracts. Patients with secondary glaucoma, iritis, corneal abrasion, or any acute inflammatory disease of the eye should not use the ophthalmic cholinergic preparations.

Precautions

These drugs are used cautiously in patients with hypertension, epilepsy, cardiac arrhythmias, bradycardia, recent coronary occlusion, and megacolon. The safety of these drugs has not been established for use during pregnancy (category C) or lactation, or in children.

Interactions

The following interactions may occur when a cholinergic drug is administered with another agent:

Interacting Drug	Common Use	Effect of Interaction
aminoglycoside antibiotics	Anti-infective agent	Increased neuromuscular blocking effect
corticosteroids	Treatment of inflammation/respiratory problems	Decreased effect of the cholinergic

When the cholinergic drugs are administered with other cholinergics, there is an increase in the effects of the drugs and greater risk for toxicity. Concurrent use of the anticholinergic drugs antagonizes the effects of the cholinergic drugs. Because of this property, atropine is considered an antidote for overdosage of the cholinergic drugs. Carbachol and pilocarpine produce an additive effect when used concurrently.

NURSING PROCESS

The Patient Receiving a Cholinergic Drug

ASSESSMENT

PREADMINISTRATION ASSESSMENT

The preadministration assessment depends on the drug and the reason for administration.

GLAUCOMA Before therapy for glaucoma is started, the primary health care provider thoroughly examines the eye. The nurse reviews the primary health care provider's diagnosis and comments, takes a general patient health history, and evaluates the patient's ability to carry out the activities of daily living, especially if the patient is elderly or has limited vision.

MYASTHENIA GRAVIS Before the nurse gives a cholinergic drug to a patient with myasthenia gravis, the primary health care provider performs a complete neurologic assessment. The nurse assesses for signs of muscle weakness, such as drooling (i.e., the lack of ability to swallow), inability to chew and swallow, drooping of the eyelids, inability to perform repetitive movements (e.g., walking, combing hair, using eating utensils), difficulty breathing, and extreme fatigue.

URINARY RETENTION If a patient receives a cholinergic drug for the treatment of urinary retention, the nurse palpates the abdomen in the pelvic area to determine if distention is present. A rounded swelling over the pelvis usually indicates retention and a distended bladder. The patient may also complain of discomfort in the lower abdomen. In addition, the nurse takes the patient's blood pressure and pulse rate.

ONGOING ASSESSMENT

While the patient is receiving a cholinergic drug it is important for the nurse to monitor for drug toxicity or cholinergic crisis.

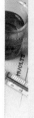

Nursing Alert

Symptoms of **cholinergic crisis** (cholinergic drug toxicity) include severe abdominal cramping, diarrhea, excessive salivation, muscle weakness, rigidity and spasm, and clenching of the jaw. Patients exhibiting these symptoms require immediate medical treatment and their condition must be immediately reported to the primary health care provider. In the case of overdosage, an antidote such as atropine is administered, and other treatment also may be prescribed. The usual dosage of atropine is 0.4 to 0.6 mg intravenously (IV).

GLAUCOMA When a cholinergic drug is used to treat glaucoma, the nurse checks the eye and the area around the eye daily for evidence of redness, inflammation, and excessive secretions, particularly if the ocular system for continuous release of the drug is used. If secretions are present around the eye, the nurse removes them with a cotton ball or gauze soaked in normal saline or other cleansing solution recommended by the primary health care provider.

MYASTHENIA GRAVIS Once therapy is under way, the nurse must document any increase in symptoms of the disease or adverse drug reactions before giving each dose of the drug. The nurse assesses the patient for the presence or absence of the symptoms of myasthenia gravis before each drug dose. In patients with severe myasthenia gravis, the nurse can carry out these assessments between drug doses, as well as immediately before drug administration. The

nurse documents each symptom, as well as the patient's response or lack of response to drug therapy.

Assessment is important because the dosage frequently has to be increased or decreased early in therapy, depending on the patient's response. Regulation of dosage is important in keeping the symptoms of myasthenia gravis from incapacitating the patient. For many patients, the symptoms are fairly well controlled with drug therapy once the optimal drug dose is determined.

URINARY RETENTION The ongoing assessment for a patient with urinary retention includes measuring and recording the fluid intake and output. The nurse must notify the primary health care provider if the patient fails to void after drug administration.

If a cholinergic drug is ordered for preventing urinary retention, the nurse measures and records the fluid intake and output. If the amount of each voiding is insufficient or the patient fails to void, the nurse palpates the bladder to determine its size and notifies the primary health care provider.

NURSING DIAGNOSES

Drug-specific nursing diagnoses are highlighted in the Nursing Diagnoses Checklist. Other nursing diagnoses applicable to these drugs are discussed in depth in Chapter 4.

Nursing Diagnoses Checklist

☑ **Disturbed Sensory Perception: Visual** related to adverse drug reactions or increased pressure within the eye

☑ **Diarrhea** related to adverse drug reaction

PLANNING

The expected outcomes of the patient depend on the reason for administration of the cholinergic drug, but may include an optimal response to therapy, support of patient needs related to the management of adverse reactions, and an understanding of and compliance with the prescribed therapeutic regimen.

IMPLEMENTATION

PROMOTING AN OPTIMAL RESPONSE TO THERAPY

The care of a patient receiving a cholinergic drug depends on the drug used, the reason for administration, and the patient's response to the drug.

MANAGING GLAUCOMA The nurse checks the primary health care provider's order and the drug label carefully when instilling any ophthalmic preparation. The drug label must indicate that the preparation is for ophthalmic use. In addition, the nurse should check the name of the drug and the drug dosage or strength as stated on the label against the primary health care provider's orders. The nurse instills the drug in the lower conjunctival sac unless the primary health care provider orders a different method of instillation. The nurse supports the hand holding the dropper against the patient's forehead. The tip of the dropper must never touch the eye.

In some instances, the patient may have been using an ophthalmic preparation for glaucoma for a long time, and the primary health care provider may allow the hospitalized patient to instill his or her own eye drops. When this is stated on the patient's order sheet, the nurse can leave the drug at the patient's bedside. Even though the drug is self-administered, the nurse checks the patient at intervals to be sure that the drug is instilled at the prescribed time using the correct technique for ophthalmic instillation.

USING A PILOCARPINE OCULAR SYSTEM Patients with glaucoma may choose administration of drug using an elliptically shaped membrane designed for continuous release of pilocarpine. If the pilocarpine ocular system is prescribed for the hospitalized patient, the nurse checks the check and eye area several times a day because the system can become displaced from the eye. The nurse questions the patient about his or her ability to self-administer the disk while in the hospital. The patient or the nurse changes the pilocarpine ocular system every 7 days unless the primary health care provider directs otherwise (Display 29-1).

Gerontologic Alert

Most patients are usually aware of displacement of the pilocarpine ocular system, but some patients, the elderly in particular, may not realize that the system has come out of the eye. If displacement does occur, the nurse inserts a new system and informs the primary health care provider of the problem.

On occasion, patients cannot insert the system by themselves or cannot retain the system in the eye for the required time. When this occurs, the nurse notifies the primary health care provider because the ocular system should remain in place until it is time for it to be changed.

If patients have a problem retaining the system, placing the system in the upper conjunctival cul-de-sac is preferable. The nurse can manipulate the system from the lower to the upper conjunctival cul-de-sac using gentle massage through the eyelid. The nurse contacts the primary health care provider if the symptoms of glaucoma increase, if the patient is unable to retain the ocular system, or if redness, eye irritation, or excessive secretions are noted.

MANAGING MYASTHENIA GRAVIS At the start of therapy, determining the dosage that will control symptoms may be difficult. In many cases, the dosage must be adjusted upward or downward until optimal drug effects are obtained. Patients with severe symptoms of the disease require the drug every 2 to 4 hours, even during the night. Sustained-released tablets are available that allow less frequent dosing and help the patient to have longer undisturbed periods during the night.

Nursing Alert

Because of the need to make frequent dosage adjustments, the nurse should observe the patient closely for symptoms of drug overdosage or underdosage. Signs of drug overdosage include muscle rigidity and spasm, salivation, and clenching of the jaw. Signs of drug underdosage are signs of the disease itself, namely, rapid fatigability of the muscles, drooping of the eyelids, and difficulty breathing. If symptoms of drug overdosage or underdosage develop, the nurse should contact the primary health care provider immediately because a change in dosage is usually necessary.

MANAGING URINARY RETENTION Voiding usually occurs in 5 to 15 minutes after subcutaneous drug administration and 30 to 90 minutes after oral administration. The nurse should place the call light and any other items the patient might need, such as the urinal or the bedpan, within easy reach. However, some patients are not able to reach or handle these aids easily, so the nurse must promptly answer their call light.

MONITORING AND MANAGING PATIENT NEEDS

When a cholinergic drug is given by the oral or parenteral route, adverse drug reactions may affect many systems of the body, such as the heart, respiratory and GI tracts, and the central nervous system. The nurse observes the patient closely for the appearance of adverse drug reactions, such as a change in vital signs or an increase in symptoms. The nurse documents any complaints the patient may have and notifies the primary health care provider.

Display 29.1 Inserting the Pilocarpine Ocular System

1. Wash hands and put on gloves. Press the disk with the fingertip until it remains on the finger as shown.

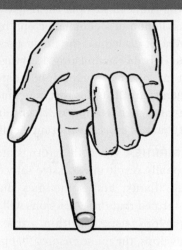

2. Have the patient look up. Pull the lower conjunctiva away from the eye and gently place the disk in the lower conjunctival sac. The disk should float on the sclera.

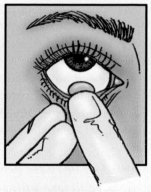

3. Pull the lower conjunctiva over the disk. Check for correct position. The disk should not be visible. If the disk is still seen, the eyelid must be repositioned by pulling the lower conjunctiva out and over the disk again.

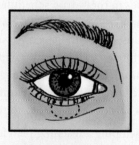

4. Use gloves when removing the disk. Pull the lower eyelid down and use the thumb and first finger of the free hand to lift the disk out of the eye as shown.

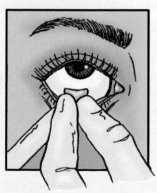

(Adapted from *Nursing94*, June, Intraocular Drug Administration, pp. 44–45, which was adapted from *Giving drugs by advanced techniques* [1993]. Springhouse, PA: Springhouse Corp.)

Cholinergic Drugs

DISTURBED SENSORY PERCEPTION: VISUAL Because drug-induced myopia (nearsightedness) may occur after instillation of a cholinergic ophthalmic drug for the treatment of glaucoma, the nurse assists the patient in getting out of bed or ambulating. Keeping the patient's room dimly lit at night is helpful because night vision may be decreased. Obstacles that may hinder ambulation or result in falls, such as slippers, chairs, and tables, are placed out of the way, especially during the night.

DIARRHEA When these drugs are used orally they occasionally result in excessive salivation, abdominal cramping, flatus, and sometimes diarrhea. The patient is informed that these reactions will continue until tolerance develops, usually within a few weeks. Until tolerance develops, the nurse ensures that proper facilities, such as a bedside commode, bedpan, or bathroom, are readily available. The patient is encouraged to ambulate to assist the passing of flatus. If needed, a rectal tube may be used to assist in the passing of flatus. The nurse keeps a record of the fluid intake and output and the number, consistency, and frequency of stools if diarrhea is present. The primary health care provider is informed if diarrhea is excessive because this may be an indication of toxicity.

EDUCATING THE PATIENT AND FAMILY

Patients required to take a drug over a long period may incur lapses in their drug schedule. For some, it is a matter of occasionally forgetting to take a drug; for others, a lapse may be caused by other factors, such as failure to understand the importance of drug therapy, inability to instill an ophthalmic drug (when the drug is prescribed for glaucoma), the cost of the drug, or unfamiliarity with the consequences associated with discontinuing the drug therapy.

When developing a teaching plan for the patient and family, the nurse emphasizes the importance of uninterrupted drug therapy. The nurse allows the patient and family time to ask questions. The nurse explores any problems that appear to be associated with the prescribed drug regimen and then reports them to the primary health care provider. The nurse reviews the purpose of the drug therapy with the patient and family, as well as the adverse reactions that may occur.

GLAUCOMA When a cholinergic drug is prescribed for glaucoma, the nurse instructs the patient and a family member in instillation of the eye drops (see Patient and Family Teaching Checklist: Instilling Liquid Eye Medications).

If a family member is to instill the drug, the nurse allows time for instruction as well as supervised practice of the procedure. The nurse warns the patient that the eye drops may sting when instilled into the eye and that this is a

---

Patient and Family Teaching Checklist

Instilling Liquid Eye Medications

The nurse:

✔ Explains the importance of keeping the bottle tightly closed.

✔ Stresses that the tip of the dropper should not be washed.

✔ States that the dropper should not be put down on a table or other surface.

✔ Demonstrates support of the hand holding the dropper against the forehead.

✔ Cautions against letting the tip of the dropper touch the eye to prevent injury or infection.

✔ States that the dropper should be put back in the bottle immediately after use.

✔ Instructs on tilting the head back and instilling the prescribed number of drops in the inner lower eyelid (lower conjunctival sac).

✔ Demonstrates applying light finger pressure to the inner corner of the eye (lacrimal sac) for about 1 minute after instillation (teaching the use of this maneuver should be approved by the primary health care provider).

✔ Explains that if the patient or caregiver is unable to instill eye drops, the primary health care provider should be contacted immediately.

---

normal, but often temporary, discomfort. The nurse advises the patient to observe caution while driving or performing any task that requires visual acuity.

Local irritation and headache may occur at the beginning of therapy. The patient is instructed to notify the primary health care provider if abdominal cramping, diarrhea, or excessive salivation occurs.

PILOCARPINE OCULAR SYSTEM If the pilocarpine ocular system is prescribed, the primary health care provider must evaluate the patient's ability to insert and remove the system. A package insert is provided with the system and the nurse reviews this with the patient. The patient should demonstrate the ability to place, adjust, and remove the device at the appointment. The nurse instructs the patient to remove and replace the system every 7 days or as instructed by the primary health care provider. Replacement is best done at bedtime (unless the primary health care provider orders otherwise) because there is some impairment of vision for a short time after insertion. The nurse tells the patient to check for unit placement before retiring at night and in the morning on arising. The nurse notifies the primary health care provider if eye secretions are excessive or irritation occurs.

MYASTHENIA GRAVIS Many patients with myasthenia gravis learn to adjust their drug dosage according to their needs because dosage needs may vary slightly from day to day. The nurse teaches the patient and family members to recognize symptoms of overdosage and underdosage, as well as what steps the primary health care provider wishes them to take if either occurs. The dosage regimen is explained and instruction is given in how to adjust the dosage upward or downward.

The nurse gives the patient a written or printed description of the signs and symptoms of drug overdosage or underdosage. The nurse instructs the patient to keep a record of the response to drug therapy (e.g., time of day, increased or decreased muscle strength, fatigue) and to bring this to each primary health care provider or clinic visit until the symptoms are well controlled and the drug dosage is stabilized. These patients must wear or carry identification (such as a Medic Alert tag) indicating that they have myasthenia gravis.

EVALUATION

- The therapeutic effect is achieved.

- Adverse reactions are identified, reported to the primary health care provider, and managed successfully through appropriate nursing interventions.

- The patient verbalizes the importance of complying with the prescribed treatment regimen.

- The patient complies with the prescribed drug regimen.

- The patient and family demonstrate understanding of the drug regimen.

Critical Thinking Exercises

1. Mr. Johnson, aged 78 years, has glaucoma and is prescribed the pilocarpine ocular system. On a visit to the outpatient clinic, Mr. Johnson tells you that he is having problems retaining the ocular system. You notice that his right eye is very red and inflamed. Determine how you can investigate this problem further with Mr. Johnson. Provide suggestions that will help Mr. Johnson to retain the system.

2. Mr. Hopkins, aged 32 years, has myasthenia gravis. Explain to Mr. Hopkins the symptoms he should be aware of that would indicate toxicity.

3. Discuss the types of ongoing assessments made when a patient takes a cholinergic drug for urinary retention.

Review Questions

1. A patient with glaucoma is prescribed pilocarpine eye drops. One adverse reaction that the nurse will expect with the use of this drug is _____.

   A. a temporary loss of visual acuity

   B. pain in the affected eye

   C. excessive tearing of both eyes

   D. mydriasis of the eyes

2. The primary care provider allows the patient to keep pilocarpine eye drops at the bedside and to self-administer the eye drops four times daily. The nurse _____.

   A. need not check with the patient concerning the eye drops because the patient is a responsible adult

   B. must check the patient to be sure the medication is used properly and at the right time

   C. is not responsible for monitoring the patient's response to the medication

   D. does not record the administration of the drug in the patient's chart

3. Ms. Martin has received a diagnosis of myasthenia gravis and begins a regimen of ambenonium. The nursing assessment is important because the dose of the drug _____.

   A. usually must be increased every 4 hours early in therapy

   B. frequently is increased or decreased early in therapy

   C. is titrated according to the patient's blood pressure

   D. is gradually decreased as a therapeutic response is achieved

Medication Dosage Problems

1. The dosage of pyridostigmine bromide (Mestinon) is 600 mg/d. How many tablets will the patient take if they are 60 mg each?

2. The primary care provider prescribes 2.5 mg of bethanechol subcutaneously. The drug is available in a solution of 5 mg/mL. The nurse administers _____.

To check your answers, see Appendix G.

Cholinergic Drugs

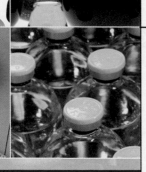

Cholinergic Blocking Drugs

Learning Objectives

On completion of this chapter, the student will:

- Discuss the uses, general drug actions, general adverse reactions, contraindications, precautions, and interactions of the cholinergic blocking drugs (also called anticholinergic drugs and cholinergic blockers).
- Discuss important preadministration and ongoing assessment activities the

nurse should perform on the patient taking cholinergic blocking drugs.

- List nursing diagnoses particular to the patient taking cholinergic blocking drugs.
- Discuss ways to promote an optimal response to therapy, how to manage common adverse reactions, and important points to keep in mind when educating patients taking a cholinergic blocking drug.

Like adrenergic blocking drugs, the cholinergic blocking drugs have an effect on the autonomic nervous system. Cholinergic blocking drugs are also called *anticholinergic drugs*, *cholinergic blockers*, or *parasympatholytic drugs*. In this chapter, these drugs are identified as cholinergic blocking drugs.

Acetylcholine is the primary neurotransmitter in the parasympathetic branch of the autonomic nervous system. **Cholinergic blocking drugs** block the action of the neurotransmitter acetylcholine in the parasympathetic nervous system. Because parasympathetic nerves influence many areas of the body, the effects of the cholinergic blocking drugs are numerous. Examples of cholinergic blocking drugs include atropine, scopolamine, and oxybutynin (Ditropan).

Actions

Cholinergic blocking drugs inhibit the activity of acetylcholine at the parasympathetic nerve synapse (see Fig. 27-1 in Chapter 27). When the activity of acetylcholine is inhibited, impulses traveling along the parasympathetic nerve cannot pass from the nerve ending to the effector organ or structure.

Two types of receptors are found in the parasympathetic nervous branch: muscarinic and nicotinic. Cholinergic blocking drugs can specifically target certain receptors. For example, antispasmodic drugs used to treat an overactive urinary bladder work because they inhibit the action of the muscarinic receptors in the parasympathetic nervous system. As a result, the detrusor muscle of the bladder does not contract, which prevents the sensations of urinary urgency. Yet, an antispasmodic drug has no effect on skeletal muscles because it does not inhibit the nicotinic receptors in the parasympathetic nervous system.

Because of the wide distribution of parasympathetic nerves, some of these drugs that inhibit nerve impulses at both muscarinic and nicotinic receptors affect many organs and structures of the body, including the eyes, the respiratory and gastrointestinal (GI) tracts, the heart, and the bladder (Display 30-1).

Display 30.1 Effects of the Cholinergic Blocking Drugs

Cholinergic blocking drugs produce the following responses:

Central nervous system—dreamless sleep, drowsiness; atropine may produce mild stimulation in some patients

Eye—**mydriasis** (dilation of the pupil), **cycloplegia** (paralysis of accommodation or inability to focus the eye)

Respiratory tract—**xerostomia** (drying of the secretions of the mouth); drying of the secretions of the nose, throat, bronchi; relaxation of smooth muscles of the bronchi resulting in slight bronchodilation

Gastrointestinal tract—decrease in secretions of the stomach, decrease in gastric and intestinal movement (motility)

Cardiovascular system—increase in pulse rate (most pronounced with atropine administration)

Urinary tract—dilation of smooth muscles of the ureters and renal pelvis

However, responses to administration of a cholinergic blocking drug vary and often depend on the drug and the dose used. For example, scopolamine may occasionally cause excitement, delirium, and restlessness. This reaction is thought to be a **drug idiosyncrasy** (an unexpected or unusual drug effect).

Uses

The primary uses of the cholinergic blocking drugs are treatment of

- Pylorospasm and peptic ulcer
- Ureteral or biliary colic and bladder overactivity
- Vagal nerve-induced bradycardia
- Parkinsonism

In addition, the cholinergic blocking drugs are administered for the preoperative reduction of oral secretions. The Summary Drug Table: Cholinergic Blocking Drugs lists the uses of specific cholinergic blocking drugs.

Adverse Reactions

The severity of many adverse reactions is often dose dependent—that is, the larger the dose, the more intense the adverse reaction. Body system adverse reactions that may occur with the administration of a cholinergic blocking drug are listed in the following sections.

Gastrointestinal Reactions

- Dry mouth, nausea, vomiting
- Difficulty in swallowing, heartburn
- Constipation

Central Nervous System Reactions

- Headache, flushing, nervousness
- Drowsiness, weakness, insomnia
- Nasal congestion, fever

Visual Reactions

- Blurred vision
- Mydriasis
- Photophobia
- Cycloplegia
- Increased ocular tension

Genitourinary Reactions

- Urinary hesitancy and retention
- Dysuria

Cardiovascular Reactions

- Palpitations
- Bradycardia (after low doses of atropine)
- Tachycardia (after higher doses of atropine)

Other

- Urticaria
- Decreased sweat production
- Anaphylactic shock
- Rash

Sometimes a secondary adverse reaction, such as drowsiness, is desirable. For example, when atropine is used before surgery to reduce the production of secretions in the respiratory tract, drowsiness is part of the desired response.

Gerontologic Alert

The nurse observes the elderly patient receiving a cholinergic blocking drug at frequent intervals for excitement, agitation, mental confusion, drowsiness, urinary retention, or other adverse effects. These effects may be seen even with small doses. If any should occur, it is important to withhold the next dose of the drug and contact the primary health care provider. The nurse ensures patient safety until these adverse reactions disappear.

Cholinergic Blocking Drugs

SUMMARY DRUG TABLE   CHOLINERGIC BLOCKING DRUGS

GENERIC NAME	TRADE NAME	USES	ADVERSE REACTIONS	DOSAGE RANGES
atropine *a'-troe-peen*	AtroPen	Pylorospasm, reduction of bronchial and oral secretions, excessive vagal-induced bradycardia, ureteral and biliary colic	Drowsiness, blurred vision, tachycardia, dry mouth, urinary hesitancy	0.4–0.6 mg orally, IM,SC, IV
belladonna alkaloids *bel-ah-dohn'-a*		Adjunctive therapy for peptic ulcer, digestive disorders, diverticulitis, pancreatitis, diarrhea	Same as atropine	0.25–0.5 mg orally TID
dicyclomine HCl *dye-sye'-kloe-meen*	Benty1	Functional bowel/ irritable bowel syndrome	Same as atropine	80–160 mg orally QID
glycopyrrolate *glye-koe-pye'-roe-late*	Robinul	Oral: peptic ulcer Parenteral: in conjunction with anesthesia to reduce bronchial and oral secretions, to block cardiac vagal inhibitory reflexes during induction of anesthesia and intubation; protection against the peripheral muscarinic effects of cholinergic agents (e.g., neostigmine)	Blurred vision, dry mouth, altered taste perception, nausea, vomiting, dysphagia, urinary hesitancy and retention	Oral: 1–2 mg BID or TID Parenteral: peptic ulcer, 0.1–0.2 mg IM, IV, TID, QID Preanesthesia: 0.002 mg/lb IM Intraoperative: 0.1 mg IV
mepenzolate bromide *meh-pen'-zoe-late*	Cantil	Adjunctive treatment of peptic ulcer	Same as atropine	25–50 mg orally TID or QID with meals and at bedtime
methscopolamine *mehth-scoe-pol'-a-meen*	Pamine	Adjunctive therapy for peptic ulcer	Same as atropine	2.5 mg 30 min before meals and 2.5–5 mg orally at bedtime
propantheline bromide *proe-pan'-the-leen*	Pro-Banthine	Adjunctive therapy for peptic ulcer	Dry mouth, constipation, hesitancy, urinary retention, blurred vision	15 mg orally 30 min before meals and at bedtime
scopolamine hydrobromide *scoe-pol'-a-meen*		Preanesthetic sedation, motion sickness	Confusion, dry mouth, constipation, urinary hesitancy, urinary retention, blurred vision	0.32–0.65 mg IM, SC, IV, diluted with sterile water for injections Transdermal: apply 1 patch 4 h before travel q3d
trihexyphenidyl *trye-hex-ee-fen'-i-dill*		Parkinsonism, extrapyramidal effects caused by antipsychotic drugs	Disorientation, confusion, lightheadedness, dizziness, blurred vision, mydriasis, dry mouth, urinary retention, flushing	1–2 mg/d; increase by 2 mg q3–5d, to a total of 6–10 mg/d; divide dose into 3–4 times/d orally
Anticholinergic Urinary Antispasmodics				
darifenacin HCl *da-ree-fen'-ah-sin*	Enablex	Overactive bladder	Dry mouth, constipation	7.5 mg orally daily

GENERIC NAME	TRADE NAME	USES	ADVERSE REACTIONS	DOSAGE RANGES
flavoxate HCl *fla-vox'-ate*	Urispas	Urinary symptoms caused by cystitis, prostatitis, and other urinary problems	Dry mouth, drowsiness, blurred vision, headache, urinary retention	100–200 mg orally 3–4 times/d
oxybutynin *ocks-ee-byoo-tie'nin*	Ditropan	Overactive bladder, neurogenic bladder	Dry mouth, nausea, headache, drowsiness, constipation, urinary retention	5 mg orally, 2–3 times/d
solifenacin *sole-ah-fen'-ah-sin*	Vesicare	Overactive bladder	Dry mouth, constipation, blurred vision, dry eyes	5 mg orally daily
tolterodine *toll-tear'-oh-dyne*	Detrol, Detrol LA (long-acting, extended-release)	Overactive bladder	Dry mouth, constipation, headache, dizziness	2 mg orally, TID; extended-release: 4 mg daily
® **trospium** *troz'-pee-um*	Sanctura	Overactive bladder	Dry mouth, constipation, headache	20 mg orally TID

® This drug should be administered at least 1 hour before or 2 hours after a meal.

The nurse should observe patients receiving a cholinergic blocking drug during the hot summer months for signs of heat prostration (e.g., fever, tachycardia, flushing, warm dry skin, mental confusion) because these drugs decrease sweating.

Contraindications

Cholinergic blocking drugs are contraindicated in patients with known hypersensitivity to the drugs or glaucoma. Other patients for whom cholinergic blocking drugs are contraindicated are those with myasthenia gravis, tachyarrhythmias, myocardial infarction, and congestive heart failure (unless bradycardia is present).

Precautions

The nurse should use these drugs with caution in patients with GI infections, benign prostatic hypertrophy, urinary retention, hyperthyroidism, hepatic or renal disease, and hypertension. The nurse should use atropine with caution in patients with asthma. The cholinergic blocking drugs are classified as pregnancy category C drugs and are used only when the benefit to the woman outweighs the risk to the fetus.

This caution applies to some over-the-counter (OTC) preparations available for the relief of allergy and cold symptoms and as aids to induce sleep. Some of these products contain atropine, scopolamine, or other cholinergic blocking drugs. Although this warning is printed on the container or package, many users fail to read drug labels carefully.

Interactions

The following interactions may occur when a cholinergic blocking drug is administered with another agent:

Interacting Drug	Common Use	Effect of Interaction
antibiotics/ antifungals	Fight infection	Decreased effectiveness of anti-infective drug
meperidine, flurazepam, phenothiazines	Preoperative sedation	Increased effect of the cholinergic blocker
tricyclic antidepressants	Management of depression	Increased effect of the cholinergic blocker
haloperidol	Antianxiety/ antipsychotic agent	Decreased effectiveness of antipsychotic drug
digoxin	Management of cardiac problems	Increased serum levels of digoxin

Cholinergic Blocking Drugs

The Patient Receiving a Cholinergic Blocking Drug

ASSESSMENT

PREADMINISTRATION ASSESSMENT

Before administering a cholinergic blocking drug to a patient for the first time, the nurse obtains a thorough health history as well as a history of the signs and symptoms of the current disorder. The focus of the initial physical assessment depends on the reason for administering the drug. In most instances, the nurse obtains the blood pressure, pulse, and respiratory rate. The nurse also may include additional assessments, such as checking the stool of the patient who has a peptic ulcer for color and signs of occult blood, determining visual acuity in the patient with glaucoma, or looking for signs of dehydration and weighing the patient if prolonged diarrhea is one of the patient's symptoms.

ONGOING ASSESSMENT

When administering a cholinergic blocking drug, the daily ongoing assessment requires that the nurse closely observe the patient. The nurse checks vital signs, observes for adverse drug reactions, and evaluates the symptoms and complaints related to the patient's diagnosis. For example, the nurse questions the patient with a peptic ulcer regarding current symptoms, then makes a comparison of these symptoms to the symptoms present before the start of therapy. The nurse reports any increase in the severity of symptoms to the primary health care provider immediately.

NURSING DIAGNOSES

Drug-specific nursing diagnoses are highlighted in the Nursing Diagnoses Checklist. Other nursing diagnoses applicable to these drugs are discussed in depth in Chapter 4.

 Nursing Diagnoses Checklist

✓ **Impaired Comfort** related to xerostomia

✓ **Constipation** related to slowing of peristalsis in the GI tract

✓ **Risk for Injury** related to dizziness, drowsiness, mental confusion, or heat prostration

✓ **Disturbed Sensory Perception: Visual** related to adverse drug reaction

✓ **Ineffective Tissue Perfusion** related to impaired heart pumping action

---

PLANNING

The expected outcomes for the patient depend on the reason for administration of a cholinergic blocking drug, but may include an optimal response to therapy, support of patient needs related to the management of adverse reactions, and an understanding of and compliance with the prescribed therapeutic regimen.

IMPLEMENTATION

PROMOTING AN OPTIMAL RESPONSE TO THERAPY

THE PATIENT RECEIVING A PREOPERATIVE DRUG If a cholinergic blocking drug is administered before surgery, the nurse instructs the patient to void before the drug is given. The nurse informs the patient that his or her mouth will become extremely dry, that this is normal, and that fluid is not to be taken. The side rails of the bed are raised, and the patient is instructed to remain in bed after administration of the preoperative drug.

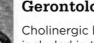 **Nursing Alert**

The nurse must administer the preoperative drug at the exact time prescribed because the cholinergic blocking drug must be given time to produce the greatest effect (i.e., the drying of upper respiratory and oral secretions) before the administration of a general anesthetic. The anesthesiologist must be notified if the preoperative drug is given late.

Gerontologic Alert

Cholinergic blocking drugs are usually not included in the preoperative drugs of patients older than 60 years because of the effects of these drugs on the eye and the central nervous system.

MONITORING AND MANAGING PATIENT NEEDS

IMPAIRED COMFORT: XEROSTOMIA When taking these drugs on a daily basis, mouth dryness may be severe and extremely uncomfortable in some patients. The patient may complain of a "cottonmouth" sensation, in which oral dryness feels like a mouthful of cotton. The patient may have moderate to extreme difficulty swallowing drugs and food. The patient's speech may be impeded and hard to understand because of the dry mouth.

The nurse encourages the patient to take a few sips of water before and while taking an oral drug and to sip

Home Care Checklist

Combating Dry Mouth

One of the most common adverse effects occurring with the use of cholinergic blocking drugs is a dry mouth. The nurse offers the following suggestions to the patient to help combat this problem:

☑ Perform frequent mouth care, including brushing, rinsing, and flossing.

☑ Keep a glass or sports bottle filled with fluid on hand at all times.

☑ Sip small amounts of cool water or fluids throughout the day and with meals.

☑ Take a few sips of water before taking any oral drugs.

☑ Suck on ice chips or frozen ices, such as Popsicles.

☑ Chew gum.

☑ Suck on sugar-free hard candies.

☑ Avoid alcohol-based mouthwashes.

water at intervals during meals. If allowed, hard candy slowly dissolved in the mouth and frequent sips of water during the day may help relieve persistent oral dryness. The nurse checks the oral cavity daily for soreness or ulcerations. Refer to the Home Care Checklist: Combating Dry Mouth for suggestions on diminishing the discomfort.

CONSTIPATION Constipation caused by decreased gastric motility can be a problem with cholinergic blocking drugs. The nurse urges the patient to increase fluid intake up to 2000 mL daily (if health conditions permit), eat a diet high in fiber, and obtain adequate exercise. Patients being treated for an overactive bladder may be hesitant to increase fluids because of fear of an episode of urinary incontinence. The nurse reassures the patient that increasing fluids will help minimize the adverse reactions of constipation and dry mouth, whereas the cholinergic blocking drug helps to eliminate the sensations of urinary frequency and urgency. The primary health care provider may prescribe a stool softener, if necessary, to prevent constipation.

RISK FOR INJURY These drugs may cause drowsiness, dizziness, and blurred vision. Patients (especially older adults) may require assistance with ambulation. Blurred vision and photophobia are commonly seen with the administration of a cholinergic blocking drug. The severity of this adverse reaction is commonly dose dependent; that is, the larger the dose, the more intense the adverse reaction. The nurse monitors the patient for any disturbance in vision.

Gerontologic Alert

The nurse advises the family of an elderly patient of possible visual and mental impairments (blurred vision, confusion, agitation) that may occur during therapy with these drugs. Objects or situations that may cause falls, such as throw rugs, footstools, and wet or newly waxed floors, are removed or avoided whenever possible. The nurse instructs the family to place against the walls any items of furniture (e.g., footstools, chairs, stands) that obstruct walkways. The nurse alerts the family to the dangers of heat prostration and explains the steps to take to avoid this problem. The patient must be closely observed during the first few days of therapy, and the primary health care provider is notified if mental changes occur.

In hot weather, sweating may decrease and may be followed by heat prostration. The nurse makes sure that the patient is observed at frequent intervals for signs of heat prostration, especially if the patient is elderly or debilitated. In cases of suspected heat prostration, the next dose of the drug is withheld and the primary health care provider contacted immediately. The older adult patient receiving a cholinergic blocking drug is also observed at frequent intervals for excitement, agitation, mental confusion, drowsiness, urinary retention, or other adverse effects. If any of these should occur, the next dose of the drug should be withheld and the primary health care provider contacted. Patient safety must be ensured until these adverse reactions subside.

Cholinergic Blocking Drugs

DISTURBED SENSORY PERCEPTION: VISUAL If photophobia is a problem, the patient may need to wear shaded glasses when going outside, even on cloudy days. Rooms are kept dimly lit and curtains or blinds closed to eliminate bright sunlight in the room. Those with photophobia may be more comfortable in a semidarkened room, especially on sunny days. It is a good idea to use overhead lights as little as possible.

Mydriasis (prolonged pupillary dilation) and **cycloplegia** (difficulty focusing resulting from paralysis of ciliary muscle), if they occur, may interfere with reading, watching television, and similar activities. If these drug effects upset the patient, the nurse discusses the problem with the primary health care provider. At times, these visual impairments will have to be tolerated because drug therapy cannot be changed or discontinued. The nurse can assist the patient to find other forms of diversional therapy, such as interaction with others or listening to the radio.

INEFFECTIVE TISSUE PERFUSION The patient receiving atropine for third-degree heart block is placed on a cardiac monitor during and after administration of the drug. The nurse watches the monitor for a change in pulse rate or rhythm. Tachycardia, other cardiac arrhythmias, or failure of the drug to increase the heart rate must be reported to the primary health care provider immediately because other drugs or medical management may be necessary.

EDUCATING THE PATIENT AND FAMILY

A cholinergic blocking drug may be prescribed for a prolonged period. Some patients may discontinue drug use, especially if their original symptoms have been relieved. The nurse must make sure that the patient and family understand the prescribed drug is to be taken even though symptoms have been relieved.

When a cholinergic blocking drug is prescribed for outpatient use, the nurse informs the patient about the more common adverse reactions associated with these drugs, such as dry mouth, drowsiness, dizziness, and visual impairments. The nurse warns the patient that if drowsiness, dizziness, or blurred vision occurs, caution must be observed while driving or performing other tasks requiring alertness and clear vision.

Some of the adverse reactions associated with the cholinergic blocking drugs may be uncomfortable or distressing. The nurse encourages the patient to discuss these problems with the primary health care provider. The nurse also makes suggestions to lessen the intensity of some of these adverse reactions.

The following is a list of adverse reactions that can be included in the teaching plan, along with the measures that may lessen their intensity or allow the patient to perform tasks at times when the adverse reactions are least likely to occur.

- **Photophobia**—Wear sunglasses when outside, even on cloudy days. Keep rooms dimly lit, and close curtains or blinds to eliminate bright sunlight in the room; soft, indirect lighting is usually more comfortable. Schedule outdoor activities (when necessary) before the first dose of the drug is taken, such as early in the morning.
- **Dry mouth**—Take frequent sips of cool water during the day, before taking the drug orally, and during meals. In addition, if allowed, chew gum or dissolve hard candy in the mouth (see Home Care Checklist: Combating Dry Mouth).
- **Constipation**—It is a good idea to drink plenty of fluids during the day, exercise if approved by the primary health care provider, and eat foods high in fiber.
- **Heat prostration**—Avoid going outside on hot, sunny days; use fans to cool the body if the day is extremely warm; sponge the skin with cool water if other cooling measures are not available; and wear loose-fitting clothes in warm weather.
- **Drowsiness**—Schedule tasks requiring alertness during times when drowsiness does not occur, such as early in the morning before the first dose of the drug is taken.

EDUCATING THE PATIENT RECEIVING A PREOPERATIVE DRUG

When one of these drugs is administered before surgery, the nurse gives the patient an explanation of the preoperative drug: namely, why the drug is being given, when the drug will be given, and when the patient is going to surgery. Sufficient time is allowed for the patient to void before the preoperative drug is administered. The nurse informs the patient and family members that drowsiness and extreme dryness of the mouth and nose will occur about 20 to 30 minutes after the drug is given. The importance of remaining in bed with the side rails raised after the drug is administered is stressed.

EDUCATING THE PATIENT WITH A PEPTIC ULCER

The nurse gives the patient with a peptic ulcer a full explanation of the treatment regimen, which may include drugs and a special diet. The patient is instructed to take the drug exactly as prescribed by the primary health care provider (e.g., 30 minutes before meals or between meals) to obtain the desired results. The nurse discusses the importance of diet in peptic ulcer treatment and gives a full explanation of the special diet (when ordered).

EVALUATION

- The therapeutic effect is achieved.
- Adverse reactions are identified, reported to the primary health care provider, and managed successfully through appropriate nursing interventions.
- Oral mucous membranes remain moist.
- The patient complies with the prescribed drug regimen.
- No evidence of injury is seen.
- The patient and family demonstrate an understanding of the drug regimen.
- The patient verbalizes the importance of complying with the prescribed therapeutic regimen.

Critical Thinking Exercises

1. Mr. Anthony is prescribed a cholinergic blocking drug for the treatment of peptic ulcer. In planning patient teaching for Mr. Anthony before dismissal from the hospital, determine what information must be included to prevent complications of therapy.

2. A nurse assistant asks you what is the purpose of preoperative drugs and why patients cannot get out of bed after receiving a preoperative drug. Describe how you would explain this to the nurse assistant.

3. Mr. Salinas is prescribed a cholinergic blocking drug for a gastric ulcer. You note in the admission interview that he states that he has a history of enlarged prostate. Discuss how Mr. Salinas's history of enlarged prostate relates to the drug therapy for a gastric ulcer.

4. Develop a teaching plan for Ms. Likens, aged 54 years, who will be taking glycopyrrolate (Robinul) for a peptic ulcer. Ms. Likens is alert, well oriented, and teaches at a local high school.

Review Questions

1. A patient taking solifenacin (Vesicare) for an overactive bladder complains of dry mouth. The nurse should _____.
   A. consider this to be unusual and contact the primary health care provider
   B. encourage the patient to take frequent sips of water
   C. give the patient salt-water mouth rinses
   D. ignore this reaction because it is only temporary

2. Which of the following adverse reactions would the nurse expect after the administration of atropine as part of a patient's preoperative medication regimen?
   A. Enhanced action of anesthesia
   B. Reduced secretions of the upper respiratory tract
   C. Prolonged action of the preoperative opioid
   D. Increased gastric motility

3. Because of the effect of cholinergic blocking drugs on intestinal motility, the nurse must monitor the patient taking these drugs for the development of _____.
   A. esophageal ulcers
   B. diarrhea
   C. heartburn
   D. constipation

4. Cholinergic blocking drugs are contraindicated in patients with _____.
   A. gout
   B. glaucoma
   C. diabetes
   D. bradycardia

Medication Dosage Problems

1. A patient is prescribed glycopyrrolate (Robinul) 0.1 mg IM. The drug is available in a solution of 0.2 mg/mL. The nurse administers _____.

2. Oral trihexyphenidyl 4 mg is ordered. The drug is available as an elixir with a strength of 2 mg/5 mL. The nurse administers _____.

To check your answers, see Appendix G.

Cholinergic Blocking Drugs

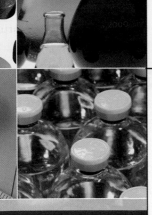

Anticonvulsants

Learning Objectives

On completion of this chapter, the student will:

- List the five types of drugs used as anticonvulsants.
- Discuss the general drug actions, uses, adverse reactions, contraindications, precautions, and interactions of anticonvulsants.
- Discuss important preadministration and ongoing assessment activities the nurse

should perform with the patient receiving an anticonvulsant.

- List nursing diagnoses particular to a patient taking an anticonvulsant.
- Discuss ways to promote an optimal response to therapy, how to manage common adverse reactions when administering the anticonvulsants, and important points to keep in mind when educating a patient about the use of anticonvulsants.

The term **convulsion** refers to a sudden, involuntary contraction of the muscles of the body, often accompanied by loss of consciousness. A **seizure** may be defined as periodic disturbances of the brain's electrical activity. The terms *convulsion* and *seizure* are often used interchangeably, with basically the same meaning. Seizure disorders are generally categorized as idiopathic, hereditary, or acquired. Idiopathic seizures have no known cause; hereditary seizures are passed from parent to child in their genetic makeup; and acquired seizure disorders have a known cause, including high fever, electrolyte imbalances, uremia, hypoglycemia, hypoxia, brain tumors, and some drug withdrawal reactions. The primary goal is to treat the underlying pathologic process to stop the seizures. Sometimes the cause is not clear and the seizures cannot be stopped; rather, the activity needs to be controlled.

Seizures caused by disease, such as epilepsy, may not be easy to eliminate. **Epilepsy** may be defined as a permanent, recurrent seizure disorder. Examples of the known causes of epilepsy include brain injury at birth, head injuries, and inborn errors of metabolism. In some patients, the cause of epilepsy is never determined. Epileptic seizures are classified according to an international system. Each different type of seizure disorder is characterized by a specific pattern of events, as well as a different pattern of motor or sensory manifestation.

Partial seizures are the most common type of epileptic seizure. They arise from a localized area in the brain and cause specific symptoms. Partial seizures include simple seizures in which consciousness is impaired and variable, and **motor seizures** with uncontrolled stiffening or jerking in one part of the body such as the finger, mouth, hand, or foot that may progress to the entire limb. Partial seizures can involve areas of the brain that interpret information; they may present as flashing lights or a change in taste or speech (**somatosensory seizure**).

Generalized seizures involve a loss of consciousness. They may or may not include convulsive movements. Manifestations of a generalized **tonic-clonic seizure** include alternate contraction (tonic phase) and relaxation (clonic phase) of muscles, a loss of consciousness, and abnormal behavior. **Myoclonic seizures** involve sudden, forceful contractions of single or multiple groups of muscles. Other classifications of epileptic seizures include localized epilepsy, generalized epilepsy, special syndromes, and unclassified.

Drugs used for managing seizure disorders are called **anticonvulsants**. Most anticonvulsants have specific uses, that is, they are of value only in treating certain types of seizure disorders. The five drug categories used as anticonvulsants are the barbiturates, benzodiazepines, hydantoins, oxazolidinediones, and the succinimides. In addition, several adjunct drugs are used as anticonvulsants. All possess the ability to depress abnormal neural discharges in the central nervous system (CNS), thereby inhibiting seizure activity.

Actions

Generally, anticonvulsants have the ability to depress abnormal nerve impulse discharges in the CNS.

- *Benzodiazepines* and *barbiturates* inhibit the uptake of GABA (gamma-aminobutyric acid) at receptors.
- *Hydantoins* stabilize the hyperexcitability postsynaptically in the motor cortex of the brain.
- *Oxazolidinediones* decrease repetitive synaptic transmissions of nerve impulses.
- *Succinimides* depress the motor cortex, creating a higher threshold before nerves react to the convulsive stimuli.

Seizures are theoretically reduced in intensity and frequency of occurrence or, in some instances, are virtually eliminated. For some patients, only partial control of the seizure disorder may be obtained with anticonvulsant drug therapy.

Uses

The anticonvulsants are used prophylactically to prevent seizures after trauma or neurosurgery or in patients with tumor, and in the treatment of

- Seizures of all types
- Neuropathic pain
- Bipolar disorders
- Anxiety disorders

Occasionally, **status epilepticus** (an emergency characterized by continual seizure activity with no interruptions) can occur. Diazepam (Valium) is the drug most often prescribed initially for this condition. However, because the effects of diazepam last less than 1 hour, a longer-lasting anticonvulsant, such as phenytoin (Dilantin) or phenobarbital, also must be given to continue to control the seizure activity.

Nursing Alert

Research suggests an association between the use of anticonvulsants by pregnant women with epilepsy and an increased incidence of birth defects in children born to these women. The use of anticonvulsants generally is not discontinued in pregnant women with a history of major seizures because of the danger of precipitating status epilepticus. However, when seizure activity poses no serious threat to the pregnant woman, the primary health care provider may consider discontinuing use of the drug during pregnancy.

Adverse Reactions

Adverse reactions that may occur with the administration of an anticonvulsant drug include

Central Nervous System Reactions

- Drowsiness, weakness, dizziness
- Headache, somnolence
- **Nystagmus** (constant, involuntary movement of the eyeball)
- Ataxia (loss of control of voluntary movements, especially gait)
- Slurred speech

Gastrointestinal Reactions

- Nausea, vomiting
- Anorexia
- Constipation, diarrhea
- **Gingival hyperplasia** (overgrowth of gum tissue)

Other

- Skin rashes, pruritus, urticaria
- Urinary frequency
- Serious skin reactions, such as Stevens-Johnson syndrome, have been associated with the use of lamotrigine (Lamictal)
- Hematologic changes, such as **pancytopenia** (decrease in all the cellular components of the blood), leukopenia, aplastic anemia, and thrombocytopenia, have occurred with administration of selected drugs, including carbamazepine (Tegretol), felbamate (Felbatol), and trimethadione (Tridione)

See the Summary Drug Table: Anticonvulsants for more information.

Anticonvulsants

SUMMARY DRUG TABLE   ANTICONVULSANTS

GENERIC NAME	TRADE NAME	USES	ADVERSE REACTIONS	DOSAGE RANGES
Barbiturates				
phenobarbital *fee-noe-bar'-bi-tal*		Status epilepticus, cortical focal seizures, tonic-clonic seizures	Somnolence, agitation, confusion, ataxia, CNS depression, nervousness, nausea, vomiting, constipation, diarrhea, rash	30–200 mg/d orally BID, TID
phenobarbital sodium	Luminal Sodium	Same as phenobarbital	Same as phenobarbital	30–320 mg IM, IV; may repeat in 6 h
Hydantoins				
ethotoin *eth'-i-toe-in*	Peganone	Tonic-clonic seizures	Ataxia, CNS depression, hypotension, nystagmus, mental confusion, slurred speech, dizziness, drowsiness, gingival hyperplasia, rash	2–3 g/d orally in 4–6 divided doses
fosphenytoin *fos-fen'-i-toe-in*	Cerebyx	Status epilepticus	Same as ethotoin	Loading dose: 15–20 mg/kg IV Maintenance dose: 4–6 mg/kg/d IV
phenytoin sodium, parenteral *fen'-i-toe-in*	Dilantin	Tonic-clonic seizures, status epilepticus, prophylactic seizure prevention	Same as ethotoin	10–15 mg/kg IV
phenytoin sodium, oral *fen'-i-toe-in*	Dilantin	Tonic-clonic seizures, prophylactic seizure prevention	Same as ethotoin	Loading dose: 1 g divided into three doses (400 mg, 300 mg, 300 mg) orally q2h Maintenance dose: started 24 h after loading dose, 300–400 mg/d orally
Succinimides				
ethosuximide *eth-oh-sux'-i-mide*	Zarontin	Partial seizures	Drowsiness, ataxia, dizziness, nausea, vomiting, urinary frequency, pruritus, urticaria, gingival hyperplasia	Up to 1.5 g/d orally in divided doses; children, 250 mg/d orally
methsuximide *meth-sux'-i-mide*	Celontin	Partial seizures	Same as ethosuximide	300–1200 mg/d orally
Oxazolidinediones				
trimethadione *trye-meth-a-dye'-on*	Tridione	Epilepsy	Dizziness, drowsiness, nausea, vomiting, photosensitivity, personality changes, increased irritability, headache, fatigue	900 mg–2.4 g/d orally in equally divided doses

GENERIC NAME	TRADE NAME	USES	ADVERSE REACTIONS	DOSAGE RANGES
Benzodiazepines				
clonazepam *clo-nay'-zeh-pam*	Klonopin	Seizure disorders, panic disorders	Drowsiness, depression, ataxia, anorexia, diarrhea, constipation, dry mouth, palpitations, visual disturbances, rash	Initial dose: do not exceed 1.5 mg/d orally in 3 divided doses; increase in increments of 0.5–1 mg q3d; do not exceed 20 mg/d
clorazepate *klore-az'-e-pate*	Tranxene	Partial seizures, anxiety disorders, alcohol withdrawal	Same as clonazepam	Initial dose: 7.5 mg orally TID, maximum dose 90 mg/d
diazepam *dye-az'-e-pam*	Valium, Diastat	Status epilepticus, seizure disorders (all forms), anxiety disorders, alcohol withdrawal	Same as clonazepam	Seizure control: 2–10 mg/d orally BID to QID Status epilepticus: 5–10 mg IV initially, maximum dose 30 mg Rectally: 0.2–0.5 mg/kg
lorazepam *lor-az'-e-pam*	Ativan	Status epilepticus, preanesthetic	Same as clonazepam	Status epilepticus: 4 mg IV over 2 min
Miscellaneous Preparations				
acetazolamide *ah-see-ta-zol'-a-myde*	Diamox	Epilepsy, altitude sickness	Drowsiness, dizziness, nausea, diarrhea, constipation, visual disturbances	8–30 mg/kg/d in divided doses
carbamazepine *kar-ba-maz'-e-peen*	Tegretol, Epitol	Epilepsy, bipolar disorder, trigeminal/postherpetic neuralgia	Dizziness, nausea, drowsiness, unsteady gait, aplastic anemia and other blood cell abnormalities	Maintenance: 800–1200 mg/d orally in divided doses
felbamate *fell'-ba-mate*	Felbatol	Partial seizures in patients who fail other drug therapy first	Insomnia, headache, anxiety, acne, rash, dyspepsia, vomiting, constipation, diarrhea, upper respiratory tract infection, fatigue, rhinitis, aplastic anemia, hepatic disorders	1200–3600 mg/d orally in divided doses
gabapentin *gab-ah-pen'-tin*	Neurontin	Partial seizures (adults), postherpetic neuralgia	Somnolence, dizziness, ataxia	900–1800 mg/d orally in 3–4 divided doses
lamotrigine *la-mo'-tri-geen*	Lamictal	Partial seizures (used with other anticonvulsants), bipolar disorder	Dizziness, insomnia, somnolence, ataxia, nausea, vomiting, diplopia, headache, Stevens-Johnson Syndrome rash	50–500 mg/d orally in 2 divided doses
magnesium sulfate *mag-nee'-ze-um*		Hypomagnesemia, seizures associated with eclampsia and acute nephritis (children)	Flushing, sweating, hypothermia, depressed reflexes, hypotension, cardiac and CNS depression	Nephritis: 20–40 mg/kg IM in a dilute solution Eclampsia: 4 g IV in dilute solution, titrate continued infusion per serum level
oxcarbazepine *ox-car-baz'-e-peen*	Trileptal	Epilepsy	Headache, dizziness, fatigue, somnolence, ataxia, diplopia, nausea, vomiting, abdominal pain	600–1200 mg orally BID

Anticonvulsants

SUMMARY DRUG TABLE *(continued)*

GENERIC NAME	TRADE NAME	USES	ADVERSE REACTIONS	DOSAGE RANGES
pregabalin *preg'-a-bal-in*	Lyrica	Partial seizures (adults), neuropathic pain, postherpetic neuralgia	Dizziness, somnolence	Seizure activity: 150 mg/d in 2–3 divided doses
primidone *pri'-mi-done*	Mysoline	Epilepsy	Dizziness, somnolence, nausea, vomiting	Up to 500 mg orally QID
tiagabine *tye-ag'-ah-been*	Gabitril	Partial seizures	Dizziness, somnolence, asthenia, nervousness, nausea	4–56 mg/d orally
topiramate *toe-pie'-rah-mate*	Topamax	Partial/tonic-clonic seizures, migraine headache	Fatigue, concentration problems, somnolence, anorexia	Seizure activity: 200–400 mg/d orally in divided doses
valproic acid *val-proe'-ik*	Depakote, Depakene	Epilepsy, migraine headache, mania	Headache, somnolence, dizziness, tremor, nausea, vomiting, diplopia	10–60 mg/kg/d orally; if dosage is more than 250 mg/d, give in divided doses
zonisamide *zoh-niss'-ah-mide*	Zonegran	Partial seizures of epilepsy	Somnolence, anorexia, dizziness, headache, rash, heat stroke	100–400 mg/d orally

CNS, central nervous system.

Contraindications

All categories of anticonvulsants are contraindicated in patients with known hypersensitivity to the drugs. Phenytoin is contraindicated in patients with sinus bradycardia, sinoatrial block, Adams-Stokes syndrome, and second- and third-degree atrioventricular (AV) block; it also is contraindicated during pregnancy and lactation (ethotoin and phenytoin are pregnancy category D drugs). Ethotoin (Peganone) is contraindicated in patients with hepatic abnormalities. The oxazolidinediones have been associated with serious adverse reactions and fetal malformations. They should be used only when other, less toxic drugs are not effective in controlling seizures. The succinimides are contraindicated in patients with bone marrow depression or hepatic or renal impairment. A higher incidence of lupus erythematosus has been found in patients taking succinimides.

Carbamazepine (Tegretol) should not be given within 14 days of monoamine oxidase inhibitor (MAOI) antidepressants. Carbamazepine is contraindicated in patients with bone marrow depression or hepatic or renal impairment and during pregnancy (category D). Valproic acid (Depakote) is not administered to patients with renal impairment or during pregnancy (category D). Oxcarbazepine (Trileptal), a miscellaneous anticonvulsant, may exacerbate dementia.

Precautions

The anticonvulsants should be used cautiously in patients with liver or kidney disease and those with neurologic disorders. The barbiturates (e.g., phenobarbital) are used with caution in patients with pulmonary disease and in hyperactive children. The benzodiazepines are used cautiously during pregnancy (category D) and in patients with psychoses, acute narrow-angle glaucoma, and elderly or debilitated patients. Phenytoin is used cautiously in patients with hypotension, severe myocardial insufficiency, and hepatic impairment. Trimethadione is used with caution in patients with eye disorders (e.g., retinal or optic nerve disease).

The miscellaneous anticonvulsants are used cautiously in patients with glaucoma or increased intraocular pressure; a history of cardiac, renal or liver dysfunction; and psychiatric disorders. In addition to hepatic failure and birth defects, valproic acid is associated with an increased risk for pancreatitis.

Interactions

The following interactions may occur when an anticonvulsant is administered with another agent:

Interacting Drug	Common Use	Effect of Interaction
antibiotics/ antifungals	Fight infection	Increased effect of the anticonvulsant
tricyclic antidepressants	Manage depression	Increased effect of the anticonvulsant
salicylates	Pain relief	Increased effect of the anticonvulsant
cimetidine	Control GI upset	Increased effect of the anticonvulsant
theophylline	Treatment of respiratory problems	Decreased serum levels of the anticonvulsant
antiseizure medications	Reduce seizure activity	May increase seizure activity
protease inhibitors	Treatment of human immunodeficiency virus (HIV) infection	Increased carbamazepine levels, resulting in toxicity
oral contraceptives	Birth control	Decreased effectiveness of birth control, resulting in breakthrough bleeding or pregnancy
analgesics or alcohol	CNS depressants	Increased depressant effect
antidiabetic medications	Manage diabetes mellitus	Increased blood glucose levels

NURSING PROCESS

The Patient Receiving an Anticonvulsant

ASSESSMENT

PREADMINISTRATION ASSESSMENT

Seizures that occur in the outpatient setting are almost always seen first by family members or friends, rather than by a member of the health care profession. The occurrence of abnormal behavior patterns or convulsive movements usually prompts the patient to visit the primary health care provider's office or a neurologic clinic. A thorough patient history is necessary to identify the type of seizure disorder.

- A description of the seizures (the motor or psychic activity occurring during the seizure)
- The frequency of the seizures (approximate number per day)
- The average length of a seizure
- A description of an aura (a subjective sensation preceding a seizure) if any has occurred
- A description of the degree of impairment of consciousness
- A description of what, if anything, appears to bring on the seizure

Information the nurse should obtain from those who have observed the seizure is listed in Display 31-1.

Additional patient information should include a family history of seizures (if any) and recent drug therapy (all drugs currently being used). Depending on the type of seizure disorder, other information may be needed, such as a history of a head or other injury or a thorough medical history.

The nurse obtains the vital signs at the time of the initial assessment to provide baseline data. The primary health care provider may order laboratory and diagnostic tests, such as an electroencephalogram, magnetic resonance imaging (MRI) scan, complete blood count, and hepatic and renal function tests, to confirm the diagnosis and identify a possible cause of the seizure disorder as well as to provide a baseline during therapy with anticonvulsants.

ONGOING ASSESSMENT

Anticonvulsants control, but do not cure, epilepsy. An accurate ongoing assessment is important for obtaining the desired effect of the anticonvulsant. The dosage of the anticonvulsant may require frequent adjustments during the initial treatment period. Dosage adjustments are based on the patient's response to therapy (e.g., the control of the seizures) as well as the occurrence of adverse reactions. Depending on the patient's response to therapy, a second anticonvulsant may be added to the therapeutic regimen, or one anticonvulsant may be changed to another. Regularly, serum plasma levels of the anticonvulsant are measured to monitor for toxicity.

The patient's seizures, along with response to drug therapy, must be observed when a hospitalized patient is receiving an anticonvulsant. The nurse must document each seizure carefully with regard to the time of occurrence, the duration, and the psychic or motor activity occurring before, during, and after the seizure. Most seizures occur without warning, and the nurse may not see the patient until after the seizure has begun or after the seizure is over. However, any observations made during and after the seizure are important and may aid in the diagnosis of the type of seizure, as well as assist the primary health care provider in evaluating the effectiveness of drug therapy.

NURSING DIAGNOSES

Drug-specific nursing diagnoses are highlighted in the Nursing Diagnoses Checklist. Other nursing diagnoses applicable to these drugs are discussed in depth in Chapter 4.

Nursing Diagnoses Checklist

✔ **Risk for Injury** related to seizure disorder, adverse drug reactions (drowsiness, ataxia)

✔ **Risk for Impaired Skin Integrity** related to adverse reactions (rash)

✔ **Impaired Oral Mucous Membranes** related to adverse drug reactions (hydantoins)

✔ **Disturbed Sensory Perception: Visual** related to adverse drug reactions

---

PLANNING

The expected outcomes for the patient depend on the type and severity of the seizure, but may include an optimal response to therapy (control of seizure), support of patient needs related to the management of adverse reactions, and an understanding of and compliance with the prescribed therapeutic regimen.

IMPLEMENTATION

PROMOTING AN OPTIMAL RESPONSE TO THERAPY

When administering an anticonvulsant, the nurse must not omit or miss a dose (except by order of the primary health care provider). An abrupt interruption in therapy by omitting a dose may result in a recurrence of the seizures.

Nursing Alert

Status epilepticus may result from abrupt discontinuation of the drug, even when the anticonvulsant is being administered in small daily doses.

The nurse supports continuity of anticonvulsant administration by making a notation on the care plan, as well as by informing all health care team members of the importance of the drug. If the primary health care provider discontinues the anticonvulsant therapy, the dosage is gradually withdrawn or another drug is gradually substituted.

BARBITURATES The barbiturate phenobarbital (Luminal) is commonly used to treat convulsive disorders. When administering the barbiturates by the intravenous (IV) route, it is important not to exceed a rate of 60 mg/min and to administer the drug within 30 minutes of preparation. The nurse monitors the patient carefully during administration of a barbiturate, taking blood pressure and observing respirations frequently. Resuscitation equipment and artificial ventilation equipment are kept nearby.

Gerontologic Alert

The barbiturates may produce marked excitement, depression, and confusion in the elderly. In some individuals the barbiturates produce excitement, rather than depression. The nurse should monitor the older adult carefully during therapy with the barbiturates and report any unusual effects to the primary health care provider.

BENZODIAZEPINES The dosage of the benzodiazepines is highly individualized, and the nurse must increase the dosage cautiously to avoid adverse reactions, particularly in elderly and debilitated patients. Intravenous (IV) diazepam may bring seizures under control quickly. However, for some patients, seizure activity may resume because of the short duration of the drug effects. The nurse must be prepared to administer another dose of the drug, and the nurse must not mix diazepam with other drugs. When used to control seizures, diazepam is administered by IV push, slowly, allowing at least 1 minute for each 5 mg of drug.

HYDANTOINS Phenytoin is the most commonly prescribed anticonvulsant because of its effectiveness and relatively low toxicity. However, a genetically linked inability to metabolize phenytoin has been identified. For this reason, it is important to monitor serum concentrations of the drug on a regular basis to detect signs of toxicity (slurred speech, ataxia, lethargy, dizziness, nausea, and vomiting). Phenytoin is administered orally and parenterally. When taken orally the drug should be taken with meals to avoid GI upset. If the drug is administered parenterally, the IV route is preferred over the intramuscular (IM) route because erratic absorption of phenytoin causes pain and muscle damage at the injection site.

OXAZOLIDINEDIONES The oxazolidinediones are used only when other, less toxic drugs have not been effective in controlling the seizure disorder because they have been associated with fetal abnormalities and serious adverse reactions.

SUCCINIMIDES The succinimides are easily absorbed in the GI tract and are effective in controlling partial seizures. These drugs are given with food to prevent GI upset.

MISCELLANEOUS ANTICONVULSANTS Valproic acid is unrelated chemically to the other anticonvulsants. This drug is absorbed rapidly when taken orally. Tablets should not be chewed but swallowed whole to avoid irritation to the mouth and throat.

MONITORING AND MANAGING PATIENT NEEDS

RISK FOR INJURY Drowsiness is a common adverse reaction to the anticonvulsant drugs, especially early in therapy. Therefore, the nurse should assist the patient with all ambulatory activities. The nurse helps the patient to rise from the bed slowly and sit for a few minutes before standing. Drowsiness decreases with continued use.

The nurse must use caution when giving an oral preparation because aspiration of the tablet, capsule, or liquid may occur if the patient experiences drowsiness. The nurse tests the swallowing ability of the patient by offering small sips of water before giving the drug. If the patient has difficulty swallowing, the nurse withholds the drug and notifies the primary health care provider as soon as possible. A different route of administration may be necessary. Because injury may occur when the patient has a seizure, the nurse takes precautions to prevent falls and other injuries until seizures are controlled by the drug.

Gerontologic Alert

Older or debilitated adults may require a decreased dosage of diazepam to reduce ataxia and oversedation. The nurse observes these patients carefully. Apnea and cardiac arrest have occurred when diazepam is administered to older adults, very ill patients, and individuals with limited pulmonary reserve.

RISK FOR IMPAIRED SKIN INTEGRITY A severe and potentially fatal rash can occur in patients taking lamotrigine, and the barbiturates also can produce a hypersensitivity rash.

Should a rash occur, the nurse must notify the primary health care provider immediately because the primary health care provider may discontinue the drug. The nurse carefully examines all affected areas and provides an accurate description. If pruritus is present, the nurse keeps the patient's nails short, applies an antiseptic cream (if prescribed), and tells the patient to avoid using soap until the rash subsides.

Nursing Alert

The nurse informs the primary health care provider immediately if a skin reaction occurs. Phenytoin is usually discontinued in such cases. If the rash is exfoliative (red rash with scaling of the skin), purpuric (small hemorrhages or bruising on the skin), or bullous (skin vesicle filled with fluid, i.e., blister), use of the drug is not resumed. If the rash is milder (e.g., acne/sunburn-like), therapy may be resumed after the rash completely disappears.

The nurse must also be alert for the signs of pancytopenia, such as sore throat, fever, general malaise, bleeding of the mucous membranes, epistaxis (bleeding from the nose), and easy bruising. Anticonvulsants such as carbamazepine may cause aplastic anemia and agranulocytosis. The succinimides are also particularly toxic. Routine laboratory tests, such as complete blood counts and differential counts, should be performed periodically. If bone marrow depression is evident (e.g., the patient's platelet count and white blood cell count decrease significantly), the primary health care provider is notified because the drug may be discontinued. When pancytopenia is present and blood cell counts are low, using a soft-bristled toothbrush may protect the mucous membranes from bleeding and easy bruising. The extremities also need to be protected from trauma or injury.

Nursing Alert

Phenytoin can cause hematologic changes (e.g., aplastic anemia, leukopenia, and thrombocytopenia). The nurse should immediately report any signs of thrombocytopenia (bleeding gums, easy bruising, increased menstrual bleeding, tarry stools) or leukopenia (sore throat, chills, swollen glands, excessive fatigue, or shortness of breath) to the primary health care provider.

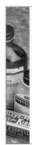

IMPAIRED ORAL MUCOUS MEMBRANE Long-term administration of the hydantoins can cause gingivitis and gingival hyperplasia (overgrowth of gum tissue). It is important periodically to inspect the mouth, teeth, and gums of patients in a hospital or long-term clinical setting who are receiving one of these drugs. Any changes in the gums or teeth are reported to the primary health care provider. Oral care needs to be given after each meal.

> ### Nursing Alert
>
> When administering phenytoin, the nurse closely monitors the patient for the following signs of drug toxicity: slurred speech, ataxia, lethargy, dizziness, nausea, and vomiting. Phenytoin plasma levels between 10 and 20 mcg/mL give optimal anticonvulsant effect. However, many patients achieve seizure control at lower serum concentration levels. Levels greater than 20 mcg/mL are associated with toxicity. Patients with plasma levels greater than 20 mcg/mL may exhibit nystagmus, and at concentrations greater than 30 mcg/mL, ataxia and mental changes are common.

DISTURBED SENSORY PERCEPTION: VISUAL Visual disturbances may occur with anticonvulsant therapy. The patient with a visual disturbance is assisted with ambulation and oriented carefully to the environment. The nurse ensures that the environment is safe. The patient may be especially sensitive to bright lights and may want the room light dimmed. Because photosensitivity can occur, the patient should stay out of the sun if possible and wear sunscreens and protective clothing as needed until the individual effects of the drug are known.

EDUCATING THE PATIENT AND FAMILY

When the patient receives a diagnosis of epilepsy, the nurse must assist the patient and the family to adjust to the diagnosis. The nurse should instruct family members in the care of the patient before, during, and after a seizure. The nurse explains the importance of restricting some activities until the seizures are controlled by drugs. Restriction of activities often depends on the age, sex, and occupation of the patient. For some patients, the restriction of activities may create problems with such activities as employment, management of the home environment, or child care. For example, the patient may be prohibited from driving while the primary health care provider attempts to control the seizure activity. The nurse should assist the patient to look for other modes of transportation in order to continue typical activities or employment. If a problem is recognized, a referral to a social worker, discharge planning coordinator, or public health nurse may be needed.

The nurse reviews adverse drug reactions associated with the prescribed anticonvulsant with the patient and family members. The patient and family members are instructed to contact the primary health care provider if any adverse reactions occur before the next dose of the drug is due. The patient must not stop taking the drug until the problem is discussed with the primary health care provider.

Some patients, once their seizures are under control (e.g., stop occurring or occur less frequently), may have a tendency to stop the drug abruptly or begin to omit a dose occasionally. The drug must never be abruptly discontinued or doses omitted. If the patient experiences drowsiness during initial therapy, a family member should be responsible for administering the drug. The nurse should include the following points in a patient and family teaching plan:

- Do not omit, increase, or decrease the prescribed dose.

- Anticonvulsant blood levels must be monitored at regular intervals, even if the seizures are well controlled.

- This drug should never be abruptly discontinued, except when recommended by the primary health care provider.

- Do not attempt to put anything in the mouth of a person having a seizure.

- If the primary health care provider finds it necessary to stop the drug, another drug usually is prescribed. Start taking this drug immediately (at the time the next dose of the previously used drug was due).

- Anticonvulsant drugs may cause drowsiness or dizziness. Observe caution when performing hazardous tasks. Do not drive unless the adverse reactions of drowsiness, dizziness, or blurred vision are not significant. Driving privileges will be approved or reinstated by the primary health care provider based on seizure control.

- Avoid the use of alcohol unless use has been approved by the primary health care provider.

- Carry medical identification, such as a MedicAlert tag or bracelet, indicating drug use and the type of seizure disorder.

- Do not use any nonprescription drug unless the preparation has been approved by the primary health care provider.

- Keep a record of all seizures (date, time, length), as well as any minor problems (e.g., drowsiness, dizziness, lethargy), and take the record to each clinic or office visit.

- Contact the local branches of agencies, such as the Epilepsy Foundation of America, for information and assistance with problems, such as legal matters, insurance, driver's license, low-cost prescription services, and job training or retraining.

HYDANTOINS

- Inform the dentist and other primary health care providers of use of this drug.

- Brush and floss the teeth after each meal and make periodic dental appointments for oral examination and care.

- Take the medication with food to reduce GI upset.

- Thoroughly shake a phenytoin suspension immediately before use.

- Do not take capsules that are discolored.

- Notify the primary health care provider if any of the following occurs: skin rash, bleeding, swollen or tender gums, yellowish discoloration of the skin or eyes, unexplained fever, sore throat, unusual bleeding or bruising, persistent headache, malaise, or pregnancy.

SUCCINIMIDES

- If GI upset occurs, take the drug with food or milk.

- Notify the primary health care provider if any of the following occurs: skin rash, joint pain, unexplained fever, sore throat, usual bleeding or bruising, drowsiness, dizziness, blurred vision, or pregnancy.

OXAZOLIDINEDIONES

- This drug may cause photosensitivity. Take protective measures (e.g., wear sunscreens and protective clothing) when exposed to ultraviolet light or sunlight until tolerance is determined.

- Notify the primary care provider if the following reactions occur: visual disturbances, excessive drowsiness or dizziness, sore throat, fever, skin rash, pregnancy, malaise, easy bruising, epistaxis, or bleeding tendencies.

- Avoid pregnancy while taking trimethadione; the drug has caused serious birth defects.

EVALUATION

- The therapeutic effect is achieved, and convulsions are controlled.

- No injury is evident.

- Adverse reactions are identified, reported to the primary health care provider, and managed successfully through appropriate nursing interventions.

- The patient verbalizes the importance of complying with the prescribed treatment regimen.

- The patient verbalizes an understanding of treatment modalities and the importance of continued follow-up care.

- The patient and family demonstrate an understanding of the drug regimen.

Critical Thinking Exercises

1. Ms. Taylor tells you that since she has been taking phenytoin she has had no seizures. In fact, she states that she has omitted one or two doses over the last month because she is "doing so well." Explain your response to Ms. Taylor's statement.

2. Mr. Parks, aged 32 years, has recently received a diagnosis of epilepsy. He has been taking the anticonvulsant carbamazepine, but his seizures are not yet under control. Mr. Parks asks you how long it will take to "cure" his epilepsy. Determine how you would respond to Mr. Parks.

3. Develop a teaching plan to educate family members on what to do when the patient has a seizure.

Review Questions

1. A patient is prescribed phenytoin for a recurrent convulsive disorder. The nurse informs the patient that the most common adverse reactions are _____.

   A. related to the gastrointestinal system

   B. associated with the reproductive system

   C. associated with kidney function

   D. related to the central nervous system

2. Which of the following adverse reactions, if observed in a patient prescribed phenytoin, would indicate that the patient may be developing phenytoin toxicity?

   A. Severe occipital headache

   B. Ataxia

   C. Hyperactivity

   D. Somnolence

Anticonvulsants

3. When administering phenobarbital to an elderly patient, the nurse should monitor the patient for unusual effects of the drug such as _____.

   A. marked excitement

   B. excessive sweating

   C. insomnia

   D. agitation

4. When caring for a patient taking a succinimide for seizure control, the nurse monitors the patient for blood dyscrasias. Which of the following symptoms would indicate that the patient may be developing a blood dyscrasia?

   A. Constipation, blood in the stool

   B. Diarrhea, lethargy

   C. Sore throat, general malaise

   D. Hyperthermia, excitement

5. Which statement would be included when educating the patient taking trimethadione for seizures?

   A. Take this drug with milk to enhance absorption.

   B. Wear a sunscreen and protective clothing when exposed to sunlight.

   C. To minimize adverse reactions, take this drug once daily at bedtime.

   D. Visit a dentist frequently because this drug increases the risk of gum disease.

Medication Dosage Problems

1. The nurse is preparing to administer an anticonvulsant for status epilepticus. The primary care provider prescribes phenobarbital sodium (Luminal) 200 mg IV. The drug is available in a dosage of 60 mg/mL. The nurse administers _____.

2. Zonisamide 200 mg is prescribed. The drug is available in 100-mg tablets. The nurse administers _____.

3. The primary care provider prescribes ethosuximide syrup 500 mg for a patient with absence seizures. The drug is available in a strength of 250 mg/5 mL. The nurse administers _____.

To check your answers, see Appendix G.

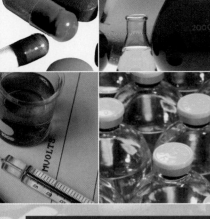

Antiparkinsonism Drugs

Learning Objectives

On completion of this chapter, the student will:

- Define the terms *Parkinson's disease* and *parkinsonism*.
- Discuss the uses, general drug action, adverse drug reactions, contraindications, precautions, and interactions of the antiparkinsonism drugs.
- Discuss important preadministration and ongoing assessment activities

the nurse should perform on the patient taking antiparkinsonism drugs.

- List nursing diagnoses particular to a patient taking antiparkinsonism drugs.
- Discuss ways to promote an optimal response to therapy, how to manage adverse reactions, and important points to keep in mind when educating patients about the use of the antiparkinsonism drugs.

Parkinsonism is a term that refers to a group of symptoms involving motor movement. These are characterized by tremors, rigidity, and slow movement (**bradykinesia**). Although Parkinson-like symptoms may be seen with the use of certain drugs, head injuries, and encephalitis, **Parkinson's disease** is the most common form of parkinsonism. Parkinson's disease is a degenerative disorder of the central nervous system (CNS). The disease is caused by an imbalance of dopamine and acetylcholine in the CNS. An area of the brain, the substantia nigra, loses cells and the supply of the neurotransmitter dopamine is decreased. As a result, too much acetylcholine affects this area of the brain, which controls muscle movement, thus causing such symptoms as trembling, rigidity, difficulty walking, and problems with balance.

Parkinson's disease has no cure, but the antiparkinsonism drugs are used to relieve the symptoms and assist in maintaining the patient's mobility and functioning capability as long as possible. Because Parkinson's disease is progressive, the symptoms worsen over time. Speech becomes slurred, the face takes on a masklike and emotionless expression, and the patient may have difficulty chewing and swallowing. The patient's gait becomes unsteady and shuffled, with the upper part of the body bent forward.

Drugs used to treat the symptoms associated with parkinsonism are called *antiparkinsonism drugs.* These drugs either supplement the dopamine in the brain, or block the excessive acetylcholine so that better transmission of nerve impulses occurs. The Summary Drug Table: Antiparkinsonism Drugs provides a listing of the drugs used to treat Parkinson's disease. Antiparkinsonism drugs discussed in the chapter are classified as dopaminergic agents (monoamine oxidase inhibitors [MAOIs] and dopamine receptor agonists), cholinergic blocking drugs (also known as anticholinergic drugs or cholinergic blockers), catechol-O-methyltransferase (COMT) inhibitors, and non-ergot dopamine receptor agonists.

SUMMARY DRUG TABLE   ANTIPARKINSONISM DRUGS

GENERIC NAME	TRADE NAME	USES	ADVERSE REACTIONS	DOSAGE RANGES
Dopaminergic Agents				
amantadine *a-man'-ta-deen*	Symmetrel	Parkinson's disease/drug-induced EPS, prevention and treatment of infection with influenza A virus	Lightheadedness, dizziness, insomnia, confusion, nausea, constipation, dry mouth, orthostatic hypotension, depression	200–400 mg/d orally in divided doses
bromocriptine *broe-moe-krip'-teen*	Parlodel, Parlodel Snap Tabs	Parkinson's disease, female endocrine imbalances	Drowsiness, sedation, dizziness, faintness, epigastric distress, anorexia	12.5–100 mg/d orally
carbidopa *kar'-bi-doe-pa*	Lodosyn	used with levodopa in the treatment of Parkinson's disease	None if given alone; adverse reactions are those of levodopa	70–100 mg/d orally
carbidopa/levodopa *kar'-bi-doe-pa/lee'-voe-doe-pa*	Sinemet, Sinemet CR, Parcopa, Carbilev	Parkinson's disease	Anorexia, nausea, vomiting, abdominal pain, dysphagia, dry mouth, mental changes, headache, dizziness, increased hand tremor, choreiform or dystonic movements	10 mg/100 mg tablet orally TID, titrated dose combination to minimize symptoms
levodopa *lee'-voe-doe-pa*		Parkinson's disease	Same as carbidopa/levodopa	0.5–1 g/d orally initially, not to exceed 8 g/d
pergolide *per'-goe-lide*	Permax	Agonist for levodopa/carbidopa in Parkinson's disease	Nausea, dyskinesia, dizziness, hallucinations, somnolence, insomnia, rhinitis, constipation	0.05–3 mg/d orally TID
selegiline *sell-eh'-geh-leen*	Eldepryl	Agonist for levodopa/carbidopa in Parkinson's disease	Nausea, dizziness	5 mg orally at breakfast and lunch
Cholinergic Blocking Drugs (Anticholinergics)				
benztropine mesylate *Benz'-tro-peen*	Cogentin	Parkinson's disease, drug-induced EPS	Dry mouth, blurred vision, dizziness, nausea, nervousness, skin rash, urinary retention, dysuria, tachycardia, muscle weakness, disorientation, confusion	0.5–6 mg/d orally Acute dystonia: 1–2 mL IM or IV
biperiden *by-per'-l-den*	Akineton	Parkinson's disease, drug-induced EPS	Same as benztropine mesylate	2 mg orally TID or QID; maximum dose 16 mg/24 h
diphenhydramine *dye-fen-hye'-dra-meen*	Benadryl	Drug-induced EPS, allergies	Same as benztropine mesylate	25–50 mg orally TID or QID
procyclidine *pro-sye'-kli-deen*	Kemadrin	Parkinsonism symptoms, drug-induced EPS	Same as benztropine mesylate	2.5–5 mg orally TID
trihexyphenidyl *trye-hex-ee-fen'-i-dill*		Parkinsonism symptoms, drug-induced EPS	Same as benztropine mesylate	1–15 mg/d orally in divided doses

GENERIC NAME	TRADE NAME	USES	ADVERSE REACTIONS	DOSAGE RANGES
COMT Inhibitors				
entacapone *en-tah-kap'-own*	Comtan	As adjunct to levodopa/carbidopa in Parkinson's disease	Dyskinesia, hyperkinesia, nausea, diarrhea, urine discoloration	200–1600 mg/d orally
tolcapone *toll-kap'own*	Tasmar	Parkinson's disease when refractory to levodopa/carbidopa	Orthostatic hypotension, dyskinesia, sleep disorders, dystonia, excessive dreaming, somnolence, dizziness, nausea, anorexia, muscle cramps	100–200 mg orally TID
Dopamine Receptor Agonists, Non-Ergot				
apomorphine HCl *ay-po-more'-feen*	Apokyn	Parkinson's disease "off" episode	Profound hypotension, nausea, vomiting	0.2 mL as needed for "off" episode
pramipexole *pram-ah-pex'-ole*	Mirapex	Parkinson's disease	Dizziness, somnolence, insomnia, hallucinations, confusion, nausea, dyspepsia, syncope	0.125–1.5 mg orally TID
ropinirole HCl *roe-pin'-o-role*	Requip	Parkinson's disease	Dizziness, somnolence, insomnia, hallucinations, confusion, nausea, dyspepsia, syncope	0.25–1 mg orally TID

EPS, extrapyramidal symptoms.

DOPAMINERGIC DRUGS

Dopaminergic drugs are drugs that affect the dopamine content of the brain. These drugs include levodopa, carbidopa (Lodosyn), amantadine (Symmetrel), and carbidopa/levodopa combination (Sinemet). Other drugs that work to enhance dopamine include agonists such as bromocriptine (Parlodel) or MAOIs such as selegiline (Eldepryl). (See Summary Drug Table: Antiparkinsonism Drugs).

Actions

The symptoms of parkinsonism are caused by a depletion of dopamine in the CNS. It is hard to supplement dopamine because of the **blood–brain barrier**. The blood–brain barrier is a meshwork of tightly packed cells in the walls of the brain's capillaries that screen out certain substances. This unique meshwork of cells in the CNS prohibits large and potentially harmful molecules from crossing into the brain. This ability to screen out certain substances has important implications for drug therapy because some drugs can pass through the blood–brain barrier more easily than others.

Levodopa is a chemical formulation found in plants and animals that is converted into dopamine by the body. Dopamine, in the form of levodopa, crosses the blood–brain barrier only in small quantities. At one time, levodopa, used alone, caused adverse reactions because too much dopamine stayed in the peripheral nervous system. Combining levodopa with another drug (carbidopa) allows more levodopa to reach the brain, which in turn permits the drug to have a better pharmacologic effect in patients with Parkinson's disease (Fig. 32-1). Carbidopa has no effect when given alone. Therefore, the combination makes more levodopa available to the brain, and as a result the dosage of levodopa may be reduced, decreasing peripheral effects. Combination tablets of carbidopa and levodopa are available in several strengths of the two drugs and as a timed-released medication.

Drugs that work to stimulate the dopamine receptors are called *agonists*. These drugs include bromocriptine (Parlodel) and pergolide (Permax). The action of amantadine (Symmetrel) is to make more of the dopamine available at the receptor site, and selegiline (Eldepryl) inhibits monoamine oxidase type B, again making more dopamine available.

Other dopamine receptor agonists are under investigation for use with Parkinson's disease and restless leg syndrome. These agents are not taken orally; instead they are manufactured as a transdermal patch to deliver the medication, which is poorly absorbed when taken by mouth.

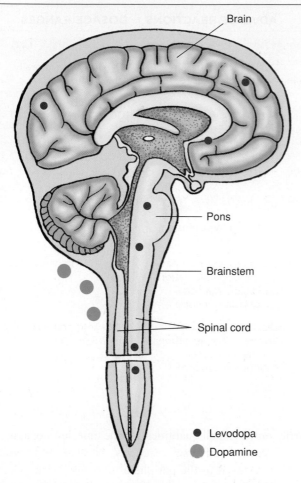

Figure 32.1 The blood–brain barrier selectively inhibits certain substances from entering the interstitial spaces of the brain and spinal fluid. It is thought that certain cells in the brain form tight junctions that prevent or slow the passage of certain substances. Levodopa passes the blood–brain barrier, whereas dopamine is unable to pass.

Uses

The dopaminergic drugs are used to treat the signs and symptoms of parkinsonism and

- Parkinson's disease
- Parkinson-like symptoms (extrapyramidal) as a result of injury, drug therapy, or encephalitis
- Restless leg syndrome
- Viral infections (amantadine)

Adverse Reactions

During early treatment with levodopa/carbidopa, adverse reactions are usually not a problem because of the resolution of Parkinson-like symptoms. As the medication's effectiveness lessens, generalized adverse reactions include

- Dry mouth and difficulty in swallowing
- Anorexia, nausea, and vomiting
- Abdominal pain and constipation
- Increased hand tremor
- Headache and dizziness

The most serious adverse reactions seen with levodopa include **choreiform movements** (involuntary muscular twitching of the limbs or facial muscles) and dystonic movements (muscular spasms most often affecting the tongue, jaw, eyes, and neck). Less common but still serious reactions include mental changes such as depression, psychotic episodes, paranoia, and suicidal tendencies.

Contraindications and Precautions

The dopaminergic drugs are contraindicated in patients with known hypersensitivity to the drugs. Levodopa is contraindicated in patients with narrow-angle glaucoma and those receiving MAOI antidepressants. The patient should be screened for unusual skin lesions because levodopa can activate malignant melanoma. Levodopa is used cautiously in patients with cardiovascular or pulmonary diseases, peptic ulcer disease, renal or hepatic disease, and psychosis. Levodopa and combination antiparkinsonism drugs (e.g., carbidopa/levodopa) are classified in pregnancy category C and are used with caution during pregnancy and lactation.

The dopamine agonist selegiline (Eldepryl) should not be used with the opioid meperidine (Demerol) because of antimetabolite conversion. Caution should be taken with any other opioid used with selegiline.

Interactions

The following interactions may occur when a dopaminergic drug is administered with another agent:

Interacting Drug	Common Use	Effect of Interaction
tricyclic antidepressants	Management of depression	Increased risk of hypertension and dyskinesia
antacids	Relief of gastrointestinal (GI) upset and heartburn	Increased effect of levodopa
anticonvulsants	Seizure control	Decreased effect of levodopa

Foods high in pyridoxine (vitamin B₆) or vitamin B₆ preparations reduce the effect of levodopa. However, when carbidopa is used with levodopa, pyridoxine has no effect on the action of levodopa. In fact, when levodopa and carbidopa are given together, pyridoxine may be prescribed to decrease the adverse effects associated with levodopa.

CHOLINERGIC BLOCKING DRUGS (ANTICHOLINERGICS)

Actions

Acetylcholine (ACh), a neurotransmitter, is produced in excess in Parkinson's disease. Drugs with cholinergic blocking activity block ACh in the CNS, enhancing dopamine transmission. Drugs with cholinergic blocking activity are generally less effective than levodopa in treating parkinsonism and are limited in dose by peripheral adverse reactions. Antihistamines, such as diphenhydramine (Benadryl), are used in elderly patients because they produce fewer adverse effects.

Uses

Drugs with cholinergic blocking activity are used as adjunctive therapy in all forms of parkinsonism and in the control of drug-induced extrapyramidal disorders. Examples of drugs with cholinergic blocking activity include benztropine mesylate (Cogentin), biperiden (Akineton), diphenhydramine, procyclidine (Kemadrin), and trihexyphenidyl. See Summary Drug Table: Antiparkinsonism Drugs for specific uses of these drugs.

Adverse Reactions

Frequently seen adverse reactions to drugs with cholinergic blocking activity include

- Dry mouth
- Blurred vision
- Dizziness, mild nausea, and nervousness

These reactions may become less pronounced as therapy progresses. Other adverse reactions may include

- Skin rash, urticaria (hives)
- Urinary retention, dysuria
- Tachycardia, muscle weakness
- Disorientation and confusion

If any of these reactions are severe, the drug may be discontinued for several days and restarted at a lower dosage, or a different antiparkinsonism drug may be prescribed.

Gerontologic Alert

Individuals older than 60 years frequently develop increased sensitivity to anticholinergic drugs and require careful monitoring. Confusion and disorientation may occur. Lower doses may be required.

Contraindications and Precautions

These drugs are contraindicated in those with a hypersensitivity to the anticholinergic drugs, those with glaucoma (angle-closure glaucoma), pyloric or duodenal obstruction, peptic ulcers, prostatic hypertrophy, **achalasia** (failure of the muscles of the lower esophagus to relax, causing difficulty swallowing), myasthenia gravis, and megacolon.

These drugs are used with caution in patients with tachycardia, cardiac arrhythmias, hypertension, or hypotension, those with a tendency toward urinary retention, those with decreased liver or kidney function, and those with obstructive disease of the urinary system or GI tract. The cholinergic blocking drugs are given with caution to the older adult.

Interactions

The following interactions may occur when a cholinergic blocking drug is administered with another agent:

Interacting Drug	Common Use	Effect of Interaction
amantadine	Treatment of parkinsonism	Increased anticholinergic effects
digoxin	Management of cardiac disease	Increased digoxin serum levels
haloperidol	Antipsychotic agent	Increased psychotic behavior
phenothiazines	Antipsychotic agent	Increased anticholinergic effects

Antiparkinsonism Drugs

COMT INHIBITORS

Another classification of antiparkinsonism drugs is the catechol-O-methyltransferase (COMT) inhibitors. Examples of the COMT inhibitors are entacapone (Comtan) and tolcapone (Tasmar).

Actions

These drugs are thought to prolong the effect of levodopa by blocking an enzyme, COMT, which eliminates dopamine. When given with levodopa, the COMT inhibitors increase the plasma concentrations and duration of action of levodopa.

Uses

The COMT inhibitors are used as adjuncts to levodopa/carbidopa in treating Parkinson's disease. Tolcapone is a potent COMT inhibitor that easily crosses the blood–brain barrier. However, the drug is associated with liver damage and liver failure. Because of the danger to the liver, tolcapone is reserved for people who are not responding to other therapies. Entacapone is a milder COMT inhibitor and is used to help manage fluctuations in the response to levodopa in individuals with Parkinson's disease.

Adverse Reactions

The adverse reactions most often associated with the administration of the COMT inhibitors include
- Dizziness
- Dyskinesias, hyperkinesias
- Nausea, anorexia, and diarrhea

  Other adverse reactions are
- Orthostatic hypotension, sleep disorders, excessive dreaming
- Somnolence and muscle cramps

A serious and possibly fatal adverse reaction that can occur with the administration of tolcapone is liver failure.

Contraindications and Precautions

These drugs are contraindicated in patients with a hypersensitivity to the drugs and during pregnancy and lactation

(pregnancy category C). Tolcapone is contraindicated in patients with liver dysfunction. The COMT inhibitors are used with caution in patients with hypertension, hypotension, and decreased hepatic or renal function.

Interactions

The following interactions may occur when a COMT inhibitor is administered with another agent:

Interacting Drug	Common Use	Effect of Interaction
MAOI antidepressants	Management of depression	Increased risk of toxicity of both drugs
adrenergic drugs	Treatment of cardiac and blood pressure problems	Increased risk of cardiac symptoms

DOPAMINE RECEPTOR AGONISTS

Actions

The exact mechanism of action of the non-ergot dopamine receptor agonists is not understood. It is thought that they act directly on postsynaptic dopamine receptors of nerve cells in the brain, mimicking the effects of dopamine in the brain.

Uses

The dopamine receptor agonists, such as pramipexole (Mirapex) and ropinirole (Requip), are used for the treatment of the signs and symptoms of Parkinson's disease. The drug apomorphine (Apokyn) is used for "on-off" hypomobility episodes. Antiemetic therapy must be initiated with this drug.

Adverse Reactions

The most common adverse reactions seen with pramipexole and ropinirole include
- Nausea, dizziness, vomiting
- Somnolence, hallucinations, confusion, visual disturbances

- Postural hypotension, abnormal involuntary movements
- Headache

Contraindications and Precautions

The dopamine receptor agonists are contraindicated in patients with known hypersensitivity to the drugs. The dopamine receptor agonists are used with caution in patients with dyskinesia, orthostatic hypotension, hepatic or renal impairment, cardiovascular disease, and a history of hallucinations or psychosis. Both ropinirole and pramipexole are pregnancy category C drugs, and safety during pregnancy has not been established.

There is an increased risk of CNS depression when the dopamine receptor agonists are administered with other CNS depressants. When administered with levodopa, the dopamine receptor agonists increase the effects of levodopa (a lower dosage of levodopa may be required). In addition, when the dopamine receptor agonists are administered with levodopa, there is an increased risk of hallucinations. When administered with ciprofloxacin, there is an increased effect of the dopamine receptor agonist.

Interactions

The following interactions may occur when a dopamine receptor agonist is administered with another agent:

Interacting Drug	Common Use	Effect of Interaction
cimetidine, ranitidine	Management of GI problems	Increased dopamine agonist effectiveness
verapamil, quinidine	Management of cardiac problems	Increased dopamine agonist effectiveness
estrogen	Female hormonal supplement	Increased dopamine agonist effectiveness
phenothiazines	Antipsychotic agent	Decreased dopamine agonist effectiveness

NURSING PROCESS

The Patient Receiving an Antiparkinsonism Drug

ASSESSMENT

PREADMINISTRATION ASSESSMENT

Because of memory impairment and alterations in thinking in some patients with parkinsonism, a history obtained from the patient may be unreliable. When necessary, the nurse obtains the health history from a family member. Important data to include are information regarding the symptoms of the disorder, the length of time the symptoms have been present, the ability of the patient to carry on activities of daily living, and the patient's current mental condition (e.g., impairment in memory, signs of depression, or withdrawal).

Before starting the drug therapy, the nurse performs a physical assessment of the patient to provide a baseline for future evaluations of drug therapy. It also is important to include an evaluation of the patient's neuromuscular status. Display 32-1 describes the assessments the nurse would make when evaluating the neurologic and musculoskeletal status.

ONGOING ASSESSMENT

The nurse evaluates the patient's response to drug therapy by observing the patient for various neuromuscular signs (see Display 32-1), and compares these observations with the data obtained during the initial physical assessment. For example, the patient is assessed for clinical improvement of the symptoms of the disease, such as improvement

Display 32.1 Neuromuscular Evaluation

The neuromuscular evaluation includes observation for the following:
- Tremors of the hands or head while the patient is at rest
- A masklike facial expression
- Changes (from the normal) in walking
- Type of speech pattern (halting, monotone)
- Postural deformities
- Muscular rigidity
- Drooling, difficulty in chewing or swallowing
- Changes in thought processes
- Ability of the patient to carry out any or all of the activities of daily living (e.g., bathing, ambulating, dressing)

Antiparkinsonism Drugs

of tremor of head or hands at rest, muscular rigidity, mask-like facial expression, and ambulation stability. Although drug response may occur slowly in some patients, these observations aid the primary health care provider in adjusting the dosage of the drug upward or downward to obtain the desired therapeutic results.

NURSING DIAGNOSES

Drug-specific nursing diagnoses are highlighted in the Nursing Diagnoses Checklist. Other nursing diagnoses applicable to these drugs are discussed in depth in Chapter 4.

Nursing Diagnoses Checklist

✓ **Imbalanced Nutrition: Less Than Body Requirements** related to adverse drug effects (nausea, dry mouth)

✓ **Constipation** related to adverse drug reactions and sluggishness of bowel

✓ **Risk for Injury** related to parkinsonism, adverse drug reactions (dizziness, lightheadedness, orthostatic hypotension, loss of balance)

✓ **Impaired Physical Mobility** related to alterations in balance, unsteady gait, dizziness

---

PLANNING

The expected outcomes for the patient may include an optimal response to drug therapy, support of patient needs related to the management of adverse reactions, absence of injury, and an understanding of and compliance with the prescribed therapeutic regimen.

IMPLEMENTATION

PROMOTING AN OPTIMAL RESPONSE TO THERAPY

Effective management of the patient with parkinsonism requires that the nurse carefully monitor the drug therapy, provide psychological support, and emphasize patient and family teaching. Optimal response to these drugs often requires titration of doses based on patient activities. To find the best response with the fewest adverse reactions, family members may be given a range of drug dosages to administer.

The antiparkinsonism drugs also may be used to treat the symptoms of parkinsonism that occur with the administration of some of the psychotherapeutic drugs. When used for this purpose, the antiparkinsonism drugs may exacerbate mental symptoms and precipitate a psychosis. The nurse must observe the patient's behavior at frequent intervals. If sudden behavioral changes are noted, the nurse withholds the next dose of the drug and immediately notifies the primary health care provider.

MONITORING AND MANAGING PATIENT NEEDS

The nurse observes the patient daily for the development of adverse reactions. All adverse reactions are reported to the primary health care provider because a dosage adjustment or change to a different antiparkinsonism drug may be necessary with the occurrence of the more serious adverse reactions.

Nursing Alert

The nurse observes patients receiving carbidopa/levodopa for the occurrence of choreiform and dystonic movements such as facial grimacing, protruding tongue, exaggerated chewing motions and head movements, and jerking movements of the arms and legs. If these occur, the nurse withholds the next dose of the drug and notifies the primary health care provider immediately because it may be necessary to reduce the dosage of levodopa or discontinue use of the drug.

IMBALANCED NUTRITION: LESS THAN BODY REQUIREMENTS Patients may experience multiple adverse reactions that can affect their dietary intake and cause them to lose weight. Some adverse reactions, although not serious, may be uncomfortable. An example of a less serious but uncomfortable adverse reaction is dryness of the mouth. The nurse can help relieve dry mouth by offering frequent sips of water, ice chips, or hard candy (if allowed). If dry mouth is so severe that there is difficulty in swallowing or speaking, or if loss of appetite and weight loss occur, the dosage of the antiparkinsonism drug may be reduced.

Some patients taking the antiparkinsonism drugs experience GI disturbances such as nausea, vomiting, or constipation. This can affect the patient's nutritional status. It is a good idea for the nurse to create a calm environment, serve small, frequent meals, and serve foods the patient prefers to help improve nutrition. The nurse also may monitor the patient's weight daily. GI disturbances are sometimes helped by taking the drug with meals. Severe nausea or vomiting may necessitate discontinuing the drug and changing to a different antiparkinsonism drug. With continued use of the drug, nausea usually decreases or resolves.

CONSTIPATION Some patients with parkinsonism may have difficulty communicating and are not able to tell the primary health care provider or nurse that problems are occurring. The nurse observes the patient with parkinsonism for outward changes that may indicate one or more adverse reactions. For example, a sudden change in the facial expression or changes in posture may indicate abdominal pain or discomfort, which may be caused by urinary retention, paralytic ileus, or constipation. If constipation is a problem, the nurse stresses the need for a diet high in fiber and increasing fluids in the diet. A stool softener may be needed to help prevent constipation.

Nursing Alert

A serious and potentially fatal adverse reaction to tolcapone is hepatic injury. Regular blood testing to monitor liver function is usually prescribed. The physician may order testing of serum aminotransferase levels at frequent intervals (e.g., every 2 weeks for the first year and every 8 weeks thereafter). Treatment is discontinued if the alanine aminotransferase (ALT; previously, serum glutamic pyruvic transaminase [SGPT]) exceeds the upper normal limit or signs or symptoms of liver failure develop. The patient is observed for persistent nausea, fatigue, lethargy, anorexia, jaundice, dark urine, pruritus, and right upper quadrant tenderness.

RISK FOR INJURY Minimizing the risk for injury is an important aspect in the care of the patient with parkinsonism. The patient with visual difficulties may need assistance with ambulation. Visual difficulties (e.g., adverse reactions of blurred vision and diplopia) may be evidenced only by the patient's sudden refusal to read or watch television or by the patient bumping into objects when ambulating. The nurse carefully evaluates any sudden changes in the patient's behavior or activity and reports them to the primary health care provider. Sudden changes in behavior may indicate hallucinations, depression, or other psychotic episodes.

Gerontologic Alert

Hallucinations occur more often in the older adult than in the younger adult receiving the antiparkinsonism drugs, especially when taking the dopamine receptor agonists. The nurse should assess the older adult for signs of visual, auditory, or tactile hallucinations. The incidence of hallucinations appears to increase with age.

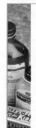

Adverse reactions such as dizziness, muscle weakness, and ataxia (lack of muscular coordination) may further increase difficulty with ambulatory activities. Patients with Parkinson's disease are especially prone to falls and other accidents because of the disease process and possible adverse drug reactions. The nurse assists the patient in getting out of the bed or a chair, walking, and other self-care activities. In addition, assistive devices such as a cane or walker may help with ambulation. The nurse may suggest that the patient wear shoes with rubber soles to minimize the possibility of slipping. The room should be kept well lighted, the use of scatter or throw rugs should be avoided, and any small pieces of furniture or objects that might increase the risk of falling should be removed. The nurse carefully assesses the environment and makes necessary adjustments to ensure the patient's safety.

Patients who are prone to orthostatic hypotension as a result of the drug regimen are instructed to arise slowly from a sitting or lying position, especially after sitting or lying for a prolonged time.

IMPAIRED PHYSICAL MOBILITY The **on-off phenomenon** may occur in patients taking levodopa. In this condition, the patient may suddenly alternate between improved clinical status and loss of therapeutic effect. This effect is associated with long-term levodopa treatment. Low doses of the drug, reserving the drug for severe cases, or the use of a "drug holiday" may be prescribed. Should symptoms occur, the primary health care provider may order a drug holiday that includes complete withdrawal of levodopa for 5 to 14 days, followed by gradually restarting drug therapy at a lower dose. Patients on a drug holiday need to be monitored for complications.

Nursing Alert

Do not abruptly discontinue use of the antiparkinsonism drugs. A neuroleptic malignant-like syndrome may occur when the antiparkinsonism drugs are discontinued or the dosage of levodopa is reduced abruptly. The nurse carefully observes the patient and reports the following symptoms: muscular rigidity, elevated body temperature, and mental changes.

EDUCATING THE PATIENT AND FAMILY

The nurse evaluates the patient's ability to understand the therapeutic drug regimen, ability to perform self-care in the home environment, and ability to comply with the prescribed drug therapy. If any type of assistance is needed, the nurse provides a referral to the discharge planning coordinator or social worker.

Antiparkinsonism Drugs

If the patient requires supervision or help with daily activities and the drug regimen, the nurse encourages the family to create a home environment that is least likely to result in accidents or falls. Changes such as removing throw rugs, installing a hand rail next to the toilet, and moving obstacles that can result in tripping or falling can be made at little or no expense to the family. The nurse should include the following information in the patient and family teaching plan:

- Take this drug as prescribed. Increase, decrease, or omit a dose only as directed by the primary health care provider. If GI upset occurs, take the drug with food.

- If dizziness, drowsiness, or blurred vision occurs, avoid driving or performing other tasks that require alertness.

- Avoid the use of alcohol unless use has been approved by the primary health care provider.

- Relieve dry mouth by sucking on hard candy (unless the patient has diabetes) or frequent sips of water. Consult a dentist if dryness of the mouth interferes with wearing, inserting, or removing dentures or causes other dental problems.

- Inform patients that orthostatic hypotension may develop with or without symptoms of dizziness, nausea, fainting, and sweating. Caution the patient against rising rapidly after sitting or lying down.

- Notify the primary health care provider if any of these problems occur: severe dry mouth, inability to chew or swallow food, inability to urinate, feelings of depression, severe dizziness or drowsiness, rapid or irregular heart beat, abdominal pain, mood changes, and unusual movements of the head, eyes, tongue, neck, arms, legs, feet, mouth, or tongue.

- Keep all appointments with the primary health care provider or clinic personnel because close monitoring of therapy is necessary.

- When taking levodopa, avoid vitamin B_6 (pyridoxine) because this vitamin may interfere with the action of levodopa.

- *Patients with diabetes:* Levodopa may interfere with urine tests for glucose or ketones, if used. Patients who test urine should report any abnormal result to the primary care provider before adjusting the dosage of the antidiabetic medication.

- *Tolcapone:* Keep all appointments with the primary health care provider. Liver function tests are performed periodically and are an important part of therapy. Report any signs of liver failure, such as persistent nausea, fatigue, lethargy, anorexia, jaundice, dark urine, pruritus, and right upper quadrant tenderness.

EVALUATION

- The therapeutic effect is achieved and the symptoms of parkinsonism are controlled.

- Adverse reactions are identified, reported to the primary health care provider, and managed successfully through appropriate nursing interventions.

- No evidence of injury is seen.

- The patient verbalizes an understanding of the treatment modalities, adverse reactions, and importance of continued follow-up care.

- The patient and family demonstrate an understanding of the drug regimen.

Critical Thinking Exercises

1. Ms. Dennis, aged 89 years, has Parkinson's disease and is taking amantadine daily. In discussing her care with the family, determine what information you would include in the teaching plan and what information would be most important for the family to understand. Explain your answer.

2. Ms. Whitman is taking two drugs for Parkinson's disease: levodopa and carbidopa. Ms. Whitman questions you about why she received two drugs while her friend with Parkinson's disease is taking only one drug. Discuss how you would explain this to Ms. Whitman.

3. Discuss the special considerations the nurse should be aware of when administering tolcapone.

4. Explain what adverse reaction would be more likely to occur in the older adult prescribed a non-ergot dopamine receptor agonist drug. Describe how you would assess for this adverse reaction.

Review Questions

1. The most serious adverse reactions seen with levodopa include _____.

   A. choreiform and dystonic movements

   B. depression

   C. suicidal tendencies

   D. paranoia

2. Elderly patients prescribed one of the dopamine receptor agonists are monitored closely for which of the following adverse reactions?

   A. Occipital headache

   B. Hallucinations

   C. Paralytic ileus

   D. Cardiac arrhythmias

3. When taking a cholinergic blocking drug for parkinsonism, the patient would mostly experience which of the following adverse reactions?

   A. Constipation, urinary frequency

   B. Muscle spasm, convulsions

   C. Diarrhea, hypertension

   D. Dry mouth, dizziness

4. The patient taking tolcapone for Parkinson's disease is monitored closely for _____.

   A. kidney dysfunction

   B. liver dysfunction

   C. agranulocytosis

   D. the development of an autoimmune disease

Medication Dosage Problems

1. Oral levodopa 0.75 g is prescribed. The drug is available in 100-mg tablets, 250-mg tablets, and 500-mg tablets. The nurse administers _____.

2. Oral ropinirole 6 mg is prescribed. The drug is available in 2-mg tablets. The nurse administers _____.

To check your answers, see Appendix G.

Antiparkinsonism Drugs

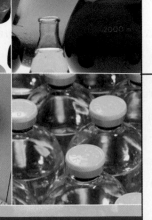

Chapter 33

Cholinesterase Inhibitors

Key Terms

alanine aminotransferase
Alzheimer's disease
dementia

Learning Objectives

On completion of this chapter, the student will:

- Discuss the clinical manifestations of Alzheimer's disease.
- List the uses, general drug actions, general adverse reactions, contraindications, precautions, and interactions associated with the administration of the cholinesterase inhibitors.
- Discuss important preadministration and ongoing assessment activities the

nurse should perform with the patient taking a cholinesterase inhibitor.

- List nursing diagnoses particular to a patient taking a cholinesterase inhibitor.
- Discuss ways to promote an optimal response to therapy, how to manage common adverse reactions, and important points to keep in mind when educating patients about the use of the cholinesterase inhibitors.

Alzheimer's disease (AD) is a progressive deterioration of emotional, physical, and cognitive abilities. Approximately 4 million Americans have the disease. Almost one half of those older than 85 years have AD. Currently it is the ninth leading cause of death in adults older than 65 years. Typically, an individual lives on average 8 years after diagnosis, yet some people have been known to live up to 20 years after AD is discovered. Close to $100 billion has been spent to care for people with AD (both direct and indirect costs).

In AD, specific pathologic changes occur in the cortex of the brain. These changes involve the degeneration of nerves into amyloid plaques and tangled nerve bundles. AD comprises a number of symptoms that become progressively worse in three stages: early, middle, and late. Display 33-1 identifies the stages of AD and their associated clinical manifestations.

Early-stage disease is characterized by difficulties with memory, poor judgment, and withdrawal behaviors. As a person progresses to the middle stage, difficult behaviors appear, such as anger, wandering, and hoarding. Late-stage or the final phase of AD finds the patient becoming increasingly immobile and dysfunctional. This stage may last from a few months to several years.

One of the most debilitating symptoms of AD is dementia. Dementia involves a decrease in cognitive functioning. Drugs that are used to treat AD do not cure the disease but are aimed at slowing the progression of dementia. Cholinesterase inhibitors are used to treat mild to moderate dementia. Examples of the cholinesterase inhibitors include donepezil (Aricept), rivastigmine tartrate (Exelon), and tacrine hydrochloride (Cognex). Other drugs are used for symptomatic relief. For example, wandering, irritability, and aggression in people with AD are treated with the antipsychotics, such as risperidone and olanzapine. Other drugs, such as the antidepressants or antianxiety drugs, may be helpful in AD for symptoms of depression and anxiety; these drugs are all discussed in previous chapters.

Display 33.1 Clinical Manifestations of Alzheimer's Disease

Early Phase–Mild Cognitive Decline

- Increased forgetfulness
- Decreased performance in social settings
- Evidence of memory deficit when interviewed
- Mild to moderate anxiety

Early Dementia Phase–Moderately Severe Cognitive Decline

- Needs assistance for activities of daily living
- Unable to recall important aspects of current life
- Difficulty making choices (e.g., what clothes to wear, what to eat)
- Able to recall major facts (e.g., their name and family members' names)
- Needs assistance for survival

Late Dementia Phase–Severe Cognitive Decline

- Incontinent of urine
- No verbal ability
- No basic psychomotor skills
- Needs assistance when bathing, toileting, and feeding

*Jagust, W. (2002). Alzheimer's disease. Retrieved December 4, 2005, from the Family Caregiver Alliance website: www.caregiver.org/caregiver/jsp/content_node.jsp?nodeid=567

Actions

Acetylcholine is the transmitter in the cholinergic neuropathway. Individuals with early AD experience degeneration of these cholinergic neuropathways. As a result, the patient experiences problems with memory and thinking. The cholinesterase inhibitors act to increase the level of acetylcholine in the central nervous system by inhibiting its breakdown and slowing neural destruction. However, the disease is progressive, and although these drugs alter the progress of the disease, they do not stop it. A newer group of drugs, N-methyl-D-aspartate (NMDA) receptor antagonists, is coming to the marketplace. One drug approved by the U.S. Food and Drug Administration, memantine (Namenda), is thought to work by decreasing the excitability of neurotransmission along GABA (gamma-aminobutyric acid) pathways.

Uses

Cholinesterase inhibitors are used to treat dementia associated with AD.

Adverse Reactions

Generalized adverse reactions include

- Anorexia, nausea, vomiting, diarrhea
- Dizziness and headache

Tacrine is particularly damaging to the liver and can result in hepatotoxicity. Patients taking tacrine should have blood drawn periodically and liver function tests performed. Family members or care providers should be instructed on adverse reactions indicating liver dysfunction such as yellow color to skin or eyes. Additional adverse reactions are listed in the Summary Drug Table: Cholinesterase Inhibitors.

Contraindications and Precautions

The cholinesterase inhibitors are contraindicated in patients with a hypersensitivity to the drugs and during pregnancy and lactation (pregnancy category B). Tacrine should not be used in patients with known liver dysfunction.

These drugs are used cautiously in patients with renal or hepatic disease, bladder obstruction, seizure disorders, sick sinus syndrome, gastrointestinal (GI) bleeding, and asthma. In individuals with a history of ulcer disease, bleeding may recur.

Interactions

The following interactions may occur when a cholinesterase inhibitor is administered with another agent:

Interacting Drug	Common Use	Effect of Interaction
anticholinergics	Decrease of bodily secretions	Decreased effectiveness of anticholinergics
nonsteroidal anti-inflammatory drugs (NSAIDs)	Pain relief	Increased risk of GI bleeding
theophylline	Breathing problems	Increased risk of theophylline toxicity

Cholinesterase Inhibitors

SUMMARY DRUG TABLE   CHOLINESTERASE INHIBITORS

GENERIC NAME	TRADE NAME	USES	ADVERSE REACTIONS	DOSAGE RANGES
donepezil HCl *doe-nep'-ah-zill*	Aricept	Mild to moderate dementia of the Alzheimer's type	Headache, nausea, diarrhea, insomnia, muscle cramps	5–10 mg/d orally
memantine *meh-man'-teen*	Namenda	Moderate to severe dementia of the Alzheimer's type	Dizziness, headache, confusion	20 mg/d orally
rivastigmine tartrate *riv-ah-stig'-meen*	Exelon	Mild to moderate dementia of the Alzheimer's type	Nausea, vomiting, diarrhea, dyspepsia, anorexia, insomnia, fatigue, dizziness, headache	1.5–12 mg/d BID orally
℞ **tacrine HCl** *tay'-krin*	Cognex	Mild to moderate dementia of the Alzheimer's type	Nausea, vomiting, diarrhea, dizziness, headache	40–80 mg/d in 4 divided doses orally

℞ This drug should be administered at least 1 hour before or 2 hours after a meal.

Herbal Alert

Ginseng has been called the "king of herbs" because of its wide use and the benefits attributed to it. In early China, the value of ginseng was as high as that of gold. Ginseng is the fourth best-selling herb in the United States, where hundreds of ginseng products (e.g., teas, chewing gum, juices) are sold. The primary use of ginseng is to improve energy and mental performance. The benefits of ginseng include improving endurance during exercise, reducing fatigue, boosting stamina and reaction times, and increasing feelings of well-being.

Adverse reactions are rare, but sleeplessness, nervousness, and diarrhea have been reported in individuals taking large amounts of the herb. The herb should not be taken in combination with stimulants, including those containing caffeine. Dosage is 200 to 500 mg daily of the standardized extract, or 1 to 4 g of powdered root a day. Ginseng is contraindicated in individuals with high blood pressure and during pregnancy.

Herbal Alert

Ginkgo, one of the oldest herbs in the world, has many beneficial effects. It is thought to improve memory and brain function and enhance circulation to the brain, heart, limbs, and eyes. Most of the research done on ginkgo has been done on standardized extract ginkgo. The recommended dose is 40 mg standardized extract ginkgo three times daily. The effects of ginkgo may not be evident until after 4 to 24 weeks of treatment. The most common adverse reactions include mild GI discomfort, headache, and rash. Excessively large doses have been reported to cause diarrhea, nausea, vomiting, and restlessness. Ginkgo is contraindicated in patients taking monoamine oxidase inhibitors (MAOIs) because of the risk of a toxic reaction. Moreover, individuals taking anticoagulants should take ginkgo only on the advice of a primary care provider.

NURSING PROCESS

The Patient Receiving a Cholinesterase Inhibitor for Mild to Moderate Dementia of Alzheimer's Disease

ASSESSMENT

PREADMINISTRATION ASSESSMENT

A patient receiving a cholinesterase inhibitor may be treated in the hospital, nursing home, or an outpatient setting. The patient's cognitive ability and functional ability are assessed before and during therapy. Cognition can be assessed by using tools such as the Folstein Mini-Mental Status Examination. Patients are assessed on items such as orientation, calculation, recall, and language. Scoring is done by comparison with a standardized answer sheet, and the likelihood of dementia is determined. The nurse assesses the patient for agitation and impulsive behavior. Functional ability, such as performing activities of daily living and self-care, also is assessed. These assessments are used by the nurse in the ongoing monitoring of the patient's improvement (if any) after taking a cholinesterase inhibitor.

Before starting therapy for the hospitalized patient, the nurse obtains a complete mental health and medical history. Often, patients with AD are unable to give a reliable history of their illness. A family member or primary caregiver may be helpful in verifying or providing information needed for an accurate assessment. When taking the history, the nurse observes the patient for any behavior patterns that appear to deviate from normal. Examples of deviations include poor eye contact, failure to answer questions completely, inappropriate answers to questions, monotone speech pattern, and inappropriate laughter, sadness, or crying signifying varying stages of decline. The nurse documents the patient's cognitive ability using Display 33-1 as a guide.

Physical assessments include obtaining blood pressure measurements on both arms with the patient in a sitting position, pulse, respiratory rate, and weight. Assessing the patient's functional ability is also important.

The initial assessments of the outpatient are basically the same as those for the hospitalized patient. The nurse obtains a complete medical history and a history of the symptoms of AD from the patient (if possible), a family member, or the patient's hospital records. During the initial interview, the nurse observes the patient for what appear to be deviations from a normal behavior pattern. The nurse asks the family about unusual behaviors, such as wandering or outbursts of angry or frustrated behavior. The nurse also should assess the patient's vital signs and body weight.

ONGOING ASSESSMENT

Ongoing assessment of patients taking the cholinesterase inhibitors includes both mental and physical assessments. Cognitive and functional abilities are assessed using Display 33-1 as a guide. Initial assessments will be compared with the ongoing assessments to monitor the patient's improvement (if any) after taking the cholinesterase inhibitors.

NURSING DIAGNOSES

Drug-specific nursing diagnoses are highlighted in the Nursing Diagnoses Checklist. Other nursing diagnoses applicable to these drugs are discussed in depth in Chapter 4.

Nursing Diagnoses Checklist

✔ **Imbalanced Nutrition: Less Than Body Requirements** related to adverse reactions (e.g., anorexia, nausea)

✔ **Risk for Injury** related to an adverse drug reaction (e.g., dizziness, syncope, clumsiness) or disease process

---

PLANNING

The expected outcomes for the patient may include an optimal response to drug therapy, support of patient needs related to the management of adverse reactions, an absence of injury, and compliance with the prescribed therapeutic regimen.

IMPLEMENTATION
PROMOTING AN OPTIMAL RESPONSE TO THERAPY

The nurse develops a care plan to meet the patient's individual needs. It is important to monitor vital signs at least daily and to report any significant change in vital signs to the primary health care provider.

Behavioral records should be written at periodic intervals (frequency depends on hospital or unit guidelines). An accurate description of the patient's behavior and cognitive ability aids the primary health care provider in planning therapy and thus becomes an important part of nursing management. Patients with poor response to drug therapy may require dosage changes, discontinuation of the drug therapy, or the addition of other therapies to the treatment regimen. However, it is important to remember that response to these drugs may take several weeks. The symptoms that the patient is experiencing may improve or remain the same, or the patient may experience only a small response to therapy. It is important to remember that a treatment that slows the progression of symptoms in AD is a successful treatment.

When administering tacrine (Cognex), the nurse must monitor the patient for liver damage. This is best accomplished by monitoring levels of **alanine aminotransferase** (ALT), an enzyme found predominantly in the liver. Disease or injury to the liver causes this enzyme to be released into the bloodstream, resulting in elevated serum ALT levels. In patients taking tacrine, ALT levels should be obtained weekly from at least week 4 to week 16 after the initiation of therapy. After week 16, ALT levels are monitored every 3 months.

Nursing Alert

The nurse immediately reports any elevated ALT level to the primary health care provider. The primary health care provider may want to continue monitoring the ALT level or discontinue use of the drug because of the danger of hepatotoxicity. However, abrupt discontinuation may cause a decline in cognitive functioning.

Within 6 weeks of the discontinuation of cholinesterase inhibitor therapy, individuals lose any benefit they have received from the drugs.

MONITORING AND MANAGING PATIENT NEEDS

IMBALANCED NUTRITION: LESS THAN BODY REQUIRE-MENTS When taking the cholinesterase inhibitors, patients may experience nausea and vomiting. Although this can occur with all of the cholinesterase inhibitors, patients taking rivastigmine (Exelon) appear to have more problems with nausea and severe vomiting. Nausea and vomiting should be reported to the primary health care provider who may discontinue use of the drug and then restart the drug therapy at the lowest dose possible. Restarting therapy at the lower dose helps to reduce the nausea and vomiting.

Attention to the dosing of medications can be helpful to decrease the adverse GI reactions and promote nutrition. Donepezil (Aricept) is administered orally once daily at bedtime. It can be taken with or without food.

Rivastigmine (Exelon) is administered as a tablet or oral solution twice daily. When rivastigmine is administered as an oral solution, the nurse removes the oral dosing syringe provided in the protective container. The syringe provided is used to withdraw the prescribed amount. The dose may be swallowed directly from the syringe or first mixed with a small glass of water, cold fruit juice, or soda.

Tacrine (Cognex) is administered orally three or four times a day, preferably on an empty stomach 1 hour before or 2 hours after meals. For best results, the drug should be administered around the clock.

Weight loss and eating problems related to the inability to swallow are two major problems in the late stage of AD. These problems, coupled with the anorexia and nausea associated with administration of the cholinesterase inhibitors, present a challenge for the nurse or caregiver. Mealtime should be simple and calm. The patient should be offered a well-balanced diet with foods that are easy to chew and digest. Frequent, small meals may be tolerated better than three regular meals. Offering foods of different consistency and flavor is important in case the patient can handle one form better than another. Fluid intake of six to eight glasses of water daily is encouraged to prevent dehydration. In later stages, the patient may be fed through a feeding syringe, or the caregiver can encourage chewing action by pressing gently on the bottom of the patient's chin and on the lips.

RISK FOR INJURY. Physical decline and the adverse reactions of dizziness and syncope place the patient at risk for injury. The patient may require assistance by the nurse when ambulating. Assistive devices such as walkers or canes may reduce falls. To minimize the risk of injury, the patient's environment should be controlled and safe. Encouraging the use of side rails, keeping the bed in low position, and using night lights, as well as frequent monitoring by the nurse or caregiver, will reduce the risk of injury. The patient should wear medical identification, such as a MedicAlert bracelet.

EDUCATING THE PATIENT AND FAMILY

Early in the disease the patient may be able to understand changes, yet suspicion and denial are classic symptoms of the disease; therefore, the patient may never comprehend the disease. As cognitive abilities decrease, the nurse focuses on educating the family and major caregiver of the patient needs. Depending on the degree of cognitive decline, the nurse discusses the drug regimen with the patient, family member, or caregiver. It is important for the nurse to evaluate accurately the patient's ability to assume responsibility for taking drugs at home. The administration of drugs to the patient with AD becomes a family responsibility when the outpatient appears to be unable to manage his or her own drug therapy.

The nurse explains any adverse reactions that may occur with a specific drug and encourages the caregiver or family members to contact the primary health care provider immediately when a serious drug reaction occurs.

The nurse includes the following points in a teaching plan for the patient or family member:

- Keep all appointments with the primary care provider or clinic because close monitoring of therapy is essential. Dose changes may be needed to achieve the best results.

- Report any unusual changes or physical effects to the primary health care provider.

- Take the drug exactly as directed. Do not increase, decrease, or omit a dose or discontinue use of this drug unless directed to do so by the primary health care provider.

- Do not drive or perform other hazardous tasks if drowsiness occurs. As soon as the diagnosis of AD is made, patients should not be permitted to drive.

- Do not take any nonprescription drug unless use of a specific drug has been approved by the primary health care provider.

- Inform physicians, dentists, and other medical personnel of therapy with this drug.

- Keep track of when the drug is taken. In the early stages of forgetfulness, a mark on the calendar each time the medicine is taken or a pill counter that holds the medicine for each day of the week may be used to help the patient remember to take the medication or determine whether the medication has been taken for the day.

- Notify the primary care provider if the following adverse reactions are experienced for more than a few days: nausea, diarrhea, difficulty sleeping, vomiting, or loss of appetite.

- Immediately report the occurrence of the following adverse reactions: severe vomiting, dehydration, changes in neurologic functioning, or yellowing of the skin or eyes.

- Notify the primary health care provider if the patient has a history of ulcers, feels faint, experiences severe stomach pains, vomits blood or material that resembles coffee grounds, or has bloody or black stools.

- Remember that these drugs do not cure AD but slow the mental and physical degeneration associated with the disease.

- Remember that during tacrine (Cognex) therapy, the ALT level must be monitored at intervals prescribed by the primary health care provider.

EVALUATION

- The therapeutic effect is achieved.

- Adverse reactions are identified, reported to the primary health care provider, and managed successfully through appropriate nursing interventions.

- No injury is evident.

- The patient (if possible), family member, or caregiver demonstrates understanding of the drug regimen.

Critical Thinking Exercises

1. A patient is prescribed tacrine (Cognex) for mild dementia related to AD. The nurse has a meeting with the patient and family. What patient assessments would you need to make before discussing the drug regimen with the patient? What would you include in a teaching plan for the patient and family?

2. A female patient with AD is taking donepezil (Aricept). She attends an adult day care center during the day. She is not eating well and recently has lost 5 pounds. If you are the nurse at the center, what actions would you take, and why would you take these particular actions?

Review Questions

1. Adverse reactions that the nurse would assess for in a patient taking rivastigmine (Exelon) include _____.

   A. occipital headache

   B. vomiting

   C. hyperactivity

   D. hypoactivity

2. When administering tacrine (Cognex) to a patient with AD, the nurse would most likely expect which laboratory tests to be prescribed?

   A. A complete blood count

   B. Cholesterol levels

   C. Liver function studies

   D. Electrolyte analysis

3. Which of the following nursing diagnoses would the nurse most likely place on the care plan of a patient with AD that is related to adverse reactions of the cholinesterase inhibitors?

   A. Imbalanced Nutrition

   B. Confusion

   C. Risk for Suicide

   D. Bowel Incontinence

4. The nurse correctly administers donepezil (Aricept) _____.

   A. three times daily around the clock

   B. twice daily 1 hour before meals or 2 hours after meals

   C. once daily in the morning

   D. once daily at bedtime

Medication Dosage Problems

1. Rivastigmine (Exelon) oral solution 6 mg is prescribed. The drug is available as an oral solution of 2 mg/mL. The nurse administers _____.

2. Oral memantine (Namenda) 10 mg is prescribed for a patient with AD. On hand are 5-mg tablets. The nurse administers _____.

To check your answers, see Appendix G.

Cholinesterase Inhibitors

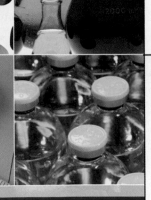
Drugs Used to Treat Disorders of the Musculoskeletal System

Learning Objectives

On completion of this chapter, the student will:

- List the types of drugs used to treat musculoskeletal disorders.

- Discuss the uses, general drug actions, adverse reactions, contraindications, precautions, and interactions of the drugs used to treat musculoskeletal disorders.

- Discuss important preadministration and ongoing assessment activities the nurse should perform on the patient taking drugs used to treat musculoskeletal disorders.

- List nursing diagnoses particular to a patient taking a drug for the treatment of musculoskeletal disorders.

- Discuss ways to promote an optimal response to therapy, how to manage adverse reactions, and important points to keep in mind when educating the patient about drugs used to treat musculoskeletal disorders.

A variety of drugs are used in treating **musculoskeletal** (bone and muscle) disorders. Examples of the drugs discussed for musculoskeletal disorders in this chapter include bone resorption inhibitors (used to treat osteoporosis), disease-modifying antirheumatic drugs (DMARDs; used to treat rheumatoid arthritis), and uric acid inhibitors (used to treat gout). A description of these and other musculoskeletal disorders is given in Table 34-1. The drug selected is based on the musculoskeletal disorder being treated, the severity of the disorder, and the patient's positive or negative response to past therapy. For example, early cases of rheumatoid arthritis may respond well to the nonsteroidal antiinflammatory drugs (NSAIDs), whereas advanced rheumatoid arthritis not responding to other drug therapies may require the use of corticosteroids or immunosuppressive drugs.

The salicylates and NSAIDs are important agents used in treating arthritic conditions. For example, the salicylates and NSAIDs are used for **rheumatoid arthritis** (a chronic disease characterized by inflammatory changes in the body's connective tissue) and **osteoarthritis** (a noninflammatory joint disease resulting in degeneration of the articular cartilage and changes in the synovial membrane), as well as for relief of pain or discomfort resulting from musculoskeletal injuries such as sprains.

Table 34.1 Selected Musculoskeletal Disorders

Disorder	Description
Synovitis	An inflammation of the synovial membrane of a joint resulting in pain, swelling, and inflammation. It occurs in disorders such as rheumatic fever, rheumatoid arthritis, and gout.
Arthritis	The inflammation of a joint. The term is frequently used to refer to any disease involving pain or stiffness of the musculoskeletal system.
Osteoarthritis or degenerative joint disease (DJD)	A noninflammatory DJD marked by degeneration of the articular cartilage, changes in the synovial membrane, and hypertrophy of the bone at the margins.
Rheumatoid arthritis (RA)	A chronic systemic disease that produces inflammatory changes throughout the connective tissue in the body. It affects joints and other organ systems of the body. Destruction of articular cartilage occurs, affecting joint structure and mobility. RA primarily affects individuals between 20 and 40 years of age.
Gout	A form of arthritis in which uric acid accumulates in increased amounts in the blood and often is deposited in the joints. The deposit or collection of urate crystals in the joints causes the symptoms (pain, redness, swelling, joint deformity).
Osteoporosis	A loss of bone density occurring when the loss of bone substance exceeds the rate of bone formation. Bones become porous, brittle, and fragile. Compression fractures of the vertebrae are common. This disorder occurs most often in postmenopausal women, but can occur in men as well.
Hypercalcemia of malignancy	Associated with advanced-stage malignant disease. It can occur with 10%–50% of tumors. It is associated with parathyroid hormone production and can be difficult to manage. Symptoms include lethargy, anorexia, nausea, vomiting, thirst, polydipsia, constipation, and dehydration. If untreated, it may lead to cognitive difficulties, confusion, obtundation (extreme dullness, near-coma), and coma.
Paget's disease (osteitis deformans)	A chronic bone disorder characterized by abnormal bone remodeling. The disease disrupts the growth of new bone tissue, causing the bone to thicken and become soft. This weakens the bone, which increases susceptibility to fracture or collapse of the bone (e.g., the vertebrae) even with slight trauma.

BONE RESORPTION INHIBITORS: BISPHOSPHONATES

The bisphosphonates are drugs used to treat musculoskeletal disorders such as osteoporosis and Paget's disease.

Actions

The bisphosphonates act primarily on the bone by inhibiting normal and abnormal bone resorption. This results in increased bone mineral density, reversing the progression of osteoporosis.

Uses

The bisphosphonates are used in the treatment of
- Osteoporosis in postmenopausal women and men
- Hypercalcemia of malignant diseases
- Paget's disease of the bone

Adverse Reactions

Adverse reactions with the bisphosphonates include
- Nausea, diarrhea
- Increased or recurrent bone pain
- Headache
- Dyspepsia, acid regurgitation, dysphagia
- Abdominal pain

Contraindications and Precautions

These drugs are contraindicated in patients who are hypersensitive to the bisphosphonates. Alendronate (Fosamax) and risedronate (Actonel) are contraindicated in patients with hypocalcemia. Alendronate is a pregnancy category C drug and is contraindicated during pregnancy. These drugs are also contraindicated in patients with delayed esophageal emptying or renal impairment. Concurrent use of these drugs with hormone replacement therapy is not recommended.

These drugs are used cautiously in patients with gastrointestinal (GI) disorders or renal impairment. Although these drugs have not been studied, if a pregnant woman presents with malignancy, their use during the pregnancy may be justified if the potential benefit outweighs the potential risk to the fetus.

Interactions

The following interactions may occur when a bisphosphonate is administered with another agent:

Interacting Drug	Common Use	Effect of Interaction
calcium supplements or antacids with magnesium and aluminum	Relief of gastric upset	Decreased effectiveness of bisphosphonates
aspirin	Pain relief	Increased risk of GI bleeding
theophylline	Breathing problems	Increased risk of theophylline toxicity

DRUGS USED TO TREAT RHEUMATOID ARTHRITIS

Rheumatoid arthritis (RA), a chronic disorder involving the inflammation and accumulation of fluid in joints, is considered an autoimmune disease. This condition is typically treated using three classifications of drugs: NSAIDs, corticosteroids, and DMARDs. The NSAIDs and corticosteroids are discussed in Chapters 18 and 50, respectively.

DISEASE-MODIFYING ANTIRHEUMATIC DRUGS
Actions and Uses

Because RA is an autoimmune disorder, antibodies are formed against one's own body. As a defense mechanism, white blood cells are mobilized and lodge in the joints, causing swelling, pain, and inflammation. When the immobility and pain of RA can no longer be controlled by pain relief agents and anti-inflammatory drugs, DMARDs

are used. These drugs have properties to produce immunosuppression, which in turn decreases the body's autoimmune response. Therefore, in RA treatment, the DMARDs are useful for their immunosuppressive ability. (DMARDs may also be used for other purposes, such as cancer therapy, in which the immunosuppression is considered an adverse reaction rather than an intended effect.)

Cytotoxic drugs, such as azathioprine (Imuran), cyclophosphamide (Cytoxan), and cyclosporine, are reserved for life-threatening problems (such as systemic vasculitis) because they are associated with a high rate of toxic adverse reactions. Gold salts and penicillamine are considered extremely toxic and used only when other drugs fail to achieve remission.

Adverse Reactions

The immunosuppressive drugs can cause
- Nausea
- Stomatitis
- **Alopecia** (hair loss)

The adverse reactions to the sulfa-based drug include ocular changes, GI upset, and mild pancytopenia. The most common adverse reaction to the drugs given by injection is skin irritation. For more information, see the Summary Drug Table: Drugs Used to Treat Musculoskeletal Disorders.

Contraindications

All categories of DMARDs are contraindicated in patients with known hypersensitivity to the drugs. Patients with renal insufficiency, liver disease, alcohol abuse, pancytopenia, or folate deficiency should not take methotrexate. Etanercept (Enbrel), adalimumab (Humira), and infliximab (Remicade) should not be used in patients with congestive heart failure or neurologic demyelinating diseases. Anakinra (Kineret) should not be used in combination with etanercept (Enbrel), adalimumab (Humira), or infliximab (Remicade).

Precautions

These drugs should be used with caution in patients with obesity, diabetes, and hepatitis B or C. Women should not become pregnant, and sexual partners should use barrier contraception to prevent transmission of the drug by semen.

SUMMARY DRUG TABLE DRUGS USED TO TREAT MUSCULOSKELETAL DISORDERS

GENERIC NAME	TRADE NAME	USES	ADVERSE REACTIONS	DOSAGE RANGES
Bone Resorption Inhibitors: Bisphosphonates				
alendronate sodium *ah-len'-dro-nate*	Fosamax	Treatment and prevention of postmenopausal osteoporosis; glucocorticoid-induced osteoporosis; osteoporosis in men; Paget's disease	Abdominal pain, esophageal reflux	35–70 mg/wk or 10 mg/d orally
Ⓡ **etidronate** *e-tid'-ro-nate*	Didronel	Hypercalcemia of malignancy, Paget's disease, prevent bone spurs after total hip replacement	Nausea, fever, fluid overload	5–20 mg/kg/d orally (treatment not to exceed 6 mo)
ibandronate *ih-ban'-dro-nate*	Boniva	Postmenopausal osteoporosis	Abdominal pain, nausea, diarrhea	2.5 mg/d orally, available in 150-mg tablet taken once monthly
pamidronate *pa-mid'-ro-nate*	Aredia	Hypercalcemia of malignancy, Paget's disease	Anxiety, headache, insomnia, nausea, vomiting, diarrhea, constipation, dyspepsia, pancytopenia, fever, fatigue, bone pain	60–90 mg in a single IV dose infused over 2–24 h
risedronate sodium *rah-sed'-ro-nate*	Actonel	Treatment and prevention of postmenopausal osteoporosis, glucocorticoid induced osteoporosis, Paget's disease	Headache, abdominal pain, arthralgia, recurrent bone pain, nausea, diarrhea	Osteoporosis: 5 mg/d orally Paget's disease: 30 mg/d orally for 2 mo
tiludronate disodium *tih-loo'-dro-nate*	Skelid	Paget's disease	Headache, nausea, diarrhea, arthralgia, pain	400 mg/d orally for no more than 3 mo
zoledronic acid *zole-eh-dron'-ic*	Zometa	Hypercalcemia of malignancy	Hypotension, confusion, anxiety, agitation, nausea, diarrhea, constipation, fatigue	4 mg in a single IV dose infused over 15 min
Disease-Modifying Antirheumatic Drugs (DMARDs)				
adalimumab	Humira	Rheumatoid arthritis	Irritation at injection site, increased risk of infections	40 mg SC every other week
anakinra *ann-ack'-in-rah*	Kineret	Rheumatoid arthritis	Headache, irritation at injection site, pancytopenia	100 mg SC daily
etanercept *ee-tah-ner'-sept*	Enbrel	Rheumatoid arthritis	Headache, rhinitis, irritation at injection site, increased risk of infections	25 mg SC twice weekly, or 50 mg SC weekly
hydroxychloroquine sulfate *hye-drox-ee-klor'-oh-kwin*	Plaquenil	Rheumatoid arthritis, antimalarial	Irritability nervousness, retinal and corneal changes, anorexia, nausea, vomiting, hematologic effects	400–600 mg/d orally

⬤ SUMMARY DRUG TABLE *(continued)*

GENERIC NAME	TRADE NAME	USES	ADVERSE REACTIONS	DOSAGE RANGES
infliximab *in-flicks'-ee-mab*	Remicade	Rheumatoid arthritis in combination with methotrexate, Crohn's disease	Fever, chills, headache	3–10 mg/kg IV infusion at specified weekly intervals
leflunomide *le-flu'-no-mide*	Arava	Rheumatoid arthritis	Hypertension, alopecia, rash, nausea, diarrhea	Initial dose: 100 mg for 3 d Maintenance dose: 20 mg/d orally
methotrexate (MTX) *meth-oh-trex'-ate*	Rheumatrex	Rheumatoid arthritis, cancer chemotherapy	Nausea, stomatitis, alopecia	7.5–20 mg orally once weekly
sulfasalazine *sul-fa-sal'-a-zeen*	Azulfidine	Rheumatoid arthritis, ulcerative colitis	Nausea, emesis, abdominal pains, crystalluria, hematuria, Stevens-Johnson syndrome, rash, headache, drowsiness, diarrhea	2–4 g/d orally in divided doses
Uric Acid Inhibitors				
allopurinol *al-oh-pure'-i-nole*	Zyloprim	Management of symptoms of gout	Rash, exfoliative dermatitis, Stevens-Johnson syndrome, nausea, vomiting, diarrhea, abdominal pain, hematologic changes	100–800 mg/d orally
colchicine *kol'-chi-seen*		Relief of acute attacks of gout, prevention of gout attacks	Nausea, vomiting, diarrhea, abdominal pain, bone marrow depression	Acute attack: initial dose 0.5–1.2 mg orally or 2 mg IV, then 0.5–1.2 mg orally q1–2h or 0.5 mg IV q6h until attack is aborted or adverse effects occur Prophylaxis: 0.5–0.6 mg/d orally
probenecid *proe-ben'-e-sid*	Benemid	Treatment of hyperuricemia of gout and gouty arthritis	Headache, anorexia, nausea, vomiting, urinary frequency, flushing, dizziness	0.25 mg orally BID for 1 wk, then 0.5 mg orally BID
sulfinpyrazone *sul-fin-peer'-a-zone*	Anturane	Treatment of gouty arthritis	Upper GI disturbances, rash	200–400 mg/d orally BID
Skeletal Muscle Relaxants				
baclofen *bak'-loe-fen*	Lioresal	Spasticity due to multiple sclerosis, spinal cord injuries (intrathecal administration)	Drowsiness, dizziness, nausea, weakness, hypotension	15–80 mg/d orally in divided doses
carisoprodol *ker-eye-soe-proe'-dol*	Soma	Relief of discomfort due to acute, painful musculoskeletal conditions	Dizziness, drowsiness, tachycardia, nausea, vomiting	350 mg orally TID or QID
chlorzoxazone *klor-zox'-a-zone*	Parafon Forte DSC	Same as carisoprodol	GI disturbances, drowsiness, dizziness, rash	250–750 mg orally TID or QID
cyclobenzaprine HCl *sye-kloe-ben'-za-preen*	Flexeril	Same as carisoprodol	Drowsiness, dizziness, dry mouth, nausea, constipation	10–60 mg/d orally in divided doses

GENERIC NAME	TRADE NAME	USES	ADVERSE REACTIONS	DOSAGE RANGES
dantrolene sodium *dan'-troe-leen*	Dantrium	Spasticity due to spinal cord injury, stroke, cerebral palsy, multiple sclerosis	Drowsiness, dizziness, weakness, constipation, tachycardia, malaise	Initial dose: 25 mg/d orally, then 50–400 mg/d orally in divided doses
diazepam *dye-az'-e-pam*	Valium	Relief of skeletal muscle spasm, spasticity due to cerebral palsy, epilepsy, paraplegia, anxiety	Drowsiness, sedation, sleepiness, lethargy, constipation, diarrhea, bradycardia, tachycardia, rash	2–10 mg orally BID–QID; 2–20 mg IM, IV Sustained release, 15–30 mg/d orally
methocarbamol *meth-oh-kar'-ba-mol*	Robaxin	Relief of discomfort due to musculoskeletal disorders	Drowsiness, dizziness, lightheadedness, confusion, headache, rash, blurred vision, GI upset	1–1.5 g QID orally; up to 3 g/d IM, IV
orphenadrine citrate *or-fen'-a-dreen*	Banflex, Flexojet, Flexon, Norflex	Discomfort due to musculoskeletal disorders	Drowsiness, dizziness, lightheadedness, confusion, headache, rash, blurred vision, GI upset	100 mg BID orally; 60 mg IV or IM q12h
tizanidine *tis-an'-i-deen*	Zanaflex	Spasticity due to spinal cord injury	Somnolence, fatigue, dizziness, dry mouth, urinary tract infections	4–8 mg orally up to TID

GI, gastrointestinal.

Ⓡ This drug should be administered at least 1 hour before or 2 hours after a meal.

Sulfasalazine is selected over methotrexate for patients with liver disease. Patients taking etanercept (Enbrel), adalimumab (Humira), or infliximab (Remicade) should be screened for preexisting tuberculosis because of the increase in opportunistic infections presenting after treatment.

Interactions

The following interactions may occur when a DMARD, such as methotrexate, is administered with another agent:

Interacting Drug	Common Use	Effect of Interaction
sulfa antibiotics	Fight infection	Increased risk of methotrexate toxicity
aspirin and NSAIDs	Pain relief	Increased risk of methotrexate toxicity

URIC ACID INHIBITORS

Gout is a condition in which uric acid accumulates in increased amounts in the blood and often is deposited in the joints. The deposit or collection of urate crystals in the joints causes the symptoms (pain, redness, swelling, joint deformity) of gout.

Actions

Allopurinol (Zyloprim) reduces the production of uric acid, thereby decreasing serum uric acid levels and the deposit of urate crystals in joints. This probably accounts for its ability to relieve the severe pain of acute gout.

The exact mechanism of action of colchicine is unknown, but it does reduce the inflammation associated with the deposit of urate crystals in the joints. Colchicine has no effect on uric acid metabolism.

In people with gout, the serum uric acid level is usually elevated. Sulfinpyrazone (Anturane) increases the excretion of uric acid by the kidneys, which lowers serum uric acid levels and consequently retards the deposit of urate crystals in the joints. Probenecid (Benemid) works in the same manner and may be given alone or with colchicine as combination therapy when there are frequent, recurrent attacks of gout. Probenecid also has been used to prolong the plasma levels of the penicillins and cephalosporins.

Drugs Used to Treat Musculoskeletal Disorders

Uses

Drugs indicated for treatment of gout may be used to manage acute attacks of gout or in preventing acute attacks of gout (prophylaxis).

Adverse Reactions

Gastrointestinal Reactions

- Nausea, vomiting, diarrhea
- Abdominal pain

Other

- Headache
- Urinary frequency

One adverse reaction associated with allopurinol is skin rash, which in some cases has been followed by serious hypersensitivity reactions, such as exfoliative dermatitis and Stevens-Johnson syndrome. Colchicine administration may result in severe nausea, vomiting, and bone marrow depression; therefore, it is used as a second line of treatment when other drugs fail.

Contraindications

The drugs used for gout are contraindicated in patients with known hypersensitivity. Sulfinpyrazone is contraindicated in patients with peptic ulcer disease and GI inflammation. Colchicine is contraindicated in patients with serious GI, renal, hepatic, or cardiac disorders and those with blood dyscrasias. Probenecid is contraindicated in patients with blood dyscrasias or uric acid kidney stones, and in children younger than 2 years.

Precautions

Uric acid inhibitors are used cautiously in patients with renal impairment and during pregnancy; these agents are either pregnancy category B or C drugs. Allopurinol is used cautiously in patients with liver impairment. Probenecid is used cautiously in patients who are hypersensitive to sulfa drugs or have peptic ulcer disease. Colchicine is used with caution in older adults.

Interactions

The following interactions may occur when a uric acid inhibitor is administered with another agent:

Interacting Drug	Common Use	Effect of Interaction
allopurinol		
ampicillin	Anti-infective agent	Increased risk of rash
theophylline	Breathing problems	Increased risk of theophylline toxicity
aluminum-based antacids	Relief of gastric upset	Decreased effectiveness of allopurinol
probenecid		
penicillins, cephalosporins, acyclovir, rifampin, and the sulfonamides	Anti-infective agent	Increased serum level of anti-infective
barbiturates and benzodiazepines	Sedation	Increased serum level of sedative
NSAIDs	Pain relief	Increased serum level of NSAID
salicylates	Pain relief	Decreased effectiveness of probenecid
sulfinpyrazone		
oral anticoagulants	Blood thinner	Increased risk of bleeding
tolbutamide	Antidiabetic agent	Increased risk of hypoglycemia
verapamil	Management of heart problems	Increased effectiveness of verapamil

SKELETAL MUSCLE RELAXANTS

Actions

The mode of action of many skeletal muscle relaxants, such as carisoprodol (Soma), baclofen (Lioresal), and chlorzoxazone (Parafon Forte), is not clearly understood. Many of these drugs do not directly relax skeletal muscles, but their ability to relieve acute painful musculoskeletal conditions may be due to their sedative action. Cyclobenzaprine (Flexeril) appears to have an effect on muscle tone, thereby reducing muscle spasm.

The exact mode of action of diazepam (Valium), an antianxiety drug (see Chapter 22), in the relief of painful musculoskeletal conditions is unknown. The drug does have a sedative action, which may account for some of its ability to relieve muscle spasm and pain.

Uses

Skeletal muscle relaxants are used in various acute painful musculoskeletal conditions, such as muscle strains and back pain.

Adverse Reactions

Drowsiness is the most common reaction seen with the use of skeletal muscle relaxants. Additional adverse reactions are given in the Summary Drug Table: Drugs Used to Treat Musculoskeletal Disorders. Some of the adverse reactions that may occur with the administration of diazepam include drowsiness, sedation, sleepiness, lethargy, constipation or diarrhea, bradycardia or tachycardia, and rash.

Contraindications

The skeletal muscle relaxants are contraindicated in patients with known hypersensitivity to the drugs. Baclofen is contraindicated in skeletal muscle spasms caused by rheumatic disorders. Carisoprodol is contraindicated in patients with a known hypersensitivity to meprobamate. Cyclobenzaprine is contraindicated in patients with a recent myocardial infarction, cardiac conduction disorders, and hyperthyroidism. In addition, cyclobenzaprine is contraindicated within 14 days of the administration of a monoamine oxidase inhibitor (MAOI). Oral dantrolene is contraindicated during lactation and in patients with active hepatic disease and muscle spasm caused by rheumatic disorders.

Precautions

The skeletal muscle relaxants are used with caution in patients with a history of cerebrovascular accident, cerebral palsy, parkinsonism, or seizure disorders and during pregnancy and lactation (pregnancy category C). Carisoprodol is used with caution in patients with severe liver or kidney disease and during pregnancy (category unknown) and lactation. Cyclobenzaprine is used cau-

tiously in patients with cardiovascular disease and during pregnancy and lactation (pregnancy category B). Dantrolene, a pregnancy category C drug, is used with caution during pregnancy.

Interactions

The following interactions may occur when a skeletal muscle relaxant is administered with another agent:

Interacting Drug	Common Use	Effect of Interaction
Central nervous system (CNS) depressants, such as alcohol, antihistamines, opiates, and sedatives	To promote a calming effect or provide pain relief	Increased CNS depressant effect
cyclobenzaprine		
MAOIs	Manage depression	Risk for high fever and convulsions
orphenadrine		
haloperidol	Treat psychotic behavior	Increased psychosis
tizanidine		
antihypertensives	Blood pressure reduction	Increased risk of hypotension

Health Supplement Alert

Glucosamine and *chondroitin* are used, in combination or alone, to treat arthritis, particularly osteoarthritis. Chondroitin acts as the flexible connecting matrix between the protein filaments in cartilage. Chondroitin can be produced in the laboratory or can come from natural sources (e.g., shark cartilage). Some studies suggest that if chondroitin sulfate is available to the cell matrix, synthesis of tissue can occur. For this reason it is used to treat arthritis. Although there is little information on chondroitin's long-term effects, it is generally not considered to be harmful.

Glucosamine is found in mucopolysaccharides, mucoproteins, and chitin. Chitin is found in various marine invertebrates and other lower animals and members of the plant family. In

Health Supplement Alert (continued)

osteoarthritis there is a progressive degeneration of cartilage glycosaminoglycans. Oral glucosamine theoretically provides a building block for regeneration of damaged cartilage. The absorption of oral glucosamine is 90% to 98%, making it widely accepted for use. However, chondroitin molecules are very large (50 to 300 times larger than glucosamine), and little (0% to 13%) chondroitin is absorbed. There is speculation that these larger molecules are undeliverable to cartilage cells. Glucosamine is generally well tolerated, and no adverse reactions have been reported with its use.

NURSING PROCESS

The Patient Receiving a Drug for a Musculoskeletal Disorder

ASSESSMENT

PREADMINISTRATION ASSESSMENT

The nurse obtains the patient's history, that is, a summary of the disorder, including onset, symptoms, and current treatment or therapy. In some instances, it may be necessary to question patients regarding their ability to carry out activities of daily living, including employment when applicable.

For the physical assessment, the nurse generally appraises the patient's physical condition and limitations. If the patient has arthritis (any type), the nurse examines the affected joints in the extremities for appearance of the skin over the joint, evidence of joint deformity, and mobility of the affected joint. Patients with osteoporosis are assessed for pain, particularly in the upper and lower back or hip. If the patient has gout, the nurse examines the affected joints and notes the appearance of the skin over the joints and any joint enlargement. Vital signs and weight are taken to provide a baseline for comparison during therapy.

The primary health care provider may order laboratory tests and bone scans to measure bone density. This is especially important for use as baseline data when a bone resorption inhibitor is prescribed for the patient.

Nursing Alert

When bisphosphonates are administered, serum calcium levels are monitored before, during, and after therapy.

ONGOING ASSESSMENT

Periodic evaluation is an important part of therapy for musculoskeletal disorders. With some disorders, such as acute gout, the patient can be expected to respond to therapy in hours. Therefore, it is important for the nurse to inspect the joints involved every 1 to 2 hours to identify immediately a response or nonresponse to therapy. At this time, the nurse questions the patient regarding the relief of pain, as well as adverse drug reactions.

In other disorders, response is gradual and may take days, weeks, and even months of treatment. Depending on the drug administered and the disorder being treated, the evaluation of therapy may be daily or weekly. These recorded evaluations help the primary health care provider plan current and future therapy, including dosage changes, changes in the drug administered, and institution of physical therapy.

When first-line treatments are not successful, sometimes drugs that are more toxic may be taken. The nurse closely observes the patient for the development of adverse reactions. Should any one or more adverse reactions occur, the nurse notifies the primary health care provider before the next dose is given.

NURSING DIAGNOSES

Drug-specific nursing diagnoses are highlighted in the Nursing Diagnoses Checklist. Other nursing diagnoses applicable to these drugs are discussed in depth in Chapter 4.

Nursing Diagnoses Checklist

✔ **Readiness for Enhanced Fluid Balance** related to need for increased fluid intake to promote excretion of urate crystals

✔ **Impaired Comfort: Gastric Distress** related to irritation of gastric lining from medication administration

✔ **Risk for Injury** related to medication-induced drowsiness and associated risk for imbalance and falls

PLANNING

The expected outcomes for the patient depend on the reason for administration but may include an optimal response to therapy, support of patient needs related to the management of adverse reactions, and an understanding of and compliance with the prescribed therapeutic regimen.

IMPLEMENTATION

PROMOTING AN OPTIMAL RESPONSE TO THERAPY

The patient with a musculoskeletal disorder may have long-standing chronic pain, which can be just as difficult to tolerate as acute pain. Along with pain, there may be skeletal deformities, such as the joint deformities seen with advanced RA. For many musculoskeletal conditions, drug therapy is a major treatment modality. In addition to drug therapy, rest, physical therapy, and other measures may be part of treatment. Including drugs as a major part of the treatment plan may keep the disorder under control (e.g., therapy for gout), improve the patient's ability to carry out activities of daily living, or make the pain and discomfort tolerable.

Patients with a musculoskeletal disorder often have anxiety related to the symptoms and the chronicity of their disorder. In addition to physical care, these patients often require emotional support, especially when a disorder is disabling and chronic. The nurse explains to the patient that therapy may take weeks or longer before any benefit is noted. When this is explained before therapy starts, the patient is less likely to become discouraged over the slow results.

Because of the toxic nature of some drugs, they are not used as frequently as newer drugs. It is important for the nurse to be aware of the adverse toxic reactions that can occur when less frequently prescribed drugs are given. The nurse closely observes the patient taking hydroxychloroquine for adverse reactions. It is important for the nurse to be alert to reactions such as skin rash, fever, cough, or easy bruising. The nurse should be attentive to specific patient complaints such as visual changes, tinnitus, or hearing loss. The nurse immediately reports these adverse reactions. Particular attention is paid to visual changes because irreversible retinal damage may occur.

Administration of penicillamine has been associated with many adverse reactions, some of which are potentially serious and even fatal. The nurse carefully evaluates any complaint or comment made by the patient and reports it to the primary health care provider. Increased skin friability (easy to tear) may occur, which may result in easy breakdown of the skin at pressure sites, such as the hips, elbows, and shoulders. If the patient cannot ambulate, the nurse changes the patient's position and inspects pressure sites for skin breakdown every 2 hours.

Administration of allopurinol may result in skin rash. A rash should be monitored carefully because it may precede a serious adverse reaction, such as Stevens-Johnson syndrome. The nurse immediately reports any rash to the primary health care provider.

Gold compounds and methotrexate are potentially toxic. Therefore, the nurse observes closely for development of adverse reactions, such as thrombocytopenia and leukopenia. Hematology, liver, and renal function studies are monitored every 1 to 3 months with methotrexate therapy. The primary care provider is notified of abnormal hematology, liver function, or kidney function findings. The nurse immediately brings all adverse reactions or suspected adverse reactions to the attention of the primary health care provider.

MONITORING AND MANAGING PATIENT NEEDS

READINESS FOR ENHANCED FLUID BALANCE When using the uric acid inhibitors, the nurse encourages liberal fluid intake and measures the intake and output. The nurse provides adequate fluids and reminds the patient frequently of the importance of increasing fluid intake. If the patient fails to increase the oral intake, the nurse informs the primary health care provider. In some instances, it may be necessary to administer intravenous fluids to supplement the oral intake when the patient fails to drink about 3000 mL of fluid per day. The daily urine output should be at least 2 L. An increase in urinary output is necessary to excrete the urates (uric acid) and prevent urate acid stone formation in the genitourinary tract.

IMPAIRED COMFORT: GASTRIC DISTRESS Adequate drug absorption and metabolism can depend on timing with meals. To facilitate delivery of the bone reabsorption inhibitor to the stomach and minimize adverse GI effects, the nurse administers the drug with 6 to 8 oz of water while the patient is in an upright position. The patient is instructed to remain upright (avoid lying down) for at least 30 minutes after taking the drug. When administering alendronate or risedronate the nurse gives the drug orally in the morning before the first food or drink of the day. Risedronate and etidronate are typically administered once daily. Many bisphosphonates are becoming available in both once-a-week and once-a-month dosing forms. The nurse should check the dosage and frequency carefully to prevent drug administration errors. Etidronate is not administered within 2 hours of food, vitamin and mineral supplements, or antacids.

The nurse administers DMARDs, uric acid inhibitors, and skeletal muscle relaxants with, or immediately after, meals to minimize gastric distress.

RISK FOR INJURY Many of these drugs may cause drowsiness. In addition, pain or deformity may hamper mobility. These two factors place the patient at risk of injury. Therefore the nurse evaluates the patient carefully before allowing the patient to ambulate alone. If drowsiness does occur, assistance with ambulatory activities is necessary. If drowsiness is severe, the nurse notifies the primary health care provider before the next dose is due.

The patient with an arthritis disorder may experience much pain or discomfort and may require assistance with activities, such as ambulating, eating, and grooming. Patients on bed rest require position changes and skin care every 2 hours. Patients with osteoporosis may require a brace or corset when out of bed.

EDUCATING THE PATIENT AND FAMILY

To ensure compliance with the treatment regimen, the patient must understand the importance of the prescribed therapy and taking the drug exactly as directed to obtain the best results. To meet this goal, the nurse develops an effective plan of patient and family teaching.

The points included in a patient and family teaching plan depend on the type and severity of the patient's musculoskeletal disorder. The nurse must explain carefully that treatment for the disorder includes drug therapy, as well as other medical management, such as diet, exercise, limitations or nonlimitations of activity, and periodic physical therapy treatments. The nurse emphasizes the importance of not taking any nonprescription drugs unless their use has been approved by the primary health care provider.

The dosing schedule can be difficult for the patient to understand when the drugs are given on an outpatient basis, particularly if the person is elderly or confused and responsible for self-administering the drug.

Dosing schedules may require taking medications on alternate days (alternate-day therapy), at specific times of the day, or weekly. The patient may not see a therapeutic response until 3 to 6 weeks of therapy and become discouraged. In some cases, a patient may stop treatment.

Nursing Alert

Alendronate is administered orally each day or as a once-a-week dose. The nurse should check the physician's order to be certain of the dosage and the times of administration. When administering the drug for treatment of osteoporosis in postmenopausal women, the dosage is 70 mg once weekly or 10 mg daily. When administering the drug for prevention of osteoporosis, 5 mg of the drug is given daily or 35 mg once a week.

Some drugs used for RA require self-administered subcutaneous injections. The nurse teaches the patient and family proper injection and disposal techniques. Teaching about site rotation should be included. The patient should demonstrate proper injection technique before this becomes a self-administered procedure. Patients need to be taught how to manage the discomfort to the site of injection and to report redness, pain, and swelling to the primary health care provider.

The following points for specific drugs are included in the teaching plan:

- *Drugs used to treat osteoporosis*

  - Take these drugs with 6 to 8 oz of water first thing in the morning.

  - Do not lie down for at least 30 minutes after taking the drug and wait at least 30 minutes before taking any other food or drink.

  - Take supplemental calcium and vitamin D if dietary intake is inadequate.

- *Drugs used to treat RA*

  - When taking methotrexate, use a calendar or some other memory device to remember to take the drug on the same day each week.

  - Notify the primary health care provider immediately if any of the following occur: sore mouth or sores in the mouth, diarrhea, fever, sore throat, easy bruising, rash, itching, or nausea and vomiting.

  - Women of childbearing age should use an effective contraceptive during therapy with methotrexate and for 8 weeks after therapy.

- *Drugs used to treat gout*

  - Drink at least 10 glasses of water a day until the acute attack has subsided.

  - Take this drug with food to minimize GI upset.

  - If drowsiness occurs, avoid driving or performing other hazardous tasks.

  - Acute gout—notify the primary health care provider if pain is not relieved in a few days.

  - Notify the primary health care provider if a skin rash occurs.

- *Drugs used for muscle spasm and cramping*

  - This drug may cause drowsiness. Do not drive or perform other hazardous tasks if drowsiness occurs.

- This drug is for short-term use. Do not use the drug for longer than 2 to 3 weeks.

- Avoid alcohol or other CNS depressants while taking this drug.

EVALUATION

- The therapeutic drug effect is achieved.

- Adverse reactions are identified, reported to the primary health care provider, and managed using appropriate nursing interventions.

- The patient verbalizes the importance of complying with the prescribed therapeutic regimen.

- The patient and family demonstrate an understanding of the drug regimen.

Critical Thinking Exercises

1. Mary is a nurse who has returned to nursing after 15 years' absence to raise a family. Mary asks you what should be included in a teaching plan for a patient who has rheumatoid arthritis and who is now taking DMARDs. Discuss what information you would suggest that Mary emphasize in a teaching plan.

2. Ms. Leeds is prescribed methotrexate for rheumatoid arthritis not responding to other therapies. She became nervous about starting the drug after she was told that the drug can cause many serious adverse reactions. Discuss what you could say to Ms. Leeds to relieve her anxiety. Identify specific instructions you would give her before she begins therapy with this drug.

3. Discuss important points the nurse should consider when administering colchicine to a patient with an acute attack of diarrhea.

4. Discuss the important points to include when educating a patient prescribed alendronate 35 mg once weekly. What suggestions could you give to help the patient remember when to take the drug?

Review Questions

1. When a patient is taking hydroxychloroquine on an outpatient basis, the nurse advises the patient to inform the primary health care provider if _____.

   A. the appetite decreases

   B. a productive cough occurs

   C. sudden ringing in the ears occurs

   D. hair loss occurs

2. When administering a skeletal muscle relaxant, the nurse observes the patient for the most common adverse reaction, which is _____.

   A. drowsiness

   B. gastrointestinal bleeding

   C. vomiting

   D. constipation

3. When a patient is prescribed alendronate (Fosamax) for osteoporosis, the nurse administers the drug _____.

   A. with food or milk

   B. by injection

   C. 30 minutes before breakfast

   D. at bedtime

4. When allopurinol (Zyloprim) is used for treating gout, the nurse _____.

   A. administers the drug with juice or milk

   B. administers the drug after the evening meal

   C. restricts fluids during evening hours

   D. encourages liberal fluid intake

5. What teaching points would the nurse include when educating the patient who will begin taking risedronate?

   A. The drug is administered once weekly.

   B. Take a daily laxative because the drug will likely cause constipation.

   C. Take the drug with antacids to decrease gastric distress.

   D. After taking the drug, remain upright for at least 30 minutes.

Medication Dosage Problems

1. A patient is to receive allopurinol 300 mg orally for gout. The nurse has 100-mg tablets available. How many tablets would the nurse administer? _____

2. The physician prescribes 1.5 g methocarbamol (Robaxin) orally for a musculoskeletal disorder. Available for administration are 500-mg tablets. The nurse administers _____.

To check your answers, see Appendix G.

Drugs Used to Treat Musculoskeletal Disorders

Drugs That Affect the Respiratory System

The respiratory system consists of the upper and lower airways, the lungs, and the thoracic cavity. The respiratory system provides a mechanism for the exchange of oxygen and carbon dioxide in the lungs. Any change in the respiratory status has the potential to affect every other body system because all cells need an adequate supply of oxygen for optimal functioning. This unit focuses on drugs used to treat some of the more common disorders affecting the respiratory system.

Among the most common conditions of humans, upper respiratory infections include allergic rhinitis, coughs, the common cold, and congestion. The drugs used to treat the discomfort associated with an upper respiratory infection include antihistamines, decongestants, antitussives, mucolytics, and expectorants. Many of these drugs are available as nonprescription (over-the-counter) drugs, whereas others are available only by prescription. Other drugs discussed are those used to treat disorders of the lower respiratory tract. These drugs include the bronchodilating drugs, which are the sympathomimetics and the xanthine derivatives. Along with the bronchodilating drugs, the antiasthma drugs include the corticosteroids, leukotriene receptor antagonists, leukotriene formation inhibitors, and the mast cell stabilizers.

Disorders of the lower respiratory tract include asthma (chronic inflammatory disease of the airways), emphysema (lung disorder in which the alveoli become enlarged and plugged with mucus), chronic bronchitis (chronic inflammation and possibly infection of the bronchi), and chronic obstructive pulmonary disease (COPD). COPD is a slowly progressive disease of the airways characterized by a gradual loss of lung function. The symptoms of COPD range from chronic cough and sputum production to severe, disabling shortness of breath. There is no known cure for COPD; the treatment is usually supportive and designed to relieve symptoms and improve quality of life.

Asthma is a chronic inflammatory condition of the lower airway with airway constriction caused by bronchospasm and bronchoconstriction. Adding to the narrowing of the airway is edema of the lining of the bronchioles and the production of thick mucus that can plug the airway. Patients with asthma may experience periods of exacerbation alternating with periods of normal lung function. Environmental exposure to such allergens as house dust mites, tobacco smoke, pets and pet dander, mold, and cockroach wastes and physical exercise are important "triggers" for an asthma attack. Anti-inflammatory drugs play an important role in treating individuals with asthma. These drugs prevent asthma attacks by decreasing the swelling and mucus production in the airways, thereby making the airways less sensitive to asthma triggers. Drug therapy for asthma is aimed at preventing attacks and reducing swelling and mucus production in the airways.

CONCEPTSin action **ANIMATION**

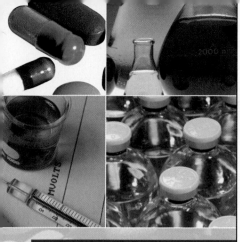

Antitussives, Mucolytics, and Expectorants

Key Terms

antitussive
coughing
expectorant
mucolytic
nonproductive cough
productive cough

Learning Objectives

On completion of this chapter, the student will:

- Define the terms *antitussive*, *mucolytic*, and *expectorant*.
- Describe the uses, general drug actions, adverse reactions, contraindications, precautions and interactions of antitussive, mucolytic, and expectorant drugs.
- Discuss important nursing preadministration and ongoing assessment activities for patients receiving an

antitussive, mucolytic, or expectorant drug.
- List nursing diagnoses particular to a patient taking an antitussive, mucolytic, or expectorant drug.
- Discuss ways to promote an optimal response to therapy, to manage common adverse reactions, and to educate the patient about the use of an antitussive, mucolytic, or expectorant drug.

Upper respiratory infections are among the most common human illnesses. The drugs used to treat the discomfort associated with an upper respiratory infection include antitussives, mucolytics, and expectorants. Many of these drugs are available as nonprescription (over-the-counter) drugs, whereas others are available only by prescription.

ANTITUSSIVES

Coughing is the forceful expulsion of air from the lungs. A cough may be productive or nonproductive. With a **productive cough**, secretions from the lower respiratory tract are expelled. A **nonproductive cough** is a dry, hacking one that produces no secretions. An **antitussive** is a drug used to relieve coughing. Many antitussive drugs are combined with another drug, such as an antihistamine or expectorant, and sold over the counter (OTC) as a nonprescription cough medicine. Other antitussives, either alone or in combination with other drugs, are available by prescription only.

Actions

Some antitussives depress the cough center located in the medulla and are called centrally acting drugs. Codeine and dextromethorphan are examples of centrally acting antitussives. Other antitussives are peripherally acting drugs, which act by anesthetizing stretch receptors in the respiratory passages, thereby decreasing coughing. An example of a peripherally acting antitussive is benzonatate (Tessalon).

Uses

Antitussives are used to relieve a nonproductive cough. When the cough produces sputum, it should be treated by the primary health care provider, who, based on a physical examination, may or may not prescribe or recommend an antitussive.

> ## Herbal Alert
>
> *Eucalyptus* is used to treat nasal congestion and is found as a component in OTC products used for the treatment of sinusitis and pharyngitis. The plant is grown throughout the world and the leaves and oil are used to treat various respiratory conditions such as asthma and chronic bronchitis. The lozenges are useful to soothe sore throats and as cough drops. Eucalyptus can also be used as a vapor bath for asthma or other bronchial conditions. The herb is available in many forms, including an essential oil, fluid extract, and aqueous solution in alcohol, as well as a component of various OTC products. Eucalyptus should not be used during pregnancy and lactation and in children younger than 2 years of age. Eucalyptus may be used topically on children and adults in combination with menthol and camphor. All products used internally should be diluted before use, and individuals with hypersensitivity to eucalyptus should avoid its use.

Adverse Reactions

Central Nervous System Reactions

- Sedation
- Dizziness
- Lightheadedness

Gastrointestinal Reactions

- Nausea
- Vomiting
- Constipation

When used as directed, nonprescription cough medicines containing two or more ingredients produce few adverse reactions. However, those that contain an antihistamine may cause drowsiness. The more common adverse reactions associated with the mucolytics and expectorants are listed in the Summary Drug Table: Antitussive, Mucolytic, and Expectorant Drugs.

Contraindications

Antitussives are contraindicated in patients with known hypersensitivity to the drugs. The opioid antitussives (those with codeine) are contraindicated in premature infants or during labor when delivery of a premature infant is anticipated.

Precautions

Antitussives are given with caution to patients with a persistent or chronic cough, a cough accompanied by excessive secretions, a high fever, rash, persistent headache, or nausea or vomiting.

Antitussives containing codeine are used with caution during pregnancy (category C) and labor (pregnancy category D), in patients with chronic obstructive pulmonary disease (COPD), acute asthmatic attack, preexisting respiratory disorders, acute abdominal conditions, head injury, increased intracranial pressure, convulsive disorders, hepatic or renal impairment, and prostatic hypertrophy.

Interactions

Other central nervous system (CNS) depressants and alcohol may cause additive depressant effects when administered with antitussives containing codeine. When dextromethorphan is administered with the monoamine oxidase inhibitors (see Chapter 24), patients may experience hypotension, fever, nausea, jerking motions to the leg, and coma.

NURSING PROCESS

The Patient Receiving an Antitussive Drug

ASSESSMENT

PREADMINISTRATION ASSESSMENT

A hospitalized patient may occasionally have an antitussive preparation prescribed, especially when a nonproductive cough causes discomfort or threatens to cause more serious problems, such as raising pressure in the eye (increased intraocular pressure) after eye surgery or increasing intracranial pressure in those with CNS disorders. During the preadministration assessment, the nurse documents the type of cough (productive, nonproductive) and describes the color and amount of any

SUMMARY DRUG TABLE ANTITUSSIVES, MUCOLYTIC, AND EXPECTORANT DRUGS

GENERIC NAME	TRADE NAME	USES	ADVERSE REACTIONS	DOSAGE RANGES
Antitussives				
Opioid Antitussives				
codeine sulfate *koe'-deen*		Suppression of nonproductive cough, relief of mild to moderate pain	Sedation, nausea, vomiting, dizziness, constipation, central nervous system depression	10–20 mg orally q4–6h; maximum dosage 120 mg/d
Nonopioid Antitussives				
benzonatate *ben-zoe'-na-tate*	Tessalon Perles	Symptomatic relief of cough	Sedation, headache, mild dizziness, constipation, nausea, GI upset, skin eruptions, nasal congestion	Adults and children older than 10 y: 100 mg TID (up to 600 mg/d)
dextromethorphan HBr *dex-troe-meth-or'-fan*	Benylin, DexAlone, Robitussin Pediatric, Delsym	Symptomatic relief of cough	Sedation, headache, mild dizziness, constipation, nausea, GI upset, skin eruptions, nasal congestion	Adults and children older than 12 y: 10–30 mg q4–8h; sustained-release (SR) 60 mg q12h orally Children 6–12 y: 5–10 mg q4h or 15 mg q6–8h; SR 30 mg q12h orally Children 2–6 y: 2.5–7.5 mg q4–8h; SR 15 mg q12h orally
dextromethorphan HBr and benzocaine *ben'-zoe-cane*	Cough-X, Tetra-Formula, Formula 44 Cough	Symptomatic relief of cough	Same as dextromethorphan HBr	Varies, depending on formulation; take as directed on package
diphenhydramine HCl *dye-fen-hye'-dra-meen*	AllerMax, Hydramine Cough, Tusstat	Symptomatic relief of cough caused by colds, allergy, or bronchial irritation	Sedation, headache, mild dizziness, constipation, nausea, GI upset, skin eruptions, postural hypotension	Adults: 25 mg q4h orally, not to exceed 150 mg/d Children 6–12 y: 12.5 mg orally q4h, not to exceed 75 mg/d Children 2–6 y: 6.25 mg q4h, not to exceed 25 mg/d
Mucolytics				
acetylcysteine *a-se-teel-sis'-tay-een*	Mucomyst	Reduction of viscosity of mucus in acute and chronic bronchopulmonary disease, tracheostomy care, atelectasis due pulmonary to mucus obstruction, complications of cystic fibrosis, diagnostic bronchial studies, acetaminophen toxicity	Stomatitis, nausea, vomiting, fever, drowsiness, bronchospasm, irritation of the trachea and bronchi	1–10 mL of 20% solution by nebulization or 2–20 mL of 10% solution q2–6h PRN Acetaminophen toxicity: initially 140 mg/kg orally, then 70 mg/kg orally q4h for 17 doses (total)

SUMMARY DRUG TABLE (continued)

GENERIC NAME	TRADE NAME	USES	ADVERSE REACTIONS	DOSAGE RANGES
Expectorants				
guaifenesin (glyceryl guaiacolate) *gwy-e-fen'-e-sin*	Hytuss, Organidin NR, Robitussin	Relief of cough associated with respiratory tract infection (sinusitis, asthma, bronchitis, pharyngitis), especially when the cough is dry and nonproductive	Nausea, vomiting, dizziness, headache, rash	Adults and children 12 y and older: 200–400 mg orally q4h Children 6–12y: 100–200 mg q4h orally Children 2–6 years: 50–100 mg q4h
potassium iodide *poe-tass'-ee-um eye-o-dide*	Pima, SSKI	Symptomatic relief of chronic pulmonary disease complicated by tenacious mucus	Iodine sensitivity or iodism (sore mouth, metallic taste, increased salivation, nausea, vomiting, epigastric pain, parotid swelling, and pain)	300–1000 mg orally after meals BID or TID, to 1.5 g orally TID
terpin hydrate *ter'-pin high'-drate*		Symptomatic relief of dry, nonproductive cough	Drowsiness, nausea, vomiting, or abdiminal pain	85–170 mg TID or QID orally

GI, gastrointestinal.

sputum present. The nurse takes and records vital signs because some patients with a productive cough may have an infection.

ONGOING ASSESSMENT

During the ongoing assessment, the nurse observes for a therapeutic effect (e.g., coughing decreases). The nurse auscultates lung sounds and takes vital signs periodically. When a patient has a cough, the nurse describes and records in the chart the type of cough (productive or nonproductive of sputum) and the frequency of coughing. The nurse also notes and records whether the cough interrupts sleep or causes pain in the chest or other parts of the body.

NURSING DIAGNOSES

A drug-specific nursing diagnosis is highlighted in the Nursing Diagnoses Checklist. Other nursing diagnoses applicable to these drugs are discussed in depth in Chapter 4.

Nursing Diagnoses Checklist

✔ **Risk for Injury** related to the adverse effects of the drugs (sedation and dizziness)

PLANNING

The expected outcomes for the patient depend on the reason for administration, but may include an optimal response to therapy, support of patient needs related to managing adverse drug reactions, and an understanding of and compliance with the prescribed treatment regimen.

IMPLEMENTATION
PROMOTING AN OPTIMAL RESPONSE TO THERAPY

The nurse administers antitussives orally. When the nurse gives the drug as a tablet, the patient should swallow the drug whole and not chew it. For example, chewing benzonatate tablets may result in a local anesthetic effect (oropharyngeal anesthesia) with possible choking.

One problem associated with the use of an antitussive is related to its drug action. Although not an adverse reaction, depression of the cough reflex can cause secretions to pool in the lungs. Pooling of the secretions that are normally removed by coughing may result in more serious problems, such as pneumonia and atelectasis. For this reason, using an antitussive for a productive cough is contraindicated in many situations.

Another problem can arise from the use of a nonprescription antitussive for self-treatment of a chronic cough. Indiscriminate use of antitussives by the general public may prevent early diagnosis and treatment of serious disorders, such as lung cancer and emphysema.

Nursing Alert

The nurse should advise the patient taking a nonprescription cough medicine that if a cough lasts more than 10 days or is accompanied by fever, chest pain, severe headache, or skin rash, the patient should consult the primary health care provider.

MONITORING AND MANAGING PATIENT NEEDS

RISK FOR INJURY Many of the antitussives cause dizziness or sedation. These effects increase the patient's risk for falling. The nurse can minimize this risk for hospitalized patients by carefully orienting each patient to the surroundings and closely supervising the patient. A night light helps the patient to see at night. The nurse encourages the patient to ask for assistance if he or she feels dizzy or unsteady.

EDUCATING THE PATIENT AND FAMILY

The nurse discourages the indiscriminate use of nonprescription antitussives, especially when coughing produces sputum. The nurse advises the patient to read the label carefully, follow the dosage recommendations, and consult the primary health care provider if the cough persists for more than 10 days or if fever or chest pain occurs. If an antitussive is prescribed for use at home, the nurse includes the following information in a teaching plan:

- Do not exceed the recommended dose.
- If chills, fever, chest pain, or sputum production occurs, contact the primary health care provider as soon as possible.
- Drink plenty of fluids (if not contraindicated by disease process). A fluid intake of 1500 to 2000 mL is recommended.
- If taking oral capsules, do not chew or break open the capsules; swallow them whole.
- If taking a lozenge, avoid drinking fluids for 30 minutes after use to avoid losing effectiveness of the drug.
- If the cough is not relieved or becomes worse, contact the primary health care provider.
- Avoid irritants, such as cigarette smoke, dust, or fumes, to decrease irritation to the throat.
- Take frequent sips of water, suck on sugarless hard candy, or chew gum to diminish coughing.

- Remember that codeine may impair mental or physical abilities required for the performance of potentially hazardous tasks. Observe caution when driving or performing tasks requiring alertness, coordination, or physical dexterity. Codeine may cause orthostatic hypotension when rising too quickly from a sitting or lying position. Do not take codeine preparations for persistent or chronic cough, such as occurs with smoking, asthma, or emphysema or when the cough is accompanied by excessive secretions, except when under the supervision of the health care provider.
- Do not use with alcohol or other CNS depressants (e.g., antidepressants, hypnotics, sedatives, tranquilizers).

EVALUATION

- The therapeutic effect is achieved and coughing is relieved.
- The patient reports no injuries related to adverse reactions.
- The patient and family demonstrate an understanding of the drug regimen.

MUCOLYTICS AND EXPECTORANTS

A **mucolytic** is a drug that loosens respiratory secretions. An **expectorant** is a drug that aids in raising thick, tenacious mucus from the respiratory passages.

Actions

A drug with mucolytic activity appears to reduce the viscosity (thickness) of respiratory secretions by direct action on the mucus. An example of a mucolytic drug is acetylcysteine (Mucomyst).

Expectorants increase the production of respiratory secretions, which in turn appears to decrease the viscosity of the mucus. This helps to raise secretions from the respiratory passages. An example of an expectorant is guaifenesin.

Uses

The mucolytic acetylcysteine is used to treat
- Acute bronchopulmonary disease (pneumonia, bronchitis, tracheobronchitis)
- Pulmonary complications of cystic fibrosis
- Pulmonary complications associated with surgery

- Post-traumatic chest conditions
- Atelectasis due to mucus obstruction
- Acetaminophen overdosage

This drug is also used for diagnostic bronchial studies such as bronchograms and bronchial wedge catheterizations. It is primarily given by nebulizer but also may be directly instilled into a tracheostomy to liquefy (thin) secretions.

Expectorants are used to help raise respiratory secretions. An expectorant may also be included along with one or more additional drugs, such as an antihistamine, decongestant, or antitussive, in some prescription and nonprescription cough medicines.

Adverse Reactions

The more common adverse reactions associated with mucolytic and expectorant drugs are listed in the Summary Drug Table: Antitussive, Mucolytic, and Expectorant Drugs.

Contraindications

The expectorants and mucolytics are contraindicated in patients with known hypersensitivity. The expectorant potassium iodide is contraindicated during pregnancy (category D).

Precautions

The expectorants are used cautiously during pregnancy and lactation (guaifenesin is a pregnancy category C drug and acetylcysteine is a pregnancy category B drug), in patients with persistent cough, severe respiratory insufficiency, or asthma, and in older adults or debilitated patients.

Interactions

No significant interactions have been reported when the expectorants are used as directed. The exception is iodine products. If used concurrently with iodine products, lithium and other antithyroid drugs may potentiate the hypothyroid effects of these drugs. When potassium-containing medications and potassium-sparing diuretics are administered with iodine products, the patient may experience hypokalemia, cardiac arrhythmias, or cardiac arrest. Thyroid function test results may also be altered by iodine.

The Patient Receiving a Mucolytic or an Expectorant

ASSESSMENT

PREADMINISTRATION ASSESSMENT

Before administering the drug, the nurse assesses the respiratory status of the patient. The nurse documents lung sounds, amount of dyspnea (if any), and consistency of sputum (if present). A description of the sputum is important as a baseline for future comparison.

ONGOING ASSESSMENT

After administering the drug, the nurse notes any increase in sputum or change in consistency. The nurse documents, on the patient's chart, a description of the sputum raised. Patients with thick, tenacious mucus may have difficulty breathing. It is important to notify the primary health care provider if the patient has difficulty breathing because of an inability to raise sputum and clear the respiratory passages.

Immediately before and after treatment with the mucolytic acetylcysteine, the nurse auscultates the lungs and records the findings of both assessments on the patient's chart. Between treatments, the nurse evaluates the patient's respiratory status and records these findings on the patient's chart. These evaluations aid the primary health care provider in determining the effectiveness of therapy. If any problem occurs during or after treatment, or if the patient is uncooperative, the nurse discusses the problem with the primary health care provider.

When expectorants are given to those with chronic pulmonary disease, the nurse evaluates the effectiveness of drug therapy (i.e., the patient's ability to raise sputum) and records this finding in the patient's chart.

NURSING DIAGNOSES

A drug-specific nursing diagnosis is highlighted in the Nursing Diagnoses Checklist. Other nursing diagnoses applicable to these drugs are discussed in depth in Chapter 4.

> **Nursing Diagnoses Checklist**
>
> ✓ **Ineffective Airway Clearance** related to thick, tenacious mucus

PLANNING

The expected outcomes for the patient depend on the reason for administration, but may include an optimal response to therapy, support of patient needs related to management of adverse drug reactions, and an understanding of and compliance with the prescribed treatment regimen.

IMPLEMENTATION

PROMOTING AN OPTIMAL RESPONSE TO THERAPY

When the mucolytic acetylcysteine is administered by nebulization, the nurse explains the treatment to the patient and demonstrates how the nebulizer will be used. The nurse remains with the patient during the first few treatments, especially when the patient is elderly or exhibits anxiety. The nurse supplies the patient with tissues and places a paper bag for disposal of the tissues within the patient's reach. If acetylcysteine is ordered to be inserted into a tracheostomy, the nurse must make sure suction equipment is at the bedside to be immediately available for aspiration of secretions.

MANAGING AND MONITORING PATIENT NEEDS

INEFFECTIVE AIRWAY CLEARANCE For the patient with thick sputum, the nurse encourages a fluid intake of up to 2000 mL per day, if this amount is not contraindicated by the patient's condition or disease process. The nurse encourages the patient to take deep, diaphragmatic breaths. The amount and consistency of sputum is monitored.

EDUCATING THE PATIENT AND FAMILY

Acetylcysteine usually is administered in the hospital but may be prescribed for the patient being discharged and renting or buying respiratory therapy equipment for use at home (see Patient and Family Teaching Checklist: Using Respiratory Equipment at Home). The nurse gives the patient or a family member full instruction in the use and maintenance of the equipment, as well as the technique of administration of acetylcysteine.

When an expectorant is prescribed, the nurse instructs the patient to take the drug as directed and to contact the primary health care provider if any unusual symptoms or other problems occur during use of the drug or if the drug appears to be ineffective.

EVALUATION

- The therapeutic effect is achieved, and secretions are thinned and easily expectorated.
- The patient has an easy, unlabored breathing pattern.
- Adverse reactions are identified, reported to the primary health care provider, and managed successfully with nursing interventions.
- The patient and family demonstrate an understanding of the drug regimen and use of equipment to administer the drug (mucolytic).

Patient and Family Teaching Checklist

Using Respiratory Equipment at Home

The nurse:

✓ Contacts the respiratory care provider to arrange for equipment delivery to the patient's home.

✓ Describes equipment, such as compressor, filter, tubing, aerosol, cup, and mask or mouthpiece, to be used for therapy, including rationale for use and need for electrical power source.

✓ Reviews the drug therapy regimen, including the prescribed drug and solution strength, dosage, amount and type of diluent, if required, and frequency of administration.

✓ Demonstrates step-by-step procedure for equipment setup and drug preparation and administration.

✓ Evaluates return demonstration of procedure.

✓ Recommends sitting or high Fowler's position to maximize lung expansion and drug dispersion.

✓ Instructs to observe for misting as evidence of proper equipment function.

✓ Encourages slow, even breathing during treatment and coughing and expectorating as necessary.

✓ Stresses the importance of continuing treatment until the entire drug has evaporated and misting has ceased.

✓ Reviews the signs and symptoms of possible adverse reactions and impaired respiratory function, including changes in cough, color, and amount of sputum, shortness of breath, or difficulty breathing, and stresses the need to notify the primary health care provider at once should any occur.

✓ Instructs to rinse equipment after each use with warm or cool water and allow to air dry.

✓ Recommends storing equipment parts in clean plastic bag or container.

✓ Reviews manufacturer's instructions for daily cleaning of equipment parts and routine maintenance of compressor.

✓ Provides written list for trouble-shooting problems such as changing filter, tightening connections, or replacing aerosol cup.

✓ Explains use of any additional drug therapy.

✓ Stresses need for fluid intake to liquefy secretions.

✓ Emphasizes importance of periodic laboratory tests and follow-up visits with primary health care provider to evaluate effectiveness of therapy.

Antitussives, Mucolytics, and Expectorants

Critical Thinking Exercises

1. Your neighbor, Mr. Peterson, tells you that he has had a chronic cough for the past several months and asks you to recommend the best over-the-counter "cough medicine." Describe the advice you would give to Mr. Peterson.

2. Ms. Moore, a patient in a nursing home, has had a cough for the past 3 weeks. Ms. Moore's primary health care provider is aware of her problem and has ordered an expectorant and has told her that she needs to cough and raise sputum. Ms. Moore's family members ask you if something can be given to stop Ms. Moore's coughing. Explain how you would discuss this problem and explain the prescribed therapy with the family.

3. Discuss any precautions the nurse would consider when the expectorants are administered. Give a rationale for your answer.

Review Questions

1. Antitussives are given with caution to patients with _____.

   A. an unproductive cough

   B. a chronic cough

   C. hypertension

   D. hypotension

2. Which of these drugs is classified as an expectorant?

   A. guaifenesin

   B. codeine

   C. dextromethorphan

   D. diphenhydramine

3. Which of the following statements is appropriate for the nurse to include in discharge instructions for a patient taking an antitussive?

   A. Increase the dosage if the drug does not relieve the cough.

   B. Limit fluids to less than 1000 mL each day.

   C. Expect the cough to worsen during the first few days of treatment.

   D. Frequent sips of water and sucking on sugarless hard candy may diminish coughing.

4. Which of these drugs would mostly likely be used in caring for a patient with a tracheostomy?

   A. acetylcysteine

   B. guaifenesin

   C. benzonatate

   D. dextromethorphan

5. When administering a mucolytic, which of the following nursing actions is appropriate to take to promote an effective airway clearance?

   A. Increase fluid intake to 2000 mL per day.

   B. Limit fluids to 200 mL per day.

   C. Monitor intake and output every 8 hours.

   D. Have the patient take the mucolytic after each coughing episode.

Medication Dosage Problems

1. A patient is prescribed 200 mg of guaifenesin syrup. The drug is available in syrup of 200 mg/ 5 mL. The nurse administers _____.

2. Codeine 10 mg is prescribed for a patient with a severe unproductive cough. The drug is available as an oral solution of 10 mg/5 mL. The nurse administers _____.

To check your answers, see Appendix G.

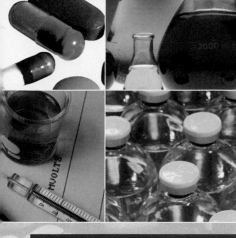

Chapter 36

Antihistamines and Decongestants

Learning Objectives

On completion of this chapter, the student will:

- Describe the uses, general drug action, general adverse reactions, contraindications, precautions, and interactions of the antihistamines and decongestants.
- Discuss important preadministration and ongoing assessment activities the nurse should perform on the patient taking an antihistamine or a decongestant.

- List nursing diagnoses particular to a patient taking an antihistamine or a decongestant.
- Discuss ways to promote an optimal response to therapy, how to manage common patient needs (e.g., adverse reactions), and important points to keep in mind when educating a patient about the use of an antihistamine or a decongestant.

This chapter focuses on drugs used to treat some of the more common disorders affecting the respiratory system, particularly allergies and the congestion associated with certain respiratory disorders.

ANTIHISTAMINES

Histamine is a substance produced from the amino acid histidine. Histamine is present in various tissues of the body, such as the heart, lungs, gastric mucosa, and skin (Fig. 36-1). The highest concentration of histamine is found in the basophil (a type of white blood cell) and the mast cells that are found near capillaries. Histamine is produced in response to injury. It acts on areas such as the vascular system and smooth muscle, producing dilation of arterioles and an increased permeability of capillaries and venules. Dilation of the arterioles results in localized redness. An increase in the permeability of small blood vessels promotes an escape of fluid from these blood vessels into the surrounding tissues, which produces localized swelling. Thus, the release of histamine produces an inflammatory response. Histamine is also released from mast cells in allergic reactions or hypersensitivity reactions, such as anaphylactic shock.

An **antihistamine** is a drug used to counteract the effects of histamine on body organs and structures. Examples of antihistamines include diphenhydramine (Benadryl), loratadine (Claritin), fexofenadine (Allegra), and cetirizine (Zyrtec). Desloratadine (Clarinex), loratadine, and fexofenadine minimally penetrate the blood–brain barrier, which means that little of the drug is distributed in the central nervous system (CNS) so that fewer of the sedating effects are felt. Topical corticosteroid nasal sprays, such as fluticasone propionate (Flonase) or triamcinolone acetonide (Nasacort), are also used for nasal allergy symptoms. See Chapter 56 for more information on the topical corticosteroids.

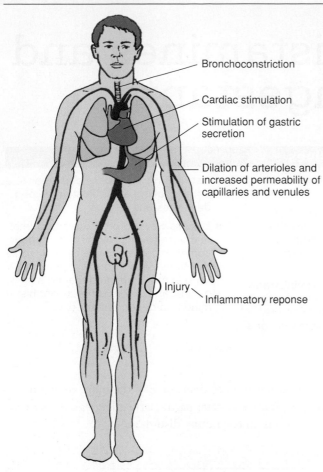

Figure 36.1 Effects of histamine in the body.

Actions

Antihistamines (or histamine type 1 [H₁] receptor antagonists) block most, but not all, of the effects of histamine. They do this by competing for histamine at histamine receptor sites throughout the body, thereby preventing histamine from entering these receptor sites and producing an effect on body tissues. First-generation antihistamines bind nonselectively to central and peripheral H₁ receptors and may result in CNS stimulation or depression. CNS depression usually occurs with higher doses and allows some of these agents to be used for sedation. Other first-generation drugs may have additional effects, such as antipruritic (anti-itching) or antiemetic (antinausea) effects. Second-generation antihistamines are selective for peripheral H₁ receptors and, as a group, are less sedating. See the Summary Drug Table: Antihistamines for a listing of first- and second-generation antihistamines.

Uses

The general uses of the antihistamines include
- Relief of the symptoms of seasonal and perennial allergies
- Allergic and vasomotor rhinitis
- Allergic conjunctivitis
- Mild and uncomplicated angioneurotic edema and urticaria
- Relief of allergic reactions to drugs, blood, or plasma
- Relief of coughs caused by colds or allergy
- Adjunctive therapy in anaphylactic shock
- Treatment of parkinsonism
- Relief of nausea and vomiting
- Relief of motion sickness
- Sedation
- Adjuncts to analgesics

Each antihistamine may be used for one or more of these reasons. The more specific uses of the various antihistamine preparations are given in the Summary Drug Table: Antihistamines.

Adverse Reactions

Central Nervous System Reactions
- Drowsiness or sedation
- Disturbed coordination

Anticholinergic (Cholinergic Blocking) Effects

Anticholinergic effects of antihistamines include
- Dryness of the mouth, nose, and throat
- Thickening of bronchial secretions

Second-generation preparations (e.g., loratadine) cause less drowsiness and fewer anticholinergic effects than some of the other antihistamines. Although these drugs are sometimes used to treat allergies, a drug allergy can occur with the use of an antihistamine. Symptoms that may indicate an allergy to these drugs include skin rash, urticaria, and anaphylactic shock.

Contraindications

Although the antihistamines are classified in pregnancy category B (chlorpheniramine, cetirizine, dexchlorpheniramine, clemastine, diphenhydramine, and loratadine)

SUMMARY DRUG TABLE ANTIHISTAMINES

GENERIC NAME	TRADE NAME	USES	ADVERSE REACTIONS	DOSAGE RANGES
First-Generation Antihistamines				
brompheniramine *brome-fen-ir'-a-meen*	LoHist 12 Hour, Bidhist, Lodrane 24, VaZol, Lodrane XR, BroveX	Temporary relief of sneezing, itchy, watery eyes, itchy nose or throat, and runny nose caused by hay fever or other respiratory allergies; VaZol also used for symptoms of the common cold; treatment of allergic reactions to blood or plasma and anaphylactic reactions	Drowsiness, sedation, dizziness, disturbed coordination, hypotension, headache, blurred vision, thickening of bronchial secretions	Adults and children 12 y and older: 6–12 mg orally q12h Sustained release: 8–12 mg orally q12h Oral liquid: 4 mg QID
chlorpheniramine maleate *klor-fen-eer'-a-meen*	Aller-Chlor, Chlor-Trimeton Allergy 8 Hour, Chlor-Trimeton Allergy 12 Hour	Temporary relief of sneezing, itchy, watery eyes, itchy throat, and runny nose caused by hay fever, other upper respiratory allergies, and the common cold	Drowsiness, sedation, hypotension, palpitations, blurred vision, dry mouth, urinary hesitancy	Adults and children 12 y and older: 4 mg q4–6h, maximum dose 24 mg in 24h Extended release: 8–12 mg orally q8–12h
clemastine fumarate *klem'-as-teen*	Tavist, Dayhist-1	Allergic rhinitis, urticaria, angioedema	Drowsiness, sedation, hypotension, palpitations, blurred vision, dry mouth, urinary hesitancy	Allergic rhinitis: 1.34 mg orally BID (not to exceed 8.04 mg/d for the syrup and 2.68 mg for the tablets) Urticaria and angioedema: 2.68 mg BID orally (not to exceed 4.02 mg/d)
diphenhydramine HCl *dye-fen-hye'-dra meen*	Benadryl, Banophen, Genahist, Tusstat	Allergic symptoms; hypersensitivity reactions, including anaphylaxis and transfusion reactions; motion sickness; sleep aid; antitussive and antiparkinsonism effects	Drowsiness, dry mouth, anorexia, blurred vision, urinary frequency	25–50 mg orally q4–6h, maximum daily dose 300 mg; 10–400 mg IM, IV
hydroxyzine *hye-drox'-i-zeen*	Vistaril	Analgesic (parenteral only), antiemetic (parenteral only), pruritus, sedation (oral only), anxiety (oral)	Drowsiness, dry mouth, dizziness, involuntary motor activity, pain at injection site	25–100 mg orally BID or TID; 25–100 mg IM q4–6h

SUMMARY DRUG TABLE *(continued)*

GENERIC NAME	TRADE NAME	USES	ADVERSE REACTIONS	DOSAGE RANGES
promethazine HCl *proe-meth'-a-zeen*	Phenergan	Antiemetic, hypersensitivity reactions, motion sickness, sedation	Excessive sedation, drowsiness, dry mouth, confusion, disorientation, dizziness, fatigue, blurred vision	Individualize dosage to smallest effective dose Allergy: 12.5–25 mg orally, 25 mg IM, IV Motion sickness: 25 mg BID Antiemetic: 12.5–25 mg orally, IM, IV Preoperative: 50 mg IM or orally the night before surgery
Second-Generation Antihistamines				
cetirizine HCl *se-tear'-i-zeen*	Zyrtec	Seasonal or perennial rhinitis, chronic urticaria	Sedation, dry mouth, pharyngitis, somnolence, dizziness	5–10 mg/d orally; maximum dosage 20 mg/d
desloratadine *des-low-rah'-tah-deen*	Clarinex, Clarinex Reditabs	Seasonal or perennial allergic rhinitis	Headache; fatigue; drowsiness; dry mouth, nose, and throat; flulike symptoms	Adults and children 12 y and older: 5 mg/d orally
fexofenadine *fecks-oh-fen'-a-deen*	Allegra	Seasonal rhinitis, urticaria	Headache, nausea, drowsiness, dyspepsia, fatigue, back pain, upper respiratory infection	30–60 mg orally BID; maximum dosage 180 mg/d
loratadine *lor-a'-ta-dine*	Claritin, Claritin Reditabs, Tavist ND, Alavert	Allergic rhinitis	Dizziness, headache, tremors, insomnia, dry mouth, fatigue	10 mg/d orally

and C (brompheniramine, desloratadine, fexofenadine, hydroxyzine, and promethazine), they are generally contraindicated during pregnancy and lactation.

The first-generation antihistamine drugs (see Summary Drug Table: Antihistamines) are contraindicated in patients with known hypersensitivity to the drugs, newborns, premature infants, and nursing mothers. These drugs are also contraindicated in individuals undergoing monoamine oxidase inhibitor (MAOI) therapy and in patients with angle-closure glaucoma, stenosing peptic ulcer, symptomatic prostatic hypertrophy, and bladder neck obstruction.

The second-generation antihistamines are contraindicated in patients with known hypersensitivity. Cetirizine is contraindicated in patients who are hypersensitive to hydroxyzine.

Precautions

The antihistamines are used cautiously in patients with bronchial asthma, cardiovascular disease, narrow-angle glaucoma, symptomatic prostatic hypertrophy, hypertension, impaired kidney function, peptic ulcer, urinary retention, pyloroduodenal obstruction, and hyperthyroidism.

Interactions

The following interactions may occur when an antihistamine is administered with another agent:

Interacting Drug	Common Use	Effect of Interaction
rifampin	Antitubercular agent	May reduce the absorption of the antihistamine (e.g., fexofenadine)
MAOIs	Antidepressant agent	Increased anticholinergic and sedative effects of the antihistamine
CNS depressants (e.g., opioid analgesics or alcohol)	Pain relief	Possible additive CNS depressant effect

| beta blockers | Management of cardiovascular disease | Risk for increased cardiovascular effects (e.g., with diphenhydramine) |
| aluminum- or magnesium-based antacids | Relief of gastrointestinal (GI) problems and upset | Decreased concentrations of drug in blood (e.g., fexofenadine) |

NURSING PROCESS

The Patient Receiving an Antihistamine

ASSESSMENT

PREADMINISTRATION ASSESSMENT

The preadministration assessment of the patient receiving these drugs depends on the reason for use. Examples of assessments the nurse may perform include an assessment of the involved areas (eyes, nose, and upper and lower respiratory tract) if the patient is receiving an antihistamine for the relief of allergy symptoms. If promethazine (Phenergan) is used with an opioid to enhance the effects and reduce the dosage of the opioid, the nurse should take the patient's blood pressure, pulse, and respiratory rate before giving the drug.

ONGOING ASSESSMENT

The nurse usually gives these drugs in the outpatient setting. If the patient is in the hospital or clinic, the nurse observes the patient for the expected effects of the antihistamine and for adverse reactions. The nurse reports adverse reactions to the primary health care provider. In some instances, drowsiness or sedation may occur. When the drug is given to relieve preoperative anxiety, these adverse reactions are expected and are allowed to occur.

If the antihistamine is given for a serious situation, such as a blood transfusion reaction or a severe drug allergy, the nurse assesses the patient at frequent intervals until the symptoms appear relieved and for about 24 hours after the incident.

NURSING DIAGNOSES

Drug-specific nursing diagnoses are highlighted in the Nursing Diagnoses Checklist. Other nursing diagnoses applicable to these drugs are discussed in depth in Chapter 4.

PLANNING

The expected outcomes for the patient depend on the reason for administration of the antihistamine, but may include an optimal response to therapy, support of

Nursing Diagnoses Checklist

✓ **Impaired Oral Mucous Membranes** related to adverse drug effects (dry mouth, nose, and throat)

✓ **Risk for Injury** related adverse drug reactions (drowsiness, dizziness, disturbed coordination)

patient needs related to managing adverse reactions, and an understanding of and compliance with the prescribed treatment regimen.

IMPLEMENTATION

PROMOTING AN OPTIMAL RESPONSE TO THERAPY

Most antihistamines are given orally with food to prevent GI upset. Loratadine or other rapidly disintegrating tablets can be administered with or without water and are placed on the tongue, where the tablet dissolves almost instantly. Fexofenadine is not administered within 2 hours of an antacid. When administering the antihistamines parenterally, the nurse should give the drug deep intramuscularly (IM) rather than subcutaneously (SC) because many of the antihistamines are irritating to subcutaneous tissue.

MONITORING AND MANAGING PATIENT NEEDS

IMPAIRED ORAL MUCOUS MEMBRANES Dryness of the mouth, nose, and throat may occur when the antihistamines are taken. The nurse offers the patient frequent sips of water or ice chips to relieve these symptoms. Sugarless gum or sugarless hard candy may also relieve these symptoms.

Gerontologic Alert

Older adults are more likely to experience anticholinergic effects (e.g., dryness of the mouth, nose, and throat), dizziness, sedation, hypotension, and confusion from the antihistamines. The primary care provider may recommend a dosage reduction if these symptoms persist.

RISK FOR INJURY If the patient experiences dizziness or drowsiness, it is important to provide assistance with ambulation. If drowsiness is severe or if other problems such as dizziness or a disturbance in muscle coordination occur, the patient may require assistance with ambulation and other activities. The nurse places the call light within easy reach and instructs the patient to call before attempting to get out of bed or ambulate. The nurse informs the patient that this adverse reaction may decrease with continued use of the drug.

> ### Gerontologic Alert
>
> Older adults are more likely to experience injury from dizziness because with age comes an increased risk for falls. The presence of sensori-motor deficits, such as hearing loss, visual impairments, or unsteady gait, increase the older adult's risk for injury.

EDUCATING THE PATIENT AND FAMILY

The nurse reviews the dosage regimen and possible adverse drug reactions with the patient. The following points are included in the patient teaching plan:

- Do not drive or perform other hazardous tasks if drowsiness occurs. This effect may diminish with continued use.

- Avoid the use of alcohol, as well as other drugs that cause sleepiness or drowsiness, while taking these drugs.

- Antihistamines may cause dryness of the mouth and throat. Frequent sips of water, sucking on hard candy, or chewing gum (preferably sugarless) may relieve this problem.

- If gastric upset occurs, take this drug with food or meals. Loratadine should be taken on an empty stomach, if possible. If the gastric upset is not relieved, discuss this with the primary health care provider.

- Do not take fexofenadine within 2 hours of taking an antacid.

- Do not crush or chew sustained-release preparations.

EVALUATION

- Mucous membranes are moist and intact.

- No injury is reported.

- The patient and family understand the drug regimen.

DECONGESTANTS

A **decongestant** is a drug that reduces swelling of the nasal passages, which, in turn, opens clogged nasal passages and enhances drainage of the sinuses. These drugs are used for the temporary relief of nasal congestion caused by the common cold, hay fever, sinusitis, and other respiratory allergies.

Actions

The nasal decongestants are sympathomimetic drugs that produce localized vasoconstriction of the small blood vessels of the nasal membranes. Vasoconstriction reduces swelling in the nasal passages (decongestive activity). Nasal decongestants may be applied topically, and a few are available for oral use. Examples of nasal decongestants include phenylephrine (Neo-Synephrine) and oxymetazoline (Afrin), which are available as nasal sprays or drops, and pseudoephedrine (Sudafed), which is taken orally. Additional nasal decongestants are listed in the Summary Drug Table: Systemic and Topical Nasal Decongestants.

Uses

Decongestants are used to treat the congestion associated with the following conditions:

- Common cold
- Hay fever
- Sinusitis
- Allergic rhinitis
- Congestion associated with rhinitis

Adverse Reactions

When used topically in prescribed doses, there are usually minimal systemic effects in most individuals. On occasion, nasal burning, stinging, and dryness may be seen. When the topical form is used frequently or if the liquid is swallowed, the same adverse reactions seen with the oral decongestants may occur. Use of oral decongestants may result in the following adverse reactions:

- Tachycardia and other cardiac arrhythmias
- Nervousness, restlessness, insomnia
- Blurred vision
- Nausea and vomiting

Contraindications

The decongestants are contraindicated in patients with known hypersensitivity and in patients taking MAOIs. Sustained-released pseudoephedrine is contraindicated in children younger than 12 years.

SUMMARY DRUG TABLE SYSTEMIC AND TOPICAL NASAL DECONGESTANTS

GENERIC NAME	TRADE NAME	USES	ADVERSE REACTIONS	DOSAGE RANGES
ephedrine *e-fed'-rin*	Pretz-D	Nasal congestion	Nasal burning, stinging, dryness, rebound nasal congestion	2–3 drops in each nostril q4h; maximum use, 3–4 d
epinephrine HCl *ep-i-nef'-rin*	Adrenalin Chloride	Nasal congestion	Same as ephedrine	2–3 drops or spray in each nostril q4–6h
naphazoline HCl *na-faz'-o-line*	Privine	Nasal congestion	Same as ephedrine	1–2 drops or sprays in each nostril no more than q6h
oxymetazoline HCl *oxy-met-az'-oh-leen*	Afrin 12 Hour, Dristan 12-Hour Nasal, Vicks Sinex	Nasal congestion	Same as ephedrine	2–3 drops or sprays q10–12h
phenylephrine HCl *fen-ill-ef'-rin*	Neo-Synephrine	Nasal congestion	Same as ephedrine	2–3 sprays of 0%–25% solution q3–4th
pseudoephedrine HCl *soo-dow-e-fed'-rin*	Sudafed	Nasal congestion	Anxiety, restlessness, anorexia, arrhythmias, nervousness, nausea, vomiting, blurred vision	60 mg orally q4–6h
tetrahydrozoline HCl *tet-rah-hi-draz'-oh-leen*	Tyzine	Nasal congestion	Same as pseudoephedrine	2–4 drops in each nostril or 3–4 sprays in each nostril q3h
xylometazoline HCl *zye-low-met-az'-oh-leen*	Otrivin, NatruVent	Nasal congestion	Same as ephedrine	2–3 drops or sprays in each nostril q8–10h

Precautions

The decongestants are used cautiously in patients with
- Thyroid disease
- Diabetes mellitus
- Cardiovascular disease
- Prostatic hypertrophy
- Coronary artery disease
- Peripheral vascular disease
- Hypertension
- Glaucoma

Safe use of the decongestants during pregnancy (category C) and lactation has not been established. Pregnant women should consult with their primary health care provider before using these drugs.

Interactions

The following interactions may occur when a decongestant is administered with another agent:

Interacting Drug	Common Use	Effect of Interaction
MAOIs	Control of depression	Severe headache, hypertension, and possibly hypertensive crisis
beta-adrenergic blocking drugs	Management of cardiovascular disease	Initial hypertension episode followed by bradycardia

NURSING PROCESS

The Patient Using a Nasal Decongestant

ASSESSMENT
PREADMINISTRATION ASSESSMENT

As part of the preadministration assessment, the nurse assesses the patient's blood pressure, pulse, and level of congestion before administering a decongestant. The nurse assesses lung sounds and bronchial secretions, which are noted in the patient's record. It is important to obtain a history of the use of these products, including the name of the product used and the frequency of use.

ONGOING ASSESSMENT

The ongoing assessment usually occurs when the patient comes to an outpatient clinic for follow-up treatment with the primary health care provider. The nurse assesses the patient's blood pressure, pulse, and level of congestion. The nurse questions the patient about attaining a therapeutic effect and the presence of any adverse reactions to the drug.

NURSING DIAGNOSES

A drug-specific nursing diagnosis is highlighted in the Nursing Diagnoses Checklist. Other nursing diagnoses applicable to these drugs are discussed in depth in Chapter 4.

Nursing Diagnoses Checklist

☑ **Ineffective Breathing Pattern** related to rebound effect of nasal congestion

---

PLANNING

The expected outcomes for the patient depend on the reason for administration of the drug, but may include an optimal response to therapy, support of patient needs related to the management of adverse reactions, and an understanding of and compliance with the prescribed treatment regimen.

IMPLEMENTATION

PROMOTING AN OPTIMAL RESPONSE TO THERAPY

Decongestants are used only occasionally in the clinical setting. Because some of these products are available without a prescription, their use may be discovered during a patient history for other medical disorders. Nonprescription nasal decongestants should not be used by those with hypertension or heart disease unless such use is approved by the primary health care provider.

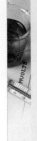

Nursing Alert

Because many decongestants can be purchased over the counter, it is important for the nurse to stress that patients who have heart disease, hypertension, hyperthyroidism, benign prostatic hypertrophy, glaucoma, and diabetes consult with their primary health care providers before using a decongestant. They should also remember to read the drug label carefully before taking a decongestant.

After administering a topical nasal decongestant, some patients may experience a mild, transient stinging sensation. This usually disappears with continued use.

Gerontologic Alert

Patients older than 60 years are at greater risk for experiencing adverse reactions to the decongestants. Overdosage may cause hallucinations, convulsion, and CNS depression.

MONITORING AND MANAGING PATIENT NEEDS

INEFFECTIVE BREATHING PATTERN Overuse of the topical form of these drugs can cause "rebound" nasal congestion. This means that the congestion becomes worse with the use of the drug. Although congestion may be relieved briefly after the drug is used, it recurs within a short time, which prompts the patient to use the drug at more frequent intervals, perpetuating the rebound congestion. The patient is taught to take the drug exactly as prescribed. A simple, but uncomfortable solution to rebound congestion is to withdraw completely from the topical medication. The primary health care provider may recommend an oral decongestant. An alternative method to minimize the occurrence of rebound nasal congestion is to discontinue the drug therapy gradually by initially discontinuing the medication in one nostril, followed by withdrawal from the other nostril.

EDUCATING THE PATIENT AND FAMILY

The nurse includes the following points in the patient teaching plan:

- Use this product as directed by the primary health care provider or on the container label.

- Understand that overuse of topical nasal decongestants can make the symptoms worse, causing rebound congestion.

- Nasal burning and stinging may occur with the topical decongestants. This effect usually disappears with use. If burning or stinging becomes severe, discontinue use and discuss this problem with the primary health care provider, who may prescribe or recommend another drug.

- If using a spray, do not allow the tip of the container to touch the nasal mucosa and do not share the container with anyone.

- To administer the spray, sit upright and sniff hard for a few minutes after administration.

- To administer drops, recline on a bed and hang your head over the edge. After using the drops, remain with the head down and turn the head from side to side.

- If using inhalers, warm the inhaler in the hand before use; wipe the inhaler after each use.

- If symptoms do not improve in 7 days or are accompanied by a high fever, consult the primary health care provider before continuing use.

EVALUATION

- The patient maintains an effective breathing pattern.

- The therapeutic effect is achieved.

- The patient demonstrates an understanding of and compliance with the drug regimen

Critical Thinking Exercises

1. A number of the antihistamines have anticholinergic effects. Discuss this term and identify nursing interactions important when caring for a patient experiencing anticholinergic effects while taking an antihistamine.

2. Discuss important teaching points that should be included in developing a teaching plan for a patient taking a nasal decongestant. Determine what teaching points would be the most important. Provide a rationale for your answer.

Review Questions

1. Which of the following is a common adverse reaction seen when administering an antihistamine?

   A. Sedation

   B. Blurred vision

   C. Headache

   D. Hypertension

2. Older adults are at increased risk for experiencing adverse reactions when taking the decongestants. Overdosage of the decongestants may cause _____.

   A. a hypotensive crisis

   B. migraine headaches

   C. hallucinations

   D. hypertension

3. When antihistamines are administered to patients receiving central nervous system depressants, the nurse monitors the patient for _____.

   A. an increase in anticholinergic effects

   B. excessive sedation

   C. seizure activity

   D. loss of hearing

4. A patient receives a prescription for phenylephrine (Neo-Synephrine). The nurse explains that overuse of this drug may _____.

   A. result in hypotensive episodes

   B. decrease sinus drainage

   C. cause rebound nasal congestion

   D. dilate capillaries in the nasal mucosa

5. Which of the following interactions would most likely occur when diphenhydramine is administered with a beta blocker drug such as propranolol (Inderal)?

   A. Increased risk for increased cardiovascular effects

   B. Increased risk for seizures

   C. Decreased risk for cardiovascular effects

   D. Decreased risk for seizures

Medication Dosage Problems

1. Loratadine 10 mg is prescribed. The drug is available in a syrup containing 1 mg/mL. The nurse prepares to administer _____.

2. A patient is to receive 50 mg of diphenhydramine HCl orally. The drug is available in 25-mg tablets. The nurse administers _____.

To check your answers, see Appendix G.

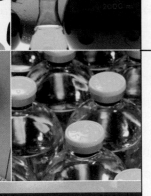

Chapter 37

Bronchodilators and Antiasthma Drugs

Key Terms

asthma
bronchodilator
leukotrienes
sympathomimetics
theophyllinization
xanthine derivatives

Learning Objectives

On completion of this chapter, the student will:

- Describe the uses, general drug action, general adverse reactions, contraindications, precautions, and interactions of the bronchodilators and antiasthma drugs.

- Discuss important preadministration and ongoing assessment activities the nurse should perform on the patient taking the bronchodilators or antiasthma drugs.

- List nursing diagnoses particular to a patient taking a bronchodilator or an antiasthma drug.

- Discuss ways to promote an optimal response to therapy, how to manage common adverse reactions, and important points to keep in mind when educating a patient about the use of a bronchodilator or an anti-asthma drug.

A bronchodilator is a drug used to relieve bronchospasm associated with respiratory disorders, such as bronchial asthma, chronic bronchitis, and emphysema. These conditions are progressive disorders characterized by a decrease in the inspiratory and expiratory capacity of the lung. The term *chronic obstructive pulmonary disease* (COPD) denotes disorders that include chronic bronchitis, chronic obstructive bronchitis, or emphysema, or a combination of these conditions. The patient with COPD experiences dyspnea (difficulty breathing) with physical exertion, has difficulty inhaling and exhaling, and may have a chronic cough.

BRONCHODILATORS

The two major types of bronchodilators are the sympathomimetics and the xanthine derivatives. The cholinergic blocking drug ipratropium bromide (Atrovent) is used for bronchospasm associated with COPD, chronic bronchitis, and emphysema. Ipratropium is featured in the Summary Drug Table: Bronchodilators. Chapter 30 provides specific information concerning the cholinergic blocking (anticholinergic) drugs.

Sympathomimetic Bronchodilators

Examples of sympathomimetic bronchodilators include albuterol (Ventolin), epinephrine (Adrenalin), salmeterol (Serevent), and terbutaline (Brethine). Many of the sympathomimetics used as bronchodilators have the subclassification of beta-2 (β_2) receptor agonists (e.g., albuterol, salmeterol, and terbutaline). Additional information concerning the various sympathomimetic drugs is given in the Summary Drug Table: Bronchodilators.

SUMMARY DRUG TABLE — BRONCHODILATORS

GENERIC NAME	TRADE NAME	USES	ADVERSE REACTIONS	DOSAGE RANGES
Sympathomimetics				
albuterol *al-byoo'-ter-ole*	Proventil, Ventolin, Volmax	Bronchospasm, prevention of EIB	Palpitations, tachycardia, hypertension, tremor, dizziness, shakiness, nervousness, nausea, vomiting	2–4 mg TID, QID orally; 1–2 inhalations q4–6h; 2 inhalations before exercise; may also be given by nebulizer Volmax: 4–8 mg q12h orally, up to 32 mg/d
bitolterol mesylate *bye-tole'-ter-ole*	Tornalate	Asthma, bronchospasm	Palpitations, hypertension, dizziness, vertigo, tremor, nervousness, headache, throat irritation	Two inhalations q8h; inhalation solution, 2.5 mg over 10–15 min with continuous-flow system or 1 mg with intermittent-flow system
ephedrine sulfate *e-fed'-rin*		Asthma, bronchospasm	Palpitations, tachycardia, hypertension, arrhythmias, dizziness, vertigo, shakiness, nervousness, headache, insomnia, nausea, vomiting	12.5–25 mg orally q3–4h PRN; 25–50 mg IM, SC, IV
epinephrine *cp-i-nef'-rin*	Adrenalin, Epinephrine Mist, Primatene Mist	Asthma, bronchospasm	Palpitations, tachycardia, hypertension, arrhythmias, dizziness, vertigo, shakiness, nervousness, headache, insomnia, nausea, vomiting, anxiety, fear, pallor	Inhalation aerosol: individualize dose Injection: Solution 1:1000, 0.3–0.5 mL SC, IM Suspension (1:200), 0.1–0.3 mL SC only
formoterol fumarate *for-moh'-te-rol*	Foradil Aerolizer Inhaler	Maintenance treatment of asthma, prevention of EIB	Palpitations, tachycardia, dizziness, nervousness	One 12–mg capsule q12h using Aerolizer Inhaler; for EIB one 12–mcg capsule 15 min before exercise using the Aerolizer Inhaler
isoetharine *eye-soe-eth'-a-reen*		Asthma, bronchospasm	Palpitations, tachycardia, hypertension, tremor, dizziness, nervousness, weakness, restlessness, hyperactivity, headache, insomnia, nausea, vomiting	Handheld nebulizer: 3–7 inhalations 1:3 dilution or 4 inhalations undiluted
isoproterenol HCl *eye-soe proe-ter'-a-nole*	Isuprel	Bronchospasm during anesthesia, vasopressor during shock	Palpitations, tachycardia, chest tightness, angina, shakiness, nervousness, weakness, hyperactivity, headache, nausea, vomiting, flushing, sweating	0.01–0.02 mg IV, repeat if necessary; dilute 1 mL of a 1:5000 solution to 10 mL with sodium chloride injections of 5% dextrose IV
levalbuterol HCl *lev-al-byoo'-ter-ole*	Xopenex	Bronchospasm	Tachycardia, nervousness, anxiety, pain, dizziness, rhinitis, cough, cardiac arrhythmias	0.63 mg TID, q6–8h by nebulization; if no response, dose may be increased to 1.25 mg TID by nebulizer

SUMMARY DRUG TABLE *(continued)*

GENERIC NAME	TRADE NAME	USES	ADVERSE REACTIONS	DOSAGE RANGES
metaproterenol sulfate *met-a-proe-ter'-e-nole*	Alupent	Asthma, bronchospasm	Tachycardia, tremor, nervousness, shakiness, nausea, vomiting	Aerosol 2–3 inhalations q3–4h; do not exceed 12 inhalations
pirbuterol acetate *peer-byoo'-ter-ole*	Maxair Autohaler, Maxair Inhaler	Asthma, bronchospasm	Shakiness, nervousness, nausea, tachycardia	Two inhalations q4–6h; do not exceed 12 inhalations
salmeterol *sal-mee'-ter-ol*	Serevent Diskus	Asthma, bronchospasm, prevention of EIB	Palpitations, tachycardia, tremor, nervousness, headache, nausea, vomiting, heartburn, GI distress, diarrhea, cough, rhinitis	Asthma/bronchospasm: aerosol, 2 inhalations BID morning and evening; inhalation powder, one (50-mcg) inhalation BID
terbutaline sulfate *ter-byoo'-ta-leen*	Brethine	Asthma, bronchospasm	Palpitations, tremor, dizziness, vertigo, shakiness, nervousness, drowsiness, headache, nausea, vomiting, GI upset	2.5–5 mg q6h orally TID during waking hours; 0.25 mg SC (may repeat once if needed)
Xanthine Derivatives				
aminophylline *am-in-off'-lin*	Phyllocontin, Truphylline	Symptomatic relief or prevention of bronchial asthma and reversible bronchospasm of chronic bronchitis and emphysema	Nausea, vomiting, restlessness, nervousness, tachycardia, tremors, headache, palpitations, hyperglycemia, electrocardiographic changes, cardiac arrhythmias	Individualize dosage: base adjustments on clinical responses, monitor serum aminophylline levels, maintain therapeutic range of 10–20 mcg/mL; base dosage on lean body mass
dyphylline *dye'-fi-lin*	Lufyllin	Same as aminophylline	Same as aminophylline	Up to 15 mg/kg orally QID; 250–500 mg IM
oxtriphylline *ox-trye'-fi-lin*	Choledyl	Same as aminophylline	Same as aminophylline	4.7 mg/kg orally q8h; sustained-action: 1 tablet orally q12h
theophylline *thee-off'-i-lin*	Theo-24, Theo-Dur, Theolair, Slo-bid, Uniphyl	Same as aminophylline	Same as aminophylline	Long-term therapy: 16 mg/kg/d or 400 mg/d in divided doses Monitor serum theophylline levels
Cholinergic Blocking Drug (Anticholinergic)				
ipratropium bromide *ih-prah-trow'-pea-um*	Atrovent	Bronchospasm associated with chronic obstructive pulmonary disease, chronic bronchitis and emphysema, rhinorrhea	Dryness of the oropharynx, nervousness, irritation from aerosol, dizziness, headache, GI distress, dry mouth, exacerbation of symptoms, nausea, palpitations	Aerosol: two inhalations (36 mcg) QID, not to exceed 12 inhalations; Solution: 500 mg (1 unit dose vial) TID, QID by oral nebulization Nasal spray: 2 sprays per nostril BID, TID of 0.03%, or 2 sprays per nostril TID, QID of 0.06%

EIB, exercise-induced bronchospasm; GI, gastrointestinal.

Actions

When bronchospasm occurs, there is a decrease in the lumen (or inside diameter) of the bronchi, which decreases the amount of air taken into the lungs with each breath. A decrease in the amount of air taken into the lungs results in respiratory distress. Use of a bronchodilating drug opens the bronchi and allows more air to enter the lungs, which, in turn, completely or partially relieves respiratory distress.

Uses

Sympathomimetics (drugs that mimic the sympathetic nervous system) are used to treat
- Bronchospasm associated with acute and chronic bronchial asthma
- Exercise-induced bronchospasm
- Bronchitis
- Emphysema
- Bronchiectasis (chronic dilation of the bronchi and bronchioles)
- Other obstructive pulmonary diseases

Adverse Reactions

Adverse effects of the sympathomimetics include
- Tachycardia, palpitations, or cardiac arrhythmias
- Nervousness, anxiety
- Hypertension
- Insomnia

When these drugs are used by inhalation, excessive use (e.g., over the recommended dose times) may result in paradoxical bronchospasm.

Contraindications

The sympathomimetic bronchodilators are contraindicated in patients with known hypersensitivity to the drug, cardiac arrhythmias associated with tachycardia, organic brain damage, cerebral arteriosclerosis, and narrow-angle glaucoma. Salmeterol is contraindicated during acute bronchospasm.

Precautions

The sympathomimetics are used cautiously in patients with hypertension, cardiac dysfunction, hyperthyroidism, glaucoma, diabetes, prostatic hypertrophy, and history of seizures.

The sympathomimetic drugs are also used cautiously during pregnancy and lactation (all are in pregnancy category C, except terbutaline, which is a pregnancy category B drug).

Interactions

The following interactions may occur when a sympathomimetic drug is used concurrently with another agent:

Interacting Drug	Common Use	Effect of Interaction
adrenergic drugs	Treatment of hypotension and shock	Possible additive adrenergic effects
monoamine oxidase inhibitors	Treatment of depression	Increased risk for severe headache, hypertension, and a hypertensive crisis
beta blockers	Treatment of hypertension	Inhibition of the cardiac, bronchodilating, and vasodilating effects of the sympathomimetic
methyldopa	Treatment of hypertension	Increased pressor response
oxytocic drugs	Uterine stimulant	Possible severe hypotension
theophylline	Treatment of asthma and COPD	Increased risk for cardiotoxicity

Xanthine Derivative Bronchodilators

Xanthine derivatives (also called *methylxanthines*) are drugs that stimulate the central nervous system (CNS) to promote bronchodilation. Examples are theophylline (Theo-Dur) and aminophylline (Phyllocontin). Additional information concerning the xanthine derivatives is found in the Summary Drug Table: Bronchodilators.

Actions

The xanthine derivatives, although a different class of drugs from the sympathomimetics, also have bronchodilating activity by means of their direct relaxation of the smooth muscles of the bronchi.

Uses

The xanthine derivatives are used for

- Symptomatic relief or prevention of bronchial asthma
- Treatment of reversible bronchospasm associated with chronic bronchitis and emphysema

Adverse Reactions

Central Nervous System Reactions

- Restlessness
- Nervousness, tremors

Cardiac

- Tachycardia
- Palpitations
- Electrocardiographic changes
- Increased respirations

Other

- Nausea, vomiting, fever
- Hyperglycemia

Contraindications

The xanthine derivatives are contraindicated in those with known hypersensitivity to the drugs, peptic ulcers, seizure disorders (unless well controlled with appropriate anticonvulsant medication), serious uncontrolled arrhythmias, and hyperthyroidism.

Precautions

The xanthine derivatives are used cautiously in patients with cardiac disease, hypoxemia, hypertension, congestive heart failure, and liver disease. They are also used cautiously in patients older than 69 years of age. Aminophylline, dyphylline, oxtriphylline, and theophylline are pregnancy category C drugs and are used cautiously during pregnancy and lactation.

Interactions

When taken with theophylline, the following agents have an effect on theophylline levels:

Interacting Agent	Common Use	Effect of Interaction
barbiturates	Sedation	Decreased theophylline levels
charcoal (in large amounts)	Broiling/grilling foods	
hydantoins	Anticonvulsant	
ketoconazole	Antifungal agent	
rifampin	Antitubercular agent	
nicotine (tobacco, nicotine gum and patches)	Used for effect from smoking tobacco or to aid smoking cessation	
adrenergic agents	Treatment of hypotension and shock	
isoniazid	Antitubercular agent	
loop diuretics	Treatment of hypertension	
allopurinol	Antigout agent	Increased theophylline levels
beta blockers	Treatment of hypertension	
calcium channel blockers	Treatment of angina and hypertension	
cimetidine	Treatment of gastrointestinal (GI) problems	
oral contraceptives	Birth control	
corticosteroids	Anti-inflammatory agents	
ephedrine	Treatment of anaphylactic shock	
Influenza virus vaccine	Prevention of flu	
macrolide antibiotics	Treatment of infections	
thyroid hormones	Treatment of hypothyroidism	
isoniazid	Antitubercular agent	
loop diuretics	Treatment of edema	

ANTIASTHMA DRUGS

Asthma is a chronic inflammatory disease of the airways. It is characterized by recurrent attacks of dyspnea (difficulty breathing) and wheezing caused by spasmodic constriction of the bronchi. With asthma, the body responds with a massive inflammation. During the inflammatory process, large amounts of histamine are released from the mast cells of the respiratory tract, causing symptoms such as increased mucus production and edema of the airway with resultant bronchospasm and inflammation. With asthma the airways become narrow, the muscles around the airways tighten, the inner lining of the bronchi swell, and extra mucus clogs the smaller airways (Fig. 37-1).

The three most common symptoms are cough, dyspnea, and wheezing. Patients with asthma may experience periods of exacerbations alternating with periods of normal respiratory function. The period of exacerbation may begin abruptly, but is usually preceded by increasing symptoms over the previous several days of the following:

- Cough (with or without mucus production)
- Generalized wheezing, dyspnea (expiration becomes prolonged)
- Generalized chest tightness
- Diaphoresis
- Tachycardia

Exercise-induced asthma (EIA), also called exercise-induced bronchospasm (EIB), is a condition that occurs when an individual develops a set of asthmatic symptoms after about 6 to 8 minutes of exercise. These symptoms include coughing, wheezing, tightness in the chest, and prolonged shortness of breath.

Along with the bronchodilators, several types of drugs are effective in treating asthma. These include corticosteroids, leukotriene formation inhibitors, leukotriene receptor agonists, and mast cell stabilizers.

Antiasthma drugs are used in various combinations to treat and manage asthma. Using several drugs may be more beneficial than using a single drug. A multidrug regimen allows smaller dosages of each drug, decreasing the number and severity of adverse reactions. Various combinations of these drugs are used depending on the patient's response.

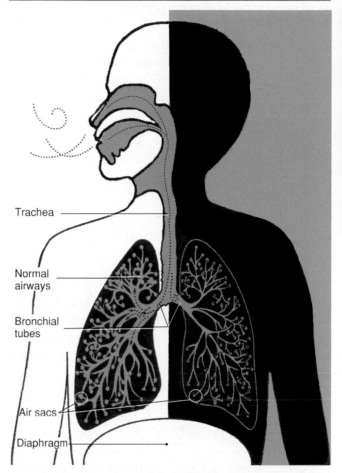

Figure 37.1 Left column. *Normal lungs*: Air comes into the body through the nose and mouth. Air then goes through the trachea into all the airways. The air reaches the tiny air sacs deep in the lungs, where gas exchange takes place. **Right column.** *Lungs in asthma*: In asthma, the patient has trouble moving air through the lungs because airways become narrow as the muscles in their walls tighten and the airway walls swell. The swollen walls give off extra mucus, which clogs the narrowed airways.

Corticosteroids
Actions

Corticosteroids, such as beclomethasone (Beclovent), flunisolide (AeroBid), and triamcinolone (Azmacort), are given by inhalation and act to decrease the inflammatory process in the airways of the patient with asthma. In addition, the corticosteroids increase the sensitivity of the β_2 receptors, which in turn increases the effectiveness of the β_2 receptor agonist drugs.

Uses

The corticosteroids are used in the management and prophylactic treatment of the inflammation associated with chronic asthma or allergic rhinitis.

Adverse Reactions

When used to manage chronic asthma, the corticosteroids are most often given by inhalation. Adverse reactions to the corticosteroids are less likely to occur when the drugs are given by inhalation rather than taken orally. Occasionally, patients may experience reactions.

Adverse Reactions

- Throat irritation
- Hoarseness
- Cough
- Fungal infection of the mouth and throat
- Vertigo
- Headache

See Chapter 50 for adverse reactions after oral administration of the corticosteroids. A more complete listing of the adverse reactions associated with the corticosteroids is found in the Summary Drug Table: Antiasthma Drugs.

Contraindications

The corticosteroids are contraindicated in patients with hypersensitivity to the corticosteroids, acute bronchospasm, status asthmaticus, or other acute episodes of asthma. Beclomethasone is contraindicated for the relief of symptoms that can be controlled by a bronchodilator and other nonsteroidal medications and in the treatment of nonasthmatic bronchitis.

Precautions

The corticosteroids are used cautiously in patients with compromised immune systems, glaucoma, kidney disease, liver disease, convulsive disorders, and diabetes. These drugs are also used with caution in those taking systemic corticosteroids and during pregnancy (category C) and lactation.

Interactions

Ketoconazole may increase plasma levels of budesonide and fluticasone.

Leukotriene Receptor Antagonists and Leukotriene Formation Inhibitors

Leukotriene receptor antagonists include montelukast sodium (Singulair) and zafirlukast (Accolate). Zileuton (Zyflo) is classified as a leukotriene formation inhibitor. Additional information concerning these drugs is found in the Summary Drug Table: Antiasthma Drugs.

Actions

Leukotrienes are bronchoconstrictive substances released by the body during the inflammatory process. When leukotriene production is inhibited, bronchodilation is facilitated. Zileuton acts by decreasing the formation of leukotrienes. Although the result is the same, montelukast and zafirlukast work in a manner slightly differently from that of zileuton. Montelukast and zafirlukast are considered leukotriene receptor antagonists because they inhibit leukotriene receptor sites in the respiratory tract, preventing airway edema and facilitating bronchodilation.

Uses

Zileuton and montelukast are used in the prophylaxis and treatment of chronic asthma in adults and children older than 12 years. Zafirlukast is used in the prophylaxis and treatment of chronic asthma in adults and in children older than 5 years.

Adverse Reactions

Zafirlukast

Adverse reactions associated with zafirlukast (Accolate) are varied. CNS reactions include
- Headache
- Dizziness

Gastrointestinal system reactions include
- Nausea, vomiting
- Diarrhea
- Abdominal pain

Other body system reactions include myalgia, pain, and fever.

SUMMARY DRUG TABLE   ANTIASTHMA DRUGS

GENERIC NAME	TRADE NAME	USES	ADVERSE REACTIONS	DOSAGE RANGES
Corticosteroids				
beclomethasone dipropionate *be-kloe-meth'-a-sone*	QVAR, Beclovent, Vanceril	Respiratory inhalant use: asthma Intranasal use: seasonal or perennial rhinitis, prevention of recurrence of nasal polyps after surgical removal	Oral, laryngeal, pharyngeal irritation, fungal infections, suppression of HPA function	Starting dose used with bronchodilators alone: 40–80 mcg BID; when used with inhaled corticosteroids: 40–60 mcg BID; maximum 320 mcg BID Children 5–12 y: 40 mcg BID when used with bronchodilators alone or with inhaled corticosteroids
budesonide *bue-des'-oh-nide*	Pulmicort Turbuhaler, Pulmicort Respules	Turbuhaler: management of chronic asthma in adults and children older than 6 y; Respules: maintenance treatment of asthma and as prophylactic therapy in children 12 mo to 8 y; Additional indication: improvement of symptoms of mild to moderate acute laryngotracheobronchitis (croup), seasonal or perennial rhinitis (nasal spray)	Oral, laryngeal, pharyngeal irritation, fungal infections, suppression of HPA function	Individualized dosage by oral inhalation Adults: 200–800 mcg BID Children 6 y and older: 200–400 mcg BID Children 12 mo to 8 y: 0.5–1 mcg total daily dose administered once or twice daily in divided doses
flunisolide *floo-niss'-oh-lide*	AeroBid, AeroBid-M	Chronic asthma Respiratory inhalant: asthma Intranasal: rhinitis	Oral, laryngeal, and pharyngeal irritation, fungal infections, suppression of HPA function	Adults: 2 inhalations BID; maximum dose, 4 inhalations BID Intranasal: 2 sprays each nostril BID (maximum dosage, 8 sprays/d) Children 6–15 y: 2 inhalations BID
fluticasone propionate *flew-tick'-ah-soan*	Flovent, Flovent Rotadisk, Flovent Diskus	Prophylactic maintenance and treatment of asthma	Oral, laryngeal, pharyngeal irritation, fungal infections, suppression of HPA function	Aerosol: 88–880 mcg BID Powder: adults and adolescents 100–1000 mcg BID; children 4–11 y, 50–100 mcg BID
mometasone furoate *moe-met'-a-soan*	Asmanex Twisthaler	Chronic asthma	Headache, allergic rhinitis, pharyngitis, upper respiratory infection, sinusitis, oral candidiasis, dysmenorrheal or musculoskeletal pain	One inhalation (220 mcg) QD in the evening for patients previously maintained on bronchodilators alone or inhaled corticosteroids; 2 inhalations (440 mcg) BID for patients previously maintained on oral corticosteroids
triamcinolone acetonide *trye-am-sin'-oh-lone*	Azmacort	Maintenance and prophylactic treatment of asthma; for patients with asthma who require systemic	Oral, laryngeal, and pharyngeal irritation, fungal infections, suppression of HPA function	Adults: 2 inhalations TID, QID; maximum daily dosage 16 inhalations Children 6–12 y: 1–2 inhalations TID, QID;

SUMMARY DRUG TABLE *(continued)*

GENERIC NAME	TRADE NAME	USES	ADVERSE REACTIONS	DOSAGE RANGES
		corticosteroid administration when adding an inhaled corticosteroid, may reduce or eliminate the need for systemic corticosteroids		maximum daily dosage, 12 inhalations
Leukotriene Receptor Antagonists				
montelukast sodium *mon-tell-oo'-kast*	Singulair	Prophylaxis and treatment of chronic asthma in adults and pediatric patients 12 mo of age and older, seasonal allergic rhinitis in adults and pediatric patients 2 y of age and older	Headache, dizziness, dyspepsia, gastroenteritis, influenza-like symptoms, cough, abdominal pain, fatigue	Adults and children older than 15 y: 10 mg orally in the evening Children 6–14 y: one 5-mg chewable tablet daily, in the evening Children 2–5 y: one 4-mg chewable tablet daily, in the evening, or one 4-mg oral granule packet daily Children 12–23 mo with asthma: 1 packet of 4-mg granules daily in the evening
zafirlukast *zah-fir'-luh-kast*	Accolate	Prophylaxis and treatment of chronic asthma in adults and children 5 y or older	Headache, dizziness, nausea, diarrhea, abdominal pain, vomiting, infection, pain, asthenia, accidental injury, myalgia, fever, ALT elevation	Adults and children older than 12 y: 20 mg orally BID Children 5–11 y: 10 mg orally BID
Leukotriene Formation Inhibitors				
zileuton *zye-loot'-on*	Zyflo	Prophylaxis and treatment of chronic asthma in adults and children 12 y or older	Dyspepsia, nausea, headache, pain, abdominal pain, asthenia, myalgia, accidental injury, ALT elevation	600 mg orally QID
Mast Cell Stabilizers				
Cromolyn *kroe'-moe-lin*	Intal, Nasalcrom, Gastrocrom	Bronchial asthma, prevention of bronchospasm; prevention of EIA Nasal preparations: prevention and treatment of allergic rhinitis	Dizziness, headache, nausea, dry and irritated throat, rash, joint swelling and pain	Inhalation solution: 20 mg (1 ampule/vial) administered by nebulizer QID Aerosol: adults and children 5 y and older: 2 metered sprays QID EIA: 2 metered sprays shortly (10–15 min but not more than 60 min) before exposure to the precipitating factor Nasal solution: 1 spray each nostril 3–6 times/d

GENERIC NAME	TRADE NAME	USES	ADVERSE REACTIONS	DOSAGE RANGES
				Oral: adults and children 13 y and older: 2 ampules QID 30 min before meals and at bedtime Children 2–12 y: 1 ampule QID before meals and at bedtime; do not exceed 40 mg/kg/d
nedocromil *nee-doc'-ro-mill*	Tilade	Maintenance therapy in mild to moderate bronchial asthma	Cough, nausea, pharyngitis, rhinitis, vomiting, dyspepsia, chest pain, headache, bronchospasm	Two inhalations QID
Miscellaneous Antiasthma Drug				
omalizumab *oh-mal-iz'-you-mab*	Xolair	Moderate to severe persistent asthma	Injection site reaction, viral infection, sinusitis, headache, pharyngitis anaphylaxis, malignancies	150–375 mg SC every 2–4 wk

ALI, alanine aminotransferase; EIA, exercise-induced asthma; HPA, hypothalamic-pituitary-adrenal.

Montelukast

Adverse reactions associated with montelukast (Singulair) are varied as well.

- CNS reactions include headache and dizziness.
- GI reactions include dyspepsia and abdominal pain.
- Respiratory reactions include flulike symptoms and cough.

Zileuton

Adverse reactions seen with the administration of zileuton (Zyflo) include headache and GI system reactions, such as

- Dyspepsia and nausea
- Abdominal pain

Contraindications and Precautions

These drugs are contraindicated in patients with known hypersensitivity, bronchospasm in acute asthma attacks, or liver disease (zileuton). They also are used cautiously in pregnancy and lactation (zafirlukast and montelukast are pregnancy category B drugs and zileuton is pregnancy category C).

Interactions

The following interactions may occur when zafirlukast is administered with another agent:

Interacting Drug	Common Use	Effect of Interaction
aspirin	Pain relief	Increased plasma levels of zafirlukast
warfarin	Anticoagulant	Increased anticoagulant effect
theophylline	Treatment of asthma and COPD	Decreased level of zafirlukast
erythromycin	Treatment of bacterial infection	Decreased level of zafirlukast

The following interactions may occur when zileuton is administered with another agent:

Interacting Drug	Common Use	Effect of Interaction
propranolol	Treatment of cardiac problems	Increased activity of the propranolol
theophylline	Treatment of asthma and COPD	Increased serum theophylline levels
warfarin	Anticoagulant	Increased prothrombin time (PT)

Administration of montelukast with other drugs has not revealed any adverse responses.

Mast Cell Stabilizers

Mast cell stabilizers include cromolyn sodium (Intal) and nedocromil sodium (Tilade).

Actions

Although their action is not fully understood, these drugs are thought to stabilize the mast cell membrane, possibly by preventing calcium ions from entering mast cells, thus preventing the release of inflammatory mediators.

Uses

The mast cell stabilizers are used in combination with other drugs in the treatment of asthma and allergic disorders, including allergic rhinitis (nasal solution). They are also used to prevent EIB.

These drugs may be given by nebulization, aerosol spray, or as an oral concentrate. The mast cell stabilizers were at one time the first choice to treat asthma in children. However, they have not been found to be as effective as inhaled corticosteroids, which are now the recommended treatment.

Adverse Reactions

Central Nervous System Reactions

- Headache
- Dizziness
- Hypotension

Other

- Nausea
- Fatigue
- Unpleasant taste sensation

These drugs may cause nasal or throat irritation when given intranasally or by inhalation. A more complete listing of the adverse reactions associated with the mast cell stabilizers is found in the Summary Drug Table: Antiasthma Drugs.

Contraindications and Precautions

The mast cell stabilizers are contraindicated in patients with known hypersensitivity to the drugs and during attacks of acute asthma because they may worsen bronchospasm during the acute asthma attack.

Mast cell stabilizers are used cautiously during pregnancy (pregnancy category B) and lactation and in patients with impaired renal or hepatic function.

Interactions

No significant drug interactions have been reported.

NURSING PROCESS

The Patient Receiving a Bronchodilator or an Antiasthma Drug

ASSESSMENT
PREADMINISTRATION ASSESSMENT

Because the bronchodilators or antiasthma drugs may be given for asthma, emphysema, or chronic bronchitis, the preadministration assessment of the patient requires careful observation and documentation. The nurse takes the blood pressure, pulse, and respiratory rate before therapy with a bronchodilator or antiasthma drug is initiated. Respiratory rates below 12 breaths/min or above 24 breaths/min are considered abnormal. It is important to assess the lung fields and carefully document the sounds heard before therapy is begun. The nurse notes any dyspnea, cough, wheezing (a musical sound of the respiratory tract caused by air passing through a narrowed bronchial tube), "noisy" respirations, or use of accessory muscles when breathing. If the patient is raising sputum, the nurse records a description of the sputum. The nurse notes and records the patient's general physical condition. It is important to record any signs of hypoxia, such as mental confusion, restlessness, anxiety, and cyanosis (bluish discoloration of the skin and mucous membranes). In some instances, the primary heath care provider may order arterial blood gas analysis or pulmonary function tests.

In patients with chronic asthma, the nurse questions the patient concerning allergies, frequency of attacks, severity of attacks, factors that cause or relieve attacks, and any antiasthma drugs used currently or taken previously.

ONGOING ASSESSMENT

During the ongoing assessment, the nurse assesses the respiratory status every 4 hours (or more often if needed) and whenever the drug is administered. The nurse notes the respiratory rate, lung sounds, and use of accessory muscles in breathing. In addition, the nurse keeps a careful record of the intake and output and reports any imbalance, which may indicate a fluid overload or excessive diuresis. It is important to monitor any patient with a history of cardiovascular problems for chest pain and changes in the electrocardiogram. The primary health care provider may order periodic pulmonary function tests, particularly for patients with emphysema or bronchitis, to help monitor respiratory status.

After administration of the drug, the nurse observes the patient for the effectiveness of drug therapy. Breathing should improve, and the patient will appear less anxious. If relief does not occur, the nurse notifies the primary health care provider because a different drug or an increase in dosage may be necessary.

NURSING DIAGNOSES

Drug-specific nursing diagnoses are highlighted in the Nursing Diagnoses Checklist. Other nursing diagnoses applicable to these drugs are discussed in depth in Chapter 4.

✔ Nursing Diagnoses Checklist

- ✔ **Anxiety** related to adverse reactions of the bronchodilators

- ✔ **Imbalanced Nutrition: Less Than Body Requirements** related to adverse reactions of the bronchodilating and antiasthma drugs

- ✔ **Impaired Oral Mucous Membranes** related to adverse reactions of the bronchodilating and antiasthma drugs

- ✔ **Ineffective Airway Clearance** related to adverse reactions of the bronchodilators and antiasthma drugs

---

PLANNING

The expected outcomes for the patient depend on the specific reason for administering the drug, but may include an optimal response to therapy, meeting patient needs related to the management of adverse drug reactions, and an understanding of and compliance with the prescribed treatment regimen.

IMPLEMENTATION
PROMOTING AN OPTIMAL RESPONSE TO THERAPY

Nursing care of the patient receiving a bronchodilating drug or an antiasthma drug requires careful monitoring of the patient and proper administration of the various drugs. These drugs may be given orally, parenterally, or topically by inhalation or nebulization. In general, the nurse gives

the drugs around the clock to maintain therapeutic blood levels. Dosages are individualized for each patient, which allows the smallest effective dose to be given. The nurse can give oral preparations with food or milk if gastric upset occurs.

PATIENTS TAKING SYMPATHOMIMETICS Some of the sympathomimetics are extremely potent drugs. The nurse exercises great care in reading the primary health care provider's order when preparing these drugs for administration. Doses of drugs such as epinephrine are measured in tenths of a milliliter. A tuberculin syringe is used for measuring and administering these drugs by the parenteral route.

Epinephrine The nurse may administer epinephrine subcutaneously for an acute bronchospasm. Therapeutic effects occur within 5 minutes after administration and last as long as 4 hours.

Salmeterol A long-acting inhaled bronchodilator, salmeterol is not used to treat acute asthma symptoms. It does not replace the fast-acting inhalers for sudden symptoms. Salmeterol is not administered more frequently than twice daily (morning and evening).

Formoterol Fumarate (Foradil Aerolizer) This drug is administered only by oral inhalation using the Aerolizer Inhaler. The usual dosage is one 12-mcg capsule of formoterol every 12 hours.

PATIENTS TAKING XANTHINE DERIVATIVES For acute respiratory symptoms, rapid theophyllinization using one of the xanthine derivatives may be required. **Theophyllinization** is accomplished by giving the patient a higher initial dose, called a *loading dose*, to bring blood levels to a therapeutic range more quickly than waiting several days for the drug to exert a therapeutic effect. The primary health care provider may prescribe loading doses to be administered orally or intravenously (IV) over 12 to 24 hours. It is important for the nurse to monitor the patient closely for signs of theophylline toxicity.

Nursing Alert

Notify the primary health care provider immediately if any of the following signs of theophylline toxicity develops: anorexia, nausea, vomiting, diarrhea, confusion, abdominal cramping, headache, restlessness, insomnia, tachycardia, arrhythmias, or seizures.

The primary health care provider may order a daily plasma theophylline level to monitor for toxicity. The therapeutic range of theophylline blood levels is 10 to 20 mcg/mL.

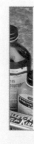

Display 37.1 Symptoms Associated With Serum Theophylline Levels

- Levels less than 20 mcg/mL adverse reactions are rare
- Levels greater than 20 mcg/mL—nausea, vomiting, diarrhea, headache, insomnia, irritability
- Levels greater than 35 mcg/mL—hyperglycemia, hypotension, cardiac arrhythmias, tachycardia, seizures, brain damage

Toxicity occurs in levels above 20 mcg/mL. In some patients, toxicity may occur with levels between 15 and 20 mcg/mL. Toxicity is more likely to occur in patients requiring high doses or during prolonged therapy. Display 37-1 identifies symptoms observed in patients with various serum theophylline levels. The nurse reports any serum theophylline levels greater than 20 mcg/mL or any symptoms associated with toxicity.

The nurse can give some of these drugs (e.g., aminophylline or theophylline) by IV infusion. When giving theophylline or aminophylline IV, the nurse monitors the patient for hypotension, cardiac arrhythmias, and tachycardia. If a bronchodilator is given IV, the nurse administers it through an infusion pump. The nurse checks the IV infusion site at frequent intervals because these patients may be extremely restless and extravasation can occur.

Gerontologic Alert

Older adults taking the sympathomimetic bronchodilators are at increased risk for adverse reactions related to both the cardiovascular system (tachycardia, arrhythmias, palpitations, and hypertension) and the CNS (restlessness, agitation, insomnia).

PATIENTS TAKING LEUKOTRIENE RECEPTOR ANTAGONISTS AND LEUKOTRIENE FORMATION INHIBITORS These drugs are used for managing asthma and are never administered during an acute asthma attack. If used during an acute attack, these drugs may worsen the attack. These drugs are administered orally.

Montelukast is administered once daily in the evening; zafirlukast is administered twice daily 1 hour before meals or 2 hours after meals. Zileuton is administered four times daily.

Zileuton may cause liver damage. Because of the danger of liver toxicity, the primary health care provider may order hepatic aminotransferase levels at the beginning of treatment and during therapy with zileuton.

PATIENTS TAKING ORAL OR INHALANT CORTICOSTEROIDS If the patient is receiving a sympathomimetic bronchodilator by inhalation and a corticosteroid by inhalation, the nurse administers the bronchodilator first, waits several minutes, and then administers the corticosteroid inhalant. When administering two inhalations of the same drug, it is advisable to wait at least 1 minute between puffs.

Pediatric Alert

When children are taking oral corticosteroids or higher doses of the inhalant form, growth should be monitored closely. A reduction in growth may occur from corticosteroid use. The primary health care provider is kept informed of the patient's growth record. It is particularly important to monitor growth in puberty and adolescence.

PATIENTS TAKING MAST CELL STABILIZERS The mast cell stabilizers, such as cromolyn (Intal), may be added to the patient's existing treatment regimen (e.g., bronchodilators). When added to the existing regimen, the other medications (e.g., corticosteroids) are decreased gradually when the patient experiences a therapeutic response to cromolyn (2 to 4 weeks) and asthma is under good control. The corticosteroids or other antiasthma drugs may be reinstituted based on the patient's symptoms. If use of the mast cell stabilizers must be discontinued for any reason, the dosage is gradually tapered.

When administered orally, cromolyn is given 1/2 hour before meals and at bedtime. The oral form of the drug comes in an ampule. The ampule is opened and the contents poured into a glass of water. The nurse stirs the mixture thoroughly. The patient must drink all of the mixture. The drug may not be mixed with any other substance (e.g., fruit juice, milk, or foods).

The drugs may be administered by a metered-dose inhaler (see Patient and Family Teaching Checklist: Teaching the Patient to Use a Metered-Dose Inhaler). If an aerosol inhaler is used for administration, the nurse teaches the patient how to use it.

MONITORING AND MANAGING PATIENT NEEDS

ANXIETY Patients who have difficulty breathing and are receiving a sympathomimetic drug may experience

Patient and Family Teaching Checklist

Teaching the Patient to Use a Metered-Dose Inhaler

To properly instruct the patient in administration of drug via a metered-dose inhaler, the nurse must be aware of general instructions for use for all metered-dose inhalers and three common methods of use: holding the lips around the mouthpiece, holding the inhaler away from the mouth, and using a spacer or extender.

General Instructions for Use for All Metered-Dose Inhalers

The nurse teaches the patient to:

✔ Shake the inhaler well, with the canister in place, for 5 to 10 seconds immediately before use.

✔ Remove the cap from the mouthpiece.

✔ Breathe out to the end of a normal breath.

✔ Hold the inhaler system upright.

✔ Place the mouthpiece into the mouth, close the lips tightly **or** position the mouthpiece 2 to 3 finger-widths from open mouth and tilt the head back.

✔ Activate the inhaler while taking a slow, deep breath for 3 to 5 seconds.

✔ Hold the breath for about 10 seconds and exhale slowly.

✔ If more than one inhalation is required, wait about 1 minute between inhalations (see manufacturer's directions for specific times). Two minutes are allowed between inhalations for metaproterenol.

✔ Gargle or rinse the mouth after each dose to relieve dry mouth and throat irritation.

✔ Rinse the extender and mouthpiece, if applicable, daily in warm water and store them away from heat.

✔ To monitor the amount of drug remaining in the canister, test the canister by placing it in a container of water.

Specific Instructions for Common Methods of Use

Holding the inhaler away from the mouth involves the use of a device called an extender or spacer attached to the inhaler. Use of the extender allows more drug to reach the lung. The nurse teaches the patient to:

✔ Place the extender over the mouth (see manufacturer's directions for specific directions).

✔ Press the chamber.

✔ When the drug passes through the extender, take four to six deep breaths to deliver the drug to the lower respiratory passages.

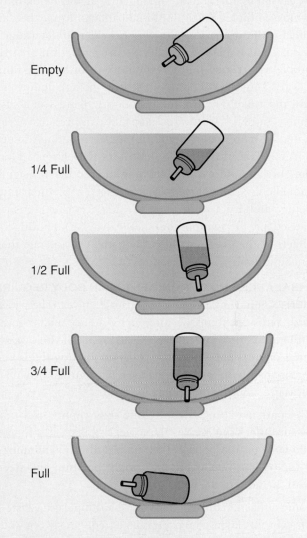

Empty

1/4 Full

1/2 Full

3/4 Full

Full

To monitor the amount of drug in a metered-dose inhaler, place the canister in a container of water. The figure shows the positioning of the canister with various amounts of medication remaining in the canister—i.e., a full canister sinks; an empty canister floats.

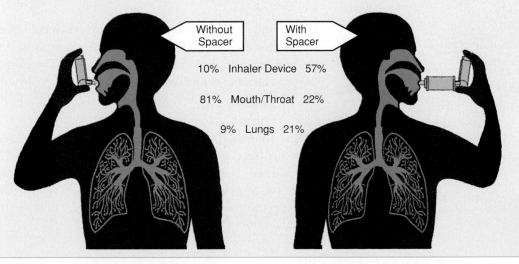

Without Spacer	Inhaler Device	With Spacer
10%	Inhaler Device	57%
81%	Mouth/Throat	22%
9%	Lungs	21%

Percentages of drug dispersal from a metered-dose inhaler without a spacer (*left*) and with a spacer (*right*).

extreme anxiety, nervousness, and restlessness, which may be caused by their breathing difficulty or the action of the sympathomimetic drug. In these patients, it may be difficult for the primary health care provider to determine if the patient is having an adverse drug reaction or if the problem is related to the respiratory disorder. The nurse can reassure the patient that the drug being administered will most likely relieve the respiratory distress in a short time. Patients who are extremely apprehensive are observed more frequently until their respirations are near normal. The nurse closely monitors the patient's blood pressure and pulse during therapy and reports any significant changes. The nurse speaks and acts in a calm manner, being careful not to increase the anxiety or nervousness caused by the sympathomimetic drug. Explaining the effects of the drug may help the patient to tolerate these uncomfortable adverse reactions.

IMBALANCED NUTRITION: LESS THAN BODY REQUIRE-MENTS Some antiasthma drugs cause nausea. The patient with nausea should be offered frequent smaller meals rather than three large meals. Meals should be followed by good mouth care. The nurse suggests limiting fluids with meals may help with the nausea. The nurse provides a pleasant, relaxed atmosphere for meals.

The patient taking theophylline may report heartburn because the drug relaxes the lower esophageal sphincter, allowing gastroesophageal reflux. Heartburn is minimized if the patient remains in an upright position and sleeps with the head of the bed elevated.

Some antiasthma drugs may cause an unpleasant taste in the mouth. Having the patient take frequent sips of water, suck on sugarless candy, or chew gum helps to alleviate the problem.

IMPAIRED ORAL MUCOUS MEMBRANES The inhalers, particularly the corticosteroid or mast cell aerosols, may cause throat irritation and promote infection with *Candida albicans*. The nurse instructs the patient to use strict oral hygiene, cleanse the inhaler as directed in the package directions, and use the proper technique when taking an inhalation. These interventions will decrease the incidence of candidiasis and help to soothe the throat. Occasionally an antifungal drug may be prescribed by the primary health care provider to manage the candidiasis.

INEFFECTIVE AIRWAY CLEARANCE Occasionally the patient may experience an acute bronchospasm either as a result of the disease, after exposure to an allergen, or as an adverse reaction to some antiasthma drugs, such as cromolyn inhalation.

Nursing Alert

Acute bronchospasm causes severe respiratory distress and wheezing from the forceful expiration of air and is considered a medical emergency. It is characterized by severe respiratory distress, dyspnea, forceful expiration, and wheezing. The nurse must report these symptoms to the primary health care provider immediately.

During an acute bronchospasm, the nurse checks the blood pressure, pulse, respiratory rate, and response to the drug every 5 to 15 minutes until the patient's condition stabilizes and respiratory distress is relieved.

EDUCATING THE PATIENT AND FAMILY

If the patient is to use an aerosol inhaler for administration of the bronchodilator, the nurse provides a thorough explanation of its use (see Patient and Family Teaching Checklist: Teaching the Patient to Use a Metered-Dose Inhaler).

Nursing Alert

The nurse should not assume that the patient understands how to use an aerosol inhaler correctly. Many patients, even with repeated instruction, do not use the proper technique to administer the drug by inhalation. Along with verbal instructions, the nurse should have the patient demonstrate the use of the inhaler to evaluate if he or she is using the proper technique. It is important to repeat instructions at each follow-up visit.

Because each brand is slightly different, the nurse carefully reviews any instruction sheets with the patient and provides information about how the unit is assembled, used, and cleaned.

In addition, the patient may use a peak flow meter at home to monitor breathing status and the effectiveness of the drug regimen. The nurse teaches the patient how to use the peak flow meter and when to notify the primary health care provider (see Home Care Checklist: Using a Peak Flow Meter).

A commonly used method to interpret peak flow rates is to relate the three zones to the traffic light colors: green, yellow, and red. See Display 37-2 for information about the three-zone system. The physician may give the patient an action plan to determine what action to take for each of the three zones (Fig. 37-2).

Home Care Checklist

Using a Peak Flow Meter

Patients receiving bronchodilators or antiasthma drugs often need to monitor their lung function at home with a peak flow meter. Doing so provides the patient and the primary health care provider with valuable information about the status of the patient's condition and the effectiveness of therapy. Often, trends in the readings can detect changes in the patient's airway and airflow even before any signs and symptoms are experienced. This allows possible intervention before a major problem arises.

Because a variety of meters are commercially available, the nurse explains about the type of meter that will be used, how often the peak flow should be checked, and the ranges for the readings along with instructions on what to do for each range. The nurse uses the following steps to instruct the patient on the use of the peak flow meter:

☑ Check to make sure that the indicator is at the lowest level of the scale.

☑ Stand upright to allow the best inhalation possible. (Be sure to remove gum or food from your mouth.)

☑ Inhale as deeply as you can and then place your lips around the mouthpiece, making sure that you have a tight seal.

☑ Exhale as forcibly and as quickly as possible in one large "huff."

☑ Watch the indicator rise on the scale, noting where it stops. The number below the indicator's position is your peak flow reading.

☑ Repeat the procedure two more times.

☑ Compare the three readings. Record the highest reading along with the date and time. Do not calculate an average.

☑ Keep a written record of your readings and bring it with you on follow-up visits.

☑ Measure the peak flow rate close to the same time each day. (Your physician may provide you with a suggested time. Some patients measure the peak flow rate twice daily between 7 and 9 AM and between 6 and 8 PM. Others measure the peak flow rate before or after taking their medication.)

☑ Follow the medication instructions written on your record sheet next to the zone color of your reading (see Display 37-2) provided by your physician.

☑ Clean your meter with mild soap and hot water after use.

Display 37.2 Monitoring Peak Flow Readings

Many primary care health providers recommend a three-zone system. This system is based on your personal best peak flow rate—the highest peak flow measurement you can achieve on a day when your asthma is under good control—and it divides peak flow readings into three zones. The green zone ranges from 80% to 100%* of your personal best, the yellow zone, from 50% to 80%, and the red zone, anything below 50%.*

*These percentages are given as an example. Your primary health care provider will tailor your zones to your individual needs and peak flow patterns.

Think of These Zones as Traffic Signals

● Green means "go." Continue your regular activities and follow your maintenance asthma medication plan.

● Yellow means "caution." Additional medication may be needed (either for an acute episode, or if your condition remains stable, as part of your maintenance plan).

● Red means "stop." This is a danger zone. Notify the primary care health provider immediately. Use the medication prescribed when peak flow readings indicate that asthma is not in good control.

The goal is to stay in the green zone as long as possible and to take action whenever you enter the yellow zone, so you **never** enter the red zone. The primary health care provider will adjust the color-coded zone indicators on your personal best peak flow meter to remind you of your red, yellow, and green zones, as well as fill out your action plan with your medication instructions.

ASTHMA ACTION PLAN FOR _____

Doctor's Name _____ Date _____

Doctor's Phone Number _____ Hospital/Emergency Room Phone Number _____

GREEN ZONE: Doing well

- No cough, wheeze, chest tightness, or shortness of breath during the day or night
- Can do usual activities

And, if peak flow meter is used,
Peak flow: more than _____
(80% or more of my best peak flow)

My best peak flow is: _____

Take These Long-Term-Control Medicines Each Day (Include an anti-inflammatory)

Medicine	How much to take	When to take it

Before exercise ☐ ☐ 2 or ☐ 4 puffs 5 to 60 minutes before exercise

YELLOW ZONE: Asthma is getting worse

- Cough, wheeze, chest tightness, or shortness of breath, or
- Waking at night due to asthma, or
- Can do some, but not all, usual activities

–Or–

Peak flow: _____ to _____
(50%–80% of my best peak flow)

FIRST → **Add: Quick-Relief Medicine—and keep taking your GREEN ZONE medicine**

_____ (short-acting beta₂-agonist) ☐ 2 or ☐ 4 puffs, every 20 minutes for up to 1 hour ☐ Nebulizer, once

SECOND → If your symptoms (and peak flow, if used) return to *GREEN ZONE* after 1 hour of above treatment:
☐ Take the quick-relief medicine every 4 hours for 1 to 2 days.
☐ Double the dose of your inhaled steroid for _____ (7-10) days.

–Or–

If your symptoms (and peak flow, if used) do not return to *GREEN ZONE* after 1 hour of above treatment:

☐ Take: _____ (short-acting beta₂-agonist) ☐ 2 or ☐ 4 puffs or ☐ Nebulizer

☐ Add: _____ (oral steroid) _____ mg. per day For _____ (3-10) days.

☐ Call the doctor ☐ before/ ☐ within _____ hours after taking the oral steroid.

RED ZONE: Medical Alert!

- Very short of breath, or
- Quick-relief medicines have not helped, or
- Cannot do usual activities, or
- Symptoms are same or get worse after 24 hours in Yellow Zone

–Or–

Peak flow: less than _____
(50% of my best peak flow)

Take this medicine:

☐ _____ (short-acting beta₂-agonist) ☐ 4 or ☐ 6 puffs or ☐ Nebulizer

☐ _____ (oral steroid) _____ mg.

Then call your doctor *NOW*. Go to the hospital or call for an ambulance if:
☐ You are still in the red zone after 15 minutes AND
☐ You have not reached your doctor.

→ Take ☐ 4 or ☐ 6 puffs of your quick-relief medicine *AND*
Go to the hospital or call for an ambulance (_____) **NOW**!

DANGER SIGNS

- Trouble walking and talking due to shortness of breath
- Lips or fingernails are blue

Figure 37.2 Example of an action plan for asthma.

The nurse also includes the following general points in the patient teaching plan:

- Take the drug exactly as prescribed by the primary health care provider.

- If symptoms become worse, do not increase the dose or frequency of use unless directed to do so by the primary health care provider.

- If GI upset occurs, take this drug with food or milk (oral form).

- Drink six to eight 8-oz glasses of water each day to decrease the thickness of secretions.

- Do not use nonprescription drugs (some may contain sympathomimetic drugs) unless use has been approved by the primary health care provider.

- Avoid smoking (when applicable). Smoking may make it difficult to adjust the dosage and may worsen breathing problems.

- Do not puncture metered-dose inhalers or store them near heat or open flame; the contents of such inhalers are under pressure. Never throw the container into a fire or incinerator. If an unusual smell or taste is noted with use of the inhaler, discontinue use and contact the primary health care provider.

Patient teaching for patients using sympathomimetic drugs includes the following points:

- Do not exceed the recommended dosage.

- These drugs may cause nervousness, insomnia, and restlessness (especially the sympathomimetics). Contact the primary health care provider if the symptoms become severe.

- Contact the primary health care provider if palpitations, tachycardia, chest pain, muscle tremors, dizziness, headache, flushing, or difficulty with urination or breathing occur.

- If using Salmeterol Diskus, do not exhale into the device. Activate and use the device only in a horizontal position. Do not use the Diskus with a spacer. Do not wash the Diskus. Notify the primary health care provider immediately if salmeterol becomes less effective for symptom relief, if more inhalations than usual are needed, or if more than the maximum number of inhalations of short-acting bronchodilators are needed.

- If salmeterol is used for preventing EIB, the drug is administered at least 30 minutes before exercise. Additional doses are not to be given for at least 12 hours.

- Formoterol fumarate (Foradil Aerolizer) is administered only by oral inhalation using the Aerolizer Inhaler. When using the Aerolizer Inhaler, do not exhale into the device. Always store formoterol capsules in the blister and remove immediately before use. Always discard the capsule and Aerolizer Inhaler by the expiration date included in the manufacturer's instructions. Do not use the device with a spacer. If using this drug for the prevention of EIB, the usual dosage is the inhalation of the contents of one 12-mcg formoterol capsule at least 15 minutes before exercise, administered as needed. Do not take an additional dose for 12 hours.

Patient teaching for patients using xanthine derivatives includes the following points:

- Follow your primary health care provider's instructions concerning monitoring of theophylline serum levels.

- Avoid foods that contain xanthine, such as colas, coffee, chocolate, and charcoal-prepared foods.

- If GI upset occurs, take the drug with food. Do not chew or crush coated or sustained-release tablets.

- Do not change from one brand to another without consulting your physician.

Patient teaching for patients using corticosteroid inhalants includes the following points:

- Corticosteroid inhalant—Rinse mouth with water without swallowing after each dose to reduce the risk of oral candidiasis. Carry a warning card indicating the need for supplemental systemic steroids in the event of stress or severe asthmatic attack that is unresponsive to bronchodilators. Do not stop therapy abruptly. These drugs are not bronchodilators and do not contain medication to provide rapid relief of breathing difficulties during an asthma attack. If taking bronchodilators by inhalation, use the bronchodilator several minutes before the corticosteroid to enhance application of the steroid into the bronchial tract (see the Patient and Family Teaching Checklist: Teaching the Patient to Use a Metered-Dose Inhaler).

- Corticosteroid inhaled powder—Hold the inhaler upright and twist off the cover. Twist the grip to the right as far as it will go, listen for the click, and then twist it back. Exhale and place the mouthpiece between lips; slightly tilt head back and inhale deeply and forcefully. Remove inhaler from the mouth and hold breath for about 10 seconds. Rinse the mouth with water after each use to help reduce dry mouth and hoarseness.

- Mometasone furoate (Asmanex Twisthaler) is a once-a-day inhaled asthma therapy given in the evening. It does not use a propellant, thereby eliminating the need for hand–breath coordination that is required by other inhalants. The medication should be taken as directed, breathing rapidly and deeply, and the patient should not breathe out through the inhaler. Another advantage is that it is equipped with a numeric dose counter that provides a visual indication of the remaining doses. The digital counter displays the doses remaining. When the counter indicates zero, the cap will lock and the unit is discarded. If the dose counter is not working correctly, the unit should not be used and should be taken back to the pharmacist. The patient should record the date of the pouch opening on the cap label, and discard the inhaler 45 days after opening the foil pouch or when the dose counter reads "00," whichever comes first. The patient is informed that maximum benefit may not occur for 1 to 2 weeks.

Patient teaching for patients using leukotriene receptor agonists and leukotriene formation inhibitors includes the following points:

- Zafirlukast—Take this drug regularly as prescribed, even during symptom-free times. Do not use to treat acute episodes of asthma.

- Montelukast—Take once daily in the evening, even when free of symptoms. Contact the primary health care provider if the asthma is not well controlled. This drug is not for the treatment of an acute attack. Avoid taking aspirin and the nonsteroidal anti-inflammatory drugs (NSAIDs) while taking montelukast.

- Zileuton—This drug is not a bronchodilator, so do not use it for an acute episode of asthma. Contact the primary health care provider if bronchodilators are needed more often than usual or if more than the maximum number of inhalations for a 24-hour period is needed. This drug can interact with other drugs; consult the primary health care provider before starting or stopping any prescription or nonprescription drug. Have liver enzyme tests monitored on a regular basis. Immediately report any symptoms of liver dysfunction, such as upper right quadrant pain, nausea, fatigue, lethargy, pruritus, and jaundice.

Patient teaching for patients using mast cell stabilizers includes the following points:

- Inform the primary health care provider if asthma symptoms do not improve within 4 weeks of initiating treatment. The primary health care provider may discontinue the drug therapy.

- Cromolyn—When taken to prevent EIA, this drug should be taken approximately 15 minutes before activity but no earlier than 1 hour before the expected activity.

- Cromolyn—When taken orally, this drug should be taken at least 30 minutes before meals and at bedtime. The drug is prepared by opening the ampule and squeezing the liquid contents into a glass of water. The nurse stirs the solution and instructs the patient to drink the entire amount. Do not mix the drug with any other food or beverage.

EVALUATION

- The therapeutic effect is achieved, and breathing is easier and more effective.

- The patient maintains adequate nutrition.

- Oral mucous membranes are intact and integrity is maintained.

- Airway is maintained with effective breathing pattern.

- Anxiety is managed successfully.

- Adverse reactions are identified, reported to the primary health care provider, and managed successfully.

- The patient demonstrates an understanding of the drug regimen and use of the aerosol inhalator.

Critical Thinking Exercises

1. Mr. Potter, aged 57, is admitted to the pulmonary unit in acute respiratory distress. The primary health care provider orders IV aminophylline. In developing a care plan for Mr. Potter, you select the nursing diagnosis Ineffective Airway Clearance. Suggest nursing interventions that would be most important in managing this problem.

2. Ms. Smith, aged 68, returned to the clinic for a follow-up visit after receiving a diagnosis of COPD. She is taking theophylline daily and using a metered-dose inhaler four times a day. Determine what assessments would be most important for you to make at this time.

3. Discuss what to include in a teaching plan for a patient taking montelukast for asthma.

Review Questions

1. Which of the following laboratory tests would the nurse expect to be ordered for a patient taking aminophylline?

   A. Thyroid hormone levels

   B. Alanine aminotransferase

   C. Electrolytes

   D. Serum aminophylline levels

2. When the sympathomimetics are administered to older adults, there is an increased risk of _____.

   A. gastrointestinal effects

   B. nephrotoxic effects

   C. neurotoxic effects

   D. cardiovascular effects

3. When mometasone furoate (Asmanex Twisthaler) is prescribed, the nurse instructs the patient to administer the drug _____.

   A. twice daily

   B. three times daily

   C. once daily, in the morning

   D. once daily, in the evening

4. When administering aminophylline, a xanthine derivative bronchodilating drug, the nurse monitors the patient for adverse reactions, which include _____.

   A. restlessness and nervousness

   B. hypoglycemia and hypothyroidism

   C. bradycardia and bronchospasm

   D. somnolence and lethargy

5. The nurse correctly administers montelukast (Singulair) _____.

   A. once daily in the evening

   B. twice daily in the morning and evening

   C. three times a day with meals

   D. once daily in the morning

Medication Dosage Problems

1. A patient is prescribed 0.25 mg of terbutaline SC. The drug is available for injection in a solution of 1 mg/mL. The nurse administers _____.

2. The patient is prescribed zafirlukast 20 mg orally BID. The drug is available in 10-mg tablets. The nurse administers _____. How many milligrams of zafirlukast will the patient receive each day?

To check your answers, see Appendix G.

Drugs That Affect the Cardiovascular System

T his unit discusses the cardiovascular system and the drugs used to treat the disorders of the cardiovascular system. The first chapter in this unit discusses the cardiotonic drugs and miscellaneous inotropic drugs. These drugs are used to treat heart failure, often referred to as *congestive heart failure*. About 4.5 million Americans have heart failure. It is the most frequent cause of hospitalization for individuals older than 65 years. With treatment, some patients may lead nearly normal lives, although more than 50% of individuals with severe heart failure die each year. The angiotensin-converting enzyme (ACE) inhibitors are considered the first-choice treatment and are the cornerstones of heart failure drug therapy. However, digoxin may be prescribed for patients with heart failure who do not respond to the ACE inhibitors and diuretics. Other drugs, such as the beta blockers, are also used in the treatment of heart failure.

The antiarrhythmic drugs are used to treat cardiac arrhythmia (a conduction disorder resulting in an abnormally slow or rapid regular heart rate, or a heart that beats with an irregular pace). Some arrhythmias do not require treatment, whereas others require immediate treatment because they are potentially fatal. Antiarrhythmic drugs are divided into four classifications:

- Class I (disopyramide, flecainide)
- Class II (acebutolol, propranolol)
- Class III (amiodarone, bretylium)
- Class IV (verapamil)

Class I drugs, comprising the largest classification, are divided into subclasses IA, IB, and IC. Unfortunately, although these drugs are used to treat arrhythmia, they are also capable of causing or worsening an arrhythmia. The benefits of treatment must be carefully weighed by the primary health care provider against the risks of treatment with the antiarrhythmic drug.

Diseases of the arteries—coronary artery disease, cerebral vascular disease, and peripheral vascular disease—can cause serious problems. Therapy for vascular diseases may include drugs that dilate blood vessels and thereby increase blood supply to an area. Atherosclerosis is a disease characterized by deposits of fatty plaques on the inner walls of arteries. These deposits narrow the lumen (inside diameter) of the artery, thereby decreasing blood supply to the area served by the artery. This unit discusses two different types of drugs whose primary purpose is to increase blood supply to an area by dilating blood vessels: the antianginal and peripheral vasodilating drugs. Vasodilating drugs relax the smooth muscle layer of arterial blood vessels, which results in vasodilation, an increase in the size of blood vessels, primarily small arteries and arterioles. Because peripheral, cerebral, or coronary artery disease usually results in decreased blood flow to an area, drugs that dilate narrowed arterial blood vessels promote an increase in blood flow to the affected area, which may result in partial or complete relief of symptoms. Vasodilating drugs sometimes relieve the symptoms of vascular disease, but in some cases drug therapy provides only minimal and temporary relief.

The vasodilating drugs are also used to treat hypertension. Hypertension is defined as a systolic blood pressure (SBP) greater than 140 mm Hg or a diastolic blood pressure (DBP) greater than 90 mm Hg, or the use of an antihypertensive medication. Patients with an SBP of 120 to 139 or a DBP of 80 to 89 are considered prehypertensive and are at an increased risk for development of hypertension. These individuals require health-promoting lifestyle modifications to prevent cardio-vascular disease. In individuals aged between 40 and 70 years, every increase of 20 mm Hg in SBP or every increase of 10 mm Hg in DBP doubles the risk of cardiovascular disease across the entire blood pressure range from 115/75 to 185/115. Treating hypertension early reduces the risk for cardiovas-cular disease and death and protects against hypertension-related complications, such as stroke, heart failure, and renal disease. In addition to the vasodilating drugs, other drugs used to treat hypertension include the adrenergic blocking drugs, centrally acting antiadrenergics, peripherally acting antiadrenergics, alpha-adrenergic blocking drugs, ACE inhibitors, angiotensin II receptor antagonists, and the drugs used for hypertensive crisis.

The last chapter in this unit discusses the cholesterol-lowering drugs or antihyperlipidemic drugs. Risk factors for hyperlipidemia, particularly elevated serum cholesterol and low-density lipoprotein (LDL) levels, play a role in the development of atherosclerotic heart disease. Other risk factors, besides elevated cholesterol levels, also play a role in the development of hyperlipidemia. Additional risk factors include

- Family history of early heart disease (father before age 45 years and mother before age 55 years)

- Tobacco smoking

- High blood pressure

- Age (men older than 45 years and women older than 55 years)

- Low high-density lipoprotein (HDL) levels

- Obesity

- Diabetes

In general, the higher the LDL level and the more risk factors involved, the greater the risk for heart disease. Lowering blood cholesterol levels can arrest or reverse atherosclerosis in the vessels and can significantly decrease the incidence of heart disease. The main goal of treatment in patients with hyperlipidemia is to lower LDL concentrations to a level that will reduce the risk of heart dis-ease. The drugs used as antihyperlipidemic drugs include bile acid sequestrants, HMG-CoA reduc-tase inhibitors, fibric acid derivatives, and niacin.

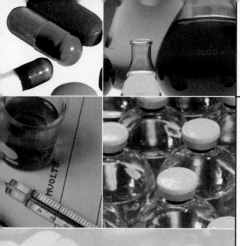

Chapter 38

Cardiotonics and Miscellaneous Inotropic Drugs

Key Terms

- atrial fibrillation
- cardiac glycosides
- cardiac output
- digitalis glycosides
- digitalis toxicity
- digitalization
- heart failure
- hypokalemia
- left ventricular dysfunction
- neurohormonal activity
- positive inotropic action
- right ventricular dysfunction

Learning Objectives

On completion of this chapter, the student will:

- Discuss heart failure in relationship to left ventricular failure, right ventricular failure, neurohormonal activity, and treatment options.

- Discuss the uses, general drug action, general adverse reactions, contraindications, precautions, and interactions of the cardiotonic and inotropic drugs.

- Discuss the use of other drugs with positive inotropic action.

- Discuss important preadministration and ongoing assessment activities

the nurse should perform on the patient taking a cardiotonic or inotropic drug.

- List nursing diagnoses particular to a patient taking a cardiotonic or inotropic drug.

- Identify the symptoms of digitalis toxicity.

- Discuss ways to promote an optimal response to therapy, how to manage common adverse reactions, and important points to keep in mind when administering a cardiotonic drug.

The cardiotonics are drugs used to increase the efficiency and improve the contraction of the heart muscle, which leads to improved blood flow to all tissues of the body. The drugs have long been used to treat congestive heart failure, a condition in which the heart cannot pump enough blood to meet the tissue needs of the body. Although the term *congestive heart failure* is commonly used, a more accurate term is simply *heart failure*.

Heart failure (HF) is a complex clinical syndrome that can result from any number of cardiac or metabolic disorders, such as ischemic heart disease, hypertension, or hyperthyroidism. Any condition that impairs the ability of the ventricle to pump blood can lead to HF. In HF, the heart fails in its ability to pump enough blood to meet the needs of the body or can do so only with an elevated filling pressure. Heart failure causes a number of neurohormonal changes as the body tries to compensate for the increased workload of the heart. Display 38-1 discusses this neurohormonal response.

CONCEPTS in action **ANIMATION**

Display 38.1 Neurohormonal Responses Affecting Heart Failure

The body activates the neurohormonal compensatory mechanisms, which result in:

- Increased secretion of the neurohormones by the sympathetic nervous system
- Activation of the renin-angiotensin-aldosterone (RAA) system
- Remodeling of the cardiac tissue

The sympathetic nervous system increases the secretion of the catecholamines (the neurohormones epinephrine and norepinephrine), which results in increased heart rate and vasoconstriction. The activation of the renin-angiotensin-aldosterone (RAA) system occurs because of decreased perfusion to the kidneys. As the RAA system is activated, angiotensin II and aldosterone levels increase, which increases the blood pressure, adding to the workload of the heart. These increases in **neurohormonal activity** cause a remodeling (restructuring) of the cardiac muscle cells, leading to hypertrophy (enlargement) of the heart, increased need for oxygen, and cardiac necrosis, which worsens the HF. The tissue of the heart is changed such that there is an increase in the cellular mass of cardiac tissue, the shape of the ventricle(s) is changed, and the heart's ability to contract effectively is reduced.

Heart failure is best described by denoting the area of initial ventricular dysfunction: left-sided (left ventricular) dysfunction or right-sided (right ventricular) dysfunction. **Left ventricular dysfunction** leads to pulmonary symptoms, such as dyspnea and moist cough with the production of frothy, pink (blood-tinged) sputum. **Right ventricular dysfunction** leads to neck vein distention, peripheral edema, weight gain, and hepatic engorgement. Because both sides of the heart work together, ultimately both sides are affected in HF. Typically the left side of the heart is affected first, followed by right ventricular involvement. The most common symptoms associated with HF include

- Left ventricular dysfunction
  - Shortness of breath with exercise
  - Dry, hacking cough or wheezing
  - Orthopnea (difficulty breathing while lying flat)
  - Restlessness and anxiety
- Right ventricular dysfunction
  - Swollen ankles, legs, or abdomen, leading to pitting edema
  - Anorexia
  - Nausea
  - Nocturia (the need to urinate frequently at night)
  - Weakness
  - Weight gain as the result of fluid retention

Other symptoms include

- Palpitations, fatigue, or pain when performing normal activities
- Tachycardia or irregular heart rate
- Dizziness or confusion

Left ventricular dysfunction, also called left ventricular systolic dysfunction, is the most common form of HF and results in decreased **cardiac output** and decreased ejection fraction (the amount of blood that the ventricle ejects per beat in relationship to the amount of blood available to eject). Typically, the ejection fraction should be greater than 60%. With left ventricular systolic dysfunction, the ejection fraction is less than 40%, and the heart is enlarged and dilated.

CARDIOTONICS

Digoxin (Lanoxin) is the most commonly used cardiotonic drug. Other terms used to identify the cardiotonics are **cardiac glycosides** or **digitalis glycosides**. The digitalis or cardiac glycosides are obtained from the leaves of the foxglove plant (*Digitalis purpurea* and *Digitalis lanata*).

Miscellaneous drugs with **positive inotropic action**, such as inamrinone and milrinone (Primacor), are nonglycosides used in the short-term management of HF. In the past the cardiotonics were the mainstay in HF treatment; currently, however, they are used in the treatment of patients who continue to experience symptoms after using the angiotensin-converting enzyme (ACE) inhibitors, diuretics, and beta blockers. See the Summary Drug Table: Cardiotonics and Miscellaneous Inotropic Drugs for information concerning these drugs.

Actions

Cardiotonics, particularly digitalis drugs, increase cardiac output through positive inotropic activity (an increase in the force of the contraction). They slow the conduction velocity through the atrioventricular (AV) node in the heart and decrease the heart rate through a negative chronotropic effect.

Uses

The cardiotonics are used to treat
- Heart failure
- Atrial fibrillation

Atrial fibrillation is a cardiac arrhythmia characterized by rapid contractions and quivering of the atrial myocardium, resulting in an irregular and often rapid ventricular rate. See Chapter 39 for more information on arrhythmias and their treatment.

SUMMARY DRUG TABLE CARDIOTONICS AND MISCELLANEOUS INOTROPIC DRUGS

GENERIC NAME	TRADE NAME	USES	ADVERSE REACTIONS	DOSAGE RANGES
Cardiotonics				
digoxin *di-jox'-in*	Digitek, Lanoxicaps, Lanoxin	HF, atrial fibrillation, atrial flutter, paroxysmal atrial tachycardia	Headache, weakness, drowsiness, visual disturbances, nausea, vomiting, anorexia, arrhythmias	Loading dose: 0.75–1.25 mg or 0.125–0.25 mg IV Maintenance: 0.125–0.25 mg/d orally Lanoxicaps: 0.1–0.3 mg/d orally
Miscellaneous Inotropic Drugs				
inamrinone lactate *in-am'-ri-none*		Short-term management of HF in patients with no response to digitalis, diuretics, or vasodilators	Arrhythmia, hypotension, nausea, vomiting, abdominal pain, anorexia, hepatotoxicity	IV: 0.75 mg/kg bolus, may repeat in 30 min Maintenance: 5–10 mg/kg/min IV, not to exceed 10 mg/kg/d
milrinone lactate *mill'-ri-none*	Primacor	HF	Ventricular arrhythmias, hypotension, angina/chest pain, headaches, hypokalemia	IV: Up to 1.13 mg/kg/d
Digoxin-Specific Antidote				
digoxin immune fab (ovine)	Digibind	Antidote for digoxin toxicity	Hypokalemia, reemergence of atrial fibrillation or HF	IV: Dosage depends on serum digoxin level or estimate of the amount of digoxin ingested; average dose up to 800 mg (20 vials)

HF, heart failure.

Adverse Reactions

Central Nervous System Reactions

- Headache
- Weakness, drowsiness
- Visual disturbances

Cardiovascular and Gastrointestinal Reactions

- Arrhythmias
- Gastrointestinal (GI) upset and anorexia

Because some patients are more sensitive to side effects of digoxin, dosage is calculated carefully and adjusted as the clinical condition indicates. There is a narrow margin of safety between the full therapeutic effects and the toxic effects of cardiotonic drugs. Even normal doses of a cardiotonic drug can cause toxic drug effects. Because substantial individual variations may occur, it is important to individualize the dosage. The term **digitalis toxicity** (digitalis intoxication) is used to describe toxic drug effects that occur when digoxin is administered.

Contraindications and Precautions

The cardiotonics are contraindicated in the presence of digitalis toxicity and in patients with known hypersensitivity, ventricular failure, ventricular tachycardia, or AV block.

The cardiotonics are given cautiously to patients with electrolyte imbalance (especially hypokalemia, hypocalcemia, and hypomagnesemia), severe carditis, heart block, myocardial infarction, severe pulmonary disease, acute glomerulonephritis and impaired renal or hepatic function.

Digoxin and digoxin immune fab are classified as pregnancy category C drugs and are used cautiously during pregnancy and lactation. Fetal toxicity and neonatal death have been reported from maternal digoxin overdosage. These drugs are used only when the potential benefit outweighs the potential harm to the fetus.

Interactions

When the cardiotonics are taken with food, absorption is slowed, but the amount absorbed is the same. However, if taken with high-fiber meals, absorption of the cardiotonics may be decreased. Certain drugs may increase or decrease plasma digitalis levels as follows:

Interacting Drug	Common Use	Effect of Interaction
amiodarone	Cardiac problems	**Increased** plasma digitalis levels leading to toxicity
benzodiazepines (diazepam)	Treatment of seizures	
indomethacin	Pain relief	
itraconazole	Fungal infections	
macrolides (erythromycin, clarithromycin)	Infections	
propafenone	Cardiac problems	
quinidine	Cardiac problems	
spironolactone	Edema	
tetracyclines	Infections	
verapamil	Cardiac problems	
oral aminoglycoside	Infections	**Decreased** plasma digitalis levels
antacids	GI problems	
antineoplastics (bleomycin, carmustine, cyclophosphamide, methotrexate, and vincristine)	Anticancer agents	

Interacting Drug	Common Use	Effect of Interaction
activated charcoal	Antidote to poisoning with certain toxic substances	**Decreased** plasma digitalis levels
cholestyramine	Agent to lower high blood cholesterol levels	
colestipol	Agent to lower high blood cholesterol levels	
neomycin	Agent to suppress GI bacteria before surgery	
rifampin	Antitubercular agent	
St. John's wort	Herb used to relieve depression	

The following interactions may occur with the cardiac glycosides:

Interacting Drug	Common Use	Effect of Interaction
thyroid hormones	Treatment of hypothyroidism	Decreased effectiveness of digitalis glycosides, requiring a larger dosage of digoxin
thiazide and loop diuretics	Management of edema and hypertension	Increased diuretic-induced electrolyte disturbances, predisposing the patient to digitalis-induced arrhythmias

MISCELLANEOUS INOTROPIC DRUGS

Inamrinone and milrinone have inotropic actions and are used in the short-term management of severe HF that is not controlled by the digitalis preparations. Milrinone is used more often than inamrinone, appears to be more effective, and has fewer adverse reactions. Both drugs are given intravenously (IV), and close monitoring is required during therapy. The nurse must monitor the patient's heart rate and blood pressure continuously with administration of either drug. If hypotension occurs, the drug is discontinued or the rate of administration is reduced. Continuous cardiac monitoring is necessary because life-threatening arrhythmias may occur. These drugs do not cure HF; rather, they control its signs and symptoms.

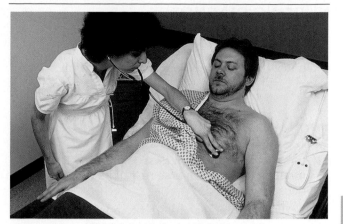

Figure 38.1 The nurse counts the apical pulse for 1 minute before administering the cardiotonic.

NURSING PROCESS

The Patient Receiving a Cardiotonic Drug

ASSESSMENT

PREADMINISTRATION ASSESSMENT

The cardiotonics are potentially toxic drugs. Therefore, the nurse must observe the patient closely, especially during initial therapy. Before therapy is started, the physical assessment should include information that will establish a database for comparison during therapy. The physical assessment should include

- Taking blood pressure, apical-radial pulse rate, respiratory rate

- Auscultating the lungs, noting any unusual sounds during inspiration and expiration

- Examining the extremities for edema

- Checking the jugular veins for distention

- Measuring weight

- Inspecting sputum raised (if any), and noting the appearance (e.g., frothy, pink-tinged, clear, yellow)

- Looking for evidence of other problems, such as cyanosis, shortness of breath on exertion (if the patient is allowed out of bed) or when lying flat, and mental changes.

The primary health care provider also may order laboratory and diagnostic tests, such as an electrocardiogram, renal and hepatic function tests, complete blood count, and serum enzyme and electrolyte levels. These tests should be reviewed before the first dose of the drug is given. Renal function is particularly important because diminished renal function could affect the prescribed dosage of digoxin. When subsequent laboratory tests are ordered, test findings also should be reviewed when the results are recorded on the patient's record. Because digoxin reacts with many medications, the nurse must take a careful drug history. Before administering the first dose of the drug, the nurse takes the patient's vital signs and documents the apical pulse rate and rhythm.

ONGOING ASSESSMENT

Before administering each dose of a cardiotonic, the nurse takes the apical pulse rate for 60 seconds (Fig. 38-1). The nurse records the apical pulse rate in the designated area on the chart or the medication administration record. If the pulse rate is below 60 beats per minute (bpm) in adults or greater than 100 bpm, the nurse withholds the drug and notifies the primary health care provider, unless there is a written order giving different guidelines for withholding the drug.

Pediatric Alert

The drug is withheld and the primary health care provider notified before administering the drug if the apical pulse rate in a child is below 70 bpm, or below 90 bpm in an infant.

Nursing Alert

The drug should be withheld and the primary health care provider contacted if there are any signs of digitalis toxicity, any change in the pulse rhythm, or a marked increase or decrease in the pulse rate since the last time it was taken, or the patient's general condition appears to be worse.

The nurse weighs patients receiving a cardiotonic drug daily, or as ordered. Intake and output are measured, especially if the patient has edema or HF or is also receiving a diuretic. Throughout therapy, the nurse assesses the patient for peripheral edema and auscultates the lungs for rales or crackles throughout therapy. Serum electrolyte levels should be assessed periodically. Hypokalemia, hypomagnesemia, or hypercalcemia may increase the risk for toxicity. Any electrolyte imbalance is reported to the primary health care provider.

NURSING DIAGNOSES

Drug-specific nursing diagnoses are highlighted in the Nursing Diagnoses Checklist. Other nursing diagnoses applicable to these drugs are discussed in depth in Chapter 4.

Nursing Diagnoses Checklist

✓ **Imbalanced Nutrition: Less Than Body Requirements** related to adverse reactions (anorexia, nausea, vomiting)

✓ **Activity Intolerance** related to adverse drug reactions (weakness and drowsiness)

PLANNING

The expected outcomes of the patient depend on the specific reason for administering the drug, but may include an optimal response to therapy, support of patient needs related to the management of adverse reactions, and an understanding of and compliance with the prescribed drug regimen.

IMPLEMENTATION
PROMOTING AN OPTIMAL RESPONSE TO THERAPY

Great care must be taken when administering a cardiotonic drug. The nurse should carefully check the primary health care provider's order and the drug container. If there is any doubt about the dosage or calculation of the dosage, the nurse checks with the primary health care provider or pharmacist before giving the drug.

DIGITALIZATION Patients started on therapy with a cardiotonic drug are being "digitalized." Digitalization may be accomplished by two general methods:

- Rapid digitalization (accomplished by administering a loading dose)

- Gradual digitalization (a maintenance dose is given, allowing therapeutic drug blood levels to accumulate gradually).

Digitalization involves giving a series of doses until the drug begins to exert a full therapeutic effect. The digitalizing, or loading dose, is administered in several doses, with approximately half the total digitalization dose administered as the first dose. Additional fractions of the digitalis dose are administered at 6- to 8-hour intervals. Once a full therapeutic effect is achieved, the primary health care provider usually prescribes a maintenance dose schedule. The ranges for digitalizing (loading) and maintenance

doses are given in the Summary Drug Table: Cardiotonics and Miscellaneous Inotropic Drugs. Digoxin injections are usually used for rapid digitalization; digoxin tablets or capsules are used for maintenance therapy.

During digitalization, the nurse takes the blood pressure, pulse, and respiratory rate every 2 to 4 hours or as ordered by the primary health care provider. This interval may be increased or decreased, depending on the patient's condition and the route used for drug administration.

Measurement of serum levels (digoxin) may be ordered daily during the period of digitalization and periodically during maintenance therapy. Any signs of digitalis toxicity are reported immediately to the primary health care provider (see Potential Complication: Digitalis Toxicity, later).

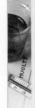

Nursing Alert

The nurse should withhold the drug and report any of the following signs of digitalis toxicity to the primary health care provider immediately: loss of appetite (anorexia), nausea, vomiting, abdominal pain, visual disturbances (blurred, yellow, or green vision and white halos, borders around dark objects), and arrhythmias (any type). The nurse also must report immediately serum digoxin levels greater than 2.0 nanograms/mL.

Periodic electrocardiograms, serum electrolytes, hepatic and renal function tests, and other laboratory studies also may be ordered. Diuretics (see Chapter 45) may be ordered for some patients receiving a cardiotonic drug. Diuretics, along with other conditions or factors, such as GI suction, diarrhea, and old age, may produce low serum potassium levels (**hypokalemia**). The primary health care provider may order a potassium salt to be given orally or IV.

Nursing Alert

Hypokalemia makes the heart muscle more sensitive to digitalis, thereby increasing the possibility of developing digitalis toxicity. At frequent intervals, the nurse must observe patients with hypokalemia closely for signs of digitalis toxicity.

Patients with hypomagnesemia (low plasma magnesium levels) are at increased risk for digitalis toxicity. If low magnesium levels are detected, the primary health care provider may prescribe magnesium replacement therapy.

PARENTERAL ADMINISTRATION The nurse may give a cardiotonic orally, IV, or intramuscularly (IM). When a cardiotonic drug is given IV, it is administered slowly and the administration site is assessed for redness or infiltration. Extravasation can lead to tissue irritation and sloughing. When giving a cardiotonic drug IM, the nurse should rotate the injection sites. To rotate injection sites correctly, the nurse inserts a diagram showing the order of rotation in the chart or the medication administration record. Each time the drug is given, the injection site is recorded in the patient's chart. However, IM injection is not recommended for these drugs.

ORAL ADMINISTRATION The nurse can administer oral preparations without regard to meals. Tablets can be crushed and mixed with food or fluids if the patient has difficulty swallowing. Do not alternate between the dosage forms (i.e., tablets and capsules) because dosages are not the same. The recommended dosage of the capsules is 80% of the dosage for tablets and elixir.

MONITORING AND MANAGING PATIENT NEEDS

IMBALANCED NUTRITION: LESS THAN BODY REQUIREMENTS The nurse must also closely observe the patient for other adverse drug reactions, such as anorexia, nausea, and vomiting. Some adverse drug reactions are also signs of digitalis toxicity, which can be serious. The nurse should carefully consider any patient complaint or comment, record it on the patient's chart, and bring it to the attention of the primary health care provider. If the nausea or anorexia is not a result of toxicity but an adverse reaction to the drug, the nurse may use nursing measures to help control the reactions. The nurse may offer frequent small meals, rather than three large meals. The nurse may suggest restricting fluids at meals and avoiding fluids 1 hour before and after meals to help control the nausea. Helping the patient to maintain good oral hygiene by brushing teeth or rinsing the mouth after ingesting food will also help with nausea. However, the nurse must always be aware that nausea and vomiting are symptoms of toxicity and must monitor the patient closely for other signs of digitalis toxicity.

ACTIVITY INTOLERANCE The patient may experience weakness or drowsiness as adverse reactions associated with digoxin, which may lead to activity intolerance. The patient is encouraged to increase daily activities gradually as tolerance increases, and the nurse plans a gradual increase in activities as tolerance increases as well. Adequate rest periods are planned during the day. The nurse assists with activities and ambulation as necessary.

POTENTIAL COMPLICATION: DIGITALIS TOXICITY The nurse observes for signs of digitalis toxicity every 2 to 4 hours during digitalization and one to two times a day when a maintenance dose is being given.

> ### Nursing Alert
>
> Plasma digoxin levels are monitored closely. Blood for plasma level measurements may be drawn 6 to 8 hours after the last dose or immediately before the next dose. Therapeutic drug levels are between 0.5 and 2 nanograms/mL. Plasma digoxin levels greater than 2 nanograms/mL are considered toxic and are reported to the primary health care provider.

Digitalis toxicity can occur even when normal doses are being administered or when the patient has been receiving a maintenance dose. Many symptoms of toxicity are similar to the symptoms of the heart conditions for which the patient is receiving the cardiotonic. This makes careful assessment of the patient by the nurse a critical aspect of care. The signs of digitalis toxicity are listed in Display 38-2. When digitalis toxicity develops, the primary health care provider may discontinue digitalis use until all signs of toxicity are gone. If severe bradycardia occurs, atropine (see Chapter 30) may be ordered. If digoxin has been given, the primary health care provider may order blood tests to determine serum drug levels.

> ### Display 38.2 Signs of Digitalis Toxicity
>
> - Gastrointestinal—anorexia (usually the first sign), nausea, vomiting diarrhea
> - Muscular—weakness
> - Central nervous system—headache, apathy, drowsiness, visual disturbances (blurred vision, disturbance in yellow green vision, halo effect around dark objects), mental depression, confusion, disorientation, delirium
> - Cardiac—changes in pulse rate or rhythm: electrocardiographic changes, such as bradycardia, tachycardia, premature ventricular contractions, bigeminal (two beats followed by a pause), or trigeminal (three beats followed by a pause) pulse. Other arrhythmias (abnormal heart rhythms) also may be seen.

Digoxin has a rapid onset and a short duration of action. Once the drug is withheld, the toxic effects of digoxin subside rapidly.

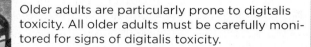

> ### Gerontologic Alert
>
> Older adults are particularly prone to digitalis toxicity. All older adults must be carefully monitored for signs of digitalis toxicity.

Most often, digoxin toxicity can be treated successfully by simply withdrawing the drug. However, severe, life-threatening toxicity is treated with digoxin immune fab (Digibind). Digoxin immune fab, composed of digoxin-specific antigen-binding fragments (fab), is used as an antidote in the treatment of digoxin overdosage. The dosage varies with the amount of digoxin ingested, and the drug is administered by the IV route during a 30-minute period. Most life-threatening states can be treated adequately with 800 mg of digoxin immune fab (20 vials). Few adverse reactions have been observed with the use of immune fab. However, the nurse should be alert for the possibility of worsening HF, low cardiac output, hypokalemia, or atrial fibrillation. Hypokalemia is of particular concern in patients taking digoxin immune fab, particularly because hypokalemia usually coexists with toxicity (see the Summary Drug Table: Cardiotonics and Miscellaneous Inotropic Drugs).

EDUCATING THE PATIENT AND FAMILY

In some instances, a cardiotonic drug may be prescribed for a prolonged period. Some patients may discontinue use of the drug, especially if they feel better and their original symptoms have been relieved. The patient and family must understand that the prescribed drug must be taken exactly as directed by the primary health care provider.

If the primary health care provider wants the patient to monitor the pulse rate daily during cardiotonic therapy, the nurse shows the patient or a family member the correct technique for taking the pulse (see Home Care Checklist: Monitoring Pulse Rate).

The primary health care provider may also want the patient to omit the next dose of the drug and call him or her if the pulse rate falls below a certain level (usually 60 bpm in an adult, 70 bpm in a child, and 90 bpm in an infant). These instructions are emphasized at the time of patient teaching. The nurse includes the following points in a teaching plan for the patient taking a cardiac glycoside drug:

- Do not discontinue use of this drug without first checking with the primary health care provider (unless instructed to do otherwise). Do not miss a dose or take an extra dose.

- Take this drug at the same time each day.

- Take your pulse before taking the drug, and withhold the drug and notify the primary health care provider if your pulse rate is less than 60 bpm or greater than 100 bpm.

- Avoid antacids and nonprescription cough, cold, allergy, antidiarrheal, and diet (weight-reducing) drugs unless their use has been approved by the primary health care provider. Some of these drugs interfere with the action of the cardiotonic drug or cause other, potentially serious problems (see Interactions, earlier).

- Contact the primary health care provider if nausea, vomiting, diarrhea, unusual fatigue, weakness, vision change (such as blurred vision, changes in colors of objects, or halos around dark objects), or mental depression occurs.

Home Care Checklist

Monitoring Pulse Rate

Monitoring a patient's pulse rate is second nature when the patient is in an acute care facility. However, when the patient goes home with digoxin, he or she will need to monitor the pulse rate to prevent possible adverse reactions. The nurse teaches the patient to perform the following steps:

☑ Have a watch with a second hand with you.

☑ Sit down and rest your nondominant arm on a table or chair armrest.

☑ Place the index and third fingers of your dominant hand just below the wrist bone on the thumb side of your nondominant arm.

☑ Feel for a beating or pulsing sensation. This is your pulse.

☑ Count the number of beats for 30 seconds (if the pulse is regular) and multiply by 2. If the pulse is irregular, count the number of beats for 60 seconds.

☑ Record the number of beats of your pulse and keep a log of your reading.

☑ If you notice the pulse rate greater than 100 bpm or less than 60 bpm, call your primary health care provider immediately.

- Carry medical identification describing the disease process and your medication regimen.
- Keep the drug in its original container.
- Follow the dietary recommendations (if any) made by the primary health care provider.
- The primary health care provider will closely monitor therapy. Keep all appointments for primary health care provider visits or laboratory or diagnostic tests.

EVALUATION

- The therapeutic effect is achieved.
- The patient maintains an adequate nutritional status.
- The patient is able to carry out activities of daily living.
- Adverse reactions are identified, reported to the primary health care provider, and managed using appropriate nursing interventions.
- The patient verbalizes the importance of continued follow-up care.
- The patient verbalizes the importance of complying with the prescribed therapeutic regimen.
- The patient and family demonstrate an understanding of the drug regimen.
- The patient complies with the prescribed drug regimen.

Critical Thinking Exercises

1. Mr. Taylor has been taking digoxin for 3 weeks and has come to the clinic for a follow-up visit. Analyze the situation to determine what questions you would ask Mr. Taylor during the interview to evaluate his knowledge of the drug regimen and to find out if he is experiencing any adverse reactions.

2. You are to participate in a team conference on the cardiac glycosides. Your topic to discuss is discharge teaching for the patient receiving a cardiac glycoside. Develop a teaching plan using the nursing process as a framework. Determine what points would be most important for you to include.

3. Discuss when you would expect the primary health care provider to order digoxin immune fab. State the assessment you feel would be most important and give a rationale.

Review Questions

1. Which of the following is commonly associated with left ventricular systolic dysfunction?
   A. Ejection fraction of 60% or more
   B. Ejection fraction below 40%

C. Increased cardiac output
D. Normal cardiac output

2. Which of the following serum digoxin levels in an adult would be most indicative that the patient may be experiencing digoxin toxicity?
   A. 0.5 nanograms/mL
   B. 0.8 nanograms/mL
   C. 1.0 nanograms/mL
   D. 2.0 nanograms/mL

3. In which of the following situations would the nurse withhold a dose of digoxin and notify the primary health care provider?
   A. A pulse rate of 50 bpm
   B. A pulse rate of 87 bpm
   C. A pulse rate of 92 bpm
   D. A pulse rate of 62 bpm

4. Which drug would the nurse expect to be prescribed for a patient with digoxin toxicity?
   A. digoxin immune fab
   B. milrinone
   C. inamrinone lactate
   D. Any inotropic drug

5. During rapid digitalization, the nurse expects the first dose to be _____.
   A. the smallest dose in case the patient is allergic to digoxin
   B. given orally, with succeeding doses given intravenously
   C. approximately half of the total digitalization dose
   D. approximately three quarters of the total digitalization dose

Medication Dosage Problems

1. Digoxin (Lanoxin) is prescribed for a patient with heart failure, and digitalization is begun. The primary health care provider prescribes digoxin (Lanoxin) 0.75 mg orally as the initial dose. Available are digoxin tablets of 0.5 and 0.25 mg. The nurse administers _____.

2. Digoxin 0.5 mg IV is prescribed. The drug is available in a solution of 0.25 mg/mL. How many milliliters will the nurse prepare?

To check your answers, see Appendix G.

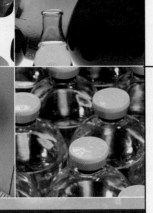

Antiarrhythmic Drugs

Learning Objectives

On completion of this chapter, the student will:

- Describe various types of cardiac arrhythmias.

- Discuss the uses, general drug actions, general adverse reactions, contraindications, precautions, and interactions of the antiarrhythmic drugs.

- Discuss important preadministration and ongoing assessments the nurse should perform on a patient taking an antiarrhythmic drug.

- List nursing diagnoses particular to a patient taking an antiarrhythmic drug.

- Discuss ways to promote an optimal response to therapy, how to manage common adverse reactions, and important points to keep in mind when educating patients about the use of antiarrhythmic drugs.

The antiarrhythmic drugs are primarily used to treat cardiac arrhythmias. A cardiac **arrhythmia** is a disturbance or irregularity in the heart rate, rhythm, or both, which requires administration of one of the antiarrhythmic drugs. Some examples of cardiac arrhythmias are listed in Table 39-1.

An arrhythmia may occur as a result of heart disease or from a disorder that affects cardiovascular function. Conditions such as emotional stress, hypoxia, and electrolyte imbalance also may trigger an arrhythmia. An electrocardiogram (ECG) provides a record of the electrical activity of the heart. Careful interpretation of the ECG along with a thorough physical assessment are necessary to determine the cause and type of arrhythmia. The goal of antiarrhythmic drug therapy is to restore normal cardiac function and prevent life-threatening arrhythmias.

Actions

The cardiac muscle (myocardium) has attributes of both nerve and muscle and therefore has the properties of both. Some cardiac arrhythmias are caused by the generation of an abnormal number of electrical impulses (stimuli). These abnormal impulses may come from the sinoatrial (SA) node or may be generated in other areas of the myocardium. The antiarrhythmic drugs are classified according to their effects on the action potential of cardiac cells and their presumed mechanism of action. As understanding of the pathophysiology of cardiac arrhythmias and the drugs used to treat these arrhythmias has increased, a method of classification has been developed that includes four basic classes and several subclasses. Drugs in each group, or class, have certain similarities, yet each drug has subtle differences that make it unique.

Table 39.1 Types of Arrhythmias

Arrhythmia	Description
Atrial flutter	Rapid contraction of the atria (up to 300 bpm) at a rate too rapid for the ventricles to pump efficiently
Atrial fibrillation	Irregular and rapid atrial contraction, resulting in a quivering of the atria and causing an irregular and inefficient ventricular contraction
Premature ventricular contractions	Beats originating in the ventricles instead of the sinoatrial node in the atria, causing the ventricles to contract before the atria and resulting in a decrease in the amount of blood pumped to the body
Ventricular tachycardia	A rapid heart beat with a rate of more than 100 bpm, usually originating in the ventricles
Ventricular fibrillation	Rapid, disorganized contractions of the ventricles resulting in the inability of the heart to pump any blood to the body, which will result in death unless treated immediately

Display 39.1 Understanding Action Potential and Refractory Period

Action Potential

All cells are electrically polarized, with the inside of the cell more negatively charged than the outside. The difference in the electrical charge is called the *resting membrane potential*. Nerve and muscle cells are excitable and can change the resting membrane potential in response to electrochemical stimuli. The **action potential** is an electrical impulse that passes from cell to cell in the myocardium, stimulating the fibers to shorten, and causing muscular contraction (systole). An action potential generated in one part of the myocardium passes almost simultaneously through all of the myocardial fibers, causing rapid contraction.

Refractory Period

Only one impulse can pass along a nerve fiber at any given time. After the passage of an impulse, there is a brief pause, or interval, before the next impulse can pass along the nerve fiber. This pause is called the **refractory period,** which is the period between the transmission of nerve impulses along a nerve fiber. Lengthening the refractory period decreases the number of impulses traveling along a nerve fiber within a given time.

Class I Antiarrhythmic Drugs

Class I antiarrhythmic drugs, such as moricizine, have a membrane-stabilizing or anesthetic effect on the cells of the myocardium, making them valuable in treating cardiac arrhythmias. Class I contains the largest number of drugs of the four antiarrhythmic drug classifications. Because their actions differ slightly, the drugs are subdivided into classes IA, IB, and IC.

Class IA

In general, class IA drugs act to

- Depress phase 0
- Prolong the action potential

The drugs disopyramide (Norpace), procainamide (Procanbid), and quinidine (Quinaglute) are examples of class IA drugs. Disopyramide decreases depolarization of myocardial fibers during the diastolic phase of the cardiac cycle, prolongs the refractory period, and increases the action potential duration of normal cardiac cells (Display 39-1).

Procainamide increases the effective refractory period of the atria and, to a lesser extent, the bundle of His-Purkinje fibers. Quinidine depresses myocardial excitability or the ability of the myocardium to respond to an electrical stimulus. By depressing the myocardium and its ability to

respond to some, but not all, electrical stimuli, the pulse rate decreases and the arrhythmia is corrected. Quinidine also depresses the conduction velocity and contractility. It prolongs the effective refractory period and increases conduction time. See Display 39-2 for a discussion of polarization, depolarization, and repolarization.

Class IB Drugs

Class IB drugs generally act to

- Slightly depress phase 0
- Shorten the action potential duration

Lidocaine (Xylocaine), the representative class IB drug, decreases diastolic depolarization, decreases automaticity of ventricular cells, and raises the threshold of the ventricular myocardium. **Threshold** is a term applied to any stimulus of the lowest intensity that will give rise to a response in a nerve fiber. A stimulus must be of a specific intensity (strength, amplitude) to pass along a given nerve fiber (Fig. 39-1).

To illustrate further the threshold phenomenon using round figures instead of precise electrical values, consider a certain nerve fiber as having a threshold of 10. If a stimulus rated as 9 reaches the fiber, it will not pass along the fiber

Display 39.2 Polarization, Depolarization, and Repolarization

Nerve cells have positive ions on the outside and negative ions on the inside of the cell membrane when they are at rest. This is called **polarization**. When a stimulus passes along the nerve, the positive ions move from outside the cell into the cell, and the negative ions move from inside the cell to outside the cell. This movement of ions is called **depolarization**. Unless positive ions move into and negative ions move out of a nerve cell, a stimulus (or impulse) cannot pass along the nerve fiber. Once the stimulus has passed along the nerve fiber, the positive and negative ions move back to their original place, that is, the positive ions on the outside and the negative ions on the inside of the nerve cell. This movement back to the original place is called **repolarization**. By decreasing the rate (or speed) of depolarization, the stimulus must literally wait for this process before it can pass along the nerve fiber. Thus, decreasing the rate (or speed) of depolarization decreases the number of impulses that can pass along a nerve fiber during a specific time period.

Polarization

When the nerve cell is polarized, positive ions (⊕) are on the outside of the cell membrane and the negative ions (⊖) are on the inside of the cell membrane.

Depolarization

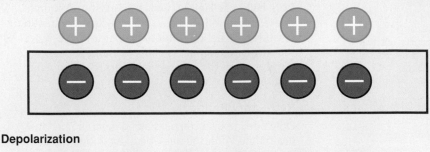

In response to a stimulus, the positive ions move from the outside to the inside of the cell membrane, while the negative ions move to the outside.

Repolarization

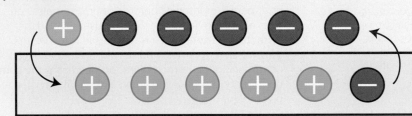

After the stimulus has passed along the nerve fiber, the ions move back to their original place until another stimulus occurs.

because its intensity is lower than the fiber's threshold of 10. If another stimulus reaches the fiber and is rated 14, it will pass along the fiber because its intensity is greater than the fiber's threshold of 10. If the threshold of a fiber is raised from 10 to 15, only stimuli greater than 15 can pass along the nerve fiber.

Some cardiac arrhythmias result from many stimuli present in the myocardium. Some of these are weak or of low intensity but are still able to excite myocardial tissue. Lidocaine, by raising the threshold of myocardial fibers, reduces the number of stimuli that will pass along these fibers and therefore decreases the pulse rate and corrects the arrhythmia.

Class IC Drugs

The general action of class IC drugs includes

- Marked depression of phase 0

- Slight effect on repolarization

- Profound slowing of conduction

Flecainide (Tambocor) and propafenone (Rythmol) are examples of class IC drugs. Specifically, flecainide depresses fast sodium channels, decreases the height and rate of rise of action potentials, and slows conduction of all areas of the heart. Propafenone, which has a direct membrane-stabilizing effect on the myocardial membrane, prolongs the refractory period.

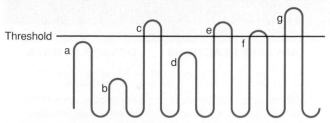

Threshold

a
b
c
d
e
f
g

A stimulus must reach the threshold to cause a response in a nerve fiber. Note that stimuli **a**, **b**, and **d** do *not* reach the threshold; therefore, they do *not* cause a response in a nerve fiber. Stimuli **c**, **e**, **f**, and **g** do reach and surpass the threshold, resulting in stimulation of nerve fiber.

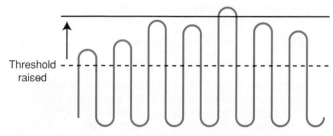

Threshold raised

After receiving lidocaine hydrochloride (Xylocaine HCl), the threshold is raised to a higher level, allowing fewer stimuli to reach the threshold. This results in decreased stimulation of the nerve fiber and prevents conduction of the nerve impulses causing the arrthythmia.

Figure 39.1 The threshold phenomenon.

Class II Antiarrhythmic Drugs

The general action of drugs in class II is depression of depolarization phase (phase 4). Class II antiarrhythmic drugs include beta-adrenergic blocking drugs, such as acebutolol (Sectral) and propranolol (Inderal). Acebutolol and propranolol act by blocking beta-adrenergic receptors of the heart and kidney, reducing the influence of the sympathetic nervous system on these areas, decreasing the excitability of the heart and the release of renin (lowering heart rate and blood pressure). These drugs have membrane-stabilizing effects that contribute to their antiarrhythmic activity.

Class III Antiarrhythmic Drugs

The general action of class III antiarrhythmic drugs is prolongation of repolarization (phase 3). Examples are amiodarone (Cordarone) and ibutilide (Corvert). Amiodarone appears to act directly on the cardiac cell membrane, prolonging the refractory period and repolarization and increasing the ventricular fibrillation threshold. Ibutilide acts by prolonging the action potential, producing a mild slowing of the sinus rate and atrioventricular (AV) conduction.

Class IV Antiarrhythmic Drugs

In general, the class IV antiarrhythmic drugs act by
- Depressing depolarization (phase 4)
- Lengthening phase 1 and 2 of repolarization

Verapamil (Calan), a class IV antiarrhythmic drug, is also classified as a calcium channel blocker. Calcium channel blockers inhibit the movement of calcium through channels across the myocardial cell membranes and vascular smooth muscle. Cardiac and vascular smooth muscle depends on the movement of calcium ions into the muscle cells through specific ion channels. When this movement is inhibited, the coronary and peripheral arteries dilate, thereby decreasing the force of cardiac contraction. This drug also reduces heart rate by slowing conduction through the SA and AV nodes. Additional information about the calcium channel blockers can be found in Chapter 41.

Uses

In general, the antiarrhythmic drugs are used to treat
- Premature ventricular contractions (PVCs)
- Ventricular tachycardia
- Premature atrial contractions
- Paroxysmal atrial tachycardia
- Other atrial arrhythmias, such as atrial fibrillation or flutter
- Tachycardia when rapid but short-term control of ventricular rate is desirable

Some of the antiarrhythmic drugs are used for other conditions. For example, propranolol, in addition to its use as an antiarrhythmic, may be used for patients with myocardial infarction. This drug has reduced the risk of death and repeated myocardial infarctions in those surviving the acute phase of a myocardial infarction. See the Summary Drug Table: Antiarrhythmic Drugs for more uses.

Adverse Reactions

Adverse reactions associated with the administration of specific antiarrhythmic drugs are given in the Summary Drug Table: Antiarrhythmic Drugs. General adverse reactions common to most antiarrhythmic drugs include the following.

Antiarrhythmic Drugs

408 Unit VI | Drugs That Affect the Cardiovascular System

SUMMARY DRUG TABLE ANTIARRHYTHMIC DRUGS

GENERIC NAME	TRADE NAME	USES	ADVERSE REACTIONS	DOSAGE RANGES
Class I				
disopyramide *dye-soe-peer'-a-mide*	Norpace, Norpace CR	Suppression and treatment of sustained ventricular tachycardia	Dry mouth, constipation, urinary hesitancy, blurred vision, nausea, fatigue, dizziness, headache, rash, hypotension, HF, proarrhythmic effect	Ventricular arrhythmias: dosage individualized, 390–800 mg/d orally in divided doses
flecainide *fle-key'-nide*	Tambocor	Paroxysmal atrial fibrillation/flutter and supraventricular tachycardia	Dizziness, headache, faintness, unsteadiness, blurred vision, headache, nausea, dyspnea, HF, fatigue, palpitations, chest pain, proarrhythmic effect	Initial dose: 100 mg orally q12h; maximum dosage, 390 mg/d
lidocaine HCl *lye'-doe-kane*	Xylocaine	Ventricular arrhythmias	Lightheadedness, nervousness, bradycardia, hypotension, drowsiness, apprehension, proarrhythmic effect	50–100 mg IV bolus; 1–4 mg/min IV infusion, 20–50 mg/kg/min; 300 mg IM
mexiletine HCl *max-ill'-i-teen*	Mexitil	Ventricular arrhythmias	Palpitations, nausea, vomiting, chest pain, heartburn, dizziness, lightheadedness, rash, agranulocytosis, proarrhythmic effect	Initial dose: 200 mg orally q8h; maximum dosage, 1200 mg/d orally
moricizine *mor-i'-siz-cen*	Ethmozine	Life-threatening ventricular arrhythmias	Cardiac rhythm disturbances, existing arrhythmias worsened, palpitations, dizziness, headache, nausea, anxiety, proarrhythmic effect	600–900 mg/d orally in three equally divided doses
procainamide HCl *proe-kane-a'-mide*	Procanbid	Life-threatening ventricular arrhythmias	Hypotension, disturbances of cardiac rhythm, urticaria, fever, chills, nausea, vomiting, rash, confusion, dizziness, weakness, anorexia, agranulocytosis, proarrhythmic effect	Oral: 50 mg/kg/d in divided doses q3h IM: 0.5–1.0 g q4–8h IV: 500–600 mg over 25–30 min, then 2–6 mg/min
propafenone HCl *proe-paf'-a-non*	Rythmol	Atrial fibrillation, ventricular arrhythmias, paroxysmal supraventricular tachycardia	Dizziness, nausea, vomiting, constipation, unusual taste, first-degree atrioventricular block, agranulocytosis, proarrhythmic effect	Initial dose: 150 mg orally q8h; may be increased to 300 mg orally q8h
quinidine gluconate *kwin'-i-deen* **quinidine sulfate** **quinidine polygalacturonate**	Quinaglute Quinidex Cardioquin	Premature atrial and ventricular contractions, atrial tachycardia and flutter, paroxysmal	Ringing in the ears, hearing loss, nausea, vomiting, dizziness, headache, rash, disturbed vision, hypotension, proarrhythmic effect, agranulocytosis atrial fibrillation, chronic atrial fibrillation	Administer test dose of 1 tablet orally or 200 mg IM to test for idiosyncratic reaction Oral: 200–300 mg TID, QID or 300–600 mg q12h if sustained release form is used. IM: 600 mg quinidine gluconate, then 390 mg q2h

GENERIC NAME	TRADE NAME	USES	ADVERSE REACTIONS	DOSAGE RANGES
				IV: 300 mg quinidine gluconate slow IV at 1 mL/min of diluted solution
Class II				
acebutolol *ah-see-byoo'-toe-lol*	Sectral	Ventricular arrhythmias, hypertension	Hypotension, nausea, diaphoresis, headache, fatigue, weakness, dizziness, impotence, bradycardia, cardiac arrhythmias, decreased exercise tolerance, proarrhythmic effect	Arrhythmias: initially 200 mg q12h orally; may increase to 1200 mg/d in 2 divided doses Hypertension: 390 mg/d in 1 or 2 doses orally Maintenance dose, 200–1200 mg in divided doses
esmolol HCl *ez'-moe-lol*	Brevibloc	Rapid, short-term treatment of ventricular rate in supraventricular arrhythmia, sinus tachycardia	Dizziness, headache, hypotension, nausea, cold extremities, bradycardia, urinary retention, proarrhythmic effect	Loading dose: 500 mg/kg/min IV for 1 min, followed by infusion of 50 mg/kg/min IV for 4 min Maintenance dose, 25 mg/kg/min IV
propranolol HCl *proe-pran'-oh-lole*	Inderal, Inderal LA	Cardiac arrhythmias, angina pectoris, hypertension, essential tremor, myocardial infarction, migraine headache, pheochromocytoma	Fatigue, weakness, nausea, vomiting, depression, bradycardia, dizziness, vertigo, rash, decreased libido, hypotension, hyperglycemia, decreased exercise tolerance, proarrhythmic effect	Cardiac arrhythmias: 10–30 mg orally TID or QID Life-threatening arrhythmias: 1–3 mg IV, may repeat once in 2 min Angina pectoris; 80–320 mg/d orally in 2–4 divided doses Hypertension: initially, 39 mg orally BID or 80 mg sustained-released QD Maintenance dose, up to 639 mg/d orally in divided doses
Class III				
amiodarone HCl *a-mee'-o-da-rone*	Cordarone, Pacerone	Life-threatening ventricular arrhythmias	Malaise, fatigue, tremor, proarrhythmic effect, nausea, vomiting, constipation, ataxia, anorexia, bradycardia, photosensitivity	Loading dose: 800–1600 mg/d orally in divided doses Maintenance dose, 390 mg/d orally; up to 1000 mg/d over 24 h IV
bretylium tosylate *bre-till'-ee-um*		Prophylaxis and treatment of ventricular fibrillation	Hypotension, nausea, vomiting, vertigo, dizziness, postural hypotension, bradycardia, proarrhythmic effect	Immediate treatment: 5–10 mg/kg (diluted) IV; maintenance, rate of 1–2 mg/min by continuous IV infusion, or infuse intermittently at 5–10 mg/kg over 10–30 min q6h
dofetilide *doe-fe'-ti-lyed*	Tikosyn	Conversion of atrial fibrillation/flutter to normal sinus rhythm, maintenance of normal sinus rhythm	Headache, chest pain, dizziness, respiratory tract infection, dyspnea, nausea, flu-like syndrome, insomnia, proarrhythmic effect	Dosage based on electrocardiogram response and creatinine clearance; range, 125–500 mg BID

SUMMARY DRUG TABLE (continued)

GENERIC NAME	TRADE NAME	USES	ADVERSE REACTIONS	DOSAGE RANGES
ibutilide fumarate *eye-byoo'-ti-lyed*	Corvert	Atrial fibrillation/flutter	Headache, nausea, hypotension or hypertension, ventricular arrhythmias, proarrhythmic effect	Adults 60 kg and more: 1 mg infused over 10 min; may repeat 10 min Adults under 60 kg: 0.1 mL/kg infused over 10 min; may repeat in 10 min
sotalol *sew'-tah-lol*	Betapace, Betapace AF	Treatment of life-threatening ventricular arrhythmias, reduction and delay of atrial fibrillation and flutter for ventricular arrhythmias (Betapace AF)	Drowsiness, difficulty sleeping, unusual tiredness or weakness, depression, decreased libido, bradycardia, HF, cold hands and feet, nausea, vomiting, nasal congestion, anxiety, life-threatening arrhythmias, proarrhythmic effect	Initially: 80 mg BID orally; may increased up to 239–320 mg/d (Betapace); up to 120 mg BID (Betapace AF)
Class IV				
Verapamil HCl *ver-ap'-ah-mill*	Calan, Covera HS, Isoptin, Verelan, Verelan PM	Supraventricular tachyarrhythmias, temporary control of rapid ventricular rate in atrial flutter/fibrillation, angina, unstable angina, hypertension	Constipation, dizziness, light-headedness, headache, asthenia, nausea, vomiting, peripheral edema, hypotension, mental depression, agranulocytosis, proarrhythmic effect	Adults: oral—initial dose 80–120 mg TID; maintenance, 320–480 mg/d Hypertension: 239 mg/d orally; sustained-release, in AM 80 mg TID; extended-release capsules, 100–300 mg orally at bedtime Parenteral: IV use only; initial dose 5–10 mg over 2 min; may repeat 10 mg 30 min later

HF, heart failure.

Central Nervous System Reactions

- Lightheadedness
- Weakness
- Somnolence

Cardiovascular Reactions

- Hypotension
- Arrhythmias
- Bradycardia

Other

- Urinary retention
- Local inflammation

All antiarrhythmic drugs may cause new arrhythmias or worsen existing arrhythmias, even though they are administered to resolve an existing arrhythmia. This phenomenon is called the **proarrhythmic effect**. This effect ranges from an increase in frequency of PVCs to the development of more severe ventricular tachycardia, to ventricular fibrillation, and the effect may lead to death. Proarrhythmic effects may occur at any time but they occur more often when excessive dosages are given, when the preexisting arrhythmia is life-threatening, or when the drug is given intravenously (IV).

Contraindications

The antiarrhythmic drugs are reserved for emergency situations and are contraindicated in patients with known hypersensitivity to these drugs. They are contraindicated during pregnancy and lactation. The antiarrhythmic drug amiodarone is a pregnancy category D drug, indicating that fetal harm can occur when the agent is administered to a pregnant woman. It is used only if the potential benefits outweigh the potential hazards to the fetus. Antiarrhythmic drugs are contraindicated in patients with second- or third-degree AV block (if the patient has no artificial pacemaker), severe congestive heart failure (CHF), aortic stenosis, hypotension, and cardiogenic shock. Quinidine and procainamide are contraindicated in patients with myasthenia gravis (see Chapter 29).

Precautions

Antiarrhythmic drugs are used cautiously in patients with hepatic disease, electrolyte disturbances, CHF (quinidine, flecainide, procainamide, and disopyramide), and renal

impairment. Most antiarrhythmics are pregnancy category B or C drugs, indicating that safe use of these drugs during pregnancy or lactation, or in children, has not been established. Disopyramide is used cautiously in patients with myasthenia gravis, urinary retention, or glaucoma, and in men with prostate enlargement.

Interactions

When antiarrhythmics are used with other medications, various interactions may occur. See Table 39-2 for more information.

Table 39.2 Interactions: Antiarrhythmics and Other Agents

Interacting Drug	Common Uses	Effect of Interaction
Disopyramide		
clarithromycin, erythromycin	Bacterial infections	Increased serum disopyramide levels
fluoroquinolones	Infections	Risk of life-threatening arrhythmias
quinidine	Cardiac problems	Increased serum levels of disopyramide
rifampin	Antitubercular agent	Decreased disopyramide serum levels
thioridazine, ziprasidone	Management of mental illness	Increased risk of life-threatening arrhythmias
Procainamide		
amiodarone	Cardiac problems	Increased serum procainamide level
cholinergic blocking drugs	GI problems	Additive antivagal effects on atrioventricular conduction
cimetidine, ranitidine	GI problems	Increased serum procainamide level
thioridazine, ziprasidone	Management of mental illness	Life-threatening cardiac arrhythmias
Quinidine		
barbiturates	Sleep aid	Possibly, decreased serum levels of quinidine
cholinergic drugs	Treatment of glaucoma	Failure to terminate paroxysmal supraventricular tachycardia
cimetidine	GI problems	Increased serum quinidine level
hydantoins	Seizure control	Decreased therapeutic effect of quinidine
nifedipine	Treatment of angina	Decreased action and serum level of quinidine
cholinergic blocking drugs	GI problems	Additive vagolytic effect
Lidocaine		
beta blockers	Hypertension and angina	Increased lidocaine levels
cimetidine	GI problems	Decreased lidocaine clearance with possible toxicity
procainamide	Cardiac problems	Additive cardiodepressant action
Flecainide		
amiodarone	Cardiac problems	Increased serum flecainide levels
cimetidine	GI problems	Increased serum flecainide levels

(continued)

Table 39.2 Interactions: Antiarrhythmics and Other Agents (continued)

Interacting Drug	Common Uses	Effect of Interaction
disopyramide, verapamil	Cardiovascular problems	May increase negative inotropic properties (see Chapter 38). Avoid using either of these drugs with flecainide.
propranolol	Cardiovascular problems	Increased serum levels of propranolol and flecainide, and additive negative inotropic effects
Propafenone		
local anesthetics	Anesthesia	Concurrent use (e.g., during pacemaker implantation, surgery or dental use) may increase the risk of central nervous system side effects
quinidine	Cardiac problems	Increased serum propafenone levels
selective serotonin reuptake inhibitors (SSRIs)	Relief of depression	Increased serum propafenone levels
anticoagulants (e.g., warfarin)	Blood thinners	Increased prothrombin time and increased plasma warfarin levels
beta blockers	Cardiovascular problems	Increased effects of the beta blockers
digoxin	Heart failure	Increased serum digoxin level
theophylline	Management of asthma and chronic obstructive pulmonary disease (COPD)	Increased serum theophylline level

GI, gastrointestinal.

NURSING PROCESS

The Patient Receiving an Antiarrhythmic Drug

ASSESSMENT

PREADMINISTRATION ASSESSMENT

Antiarrhythmic drugs are used to treat various types of cardiac arrhythmias. Certain initial preadministration assessments the nurse performs before starting therapy are the same for all antiarrhythmic drugs. These assessments include

- Taking and recording the blood pressure, apical and radial pulses, and respiratory rate. This provides a database for comparison during therapy.

- Assessing the patient's general condition and including observations such as skin color (pale, cyanotic, flushed), orientation, level of consciousness, and the patient's general status (e.g., appears acutely ill or appears somewhat ill). All observations must be recorded to provide a means of evaluating the response to drug therapy.

- Recording any symptoms (subjective data) described by the patient.

Because all antiarrhythmic drugs may produce proarrhythmic effects, a careful preadministration assessment is essential. It is often difficult to distinguish a proarrhythmic effect from the patient's underlying rhythm disorder, so it is important that the nurse assess each patient taking an antiarrhythmic drug through the use of cardiac monitoring before therapy begins and in the ongoing assessment to determine if the patient is experiencing a therapeutic response to the drug, developing another arrhythmia, or experiencing worsening of the original arrhythmia.

The primary health care provider may also order laboratory and diagnostic tests, renal and hepatic function tests, complete blood count, and serum enzymes and electrolyte analyses. The nurse reviews these test results before the first dose of an antiarrhythmic drug is given and reports any abnormalities to the primary health care provider. The patient is usually placed on a cardiac monitor before antiarrhythmic drug therapy is initiated. In addition, the primary health care provider may order an ECG to provide baseline data for comparison during therapy.

ONGOING ASSESSMENT

During ongoing therapy with the antiarrhythmic drugs, the nurse takes the patient's blood pressure, apical and radial pulses, and respiratory rate at periodic intervals, usually every 1 to 4 hours. Specific intervals depend on the primary health care provider's order or on nursing judgment and are based on the patient's general condition. The nurse closely observes the patient for a response to drug therapy, signs of CHF, the development of a new cardiac arrhythmia, or worsening of the arrhythmia being treated.

The nurse should immediately report to the primary health care provider any significant changes in the blood pressure, pulse rate or rhythm, respiratory rate or rhythm, or the patient's general condition.

> ### Nursing Alert
>
> When giving an oral antiarrhythmic drug, the nurse withholds the drug and notifies the primary health care provider immediately when the pulse rate is above 120 beats per minute (bpm) or below 60 bpm. In some instances, the primary health care provider may establish additional or different guidelines for withholding the drug.

Continual cardiac monitoring assists the nurse in assessing the patient for adverse drug reactions. If the patient is acutely ill or is receiving one of the antiarrhythmics parenterally, the nurse measures and records the fluid intake and output. The primary health care provider may order subsequent laboratory tests to monitor the patient's progress for comparison with tests performed in the preadministration assessment, such as an ECG, renal and hepatic function tests, complete blood count, and serum enzyme and electrolyte analyses. The nurse reports to the primary health care provider any abnor-

malities or significant interval changes of the ECG, such as prolongation of the PR or QT interval or widening of the QRS complex. Prolongation of the QT interval is particularly associated with life-threatening ventricular arrhythmias (see Fig. 39-2 for a diagram of a normal QRS complex). In addition, when subsequent laboratory tests are ordered, the nurse reviews the results and reports any abnormalities to the primary health care provider.

NURSING DIAGNOSES

Drug-specific nursing diagnoses are highlighted in the Nursing Diagnoses Checklist. Other nursing diagnoses applicable to these drugs are discussed in depth in Chapter 4.

> ### Nursing Diagnoses Checklist
>
> ✓ **Nausea** related to adverse drug reactions of antiarrhythmic drugs
>
> ✓ **Urinary Retention** related to adverse reactions (cholinergic blocking effects)
>
> ✓ **Impaired Oral Mucous Membranes** related to adverse drug reactions (dry mouth)
>
> ✓ **Risk for Injury** related to adverse drug reactions (dizziness, light-headedness)
>
> ✓ **Risk for Infection** related to adverse drug effects (agranulocytosis)

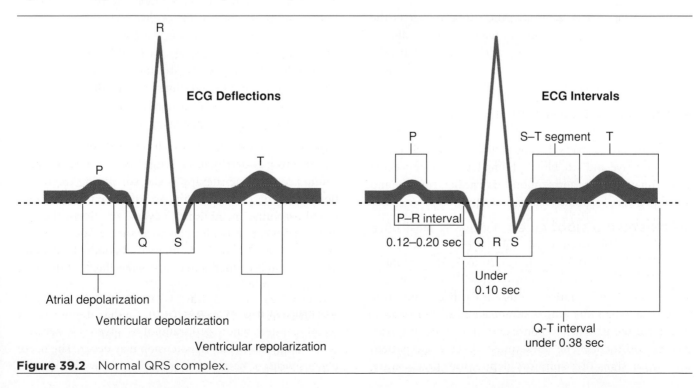

Figure 39.2   Normal QRS complex.

PLANNING

The expected outcomes for the patient depend on the reason for administration of the antiarrhythmic drug, but may include obtaining an optimal therapeutic response to drug therapy, meeting patient needs related to the management of adverse drug reactions, and an understanding of and compliance with the prescribed drug regimen.

IMPLEMENTATION
PROMOTING AN OPTIMAL RESPONSE TO THERAPY

ADMINISTERING QUINIDINE When quinidine is administered orally, the drug is not crushed or chewed. Gastrointestinal (GI) upset can be reduced if the drug is given with food. The nurse must monitor serum quinidine levels during administration of the drug. Normal therapeutic levels range between 2 and 6 mcg/mL.

ADMINISTERING PROCAINAMIDE If procainamide is given IV, the nurse maintains continuous and close cardiac monitoring. Hypotension may occur with IV administration; therefore, the blood pressure must be monitored every 15 minutes while the drug is being infused. The nurse may keep the patient supine during IV administration to minimize hypotension. If hypotension should occur, the primary health care provider is notified immediately. Although not the route of choice, the drug may be administered by intramuscular (IM) injection. When the drug is given IM, the gluteus muscle is used and the injection sites are rotated.

When the drug is given orally, the nurse instructs the patient not to chew the capsule or tablet but to swallow it whole. If GI upset occurs, the nurse can administer the drug with or immediately after meals. Sustained-released tablets should not be crushed or divided.

ADMINISTERING DISOPYRAMIDE Oral disopyramide is administered to the patient with a full 8-oz glass of water every 6 hours, or every 12 hours if in controlled-release form. Effective and safe blood plasma levels are between 2 and 8 mcg/mL. The nurse monitors cardiac rhythm and blood pressure frequently during therapy.

ADMINISTERING LIDOCAINE Lidocaine is most often administered IV continuously diluted in dextrose 5% in water (D_5W) at 1 to 4 mg/min (or 20 to 50 mcg/kg/min). The arrhythmia is usually controlled within 24 hours of continuous administration. Constant cardiac monitoring is essential when this drug is administered IV. Lidocaine is titrated to the patient's response and in accord with institutional protocols. The nurse must observe the patient closely for signs of respiratory depression, bradycardia, change in mental status, respiratory arrest, convulsions, and hypotension. The infusion is discontinued when the heart rhythm is stable or at the earliest sign of lidocaine toxicity. Blood concentration levels exceeding 6 mcg/mL are associated with significant risk of central nervous system (CNS) and cardiovascular depression. An oropharyngeal airway and suction equipment are kept at the bedside in case convulsions occur. Life support equipment and vasopressors are also readily available in case of adverse reaction. Any sudden change in mental state should be reported to the primary health care provider immediately because a decrease in the dosage may be necessary.

ADMINISTERING MEXILETINE Mexiletine is administered at 8-hour intervals and with food (or an antacid) to prevent GI upset. The dosage of mexiletine must be individualized; therefore, the nurse monitors vital signs at frequent intervals during initial therapy. The nurse reports any changes in the pulse rate or rhythm to the primary health care provider. Onset of tremors indicates that the maximum dosage of mexiletine has been reached. Adverse effects related to the CNS or GI tract may occur during initial therapy and must be reported to the primary health care provider.

ADMINISTERING FLECAINIDE AND PROPAFENONE It is advisable to hospitalize the patient during withdrawal of a previously given antiarrhythmic drug before initiating flecainide therapy because life-threatening arrhythmias may occur. When administering flecainide, the nurse must carefully monitor the patient for cardiac arrhythmias. Therapeutic serum levels fall between 0.2 and 1 mcg/mL. Life support equipment, including a pacemaker, should be kept on standby during administration. The nurse closely observes the patient for a response to drug therapy, signs of CHF, the development of a new cardiac arrhythmia, or worsening of the arrhythmia being treated.

Propafenone is administered orally every 8 hours. Any previously given antiarrhythmic drug should be discontinued before propafenone therapy is started. During the initiation of therapy, patients taking propafenone must be monitored carefully. To minimize adverse reactions, the primary health care provider may increase the dosage slowly at a minimum of 3- to 4-day intervals. Periodic ECG monitoring is usually ordered to evaluate the effects of the drug on cardiac conduction.

ADMINISTERING PROPRANOLOL Cardiac monitoring is recommended when propranolol is given IV because severe bradycardia and hypotension may occur. The nurse obtains written instructions from the primary health care provider for propranolol administration. For example, the primary health care provider may want the drug to be withheld for a systolic blood pressure less than 90 mm Hg or a pulse rate less than 50 bpm. The nurse monitors the ECG frequently for cardiac arrhythmias. Patients receiving IV propranolol must have continuous cardiac monitoring. The nurse must monitor the blood pressure and pulse frequently during the dosage adjustment period and periodically throughout therapy.

ADMINISTERING BRETYLIUM Bretylium is used in the emergency treatment of life-threatening ventricular arrhythmias. Because of its adverse reactions, bretylium is used only when the arrhythmia is unresponsive to the other antiarrhythmic drugs. Baseline data come from routine assessments made before the emergency. The nurse administers this drug IM or IV and uses continuous cardiac monitoring. The patient is placed in a supine position with suction equipment readily available in case vomiting occurs.

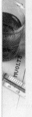

Nursing Alert

A transient increase in arrhythmias and hypertension may occur within 1 hour after initial therapy with bretylium is begun. The nurse should take the blood pressure and respiratory rate every 5 to 15 minutes and obtain the pulse rate from the cardiac monitor. These activities are continued until the arrhythmia is corrected.

The nurse monitors cardiac rhythm and blood pressure continuously during administration. Hypotension and postural hypotension occur in about 50% of the patients receiving bretylium. If systolic pressure is less than 75 mm Hg, the nurse should notify the primary health care provider. The patient remains supine until tolerance of postural hypotension develops. The nurse instructs the patient to change position slowly. Most individuals adjust to blood pressure changes within a few days.

To discontinue use of the drug, dosage should be reduced gradually over 3 to 5 days. After administering the drug, the nurse observes the patient closely. An oral antiarrhythmic drug may be prescribed to provide continued stability to the cardiac muscle.

ADMINISTERING VERAPAMIL This drug is used to manage supraventricular arrhythmias and rapid ventricular rates in atrial flutter or fibrillation. Continuous cardiac monitoring is necessary during IV administration. The nurse monitors the patient's blood pressure and cardiac rhythm carefully while the drug is being titrated (dosage increased or decreased based on criteria established by the

primary health care provider). The dosage may be increased more rapidly in a hospital setting. The nurse notifies the primary health care provider if bradycardia or hypotension occurs. When verapamil is administered orally, it may be given with food to minimize gastric upset.

MONITORING AND MANAGING PATIENT NEEDS

NAUSEA Most of the antiarrhythmic drugs cause nausea. The nurse advises the patient that eating small meals frequently may be better tolerated than three full meals daily. The nurse tells the patient to avoid lying flat for approximately 2 hours after meals. When the patient rests or reclines, the head should be at least 4 inches higher than the feet. The nurse administers the drug with meals to decrease GI effects.

URINARY RETENTION Because of the cholinergic blocking effects of disopyramide (see Chapter 30), urinary retention may occur. The nurse monitors the urinary output closely, especially during the initial period of therapy. If the patient's intake is sufficient but the output is low, the lower abdomen is palpated for bladder distention. If urinary retention occurs, the nurse notifies the primary health care provider because catheterization may be necessary.

IMPAIRED ORAL MUCOUS MEMBRANES Dryness of the mouth and throat caused by the cholinergic blocking action of disopyramide may occur. The nurse provides an adequate amount of fluid and instructs the patient to take frequent sips of water to relieve this problem. The nurse instructs the patient that sucking on hard candy (preferably sugarless) will help to keep the mouth moist.

RISK FOR INJURY Many of the antiarrhythmic drugs may cause dizziness and lightheadedness, especially during early therapy. This places the patient at risk for injury from falling. The nurse assists patients who are not on complete bed rest to ambulate until these symptoms subside.

Postural hypotension also may occur during the first few weeks of disopyramide therapy. The patient is advised to make position changes slowly. In some instances, the patient may require assistance in getting out of the bed or chair.

RISK FOR INFECTION Some antiarrhythmic drugs such as quinidine, procainamide, mexiletine, or verapamil may cause agranulocytosis. The nurse reports any signs of agranulocytosis such as fever, chills, sore throat, or unusual bleeding or bruising. A complete blood count is usually ordered every 2 to 3 weeks during the first

3 months of therapy. If a decrease in the blood levels of leukocytes or platelets occurs or the hematocrit falls, the nurse reports this to the primary health care provider immediately because the drug may be discontinued. Blood levels usually return to normal within 1 month after discontinuing the antiarrhythmic drug.

POTENTIAL COMPLICATION: PROARRHYTHMIC EFFECTS
Proarrhythmic effects may occur, such as ventricular tachycardia or ventricular fibrillation. It is often difficult to distinguish proarrhythmic effects from the patient's preexisting arrhythmia.

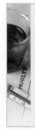

Nursing Alert

Antiarrhythmic drugs are capable of causing new arrhythmias, as well as exacerbating existing arrhythmias. The nurse must report any new arrhythmia or exacerbation of an existing arrhythmia to the primary health care provider immediately.

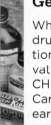

Gerontologic Alert

When older adults take the antiarrhythmic drugs, they are at greater risk for adverse reactions such as additional arrhythmias or aggravation of existing arrhythmias, hypotension, and CHF. A dosage reduction may be indicated. Careful monitoring by the nurse is necessary for early identification and management of adverse reactions. The nurse monitors the intake and output and reports any signs of CHF, such as increase in weight, decrease in urinary output, or shortness of breath.

POTENTIAL COMPLICATION: QUINIDINE TOXICITY The nurse monitors the patient for the most common adverse reactions associated with quinidine (nausea, vomiting, abdominal pain, diarrhea, or anorexia). **Cinchonism** is the term used to describe quinidine toxicity. Cinchonism occurs with high blood levels of quinidine (greater than 6 mcg/mL). The nurse must report any quinidine levels greater than 6 mcg/mL and the occurrence of any of the following signs or symptoms of cinchonism: ringing in the ears (tinnitus), hearing loss, headache, nausea, dizziness, vertigo, and lightheadedness. These symptoms may be experienced after a single dose.

EDUCATING THE PATIENT AND FAMILY

The nurse discusses with the patient and family the adverse drug effects that may occur. To ensure compliance

---

Patient and Family Teaching Checklist

Self-Monitoring Pulse Rate With Antiarrhythmic Therapy

The nurse:

☑ Explains the purpose of self-monitoring of pulse rate when receiving antiarrhythmic therapy.

☑ Instructs in importance of drug therapy and taking drug exactly as prescribed.

☑ Provides written instruction for monitoring pulse rate

☑ Encourages self-monitoring before each dose.

☑ Reviews acceptable pulse rate ranges for taking the drug, both verbally and in writing.

☑ Encourages recording of pulse rates in a log.

☑ Emphasizes need to notify primary health care provider should rate fall outside acceptable range or rhythm changes.

☑ Reassures that results of therapy will be monitored by periodic laboratory and diagnostic tests and follow-up visits with primary health care provider.

☑ Assists with arrangements for follow-up as necessary.

---

with the prescribed drug regimen, the nurse emphasizes the importance of taking these drugs exactly as prescribed. If necessary, the nurse may teach the patient or a family member how to take the pulse and report any changes in the pulse rate or rhythm to the primary health care provider (see Patient and Family Teaching Checklist: Self-Monitoring Pulse Rate With Antiarrhythmic Therapy).

The nurse emphasizes the following points when teaching the patient and the family:

• Take the drug at the prescribed intervals. Do not omit a dose or increase or decrease the dose unless advised to do so by the primary health care provider. Do not stop taking the drug unless advised to do so by the primary health care provider.

• Do not take any nonprescription drug unless the use of a specific drug is approved by the primary health care provider.

• Avoid drinking alcoholic beverages or smoking unless these have been approved by the primary health care provider.

- Follow the directions on the drug label, such as taking the drug with food.

- Do not chew tablets or capsules; instead, swallow them whole.

- Do not attempt to drive or perform hazardous tasks if lightheadedness or dizziness occur.

- Notify the primary health care provider as soon as possible if any adverse effects occur.

- To relieve dry mouth, take frequent sips of water, allow ice chips to dissolve in the mouth, or chew (sugar-free) gum.

- Remember that the tablet matrix of sustained-release tablets of procainamide is not absorbed by the body and may be found in the stool. This is normal.

- Keep all appointments with the primary health care provider, clinic, or laboratory because therapy will be closely monitored.

- If you have diabetes and are taking propranolol, adhere to the prescribed diet and check the blood glucose levels one to two times a day (or as recommended by the primary health care provider). Report elevated glucose levels to the primary health care provider as soon as possible because an adjustment in the dosage of insulin or oral hypoglycemic drugs may be necessary.

EVALUATION

- The therapeutic response is achieved and the arrhythmia is controlled.

- Adverse reactions are identified, reported to the primary health care provider, and managed successfully with appropriate nursing interventions:

  - The patient reports no nausea.

  - The patient reports no urinary retention.

  - Oral mucous membranes are intact and moist.

  - No symptoms of infection are experienced.

  - No evidence of injury is seen.

- The patient and family demonstrate an understanding of the drug regimen.

- The patient verbalizes the importance of continued follow-up care.

- The patient verbalizes the importance of complying with the prescribed treatment regimen.

- The patient complies with the prescribed drug regimen.

Critical Thinking Exercises

1. Mr. Parker is at an outpatient clinic for a follow-up visit. He has been taking quinidine for several months for a cardiac arrhythmia. Analyze what assessments you would make on Mr. Parker to determine the effectiveness of quinidine therapy. Discuss what questions you would ask to determine the presence of any adverse reactions.

2. Ms. Grady, aged 48 years, will be discharged in 2 days. The primary health care provider has prescribed propranolol to treat her arrhythmia. Develop a patient educational handout for Ms. Grady to take home, explaining the most important points for her to know when taking propranolol.

3. Mr. Summers has a ventricular arrhythmia and cardiac monitoring is ordered. The primary health care provider prescribes IV lidocaine. Discuss preadministration assessments you would perform for Mr. Summers. Analyze which adverse reactions would be most important to watch for during the ongoing assessment. Determine what reactions should be reported immediately.

Review Questions

1. Which of the following adverse reactions of lidocaine (Xylocaine) should be reported immediately to the primary health care provider?

   A. Sudden change in mental status

   B. Dry mouth

   C. Occipital headache

   D. Lightheadedness

2. Which of the following drugs, when given with disopyramide (Norpace), would possibly increase the serum disopyramide levels?

   A. verapamil (Calan)

   B. propranolol (Inderal)

   C. flecainide (Tambocor)

   D. quinidine (Quinidex)

3. Common adverse reactions of the antiarrhythmic drugs include _____.

   A. lightheadedness, hypotension, and weakness

   B. headache, hypertension, and lethargy

   C. weakness, lethargy, and hyperglycemia

   D. anorexia, gastrointestinal upset, and hypertension

4. When administering quinidine (Quinidex), the nurse reports a blood level greater than _____.

    A. 2 mcg/mL

    B. 3 mcg/mL

    C. 4 mcg/mL

    D. 6 mcg/mL

5. Which of the following statements would the nurse include in a teaching plan for the patient taking an antiarrhythmic drug on an outpatient basis?

    A. Take the drug without regard to meals.

    B. Limit fluid intake during the evening hours.

    C. Avoid drinking alcoholic beverages unless their consumption has been approved by the primary health care provider.

    D. Eat a diet high in potassium.

Medication Dosage Problems

1. The primary health care provider prescribes verapamil 80 mg orally. The drug is available in 40-mg tablets. The nurse prepares _____.

2. Disopyramide 200 mg orally is prescribed. The pharmacy sends disopyramide (Norpace) 100-mg tablets. The nurse administers _____.

To check your answers, see Appendix G.

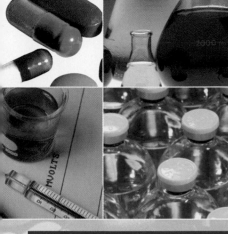

Chapter 40

Antianginal and Peripheral Vasodilating Drugs

Learning Objectives

On completion of this chapter, the student will:

- List the two types of antianginal drugs.

- Discuss the general actions, uses, adverse reactions, contraindications, precautions, and interactions of antianginal and peripheral vasodilating drugs.

- Discuss important preadministration and ongoing assessment activities the nurse should perform on the

patient taking an antianginal or peripheral vasodilating drug.

- List nursing diagnoses particular to a patient taking an antianginal or peripheral vasodilating drug.

- Discuss ways to promote an optimal response to therapy, how to manage common adverse reactions, and important points to keep in mind when educating patients about the use of antianginal and peripheral vasodilating drugs.

D iseases of the arteries can cause serious problems, namely, coronary artery disease, cerebral vascular disease, and peripheral vascular disease. Drug therapy for vascular diseases may include drugs that dilate blood vessels and thereby increase blood supply to an area.

Atherosclerosis is a disease characterized by deposits of fatty plaques on the inner wall of arteries. These deposits result in a narrowing of the **lumen** (inside diameter) of the artery and a decrease in blood supply to the area served by the artery.

This chapter discusses two different types of drugs whose primary purpose is to increase blood supply to an area by dilating blood vessels: the antianginal and peripheral vasodilating drugs. Vasodilating drugs relax the smooth muscle layer of arterial blood vessels, which results in **vasodilation**, an increase in the size of blood vessels, primarily small arteries and arterioles. Because peripheral, cerebral, or coronary artery disease usually results in decreased blood flow to an area, drugs that dilate narrowed arterial vessels will permit the vessels to carry more blood, resulting in an increase in blood flow to the affected area. Increasing the blood flow to an area may result in complete or partial relief of symptoms. Vasodilating drugs sometimes relieve the symptoms of vascular disease. In some cases, however, drug therapy provides only minimal and temporary relief. Many of the vasodilating drugs are also used to treat hypertension. Their use as antihypertensives is discussed in Chapter 41.

ANTIANGINAL DRUGS

Angina is a disorder characterized by atherosclerotic plaque formation in the coronary arteries, which causes decreased oxygen supply to the heart muscle and results in chest pain or pressure. Any activity that increases the workload of the heart, such as exercise or simply climbing stairs, can precipitate an angina attack.

Antianginal drugs relieve chest pain or pressure by dilating coronary arteries, increasing the blood supply to the myocardium.

The antianginal drugs include the nitrates and the calcium channel blockers. Chapter 28 and its Summary Drug Table: Adrenergic Blocking Drugs discuss the adrenergic blocking drugs that are also used to treat angina and other disorders.

Actions

Nitrates

The nitrates act by relaxing the smooth muscle layer of blood vessels, increasing the lumen of the artery or arteriole and increasing the amount of blood flowing through the vessels. An increased blood flow results in an increase in the oxygen supply to surrounding tissues.

Calcium Channel Blockers

Systemic and coronary arteries are influenced by movement of calcium across cell membranes of vascular smooth muscle. The contractions of cardiac and vascular smooth muscle depend on movement of extracellular calcium ions into these walls through specific ion channels.

Calcium channel blockers act by inhibiting the movement of calcium ions across cell membranes of cardiac and arterial muscle cells. This results in less calcium available for the transmission of nerve impulses (Fig. 40-1).

This drug action of the calcium channel blockers has several effects on the heart:

- Slowing the conduction velocity of the cardiac impulse
- Depressing myocardial contractility
- Dilating coronary arteries and arterioles, which in turn deliver more oxygen to cardiac muscle

Dilation of peripheral arteries reduces the workload of the heart. The end effect of these drugs is the same as that of the nitrates.

Uses

Nitrates

The nitrates are used to
- Relieve pain of acute anginal attacks
- Prevent (**prophylaxis**) angina attacks
- Treat chronic stable angina pectoris
- Control perioperative hypertension associated with surgical procedures (intravenous [IV] nitroglycerin)

See the Summary Drug Table: Antianginal Drugs for additional uses of the nitrates.

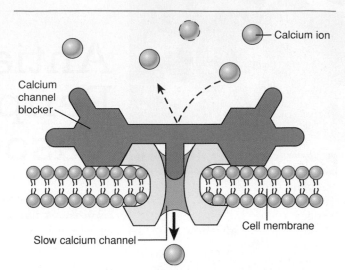

Figure 40.1 Calcium channel blockers increase the myocardial oxygen supply and slow the heart rate by blocking the slow calcium channel, which inhibits the influx of extracellular calcium ions across myocardial and vascular smooth muscle cell membranes. They achieve this blockade without changing the calcium level. The calcium blockade causes the coronary arteries (and, to a lesser extent, the peripheral arteries and arterioles) to dilate, decreasing afterload and increasing myocardial oxygen supply. The blockade also slows sinoatrial and atrioventricular node conduction, slightly reducing the heart rate. (Adapted from *Pharmacology: A 2-in-1 Reference for Nurses*. [2005]. p. 185. Ambler, PA: Lippincott Williams & Wilkins.)

Calcium Channel Blockers

Calcium channel blockers are primarily used to treat

- Anginal pain associated with certain forms of angina, such as vasospastic (Prinzmetal's or variant) angina
- Chronic stable angina
- Hypertension (see Chapter 41)

Calcium channel blockers used as antianginals are listed in the Summary Drug Table: Antianginal Drugs. Some calcium channel blocking drugs have additional uses. For example, verapamil affects the conduction system of the heart and is used to treat cardiac arrhythmias.

Adverse Reactions

Nitrates

Adverse reactions associated with the nitrates include
- Central nervous system (CNS) reactions, such as headache (may be severe and persistent), dizziness, weakness, and restlessness

SUMMARY DRUG TABLE   ANTIANGINAL DRUGS

GENERIC NAME	TRADE NAME	USES	ADVERSE REACTIONS	DOSAGE RANGES
Nitrates				
amyl nitrite *am'-il-nye'-trite*	Amyl Nitrate Vaporole	Relief of angina pectoris	Headache, hypotension, dizziness, weakness, flushing, restlessness, rash	Crush capsule and wave under nose, taking 1–6 inhalations; may repeat in 3–5 min
isosorbide mononitrate, oral *eye-soe-sor'-bide*	ISMO, Imdur, Monoket	Prevention of angina pectoris	Same as amyl nitrite	20 mg BID orally with the 2 doses given 7 h apart Extended-release tablets: 30–60 mg QD orally may be increased to 240 mg/d orally
isosorbide dinitrate, sublingual and chewable	Isordil, Sorbitrate	Treatment and prevention of angina pectoris	Same as amyl nitrite	Treatment: 2.5–5 mg sublingually Prevention: 5–10 mg sublingually, 5 mg chewable
isosorbide dinitrate, oral	Dilatrate SR, Isordil Tembids, Isordil Titradose, Sorbitrate	Treatment and prevention of angina pectoris	Same as amyl nitrite	Initial dose 5–20 mg orally; maintenance dose 10–40 mg BID, TID Sustained-release: 40 mg/d Daily maximum dose, 160 mg/d orally
nitroglycerin, intravenous *nye-troe-gli'-ser-in*	Nitro-Bid IV, Tridil	Control of blood pressure in perioperative hypertension and in immediate postoperative period, congestive heart failure associated with acute myocardial infarction, angina pectoris unresponsive to recommended doses of nitrates or beta blockers	Same as amyl nitrite	Initially 5 mcg/min by IV infusion pump, may increase to 20 mcg/min
nitroglycerin, sublingual	NitroQuick, Nitrostat	Acute relief of an attack or prophylaxis of angina pectoris	Same as amyl nitrite	I tablet under tongue or in buccal pouch at first sign of an acute anginal attack; may repeat every 5 min until relief or 3 tablets have been taken
nitroglycerin, sustained release	Nitroglyn, Nitrong, Nitro-Time	Prevention of angina pectoris	Same as amyl nitrite	2.5–2.6 mg TID, QID orally, up to 26 mg QID
nitroglycerin, translingual	Nitrolingual	Acute relief of an attack or prophylaxis of angina pectoris	Same as amyl nitrite	1–2 metered-dose sprays onto or under the tongue; maximum of 3 metered doses in 15 min
nitroglycerin, transmucosal	Nitrogard	Prevention of angina pectoris	Same as amyl nitrite	1 tablet q3–5h between lip and gum or between cheek and gum

Antianginal and Peripheral Vasodilating Drugs

SUMMARY DRUG TABLE *(continued)*

GENERIC NAME	TRADE NAME	USES	ADVERSE REACTIONS	DOSAGE RANGES
nitroglycerin, topical	Nitro-Bid, Nitrol	Prevention and treatment of angina pectoris	Same as amyl nitrite	1–5 inches q4–8h
nitroglycerin transdermal systems	Deponit, Minitran, Nitro–Dur, Transderm-Nitrol	Prevention of angina pectoris	Same as amyl nitrite	One system daily, 0.2–0.8 mg/h
Calcium Channel Blockers				
amlodipine *am-low'-dih-peen*	Norvasc	Hypertension, chronic stable angina, vasospastic angina (Prinzmetal's angina)	Dizziness, light-headedness, headache, nervousness, nausea, constipation, peripheral edema, asthenia bradycardia, atrioventricular block, arrhythmias, flushing, rash	Individualize dosage; 5–10 mg/d orally
bepridil HCl *be'-pri-dil*	Vascor	Chronic stable angina	Same as amlodipine	Individualize dosage; 200–400 mg/d orally
diltiazem HCl hydrochloride *dil-tye'-a-zem*	Cardizem, Cardizem CD, Dilacor XR	Oral: Angina pectoris, chronic stable angina Extended-release forms: essential hypertension Parenteral: atrial fibrillation or flutter, paroxysmal supraventricular tachycardia	Same as amlodipine	Tablets: 30–360 mg/d in divided doses Sustained release: Cardizen SR 120–360 mg/d; Cardizem CD angina 120–240 mg QD Dilacor XR, 180–480 mg QD orally Parenteral: 0.25 mg/kg IV bolus; 5–15 mg/h IV
felodipine *fell-oh'-di-peen*	Plendil	Essential hypertension	Same as amlodipine	2.5–10 mg/d orally
nicardipine HCl *nye-kar'-de-peen*	Cardene, Cardene IV, Cardene SR	Chronic stable angina, hypertension, short-term treatment of hypertension when oral therapy is not desirable	Same as amlodipine	Angina: individulize dosage; immediate-release only, 20–40 mg TID orally
nifedipine *nye-fed'-i-peen*	Adalat, Procardia, Procardia XL	Vasospastic angina (Prinzmetal's variant angina), chronic stable angina, hypertension (sustained-release only)	Same as amlodipine	10–20 mg TID orally; may increase to 120 mg/d Sustained-release: 30–60 mg/d orally; may increase to 120 mg/d
nisoldipine *nye- sole'-di-peen*	Sular	Essential hypertension	Same as amlodipine	20–40 mg/d orally
verapamil HCl *ver-ap'-a-mil*	Calan, Calan SR, Isoptin, Isoptin SR, Verelan	Angina pectoris, arrhythmias, essential hypertension, supraven-tricular tachycardia (parenteral only), atrial flutter or fibrillation (parenteral only)	Same as amlodipine	Individualize dosage; do not exceed 480 mg/d orally in divided doses Sustained-release: 120–180 mg/d orally; maximum dose, 480 mg Extended-release: 120–180 mg/d orally, maximum dose, 480 mg/d Parenteral: 5–10 mg IV over 2 min

- Other body system reactions, such as hypotension, flushing (caused by dilation of small capillaries near the surface of the skin), and rash

The nitrates are available in various forms (e.g., sublingual, transmucosal, translingual spray, and inhalation). Some adverse reactions are a result of the method of administration. For example, sublingual nitroglycerin may cause a local burning or tingling in the oral cavity. However, the patient must be aware that an absence of this effect does not indicate a decrease in the drug's potency. Contact dermatitis may occur from use of the transdermal delivery system.

In many instances, the adverse reactions associated with the nitrates lessen and often disappear with prolonged use of the drug. However, for some patients, these adverse reactions become severe, and the primary health care provider may lower the dose until symptoms subside. The dose may then be slowly increased if the lower dosage does not provide relief from the symptoms of angina. See the Summary Drug Table: Antianginal Drugs for more information.

Calcium Channel Blockers

Adverse reactions associated with the calcium channel blockers include

- CNS reactions such as dizziness, lightheadedness, headache, nervousness, asthenia (loss of muscular strength), and fatigue
- Gastrointestinal (GI) reactions such as nausea, constipation, and abdominal discomfort
- Cardiovascular reactions such as peripheral edema, hypotension, arrhythmias, and bradycardia
- Other body system reactions, including rash, flushing, nasal congestion, and cough

Adverse reactions to the calcium channel blocking drugs usually are not serious and rarely require discontinuation of the drug therapy.

Contraindications and Precautions

Nitrates

The nitrates are contraindicated in patients with known hypersensitivity to the drugs, severe anemia, closed-angle glaucoma, postural hypertension, early myocardial infarction (sublingual form), head trauma, cerebral hemorrhage (may increase intracranial hemorrhage), allergy to adhesive (transdermal system), or constrictive pericarditis. Amyl nitrite is contraindicated during pregnancy (category X).

The nitrates are used cautiously in patients with

- Severe hepatic or renal disease
- Severe head trauma
- Hypothyroidism

These drugs are used cautiously during pregnancy and lactation (pregnancy category C, except for amyl nitrite).

Calcium Channel Blockers

Calcium channel blockers are contraindicated in patients who are hypersensitive to the drugs and those with sick sinus syndrome, second- or third-degree atrioventricular (AV) block (except with a functioning pacemaker), hypotension (systolic pressure less than 90 mm Hg), ventricular dysfunction, or cardiogenic shock.

The calcium channel blockers are used cautiously in patients with

- Heart failure (HF)
- Renal impairment
- Hepatic impairment

The calcium channel blockers are used cautiously during pregnancy (category C) and lactation.

Interactions

Nitrates

The following interactions may occur when the nitrates are used with another agent:

Interacting Drug	Common Use	Effect of Interaction
alcohol	Recreational drug	Severe hypotension and cardiovascular collapse may occur
aspirin	Pain reliever	Increased nitrate plasma concentrations and action may occur
calcium channel blockers	Treatment of angina	Increased symptomatic orthostatic hypotension
dihydroergotamine	Migraine headache treatment	Increased risk of hypertension and decreased antianginal effect
heparin	Anticoagulant	Decreased effect of heparin

Calcium Channel Blockers

The following interactions may occur when the calcium channel blockers are used with another agent:

Interacting Drug	Common Use	Effect of Interaction
cimetidine or ranitidine	GI disorders	Increased effects of calcium channel blockers
theophylline	Control of asthma and chronic obstructive pulmonary disease	Increased pharmacologic and toxic effects of theophylline
St. John's wort	Herb used to treat depression	Reduced serum concentrations of calcium channel blocker (e.g., nifedipine)
digoxin	Heart failure	Increased risk for digitalis toxicity
rifampin	Antitubercular agent	Decreased effect of calcium channel blocker

NURSING PROCESS

The Patient Receiving an Antianginal Drug

ASSESSMENT

PREADMINISTRATION ASSESSMENT

Before administering an antianginal drug, the nurse obtains and records a thorough description of the patient's anginal pain as well as a history of allergy to the nitrates or calcium channel blockers and of other disease processes that would contraindicate administration of the drug (Display 40-1). The nurse also assesses the physical appearance of the patient (e.g., skin color, lesions), auscultates the lungs for adventitious sounds, and obtains a baseline electrocardiogram and vital signs. Any problem with orthostatic hypotension is noted.

ONGOING ASSESSMENT

As a part of the ongoing assessment, the nurse monitors the patient for the frequency and severity of any episodes of anginal pain. With treatment, episodes of angina should be eliminated or decrease in frequency and severity. The nurse should report to the primary health care provider any chest pain that does not respond to three doses of nitroglycerin given every 5 minutes for 15 minutes.

Display 40.1 Information Regarding Anginal Pain

History

- Description of the type of pain (e.g., sharp, dull, squeezing)
- Whether the pain radiates and to where
- Events that appear to cause anginal pain (e.g., exercise, emotion)
- Events that appear to relieve the pain (e.g., resting)

Physical Assessment

- Blood pressure
- Apical and radial pulse rates
- Respiratory rate (after the patient has been at rest for about 10 minutes)
- Weight*
- Inspection of the extremities for edema*
- Auscultation of the lungs*

*These assessments may be appropriate, depending on the type of heart disease.

The nurse takes the patient's vital signs before the drug is administered and frequently during administration of the antianginals or calcium channel blockers. If the patient's heart rate falls below 50 beats per minute or the systolic blood pressure drops below 90 mm Hg, the drug is withheld and the primary health care provider notified. A dosage adjustment may be necessary.

The nurse should assess patients receiving the calcium channel blockers for signs of CHF: dyspnea, weight gain, peripheral edema, abnormal lung sounds (crackles/rales), and jugular vein distention. Any symptoms of CHF are reported immediately to the primary health care provider.

The patient is monitored carefully; vital signs are taken frequently, and the patient is placed on a cardiac monitor while the drug is being titrated to a therapeutic dose. The dosage may be increased more rapidly in hospitalized patients under close supervision.

NURSING DIAGNOSES

Drug-specific nursing diagnoses are highlighted in the Nursing Diagnoses Checklist. Other nursing diagnoses applicable to these drugs are discussed in depth in Chapter 4.

Nursing Diagnoses Checklist

✔ **Risk for Injury** related to hypotension, dizziness, lightheadedness secondary to drug actions
✔ **Pain** related to narrowing of peripheral arteries, decreased blood supply to the extremities

PLANNING

The expected outcomes for the patient depend on the specific reason for administration of an antianginal drug, but may include an optimal response to drug therapy, meeting of patient needs related to the management of common adverse drug reactions, and an understanding of the postdischarge drug regimen.

IMPLEMENTATION

PROMOTING AN OPTIMAL RESPONSE TO THERAPY

NITRATES The nitrates may be administered by the **sublingual** (under the tongue), **buccal** (between the cheek and gum), oral, **IV**, or transdermal route. Nitroglycerin may be administered by the sublingual, buccal, topical, transdermal, oral, or **IV** route. If the buccal form of nitroglycerin has been prescribed, the nurse instructs the patient to place the buccal tablet between the cheek and gum or between the upper lip and gum above the incisors and allow it to dissolve. The nurse shows the patient how and where to place the tablet in the mouth. Absorption of sublingual and buccal forms depends on salivary secretion. Dry mouth decreases absorption.

Nitroglycerin may also be administered by a metered spray canister that is used to abort an acute anginal attack. The spray is directed from the canister onto or under the tongue. Each dose is metered so that when the canister top is depressed, the same dose is delivered each time. The nurse instructs the patient not to inhale the spray. For some individuals, this is more convenient than placing small tablets under the tongue.

Nursing Alert

The dose of sublingual nitroglycerin may be repeated every 5 minutes until pain is relieved or until the patient has received three doses in a 15-minute period. One to two sprays of translingual nitroglycerin may be used to relieve angina, but no more than three metered doses are recommended within a 15-minute period.

The nurse instructs the patient to call the nurse if the pain is not relieved after three doses. The primary health care provider is notified if the patient frequently has anginal pain, if the pain worsens, or if the pain is not relieved after three doses within a 15-minute period because a change in the dosage of the drug or other treatment may be necessary.

Administering Topical Nitroglycerin The dose of **topical** (ointment) nitroglycerin is measured in inches or millimeters (mm); 1 inch (25 mm) of ointment equals about 15 mg nitroglycerin. Before the drug is measured and applied and after the ambulatory patient has rested for 10 to 15 minutes,

the nurse obtains the patient's blood pressure and pulse rate and compares the results with the baseline and previous vital signs. If the blood pressure is appreciably lower or the pulse rate higher than the resting baseline, the nurse contacts the primary health care provider before applying the drug. Applicator paper is supplied with the drug; one paper is used for each application. While holding the paper, the nurse expresses the prescribed amount of ointment from the tube onto the paper. The nurse must remove the paper from the previous application and cleanse the area as needed. The nurse uses the applicator or dose-measured paper to gently spread a thin uniform layer over at least a 2-1/4 by 3-1/2-inch area. The ointment is usually applied to the chest or back. Application sites are rotated to prevent inflammation of the skin. Areas that may be used for application include the chest (front and back), abdomen, and upper arms and legs.

Nursing Alert

The nurse must not rub the nitroglycerin ointment into the patient's skin because this will immediately deliver a large amount of the drug through the skin. Exercise care in applying topical nitroglycerin and do not allow the ointment to come in contact with the fingers or hands while measuring or applying the ointment because the drug will be absorbed through the skin of the person applying the drug. The nurse should wear disposable plastic gloves if drug contact is a problem. After application of the ointment, the nurse may secure the paper with nonallergenic tape.

Administering Transdermal Nitroglycerin For most people, nitroglycerin transdermal systems are more convenient and easier to use because the drug is absorbed through the skin. A **transdermal system** has the drug impregnated in a pad. The primary health care provider may prescribe the pad to be applied to the skin once a day for 10 to 12 hours. Tolerance to the vascular and antianginal effects of the nitrates may develop, particularly in patients taking higher dosages, those who are prescribed longer-acting products, or those who are on more frequent dosing schedules. Patients using the transdermal nitroglycerin patches are particularly prone to tolerance because the nitroglycerin is released at a constant rate, and steady plasma concentrations are maintained. Applying the patch in the morning and leaving it in place for 10 to 12 hours, followed by leaving the patch off for 10 to 12 hours, typically yields better results and delays tolerance to the drug.

When applying the transdermal system, the nurse inspects the skin site to be sure it is dry, free of hair, and not subject to excessive rubbing or movement. If needed, the nurse shaves the application site. The nurse applies the transdermal system at the same time each day and rotates the placement sites. Optimal sites include the chest, abdomen, and thighs. The system is not applied to distal extremities. The best time to apply the transdermal system is after morning care (bed bath, shower, tub bath) because it is important that the skin be thoroughly dry before applying the system. When removing the pad, the nurse cleanses the area as needed. To avoid errors in applying and removing the patch, the person applying the patch can use a fiber-tipped pen to write his or her name (or initials), date, and time of application on the top side of the patch. Patches should be removed before cardioversion or defibrillation to prevent patient burns.

Administering Oral Nitroglycerin Nitroglycerin is also available as oral tablets that are swallowed. The nurse gives this form of nitroglycerin to the patient whose stomach is empty, unless the primary health care provider orders otherwise. If nausea occurs after administration, the nurse notifies the primary health care provider. Taking the tablet or capsule with food may be ordered to relieve nausea. The sustained-released preparation may not be crushed or chewed.

Because of the risk of tolerance to oral nitrates developing, the primary care provider may prescribe the short-acting preparations two to three times daily, with the last dose no later than 7 PM, and the sustained-release preparations once daily or twice daily at 8 AM and 2 PM.

Administering IV Nitroglycerin The nurse administers IV nitroglycerin diluted in normal saline solution or 5% dextrose in water (D_5W) by continuous infusion using an infusion pump to ensure an accurate rate. The nurse administers the drug by using the glass IV bottles and administration sets provided by the manufacturer. The nurse regulates the dosage according to the patient's response and the primary health care provider's instructions.

CALCIUM CHANNEL BLOCKERS With a few exceptions, the calcium channel blockers may be taken without regard to meals. If GI upset occurs, the drug may be taken with meals. Verapamil and bepridil frequently cause gastric upset, and the nurse should routinely give them with meals. Verapamil tablets may be opened and sprinkled on foods or mixed in liquids. Sometimes the tablet coverings of verapamil are expelled in the stool. This causes no change in the effect of the drug and need not cause the patient concern.

For patients who have difficulty swallowing diltiazem (except Dilacor XR), tablets can be crushed and mixed with food or liquids. However, the patient should swallow the sustained-released tablets whole and not chew or divide them.

MONITORING AND MANAGING PATIENT NEEDS

The nurse must observe carefully patients receiving these drugs for adverse reactions. Hypotension may be accompanied by paradoxical bradycardia and increased angina pectoris. Adverse reactions such as headache, flushing, and postural hypotension that are seen with the administration of the antianginal drugs often become less severe or even disappear after a period of time.

RISK FOR INJURY The nurse assists patients having episodes of postural hypotension with all ambulatory activities. The nurse instructs those with episodes of postural hypotension to take the drug in a sitting or supine position and to remain in that position until symptoms disappear. The nurse monitors the blood pressure frequently in the patient with dizziness or lightheadedness. The patient may need help during ambulation if dizziness occurs.

> ### Gerontologic Alert
>
> The older adult may experience a greater hypotensive effect after taking the antianginal drugs than younger adults. The nurse must monitor the older adult closely during dosage adjustments. Blood pressure and ability to ambulate should be monitored closely.

PAIN The nurse must evaluate the patient's response to therapy by questioning the patient about the anginal pain. In some patients, the pain may be entirely relieved, whereas in others it may be less intense or less frequent or may occur only with prolonged exercise. The nurse records all information in the patient's chart because this helps the primary health care provider plan future therapy, as well as make dosage adjustments if required.

> ### Nursing Alert
>
> If the administration of sublingual or transmucosal nitrate fails to abort an anginal attack, the nurse must immediately notify the primary health care provider because additional therapy or tests may be necessary. Also, if an antianginal drug is used to prevent angina but the angina continues to occur, the nurse immediately notifies the primary health care provider. If anginal attacks occur while the patient is receiving a calcium channel blocking drug, the nurse informs the primary health care provider of this problem because a different approach to therapy may be necessary.

EDUCATING THE PATIENT AND FAMILY

The patient and family must have a thorough understanding of the treatment of chest pain with an antianginal drug. These drugs are used either to prevent angina from occurring or to relieve the pain of angina. The nurse explains the therapeutic regimen (dose, time of day the drug is taken, how often to take the drug, how to take or apply the drug) to the patient. The nurse adapts a teaching plan to the type of prescribed antianginal drug. The nurse should include the following general areas, as well as those points relevant to specific routes of administration of the drug, in a teaching plan:

- Avoid the use of alcohol unless use has been permitted by the primary health care provider.

- Notify the primary health care provider if the drug does not relieve pain or if pain becomes more intense despite use of this drug.

- Follow the recommendations of the primary health care provider regarding frequency of use.

- Take oral capsules or tablets (except sublingual) on an empty stomach unless the primary health care provider directs otherwise.

- Keep an adequate supply of the drug on hand for events, such as vacations, bad weather conditions, and holidays.

- Keep a record of the frequency of acute anginal attacks (date, time of the attack, drug, and dose used to relieve the acute pain), and bring this record to each primary health care provider or clinic visit.

For more teaching points related specifically to administration routes of nitrates and calcium channel blockers, see the Patient and Family Teaching Checklist: Directions for Administering Nitrates and Calcium Channel Blockers.

EVALUATION

- The therapeutic effect is achieved and pain is relieved.
- Adverse reactions are identified, reported to the primary health care provider, and managed successfully through nursing interventions.
- The patient verbalizes an understanding of the treatment modalities.
- The patient and family demonstrate an understanding of the drug regimen.

PERIPHERAL VASODILATING DRUGS

In contrast to the antianginal drugs, which are used primarily for angina, the peripheral vasodilating drugs are given for disorders that affect blood vessels of the extremities. Unfortunately, although these drugs increase blood flow to nonischemic areas (areas with adequate blood flow), there is no conclusive evidence that blood flow is increased in ischemic areas (areas that lack adequate blood flow) that are in critical need of improved perfusion. Because the effectiveness of the peripheral vasodilating drugs is unproved, most are labeled as "possibly effective" in treating peripheral vascular disorders. These drugs are not as widely used today as they were in the past. Many of the peripheral vasodilating drugs are used for hypertension and are discussed in Chapter 41.

Actions

Peripheral vasodilating drugs act on the smooth muscle layers of peripheral blood vessels, primarily by blocking alpha-adrenergic nerves and stimulating beta-adrenergic nerves. They also inhibit platelet aggregation and dilate vascular beds, particularly in the femoral area; cilostazol (Pletal) is an example of a drug that does this. For a review of the effects of stimulation and blocking (or blockade) on adrenergic nerve fibers, see Chapters 27 and 28.

Uses

Peripheral vasodilating drugs are used for treating
- Peripheral vascular diseases, such as arteriosclerosis obliterans, Raynaud's phenomenon, and spastic peripheral vascular disorders
- Symptoms associated with cerebral vascular insufficiency
- Circulatory disturbances of the inner ear

Other uses of individual peripheral vasodilating drugs are given in the Summary Drug Table: Peripheral Vasodilators and Miscellaneous Vasodilating Drugs.

Intermittent claudication is a group of symptoms characterized by pain in the calf muscle of one or both legs, caused by walking and relieved by rest. It is a manifestation of peripheral vascular disease, in which atherosclerotic lesions develop in the femoral artery, diminishing blood supply to the lower leg. Cilostazol, a phosphodiesterase II inhibitor, is used to treat intermittent claudication. Cilostazol reduces the symptoms of intermittent claudication associated with peripheral vascular disease. This drug increases the walking distance in those with intermittent claudication. This drug is listed under Miscellaneous Drugs in the Summary Drug Table: Peripheral Vasodilators and Miscellaneous Vasodilating Drugs.

Patient and Family Teaching Checklist
Directions for Administering Nitrates and Calcium Channel Blockers

NITRATES

☑ Explain that headache is a common adverse reaction but should decrease with continued therapy. If headache persists or becomes severe, notify the primary health care provider because a change in dosage may be needed. In patients who get headaches, the headaches may be a marker of the drug's effectiveness. Patients should not try to avoid headaches by altering the treatment schedule because loss of headache may be associated with simultaneous loss of drug effectiveness. Aspirin or acetaminophen may be used for headache relief.

☑ Advise the patient not to change from one brand of nitrates to another without consulting the pharmacist or primary care provider. Products manufactured by different companies may not be equally effective.

Oral Nitrates

☑ Advise patients taking nitroglycerin for an acute attack of angina to sit or lie down. To relieve severe light-headedness or dizziness, lie down, elevate the extremities, move the extremities, and breathe deeply.

☑ Store capsules and tablets in their original containers because nitroglycerin must be kept in a dark container and protected from exposure to light. Never mix this drug with any other drug in a container. Nitroglycerin will lose its potency if stored in containers made of plastic or if mixed with other drugs.

☑ Always replace the cover or cap of the container as soon as the oral drug or ointment is removed from the container or tube. Replace caps or covers tightly because the drug deteriorates on contact with air.

☑ Seek prompt medical attention if chest pain persists, changes character, increases in severity, or is not relieved by following the recommended dosing regimen.

Sublingual or Buccal Nitrates

☑ Do not handle the tablets labeled as sublingual any more than necessary.

☑ Check the expiration date on the container of sublingual tablets. If the expiration date has passed, do not use the tablets. Instead, purchase a new supply.

☑ Do not swallow or chew sublingual or transmucosal tablets; allow them to dissolve slowly. The tablet may cause a burning or tingling in the oral cavity. Absence of this effect does not indicate a decrease in potency. Older adults are less likely to report a burning or tingling sensation on administration.

Translingual or Transmucosal Nitrates

☑ The directions for use of translingual nitroglycerin are supplied with the product. Follow the instructions regarding using and cleaning the canister.

☑ This drug may be used prophylactically 5 to 10 minutes before engaging in activities that precipitate an anginal attack.

☑ At the onset of an anginal attack, spray 1 to 2 metered doses onto or under the tongue. Do not exceed 3 metered doses within 15 minutes.

☑ When using the transmucosal form, insert the tablet between the lip and gum above the incisors or between the cheek and gum.

Topical Ointment or Transdermal System

☑ Instructions for application of the topical ointment or transdermal system are available with the product. Read these instructions carefully.

☑ Apply the topical ointment or topical transdermal system at approximately the same time each day.

☑ Be sure the area is clean and thoroughly dry before applying the topical ointment or transdermal system, and rotate the application sites. Apply the transdermal system to the chest (front and back), abdomen, and upper or lower arms and legs. Firmly press the patch to ensure contact with the skin. If the transdermal system comes off or becomes loose, apply a new system. Apply the topical ointment to the front or the back of the chest. If applying to the back, another person should apply the ointment.

☑ When using the topical ointment form or transdermal system, cleanse old application sites with soap and warm water as soon as the ointment or transdermal system is removed.

☑ To use the topical ointment, apply a thin layer on the skin using the paper applicator (the patient or family member may need instructions regarding this technique). Avoid finger contact with the ointment.

☑ Wash hands before and after applying the ointment.

CALCIUM CHANNEL BLOCKERS

☑ Do not chew or divide sustained-released tablets. Swallow them whole.

Patient and Family Teaching Checklist (continued)

✔ Notify the primary health care provider if any of the following occurs: increased severity of chest pain or discomfort, irregular heartbeat, palpitations, nausea, shortness of breath, swelling of the hands or feet, or severe and prolonged episodes of light-headedness and dizziness.

✔ If the primary health care provider prescribes one of these drugs plus a nitrate, take both

drugs exactly as directed to obtain the best results of the combined drug therapy.

✔ Make position changes slowly to minimize hypotensive effects.

✔ Because these drugs can cause dizziness or drowsiness, do not drive or engage in hazardous activities until response to the drug is known.

Adverse Reactions

Central Nervous System Reactions

- Hypotension
- Physiologic increase in the pulse rate (tachycardia)
- Headache and excessive sedation

Other

- Nausea, abdominal distress
- Flushing of the skin, which can range from mild to moderately severe, rash, and sweating

Adverse reactions associated with cilostazol (Pletal) include CNS reactions, such as headache and dizziness, as

well as cardiac reactions such as palpitations, hypotension, and cardiac arrhythmias. Other body system reactions include nausea, diarrhea, flatulence, and pharyngitis.

Contraindications, Precautions, and Interactions

The peripheral vasodilating drugs are contraindicated in patients with known hypersensitivity to the drugs, women in the immediate postpartum period (isoxsuprine causes uterine relaxation), and in patients with arterial bleeding. Cilostazol is contraindicated in patients with CHF. These drugs are used cautiously in patients with bleeding tendencies, severe cerebrovascular or cardiovascular disease,

SUMMARY DRUG TABLE PERIPHERAL VASODILATORS AND MISCELLANEOUS VASODILATING DRUGS

GENERIC NAME	TRADE NAME	USES	ADVERSE REACTIONS	DOSAGE RANGES
Peripheral Vasodilators				
isoxsuprine HCl *eye-soks-u'-preen*	Vasodilan, Voxsuprine	Peripheral vascular disease, Raynaud's disease	Hypotension, tachycardia, chest pain, nausea, vomiting, abdominal distress, palpitations, rash	10–20 mg orally TID, QID
papaverine HCl *pa-pav'-er-reen*	Pavabid Plateau, Pavagen	Relief of cerebral and peripheral ischemia associated with arterial spasm, myocardial ischemia complicated by arrhythmias	Nausea, abdominal distress, anorexia, vertigo, sweating, flushing, rash, excessive sedation, headache	150–300 mg orally q12h
Miscellaneous Drugs				
cilostazol *sill-oh-stay'-zole*	Pletal	Reduction of symptoms of intermittent claudication	Headache, dizziness, diarrhea, nausea, flatulence, dyspepsia, rhinitis, abdominal pain, tachycardia	100 mg orally BID

after a myocardial infarction, and during pregnancy (category C). There are no significant drug–drug interactions.

Herbal Alert

L-Arginine has been beneficial in several disorders, such as heart failure, peripheral artery disease, hypertension, hyperlipidemia, and type 2 diabetes. The herb appears to increase nitric oxide concentrations. Abnormalities of the vascular endothelial cells may cause vasoconstriction, inflammation, and thrombolytic activity. These abnormalities are partially attributable to degradation of nitric oxide. L-Arginine's ability to increase nitric oxide is the basis for its effectiveness in improving some vascular disease states. In a study conducted by Lerman and colleagues (1998, *Circulation, 97,* 2123–2128), oral doses of 9 to 30 g/d were well tolerated. No adverse reactions were reported in those taking 9 g/d. Higher doses may cause nausea and mild diarrhea. L-Arginine may exacerbate sickle cell crisis and should be used with caution in those with sickle cell anemia. As with all herbal therapy, the primary health care provider should be notified of all herbs being taken.

NURSING PROCESS

The Patient Receiving a Peripheral Vasodilating Drug

ASSESSMENT

PREADMINISTRATION ASSESSMENT

Before administering the first dose of a peripheral vasodilating drug, the nurse obtains a thorough history of the patient's symptoms. The physical assessment is based on the patient's diagnosis. If cerebral vascular disease is present, the nurse evaluates the patient's mental status. If the diagnosis is a peripheral vascular disorder, the nurse examines the involved areas for general appearance, such as the color of the skin and evidence of drying or scaling. The nurse notes the skin temperature (warm, cool, cold) of the involved area and compares it with other areas of the body and with the extremities not affected by peripheral vascular disease. The nurse then records these findings in the patient's record. The nurse palpates the peripheral pulses in the affected extremities and records the strength and amplitude of each peripheral pulse. Vital signs are obtained and recorded. For patients taking cilostazol for intermittent claudication, a "baseline walking distance" is assessed to monitor drug effectiveness.

ONGOING ASSESSMENT

Therapeutic results obtained from the administration of a peripheral vasodilating drug may not occur immediately.

In some instances, results are minimal. The nurse assesses involved extremities daily for changes in color and temperature and records the patient's comments regarding relief from pain or discomfort. The nurse should monitor the blood pressure and pulse one to two times daily because these drugs may cause a decrease in blood pressure. The anticipated result of therapy for cerebral vascular disease is an improvement in the patient's mental status. When the drug is taken for intermittent claudication, the nurse assesses the patient to determine capacity for increased walking distance without leg pain.

NURSING DIAGNOSES

A common nursing diagnosis associated with peripheral vasodilator therapy is Risk for Injury related to hypotension, dizziness, and lightheadedness secondary to drug actions. Other nursing diagnoses applicable to these drugs are discussed in depth in Chapter 4.

PLANNING

The expected outcomes for the patient may include relief of pain, management of common adverse drug reactions, absence of injury, and an understanding of and compliance with the prescribed therapeutic regimen.

IMPLEMENTATION

PROMOTING AN OPTIMAL RESPONSE TO THERAPY

Peripheral vasodilators are often prescribed for outpatient use. Positive results of therapy for a peripheral vascular disorder may include a decrease in pain, discomfort, and cramping; increased warmth in the extremities; and an increase in amplitude of the peripheral pulses. In many cases, patients taking these drugs for relief of symptoms associated with peripheral vascular disorders become discouraged about the lack of effectiveness of drug therapy. The nurse encourages the patient to continue with the prescribed drug regimen and to follow the primary health care provider's recommendations regarding additional methods of treating the disorder.

The patient is reminded that sometimes signs of improvement may be rapid, but improvement usually occurs slowly over the course of many weeks. The nurse examines the patient's affected areas at the time of each visit to a primary health care provider's office or outpatient clinic and records the findings in the patient's record. In the case of cilostazol, the nurse advises the patient to take this drug at least 30 minutes before or 2 hours after meals. The drug is not administered with grapefruit juice because the juice may increase blood concentrations of the drug.

MONITORING AND MANAGING PATIENT NEEDS

If adverse reactions occur, the nurse should notify the primary health care provider. It is important to note the severity of the adverse reactions on the patient's record. In some instances, adverse reactions are mild and the patient may need to tolerate them.

RISK FOR INJURY Some patients may experience dizziness and lightheadedness, especially during early therapy. If these effects occur, the nurse assists the patient with all ambulatory activities and instructs the patient to ask for help when getting out of bed or ambulating. Encouraging the patient to dangle the legs over the side of the bed for a few minutes before getting up in the morning or after lying down will decrease the feelings of lightheadedness when arising.

EDUCATING THE PATIENT AND FAMILY

To ensure compliance with the drug regimen, the nurse tells the patient and family that improvement will most likely be gradual, although some improvement may be noted in a few days. The nurse encourages the patient to continue with drug therapy and to follow the primary health care provider's recommendations regarding care of the affected extremities, even though improvement may be slow. The nurse includes the following in a teaching plan:

- If nausea, vomiting, or diarrhea occurs, contact the primary health care provider. These drugs may also cause flushing, sweating, headache, tiredness, jaundice, skin rash, anorexia, and abdominal distress. Notify the primary health care provider if these effects become pronounced.

- Dizziness may occur. Use caution when driving and when performing other potentially dangerous tasks, as well as when making sudden changes in position. Dangle the legs over the side of the bed for a few minutes when getting up in the morning or after lying down. If dizziness persists, contact the primary health care provider.

- Use caution when walking up or down stairs or when walking on ice, snow, a slick pavement, or slippery floors.

- Stop smoking (if applicable).

- For peripheral vascular disease, follow the primary health care provider's recommendations regarding exercise, avoiding exposure to cold, keeping the extremities warm, and avoiding injury to the extremities.

- Therapeutic effects when taking the drugs for peripheral vascular disease may not be seen for 2 weeks and may take up to 12 weeks.

- Take cilostazol 30 minutes before or 2 hours after meals. Do not take the drug with grapefruit juice.

EVALUATION

- The therapeutic effect is achieved and pain is relieved.

- Adverse reactions are identified, reported to the primary health care provider, and managed successfully through appropriate nursing interventions.

- No evidence of injury is seen.

- The patient and family demonstrate an understanding of the drug regimen.

- The patient verbalizes the importance of complying with the prescribed therapeutic regimen.

Critical Thinking Exercises

1. Ms. Moore is admitted with severe chest pain and a possible myocardial infarction. After tests are done, her primary health care provider prescribes transdermal nitroglycerin for her angina. Develop a teaching plan that will show Ms. Moore how and when to apply the transdermal form of nitroglycerin.

2. Mr. Billings is prescribed sublingual nitroglycerin for his angina. What information would Mr. Billings need to know about when and how to take the drug and what precautions he should take regarding handling and storage of the drug?

3. Mr. Crawford has peripheral vascular disease and is prescribed isoxsuprine hydrochloride (Vasodilan). Discuss the important aspects of the preadministration and ongoing assessment for Mr. Crawford.

Review Questions

1. When administering the nitrates for angina pectoris, the nurse monitors the patient for which common adverse reaction?

   A. Hyperglycemia

   B. Headache

   C. Fever

   D. Anorexia

2. When teaching a patient about prescribed sublingual nitroglycerin, the nurse informs the patient that if pain is not relieved, the dose can be repeated in _____ minute(s).

   A. 1

   B. 5

   C. 15

   D. 30

3. When administering nitroglycerin ointment, the nurse _____.

   A. rubs the ointment into the skin

   B. applies the ointment every hour or until the angina is relieved

   C. applies the ointment to a clean, dry area

   D. rubs the ointment between his or her palms and then spreads it evenly onto the patient's chest

4. A patient taking a calcium channel blocker experiences orthostatic hypotension. The nurse instructs the patient with orthostatic hypotension to _____.

   A. remain in a supine position until the effects subside

   B. make position changes slowly to minimize hypotensive effects

   C. increase the dosage of the calcium channel blocker

   D. discontinue use of the calcium channel blocker until the hypotensive effects diminish

5. When administering cilostazol, the nurse instructs the patient _____.

   A. that drugs used to treat peripheral vascular disease may take up to 4 weeks before improvement is seen

   B. to take the drug with food to enhance absorption

   C. to increase the dose if no response is seen within the first week

   D. that the drug must be given for short periods only (up to 4 to 8 weeks)

6. The peripheral vasodilating drugs are contraindicated in patients _____.

   A. with arthritis

   B. with hypertension

   C. with elevated blood cholesterol levels

   D. during the immediate postpartum period

Medication Dosage Problems

1. The primary care provider prescribed verapamil hydrochloride (Calan) 120 mg TID orally. The drug is available in 40-mg tablets. The nurse administers _____.

2. The patient is prescribed isosorbide (Isordil) 40 mg orally BID. The drug form available is 20-mg tablets. The nurse administers _____.

To check your answers, see Appendix G.

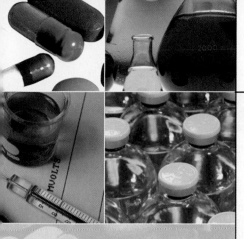

Chapter 41

Antihypertensive Drugs

Key Terms

- aldosterone
- angiotensin-converting enzyme
- blood pressure
- endogenous
- essential hypertension
- hypertension
- hypertensive emergency
- hypokalemia
- hyponatremia
- isolated systolic hypertension
- lumen
- orthostatic hypotension
- prehypertension
- secondary hypertension
- vasodilation

Learning Objectives

On completion of this chapter, the student will:

- Discuss the various types of hypertension and risk factors involved.
- Identify normal and abnormal blood pressure levels for adults.
- List the various types of drugs used to treat hypertension.
- Discuss the general drug actions, uses, adverse reactions, contraindications, precautions, and interactions of the antihypertensive drugs.
- Discuss important preadministration and ongoing assessment activities the

nurse should perform for the patient taking an antihypertensive drug.

- Explain why blood pressure determinations are important during therapy with an antihypertensive drug.
- List nursing diagnoses particular to a patient taking an antihypertensive drug.
- Discuss ways to promote an optimal response to therapy, how to manage adverse reactions, and important points to keep in mind when educating patients about the use of an antihypertensive drug.

Blood pressure is the force of the blood against the walls of the arteries. Blood pressure rises and falls throughout the day. The condition in which blood pressure stays elevated over time is known as **hypertension**. A systolic blood pressure less than 120 mm Hg and a diastolic blood pressure less than 80 mm Hg (120/80) are considered normal. **Prehypertension** is defined as a systolic pressure between 120 and 139 mm Hg or a diastolic pressure between 80 and 89 mm Hg. Individuals with prehypertensive blood pressures are at risk for developing hypertension and should begin health-promoting lifestyle modifications. Table 41-1 identifies blood pressure levels for adults and implications of diagnosis.

CONCEPTSin action **ANIMATION**

Risks and Effects of Hypertension

Hypertension is serious because it causes the heart to work too hard and contributes to atherosclerosis. It also increases the risk of heart disease, congestive heart failure, kidney disease, blindness, and stroke. Most cases of hypertension have no known cause. When there is no known cause of hypertension, the term **essential hypertension** is used. Essential hypertension has been linked to certain risk factors, such as diet and lifestyle. Display 41-1 identifies the risk factors associated with hypertension.

In the United States, African Americans are twice as likely as whites to experience hypertension. After age 65, African-American women have the highest incidence of hypertension. Essential hypertension cannot be cured but can be controlled. Many individuals experience hypertension as they grow older, but

433

Table 41.1 Blood Pressure Levels for Adults

Blood Pressure Category	Systolic Pressure* (in mm Hg)		Diastolic Pressure* (in mm Hg)
Normal	less than 120	And	less than 80
Prehypertension†	120–139	Or	80–89
Hypertension			
Stage 1‡	140–159	Or	90–99
Stage 2‡	160 or greater	Or	100 or higher

*If systolic and diastolic pressures fall into different categories, the patient's status is the higher category.

†Requires health-promoting lifestyle modifications to prevent cardiovascular disease.

‡Requires the average of two or more blood pressure readings taken at each of two or more visits after an initial screening, and health-promoting lifestyle modifications.

From U.S. Department of Health and Human Services, National Institutes of Health, National Heart, Lung and Blood Institute, available at www.nhlbi.nih.gov/health/dci/Diseases/Hbp/HBP_WhatIs.html.

hypertension is not a part of healthy aging. For many older individuals, the systolic pressure gives the most accurate diagnosis of hypertension. Display 41-2 discusses the importance of the systolic pressure.

Nondrug Management of Hypertension

Once essential hypertension develops, management of the disorder becomes a lifetime task. When a direct cause of

Display 41.1 Risk Factors in Hypertensive Patients

- Cigarette smoking
- Age and sex (women older than 55 years and men older than 45 years of age)
- Obesity
- Diabetes
- Lack of physical activity
- Chronic alcohol consumption
- Excessive dietary intake of salt and too little intake of potassium
- Family history of high blood pressure and/or cardiovascular disease
- Current situation of prehypertension (120–139/80–89)

Display 41.2 Importance of the Systolic Blood Pressure

In most individuals, systolic pressure increases sharply with age, whereas diastolic pressure increases until about age 55 and then declines. Older individuals with an elevated systolic pressure have a condition known as **isolated systolic hypertension** (ISH). In ISH systolic blood pressure is 140 mm Hg or greater with diastolic blood pressure less than 90 mm Hg. When the systolic pressure is high, blood vessels become less flexible and stiffen, leading to cardiovascular disease and kidney damage. Research indicates that treating ISH saves lives and reduces illness. The treatment is the same for ISH as for other forms of hypertension.

the hypertension can be identified, the condition is described as **secondary hypertension**. Among the known causes of secondary hypertension, kidney disease ranks first, with tumors or other abnormalities of the adrenal glands following. Most primary health care providers prescribe lifestyle changes to reduce risk factors before prescribing drugs. The primary health care provider may recommend measures such as

- Weight loss (if the patient is overweight)
- Stress reduction (e.g., relaxation techniques, meditation, and yoga)
- Regular aerobic exercise
- Smoking cessation (if applicable)
- Moderation of alcohol consumption
- Dietary changes, such as a decrease in sodium (salt) intake

Many people with hypertension are "salt sensitive," in that any salt or sodium more than the minimal bodily need is too much for them and leads to an increase in blood pressure. Dietitians usually recommend the Dietary Approaches to Stop Hypertension (DASH) diet. Studies indicate that blood pressure was reduced by eating a diet low in saturated fat, total fat, and cholesterol and rich in fruits, vegetables, and low-fat dairy foods. The DASH diet includes whole grains, poultry, fish, and nuts and has reduced amounts of fats, red meats, sweets and sugared beverages.

Drug Therapy for Hypertension

When nondrug measures do not control high blood pressure, drug therapy usually begins, and the primary health care provider may first prescribe a diuretic (see Chapter 45)

Table 41.2 Compelling Indicators for Hypertensive Drug Therapy

Compelling Indicator	Anticipated Drug Therapy
Heart failure	Thiazide, BB, ACEI, ARB, ALDO ant
High risk for cardiovascular disease	Thiazide, BB, ACEI, CCB
Post-myocardial infarction	BB, ACEI, ALDO ant
Diabetes	Thiazide, BB, ACEI, ARB, CCB
Stroke prevention (recurrent)	Thiazide, ACEI
Chronic kidney disease	ACEI, ARB

ACEI, angiotensin-converting enzyme inhibitor; ARB, angiotensin receptor blocker; ALDO ant, aldosterone antagonist receptor blocker; BB, beta blockers; CCB, calcium channel blocker.
From *The seventh report of the Joint National Committee on Prevention, Detection, Evaluation, and Treatment of High Blood Pressure* (2003). Bethesda, MD: National Institutes of Health.

or beta (β)-adrenergic blocker (see Chapter 28) because these drugs have been highly effective (see Table 41-2 for indicators suggesting that drug therapy for hypertension should begin). However, as in many other diseases and conditions, there is no "best" single drug, drug combination, or medical regimen for hypertension treatment. After examination and evaluation of the patient, the primary health care provider selects the antihypertensive drug and therapeutic regimen that will probably be most effective. Figure 41-1 shows an algorithm for the treatment of hypertension.

In some instances, it may be necessary to change to another antihypertensive drug or add a second antihypertensive drug when the patient does not experience a response to therapy. The primary health care provider also recommends that the patient continue with stress reduction, dietary modifications, and other lifestyle modifications needed for controlling hypertension. The types of drugs used for the treatment of hypertension include

- Vasodilating drugs—for example, hydralazine and minoxidil

- Beta-adrenergic blocking drugs—for example, atenolol and propranolol

- Antiadrenergic drugs (centrally acting)—for example, guanabenz and guanfacine

- Antiadrenergic drugs (peripherally acting)—for example, guanadrel and guanethidine

- Alpha-adrenergic blocking drugs—for example, doxazosin and prazosin

- Calcium channel blocking drugs—for example, amlodipine and diltiazem

- Angiotensin-converting enzyme inhibitors (ACEIs)—for example, captopril and enalapril

- Angiotensin II receptor antagonists—for example, irbesartan and losartan

- Diuretics—for example, furosemide and hydrochlorothiazide

For additional information concerning the anti-adrenergic drugs (both centrally and peripherally acting), and the alpha- and beta-adrenergic blocking drugs, see Chapter 28. For more information on the calcium channel blockers see Chapter 40. Information on the vasodilating drugs and the diuretics can be found in Chapters 40 and 45, respectively. The ACEIs and the angiotensin II receptor antagonists are discussed in this chapter.

In addition to these antihypertensive drugs, many antihypertensive combinations are available, such as Ser-Ap-Es, Timolide 10-25, Aldoril 15, and Lopressor 100/50 (Table 41-3). Most combination antihypertensive drugs combine antihypertensive and diuretic agents.

Actions

Many antihypertensive drugs lower the blood pressure by dilating or increasing the size of the arterial blood vessels (**vasodilation**). Vasodilation creates an increase in the **lumen** (the space or opening within a blood vessel) of the arterial blood vessels, which in turn increases the amount of space available for the blood to circulate. Because blood volume (the amount of blood) remains relatively constant, an increase in the space in which the blood circulates (i.e., the blood vessels) lowers the pressure of the fluid (measured as blood pressure) in the blood vessels. Although the method by which antihypertensive drugs dilate blood vessels varies, the result remains basically the same. Antihypertensive drugs that have vasodilating activity include

- Adrenergic blocking drugs

- Antiadrenergic drugs

- Calcium channel blocking drugs

- Vasodilating drugs

Another type of antihypertensive drug is the diuretic. The mechanism by which the diuretics reduce elevated blood pressure is unknown, but it is thought to be based, in part, on their ability to increase the excretion of sodium

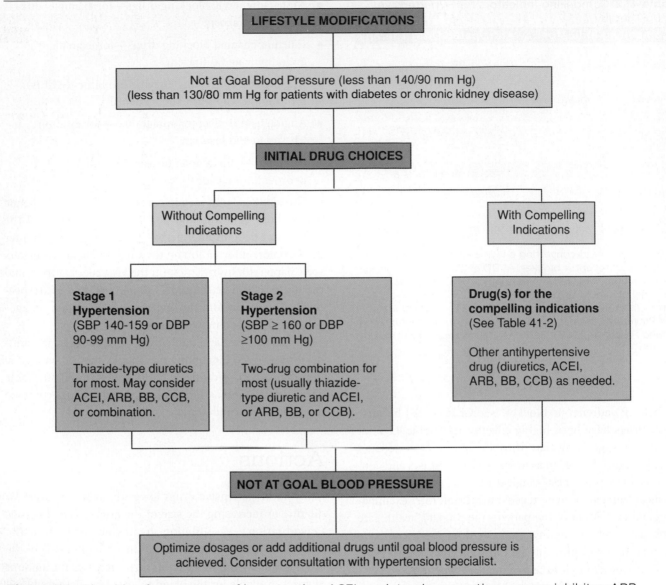

Figure 41.1 Algorithm for treatment of hypertension. ACEI, angiotensin-converting enzyme inhibitor; ARB, angiotensin receptor blocker; BB, beta blocker; CCB, calcium channel blocker; DBP, diastolic blood pressure; SBP, systolic blood pressure. (From *The seventh report of the Joint National Committee on Prevention, Detection, Evaluation, and Treatment of High Blood Pressure* (2003). Bethesda, MD: National Institutes of Health.)

from the body. The actions and uses of diuretics are discussed in Chapter 45.

Action of Angiotensin-Converting Enzyme Inhibitors

The ACEIs appear to act primarily through suppression of the renin-angiotensin-aldosterone system. These drugs prevent (or inhibit) the activity of **angiotensin-converting enzyme**, which converts angiotensin I to angiotensin II, a powerful vasoconstrictor. Both angiotensin I and ACE

normally are manufactured by the body and are called **endogenous** substances. The vasoconstricting activity of angiotensin II stimulates the secretion of the endogenous hormone aldosterone by the adrenal cortex. **Aldosterone** promotes the retention of sodium and water, which may contribute to a rise in blood pressure. By preventing the conversion of angiotensin I to angiotensin II, this chain of events is interrupted, sodium and water are not retained, and the blood pressure decreases (Fig. 41-2)

Table 41.3 Examples of Selected Antihypertensive Combinations

Trade Name	Diuretic Constituent	Antihypertensive
Aldoril-15	hydrochlorothiazide (15 mg)	methyldopa (250 mg)
Apresazide	hydrochlorothiazide (50 mg)	hydralazine (50 mg)
Combipres	chlorthalidone (15 mg)	clonidine (0.1 mg)
Hydropres-50	hydrochlorothiazide (50 mg)	reserpine (0.125 mg)
Lopressor 100/50	hydrochlorothiazide (50 mg)	metoprolol (100 mg)
Minizide 5	polythiazide (0.5 mg)	prazosin (5 mg)
Ser-Ap-Es	hydrochlorothiazide (15 mg)	reserpine (0.1 mg)
	hydralazine (25 mg)	
Tenoretic 100	chlorthalidone (25 mg)	atenolol (100 mg)
Timolide 10–25	hydrochlorothiazide (25 mg)	timolol maleate (10 mg)
Zestoretic	hydrochlorothiazide (12.5 mg)	lisinopril (20 mg)

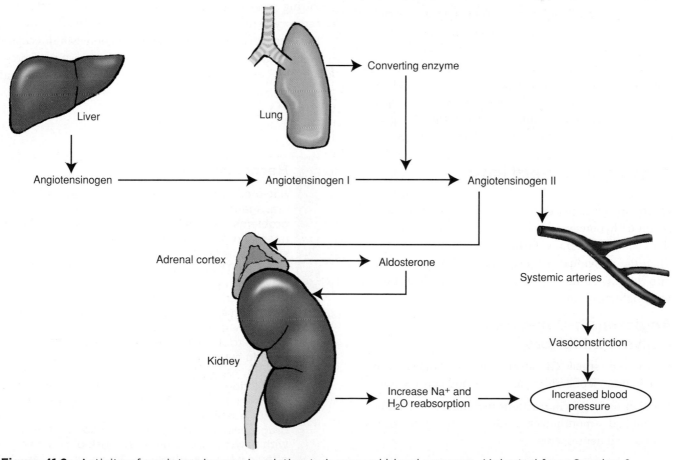

Figure 41.2   Activity of angiotensinogen in relation to increased blood pressure. (Adapted from Scanlon & Sanders. [1999]. *Essentials of anatomy and physiology* [3rd ed., p. 295]. Philadelphia: FA Davis.)

Action of the Angiotensin II Receptor Antagonists

These drugs act to block the binding of angiotensin II at various receptor sites in the vascular smooth muscle and adrenal gland, which blocks the vasoconstrictive effect of the renin-angiotensin system and the release of aldosterone, resulting in a lowering of the blood pressure.

Uses

Antihypertensive drugs are used in the treatment of hypertension. Although many antihypertensive drugs are available, not all drugs work equally well in a given patient. In some instances, the primary health care provider may find it necessary to prescribe a different antihypertensive drug when the patient experiences no response to therapy. Some antihypertensive drugs are used only in severe cases of hypertension and when other, less potent drugs fail to lower the blood pressure. At times, two antihypertensive drugs may be given together to achieve a better response (see Fig. 41-1).

Diazoxide (Hyperstat IV) and nitroprusside (Nitropress) are examples of intravenous (IV) drugs that may be used to treat hypertensive emergencies. A **hypertensive emergency** is a case of extremely high blood pressure in which blood pressure must be lowered immediately to prevent damage to the target organs. Target organs of hypertension include the heart, kidney, and eyes (retinopathy). Additional uses of the antihypertensive drugs are given in the Summary Drug Table: Antihypertensive Drugs.

Adverse Reactions

When any antihypertensive drug is given, orthostatic (or postural) hypotension may result in some patients, especially early in therapy. **Orthostatic hypotension** occurs when the individual has a significant drop in blood pressure (usually 10 mm Hg systolic or more) when assuming an upright position.

Angiotensin-Converting Enzyme Inhibitors

- Gastrointestinal (GI) adverse effects include gastric irritation, peptic ulcers, anorexia, and constipation

- Other body system reactions include rash, pruritus, cough, dry mouth, tachycardia, hypotension, proteinuria, and neutropenia

Angiotensin II Receptor Blocker Drugs

- Central nervous system (CNS) adverse effects include fatigue, depression, dizziness, headache, and syncope

- GI reactions may include abdominal pain, nausea, diarrhea, and constipation

- Other body system effects may be hypotension, symptoms like those of upper respiratory infections, and cough.

Additional adverse reactions that may occur when an antihypertensive drug is administered are listed in the Summary Drug Table: Antihypertensive Drugs. For the adverse reactions that may result when a diuretic is used as an antihypertensive drug, see the Summary Drug Table: Diuretics in Chapter 45.

Contraindications

Antihypertensive drugs are contraindicated in patients with known hypersensitivity to the individual drugs.

The ACEIs and angiotensin II receptor blockers are contraindicated if the patient has impaired renal function, congestive heart failure, salt or volume depletion, bilateral stenosis, or angioedema. They are also contraindicated during pregnancy (category C during first trimester and category D in the second and third trimesters) or during lactation. Use of the ACEIs and the angiotensin II receptor blockers during the second and third trimesters of pregnancy is contraindicated because use may cause fetal and neonatal injury or death.

Herbal Alert

Hawthorn, one of the most commonly used natural agents to treat various cardiovascular problems such as hypertension, angina, arrhythmias, and heart failure, is known for its white, strong-smelling flowers that grow in large bunches. They are used, along with the fruit and leaves of the plant, in the form of capsules, fluid extract, tea, tinctures, and topical creams. Hawthorn should not be administered to individuals who are pregnant, breastfeeding, or allergic to the agent. Possible adverse reactions include hypotension, arrhythmias, sedation, nausea, and anorexia. Possible drug–hawthorn interactions include a risk of hypotension when hawthorn is used with other antihypertensive drugs; possibly increased effects of inotropic drugs when inotropic drugs are administered with hawthorn; and increased risk of sedative effects when hawthorn is administered with other CNS depressants. As with all substances, hawthorn should be used only under the supervision of the primary health care provider.

SUMMARY DRUG TABLE   ANTIHYPERTENSIVE DRUGS

GENERIC NAME	TRADE NAME	USES	ADVERSE REACTIONS	DOSAGE RANGES
Peripheral Vasodilators				
hydralazine HCl *hy-dral'-a-zeen*	Apresoline	Essential hypertension (oral) When need to lower blood pressure is urgent (parenteral)	Dizziness, palpitations, tachycardia, angina, anorexia, nausea, vomiting, headache, hypotension, diarrhea, rash, nasal congestion	10–50 mg QID orally, up to 300 mg/d; 20–40 mg IM or IV
minoxidil *mi-nox'-i-dill*	Loniten	Severe hypertension	Headache, hypotension, electrocardiogram changes, tachycardia, rash, fatigue, sodium and water retention, nausea, hair growth, changes in direction and magnitude of T waves	5–100 mg/d orally; dose greater than 5 mg given in divided doses
Beta-Adrenergic Blocking Drugs				
acebutolol HCl *a-se-byoo'-toe-lole*	Sectral	Hypertension	Dizziness, vertigo, fatigue, bradycardia, CHF, arrhythmias, tachycardia, sinoatrial or atrioventricular block, gastric pain, flatulence, constipation, diarrhea, nausea, vomiting, impotence, decreased libido, decreased exercise tolerance, rash, eye irritation	400–1200 mg/d orally in single or divided doses
atenolol *a-ten'-oh-lole*	Tenormin	Angina pectoris, hypertension, MI	Same as acebutolol	50–100 mg/d orally in single dose, may increase to 200 mg/d orally; 5 mg IV; may repeat every 10 min up to two times
betaxolol HCl *be-tax'-oh-lol*	Kerlone	Hypertension	Same as acebutolol	10–20 mg QD orally
bisoprolol fumarate *bis-oh'-pro-lole*	Zebeta	Hypertension	Same as acebutolol	2.5–20 mg QD orally
carteolol HCl *kar'-tee-oh-lole*	Cartrol	Hypertension	Same as acebutolol	2.5–10 mg QD orally
metoprolol *me-toe'-proe-lole*	Lopressor, Toprol-XL	Hypertension	Same as acebutolol	100–450 mg/d orally; extended-release products are given once daily
nadolol *nay'-doe-lole*	Corgard	Hypertension	Same as acebutolol	Hypertension: 40–80 mg QD orally; may increase to 320 mg/d
penbutolol sulfate *pen-byoo'-toe-lole*	Levatol	Hypertension	Same as acebutolol	20 mg QD orally
pindolol *pin'-doe-lole*	Visken	Hypertension	Same as acebutolol	5–60 mg/d BID orally

⬤ SUMMARY DRUG TABLE   *(continued)*

GENERIC NAME	TRADE NAME	USES	ADVERSE REACTIONS	DOSAGE RANGES
propranolol HCl *proe-pran'-oh-lole*	Inderal, Inderal LA	Hypertension	Same as acebutolol	Hypertension: 80–240 mg/d orally in divided doses; doses up to 640 mg have been given
timolol maleate *tim'-oh-lole*	Blocadren	Hypertension	Same as acebutolol	Hypertension: 20 mg/d orally in divided doses, up to 60 mg/d
Antiadrenergic Drugs—Centrally Acting				
clonidine HCl oral *kloe'-ni-deen*	Catapres	Hypertension	Drowsiness, sedation dizziness, headache, fatigue that tends to diminish within 4–6 wk, dry mouth, constipation, impotence, decreased sexual activity	Individualize dosage, 0.1–0.8 mg/d orally in divided doses; maximum dosage, 2.4 mg/d
clonidine HCl, transdermal	Catapres-TTS-1, Catapres-TTS-2, Catapres-TTS-3	Hypertension	Drowsiness, dry mouth, transient localized skin reactions, fatigue, headache, constipation, nausea	0.1-mg system–0.3-mg system every 7 d, may increase up to two 0.3-mg systems per 24 h
guanabenz acetate *gwahn'-a-benz*	Wytensin	Hypertension	Dizziness, weakness, lassitude, syncope, postural or exertional hypotension, diarrhea, bradycardia, fluid retention and edema, inhibition of ejaculation, CHF	Individualize dosage, 4–8 mg BID orally; may increase up to 64 mg/d
guanfacine HCl *gwahn'-fa-seen*	Tenex	Hypertension	Sedation, weakness, dizziness, dry mouth, constipation, impotence	1–3 mg orally at bedtime
methyldopa and methyldopate HCl *meth-ill-doe'-pa*	Aldomet	Hypertension	Sedation, headache, asthenia, weakness, nausea, vomiting, abdominal discomfort, constipation, bradycardia	methyldopa: 250 mg–3.0 g/d orally in divided doses methyldopate: 250 mg–1 g q6h IV
Antiadrenergic Drugs—Peripherally Acting				
doxazosin *dox-ay'-zoe-sin*	Cardura	Mild to moderate hypertension	Headache, fatigue dizziness, orthostatic hypotension, dizziness, lethargy, vertigo, tachycardia, palpitations, edema, orthostatic hypotension, nausea, dyspepsia, diarrhea, sexual dysfunction	1–16 mg/d orally
guanadrel *gwahn'-a-drel*	Hylorel	Hypertension	Fatigue, headache, faintness, drowsiness, visual disturbances,	10–75 mg/d orally

GENERIC NAME	TRADE NAME	USES	ADVERSE REACTIONS	DOSAGE RANGES
			confusion, increased bowel movements, indigestion, constipation, anorexia, shortness of breath on exertion, palpitations, chest pain, coughing, nocturia, urinary urgency or frequency, peripheral edema, ejaculation disturbances, weight loss or gain	
guanethidine monosulfate *gwahn-eth'-i-deen*	Ismelin	Hypertension	Dizziness, weakness, lassitude, syncope, postural or exertional hypotension, diarrhea, bradycardia, fluid retention and edema, CHF, inhibition of ejaculation	10–50 mg/d orally
reserpine *re-ser'-peen*		Hypertension	Drowsiness, sedation, lethargy, respiratory depression, edema, orthostatic hypotension, nasal congestion	0.5–1 mg/d orally

Alpha-Adrenergic Blocking Drugs

GENERIC NAME	TRADE NAME	USES	ADVERSE REACTIONS	DOSAGE RANGES
doxazosin mesylate *dox-ay'-zoe-sin*	Cardura	Hypertension	Headache, fatigue, dizziness, orthostatic hypotension, dizziness, lethargy, vertigo, nausea, dyspepsia, diarrhea, tachycardia, palpitations, edema, sexual dysfunction	1–16 mg/d orally
mecamylamine HCl *mek-a-mill'-a-meen*	Inversine	Severe hypertension	Weakness, fatigue, sedation, anorexia, dry mouth, glossitis, nausea, orthostatic hypotension	5–25 mg/d orally in 2 or 3 doses
prazosin *pra'-zoe-sin*	Minipress	Hypertension	Dizziness, headache, drowsiness, lethargy, weakness, nausea, palpitations	1–20 mg/d orally in divided doses
terazosin *ter-ay'-zoe-sin*	Hytrin	Hypertension	Dizziness, headache, drowsiness, lack of energy, weakness, somnolence, nausea, palpitations, edema, dyspnea, nasal congestion, sinusitis	1–20 mg/d orally at bedtime

Alpha- and Beta-Adrenergic Blocking Drugs

GENERIC NAME	TRADE NAME	USES	ADVERSE REACTIONS	DOSAGE RANGES
carvedilol *kar-ve'-di-lole*	Coreg	Essential hypertension, CHF, left ventricular dysfunction	Dizziness, tinnitus, fatigue, bradycardia, orthostatic hypotension, CHF, cardiac arrhythmias, gastric pain, flatulence, constipation, diarrhea, rhinitis	Hypertension: 6.25–25 mg BID orally CHF: 3.125–25 mg BID orally

⬤ SUMMARY DRUG TABLE   *(continued)*

GENERIC NAME	TRADE NAME	USES	ADVERSE REACTIONS	DOSAGE RANGES
labetalol HCl *la-bet'-oh-lole*	Normodyne, Trandate	Hypertension, severe hypertension (parenteral preparations)	Same as acebutolol	Oral: 200–400 mg BID (up to 2400 mg) in divided doses TID Parenteral: 20 mg slowly IV over 2 min at 10-min intervals, or continuous IV infusion at the rate of 2 mg/min for a total dosage of 300 mg
Angiotensin-Converting Enzyme Inhibitors				
benazepril HCl *ben-a'-za-pril*	Lotensin	Hypertension	Nausea, cough, vomiting, constipation, hypotension, palpitations, rash	10–40 mg/d orally in single dose or two divided doses, maximum dose 80 mg
ⓡ **captopril** *kap'-toe-pril*	Capoten	Hypertension, HF, LVD after MI, diabetic nephropathy	Tachycardia, gastric irritation, peptic ulcer, proteinuria, rash, pruritus, cough	Hypertension: 50–450 mg/d orally in divided doses
enalapril *e-nal'-a-pril*	Vasotec, Vasotec IV	Hypertension, CHF, asymptomatic LVD	Headache, dizziness, fatigue, nausea, diarrhea, decreased hematocrit and hemoglobin, cough	Hypertension: 5–40 mg/d orally as a single dose or in two divided doses; 0.625–1.25 mg q6h IV
fosinopril sodium *foh-sin'-oh-pril*	Monopril	Hypertension, CHF	Nausea, cough, abdominal pain, vomiting, orthostatic hypotension, palpitations, rash	10–40 mg/d orally in a single dose or two divided doses
lisinopril *lyse-in'-oh-pril*	Prinivil, Zestril	Hypertension	Headache, dizziness, insomnia, fatigue, gastric irritation, nausea, diarrhea, orthostatic hypotension, proteinuria, angioedema, cough	Hypertension: 10–40 mg/d orally as a single dose
ⓡ **moexipril HCl** *mo-ex'-ah-pril*	Univasc	Hypertension	Tachycardia, gastric irritation, peptic ulcers, diarrhea, proteinuria, rash, pruritus, flushing, flulike syndrome, dizziness, cough	7.5–30 mg orally as a single dose or two divided doses
perindopril erbumine *pur-in'-doh-pril*	Aceon	Essential hypertension	Orthostatic hypotension, headache, dizziness, insomnia, fatigue, proteinuria, gastric irritation, nausea, cough	4–16 mg/d orally
quinapril HCl *kwin'-ah-pril*	Accupril	Hypertension, CHF	Nausea, cough, abdominal pain, vomiting, orthostatic hypotension, palpitations, rash	Hypertension: 10–80 mg/d orally as a single dose or two divided doses

GENERIC NAME	TRADE NAME	USES	ADVERSE REACTIONS	DOSAGE RANGES
ramipril *ra-mi'-prill*	Altace	Hypertension, CHF, decrease risk of cardiovascular disease, coronary artery disease	Nausea, cough, abdominal pain, vomiting, orthostatic hypotension, palpitations, rash	Hypertension: 2.5–20 mg/d orally as a single dose or two divided doses
trandolapril *tran-dole'-ah-pril*	Mavik	Hypertension, patients post-MI with symptoms of CHF and LVD	Headache, cough, dizziness, fatigue, tachycardia, rash, CHF, hypotension	Hypertension: 1–4 mg/d orally

Angiotensin II Receptor Antagonists

GENERIC NAME	TRADE NAME	USES	ADVERSE REACTIONS	DOSAGE RANGES
candesartan cilexetil *can-dah-sar'-tan*	Atacand	Hypertension	Diarrhea, abdominal pain, nausea, headache, dizziness, URI symptoms, hypotension, rash	16–32 mg/d orally in divided doses
eprosartan mesylate *ep-row-sar'-tan*	Teveten	Hypertension	Abdominal pain, fatigue, depression, URI symptoms, hypotension	400–800 mg/d orally in two divided doses
irbesartan *er-bah-sar'-tan*	Avapro	Hypertension, nephropathy in type 2 diabetes	Headache, dizziness, diarrhea, abdominal pain, nausea, hypotension, URI symptoms, cough, fatigue	150–300 mg/d orally as one dose
losartan potassium *low-sar'-tan*	Cozaar	Hypertension, hypertension in patients with left ventricular hypertrophy, nephropathy in type 2 diabetes	Diarrhea, abdominal pain, nausea, headache, dizziness, hypotension, URI symptoms, cough	25–100 mg/d orally in one or two doses
olmesartan *ol-ma-sar'-tan*	Benicar	Hypertension	Headache, diarrhea, abdominal pain, nausea, URI symptoms, bronchitis, back pain, flulike symptoms, dizziness, hypotension, rash	20–40 mg/d orally
telmisartan *tell-mah-sar'-tan*	Micardis	Hypertension	Diarrhea, abdominal pain, nausea, headache, dizziness, lightheadedness, URI symptoms, cough	40–80 mg/d orally
valsartan *val-sar'-tan*	Diovan	Hypertension, CHF	Headache, dizziness, diarrhea, abdominal pain, nausea, URI symptoms, cough	Hypertension: 80–320 mg/d orally

Antihypertensive Drugs

⬤ SUMMARY DRUG TABLE   *(continued)*

GENERIC NAME	TRADE NAME	USES	ADVERSE REACTIONS	DOSAGE RANGES
Drugs Used for Hypertensive Emergency				
diazoxide, parenteral *di-az-ok'-side*	Hyperstat IV	Hypertensive emergency/crisis	Dizziness, weakness, nausea, vomiting, sodium and water retention, hypotension, myocardial ischemia	1–3 mg/kg IV bolus; maximum dosage, 150 mg
nitroprusside sodium *nye-troe-pruss'-ide*	Nitropress	Hypertensive crisis	Apprehension, headache, restlessness, nausea, vomiting, palpitations, diaphoresis	3 mcg/kg/min, not to exceed infusion rate of 10 mcg/min (if blood pressure is not reduced within 10 min, discontinue administration)

Ⓡ This drug should be administered at least 1 hour before or 2 hours after a meal.
CHF, congestive heart failure; LVD, left ventricular dysfunction; MI, myocardial infarction; URI, upper respiratory infection.

Precautions

Antihypertensive drugs are used cautiously in patients with renal or hepatic impairment or electrolyte imbalances, during lactation and pregnancy, and in older patients. ACEIs are used cautiously in patients with sodium depletion, hypovolemia, or coronary or cerebrovascular insufficiency and in those receiving diuretic therapy or dialysis. The angiotensin II receptor agonists are used cautiously in patients with renal or hepatic dysfunction, hypovolemia, or volume or salt depletion, and in patients receiving high doses of diuretics.

Interactions

The hypotensive effects of most antihypertensive drugs are increased when administered with diuretics and other antihypertensives. Many drugs can interact with the antihypertensive drugs and decrease their effectiveness (e.g., antidepressants, monoamine oxidase inhibitors, antihistamines, and sympathomimetic bronchodilators).

The following interactions may occur when ACEI drugs are administered with another agent:

Interacting Drug	Common Use	Effect of Interaction
nonsteroidal anti-inflammatory drugs (NSAIDs)	Relief of pain and inflammation	Reduced hypotensive effects of the ACEIs
rifampin	Antitubercular agent	Decreased pharmacologic effect of ACEIs (particularly of enalapril)
allopurinol	Antigout agent	Higher risk of hypersensitivity reaction
digoxin	Management of heart failure	Increased or decreased plasma digoxin levels
loop diuretics	Reduce/ eliminate edema	Decreased diuretic effects
lithium	Management of bipolar disorder	Increased serum lithium levels, possible lithium toxicity
hypoglycemic agents and insulin	Management of diabetes	Increased risk of hypoglycemia
potassium-sparing diuretics or potassium preparations	Diuretics: management of blood pressure; reduce edema Potassium preparations: control of low serum potassium levels	Elevated serum potassium level

The following interactions may occur when angiotensin II receptor antagonists are administered with other agents:

Interacting Drug	Common Use	Effect of Interaction
fluconazole	Antifungal agent	Increased antihypertensive and adverse effects (particularly with losartan)
indomethacin	Pain relief	Decreased hypotensive effect (particularly with losartan)

NURSING PROCESS

The Patient Receiving an Antihypertensive Drug

ASSESSMENT

PREADMINISTRATION ASSESSMENT

Before therapy with an antihypertensive drug starts, the nurse assesses the blood pressure (Fig. 41-3) and pulse rate on both arms with the patient in standing, sitting, and lying positions. The nurse correctly identifies all pressures (e.g., the pressure readings on each arm and the three positions used to obtain the readings) and records these on the patient's chart. The nurse also obtains the patient's weight, especially if a diuretic is part of therapy or if the primary health care provider prescribes a weight-loss regimen.

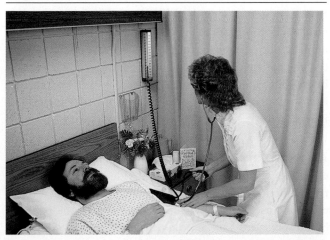

Figure 41.3 The nurse takes the patient's blood pressure before administering an antihypertensive drug.

ONGOING ASSESSMENT

Monitoring and recording the blood pressure is an important part of the ongoing assessment, especially early in therapy. The primary health care provider may need to adjust the dose of the drug upward or downward, try a different drug, or add another drug to the therapeutic regimen if the patient's response to drug therapy is inadequate.

Each time the blood pressure is measured, the nurse uses the same arm with the patient in the same position (e.g., standing, sitting, or lying down). In some instances, the primary health care provider may order the blood pressure taken in one or more positions, such as standing and lying down. The nurse monitors the blood pressure and pulse every 15 to 30 minutes if the patient has severe hypertension, does not have the expected response to drug therapy, or is critically ill.

Nursing Alert

The blood pressure and pulse rate must be obtained immediately before each administration of an antihypertensive drug and compared with previous readings. If the blood pressure is significantly decreased from baseline values, the nurse should not give the drug but should notify the primary health care provider. In addition, the primary health care provider must be notified if there is a significant increase in the blood pressure.

The nurse obtains daily weights during the initial period of drug therapy. Patients taking an antihypertensive drug occasionally retain sodium and water, resulting in edema and weight gain. The nurse assesses the patient's weight and examines the extremities for edema. The nurse reports a weight gain of 2 lb or more per day and any evidence of edema in the hands, fingers, feet, legs, or sacral area. The patient is also weighed at regular intervals if a weight-reduction diet is used to lower the blood pressure or if the patient is receiving a thiazide or related diuretic as part of antihypertensive therapy.

NURSING DIAGNOSES

Drug-specific nursing diagnoses are highlighted in the Nursing Diagnoses Checklist. Other nursing diagnoses applicable to these drugs are discussed in depth in Chapter 4.

PLANNING

The expected outcomes for the patient may include an optimal response to therapy (blood pressure maintained in an acceptable range), patient needs met in relation to management of adverse drug reactions, and an understanding of and compliance with the prescribed therapeutic regimen.

IMPLEMENTATION
PROMOTING AN OPTIMAL RESPONSE TO THERAPY

ADMINISTERING ANTIADRENERGIC DRUGS Clonidine is available as an oral tablet (Catapres) and transdermal patch (Catapres-TTS). The nurse applies the transdermal patch to a hairless area of intact skin on the upper arm or torso; the patch is kept in place for 7 days. The adhesive overlay is applied directly over the system to ensure the patch remains in place for the required time. A different body area is selected for each application. If the patch loosens before 7 days, the edges can be reinforced with nonallergenic tape. The date the patch was placed and the date the patch is to be removed can be written on the surface of the patch with a fiber-tipped pen. (See Chapter 28 for additional information concerning the antiadrenergic drugs.)

ADMINISTERING VASODILATING DRUGS The nurse must carefully monitor the patient receiving minoxidil because the drug increases the heart rate. The primary health care provider is notified if any of the following occur:

• Heart rate of 20 bpm or more above the normal rate

• Rapid weight gain of 5 lb or more

• Unusual swelling of the extremities, face, or abdomen

• Dyspnea, angina, severe indigestion, or fainting

ADMINISTERING CALCIUM CHANNEL BLOCKERS The nurse may give these drugs without regard to meals. If GI upset occurs, the drug may be administered with meals. Bepridil and verapamil are best given with meals because of the tendency of these two drugs to cause gastric upset. The sustained-release capsules should not be crushed, opened, or chewed. Verapamil capsules (not sustained-release) may be opened and the contents sprinkled in liquid or on soft foods. Diltiazem may be crushed and mixed with food or fluids for patients who have difficulty swallowing. See Chapter 40 for more information on the calcium channel blockers.

ADMINISTERING ACEIs The nurse administers captopril and moexipril 1 hour before or 2 hours after meals to enhance absorption. Some patients taking an ACEI experience a dry cough that does not subside until the drug therapy is discontinued. This reaction may need to be tolerated. If the cough becomes too bothersome, the primary health care provider may discontinue use of the drug. The nurse should ensure that the patient is not pregnant before beginning therapy. The patient should use a reliable birth control method such as barrier birth control while taking these drugs. If pregnancy is suspected, the primary health care provider is notified immediately.

The ACEIs may cause a significant drop in blood pressure after the first dose. This effect can be minimized if the primary health care provider discontinues the diuretic therapy (if the patient is taking a diuretic) or begins treatment with small doses. After the first dose of an ACEI, the nurse monitors the blood pressure every 15 to 30 minutes for at least 2 hours and afterward until the blood pressure is stable for 1 hour.

ADMINISTERING ANGIOTENSIN II RECEPTOR ANTAGONISTS These drugs can be administered without regard to meals. It is important to ensure that the patient is not pregnant before beginning therapy. The nurse recommends that the patient use a reliable birth control method such as barrier birth control while taking these drugs. If pregnancy is suspected, the primary health care provider is notified immediately.

ADMINISTERING DRUGS FOR HYPERTENSIVE EMERGENCIES Nitroprusside and diazoxide are drugs used to treat patients with a hypertensive emergency. When these drugs are used, hemodynamic monitoring of the patient's blood pressure and cardiovascular status is required throughout the course of therapy.

Nursing Alert

When diazoxide or nitroprusside is used for a hypertensive emergency, the rate of infusion (nitroprusside) or rate of direct IV administration (diazoxide) and the patient's blood pressure are monitored closely during and after administration of the drug because severe hypotension can occur. The blood pressure and pulse rate may need to be monitored every 5 to 15 minutes until the blood pressure is reduced to safe levels. A precipitous drop in blood pressure can occur, which would require immediate action to restore blood pressure to an acceptable level.

Gerontologic Alert

Older adults are particularly sensitive to the hypotensive effects of nitroprusside. To minimize the hypotensive effects, the drug is initially given in lower dosages. Older adults require more frequent monitoring during the administration of nitroprusside.

MONITORING AND MANAGING PATIENT NEEDS

The nurse observes the patient for adverse drug reactions because their occurrence may require a change in the dose of the drug. The nurse should notify the primary health care provider if any adverse reactions occur. In some instances, the patient may have to tolerate mild adverse reactions, such as dry mouth or mild anorexia.

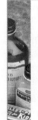

Nursing Alert

If it becomes necessary to discontinue antihypertensive therapy, the nurse should never discontinue use of the drug abruptly. The primary health care provider will prescribe the parameters by which the dosage is to be discontinued. The dosage is usually gradually reduced over 2 to 4 days to avoid rebound hypertension (a rapid rise in blood pressure).

RISK FOR DEFICIENT FLUID VOLUME The patient receiving a diuretic is observed for dehydration and electrolyte imbalances. A fluid volume deficit is most likely to occur if the patient fails to drink a sufficient amount of fluid. This is especially true in the elderly or confused patient. To prevent a fluid volume deficit, the nurse encourages patients to drink adequate oral fluids (up to 2000 mL/d, unless contraindicated because of a medical condition).

Electrolyte imbalances that may occur during therapy with a diuretic include **hyponatremia** (low blood sodium level) and **hypokalemia** (low blood potassium level), although other imbalances may also be seen. (See Chapter 58 for the signs and symptoms of electrolyte imbalances.) The primary health care provider is notified if any signs or symptoms of an electrolyte imbalance occur.

RISK FOR INJURY Dizziness or weakness along with orthostatic hypotension can occur with the administration of antihypertensive drugs. If orthostatic hypotension occurs, the nurse advises the patient to rise slowly from a sitting or lying position. The nurse explains that when rising from a lying position, sitting on the edge of the bed for 1 or 2 minutes often minimizes these symptoms. In addition, rising slowly from a chair and then standing for 1 to 2 minutes also minimizes the symptoms of orthostatic hypotension. When symptoms of orthostatic hypotension, dizziness, or weakness do occur, the nurse can assist the patient in getting out of bed or a chair and with ambulatory activities.

RISK FOR INEFFECTIVE SEXUALITY PATTERNS The antihypertensive drugs can cause sexual dysfunction ranging from impotence to inhibition of ejaculation. The nurse must provide an open and understanding atmosphere when discussing sexuality. The nurse explains potential problems with sexual patterns that can occur with these drugs. If sexual patterns are affected negatively, suggest that the partners use other means of expressing caring, such as touching, massage, and personal closeness. The nurse can suggest that sexual activity need not always end with intercourse. The nurse allows the patient time to express feelings and concerns and encourages the patient and partner to discuss ways to satisfy intimacy needs.

RISK FOR ACTIVITY INTOLERANCE Some patients on the antihypertensive drugs have decreased exercise tolerance and feel fatigued, weak, and lethargic. In addition, patients with hypertension may have other health problems (either cardiovascular or respiratory problems) that may affect their ability to perform activities. The patient is encouraged to walk and ambulate as he or she can tolerate. Assistive devices may be used if needed. Gradually increase tolerance by increasing the daily amount of activity. Plan rest periods according to the individual's tolerance. Rest can take many forms, such as sitting in a chair, napping, watching television, or sitting with legs elevated. The nurse should inform the patient that often the fatigue diminishes after 4 to 6 weeks of therapy.

Antihypertensive Drugs

ACUTE PAIN Patients taking the antihypertensive drugs may complain of a headache that could be an adverse reaction to the drugs, particularly antiadrenergics or the angiotensin II receptor blocking drugs. It the headache is acute the patient may need to remain in bed with a cool cloth on the forehead, or the nurse may give the patient a back and neck rub. Relaxation techniques such as guided imagery or progressive body relaxation may prove helpful. If nursing measures are not successful, the primary health care provider is notified because an analgesic may be required.

EDUCATING THE PATIENT AND FAMILY

Nurses can do much to educate others on the importance of having their blood pressure checked at periodic intervals. This includes people of all ages because hypertension is not a disease that affects only older individuals. Once hypertension is detected, patient teaching becomes an important factor in successfully returning the blood pressure to normal or near-normal levels.

To ensure lifetime compliance with the prescribed therapeutic regimen, the nurse emphasizes the importance of drug therapy, as well as other treatments recommended by the primary health care provider. The nurse describes the adverse reactions from a particular antihypertensive drug and advises the patient to contact the primary health care provider if any should occur.

The primary health care provider may want the patient or family to monitor blood pressure during therapy. The nurse teaches the technique of taking a blood pressure and pulse rate to the patient or family member, allowing sufficient time for supervised practice. The nurse instructs the patient to keep a record of the blood pressure and to bring this record to each visit to the primary health care provider's office or clinic.

The nurse includes the following points in a teaching plan for the patient receiving an antihypertensive drug:

- Never discontinue use of this drug except on the advice of the primary health care provider. These drugs control but do not cure hypertension. Skipping doses of the drug or voluntarily discontinuing the drug may cause severe rebound hypertension.

- Avoid the use of any nonprescription drugs (some may contain drugs that can increase the blood pressure) unless approved by the primary health care provider.

- Avoid alcohol unless its use has been approved by the primary health care provider.

- This drug may produce dizziness or lightheadedness when rising suddenly from a sitting or lying position. To avoid these effects, rise slowly from a sitting or lying position (see Home Care Checklist: Preventing Orthostatic Hypotension).

- If the drug causes drowsiness, avoid hazardous tasks such as driving or performing tasks that require alertness. Drowsiness may disappear with time.

- If unexplained weakness or fatigue occurs, contact the primary health care provider.

- Contact the primary health care provider if adverse drug effects occur.

- Follow the diet restrictions recommended by the primary health care provider. Do not use salt substitutes unless a particular brand of salt substitute is approved by the primary health care provider.

- Notify the primary health care provider if the diastolic pressure suddenly increases to 130 mm Hg or higher; this may signal a hypertensive emergency.

Home Care Checklist

Preventing Orthostatic Hypotension

Many patients receiving antihypertensive therapy commonly receive more than one drug, placing them at risk for orthostatic hypotension. If it occurs, the patient may fall and be injured, so teach the following measures to follow while in the acute care facility and at home:

☑ Change your position slowly.

☑ Sit at the edge of the bed or chair for a few minutes before standing up.

☑ Stand for a few minutes before starting to walk.

☑ Ask for assistance when necessary.

☑ If you feel dizzy or lightheaded, sit or lie down immediately.

☑ Make sure to drink adequate amounts of fluid throughout the day.

EVALUATION

- The therapeutic effect is achieved and blood pressure controlled.

- Adverse reactions are identified, reported to the primary health care provider, and managed successfully through nursing interventions.

- Fluid volume deficit is corrected (when appropriate).

- No evidence of injury is apparent.

- The patient resumes previous sexual activity or engages in alternative satisfying sexual activity.

- The patient reports no decrease in activity tolerance.

- The patient reports no headache or headache is controlled.

- The patient complies with the prescribed drug regimen.

- The patient and family demonstrate an understanding of the drug regimen.

- The patient verbalizes the importance of complying with the prescribed therapeutic regimen.

Critical Thinking Exercises

1. Discuss important preadministration assessments that should be performed with a patient prescribed captopril for hypertension.

2. While working in the medical clinic of a hospital-associated health care satellite, the primary health care provider asks you to explain to a patient what can be done to avoid dizziness and lightheadedness when rising from a sitting or lying down position. When talking to the patient, you discover that he understands little English. Discuss how you might communicate to this patient what he can do to decrease the symptoms of orthostatic hypotension.

3. Mr. Bates, who has been treated for hypertension, is admitted for treatment of a kidney stone. On admission, he had severe pain and his blood pressure was 160/96 mm Hg. For the past 2 days, his blood pressure has been between 140/92 and 148/98 mm Hg. When taking his blood pressure before giving him an oral antihypertensive drug, you find that it now is 118/82 mm Hg. Analyze the situation and discuss what actions you would take.

4. Develop a teaching plan for a patient for whom verapamil has been prescribed for hypertension. Discuss what information you would need from the patient before developing this plan. Identify important points to include in the plan.

5. Ms. Jones is admitted to the emergency department with a hypertensive emergency. Nitroprusside therapy is begun, and you are asked to monitor this patient. Discuss important points that must be kept in mind when administering this drug. Identify methods you would use to monitor the patient and prevent complications.

Review Questions

1. The nurse instructs the patient using the transdermal system Catapres TTS to _____.
   - A. place the patch on the torso and keep it in place for 24 hours
   - B. change placement of the patch every day after bathing
   - C. place the patch on the upper arm or torso and keep it in place for 7 days
   - D. avoid getting the patch wet because it might detach from the skin

2. To avoid symptoms associated with orthostatic hypotension, the nurse advises the patient to _____.
   - A. sleep in a side-lying position
   - B. avoid sitting for prolong periods
   - C. change position slowly
   - D. get up from a sitting position quickly

3. After the first dose of an ACEI, the nurse monitors _____.
   - A. the patient for a hypotensive crisis
   - B. the vital signs every 4 hours or more often if the patient reports being dizzy
   - C. the blood pressure every hour until it is stable
   - D. the blood pressure every 15 to 30 minutes for at least 2 hours

4. When discontinuing use of an antihypertensive drug, the nurse _____.
   - A. monitors the blood pressure every hour for 8 hours after the drug therapy is discontinued
   - B. expects the primary health care provider to order that the drug dosage be gradually decreased over a period of 2 to 4 days to avoid rebound hypertension
   - C. checks the blood pressure and pulse every 30 minutes after discontinuing the drug therapy
   - D. expects to taper the dosage of the drug over a period of 2 weeks to avoid a return of hypertension

5. During the preadministration assessment of a patient prescribed an antihypertensive drug, the nurse _____.

    A. places the patient in a high Fowler's position

    B. places the patient in a supine position

    C. darkens the room to decrease stimuli

    D. takes the patient's blood pressure

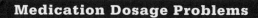

Medication Dosage Problems

1. Oral nadolol 80 mg is prescribed. The drug is available in 20-mg tablets. The nurse administers _____.

2. Diltiazem 180 mg is prescribed. The drug is available in 60-mg, 90-mg, and 120-mg tablets.

Which tablet would you select? _____

How many tablets would you administer? _____

To check your answers, see Appendix G.

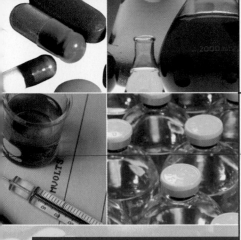

Antihyperlipidemic Drugs

Learning Objectives

On completion of this chapter, the student will:

- Discuss cholesterol, HDL, LDL, and triglyceride levels and how they contribute to the development of heart disease.

- Discuss therapeutic life changes and how they affect cholesterol levels.

- Discuss the general actions, uses, adverse reactions, contraindications, precautions, and interactions of anti-hyperlipidemic drugs.

- Discuss important preadministration and ongoing assessment activities the nurse should perform on the patient taking an antihyperlipidemic drug.

- List nursing diagnoses particular to a patient taking an antihyperlipidemic drug.

- Discuss ways to promote an optimal response to therapy, how to manage common adverse reactions, and important points to keep in mind when educating patients about the use of an antihyperlipidemic drug.

yperlipidemia is an increase (*hyper*) in the **lipids**, which are a group of fats or fatlike substances in the blood (*emia*). **Cholesterol** and the **triglycerides** are the two lipids in the blood. Elevation of one or both of these lipids occurs in hyperlipidemia. Serum cholesterol levels above 240 mg/dL and triglyceride levels above 150 mg/dL are associated with atherosclerosis. **Atherosclerosis** is a disorder in which lipid deposits accumulate on the lining of the blood vessels, eventually producing degenerative changes and obstructing blood flow. Atherosclerosis is considered to be a major contributor in the development of heart disease.

Triglycerides and cholesterol are insoluble in water and must be bound to a lipid-containing protein (**lipoprotein**) for transportation throughout the body. Although several lipoproteins are found in the blood, this chapter focuses on the low-density lipoproteins, the high-density lipoproteins, and cholesterol.

Lipoproteins

Low-density lipoproteins (LDL) transport cholesterol to the peripheral cells. When the cells have all the cholesterol they need, the excess cholesterol is discarded into the blood. This can result in an excess of cholesterol, which can penetrate the walls of the arteries, resulting in atherosclerotic plaque formation. Elevation of the LDL increases the risk for heart disease. **High-density lipoproteins (HDL)** take cholesterol from the peripheral cells and transport it to the liver, where it is metabolized and excreted. The higher the HDL, the lower the risk for development of atherosclerosis. Therefore, it is desirable to see an increase in the HDL (the "good" lipoprotein) level because of the protective nature of its properties against the development of atherosclerosis, and a decrease in the LDL level. A laboratory

Table 42.1 Cholesterol Level Analysis

Level	Category
Total Cholesterol*	
Less than 200 mg/dL	Desirable
200–239 mg/dL	Borderline
240 mg/dL and above	High
Low-Density Lipoprotein (LDL) Cholesterol*	
Less than 100 mg/dL	Optimal
100–129 mg/dL	Near optimal/above optimal
130–159 mg/dL	Borderline
160–189 mg/dL	High
190 mg/dL and above	Very high
High-Density Lipoprotein (HDL) Cholesterol*	
Less than 40 mg/dL	Low
60 mg/dL and above	High

*Cholesterol levels are measured in milligrams (mg) of cholesterol per deciliter (dL) of blood.

examination of blood lipids, called a *lipoprotein profile,* provides valuable information on the important cholesterol levels, such as

- Total cholesterol
- LDL (the harmful lipoprotein)
- HDL (the protective lipoprotein)
- Triglycerides

Table 42-1 provides an analysis of cholesterol levels.

Cholesterol Levels

High-density lipoprotein cholesterol protects against heart disease, so the higher its numbers (i.e., blood level), the better. An HDL level less than 40 mg/dL is low and considered a major risk factor for heart disease. Triglyceride levels that are borderline (150–190 mg/dL) or high (above 190 mg/dL) may need treatment in some individuals.

In general, the higher the LDL level and the more risk factors involved, the greater the risk for heart disease. The main goal of treatment in patients with hyperlipidemia is to lower the LDL to a level that will reduce the risk of heart disease.

The primary health care provider may initially seek to control the cholesterol level by encouraging therapeutic

life changes (TLC). This includes a cholesterol-lowering diet (the TLC diet), physical activity, quitting smoking (if applicable), and weight management. The TLC diet is a low–saturated fat and low-cholesterol eating plan that includes less than 200 mg of dietary cholesterol per day. In addition, 30 minutes of physical activity each day is recommended for TLC. Walking at a brisk pace for 30 minutes a day 5 to 7 days a week can help raise the HDL and lower the LDL. Added benefits of a healthy diet and exercise program include a reduction of body weight. If TLC does not result in bringing blood lipids to therapeutic levels, the primary health care provider may add one of the antihyperlipidemic drugs to the treatment plan. TLC is continued along with the drug regimen.

In addition to control of the dietary intake of fat, particularly saturated fatty acids, antihyperlipidemic drug therapy is used to lower serum levels of cholesterol and triglycerides. The primary health care provider may use one drug or, in some instances, more than one antihyperlipidemic drug for those with poor response to therapy with a single drug. Three types of antihyperlipidemic drugs are currently in use, as well as miscellaneous antihyperlipidemic drugs (see Summary Drug Table: Antihyperlipidemic Drugs for a complete listing of the drugs). The various types of drugs used to treat hyperlipidemia are

- Bile acid sequestrants
- HMG-CoA reductase inhibitors
- Fibric acid derivatives
- Niacin

The target LDL level for treatment is less than 130 mg/dL. If the response to drug treatment is adequate, lipid levels are monitored every 4 months. If the response is inadequate, another drug or a combination of two drugs is used. Antihyperlipidemic drugs decrease cholesterol and triglyceride levels in several ways. Although the end result is a lower lipid blood level, each has a slightly different action.

BILE ACID SEQUESTRANTS

Actions

Bile, which is manufactured and secreted by the liver and stored in the gallbladder, emulsifies fat and lipids as these products pass through the intestine. Once emulsified, fats and lipids are readily absorbed in the intestine. The **bile acid sequestrants** bind to bile acids to form an insoluble substance that cannot be absorbed by the intestine, so it is secreted in the feces. With increased loss of bile acids, the liver uses cholesterol to manufacture more bile. This is followed by a decrease in cholesterol levels.

SUMMARY DRUG TABLE ANTIHYPERLIPIDEMIC DRUGS

GENERIC NAME	TRADE NAME	USES	ADVERSE REACTIONS	DOSAGE RANGES
Bile Acid Sequestrants				
cholestyramine *koe-less'-tir-a-meen*	LoCHOLEST, Prevalite, Questran, Questran Light	Hyperlipidemia, relief of pruritus associated with partial biliary obstruction	Constipation (may lead to fecal impaction), exacerbation of hemorrhoids, abdominal pain, distention and cramping, nausea, increased bleeding related to vitamin K malabsorption, vitamin A and D deficiencies	4 g orally 1–6 times/d; individualize dosage based on response
colestipol HCl *koe-les'-ti-pole*	Colestid	Hyperlipidemia	Same as cholestyramine	Granules: 5–30 g/d orally in divided doses Tablets: 2–16 g/d
colesevelam HCl *ko-leh-sev'-eh-lam*	WelChol	Used alone or as adjunctive therapy with an HMG CoA inhibitor to decrease elevated LDL cholesterol	Same as cholestyramine	3–7 tablets/d orally
HMG-CoA Reductase Inhibitors				
atorvastatin *ah-tor'-va-stah-tin*	Lipitor	Primary hyperlipidemia, reduction of elevated total and LDL cholesterol levels and serum triglycerides	Headache (usually mild), flatulence, abdominal pain, cramps, constipation, nausea, dyspepsia, rhabdomyolysis with acute renal failure	10–80 mg/d orally
fluvastatin *flue-va-sta'-tin*	Lescol, Lescol XL	Hyperlipidemia and mixed dyslipidemia, reduction of elevated total and LDL cholesterol levels; slow progression of CAD, along with diet and exercise; secondary prevention of coronary events	Headache (usually mild), blurred vision, dizziness, flatulence, abdominal pain, cramps, constipation, nausea, dyspepsia, rhabdomyolysis	20–80 mg/d orally
lovastatin *loe-va-sta'-tin*	Mevacor	Treatment of familial hypercholesterolemia, hyperlipidemia, reduction of elevated total and LDL cholesterol levels, primary prevention of coronary heart disease in patients with symptomatic disease, secondary prevention of cardiovascular events; adolescents 10–17 y of age with hypercholesterolemia who have heterozygous familial hypercholesterolemia	Same as Fluvastatin	Immediate-release: 10–80 mg/d orally in single or divided doses Extended-release: 10–60 mg/d orally in single dose Adolescent boys and postmenarchal girls: 20–40 mg/d orally

SUMMARY DRUG TABLE   *(continued)*

GENERIC NAME	TRADE NAME	USES	ADVERSE REACTIONS	DOSAGE RANGES
pravastatin *prah-va-sta'-tin*	Pravachol	Hyperlipidemia, reduction of elevated total and LDL cholesterol levels, primary prevention of coronary events (prevention of first MI, to slow progression of CAD, reduce risk of stroke, TIA, and MI), prevention of secondary coronary events; treatment of children 8 y of age or older with heterozygous familial hypercholesterolemia	Headache (usually mild), blurred vision, dizziness, flatulence, abdominal pain, cramps, constipation, nausea	10–40 mg/d orally Children 8–13 y: 20 mg/d orally Adolescents 14–18 y: 40 mg/d orally
rosuvastatin calcium *row-sue'-va-stah-tin*	Crestor	Hyperlipidemia, hypercholesterolemia (heterozygous familial and nonfamilial and mixed dyslipidemia), concomitant lipid-lowering therapy, renal insufficiency	Headache, dizziness, nausea, diarrhea, constipation, pharyngitis, rhinitis, sinusitis, flulike symptoms	5–40 mg/d orally
simvastatin *sim-va-stah'-tin*	Zocor	Hyperlipidemia, reduction of elevated total and LDL cholesterol levels	Headache (usually mild), flatulence, abdominal pain, cramps, constipation, nausea	5–80 mg/d orally
Fibric Acid Derivatives				
clofibrate *klo-fye'-brate*	Atromid-S	Hyperlipidemia	Nausea, vomiting, GI upset, impotence, myalgia (muscle cramping and aching), rash, fatigue, cardiac arrhythmias, cholecystitis, cholelithiasis	2 g/d orally in divided doses
fenofibrate *fen-oh-fye'-brate*	Tricor, Antara, Lofibra	Hyperlipidemia, hypertriglyceridemia	Nausea, constipation, diarrhea, abnormal liver function test results, respiratory problems, GI upset, abdominal pain, back pain, headache, flulike syndrome, cholecystitis, cholelithiasis	Tablet: 48–145 mg/d orally Capsule: 67–200 mg/d orally
gemfibrozil *jem-fye'-broe-zil*	Lopid	Hyperlipidemia hypertriglyceridemia, reduction of CAD risk	Dyspepsia, abdominal pain, diarrhea, nausea, vomiting, rash, vertigo, headache, cholecystitis, cholelithiasis	1200 mg/d orally in two divided doses 30 min before morning and evening meals

GENERIC NAME	TRADE NAME	USES	ADVERSE REACTIONS	DOSAGE RANGES
Miscellaneous Preparations				
ezetimibe *ee-zet'-ah-mibe*	Zetia	Primary hypercholesterolemia	Diarrhea, back pain, sinusitis, dizziness, abdominal pain, arthralgia, coughing, fatigue	10 mg/d orally
niacin (nicotinic acid) *nye'-a-sin*	Niaspan, Niacor	Adjunctive treatment for hyperlipidemia	Generalized flushing sensation of warmth, severe itching and tingling, nausea, vomiting, abdominal pain	Immediate-release: 1–2 g orally BID, TID Extended-release: 500–2000 mg/d orally

CAD, coronary artery disease; GI, gastrointestinal; LDL, low-density lipoprotein; MI, myocardial infarction; TIA, transient ischemic attack.

Uses

The bile acid sequestrants are used to treat

- Hyperlipidemia (in patients who do not have an adequate response to a diet and exercise program)
- Pruritus associated with partial biliary obstruction (cholestyramine only)

Adverse Reactions

- Constipation (may be severe and occasionally result in fecal impaction), aggravation of hemorrhoids, abdominal cramps, flatulence, nausea
- Increased bleeding tendencies related to vitamin K malabsorption, and vitamin A and D deficiencies

Contraindications and Precautions

The bile acid sequestrants are contraindicated in patients with known hypersensitivity to the drugs. Bile acid sequestrants are also contraindicated in those with complete biliary obstruction.

These drugs are used cautiously in patients with liver and kidney disease; they are also used cautiously during pregnancy (category C) and lactation (decreased absorption of vitamins may affect the infant).

Interactions

The following interactions may occur when the bile acid sequestrants are administered with another agent:

Interacting Drug	Common Use	Effect of Interaction
anticoagulants	Blood thinners	Decreased effect of the anticoagulant (cholestyramine)
thyroid hormone	Treatment of hypothyroidism	Loss of efficacy of thyroid; also hypothyroidism (particularly with cholestyramine)
ursodiol	Treatment and prevention of gallstones	Reduced absorption of ursodiol (particularly cholestyramine and colestipol)

When administered with the bile acid sequestrants, a decreased serum level or decreased gastrointestinal (GI) absorption of the following drugs may occur:

- aspirin (used to treat pain)
- clindamycin, penicillin G, and tetracycline (used to treat infection)
- clofibrate and niacin (used to treat elevated cholesterol levels)
- digitalis glycosides (used to treat heart failure)
- furosemide and thiazide diuretics (used to treat edema)
- glipizide (used to treat diabetes)
- hydrocortisone (used to treat inflammation)
- methyldopa and propranolol (used to treat hypertension and cardiovascular problems, respectively)
- phenytoin (used to treat seizures)

Because the bile acids sequestrants, particularly cholestyramine, can decrease the absorption of numerous drugs, the bile acid sequestrants should be administered alone and other drugs given at least 1 hour before or 4 hours after administration of the bile acid sequestrants.

HMG-CoA REDUCTASE INHIBITORS

Actions

Another group of antihyperlipidemic drugs is called **HMG-CoA reductase inhibitors**. HMG-CoA (3-hydroxy-3-methylglutaryl coenzyme A) reductase is an enzyme that is a **catalyst** (a substance that accelerates a chemical reaction without itself undergoing a change) in the manufacture of cholesterol. These drugs appear to have one of two activities, namely, inhibiting the manufacture of cholesterol or promoting the breakdown of cholesterol. Either drug activity lowers the blood levels of cholesterol and serum triglycerides and increases blood levels of HDLs. Examples of these drugs can be found in the Summary Drug Table: Antihyperlipidemic Drugs.

Uses

These drugs, along with a diet restricted in saturated fat and cholesterol, are used

- As adjunct to diet in the treatment of hyperlipidemia when diet and other nonpharmacologic treatments alone have not lowered cholesterol levels.

- For primary prevention of coronary events (in patients with hyperlipidemia without clinically evident coronary heart disease to reduce the risk of myocardial infarction and death from other cardiovascular events, including strokes, transient ischemic attacks, and cardiac revascularization procedures).

- For secondary prevention of cardiovascular events (in patients with hyperlipidemia with evident coronary heart disease to reduce the risk of coronary death, slow the progression of coronary atherosclerosis, and reduce risk of death from stroke/transient ischemic attack; and in those undergoing myocardial revascularization procedures).

Adverse Reactions

The HMG-CoA reductase inhibitors are usually well tolerated. Adverse reactions, when they do occur, are often mild and transient and do not require discontinuing therapy. These reactions may include the following.

Central Nervous System Reactions

- Headache, blurred vision
- Dizziness
- Insomnia

Gastrointestinal Reactions

- Flatulence, abdominal pain, cramping
- Constipation, nausea

Other

- Elevated creatine phosphokinase (CPK) level
- Rhabdomyolysis with possible renal failure

Contraindications and Precautions

The HMG-CoA reductase inhibitors are contraindicated in individuals with hypersensitivity to the drugs or serious liver disorders, and during pregnancy (category X) and lactation.

These drugs are used cautiously in patients with a history of alcoholism, acute infection, hypotension, trauma, endocrine disorders, visual disturbances, and myopathy.

Interactions

The following interactions may occur when the HMG-CoA reductase inhibitors are administered with another agent:

Interacting Drug	Common Use	Effect of Interaction
macrolides, erythromycin, clarithromycin	Treatment of infections	Increased risk of severe myopathy or rhabdomyolysis
amiodarone	Cardiovascular problems	Increased risk of myopathy
niacin	Used to lower elevated cholesterol	Increased risk of severe myopathy or rhabdomyolysis
protease inhibitors	Treatment of human immunodeficiency virus (HIV) infection and acquired immunodeficiency syndrome (AIDS)	Elevated plasma levels of HMG-CoA reductase inhibitors

| verapamil | Treatment of cardiovascular problems and hypertension | Increased risk of myopathy |
| warfarin | Blood thinner (anticoagulant) | Increased anticoagulant effect |

The HMG-CoA reductase inhibitors have an additive effect when used with the bile acid sequestrants, which may provide an added benefit in treating hypercholesterolemia that does not respond to a single-drug regimen.

FIBRIC ACID DERIVATIVES

Actions

Fibric acid derivatives, the third group of antihyperlipidemic drugs, work in a variety of ways. Clofibrate acts to stimulate the liver to increase breakdown of very–low-density lipoproteins (VLDLs) to LDLs, decreasing liver synthesis of VLDLs and inhibiting cholesterol formation. Fenofibrate acts by reducing VLDL and stimulating the catabolism of triglyceride-rich lipoproteins, resulting in a decrease in plasma triglycerides and cholesterol. Gemfibrozil increases the excretion of cholesterol in the feces and reduces the production of triglycerides by the liver, thus lowering serum lipid levels.

Uses

Although the fibric acid derivatives have antihyperlipidemic effects, their use varies depending on the drug. For example, clofibrate and gemfibrozil are used to treat individuals with very high serum triglyceride levels who are at risk for abdominal pain and pancreatitis and who do not experience a response to dietary modifications. Clofibrate is not used for the treatment of other types of hyperlipidemia and is not thought to be effective for preventing coronary heart disease. Fenofibrate is used as adjunctive treatment for reducing LDL, total cholesterol, and triglycerides in patients with hyperlipidemia.

Adverse Reactions

The adverse reactions associated with fibric acid derivatives include

- Nausea, vomiting, and GI upset
- Diarrhea

- Cholelithiasis (stones in the gallbladder) or cholecystitis (inflammation of the gallbladder)

If cholelithiasis is found, the primary health care provider may discontinue the drug. See the Summary Drug Table: Antihyperlipidemic Drugs for additional adverse reactions.

Contraindications and Precautions

The fibric acid derivatives are contraindicated in patients with hypersensitivity to the drugs and in those with significant hepatic or renal dysfunction or primary biliary cirrhosis because these drugs may increase the already elevated cholesterol. The drugs are used cautiously during pregnancy (category C) and lactation and in patients with peptic ulcer disease or diabetes.

Interactions

The following interactions may occur when the fibric acid derivatives are administered with another agent:

Interacting Drug	Common Use	Effect of Interaction
anticoagulants	Blood thinners	Enhanced effects of the anticoagulants (particularly with gemfibrozil and fenofibrate)
cyclosporine	Immunosuppression after organ transplantation	Decreased effects of cyclosporine (particularly with gemfibrozil)
HMG-CoA reductase inhibitors	Treatment of elevated blood cholesterol levels	Increased risk of rhabdomyolysis (particularly with gemfibrozil and fenofibrate)
sulfonylureas	Treatment of diabetes	Increased hypoglycemic effects (particularly with gemfibrozil)

MISCELLANEOUS ANTIHYPERLIPIDEMIC DRUGS

Miscellaneous antihyperlipidemic drugs include niacin and ezetimibe. Niacin is discussed in the text; refer to the

Summary Drug Table: Antihyperlipidemic Drugs for information on ezetimibe.

Actions

The mechanism by which niacin (nicotinic acid) lowers blood lipid levels is not fully understood.

Uses

Niacin is used as adjunctive therapy for lowering very high serum triglyceride levels in patients who are at risk for pancreatitis (inflammation of the pancreas) and whose response to dietary control is inadequate.

Adverse Reactions

Gastrointestinal Reactions

- Nausea, vomiting, abdominal pain
- Diarrhea

Other

- Severe, generalized flushing of the skin, sensation of warmth
- Severe itching or tingling

Contraindications, Precautions, and Interactions

Niacin is contraindicated in patients with known hypersensitivity to niacin, active peptic ulcer, hepatic dysfunction, and arterial bleeding. The drug is used cautiously in patients with renal dysfunction, high alcohol consumption, unstable angina, gout, and pregnancy (category C).

> **Herbal Alert**
>
> *Garlic* has been used for many years throughout the world. The benefits of garlic on cardiovascular health are the best known and most extensively researched benefits of the herb. Its benefits include lowering serum cholesterol and triglyceride levels, improving the ratio of HDL to LDL cholesterol, lowering blood pressure, and helping to prevent the development of atherosclerosis. The recommended dosages of garlic are 600 to 900 mg/d of the garlic powder tablets, 10 mg of garlic oil "perles," or one

> **Herbal Alert** *(continued)*
>
> moderate-sized fresh clove of garlic a day. Adverse reactions include mild stomach upset or irritation that can usually be alleviated by taking garlic supplements with food. There is an increased risk of bleeding when garlic is taken with warfarin. Although no serious reactions have occurred in pregnant women taking garlic, its use is not recommended. Garlic is excreted in breast milk and may cause colic in some infants. As with all herbal therapy, when garlic is used for therapeutic purposes the primary health care provider should be aware of its use.

NURSING PROCESS

The Patient Receiving an Antihyperlipidemic Drug

ASSESSMENT

PREADMINISTRATION ASSESSMENT

Many individuals with hyperlipidemia have no symptoms and the disorder is not discovered until laboratory tests reveal elevated cholesterol and triglyceride levels, elevated LDL levels, and decreased HDL levels. Often, these drugs are initially prescribed on an outpatient basis, but initial administration may occur in the hospitalized patient. Serum cholesterol levels (i.e., a lipid profile) and liver functions tests are obtained before the drugs are administered.

The nurse takes a dietary history, focusing on the types of foods normally included in the diet. Vital signs and weight are recorded. The skin and eyelids are inspected for evidence of xanthomas (flat or elevated yellowish deposits) that may be seen in the more severe forms of hyperlipidemia.

ONGOING ASSESSMENT

Patients usually take these drugs on an outpatient basis and come to the clinic or the primary health care provider's office for periodic monitoring. The primary health care provider usually prescribes frequent monitoring of blood cholesterol and triglyceride levels as a part of the ongoing assessment.

> **Nursing Alert**
>
> Sometimes a paradoxical elevation of blood lipid levels occurs. Should this happen, the primary health care provider is notified because he or she may prescribe a different antihyperlipidemic drug.

During the ongoing assessment, the nurse checks vital signs and assesses bowel functioning because an adverse reaction to these drugs is constipation. Constipation may become serious if not treated.

When administering the HMG-CoA reductase inhibitors and the fibric acid derivatives, the primary health care provider may prescribe liver function tests, such as serum aminotransferase levels, before the drug regimen is started, at 6 and 12 weeks, then periodically thereafter because of the possibility of liver dysfunction with the drugs. The nurse monitors these levels. Any increase in these levels is reported to the primary health care provider. If aspartate aminotransferase (AST) levels increase to three times normal, the primary health care provider may discontinue drug therapy.

Because the maximum effects of these drugs are usually evident within 4 weeks, periodic lipid profiles are ordered to determine the therapeutic effect of the drug regimen. The primary health care provider may increase the dosage, add another antihyperlipidemic drug, or discontinue the drug therapy, depending on the patient's response to therapy.

Herbal Alert

The medicinal uses of the *flax* plant have been wide and varied, ranging from a topical emollient to a laxative. Limited research seems to support its current popular use in improving the blood lipid profile. Flax is available in capsules, oil, powder, soft gel capsules, and the seed form. Until more research is conducted, the herb should not be taken during pregnancy or by lactating women and should not be given to children. Possible adverse reactions include nausea, vomiting, flatulence, diarrhea, and hypersensitivity reactions. Possible toxic reactions include weakness, tachycardia, dyspnea, paralysis, and death. Flax may decrease the absorption of all other medications. The primary health care provider should be aware of the use of any natural supplement.

NURSING DIAGNOSES

Drug-specific nursing diagnoses are highlighted in the Nursing Diagnoses Checklist. Other nursing diagnoses applicable to these drugs are discussed in depth in Chapter 4.

Nursing Diagnoses Checklist

✔ **Constipation** related to adverse drug reactions to antihyperlipidemic drugs

✔ **Risk for Imbalanced Nutrition: Less than Body Requirements** related to adverse drug reactions to antihyperlipidemic drugs

✔ **Risk for Impaired Skin Integrity** related to adverse reactions to antihyperlipidemic drugs (rash, flushing)

✔ **Nausea** related to adverse reactions to antihyperlipidemic drugs

✔ **Risk for Injury** related to adverse reactions to antihyperlipidemic drugs

PLANNING

The expected outcomes for the patient may include an optimal response to therapy (lowered blood lipid levels), meeting patient needs related to the management of common adverse drug reactions, and an understanding of the dietary measures necessary to reduce lipid and lipoprotein levels.

IMPLEMENTATION
PROMOTING AN OPTIMAL RESPONSE TO THERAPY

Because hyperlipidemia is often treated on an outpatient basis, the nurse explains the drug regimen and possible adverse reactions. If printed dietary guidelines are given to the patient, the nurse emphasizes the importance of following these recommendations. Drug therapy usually is discontinued if the antihyperlipidemic drug is not effective after 3 months of treatment.

MONITORING AND MANAGING PATIENT NEEDS

CONSTIPATION Patients taking the antihyperlipidemic drugs, particularly the bile acid sequestrants, may experience constipation. The drugs can produce or severely worsen preexisting constipation. The nurse instructs the patient to increase fluid intake, eat foods high in dietary fiber, and exercise daily to help prevent constipation. If the problem persists or becomes severe, a stool softener or laxative may be required. Some patients require decreased dosage or discontinuation of the drug therapy.

Gerontologic Alert

Older adults are particularly prone to constipation when taking the bile acid sequestrants. The nurse should monitor older adults closely for hard, dry stools, difficulty passing stools, and any complaints of constipation. An accurate record of bowel movements must be kept.

Antihyperlipidemic Drugs

RISK FOR IMBALANCED NUTRITION: LESS THAN BODY REQUIREMENTS Bile acid sequestrants may interfere with the digestion of fats and prevent the absorption of the fat-soluble vitamins (vitamins A, D, E, and K) and folic acid. When the bile acid sequestrants are used for long-term therapy, vitamins A and D may be given in a water-soluble form or administered parenterally.

RISK FOR IMPAIRED SKIN INTEGRITY Patients taking nicotinic acid may experience moderate to severe, generalized flushing of the skin, a sensation of warmth, and severe itching or tingling. Although these reactions are most often seen at higher dose levels, some patients may experience them even when small doses of nicotinic acid are administered. The sudden appearance of these reactions may frighten the patient.

> ### Nursing Alert
>
> The nurse should advise the patient taking nicotinic acid to put the call light on if discomfort is experienced. If the patient is in severe discomfort, the nurse should contact the primary health care provider immediately. The nurse advises outpatients to contact their primary health care provider if these reactions are severe or cause extreme discomfort.

NAUSEA Some of the antihyperlipidemic drugs cause nausea (e.g., fibric acid derivatives, bile acid sequestrants, HMG-CoA reductase inhibitors). If nausea occurs, the drug should be taken with meals or with food. Other measures to help alleviate the nausea include providing a relaxed atmosphere for eating with no unpleasant odors or sights. The nurse can provide the patient with several small meals rather than three large meals. If nausea is severe or vomiting occurs, the primary health care provider is notified.

RISK FOR INJURY Injury can occur when the patient falls as the result of dizziness as an adverse reaction from the fibric acid derivatives or HMG-CoA reductase inhibitors. The nurse monitors the hospitalized patient carefully, placing the call light within easy reach. The patient may require assistance with ambulation until the effects of the medication are known, especially if the nurse is administering the initial doses of the antihyperlipidemic.

POTENTIAL COMPLICATION: VITAMIN K DEFICIENCY The nurse checks the patients for bruises over the body. The patient is encouraged to include foods high in vitamin K in the diet, such as asparagus, broccoli, green beans, lettuce, turnip greens, beef liver, collard greens, green tea,

and spinach. If bruising is observed or if bleeding tendencies occur as the result of vitamin K deficiency, the nurse reports this to the primary health care provider. Parenteral vitamin K may be prescribed by the primary health care provider for immediate treatment, and oral vitamin K for preventing a deficiency in the future.

POTENTIAL COMPLICATION: RHABDOMYOLYSIS The antihyperlipidemic drugs, particularly the HMG-CoA reductase inhibitors, have been associated with skeletal muscle effects leading to rhabdomyolysis. **Rhabdomyolysis** is a very rare condition in which muscle damage results in the release of muscle cell contents into the bloodstream. Rhabdomyolysis may precipitate renal dysfunction or acute renal failure. The nurse is alert for unexplained muscle pain, muscle tenderness, or weakness, especially if accompanied by malaise or fever. These symptoms should be reported to the primary health care provider because the drug may need to be discontinued.

EDUCATING THE PATIENT AND FAMILY

The nurse stresses the importance of following the diet recommended by the primary health care provider because drug therapy alone will not significantly lower cholesterol and triglyceride levels. The nurse provides a copy of the recommended diet and reviews the contents of the diet with the patient and family. If necessary, the nurse refers the patient or family member to a teaching dietitian, a dietary teaching session, or a lecture provided by a hospital or community agency (see Patient and Family Teaching Checklist: Using Diet and Drugs to Control High Blood Cholesterol Levels). The nurse also develops a teaching plan to include various important points for the various kinds of agents used to manage cholesterol levels.

BILE ACID SEQUESTRANTS The nurse advises the patient to take the drug before meals unless the primary health care provider directs otherwise. For the various forms of bile acid sequestrants, the nurse may add teaching points such as the following:

- *Cholestyramine powder*: The prescribed dose must be mixed in 2 to 6 fluid ounces of water or noncarbonated beverage and shaken vigorously. The powder can also be mixed with highly fluid soups or pulpy fruits (e.g., applesauce, crushed pineapple). The powder should not be ingested in the dry form. Other drugs are taken 1 hour before or 4 to 6 hours after cholestyramine. Cholestyramine is available combined with the artificial sweetener aspartame (Questran Light) for patients with diabetes or those who are concerned with weight gain.

Patient and Family Teaching Checklist

Using Diet and Drugs to Control High Blood Cholesterol Levels

The nurse:

☑ Reviews the reasons for the drug and prescribed drug therapy, including drug name, form and method of preparation, correct dose, and frequency of administration.

☑ Emphasizes that drug therapy alone will not significantly lower blood cholesterol levels.

☑ Stresses importance of taking drug exactly as prescribed.

☑ Reinforces the importance of adhering to prescribed diet.

☑ Provides a written copy of dietary plan and reviews contents.

☑ Contacts dietitian for assistance with diet teaching.

☑ Answers questions and offers suggestions for ways to reduce dietary fat intake.

☑ Instructs in possible adverse reactions and signs and symptoms to report to primary health care provider.

☑ Reviews measures to minimize gastrointestinal upset.

☑ Explains possible need for vitamin A and D therapy and high-fiber foods if patient is receiving bile acid sequestrant.

☑ Reassures that results of therapy will be monitored by periodic laboratory and diagnostic tests and follow-up with primary health care provider.

- *Colestipol granules*: The prescribed dose must be mixed in liquids, soup, cereals, carbonated beverages, or pulpy fruits. Use approximately 90 mL of liquid and, when mixing with a liquid, slowly stir the preparation until ready to drink. The granules will not dissolve. Take the entire drug, rinse the glass with a small amount of water, and drink to ensure that all the medication is taken.

- *Colestipol tablets*: Tablets should be swallowed whole, one at a time, with a full glass of water or other fluid—not chewed, cut, or crushed.

- *Colesevelam tablets*: This drug formulation is taken once or twice daily with meals.

- Constipation, nausea, abdominal pain, and distention may occur and may subside with continued therapy.

The primary health care provider is notified if these effects become bothersome or if unusual bleeding or bruising occurs.

HMG-CoA REDUCTASE INHIBITORS Typically, lovastatin is taken once daily, preferably with the evening meal. Fluvastatin, simvastatin, and pravastatin are taken once daily in the evening or at bedtime. The patient should not drink grapefruit juice while taking these drugs. On the other hand:

- Advise taking rosuvastatin calcium as a single dose once daily in the evening. If the patient is taking antacids, they should be taken at least 2 hours after the rosuvastatin.

- Inform the patient that if fluvastatin or pravastatin is prescribed with a bile acid sequestrant, the fluvastatin should be taken 2 hours after the bile acid sequestrant and pravastatin at least 4 hours afterward.

- Explain that these drugs cannot be used during pregnancy (category X). Use a barrier contraceptive while taking these drugs. If the patient wishes to become pregnant while taking these drugs, the primary health care provider should be consulted before efforts at conception.

- Advise the patient to contact the primary health care provider as soon as possible if nausea; vomiting; muscle pain, tenderness, or weakness; fever; upper respiratory infection; rash; itching; or extreme fatigue occurs.

FIBRIC ACID DERIVATIVES Some important teaching points for fibric acid derivatives follow:

- *Clofibrate*: If GI upset occurs, instruct the patient to take the drug with food and notify the primary health care provider if chest pain, shortness of breath, palpitations, nausea, vomiting, fever, chills, or sore throat occurs.

- *Gemfibrozil*: Explain that dizziness or blurred vision may occur. Observe caution when driving or performing hazardous tasks. Notify the primary health care provider if epigastric pain, diarrhea, nausea, or vomiting occurs.

MISCELLANEOUS PREPARATIONS Teaching points to cover regarding nicotinic acid and ezetimibe include the following:

- *Nicotinic acid*: Advise the patient to take this drug with meals. This drug may cause mild to severe facial flushing, a sensation of warmth, severe itching, or headache. These symptoms usually subside with continued therapy, but contact the primary health care provider as soon as possible if symptoms are severe. The primary health care provider may prescribe aspirin (325 mg) to be taken about 30 minutes before nicotinic acid to decrease the flushing reaction. If dizziness occurs, avoid sudden changes in posture.

- *Ezetimibe*: Explain that ezetimibe should be taken at least 2 hours before or 4 hours after a bile acid sequestrant. Report unusual muscle pain, weakness, or tenderness, severe diarrhea, or respiratory infections.

EVALUATION

- The therapeutic effect is achieved and serum lipid levels are decreased.

- Adverse reactions are identified, reported to the primary health care provider, and managed successfully through nursing interventions.

- The patient reports improved bowel movements.

- Nutritional needs for vitamins are met.

- Skin remains intact.

- Nausea is controlled.

- The patient reports no injury related to dizziness or falls.

- The patient and family demonstrate an understanding of the treatment regimen.

Critical Thinking Exercises

1. A patient in the medical clinic is taking cholestyramine (Questran) for hyperlipidemia. The primary health care provider has prescribed therapeutic life changes for the patient. The patient is on a low-fat diet and walks daily for exercise. His major complaint at this visit is constipation, which is very bothersome to him. Discuss how you would approach this situation with the patient. What information would you give the patient concerning his constipation?

2. Discuss the important points to include in a teaching plan for a patient who is prescribed atorvastatin (Lipitor).

3. Describe the important aspects of the ongoing assessment when administering fluvastatin to a patient.

Review Questions

1. Which of the following adverse reactions is most common in a patient taking a bile acid sequestrant?

   A. Anorexia

   B. Vomiting

   C. Constipation

   D. Headache

2. Lovastatin is best taken _____.

   A. once daily, preferably with the evening meal

   B. three times daily with meals

   C. at least 1 hour before or 2 hours after meals

   D. twice daily without regard to meals

3. When assessing a patient taking cholestyramine (Questran) for vitamin K deficiency, the nurse would _____.

   A. check the patient for bruising

   B. keep a record of the patient's intake and output

   C. monitor the patient for myalgia

   D. keep a dietary record of foods eaten

4. A patient taking niacin reports flushing after each dose of the niacin. Which of the following drugs would the nurse expect to be prescribed to help alleviate the flushing?

   A. meperidine (Demerol)

   B. aspirin

   C. vitamin K

   D. diphenhydramine (Benadryl)

5. Which of the following points would the nurse include when teaching a patient about drug and diet therapy for hyperlipidemia?

   A. Fluids are taken in limited amounts when eating a low-fat diet.

   B. The medication should be taken at least 1 hour before meals.

   C. Medication alone will not lower cholesterol.

   D. Meat is not allowed on a low-fat diet.

Medication Dosage Problems

1. A patient is prescribed 10 mg simvastatin orally daily for high cholesterol. The drug is available in 5-mg tablets. The nurse administers _____.

2. The primary health care provider prescribes fenofibrate for the treatment of hypertriglyceridemia. The patient is now taking 200 mg/d orally. Is this an appropriate dosage? If not, what action would you take? If the dose is appropriate, how many capsules would you administer if the drug is available in 67-mg capsules? _____

To check your answers, see Appendix G.

Drugs That Affect the Hematologic System

*H*eme is an ancient word referring to iron-binding groups that carry oxygen. This is how the hematologic system gets its name because one of the primary purposes of the system is to carry oxygen from the lungs to the cells by way of the blood. The red cells (erythrocytes) of the blood are the vehicles used to carry oxygen in the body. When adequate oxygen is not delivered to the tissues, anemia results. The system of channels used for this transportation is the vascular system: the arteries, veins, and capillaries. The chapters in Unit VII discuss drugs used to maintain the system (blood vessels) and drugs used to treat anemias.

Blockage of the vessels in the form of blood clots can occur in the hematologic system. Chapter 43 discusses the drugs used to prevent (anticoagulants or antiplatelets) and the drugs used to remove (thrombolytics) blood clots from the blood vessels.

Various diseases can cause the body to reduce the number of red blood cells that carry oxygen. Drugs used to enhance the production of red blood cells, or components of the cells, such as iron and folic acid, are covered in Chapter 44.

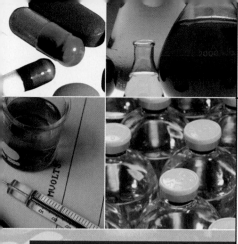

Anticoagulant and Thrombolytic Drugs

embolus
fibrolytic
hemostasis
heparin lock
lysis
prothrombin
thrombolytic
thrombosis
thrombus

Learning Objectives

On completion of this chapter, the student will:

- Describe hemostasis and thrombosis.

- Discuss the uses, general drug actions, adverse reactions, contraindications, precautions, and interactions of anticoagulant, antiplatelet, and thrombolytic drugs.

- Discuss important preadministration and ongoing assessment activities the nurse should perform on the

patient taking an anticoagulant, antiplatelet, or thrombolytic drug.

- List nursing diagnoses particular to a patient taking an anticoagulant, antiplatelet, or thrombolytic drug.

- Discuss ways to promote an optimal response to therapy, how to manage common adverse reactions, and important points to keep in mind when educating patients about the use of an anticoagulant, antiplatelet, or thrombolytic drug.

When a blood vessel is injured, a series of events occurs to form a clot and stop the bleeding. This process is called **hemostasis**. It involves a complex process also called the *coagulation cascade*. Figure 43-1 shows the blood clotting pathway and the extrinsic and intrinsic factors involved. The blood clotting or coagulation cascade is so named because as each factor is activated, it acts as a catalyst that enhances the next reaction, with the net result being a large collection of fibrin (the clot) that forms a plug in the vessel, thus stopping the bleeding. This is a normal event, taking a few minutes, that happens daily in response to tears and leaks in blood vessels throughout the body. **CONCEPTS**in action**ANIMATION**

Thrombosis is the formation of a blood clot, or **thrombus**. A thrombus may form in any vessel (artery or vein), impeding blood flow. For example, a venous thrombus can develop as the result of venous stasis (decreased blood flow), injury to the vessel wall, or altered blood coagulation. Venous thrombosis most often occurs in the lower extremities and is associated with venous stasis. Deep vein thrombosis (DVT) occurs in the lower extremities and is the most common type of venous thrombosis.

Arterial thrombosis can occur because of atherosclerosis or arrhythmias, such as atrial fibrillation. The thrombus may begin small, but fibrin, platelets, and red blood cells attach to the thrombus, increasing its size. When a thrombus detaches itself from the wall of the vessel and is carried along through the bloodstream, it becomes an **embolus**. The embolus travels until it reaches a vessel that is too small to permit its passage. If the embolus goes to the lung and obstructs a pulmonary vessel, it is called a *pulmonary embolism* (PE). Similarly, if the embolus detaches and occludes a vessel supplying blood to the heart, it can cause a myocardial infarction (MI).

The type of drugs discussed in this chapter include drugs that prevent the formation of blood clots (anticoagulants), drugs that suppress platelet aggregation (antiplatelets), and drugs that help to eliminate the clot (thrombolytics).

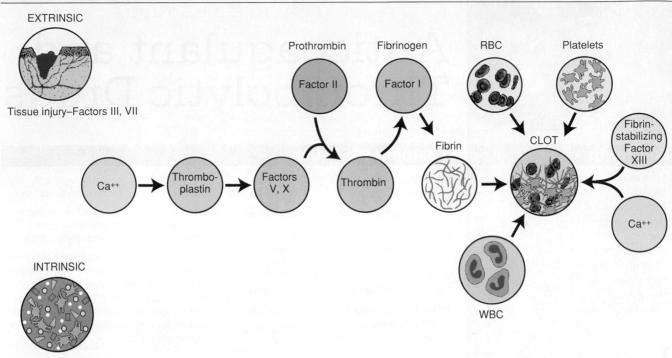

EXTRINSIC

Tissue injury—Factors III, VII

INTRINSIC

Platelets Thromboplastin Precursors
Factors VIII, IX, XI, XII

Figure 43.1 The blood clotting pathway. Blood coagulation results in the formation of a stable fibrin clot. Formation of this clot involves a cascade of interactions of clotting factors, platelets, and other substances. Clotting factors exist in the blood in inactive form and must be converted to an active form before the next step in the clotting pathway can occur. Each factor is stimulated in turn until the process is complete and a fibrin clot is formed. In the intrinsic pathway, all of the components necessary for clot formation are in the circulating blood. Clot formation in the intrinsic pathway is initiated by factor XII. In the extrinsic pathway, coagulation is initiated by release of tissue thromboplastin, a factor not found in circulating blood. RBC, red blood cell; WBC, white blood cell.

ORAL AND PARENTERAL
ANTICOAGULANTS

Anticoagulants are used to prevent the formation and extension of a thrombus. Anticoagulants have no direct effect on an existing thrombus and do not reverse any damage from the thrombus. However, once the presence of a thrombus has been established, anticoagulant therapy can prevent additional clots from forming. Although they do not thin the blood, they are commonly called *blood thinners* by patients. The anticoagulant group of drugs includes warfarin (a coumarin derivative), anisindione (an indandione derivative), and fractionated and unfractionated heparin. The anticoagulant drugs are used prophylactically in patients who are at high risk for clot formation.

Warfarin (Coumadin), a coumarin derivative, is the oral anticoagulant most commonly prescribed. Although

primarily given by the oral route, warfarin is also available for parenteral administration. Because it can be given orally, it is the drug of choice for patients requiring long-term therapy with an anticoagulant. Peak activity is reached 1.5 to 3 days after therapy is initiated. Anisindione (Miradon), an indandione derivative, is less frequently used but is an effective anticoagulant.

Heparin preparations are available as heparin sodium and the low–molecular-weight heparins (LMWHs; fractionated heparins). Heparin is not a single drug, but rather a mixture of high– and low–molecular-weight drugs. Examples of LMWH include dalteparin (Fragmin), enoxaparin (Lovenox), and tinzaparin (Innohep). LMWHs produce very stable responses when administered at recommended dosages. Because of this stability, frequent laboratory monitoring, as with heparin, is not necessary. In addition, bleeding is less likely to occur with LMWHs than with heparin.

Actions

All anticoagulants interfere with the clotting mechanism of the blood. Warfarin and anisindione interfere with the manufacturing of vitamin K–dependent clotting factors by the liver. This results in the depletion of clotting factors II (**prothrombin**), VII, IX, and X. It is the depletion of prothrombin (see Fig. 43-1), a substance that is essential for the clotting of blood, that accounts for most of the action of warfarin.

By comparison, heparin inhibits the formation of fibrin clots, inhibits the conversion of fibrinogen to fibrin, and inactivates several of the factors necessary for the clotting of blood. Heparin cannot be taken orally because it is inactivated by gastric acid in the stomach; therefore, it must be given by injection. The LMWHs act to inhibit clotting reactions by binding to antithrombin III, which inhibits the synthesis of factor X and the formation of thrombin. These drugs have no effect on clots that have already formed and aid only in preventing the formation of new blood clots.

Uses

The anticoagulants are used for

- Prevention (prophylaxis) and treatment of DVT
- Prevention and treatment of atrial fibrillation with embolization
- Prevention and treatment of PE
- Adjuvant treatment of MI
- Prevention of thrombus formation after valve replacement surgery

Parenteral anticoagulants are used specifically for

- Prevention of postoperative DVT and PE in certain patients undergoing surgical procedures, such as major abdominal surgery
- Prevention of clotting in arterial and heart surgery, in the equipment used for extracorporeal (occurring outside the body) circulation (e.g., in dialysis procedures), in blood transfusions, and in blood samples for laboratory purposes
- Prevention of a repeat cerebral thrombosis in some patients who have experienced a stroke
- Treatment of coronary occlusion, acute MI, and peripheral arterial embolism
- Diagnosis and treatment of disseminated intravascular coagulation (DIC), a severe hemorrhagic disorder
- Maintaining patency of intravenous (IV) catheters (very low doses of 10 to 100 units)

Adverse Reactions

The principal adverse reaction associated with anticoagulants is *bleeding*, which may range from very mild to severe. Bleeding may be seen in many areas of the body, such as the skin (bruising and petechiae), bladder, bowel, stomach, uterus, and mucous membranes. Other adverse reactions are rare but may include

- Nausea, vomiting, abdominal cramping, diarrhea
- Alopecia (loss of hair)
- Rash or urticaria (severe skin rash)
- Hepatitis (inflammation of the liver), jaundice (yellowish discoloration of the skin and mucous membranes), thrombocytopenia (low platelet count), and blood dyscrasias (disorders)

Additional adverse reactions include local irritation when heparin is given by the subcutaneous (SC) route. Hypersensitivity reactions may also occur with any route of administration and include fever and chills. More serious hypersensitivity reactions include an asthma-like reaction and an anaphylactic reaction. See the Summary Drug Table: Anticoagulant, Antiplatelet, and Thrombolytic Agents for additional adverse reactions.

Contraindications

Anticoagulants are contraindicated in patients with known hypersensitivity to the drugs, active bleeding (except when caused by DIC), hemorrhagic disease, tuberculosis, leukemia, uncontrolled hypertension, gastrointestinal (GI) ulcers, recent surgery of the eye or central nervous system, aneurysms, or severe renal or hepatic disease, and during lactation. Use during pregnancy can cause fetal death (oral agents are in pregnancy category X and parenteral agents are in pregnancy category C). The LMWHs are also contraindicated in patients with a hypersensitivity to pork products.

Precautions

Anticoagulants are used cautiously in patients with fever, heart failure, diarrhea, diabetes, malignancy, hypertension, renal or hepatic disease, psychoses, or depression. Women of childbearing age must use a reliable contraceptive to prevent pregnancy. These drugs are used with caution in all patients with a potential site for bleeding or hemorrhage.

SUMMARY DRUG TABLE ANTICOAGULANT, ANTIPLATELET, AND THROMBOLYTIC AGENTS

GENERIC NAME	TRADE NAME	USES	ADVERSE REACTIONS	DOSAGE RANGES
Oral Anticoagulants				
anisindione *ah-nis-in-dye'-on*	Miradon	Prophylaxis/treatment of venous thrombosis	Bleeding, fatigue, dizziness, abdominal cramping	25–300 mg/d orally, individualized dose based on PT or INR
warfarin sodium *war'-far-in*	Coumadin	Prophylaxis/treatment of venous thrombosis	Same as anisindione	2–10 mg/d orally, individualized dose based on PT or INR: IV form for injection
Parenteral Anticoagulants				
heparin *hep'-ah-rin*		Thrombosis/embolism, diagnosis and treatment of disseminated intravascular coagulation, prophylaxis of DVT, clotting prevention	Bleeding, chills, fever, urticaria, local irritation, erythema, mild pain, hematoma or bruising at the injection site (SC)	10,000–20,000 Units SC in divided doses q8–12h; 5000–10,000 Units - q4–6h intermittent IV; 5000–40,000 Units/d IV infusion
heparin sodium lock flush solution		Clearing intermittent infusion lines (heparin lock) to prevent clot formation at site	None significant	10–100 Units/mL heparin solution
Parenteral Anticoagulants: Low–Molecular-Weight Heparins				
dalteparin sodium *dal-tep'-a-rin*	Fragmin	Unstable angina/ non–Q-wave MI, DVT prophylaxis	Bleeding, bruising, rash, fever, erythema and irritation at site of injection	Angina/MI: 120 Units/kg SC q12h with concurrent oral aspirin DVT: 2500 Units/d SC
enoxaparin sodium *en-ocks'-a-par-in*	Lovenox	DVT and presurgical prophylaxis, PE treatment, unstable angina/ non–Q-wave MI	Same as dalteparin sodium	DVT prophylaxis: 30–40 mg SC q12h Treatment: 1 mg/kg SC q12h
tinzaparin sodium *ten-zah'-pear-in*	Innohep	DVT treatment	Same as dalteparin sodium	12,000–17,000 Units/d SC
Antiplatelet Agents				
abciximab *ab-sicks'-ih-mab*	ReoPro	Adjunct in coronary angioplasty	Bleeding, pain	0.125 mcg/kg/min IV during procedure
cilostazol *sill-ahs'-tah-zoll*	Pletal	Intermittent claudication	Heart palpitations, dizziness, diarrhea, headache	100 mg orally BID
clopidogrel *cloe-pid'-oh-grel*	Plavix	Recent MI, stroke, and acute coronary syndrome	Dizziness, skin rash, chest pain, constipation	Single loading dose: 300 mg; 75 mg/d orally

GENERIC NAME	TRADE NAME	USES	ADVERSE REACTIONS	DOSAGE RANGES
eptifibatide *ep-tiff-ib'-ah-tide*	Integrilin	Adjunct in coronary angioplasty, acute coronary syndrome	Bleeding, pain	1 mcg/kg/min IV infusion
ticlopidine *tye-kloh'-pih-deen*	Ticlid	Thrombotic stroke	Nausea, dyspepsia, diarrhea	250 mg orally BID
tirofiban *tye-row-feye-ban*	Aggrastat	Acute coronary syndrome	Bleeding, pain	0.4–0.1 mcg/kg/min IV infusion
treprostinil *treh-pros'-tin-ill*	Remodulin	Pulmonary arterial hypertension	Dyspnea, fatigue, chest pain, pallor, headache, rash, nausea, diarrhea	0.625–1.25 nanogram/kg/min (very small doses) IV or SC infusion
Thrombolytics				
alteplase, recombinant *al'-te-plaze*	Activase, Cathflo Activase (for IV catheter occlusions only)	Acute MI, acute ischemic stroke, PE, IV catheter clearance	Bleeding (GU, gingival, intracranial) and epistaxis, ecchymosis	Total dose of 90–100 mg IV, given as a 2- to 3-h infusion
reteplase, recombinant *ret'-ah-plaze*	Retavase	Acute MI	Bleeding (GI, GU, or at injection site), intracranial hemorrhage, anemia	Prepackaged: 2- to 10-Unit IV bolus injections
streptokinase *strep-toe-kye'-nase*	Streptase	Acute MI, DVT, PE, embolism	Minor bleeding (superficial and surface) and major bleeding (internal and severe)	250,000 Units IV loading dose, followed by 100,000 Units for 24–72 h
tenecteplase *teh-nek'-ti-plaze*	TNKase	Acute MI	Bleeding (GI, GU, or at injection site), intracranial hemorrhage, anemia	Dosage based on weight, not to exceed 50 mg IV
urokinase *yoor-oh'-kye-nase*	Abbokinase	PE, lysis of coronary artery thrombi, IV catheter clearance	Minor bleeding (superficial and surface) and major bleeding (internal and severe)	PE: 4400 Units/kg IV over 10 min, followed by 4400 Units/kg/h for 12 h
Anticoagulant Antagonists				
phytonadione (vitamin K) *fye-toe-na-dye'-on*	Aqua-Mephyton, Mephyton	Treatment of warfarin overdosage	Gastric upset, unusual taste, flushing, rash, urticaria, erythema, pain and/or swelling at injection site	2.5–10 mg oral, IM, may repeat orally in 12–48 h or in 6–8 h after parenteral dose
protamine sulfate *proe'-ta-meen*		Treatment of heparin overdose	Flushing and warm feeling, dyspnea, bradycardia, hypotension	Dose is determined by amount of heparin to be neutralized; generally, 1 mg IV neutralizes 100 Units of heparin

DVT, deep vein thrombosis; GI, gastrointestinal; GU, genitourinary; INR, international normalized ratio; MI, myocardial infarction; PE, pulmonary embolism; PT, prothrombin time.

Anticoagulant and Thrombolytic Drugs

Interactions

The following interactions may occur when an anticoagulant is administered with another agent:

Interacting Drug	Common Use	Effect of Interaction
aspirin, acetaminophen, nonsteroidal anti-inflammatory drugs (NSAIDs), and chloral hydrate	Pain relief and sedation	Increased risk for bleeding
penicillin, aminoglycosides, isoniazid, tetracyclines, and cephalosporins	Anti-infective agents	Increased risk for bleeding
beta blockers and loop diuretics	Treatment of cardiac problems	Increased risk for bleeding
disulfiram and cimetidine	Management of GI distress	Increased risk for bleeding
oral contraceptives, barbiturates, diuretics, and vitamin K	Birth control, sedation, treatment of cardiac problems and bleeding disorders, respectively	Decreased effectiveness of the anticoagulant

Herbal Alert

Warfarin, a drug with a narrow therapeutic index, has the potential to interact with many herbal remedies. For example, warfarin should not be combined with any of the following substances because they may have additive or synergistic activity and increase the risk for bleeding: celery, chamomile, clove, dong quai, feverfew, garlic, ginger, ginkgo biloba, ginseng, green tea, onion, passion flower, red clover, St. John's wort, and turmeric. Any herbal remedy should be used with caution in patients taking warfarin.

Because the absorption, metabolism, distribution, and elimination characteristics of most herbal products are poorly understood, much of the information on herb–drug interactions is speculative. Herb–drug interactions are sporadically reported and difficult to determine.

Because herbal supplements are not regulated by the U.S. Food and Drug Administration (FDA), products lack standardization with regard to purity and potency. In addition, multiple ingredients in products and batch-to-batch variation make it difficult to determine if reactions occur as the result of the herb itself. To assist with the identification of herb–drug interactions, nurses should report any potential interactions to the FDA through its MedWatch program (see Appendix A). It is especially important to take special care when patients are taking any drugs with a narrow therapeutic index (the difference between the minimum therapeutic and minimum toxic drug concentrations is small—such as warfarin) and herbal supplements.

ANTIPLATELET DRUGS

Thrombi forming in the venous system are composed primarily of fibrin and red blood cells. In contrast, it is believed that arterial thrombosis formation is due to clumping of platelet aggregates. Therefore, anticoagulant drugs prevent thrombosis in the venous system and the antiplatelet drugs prevent thrombus formation in the arterial system. In addition to aspirin therapy, the antiplatelet drugs include adenosine diphosphate (ADP) receptor blockers and glycoprotein receptor blockers.

Actions and Uses

These drugs work by decreasing the platelets' ability to stick together (aggregate) in the blood, thus forming a clot. Aspirin works by prohibiting the aggregation of the platelets for the lifetime of the platelet. The ADP blockers alter the platelet cell membrane, preventing aggregation. Glycoprotein receptor blockers work to prevent enzyme production, again inhibiting platelet aggregation. Antiplatelet drug therapy is designed primarily to treat patients at risk for acute coronary syndrome, MI, stroke, and intermittent claudication.

Adverse Reactions

Some of the more common adverse reactions include
- Heart palpitations
- Bleeding
- Dizziness and headache
- Nausea, diarrhea, constipation, dyspepsia

Contraindications and Precautions

Antiplatelet drugs are contraindicated in pregnant or lactating patients and those with known hypersensitivity to the drugs, congestive heart failure, active bleeding, or thrombotic thrombocytopenic purpura (TTP). These drugs are to be used cautiously in elderly patients, pancytopenic patients, or those with renal or hepatic impairment. If TTP is diagnosed, the antiplatelet treatment should be stopped immediately. Antiplatelet drugs should be discontinued 1 week before any surgical procedure.

Interactions

The following interactions may occur when an antiplatelet is administered with another agent:

Interacting Drug	Common Use	Effect of Interaction
aspirin and NSAIDs	Pain relief	Increased risk of bleeding
macrolide antibiotics	Anti-infective agents	Increased effectiveness of anti-infective
digoxin	Management of cardiac problems	Decreased digoxin serum levels
phenytoin	Control of seizure activity	Increased phenytoin serum levels

THROMBOLYTIC DRUGS

Whereas the anticoagulant agents prevent thrombus formation, the **thrombolytic** class of drugs dissolves blood clots that have already formed within the walls of a blood vessel. These drugs reopen blood vessels after they become occluded. Another term used to describe the thrombolytic drugs is **fibrolytic**. Examples of the thrombolytics include alteplase recombinant (Activase), streptokinase (Streptase), and tenecteplase (TNKase).

Actions

Although the exact action of each of the thrombolytic drugs is slightly different, these drugs break down fibrin clots by converting plasminogen to plasmin. Plasmin is an enzyme that breaks down the fibrin of a blood clot. This reopens blood vessels after their occlusion and prevents tissue necrosis. Because thrombolytic drugs dissolve all clots encountered (both occlusive and those repairing vessel leaks), bleeding is a great concern when using these agents. Before these drugs are used, their potential benefits must be weighed carefully against the potential dangers of bleeding.

Uses

These drugs are used to treat

- Acute MI by **lysis** (breaking up) of blood clots in the coronary arteries
- Blood clots causing pulmonary emboli and DVT
- Suspected occlusions in central venous catheters

See the Summary Drug Table: Anticoagulant, Antiplatelet, and Thrombolytic Agents for a more complete listing of the use of these drugs.

Adverse Reactions

Bleeding is the most common adverse reaction seen with the use of these drugs. Bleeding may be internal and involve areas such as the GI tract, genitourinary tract, and the brain. Bleeding may also be external (superficial) and seen at areas of broken skin, such as venipuncture sites and recent surgical wounds. Allergic reactions may also be seen.

Contraindications and Precautions

Thrombolytic drugs are contraindicated in patients with known hypersensitivity to the drugs, active bleeding, history of stroke, aneurysm, and recent intracranial surgery.

These drugs are used cautiously in patients who have recently undergone major surgery (within 10 days), such as coronary artery bypass grafting; who experienced stroke, trauma, vaginal or cesarean section delivery, GI bleeding, or trauma within the last 10 days; or who have hypertension, diabetic retinopathy, or any condition in which bleeding is a significant possibility; and in patients currently receiving oral anticoagulants. All of the thrombolytic drugs discussed in this chapter are classified in pregnancy category C, with the exception of urokinase, which is a pregnancy category B drug.

Interactions

When a thrombolytic is administered with medications that prevent blood clots, such as aspirin, dipyridamole, or an anticoagulant, the patient is at increased risk for bleeding.

NURSING PROCESS

The Patient Receiving Anticoagulant, Antiplatelet, or Thrombolytic Drugs

ASSESSMENT

PREADMINISTRATION ASSESSMENT

Before administering the first dose of an anticoagulant or thrombolytic, the nurse questions the patient about all drugs taken during the previous 2 to 3 weeks (if the patient was recently admitted to the hospital). If the patient took any drugs before admission, the nurse notifies the primary health care provider before the first dose is administered. Usually, the prothrombin time (PT) is assessed and the international normalized ratio (INR) determined before therapy begins. The first dose of warfarin is not given until blood is drawn for a baseline PT/INR test. The dosage is individualized based on the results of the PT or the INR.

Before administering the first dose of heparin, the nurse obtains the patient's vital signs. The most commonly used test to monitor heparin is the activated partial thromboplastin time (APTT). To obtain baseline data, blood is drawn for laboratory studies before giving the first dose of heparin.

If the patient has a DVT, it usually occurs in a lower extremity. The nurse examines the extremity for color and skin temperature. The nurse also checks for a pedal pulse, noting the rate and strength of the pulse. It is important to record any difference between the affected extremity and the unaffected extremity. The nurse notes areas of redness or tenderness and asks the patient to describe current symptoms. The affected extremity may appear edematous and a positive Homans' sign (pain in the calf when the foot is dorsiflexed) may be elicited. A positive Homans' sign suggests DVT.

Blood for a complete blood count is usually drawn before the administration of the thrombolytic agents. Most patients receiving a thrombolytic agent are admitted or transferred to an intensive care unit because close monitoring is necessary for 48 hours or more after therapy. If the patient is experiencing pain because of the blood clot, the nurse does a thorough pain assessment.

ONGOING ASSESSMENT

In the ongoing assessment, a patient receiving an anticoagulant, antiplatelet, or thrombolytic drug requires close observation and careful monitoring. During the course of therapy for both oral and parenteral drugs, the nurse continually assesses the patient for any signs of bleeding and hemorrhage. Areas of assessment include the gums, nose, stools, urine, or nasogastric drainage. Level of consciousness should be assessed on a routine basis to monitor for intracranial bleeding.

Patients receiving warfarin for the first time often require daily adjustment of the dose, which is based on the daily PT/INR results. The nurse withholds the drug and notifies the primary health care provider if the PT exceeds 1.2 to 1.5 times the control value or the INR ratio exceeds 3. A daily PT is performed until it stabilizes and when any other drug is added to or removed from the patient's drug regimen. After the PT has stabilized, it is monitored every 4 to 6 weeks. See Display 43-1 for more information on the laboratory tests for monitoring warfarin.

The dosage of heparin is adjusted according to daily APTT monitoring. A therapeutic dosage is attained when the APTT is 1.5 to 2.5 times the normal. The LMWHs have little or no effect on the APTT values. Special monitoring of clotting times is not necessary when administering the drugs. Periodic platelet counts, hematocrit, and tests for occult blood in the stool should be performed throughout the course of heparin therapy.

> ### Nursing Alert
>
> Blood coagulation tests for those receiving heparin by continuous IV infusion are taken at periodic intervals (usually every 4 hours) determined by the primary health care provider. If the patient is receiving long-term heparin therapy, blood coagulation tests may be performed at less frequent intervals.

It is also important that the nurse monitor for any indication of hypersensitivity reaction. The nurse reports reactions, such as chills, fever, or hives, to the primary health care provider. The nurse examines the skin temperature and color in the patient with a DVT for signs of improvement. The nurse takes and records vital signs every 4 hours or more frequently, if needed. When heparin is given to prevent the formation of a thrombus, the nurse observes the patient for signs of thrombus formation every 2 to 4 hours. Because the signs and symptoms of thrombus formation vary and depend on the area or organ involved, the nurse should evaluate and report any complaint the patient may have or any change in the patient's condition to the primary health care provider.

Display 43.1 Understanding Prothrombin Time and International Normalized Ratio

Prothrombin time (also called protime) and the international normalized ratio (INR) are used to monitor the patient's response to warfarin therapy. The daily dose of the oral anticoagulant is based on the patient's daily PT/INR. In the past, recommended therapeutic ranges for PT were 1.5 to 2.5 times the control value. However, today most laboratories use less sensitive substances for testing, and adjustments must be made to reflect this decreased sensitivity. When using the less sensitive substance, the therapeutic range of the PT is 1.2 to 1.5 times the control value. Studies indicate that levels greater than 2 times the control value do not provide additional therapeutic effects in most patients and are associated with a higher incidence of bleeding.

Most laboratories report results for the INR along with the patient's PT and the control value. The INR was devised as a way to standardize PT values and represents a way to "correct" the routine PT results from different laboratories using various sources of thromboplastin and methods of preparation for the test. The INR is determined by a mathematical equation comparing the patient's PT with the standardized PT value. Some institutions may use only PT, others PT/INR, and some may use INR. The INR is maintained between 2 and 3.

NURSING DIAGNOSES

Drug-specific nursing diagnoses are highlighted in the Nursing Diagnoses Checklist. Other nursing diagnoses applicable to these drugs are discussed in depth in Chapter 4.

Nursing Diagnoses Checklist

✓ **Risk for Injury** related to excessive bleeding due to drug therapy

✓ **Individual Effective Therapeutic Regimen Management** related to inability to communicate drug use if incapacitated

✓ **Anxiety** related to fear of atypical bleeding during thrombolytic drug therapy

PLANNING

The expected outcomes for the patient may include an optimal response to therapy, support of patient needs related to the management of adverse reactions, and an understanding of the postdischarge drug regimen.

IMPLEMENTATION
PROMOTING AN OPTIMAL RESPONSE TO THERAPY

ORAL ADMINISTRATION OF ANTICOAGULANTS Before administering each dose of warfarin, the nurse checks the prothrombin flow sheet or the laboratory report to review the current PT/INR results. The nurse notifies the primary health care provider before administering the drug if these results are outside of the acceptable parameters.

To hasten the onset of the therapeutic effect, a higher dosage (loading dose) may be prescribed for 2 to 4 days, followed by a maintenance dosage adjusted according to the daily PT/INR. Otherwise, the drug takes 3 to 5 days to reach therapeutic levels. When rapid anticoagulation is required, heparin is preferred as a loading dose, followed by maintenance dose of warfarin based on the PT or INR.

Nursing Alert

Optimal therapeutic results are obtained when the patient's PT is 1.2 to 1.5 times the control value. In certain instances, such as in recurrent systemic embolism, a PT of 1.5 to 2 may be prescribed. Studies indicate that diet can influence the PT/INR values. Patients whose PT/INR levels fluctuate should be asked about their food intake and any recent dietary changes. In patients receiving warfarin, a diet high in vitamin K may decrease the PT/INR and increase the risk of clot formation. A diet low in vitamin K may prolong the PT/INR and increase the risk of hemorrhage. Significant changes in vitamin K intake may necessitate a warfarin dosage adjustment. The key to vitamin K management for patients receiving warfarin is maintaining a consistent daily intake of vitamin K. To avoid large fluctuations in vitamin K intake, patients receiving warfarin should be aware of the vitamin K content of food (see Home Care Checklist: Ensuring Appropriate Vitamin K Intake). For example, green leafy vegetables and some vegetable oils (soybean and canola oil) are high in vitamin K. The use of these oils in food preparation may increase the intake of vitamin K enough to cause the PT/INR results to fluctuate. Root vegetables, fruits, cereals, dairy products, and meats are generally low in vitamin K.

PARENTERAL ADMINISTRATION OF ANTICOAGULANTS Heparin preparations, unlike warfarin, must be given by the parenteral route, preferably SC or IV. The onset of

Home Care Checklist

Ensuring Appropriate Vitamin K Intake

Patients receiving oral anticoagulants need to avoid eating excessive amounts of food containing vitamin K. Otherwise, the anticoagulant will not be effective. Be sure your patient knows what foods contain vitamin K. Include the following list in your teaching plan:

☑ Cabbage

☑ Cauliflower

☑ Cheese

☑ Egg yolk

☑ Green leafy vegetables (e.g., spinach)

☑ Liver

☑ Molasses

☑ Yogurt

Nursing Alert

If the patient is receiving heparin by intermittent or continuous IV infusion, other drugs administered by the IV route are not given through the IV tubing or injection port or piggybacked into the continuous IV line unless the primary health care provider orders the drug given in this manner. In addition, the nurse should never mix other drugs with heparin when heparin is given by any route.

---

anticoagulation is almost immediate after a single dose. Maximum effects occur within 10 minutes of administration. Clotting time returns to normal within 4 hours unless subsequent doses are given. Although warfarin is most often administered orally, an injectable form may be used as an alternative route for patients who are unable to receive oral drugs.

Heparin may be given by intermittent IV administration, continuous IV infusion, and the SC route. Intramuscular (IM) administration is avoided because of the possibility of the development of local irritation, pain, or hematoma (a collection of blood in the tissue). The dosage of heparin is measured in units and is available in various dosage strengths as Units per milliliter (e.g., 10,000 Units/mL). When selecting the strength used for administration, choose the strength closest to the prescribed dose. For example, if 5000 Units are ordered, and the available strengths are 1000, 5000, 7500, 20,000, and 40,000 Units/mL, use 1 mL of the 5000 Units/mL for administration.

An infusion pump must be used for the safe administration of heparin by continuous IV infusion. The nurse checks the infusion pump every 1 to 2 hours to ensure that it is working properly. The needle site is inspected for signs of inflammation, pain, and tenderness along the pathway of the vein. If these occur, the infusion is discontinued and restarted in another vein.

When heparin is given by the SC route, administration sites are rotated and the site used is recorded on the patient's chart. The recommended sites of administration are those on the abdomen, but areas within 2 inches of the umbilicus are avoided because of the increased vascularity of that area. Other areas of administration are the buttocks and lateral thighs.

Bruising may be decreased by applying an ice cube to the site before injection of the drug. The nurse inserts the needle into the tissue at a 90-degree angle and injects the drug. It is not necessary to aspirate before injecting the drug. The application of firm pressure after the injection helps to prevent hematoma formation. Each time heparin is given by this route, the nurse inspects all recent injection sites for signs of inflammation (redness, swelling, tenderness) and hematoma formation.

Blood coagulation tests are usually ordered before and during heparin therapy, and the dose of heparin is adjusted to the test results. Coagulation tests are usually performed 30 minutes before the scheduled dose and from the extremity opposite the infusion site. When administering heparin by the SC route, an APTT test is performed 4 to 6 hours after the injection. Optimal results of therapy are obtained when the APTT is 1.5 to 2.5 times the control value. The LMWHs do not require close monitoring of blood coagulation tests.

A complete blood count, platelet count, and stool analysis for occult blood may be ordered periodically throughout therapy. Thrombocytopenia may occur during heparin or antiplatelet administration. A mild, transient thrombocytopenia may occur 2 to 3 days after heparin therapy is begun. This early development of thrombocytopenia tends to resolve itself despite continued therapy. The nurse reports a platelet count of less than 100,000 mm^3 immediately because the primary health care provider may choose to discontinue the heparin therapy. Overdose of antiplatelet drugs is typically managed by withholding treatment or by infusion of platelets.

Nursing Alert

The nurse should withhold the drug and contact the primary health care provider immediately if any of the following occurs:

- The PT exceeds 1.5 times the control value.
- There is evidence of bleeding.
- The INR is greater than 3.

ADMINISTRATION OF THROMBOLYTICS For optimal therapeutic effect, the thrombolytic drugs are used as soon as possible after the formation of a thrombus, preferably within 4 to 6 hours or as soon as possible after the symptoms are identified. The greatest benefit follows drug administration within 4 hours, but significant benefits occur when the agents are used within the first 24 hours. The nurse must follow the primary health care provider's orders precisely regarding dosage and time of administration. These drugs are available in powder form and must be reconstituted according to the directions in the package insert.

The nurse must assess the patient for bleeding every 15 minutes during the first 60 minutes of therapy, every 15 to 30 minutes for the next 8 hours, and at least every 4 hours until therapy is completed. Vital signs are taken at least every 4 hours for the duration of therapy.

If pain is present, the primary health care provider may order an opioid analgesic. Once the clot dissolves and blood flows freely through the obstructed blood vessel, severe pain usually decreases.

DRUGS USED TO MAINTAIN INTRAVENOUS LINE PATENCY Intermittent IV administration may require ready access to a vein without having to maintain a continuous infusion. The use of an adapter and tubing that stays in the vein is called a **heparin lock**. A solution of dilute heparin consisting of 10 to 100 Units/mL may be ordered for injection into the heparin lock before and after the administration of the dose of a drug administered by the intermittent IV route. This is called a heparin lock flush. The flush solution aids in preventing small clots from obstructing the needle of the intermittent IV administration set. To prevent incompatibility of heparin with other drugs, the heparin lock set is flushed with sterile water or sterile normal saline solution before and after any drug is given through the IV line. The primary health care provider or institutional policy dictates the use and type of heparin lock flush solution.

Each time heparin is given, the nurse inspects the needle site for signs of inflammation, pain, and tenderness along the pathway of the vein. If these should occur, the use of this site is discontinued and a new intermittent set is inserted at a different site.

If peripheral IV catheters become troublesome, typically they are removed and a new site is initiated; however, this is not possible with central venous catheters. These catheters can become blocked at the opening by fibrin, which causes an occlusion. Only nurses trained specifically in the technique of clearing catheter occlusions should attempt this intervention. When using thrombolytics to clear an occluded IV catheter, the nurse follows the manufacturer's instructions in the packaged insert. The nurse avoids using excessive pressure when the drug is injected into the catheter. Excessive force could rupture the catheter or expel the clot into the circulation. It is important to remember that if the catheter is occluded by substances other than blood fibrin clots, such as drug precipitates, thrombolytics are not effective.

Nursing Alert

Streptokinase is not used for restoring IV catheter patency. Serious adverse reactions, including hypotension, hypersensitivity, apnea, and bleeding, have occurred when the drug is used for this purpose.

MONITORING AND MANAGING PATIENT NEEDS

RISK FOR INJURY Bleeding can occur any time during therapy with warfarin or the heparin preparations, even when the PT appears to be within a safe limit (e.g., 1.2 to 1.5 times the control value). All nursing personnel and medical team members should be made aware of any patient receiving warfarin and the observations necessary with administration. If bleeding should occur, the primary health care provider may decrease the dose, discontinue the heparin therapy for a time, or order the administration of protamine sulfate. The nurse makes the following checks for signs of bleeding:

- If a decided drop in blood pressure or rise in the pulse rate occurs, the nurse notifies the primary health care provider because this may indicate internal bleeding. Because hemorrhage may begin as a slight bleeding or bruising tendency, the nurse frequently observes the patient for these occurrences. Sometimes, hemorrhage occurs without warning.

- Urinal, bedpan, catheter drainage unit—Inspect the urine for a pink to red color and the stool for signs of GI bleeding (bright red to black stools). Visually check the catheter drainage every 2 to 4 hours and when the unit is emptied. Oral anticoagulants may impart a red-orange color to alkaline urine, making hematuria difficult to detect visually. A urinalysis may be necessary to determine if blood is in the urine.

- Emesis basin, nasogastric suction units—Visually check the nasogastric suction unit every 2 to 4 hours and when the unit is emptied. Check the emesis basin each time it is emptied.

- Skin, mucous membranes—Inspect the patient's skin daily for evidence of easy bruising or bleeding. Be alert for bleeding from minor cuts and scratches, nosebleeds, or excessive bleeding after IM, SC, or IV injections or after a venipuncture. After oral care, check the toothbrush and gums for signs of bleeding.

INDIVIDUAL EFFECTIVE THERAPEUTIC REGIMEN MANAGEMENT The patient needs to be aware of the many food and drug interactions that can cause a higher risk for bleeding when taking anticoagulants, or make the drugs less effective. Should the patient become incapacitated by accident or illness, other care providers need to know that anticoagulant or antiplatelet drugs are being taken. The nurse should instruct the patient to wear medical identification that states he or she is receiving anticoagulant or antiplatelet therapy.

The patient is instructed to notify all health care providers of the anticoagulant or antiplatelet therapy when diagnostic tests or other treatments are performed. The patient should understand why the nurse must apply prolonged pressure to needle or catheter sites after venipuncture, removal of central or peripheral IV lines, and IM and SC injections. Laboratory personnel or those responsible for drawing blood for laboratory tests are made aware of anticoagulant therapy because prolonged pressure on the venipuncture site is necessary. All laboratory requests should have a notation stating the patient is receiving anticoagulant therapy.

ANXIETY Bleeding is the most common adverse reaction when thrombolytic drugs are administered. Conditions requiring thrombolytic treatment are typically of an urgent nature and treatment occurs in special care units of the hospital such as the intensive care unit or operating room. Combined with the potential for bleeding, all this can be frightening and anxiety producing to the patient and any family members present. As the nurse monitors the patient's status, it is important to reassure the patient and communicate with family members that measures are being taken to diagnose and intervene early for any adverse reactions.

Throughout administration of the thrombolytic drug, the nurse assesses for signs of bleeding and hemorrhage. Internal

bleeding may involve the GI tract, genitourinary tract, intracranial sites, or respiratory tract. Signs and symptoms of internal bleeding may include abdominal pain, coffee-ground emesis, black, tarry stools, hematuria, joint pain, and spitting or coughing up blood.

Superficial bleeding may occur at venous or arterial puncture sites or recent surgical incision sites. Again, this can be disturbing to the patient and family and they may become anxious. Because fibrin is lysed during therapy, bleeding from recent injection sites may occur. The nurse must carefully monitor all potential bleeding sites (including catheter insertion sites, arterial and venous puncture sites, cutdown sites, and needle puncture sites). The nurse reassures the patient that bleeding will be reported to the primary health care provider and steps taken to minimize the bleeding. Minor bleeding at a puncture site can usually be controlled by applying pressure for at least 30 minutes at the site, followed by the application of a pressure dressing. The puncture site is checked frequently for evidence of further bleeding. IM injections and nonessential handling of the patient are avoided during treatment. Venipunctures are done only when absolutely necessary.

>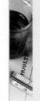
> **Nursing Alert**
>
> Heparin may be given along with or after administration of a thrombolytic drug to prevent another thrombus from forming. However, administration of an anticoagulant increases the risk for bleeding. The patient must be monitored closely for internal and external bleeding.

If uncontrolled bleeding is noted or the bleeding appears to be internal, the nurse stops the drug and immediately contacts the primary health care provider because whole blood, packed red cells, or fresh frozen plasma may be required. Vital signs are monitored every hour or more frequently for at least 48 hours after the drug is discontinued. The nurse contacts the primary health care provider if there is a marked change in one or more of the vital signs. Any signs of an allergic (hypersensitivity) reaction, such as difficulty breathing, wheezing, hives, skin rash, and hypotension, are reported immediately to the primary health care provider.

MANAGING ANTICOAGULANT OVERDOSAGE

ORAL ANTICOAGULANTS Symptoms of warfarin overdosage include blood in the stool (melena); petechiae (pinpoint-sized red hemorrhagic spots on the skin); oozing from superficial injuries, such as cuts from shaving or bleeding from the gums after brushing the teeth; or excessive menstrual bleeding. The nurse must immediately report to the primary health care provider any of these adverse reactions or evidence of bleeding.

If bleeding occurs, if the PT exceeds 1.5 times the control value, or the INR exceeds 3, the primary health care provider may either discontinue the anticoagulant therapy for a few days or order vitamin K_1 (phytonadione), an oral anticoagulant antagonist, which should be readily available when a patient is receiving warfarin. Because warfarin interferes with the synthesis of vitamin K_1–dependent clotting factors, the administration of vitamin K_1 reverses the effects of warfarin by providing the necessary ingredient to enhance clot formation and stop bleeding. However, withholding one or two doses of warfarin may quickly bring the PT to an acceptable level.

The nurse must assess the patient for additional evidence of bleeding until the PT is below 1.5 times the control value or until the bleeding episodes cease. The PT generally returns to a safe level within 6 hours of administration of vitamin K_1. Administration of whole blood or plasma may be necessary if severe bleeding occurs because of the delayed onset of action of vitamin K_1.

PARENTERAL ANTICOAGULANT In most instances, discontinuation of the drug is sufficient to correct overdosage because the duration of action of heparin is brief. However, if hemorrhaging is severe, the primary health care provider may order protamine sulfate, the specific heparin antagonist or antidote. Protamine sulfate is also used to treat overdosage of the LMWHs. Protamine sulfate has an immediate onset of action and a duration of 2 hours. It counteracts the effects of heparin and brings blood coagulation test results to within normal limits. The drug is given slowly by the IV route over a period of 10 minutes.

If administration of this drug is necessary, the nurse monitors the patient's blood pressure and pulse rate every 15 to 30 minutes for 2 hours or more after administration of the heparin antagonist. The nurse immediately reports to the primary health care provider any sudden decrease in blood pressure or increase in the pulse rate. The nurse observes the patient for new evidence of bleeding until blood coagulation test results are within normal limits. To replace blood loss, the primary health care provider may order blood transfusions or fresh frozen plasma.

EDUCATING THE PATIENT AND FAMILY

The nurse provides a full explanation of the drug regimen to patients taking an anticoagulant, antiplatelet, or thrombolytic drug, including an explanation of the problems that can occur during therapy. A thorough review of the dosage regimen, possible adverse drug reactions, and early signs of bleeding tendencies help the patient cooperate with the prescribed therapy. The nurse should include the following points in a patient and family teaching plan:

- Follow the dosage schedule prescribed by the primary health care provider, and report any signs of active bleeding immediately.

- The PT or INR will be monitored periodically. Keep all primary health care provider and laboratory appointments because dosage changes may be necessary during therapy.

- Do not take or stop taking other drugs except on the advice of the primary health care provider. This includes nonprescription drugs, as well as those prescribed by a primary health care provider or dentist.

- Inform the dentist or other primary health care providers of therapy with this drug before any treatment or procedure is started or drugs are prescribed.

- Take the drug at the same time each day.

- Do not change brands of anticoagulants without consulting a physician or pharmacist.

- Avoid alcohol unless use has been approved by the primary health care provider. Advise the patient to limit foods high in vitamin K, such as leafy green vegetables, beans, broccoli, cabbage, cauliflower, cheese, fish, and yogurt. Vegetables with large amounts of vitamin K can interfere with the anticoagulant's effect (see Home Care Checklist: Ensuring Appropriate Vitamin K Intake).

- Keep in mind that antiplatelet drugs can lower all blood counts, including the white cell count. Patients may be at greater risk of infection during the first 3 months of treatment.

- If evidence of bleeding occurs, such as unusual bleeding or bruising, bleeding gums, blood in the urine or stool, black stool, or diarrhea, omit the next dose of the drug and contact the primary health care provider immediately (anisindione may cause a red-orange discoloration of alkaline urine).

- Use a soft toothbrush and consult a dentist regarding routine oral hygiene, including the use of dental floss. Use an electric razor when possible to avoid small skin cuts.

- Women of childbearing age should use a reliable contraceptive to prevent pregnancy.

- Wear or carry medical identification, such as a MedicAlert bracelet, to inform medical personnel and others of therapy with this drug.

EVALUATION

- The therapeutic drug effect is achieved.

- Adverse reactions are identified, reported to the primary health care provider, and managed successfully using appropriate nursing interventions.

- The patient demonstrates an understanding of the drug regimen.

- The patient verbalizes the importance of complying with the prescribed therapeutic regimen.

- The patient lists or describes early signs of bleeding.

Critical Thinking Exercises

1. Ms. Jackson, aged 56 years, is hospitalized with a venous thrombosis. The primary health care provider orders SC heparin. In developing a care plan for Ms. Jackson, discuss the nursing interventions that would be most important to prevent complications while administering heparin. Provide a rationale for each intervention.

2. Mr. Harris, aged 72 years, is a widower who has lived alone since his wife died 5 years ago. He has been prescribed warfarin to take at home after his dismissal from the hospital. Determine which questions concerning the home environment would be important to ask Mr. Harris to prepare him to care for himself and prevent any complications associated with the warfarin.

3. A patient enters the emergency department with an acute MI. Thrombolytic therapy is begun with streptokinase. Discuss ongoing assessments that are important for the nurse to perform.

4. Discuss the use of laboratory tests in monitoring heparin administration.

Review Questions

1. The patient is receiving oral anticoagulant drug therapy. Before administering the drug, the nurse _____.

   A. administers a loading dose of heparin

   B. has the laboratory draw blood for a serum potassium level

   C. takes the apical pulse

   D. sees that blood has been drawn for a baseline prothrombin time evaluation

2. Optimal prothrombin time (PT) during therapy is _____.

   A. more than 15 seconds

   B. less than 25 seconds

   C. 1.8 to 2 times the control value

   D. 1.2 to 1.5 times the control value

3. There is an increased risk for bleeding when the patient receiving heparin is also taking _____.

   A. allopurinol

   B. NSAIDs

   C. digoxin

   D. furosemide

4. In which of the following situations would the nurse expect an LMWH to be prescribed?

   A. To prevent a DVT

   B. For a patient with DIC

   C. To prevent hemorrhage

   D. For a patient with atrial fibrillation

5. If bleeding is noted while a patient is receiving a thrombolytic drug, the patient may receive _____.

   A. heparin

   B. whole blood or fresh frozen plasma

   C. a diuretic

   D. protamine sulfate

Medication Dosage Problems

1. The patient is prescribed 5000 Units of heparin. The drug is available as a solution of 7500 Units/mL. The nurse administers _____.

2. Oral warfarin 5 mg is prescribed. On hand are 2.5-mg tablets. The nurse administers _____.

To check your answers, see Appendix G.

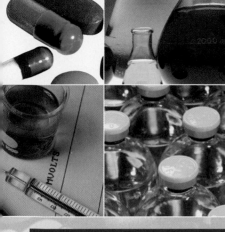

Chapter 44

Agents Used in the Treatment of Anemia

Key Terms

anemia
erythropoiesis
folinic acid rescue
intrinsic factor
iron deficiency anemia
leucovorin rescue
macrocytic anemia
megaloblastic anemia

Learning Objectives

On completion of this chapter, the student will:

- Describe the different types of anemia.
- List the drugs used in the treatment of anemia.
- Discuss the actions, uses, general adverse reactions, contraindications, precautions, and interactions of the agents used to treat anemia.
- Discuss important preadministration and ongoing assessment activities

the nurse should perform on a patient receiving an agent used to treat anemia.

- Identify nursing diagnoses particular to a patient receiving an agent used to treat anemia.
- Discuss ways to promote an optimal response to therapy and important points to keep in mind when educating patients about the use of an agent used to treat anemia.

A nemia is a condition caused by an insufficient amount of hemoglobin delivering oxygen to the tissues. Causes of anemia include a decrease in the number of red blood cells (RBCs), a decrease in the amount of hemoglobin in RBCs, or both. There are various types and causes of anemia. For example, anemia can result from blood loss, excessive destruction of RBCs, inadequate production of RBCs, and deficits in various nutrients, as in iron deficiency anemia. Once the type and cause have been identified, the primary health care provider selects a method of treatment.

The anemias discussed in this chapter include iron deficiency anemia, anemia in patients with chronic illness such as renal disease, pernicious anemia, and anemia resulting from a folic acid deficiency. Table 44-1 defines these anemias.

DRUGS USED IN TREATING IRON DEFICIENCY ANEMIA

When the body does not have enough iron to supply its own needs, the resulting condition is **iron deficiency anemia**. Iron is the component in hemoglobin that picks up oxygen from the lungs and carries it to the body tissues. Iron deficiency anemia is a very common type of anemia. Approximately 50% of pregnant women and 20% of all women experience anemia. Decreased iron stores result from a decrease in RBCs; causes include heavy menstrual bleeding and poor absorption or lack of iron in the diet.

Actions and Uses

Iron preparations act by elevating the serum iron concentration, which replenishes hemoglobin and depleted iron stores. Oral iron supplements are typically used.

Table 44.1 Anemias

Type of Anemia	Description
Iron deficiency	Anemia characterized by an inadequate amount of iron in the body to produce hemoglobin
Anemia in chronic renal failure	Anemia resulting from a reduced production of erythropoietin, a hormone secreted by the kidney that stimulates the production of RBCs
Pernicious anemia	Anemia resulting from lack of secretion by the gastric mucosa of the intrinsic factor essential to the formation of RBCs and the absorption of vitamin B_{12}
Folic acid deficiency	Anemia occurring because of a dietary lack of folic acid, a component necessary in the formation of RBCs

RBCs, red blood cells.

Iron is best absorbed on an empty stomach. Supplemental iron is needed during pregnancy and lactation because normal dietary intake rarely supplies the required amount.

Parenteral iron is used when the patient cannot take oral drugs or when the patient experiences gastrointestinal (GI) intolerance to oral iron administration. Other iron preparations, both oral and parenteral, used in treating iron deficiency anemia can be found in the Summary Drug Table: Drugs Used in the Treatment of Anemia.

Adverse Reactions

Gastrointestinal Reactions

- GI irritation
- Nausea, vomiting
- Constipation, diarrhea
- Darker (black) stools

Generalized System Reactions

- Headache
- Backache
- Allergic reactions

When given parenterally, additional adverse reactions include soreness, inflammation, and sterile abscesses at the intramuscular (IM) injection site. When iron is administered by the IM route, a brownish discoloration of the skin may occur. Intravenous (IV) administration may result in phlebitis at the injection site.

Contraindications and Precautions

Iron supplements are contraindicated in patients with known hypersensitivity to the drug or any component of the drug. Iron compounds are contraindicated in patients with hemochromatosis or hemolytic anemia. Iron compounds are used cautiously in patients with hypersensitivity to aspirin because these patients may have a hypersensitivity to the tartrazine or sulfite content of some iron compounds.

The parenteral form of iron can cause anaphylactic-type reactions and should be used only when oral supplement is contraindicated.

Interactions

The following interactions may occur when an iron preparation is administered with another agent:

Interacting Drug	Common Use	Effect of Interaction
antibiotics	Fight infection	Decreased GI absorption of the antibiotic
levothyroxine	Treatment of hypothyroidism	Decreased absorption of levothyroxine
levodopa, methyldopa	Treatment of Parkinson's disease	Decreased effect of antiparkinsonism medication
ascorbic acid (vitamin C)	Vitamin supplement	Increased absorption of iron

DRUGS USED IN TREATING ANEMIA ASSOCIATED WITH CHRONIC ILLNESS

Anemia may occur in patients with chronic illness as a result of disease treatment. Cancer and chronic renal failure are two diseases that produce disease- or treatment-related anemia. Erythropoietin is a glycoprotein that stimulates and regulates the production of erythrocytes (RBCs). Chronic renal failure reduces the kidney's ability to produce erythropoietin. Cancer treatment reduces the bone marrow's ability to produce RBCs. Two examples of drugs used to treat anemia associated with chronic illness are epoetin alfa (Epogen) and darbepoetin alfa (Aranesp).

SUMMARY DRUG TABLE   DRUGS USED IN THE TREATMENT OF ANEMIA

GENERIC NAME	TRADE NAME	USES	ADVERSE REACTIONS	DOSAGE RANGES
darbepoetin alfa *dar-bah-poe-e'-tin*	Aranesp	Anemia associated with CRF and nonmyeloid cancers	Hypertension, hypotension, headache, diarrhea, vomiting, nausea, myalgia, arthralgia, cardiac arrhythmias, cardiac arrest	CRF: 0.45 mcg/kg IV, SC weekly Cancer: 2.25 mcg/kg SC weekly
epoetin alfa (erythropoietin; EPO) *e-po-e'-tin*	Epogen, Procrit	Anemias associated with CRF, zidovudine therapy in human immunodeficiency virus–infected patients, patients with cancer receiving chemotherapy, patients undergoing elective nonvascular surgery	Hypertension, headache, nausea, vomiting, fatigue, skin reaction at injection site	50–150 Units/kg 3 times weekly SC (IV if dialysis machine used)
ferrous fumarate *fair'-us*	Feostat	Prevention and treatment of iron deficiency anemia	GI irritation, nausea, vomiting, constipation, diarrhea, allergic reactions	Daily requirements: males, 10 mg/d orally; females, 18 mg/d orally; during pregnancy and lactation, 30–60 mg/d orally Replacement in deficiency states; 90–300 mg/d (6 mg/kg/d) orally for 6–10 mo
ferrous gluconate	Fergon	Prevention and treatment of iron deficiency anemia	Same as ferrous fumarate	Same as ferrous fumarate
ferrous sulfate	Feosol, Fer-In-Sol	Prevention and treatment of iron deficiency anemia	Same as ferrous fumarate	Same as ferrous fumarate
folic acid *foe'-lik*	Folvite	Megaloblastic anemia due to deficiency of folic acid	Allergic sensitization	Up to 1 mg/d orally, IM, IV, SC
iron dextran	DexFerrum, InFeD	Iron deficiency anemia (only when oral form is contraindicated)	Anaphylactoid reactions, soreness and inflammation at injection site, chest pain, arthralgia, backache, convulsions, pruritus, abdominal pain, nausea, vomiting, dyspnea	Dosage (IV, IM) based on body weight and grams percent (g/dL) of hemoglobin
iron sucrose	Venofer	Iron deficiency anemia in renal failure, via dialysis machine	Hypotension, cramps, leg cramps, nausea, headache, vomiting, diarrhea, dizziness	100 mg elemental iron by slow IV infusion or during dialysis session
leucovorin calcium *loo-koe-vor'-in*	Wellcovorin	Treatment of megaloblastic anemia; leucovorin rescue after high-dose methotrexate therapy	Allergic sensitization, urticaria, anaphylaxis	See cancer therapy

Agents Used in the
Treatment of Anemia

SUMMARY DRUG TABLE *(continued)*

GENERIC NAME	TRADE NAME	USES	ADVERSE REACTIONS	DOSAGE RANGES
sodium ferric gluconate complex	Ferrlecit	Iron deficiency	Flushing, hypotension, syncope, tachycardia, dizziness, pruritus, dyspnea, conjunctivitis, hyperkalemia	125 mg of elemental iron IV over at least 10 min
vitamin B₁₂ (cyanocobalamin) *sye-an-oh-koe-bal'-a-min*		Vitamin B₁₂ deficiencies, GI pathology; Schilling's test	Mild diarrhea, itching, edema, anaphylaxis	Schilling's test: 100–1000 mcg/d for 2 wk, then 100–1000 mcg IM every month

CRF, chronic renal failure; GI, gastrointestinal.

Actions and Uses

Epoetin alfa is a drug that stimulates **erythropoiesis**. Erythropoiesis is the process of making RBCs. The drug acts in a manner similar to that of natural erythropoietin. Epoetin alfa is used to treat anemia associated with

- Chronic renal failure
- Chemotherapy for cancer treatment
- Zidovudine (AZT) therapy for human immunodeficiency virus infection
- Postsurgical blood replacement in place of allogeneic transfusions

Darbepoetin alfa is an erythropoiesis-stimulating protein used to treat anemia associated with chronic renal failure in patients receiving dialysis, as well as in patients who are not receiving dialysis. These drugs elevate or maintain RBC levels and decrease the need for transfusions.

Chronic illness treatment can cause the reduction of other blood elements, such as white blood cells (WBCs) and platelets. A group of drugs called hematopoietic growth factors help to stimulate the bone marrow to increase production of RBCs, WBCs, and platelets. Table 44-2 presents

Table 44.2 Hematopoietic Growth Factors

Generic Name	Trade Name	Cell Line Stimulated
epoetin alfa	Epogen, Procrit	Red blood cells
darbepoetin alfa	Aranesp	Red blood cells
filgrastim	Neupogen	White blood cells (neutrophils)
pegfilgrastim	Neulasta	White blood cells (neutrophils)
sargramostim	Leukine	White blood cells
oprelvekin	Neumega	Platelets

other hematopoietic growth factors in addition to epoetin alfa and darbepoetin alfa.

Adverse Reactions

Epoetin alfa (erythropoietin; EPO) and darbepoetin alfa are usually well tolerated. The most common adverse reactions include

- Hypertension
- Headache
- Nausea, vomiting, diarrhea
- Rashes
- Fatigue
- Arthralgia, and skin reaction at the injection site

See the Summary Drug Table: Drugs Used in the Treatment of Anemia for more information on these drugs.

Contraindications and Precautions

Epoetin alfa is contraindicated in patients with uncontrolled hypertension, those needing an emergency transfusion, and those with a hypersensitivity to human albumin. Darbepoetin alfa (Aranesp) is contraindicated in patients with uncontrolled hypertension or in those allergic to the drug. Polycythemia (an overload of RBCs in the circulation) can occur if the hemoglobin is not carefully monitored and the dosage is too high.

Epoetin alfa and darbepoetin alfa are used with caution in patients with hypertension, heart disease, congestive heart failure, or a history of seizures. Both of these drugs are pregnancy category C drugs and are used cautiously during pregnancy and lactation.

DRUGS USED IN TREATING FOLIC ACID DEFICIENCY ANEMIA

Folic acid (folate) is required for the manufacture of RBCs in the bone marrow. Folic acid is found in leafy green vegetables, fish, meat, poultry, and whole grains. A deficiency of folic acid results in **megaloblastic anemia**. Megaloblastic anemia is characterized by the presence of large, abnormal, immature erythrocytes circulating in the blood.

Actions and Uses

Folic acid is used in treating megaloblastic anemias that are caused by a deficiency of folic acid. Although neural tube defects are not related to anemia, studies indicate there is a decreased risk for embryonic neural tube defects if folic acid is taken before conception and during early pregnancy. Neural tube defects occur during early pregnancy, when the embryonic folds forming the spinal cord and brain join together. Defects of this type include anencephaly (congenital absence of brain and spinal cord), spina bifida (defect of the spinal cord), and meningocele (a saclike protrusion of the meninges in the spinal cord or skull). The U.S. Public Health Service recommends the use of folic acid for all women of childbearing age to decrease the incidence of neural tube defects. Dosages during pregnancy and lactation are as great as 0.8 mg/d.

Oral supplements are the first choice for megaloblastic anemia and folic acid deficiency treatment. If a patient is unable to take oral medications, leucovorin may be used. This drug is a derivative (an active reduced form) of folic acid. Leucovorin is more commonly used to diminish the hematologic effects of methotrexate, a drug used in treating certain types of cancer (see Chapter 55). Leucovorin "rescues" normal cells from the destruction caused by methotrexate and allows them to survive. This technique of administering leucovorin after a large dose of methotrexate is called **folinic acid rescue** or **leucovorin rescue**.

Adverse Reactions

Few adverse reactions are associated with the administration of folic acid. Rarely, parenteral administration may result in allergic hypersensitivity.

Contraindications and Precautions

Folic acid and leucovorin are contraindicated for treating pernicious anemia or for other anemias in which vitamin B$_{12}$ is deficient. Folic acid is a pregnancy category A drug and is generally considered safe for use during pregnancy. Pregnant women are more likely to experience folate deficiency because folic acid requirements are increased during pregnancy. Pregnant women with a folate deficiency are at increased risk for complications of pregnancy and fetal abnormalities. The recommended dietary allowance (RDA) of folate during pregnancy is 0.4 mg/d, and during lactation, 0.26 to 0.28 mg/d. Although the potential for fetal harm appears remote, the drug should be used cautiously and only within the RDA guidelines.

Interactions

Signs of folate deficiency may occur when sulfasalazine is administered concurrently. An increase in seizure activity may occur when folic acid is administered with the hydantoins (antiseizure drugs).

DRUGS USED IN TREATING VITAMIN B$_{12}$ DEFICIENCY ANEMIA

Vitamin B$_{12}$ is essential to growth, cell reproduction, the manufacture of myelin (which surrounds some nerve fibers), and blood cell manufacture. The **intrinsic factor**, which is produced by cells in the stomach, is necessary for the absorption of vitamin B$_{12}$ in the intestine. A deficiency of the intrinsic factor results in abnormal formation of erythrocytes because of the body's failure to absorb vitamin B$_{12}$, a necessary component for blood cell formation. The resulting anemia is called **macrocytic anemia**.

Actions and Uses

Vitamin B$_{12}$ (cyanocobalamin) is used to treat patients with a vitamin B$_{12}$ deficiency; this condition is seen in those who have

- A strict vegetarian (vegan) lifestyle

- Total gastrectomy or subtotal gastric resection (in which the cells producing the intrinsic factor are totally or partially removed)

- Intestinal diseases, such as ulcerative colitis or sprue

- Gastric carcinoma

- Congenital decrease in the number of gastric cells that secrete intrinsic factor

Vitamin B$_{12}$ is also used to perform the Schilling test, which is used to diagnose pernicious anemia.

Nursing Alert

Pernicious anemia must be diagnosed and treated as soon as possible because vitamin B_{12} deficiency that is allowed to progress for more than 3 months may result in degenerative lesions of the spinal cord.

A deficiency of vitamin B_{12} caused by a low dietary intake is rare because the vitamin is found in meats, milk, eggs, and cheese. The body is also able to store this vitamin. A deficiency, for any reason, will not occur for 5 to 6 years from birth. Patients should be assessed for a history of vegan diet or gastric bypass surgery.

Adverse Reactions

Mild diarrhea and itching have been reported with the administration of vitamin B_{12}. Other adverse reactions that may be seen include a marked increase in RBC production, acne, peripheral vascular thrombosis, congestive heart failure, and pulmonary edema.

Contraindications, Precautions, and Interactions

Vitamin B_{12} is contraindicated in patients who are allergic to cyanocobalamin. Vitamin B_{12} is a pregnancy category A drug if administered orally and a pregnancy category C drug if given parenterally. Vitamin B_{12} is administered cautiously during pregnancy and in patients with pulmonary disease and anemia. Alcohol, neomycin, and colchicine may decrease the absorption of oral vitamin B_{12}.

NURSING PROCESS

The Patient Receiving a Drug Used in the Treatment of Anemia
ASSESSMENT
PREADMINISTRATION ASSESSMENT
The nurse obtains a general health history and asks about the symptoms of the anemia. The primary health care provider may order laboratory tests to determine the type, severity, and possible cause of the anemia. At times, it may be easy to identify the cause of the anemia, but there are also instances where the cause of the anemia is obscure.

The nurse takes the vital signs to provide a baseline during therapy. Other physical assessments may include the patient's general appearance and, in the severely anemic patient, an evaluation of the patient's ability to carry out the activities of daily living. General symptoms of anemia include fatigue, shortness of breath, sore tongue, headache, and pallor.

If iron dextran is to be given, an allergy history is necessary because this drug is given with caution to those with significant allergies or asthma. The patient's weight and hemoglobin level are required for calculating the dosage.

ONGOING ASSESSMENT
During the ongoing assessment the nurse takes the vital signs daily; more frequent monitoring may be needed if the patient is moderately to acutely ill. The nurse monitors the patient for adverse reactions and reports any occurrence of adverse reactions to the primary health care provider before the next dose is due. However, the nurse immediately reports severe adverse reactions.

When the patient is receiving oral iron supplements, the nurse informs the patient that the color of the stool will become darker or black. If diarrhea or constipation occurs, the nurse notifies the primary health care provider.

If parenteral iron dextran is administered, the nurse informs the patient that soreness at the injection site may occur. Injection sites are checked daily for signs of inflammation, swelling, or abscess formation.

The nurse assesses the patient for relief of the symptoms of anemia (fatigue, shortness of breath, sore tongue, headache, pallor). Some patients may note a relief of symptoms after a few days of therapy. Periodic laboratory tests are necessary to monitor the results of therapy.

NURSING DIAGNOSES
Drug-specific nursing diagnoses are highlighted in the Nursing Diagnoses Checklist. Other nursing diagnoses applicable to these drugs are discussed in depth in Chapter 4.

Nursing Diagnoses Checklist

✔ **Imbalanced Nutrition: Less Than Body Requirements** related to lack of iron, folic acid, other (specify) in the diet
✔ **Constipation** related to adverse reaction to iron therapy

PLANNING

The expected outcomes for the patient may include an optimal response to therapy, supporting the patient needs related to the management of adverse reactions, and an understanding of and compliance with the prescribed treatment regimen.

IMPLEMENTATION

PROMOTING AN OPTIMAL RESPONSE TO THERAPY

IRON Iron supplements are preferably given between meals with water, but many people cannot tolerate this and may need to take them with food. Milk and antacids may interfere with absorption of iron and should not be taken at the same time as iron supplements. If the patient is receiving other drugs, the nurse checks with the hospital pharmacist regarding the simultaneous administration of iron salts with other drugs.

Iron dextran is given by the IM or IV route. Before iron dextran is administered, a test dose (0.5 mL iron dextran) may be administered IV at a gradual rate over a period of 30 seconds or more. A test dose is also given before administering the first dose of iron dextran IM by injecting 0.5 mL into the upper outer quadrant of the buttocks. The nurse monitors the patient for an allergic response for at least 1 hour after the test dose and before administering the remaining dose. Epinephrine is kept on standby in the event of severe anaphylactic reaction.

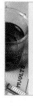

Nursing Alert

Parenteral administration of iron has resulted in fatal anaphylactic-type reactions. The nurse reports any of the following adverse reactions: dyspnea, urticaria, rashes, itching, and fever.

After the test dose, the prescribed dose of iron is administered IM. The drug is given into the muscle mass of the buttocks upper outer quadrant (never into an arm or other area) using the Z-track method (Fig. 44-1) to prevent leakage into the subcutaneous tissue. A large-bore needle is required. If the patient is standing, have the patient place weight on the leg not receiving the injection.

VITAMIN B$_{12}$ Patients with vitamin B$_{12}$ anemia are treated with vitamin B$_{12}$ administered by the parenteral route (IM) weekly. The parenteral route is used because the vitamin is ineffective orally owing to the absence of the intrinsic factor in the stomach, which is necessary for utilization of vitamin B$_{12}$. After stabilization, maintenance (usually monthly) injections may be necessary for life. Vitamin B$_{12}$ is available in an intranasal form for those who are on maintenance therapy.

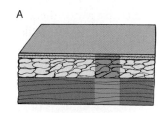
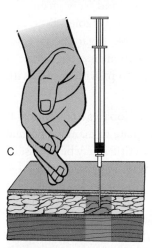

Figure 44.1 Parenteral iron may be injected intramuscularly using the Z-track (zigzag) technique in which the skin (**A**) is pulled to one side (**B**). The nurse then inserts the needle at a 90-degree angle and aspirates for blood before injecting the iron solution (**C**). When the needle is withdrawn, the displaced tissue returns to its normal position (**D**). This prevents the solution from escaping the muscle tissue.

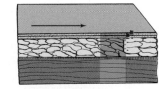

EPOETIN ALFA When epoetin alfa is administered to a patient with hypertension, the nurse monitors the blood pressure closely. The nurse reports any rise of 20 mm Hg or more in the systolic or diastolic pressure to the primary health care provider. The hematocrit is usually measured before each dose during therapy with epoetin alfa.

The drug is given three times weekly IV or SC; if the patient is receiving dialysis, the drug is administered into the venous access line. The drug is mixed gently during preparation for administration. Shaking may denature the glycoprotein. The vial is used for only one dose; any remaining or unused portion is discarded.

Agents Used in the
Treatment of Anemia

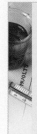

> **Nursing Alert**
>
> When monitoring the patient taking epoetin, the nurse reports any increase in the hematocrit of 4 points within any 2-week period because an exacerbation of hypertension is associated with an excessive rise of hematocrit. Hematocrit is decreased by decreasing or withholding the epoetin alfa dose.

MONITORING AND MANAGING PATIENT NEEDS

IMBALANCED NUTRITION: LESS THAN BODY REQUIRE-MENTS The nurse recommends a balanced diet with an emphasis on foods that are high in iron (e.g., organ meats, lean red meats, cereals, dried beans, and leafy green vegetables), folic acid (e.g., green leafy vegetables, liver, and yeast), or vitamin B_{12} (e.g., beef, pork, organ meats, eggs, milk, and milk products). If the patient is a vegetarian, a dietitian may need to be consulted to provide menus with appropriate iron-rich foods.

The nurse monitors the amount of food eaten at meals. If appetite is poor or eating is inadequate to maintain normal nutrition, consultation with the dietitian may be necessary. Small portions of food may be more appealing than large or moderate portions. The nurse provides a pleasant atmosphere and allows ample time for eating. If the diet is taken poorly, the nurse notes this on the patient's chart and discusses the problem with the primary health care provider.

CONSTIPATION Constipation may be a problem when a patient is taking oral iron preparations. The nurse instructs the patient to increase fluid intake to 10 to 12 glasses of water daily (if the condition permits), eat a diet high in fiber, and increase activity. An active lifestyle and regular exercise (if condition permits) help to decrease the constipating effects of iron. If constipation persists, the primary health care provider may prescribe a stool softener.

EDUCATING THE PATIENT AND FAMILY

The nurse explains the medical regimen thoroughly to the patient and family and emphasizes the importance of following the prescribed treatment regimen. The nurse includes the following points in a patient and family teaching plan:

IRON

- Take this drug with water on an empty stomach. If GI upset occurs, take the drug with food or meals.

- Do not take antacids, tetracyclines, penicillamine, or fluoroquinolones at the same time or 2 hours before or after taking iron without first checking with the primary health care provider.

- This drug may cause a darkening of the stools, constipation, or diarrhea. If constipation or diarrhea becomes severe, contact the primary health care provider.

- Mix the liquid iron preparation with water or juice and drink through a straw to prevent staining the teeth.

- Avoid the indiscriminate use of advertised iron products. If a true iron deficiency occurs, the cause must be determined and therapy should be under the care of a health care provider.

- Have periodic blood tests during therapy to determine the therapeutic response.

EPOETIN ALFA

- Keep all appointments with the primary health care provider. The drug is administered three times per week (by the SC or IV route or through a dialysis access line). Periodic blood tests are performed to determine the effects of the drug and to determine dosage.

- Strict compliance with the antihypertensive drug regimen is important in patients with known hypertension during epoetin alfa therapy.

- The following adverse reactions may occur: dizziness, headache, fatigue, joint pain, nausea, vomiting, or diarrhea. Report any of these reactions.

FOLIC ACID

- Avoid the use of multivitamin preparations unless it has been approved by the primary health care provider.

- Follow the diet recommended by the primary health care provider because diet and drug are necessary to correct a folic acid deficiency.

LEUCOVORIN

- Megaloblastic anemia—Adhere to the diet prescribed by the primary health care provider. If the purchase of foods high in protein (which can be expensive) becomes a problem, discuss this with the primary health care provider.

VITAMIN B_{12}

- Nutritional deficiency of vitamin B_{12}—Eat a balanced diet that includes seafood, eggs, meats, and dairy products.

- Pernicious anemia—Lifetime therapy is necessary. Eat a balanced diet that includes seafood, eggs, meats, and dairy products. Avoid contact with infections, and report any signs of infection to the primary health care provider immediately because an increase in dosage may be necessary.

- Adhere to the treatment regimen and keep all appointments with the clinic or primary health care provider. The drug is given at periodic intervals (usually monthly for life). In some instances, parenteral or intranasal self-administration or parenteral administration by a family member is allowed (instruction in administration is necessary).

EVALUATION

- The therapeutic effect of the drug is achieved.

- The patient has normal bowel movements.

- An adequate nutritional intake is achieved.

- The patient and family demonstrate an understanding of the drug regimen.

- The patient verbalizes the importance of complying with the prescribed treatment regimen.

Critical Thinking Exercises

1. Ms. Clepper, aged 32 years, has received a diagnosis of pernicious anemia. Although the primary health care provider has explained the diagnosis and the treatment, the patient is confused and frightened. She questions you, stating, "I just don't understand what is happening in my body to cause me to feel so weak and tired. How is the treatment going to work?" Discuss ways in which you would handle this situation with Ms. Clepper. Determine what to tell her that would decrease her anxiety and increase her understanding.

2. Mr. Garcia, aged 54 years, has chronic renal failure. He undergoes dialysis three times a week. The physician orders epoetin alfa to be administered. Discuss the preadministration and ongoing assessments for Mr. Garcia. During a discussion with you, Mr. Garcia asks why he is receiving this drug. Discuss how you would answer Mr. Garcia's question.

Review Questions

1. Which is the most common type of anemia?

   A. Iron deficiency anemia

   B. Folic acid anemia

   C. Pernicious anemia

   D. Megaloblastic anemia

2. Which of the following substances would decrease the absorption of oral iron?

   A. antacids

   B. levothyroxine

   C. ascorbic acid

   D. vitamin B$_{12}$

3. Folic acid and leucovorin are contraindicated in which of the following conditions?

   A. Hypothyroidism

   B. Hyperthyroidism

   C. Pernicious anemia

   D. Pregnancy

4. When monitoring a patient taking epoetin alfa, which of the following laboratory results would be most important for the nurse to report immediately?

   A. Any increase in hematocrit of 4 points within a 2-week period

   B. Any increase in hematocrit of 2 points within a 2-week period

   C. A daily change in the hematocrit of 1 point or more

   D. A stabilization in the hematocrit in any 2-day period

5. When teaching a patient about the use of vitamin B$_{12}$, the nurse would include which of the following statements?

   A. Take the oral form of vitamin B$_{12}$ daily at bedtime on an empty stomach.

   B. Take the oral form of vitamin B$_{12}$ when you begin to feel weak or experience a headache.

   C. You will require vitamin B$_{12}$ injections monthly for life.

   D. You will require vitamin B$_{12}$ injections every 2 weeks until remission occurs.

Medication Dosage Problems

1. The physician prescribes 25 mg iron dextran IM. The drug is available in a vial with 50 mg/mL. The nurse administers _____.

2. Folvite (folic acid) 1 mg SC is prescribed. The drug is available in a vial with 5 mg/mL. The nurse administers _____.

To check your answers, see Appendix G.

Drugs That Affect the Gastrointestinal and Urinary Systems

The urinary system is responsible for the regulation and elimination body fluids. It comprises the kidneys, ureters, bladder, and urethra. The nephron is the functional unit of the kidney (see Chapter 45). Each kidney contains about one million nephrons, which filter the bloodstream to remove waste products. During this process, water and electrolytes are also selectively removed. The filtrate (i.e., the fluid removed from the blood) normally contains ions (potassium, sodium, chloride), waste products (ammonia, urea), water, and at times other substances that are being excreted from the body, such as drugs. The filtrate then passes through the proximal tubule, the loop of Henle, and the distal tubules. At these points, selective reabsorption of amino acids, glucose, some electrolytes, and water occurs. Ions and water that are required by the body to maintain fluid and electrolyte balance are returned to the bloodstream through the minute capillaries that surround the distal and proximal tubules and the loop of Henle. Ions and water that are not needed by the body are excreted in the urine. Drugs used to control the amount and composition of the fluid excreted or reabsorbed are covered in Chapter 45.

The bladder is the storage area for urine before it is excreted from the body. The nature of the bladder and its contents make it susceptible to infection. Chapter 46 discusses drugs used specifically for treating urinary tract infections and the discomfort associated with those infections.

The gastrointestinal (GI) system is responsible for the ingestion and exchange of body nutrients. Food and fluids are broken down in the oral cavity to begin the process of digestion in the GI system. In the stomach, foodstuffs are broken down by gastric acids and enzymes to prepare for absorption in the small intestine. Nutrients are absorbed in the small intestine. The large intestine is responsible for the reabsorption of water and the elimination of waste materials in the form of feces.

The health focus on this body system increases as people age. Chronic illness, such as inflammatory bowel diseases, can affect how water and nutrients are absorbed. As aging occurs, individuals experience wear and tear on their teeth and the ability to produce saliva decreases; this changes the taste of foods. Also as the body ages, motility and absorption in the GI system slow. Drugs are used to assist in the absorption of nutrients either by altering the gastric acids for purposes of protection or by controlling the transit of food though the system by speeding up or slowing down the process. Chapter 47 describes drugs used for protecting the structures of the upper GI system—mouth, esophagus, and stomach—from the effects of gastric acid. Drugs used to slow down or facilitate transit in the lower GI system—the small and large intestines—are covered in Chapter 48. The drugs used in the treatment of chronic GI diseases are also presented.

An area of concern to the nurse is the availability of nonprescription drugs for the GI system, thereby creating the potential problems of misuse and overuse of the drugs and the disguising of more serious medical problems. This issue is addressed in Chapter 48 as well.

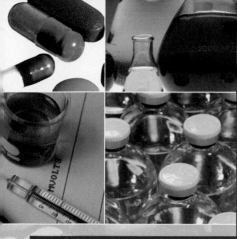

Diuretics

Learning Objectives

On completion of this chapter, the student will:

- List the five general types of diuretics.

- Discuss the uses, general drug actions, adverse reactions, contraindications, precautions, and interactions of the diuretics.

- Describe important preadministration and ongoing assessment activities

the nurse should perform with the patient taking a diuretic.

- List nursing diagnoses particular to a patient taking a diuretic.

- Discuss ways to promote an optimal response to therapy, how to manage common adverse reactions, and important points to keep in mind when educating patients about the use of diuretics.

Many conditions or diseases, such as congestive heart failure (CHF), endocrine disturbances, and kidney and liver diseases can cause **edema** (retention of excess fluid). When the patient shows signs of excess fluid retention, the primary health care provider may order a diuretic to reduce the edema. A **diuretic** is a drug that increases the excretion of urine (i.e., water, electrolytes, and waste products) by the kidneys. There are various types of diuretic drugs, and the primary health care provider selects the one that best suits the patient's needs and effectively reduces the amount of excess fluid in body tissues. The different types of diuretic drugs are

- Carbonic anhydrase inhibitors

- Loop diuretics

- Osmotic diuretics

- Potassium-sparing diuretics

- Thiazides and related diuretics

The Summary Drug Table: Diuretics lists examples of the different types of diuretic drugs. Diuretics are used in a variety of medical disorders. The primary health care provider selects the type of diuretic that will most likely be effective for treatment of a specific disorder. In some instances, hypertension may be treated with the administration of an antihypertensive drug and a diuretic. The diuretics used for this combination therapy include the loop diuretics and the thiazides and related diuretics. The specific uses of each type of diuretic drug are discussed in the following sections.

Actions

Refer to the illustration of the kidney nephron (Fig. 45-1) for a better understanding of the actions of the diuretics.

SUMMARY DRUG TABLE   DIURETICS

GENERIC NAME	TRADE NAME	USES	ADVERSE REACTIONS	DOSAGE RANGES
Carbonic Anhydrase Inhibitors				
acetazolamide *a-set-a-zole'-a-mide*	Diamox	Open-angle glaucoma, secondary glaucoma, preoperatively to lower IOP, edema due to CHF, drug-induced edema, centrencephalic epilepsy	Weakness, fatigue, anorexia, nausea, vomiting, rash, paresthesias, photosensitivity	Glaucoma: up to 1 g/d orally in divided doses Acute glaucoma: 500 mg initially then 125–250 mg orally q4h Epilepsy: 8–30 mg kg/d in divided doses CHF and edema: 250–375 mg/d orally
methazolamide *meth-a-zole'-a-mide*		Glaucoma	Same as acetazolamide	50–100 mg orally BID, TID
Loop Diuretics				
bumetanide *byoo-met'-a-nide*	Bumex	Edema due to CHF, cirrhosis of the liver, renal disease, acute pulmonary edema	Electrolyte and hematologic imbalances, anorexia, nausea, vomiting, dizziness, rash, photosensitivity, orthostatic hypotension, glycosuria	0.5–10 mg/d orally, IV, IM
ethacrynic acid *eth-a-kriń-ik*	Edecrin, Edecrin Sodium	Same as bumetanide plus ascites due to malignancy, idiopathic edema, lymphedema	Same as bumetanide plus diarrhea	50–200 mg/d orally, IV
furosemide *fur-oh'-se-mide*	Lasix	Same as bumetanide plus hypertension	Same as bumetanide	Edema: 20–80 mg/d, may go up to 600 mg/d for severe edema Hypertension: 40 mg orally BID CHF/renal failure: up to 2.5 gd
torsemide *tor'-se-myde*	Demadex	Same as bumetanide plus hypertension	Same as bumetanide plus headache	CHF/renal failure: 10–20 mg/d orally, IV Cirrhosis/hypertension: 5–10 mg/d orally, IV
Osmotic Diuretics				
glycerin (glycerol) *glí-ser-in*		Glaucoma, before and after surgery	Headache, nausea, vomiting	1–2 g/kg orally in solution
isosorbide *eye-soe-sor'-bide*		Same as glycerin	Same as glycerin	1–3 mg/kg orally, BID–QID
mannitol *man'-i-tole*	Osmitrol	To promote diuresis in acute renal failure, reduction of IOP, treatment of cerebral edema, irrigation solution in prostate surgical procedures	Edema, fluid and electrolyte imbalance, headache, blurred vision, nausea, vomiting, diarrhea, urinary retention	Diuresis: 50–200 g/24 h IV IOP: 1.5–2 g/kg IV

GENERIC NAME	TRADE NAME	USES	ADVERSE REACTIONS	DOSAGE RANGES
urea *your-ee'-a*	Ureaphil	Reduction of IOP, reduction of intracranial pressure	Headache, nausea, vomiting, fluid and electrolyte imbalance, syncope	Up to 120 g/d IV
Potassium-Sparing Diuretics				
amiloride HCl *a-mill'-oh-ride*	Midamor	CHF, hypertension, prevention of hypokalemia in at-risk patients, polyuria prevention with lithium use	Headache, dizziness, nausea, anorexia, diarrhea, vomiting, weakness, fatigue, rash, hypotension	5–20 mg/d orally
spironolactone *speer-on-oh-lak'-tone*	Aldactone	Hypertension, edema due to CHF, cirrhosis, renal disease; hypokalemia, prophylaxis of hypokalemia in at-risk patients, hyperaldosteronism	Headache, diarrhea, drowsiness, lethargy, hyperkalemia, cramping, gastritis, erectile dysfunction, gynecomastia	Up to 400 mg/d orally in single dose or divided doses
triamterene *trye-am'-ter-een*	Dyrenium	Prevention of hypokalemia, edema due to CHF, cirrhosis, renal disease, hyperaldosteronism	Diarrhea, nausea, vomiting, hyperkalemia, photosensitivity	Up to 300 mg/d orally in divided doses
Thiazides and Related Diuretics				
bendroflumethiazide *ben-droe-floo-me-thye'-a-zide*	Naturetin	Edema associated with CHF, hypertension	Orthostatic hypotension, dizziness, vertigo, lightheadedness, weakness, anorexia, gastric distress, nausea, diarrhea, constipation, hematologic changes, rash, photosensitivity reactions, hyperglycemia, fluid and electrolyte imbalances, reduced libido	Edema: 2.5–5 mg/d Hypertension: 2.5–15 mg/d orally
chlorothiazide *klor-oh-thye'-a-zide*	Diuril	Hypertension, edema due to CHF, cirrhosis, corticosteroid and estrogen therapy	Same as bendroflumethiazide	0.5–2 g orally or IV, QID or BID
chlorthalidone *klor-thal'-i-done*	Thalitone	Same as chlorothiazide	Same as bendroflumethiazide	Edema: 50–120 mg/d orally Hypertension: 25–100 mg/d orally
hydrochlorothiazide *hye-droe-klor-oh-thye'-a-zide*	HydroDIURIL, Esidrix, Microzide, Oretic	Same as chlorothiazide	Same as bendroflumethiazide	Edema: 25–200 mg/d orally Hypertension: 12.5–50 mg/d orally

Diuretics

SUMMARY DRUG TABLE (continued)

GENERIC NAME	TRADE NAME	USES	ADVERSE REACTIONS	DOSAGE RANGES
hydroflumethiazide *hye-droe-floo-me-thye'-a-zide*	Saluron	Same as chlorothiazide	Same as bendroflumethiazide	Edema: 25–200 mg/d orally Hypertension: 50–100 mg/d orally
indapamide *in-dap'-a-mide*	Lozol	Hypertension, edema due to CHF	Same as bendroflumethiazide	Edema: 2.5–5 mg/d orally Hypertension: 1.25–5 mg/d orally
metolazone *me-tole'-a-zone*	Zaroxolyn	Edema in CHF, cirrhosis, corticosteroids, estrogen therapy, renal dysfunction	Same as bendroflumethiazide	2.5–20 mg/d orally
methyclothiazide *meth-i-kloe-thye'-a-zide*	Enduron	Same as chlorothiazide	Same as bendroflumethiazide	Edema: 2.5–10 mg/d orally Hypertension: 2.5–5 mg/d orally
polythiazide *pol-i-thye'-a-zide*	Renese	Same as chlorothiazide	Same as bendroflumethiazide	Edema: 1–4 mg/d orally Hypertension: 2–4 mg/d orally

CHF, congestive heart failure; IOP, intraocular pressure.

Carbonic Anhydrase Inhibitors

These drugs are sulfonamides, with nonbacteriostatic action, that inhibit the enzyme carbonic anhydrase. The carbonic anhydrase enzyme produces free hydrogen ions, which are then exchanged for sodium ions in the kidney tubules. Carbonic anhydrase inhibition results in the excretion of sodium, potassium, bicarbonate, and water. Glaucoma, a condition of increased pressure in the eye from excess aqueous humor, is treated with carbonic anhydrase inhibitors. These diuretics decrease the production of aqueous humor in the eye, which in turn decreases intraocular pressure (IOP; i.e., pressure within the eye).

Loop Diuretics

The loop diuretics furosemide (Lasix) and ethacrynic acid (Edecrin) increase the excretion of sodium and chloride by inhibiting reabsorption of these ions in the distal and proximal tubules and in the loop of Henle. These drugs act at three sites, thereby increasing their effectiveness as diuretics. Torsemide (Demadex) also increases urinary excretion of sodium, chloride, and water but acts primarily in the ascending portion of the loop of Henle. Bumetanide (Bumex) primarily increases the excretion of chloride but also has some sodium-excreting ability. This drug acts primarily on the proximal tubule of the nephron.

Osmotic Diuretics

Osmotic diuretics increase the density of the filtrate in the glomerulus. This prevents selective reabsorption of water, which allows the water to be excreted. Sodium and chloride excretion is also increased.

Potassium-Sparing Diuretics

Potassium-sparing diuretics work in either of two ways. Triamterene (Dyrenium) and amiloride (Midamor) depress the reabsorption of sodium in the kidney tubules, thereby increasing sodium and water excretion. Both drugs additionally depress the excretion of potassium and therefore are called *potassium-sparing* (or *potassium-saving*) diuretics. Spironolactone (Aldactone), also a potassium-sparing diuretic, antagonizes the action of aldosterone. Aldosterone, a hormone produced by the adrenal cortex, enhances the reabsorption of sodium in the distal convoluted tubules of the kidney. When this activity of aldosterone is blocked, sodium (but not potassium) and water are excreted.

Thiazides and Related Diuretics

Thiazides and related diuretics inhibit the reabsorption of sodium and chloride ions in the ascending portion of the

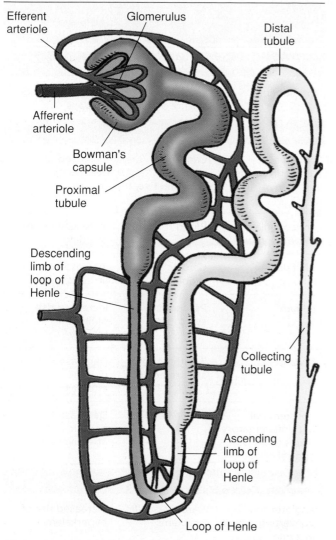

Figure 45.1 The nephron is the functional unit of the kidney. Note the various tubules, the site of most diuretic activity. The loop of Henle is the site of action for the loop diuretics. Thiazide diuretics act at the ascending portion of the loop of Henle and the distal tube of the nephron.

loop of Henle and the early distal tubule of the nephron. This action results in the excretion of sodium, chloride, and water.

Uses

The diuretic drugs are used in the treatment of

- Edema (fluid retention) associated with CHF, corticosteroid/estrogen therapy, and cirrhosis of the liver

- Hypertension

- Renal disease (acute failure, renal insufficiency, and nephrotic syndrome)

- Cerebral edema

- Acute glaucoma and increased IOP (before and after eye surgery)

Ethacrynic acid (a loop diuretic) is also used for the short-term management of ascites caused by a malignancy, idiopathic edema, or lymphedema. When patients are at risk for potassium loss, the potassium-sparing diuretics may be used with or in place of other categories of diuretics.

Adverse Reactions

Adverse reactions associated with any category of diuretics involve various body systems.

Neuromuscular Reactions
- Dizziness, lightheadedness, headache
- Weakness, fatigue

Cardiovascular Reactions
- Orthostatic hypotension
- Electrolyte imbalances, glycosuria

Gastrointestinal Reactions
- Anorexia
- Nausea, vomiting

Other

Dermatologic reactions include rash and photosensitivity. Extremity paresthesias (numbness or tingling) or flaccid muscles may indicate **hypokalemia** (low blood potassium). **Hyperkalemia** (an increase in potassium in the blood), a serious event, may occur with the administration of potassium-sparing diuretics. Hyperkalemia is most likely to occur in patients with an inadequate fluid intake and urine output, those with diabetes or renal disease, the elderly, and those who are severely ill. In male patients taking spironolactone, **gynecomastia** (breast enlargement) may occur. This reaction appears to be related to both dosage and duration of therapy. The gynecomastia is usually reversible when therapy is discontinued, but in rare instances some breast enlargement may remain.

Additional adverse reactions of these drugs are listed in the Summary Drug Table: Diuretics. When a potassium-

Diuretics

sparing diuretic and another diuretic are given together, the adverse reactions associated with both drugs may be evident.

Contraindications

The diuretics are contraindicated in patients with known hypersensitivity to the drugs, electrolyte imbalances, severe kidney or liver dysfunction, and **anuria** (cessation of urine production). Mannitol (an osmotic diuretic) is contraindicated in patients with active intracranial bleeding (except during craniotomy). The potassium-sparing diuretics are contraindicated in patients with hyperkalemia and are not recommended for children.

Precautions

Diuretics are used cautiously in patients with renal dysfunction. Most of the diuretics are pregnancy category C drugs (although ethacrynic acid, torsemide, isosorbide, amiloride, and triamterene are in pregnancy category B) and must be used cautiously during pregnancy and lactation. All of the thiazide diuretics are pregnancy category B drugs, with the exception of bendroflumethiazide, benzthiazide, hydroflumethiazide, methyclothiazide, which are pregnancy category C drugs. The safety of these drugs for use during pregnancy and lactation has not been established, so they should be used only when the drug is clearly needed and when the potential benefits to the patient outweigh the potential hazards to the fetus.

The thiazide and loop diuretics are used cautiously in patients with liver disease, diabetes, lupus erythematosus (may exacerbate or activate the disease), or diarrhea. A cross-sensitivity reaction may occur with the thiazides and sulfonamides. Some of the thiazide diuretics contain tartrazine, which may cause allergic-type reactions or bronchial asthma in individuals sensitive to tartrazine. Patients with sensitivity to the sulfonamides may show allergic reactions to loop diuretics (furosemide, torsemide, or bumetanide). The potassium-sparing diuretics should be used cautiously in patients with liver disease, diabetes, or gout.

Interactions

All the diuretics may cause increased hypotension when taken with antihypertensive drugs. The interactions for specific diuretic categories are listed here.

Interacting Drug	Common Use	Effect of Interaction
Carbonic Anhydrase Inhibitors		
primidone	Treatment of seizure activity	Decreased effectiveness
Loop Diuretics		
cisplatin, aminoglycosides	Cancer treatment, anti-infective, respectively	Increased risk of ototoxicity
anticoagulants or thrombolytics	Blood thinner	Increased risk of bleeding
digitalis	Cardiac problems	Increased risk of arrhythmias
lithium	Psychotic symptoms	Increased risk of lithium toxicity
hydantoins	Treatment of seizure activity	Decreased diuretic effectiveness
nonsteroidal anti-inflammatory drugs (NSAIDs) and salicylates	Pain relief	Decreased diuretic effectiveness
Potassium-Sparing Diuretics		
angiotensin-converting enzyme inhibitors or potassium supplements	Cardiovascular problems	Increased risk of hyperkalemia
NSAIDs and salicylates; anticoagulants	Pain relief and blood thinner, respectively	Decreased diuretic effectiveness
Thiazides and Related Diuretics		
allopurinol	Treatment of gout	Increased risk of hypersensitivity to allopurinol
anesthetics	Surgical anesthesia	Increased anesthetic effectiveness
antineoplastic drugs	Cancer treatment	Extended leukopenia
antidiabetic drugs	Control of diabetes	Hyperglycemia

Herbal Alert

Numerous *herbal diuretics* are available as over-the-counter (OTC) products. Most plant and herbal extracts available as OTC diuretics are nontoxic. However, most are either ineffective or no more effective than caffeine. The following are selected herbals reported to possess diuretic activity: *celery, chicory, sassafras, juniper berries, St. John's wort, foxglove, horsetail, licorice, dandelion, digitalis purpurea, ephedra, hibiscus, parsley,* and *elderberry*.

There is very little and in many instances no scientific evidence to justify the use of these plants as diuretics. For example, dandelion root is a popular preparation once thought to be a strong diuretic. However, scientific research has found dandelion root safe but ineffective as a diuretic. No herbal diuretic should be taken unless approved by the primary health care provider.

Diuretic teas such as juniper berries and shave grass or horsetail are contraindicated. Juniper berries have been associated with renal damage, and horsetail contains severely toxic compounds. Teas with ephedrine should be avoided, especially by individuals with hypertension.

NURSING PROCESS

The Patient Receiving a Diuretic

ASSESSMENT

PREADMINISTRATION ASSESSMENT

Before administering a diuretic, the nurse takes the vital signs and weighs the patient. Current laboratory test results, especially the levels of serum electrolytes, are carefully reviewed. Patients with renal dysfunction should have blood urea nitrogen (BUN) and creatinine clearance levels monitored as well. If the patient has peripheral edema, the nurse inspects the involved areas and records in the patient's chart the degree and extent of edema. If the patient is receiving a carbonic anhydrase inhibitor for increased IOP, the patient's description of pain and vital signs are obtained. The preadministration physical assessment of the patient receiving a diuretic for epilepsy includes vital signs and weight. The nurse reviews the patient's chart for a description of the seizures and their frequency.

If the patient is to receive an osmotic diuretic, the focus of the assessment is on the patient's disease or disorder and the symptoms being treated. For example, if the patient has a low urinary output and the osmotic diuretic is given to increase urinary output, the nurse reviews the intake and output ratio

and symptoms the patient is experiencing. In addition, the nurse weighs the patient and takes the vital signs as part of the physical assessment before drug therapy starts.

ONGOING ASSESSMENT

During initial therapy, the nurse observes the patient for the effects of drug therapy. The type of assessment depends on such factors as the reason for the administration of the diuretic, the type of diuretic administered, the route of administration, and the condition of the patient. The nurse measures and records fluid intake and output and reports to the primary health care provider any marked decrease in the output. During ongoing therapy, the nurse weighs the patient at the same time daily, making certain that the patient is wearing the same amount or type of clothing. Depending on the specific diuretic, frequent serum electrolyte, uric acid, and liver and kidney function tests may be performed during the first few months of therapy and periodically thereafter.

NURSING DIAGNOSES

Drug-specific nursing diagnoses are highlighted in the Nursing Diagnoses Checklist. Other nursing diagnoses applicable to these drugs are discussed in depth in Chapter 4.

Nursing Diagnoses Checklist

✓ **Impaired Urinary Elimination** related to action of the diuretics causing increased frequency

✓ **Risk for Deficient Fluid Volume** related to excessive diuresis secondary to administration of a diuretic

✓ **Risk for Injury** related to lightheadedness, dizziness, or cardiac arrhythmias

PLANNING

The expected outcomes for the patient depend on the reason for administration of the diuretic, but may include an optimal response to drug therapy, management of patient needs related to adverse drug reactions, correction of a fluid volume deficit, absence of injury, and an understanding of and compliance with the postdischarge drug regimen.

IMPLEMENTATION

PROMOTING AN OPTIMAL RESPONSE TO THERAPY

Diuretics are used to treat many different types of conditions. Therefore, promoting an optimal response to therapy for patients taking diuretics often depends on the specific diuretic and the patient's condition.

THE PATIENT WITH EDEMA Patients with edema caused by CHF or other causes are weighed daily or as ordered by the primary health care provider. A daily weight is taken to monitor fluid loss. Weight loss of about 2 lb daily is desirable to prevent dehydration and electrolyte imbalances. The nurse carefully measures and records the fluid intake and output every 8 hours. The critically ill patient or the patient with renal disease may require more frequent measurements of urinary output. The nurse assesses the blood pressure, pulse, and respiratory rate every 4 hours or as ordered by the primary health care provider. An acutely ill patient may require more frequent monitoring of the vital signs.

The nurse examines areas of edema daily to evaluate the effectiveness of drug therapy and records the findings in the patient's chart. The nurse examines the patient's general appearance and condition daily or more often if the patient is acutely ill.

THE PATIENT WITH HYPERTENSION The nurse monitors the blood pressure, pulse, and respiratory rate of patients with hypertension receiving a diuretic, or a diuretic along with an antihypertensive drug, before the administration of the drug. More frequent monitoring may be necessary if the patient is critically ill or the blood pressure excessively high.

THE PATIENT WITH ACUTE GLAUCOMA If a carbonic anhydrase inhibitor is given for glaucoma, the nurse evaluates the patient's response to drug therapy (relief of eye pain) every 2 hours. If the patient is ambulatory and has reduced vision because of glaucoma, the nurse may need to assist the patient with ambulatory and self-care activities.

Nursing Alert

The nurse notifies the primary health care provider immediately if eye pain increases or if it has not begun to decrease 3 to 4 hours after the first dose of diuretic. If the patient has acute closed-angle glaucoma, the nurse checks the pupil of the affected eye every 2 hours for dilation and response to light.

THE PATIENT WITH SEIZURE ACTIVITY If a carbonic anhydrase inhibitor is being given for absence or nonlocalized epileptic seizures, the nurse assesses the patient at frequent intervals for the occurrence of seizures, especially early in therapy and in patients known to experience seizures at frequent intervals. If a seizure does occur, the nurse records a description of the seizure in the patient's chart, including time of onset and duration. Accurate descriptions of the pattern and the number of seizures occurring each day help the primary health care provider plan future therapy and adjust drug dosages as needed.

THE PATIENT WITH INCREASED INTRACRANIAL PRESSURE Mannitol is administered only by the intravenous (IV) route. The nurse inspects the solution carefully before administration because, when exposed to low temperatures, mannitol solution may crystallize. Should this happen, the nurse withholds the drug, returns the solution to the pharmacy, and requests another dose. The rate of administration and concentration of the drug are individualized. The nurse must monitor the urine output hourly because the rate of administration is adjusted to maintain a urine flow of at least 30 to 50 mL/h.

When a patient is receiving the osmotic diuretic mannitol or urea for treatment of increased intracranial pressure caused by cerebral edema, the nurse monitors the blood pressure, pulse, and respiratory rate every 30 to 60 minutes or as ordered by the primary health care provider. The nurse immediately reports to the primary health care provider any increase in blood pressure, decrease in the pulse or respiratory rate, or any changes in the neurologic status. The nurse performs neurologic assessments (e.g., vital signs, response of the pupils to light, level of consciousness, or response to a painful stimulus) at the time intervals ordered by the primary health care provider. The nurse evaluates and records the patient's response to the drug, that is, the signs and symptoms that may indicate a decrease in intracranial pressure.

THE PATIENT WITH RENAL COMPROMISE When the thiazide diuretics are administered, renal function should be monitored periodically. These drugs may precipitate azotemia (accumulation of nitrogenous wastes in the blood). If nonprotein nitrogen (NPN) or BUN rises, the primary health care provider may consider withholding the drug or discontinuing its use. In addition, serum uric acid concentrations are monitored periodically during treatment with the thiazide diuretics because these drugs may precipitate an acute attack of gout. The patient also is monitored for any joint pain or discomfort. Because hyperglycemia may occur, insulin or oral antidiabetic drug dosages may require alterations. Serum glucose concentrations are monitored periodically.

THE PATIENT AT RISK FOR HYPOKALEMIA Patients who experience cardiac arrhythmias or who are being "digitalized" (initiating digoxin therapy) may be more susceptible to significant potassium loss resulting in hypokalemia when taking diuretics. The potassium-sparing diuretics are recommended for these patients. The nurse should monitor patients taking potassium-sparing diuretics because they are at a risk for hyperkalemia. Serum potassium levels are monitored frequently, particularly during initial treatment.

The drug is discontinued and the primary health care provider is notified immediately if the patient experiences these symptoms or if the serum potassium levels exceed 5.3 mEq/mL. Treatment includes administration of IV bicarbonate (if the patient is acidotic) or oral or parenteral glucose with rapid-acting insulin. Persistent hyperkalemia may require dialysis.

Nursing Alert

Symptoms of hyperkalemia include paresthesia (numbness, tingling, or prickling sensation), muscular weakness, fatigue, flaccid paralysis of the extremities, bradycardia, shock, and electrocardiographic abnormalities (see Display 45-1 for additional symptoms).

MONITORING AND MANAGING PATIENT NEEDS

IMPAIRED URINARY ELIMINATION Before the first dose of a diuretic is given, the nurse informs the patient of the drug's purpose (i.e., to rid the body of excess fluid); when diuresis may be expected to occur; and how long diuresis will last (Table 45-1). These drugs are administered early in the day to prevent any nighttime sleep disturbance caused by increased urination.

Some patients may exhibit anxiety related to the fact that it will be necessary to urinate at frequent intervals. To reduce anxiety, the nurse explains the purpose and effects of the drug. The nurse tells the patient that the need to urinate frequently will probably decrease. For some patients, the need to urinate frequently decreases after a few weeks of therapy. The nurse makes sure that the patient on bed rest has a call light and, when necessary, a bedpan or urinal within easy reach. The nurse informs the patient that the drug will be given early in the day so nighttime sleep will not be interrupted. Although the duration of activity of most diuretics is about 8 hours or

Display 45.1 Signs and Symptoms of Common Fluid and Electrolyte Imbalances Associated With Diuretic Therapy

Dehydration (Excessive Water Loss)
- Thirst
- Poor skin turgor
- Dry mucous membranes
- Weakness
- Dizziness
- Fever
- Low urine output

Hyponatremia (Excessive Loss of Sodium)
Note: Sodium—normal laboratory values 132–145 mEq/L
- Cold, clammy skin
- Decreased skin turgor
- Confusion
- Hypotension
- Irritability
- Tachycardia

Hypomagnesemia (Low Levels of Magnesium)
Note: Magnesium—normal laboratory values 1.5–2.5 mEq/L or 1.8–3 mg/dL
- Leg and foot cramps
- Hypertension
- Tachycardia
- Neuromuscular irritability

- Tremor
- Hyperactive deep tendon reflexes
- Confusion
- Visual or auditory hallucinations
- Paresthesias

Hypokalemia (Low Blood Potassium)
Note: Potassium—normal laboratory values 3.5–5 mEq/L
- Anorexia
- Nausea
- Vomiting
- Depression
- Confusion
- Cardiac arrhythmias
- Impaired thought processes
- Drowsiness

Hyperkalemia (High Blood Potassium)
- Irritability
- Anxiety
- Confusion
- Nausea
- Diarrhea
- Cardiac arrhythmias
- Abdominal distress

Table 45.1 Examples of Onset and Duration of Activity of Diuretics

Drug	Onset	Duration of Activity
acetazolamide		
tablets	1–1.5 h	8–12 h
sustained-release capsules	2 h	18–24 h
IV	2 min	4–5 h
amiloride	2 h	24 h
bumetanide		
oral	30–60 min	4–6 h
IV	Within a few minutes	Less than 1 h
ethacrynic acid		
oral	Within 30 min	6–8 h
IV	Within 5 min	2 h
furosemide		
oral	Within 1 h	6–8 h
IV	Within 5 min	2 h
mannitol (IV)	30–60 min	6–8 h
spironolactone	24–48 h	48–72 h
thiazides and related diuretics	1–2 h	Varies*
triamterene	2–4 h	12–16 h
urea (IV)	30–45 min	5–6 h

*Duration varies with drug used. Average duration is 12–24 h. Indapamide has a duration of more than 24 h.

less, some diuretics have a longer activity, which may result in a need to urinate during nighttime hours. This is especially true early in therapy.

RISK FOR DEFICIENT FLUID VOLUME The most common adverse reaction associated with the administration of a diuretic is the loss of fluid and electrolytes (see Display 45-1), especially during initial therapy with the drug. In some patients, the diuretic effect is moderate, whereas in others a large volume of fluid is lost. Regardless of the amount of fluid lost, there is always the possibility of excessive electrolyte loss, which is potentially serious.

The most common imbalances are a loss of potassium and water. Other electrolytes, particularly magnesium, sodium, and chloride, are also lost. When too much potassium is lost, hypokalemia occurs (see Home Care Checklist: Preventing Potassium Imbalances). In certain patients, such as those also receiving a digitalis glycoside or those who currently have a cardiac arrhythmia, hypokalemia has the potential to create a more serious arrhythmia.

Home Care Checklist

Preventing Potassium Imbalances

Diuretics increase the excretion of water and sodium. Some of these drugs also increase the excretion of potassium, which places your patient at risk for hypokalemia, a possibly life-threatening condition. Therefore, be sure your patient knows what foods to eat to replace the potassium lost. Patients should be taught about the following potassium-rich foods:

☑ **Meats:** Beef, chicken, pork, turkey, veal

☑ **Fish:** Flounder, haddock, halibut, salmon, sardines (canned), scallops, tuna

☑ **Fruits:** Apricots, avocado, bananas, cantaloupe, dates, dried fruit, plums, raisins, oranges and fresh orange juice, peaches, prunes, tomatoes and tomato juice (see also vegetables)

☑ **Vegetables:** Carrots, lima beans, potatoes, radishes, spinach, sweet potatoes, tomatoes

☑ **Other sources:** Coffee, gingersnaps, graham crackers, molasses, nuts, peanuts, peanut butter, tea

Hypokalemia is treated with potassium supplements or foods with high potassium content or by changing the diuretic to a potassium-sparing diuretic. In addition to hypokalemia, patients taking the loop diuretics are prone to magnesium deficiency (see Display 45-1). If too much water is lost, dehydration occurs, which also can be serious, especially in elderly patients.

Whether a fluid or electrolyte imbalance occurs depends on the amount of fluid and electrolytes lost and the ability of the individual to replace them. For example, if a patient receiving a diuretic eats poorly and does not drink extra fluids, an electrolyte and water imbalance is likely to occur, especially during initial therapy with the drug. However, even when a patient drinks adequate amounts of fluid and eats a balanced diet, an electrolyte imbalance may still occur and require electrolyte replacement (see Chapter 58 and Display 58-2 for additional discussion of fluid and electrolyte imbalances).

Gerontologic Alert

Older adults are particularly prone to fluid volume deficit and electrolyte imbalances while taking a diuretic (see Display 45-1). The older adult is carefully monitored for hypokalemia (when taking the loop or thiazide diuretics) and hyperkalemia (with the potassium-sparing diuretics).

To prevent a fluid volume deficit, the nurse encourages oral fluids at frequent intervals during waking hours. A balanced diet may help prevent electrolyte imbalances. The nurse encourages patients to eat and drink all food and fluids served at mealtime. The nurse also encourages all patients, especially the elderly, to eat or drink between meals and in the evening (when allowed). The nurse monitors the fluid intake and output and notifies the primary health care provider if the patient fails to drink an adequate amount of fluid, if the urinary output is low, if the urine appears concentrated, if the patient appears dehydrated, or if signs and symptoms of an electrolyte imbalance are apparent.

Nursing Alert

Warning signs of a fluid and electrolyte imbalance include dry mouth, thirst, weakness, lethargy, drowsiness, restlessness, muscle pains or cramps, confusion, gastrointestinal (GI) disturbances, hypotension, oliguria, tachycardia, and seizures.

The nurse must closely observe patients receiving a potassium-sparing diuretic for signs of hyperkalemia (see Display 45-1), a serious and potentially fatal electrolyte imbalance. Sometimes a potassium-sparing diuretic is prescribed along with a thiazide diuretic to keep potassium levels within normal limits. If excessive electrolyte loss occurs, the primary health care provider may reduce the dosage or withdraw the drug temporarily until the electrolyte imbalance is corrected.

RISK FOR INJURY Patients receiving a diuretic (particularly a loop or thiazide diuretic) and a digitalis glycoside concurrently require frequent monitoring of the pulse rate and rhythm because of the possibility of cardiac arrhythmias. Any significant changes in the pulse rate and rhythm are immediately reported to the primary health care provider.

Some patients experience dizziness or lightheadedness, especially during the first few days of therapy or when a rapid diuresis has occurred. Patients who are dizzy, but allowed out of bed, are assisted by the nurse with ambulatory activities until these adverse drug effects disappear.

EDUCATING THE PATIENT AND FAMILY

The patient and the family require a full explanation of the prescribed drug therapy, including when to take the drug (diuretics taken once a day are best taken early in the morning), if the drug is to be taken with food, and the importance of following the dosage schedule printed on the container label. The nurse also explains the onset and duration of the drug's diuretic effect. The patient and family must also be made aware of the signs and symptoms of fluid and electrolyte imbalances and adverse reactions that may occur when using a diuretic.

To ensure compliance with the prescribed drug regimen, the nurse stresses the importance of diuretic therapy in treating the patient's disorder. If the patient states that taking a diuretic at a specific time will be a problem, the nurse helps the patient identify the difficulty associated with drug therapy, after which the nurse can suggest ways to overcome the barrier. The nurse includes the following points in a patient teaching plan:

- Do not stop taking the drug or omit doses, except on the advice of a primary health care provider.

- If GI upset occurs, take the drug with food or milk.

- Take the drug early in the morning (once-a-day dosage) unless directed otherwise to minimize the effects on nighttime sleep. Twice-a-day dosing should be administered early in the morning (e.g., 7:00 AM) and early afternoon (e.g., 2:00 PM) or as directed by the primary health care provider. These drugs initially cause an increase in urination, which should subside after a few weeks.

- Do not reduce fluid intake to reduce the need to urinate. Be sure to continue the fluid intake recommended by the primary health care provider.

- Avoid alcohol and nonprescription drugs unless their use has been approved by the primary health care provider. Hypertensive patients should be careful to avoid medications that increase blood pressure, such as OTC drugs for appetite suppression and cold symptoms.

- Notify the primary health care provider if any of the following occur: muscle cramps or weakness, dizziness, nausea, vomiting, diarrhea, restlessness, excessive thirst, general weakness, rapid pulse, increased heart rate or pulse, or GI distress.

- If dizziness or weakness occurs, observe caution while driving or performing hazardous tasks, rise slowly from a sitting or lying position, and avoid standing in one place for an extended time.

- Weigh yourself weekly or as recommended by the primary health care provider. Keep a record of these weekly weights and contact the primary health care provider if weight loss exceeds 3 to 5 lb a week.

- If foods or fluids high in potassium are recommended by the primary health care provider, eat the amount recommended. Do not exceed this amount or eliminate these foods from the diet for more than 1 day, except when told to do so by the primary health care provider (see Home Care Checklist: Preventing Potassium Imbalances).

• After a time, the diuretic effect of the drug may be minimal because most of the body's excess fluid has been removed. Continue therapy to prevent further accumulation of fluid.

• If taking thiazide or related diuretics, loop diuretics, potassium-sparing diuretics, carbonic anhydrase inhibitors, or triamterene, avoid exposure to sunlight or ultraviolet light (sunlamps, tanning beds) because exposure may cause exaggerated sunburn (a photosensitivity reaction). Wear sunscreen and protective clothing until tolerance is determined.

• *For patients who have diabetes mellitus and who take loop or thiazide diuretics:* Know that blood glucometer test results for glucose may be elevated (blood) or urine may test positive for glucose. Contact the primary health care provider if home-tested blood glucose levels increase or if urine tests positive for glucose.

• *For patients who take potassium-sparing diuretics:* Avoid eating foods high in potassium and avoid the use of salt substitutes containing potassium. Read food labels carefully. Do not use a salt substitute unless a particular brand has been approved by the primary health care provider. Also avoid the use of potassium supplements. Male patients who take spironolactone may experience gynecomastia. This is usually reversible when therapy is discontinued.

• *For patients who take thiazide diuretics:* These agents may cause gout attacks. Contact the primary health care provider if significant, sudden joint pain occurs.

• *For patients who take carbonic anhydrase inhibitors:* During treatment for glaucoma, contact the primary health care provider immediately if eye pain is not relieved or if it increases. When a patient with epilepsy is being treated for seizures, a family member of the patient should keep a record of all seizures witnessed and bring this to the primary health care provider at the time of the next visit. Contact the primary health care provider immediately if the number of seizures increases.

EVALUATION

• The therapeutic effect is achieved.

• Adverse reactions are identified, reported to the primary health care provider, and managed successfully through appropriate nursing interventions.

• Fluid volume problems are corrected.

• No injury is evident.

• The patient verbalizes the importance of complying with the prescribed treatment regimen.

• The patient and family demonstrate an understanding of the drug regimen.

Critical Thinking Exercises

1. Mr. Walsh, aged 46 years, sees his primary health care provider and is prescribed a thiazide diuretic for hypertension. He tells you that it will be inconvenient for him to take his drug in the morning and he would prefer to take it at night. Other than asking him why taking the drug in the evening is more convenient, discuss what other questions you would ask Mr. Walsh. Analyze the situation to determine what explanation regarding present and future actions of this diuretic you would tell this patient.

2. Mr. Rodriguez, aged 78 years, is taking amiloride for hypertension. He and his wife came to the clinic for a routine blood pressure check. Mrs. Rodriguez states that her husband has been confused and very irritable for the last 2 days. He complains of nausea and has had several "loose" stools. Discuss what actions you would take. Give your rationale for each action.

3. Ms. Palmer, aged 88 years, is a resident in a nursing home. Her primary health care provider prescribes a thiazide diuretic for CHF. The nurse in charge advises you to evaluate Ms. Palmer for signs and symptoms of dehydration and hyponatremia. Discuss the assessment you would make. Identify which of these signs and symptoms might be difficult to evaluate considering the patient's age.

Review Questions

1. When evaluating the effectiveness of acetazolamide (Diamox) given for acute glaucoma, the nurse questions the patient about _____.

   A. the amount of urine each time the patient voids

   B. the relief of eye pain

   C. the amount of fluid being taken

   D. occipital headaches

2. When a patient taking mannitol for increased intracranial pressure is being assessed, which of the following findings would be most important for the nurse to report?

A. A serum potassium of 3.5 mEq/mL

B. Urine output of 20 mL for the last 2 hours

C. A blood pressure of 140/80 mm Hg

D. A heart rate of 72 bpm

3. When administering spironolactone (Aldactone), the nurse monitors the patient closely for which of the following electrolyte imbalances?

A. Hypernatremia

B. Hyponatremia

C. Hyperkalemia

D. Hypokalemia

4. When a diuretic is being administered for heart failure, which of the following would be most indicative of an effective response of diuretic therapy?

A. Output of 30 mL/h

B. Daily weight loss of 2 lb

C. An increase in blood pressure

D. Increasing edema of the lower extremities

5. Which electrolyte imbalance would the patient receiving a loop or thiazide diuretic most likely develop?

A. Hypernatremia

B. Hyponatremia

C. Hyperkalemia

D. Hypokalemia

6. Which of the following foods would the nurse most likely recommend the patient include in the daily diet to prevent hypokalemia?

A. Green beans

B. Apples

C. Bananas

D. Corn

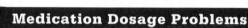
Medication Dosage Problems

1. The primary health care provider prescribes spironolactone (Aldactone) 100 mg orally. The drug is available in 50-mg tablets. The nurse administers _____.

2. Furosemide (Lasix) 20 mg oral solution is prescribed. The oral solution is available in a concentration of 40 mg/5 mL. The nurse administers

_____.

To check your answers see Appendix G.

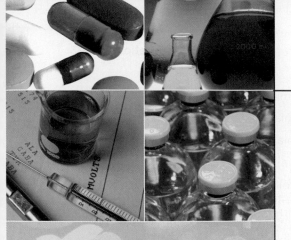

Chapter 46

Urinary Tract Anti-Infectives, Antispasmodics, and Other Urinary Drugs

Learning Objectives

On completion of this chapter, the student will:

- Discuss the uses, general drug actions, adverse reactions, contraindications, precautions, and interactions of the drugs used to treat infections and symptoms associated with urinary tract infections or an overactive bladder.

- Discuss important preadministration and ongoing assessment activities the nurse should perform with the patient taking a drug for a urinary tract infection or an overactive bladder.

- List nursing diagnoses particular to a patient taking a drug for a urinary tract infection or an overactive bladder.

- Discuss ways to promote an optimal response to therapy, how to manage adverse reactions, and important points to keep in mind when educating patients about the use of drugs used to treat a urinary tract infection or symptoms associated with an overactive bladder.

Urinary tract infection (UTI) is an infection caused by pathogenic microorganisms of one or more structures of the urinary tract. Because the female urethra is considerably shorter than the male urethra, women are affected by UTIs much more frequently than men. The most common structure affected is the bladder. Clinical manifestations of a UTI of the bladder (**cystitis**) include urgency, frequency, pressure, burning and pain on urination, and pain caused by spasm in the region of the bladder and the suprapubic area. With chronic UTIs, the urethra, prostate, and kidney may also be affected (Fig. 46-1). Display 46-1 identifies the inflammatory disorders most frequently associated with each of these structures in the urinary system.

Overactive bladder (involuntary contractions of the detrusor or bladder muscle) is estimated to affect more than 16 million individuals in the United States.

Display 46.1 Common Inflammatory Disorders Associated With the Urinary System

Cystitis—inflammation of the bladder
Urethritis—inflammation of the urethra
Prostatitis—inflammation of the prostate gland
Pyelonephritis—inflammation of the kidney and renal pelvis

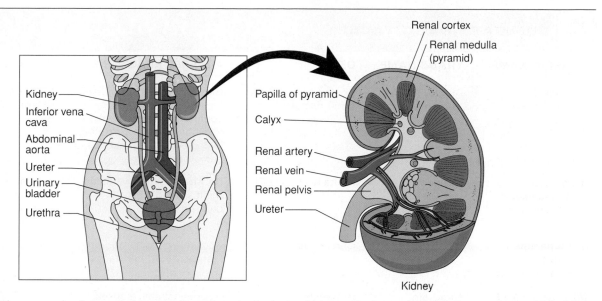

Figure 46.1 The normal urinary system, male or female, includes kidneys (enlarged at right), ureters, and bladder.

This problem sometimes results from such disorders as cystitis or prostatitis, or from abnormalities related to affected structures, such as the kidney or the urethra. Symptoms of an overactive bladder include **urinary urgency** (a strong and sudden desire to urinate), frequent urination throughout the day and night, and **urge incontinence** (involuntary urination after sudden sensation to void).

This chapter discusses drugs used to treat UTIs and drugs used to relieve the symptoms associated with an overactive bladder. When infection is present, structures of the urinary system that may be affected include the bladder (cystitis), prostate gland (**prostatitis**), the kidney (**pyelonephritis**), and the urethra (see Fig. 46-1). The drugs discussed in this chapter are anti-infectives. They are used in the treatment of UTIs and they have an effect on bacteria in the urinary tract. Although administered systemically, that is, by the oral or parenteral routes, they do not achieve significant levels in the bloodstream and are of no value in treating systemic infections. They are primarily excreted by the kidneys and exert their major antibacterial effects in the urine.

Some drugs used in the treatment of UTIs, such as nitrofurantoin, do not belong to the antibiotic or sulfonamide groups of drugs. Examples of the most common drugs used in treating UTIs include amoxicillin (broad-spectrum penicillins; see Chapter 7), trimethoprim (sulfonamides; see Chapter 6), and nitrofurantoin. The anti-infective drugs known as fluoroquinolones (see Chapter 10) were initially approved for UTI treatment, but have become of greater use in systemic infection treatment.

Combination drugs such as trimethoprim and sulfamethoxazole (Bactrim or Septra) are also used. The Summary Drug Table: Urinary Anti-infectives gives examples of the drugs used for UTIs.

Other drugs that treat UTIs include the antispasmodic drugs, which help control the discomfort associated with irritation of the lower urinary tract mucosa caused by infection, trauma, surgery, and endoscopic procedures. Phenazopyridine (Pyridium), a urinary analgesic, is another drug used to relieve discomfort associated with UTI. (See Summary Drug Table: Urinary Anti-infectives for a list of drugs used to treat problems associated with the urinary system.)

Actions and Uses

Anti-Infectives

These drugs are used for UTIs that are caused by susceptible bacterial microorganisms. Many of the anti-infective drugs used for treating UTIs are chosen because of the rapid excretion rate of the drugs rather than the way they act inside the body. As a result, these anti-infectives have a high concentration in the urine and appear to act by interfering with bacterial multiplication in the urine. Nitrofurantoin (Macrodantin) may be **bacteriostatic** (slows or retards the multiplication of bacteria) or **bactericidal** (destroys bacteria), depending on the concentration of the drug in the urine. See the specific anti-infective chapters for the manner in which other anti-infective drugs work.

SUMMARY DRUG TABLE   URINARY TRACT ANTI-INFECTIVES

GENERIC NAME	TRADE NAME	USES	ADVERSE REACTIONS	DOSAGE RANGES
amoxicillin *a-mox-i-sill'-in*	Amoxil, Trimox, Wymox	Acute bacterial UTIs, other bacterial infections	Glossitis, stomatitis, gastritis, furry tongue, nausea, vomiting, diarrhea, rash, fever, pain at injection site, hypersensitivity reactions, hematopoietic changes	250–500 mg orally q8h or 875 mg orally BID
fosfomycin tromethamine *foss-fo-my'-sin tro-meth-a-meen*	Monurol	Acute bacterial UTIs	Nausea, diarrhea, vaginitis, rhinitis, headache, back pain	3-g packet orally, provided in powder that must be mixed with fluid
methenamine hippurate *meth-en'-a-meen*	Hiprex, Urex	Chronic bacterial UTIs	Nausea, vomiting, abdominal cramps, bladder irritation	1 g orally BID
℞ nalidixic acid *nal-i-dix'-ic*	NegGram	Acute/chronic bacterial UTIs	Abdominal pain, nausea, vomiting, anorexia, diarrhea, rash, drowsiness, dizziness, photosensitivity reactions, blurred vision, weakness, headache	1 g orally QID for 1–2 wk; may reduce to 2 g/d for prolonged therapy
nitrofurantoin *nye-troe-fyoor-an'-toyn*	Furadantin, Macrobid, Macrodantin	Acute bacterial UTIs	Nausea, anorexia, peripheral neuropathy, headache, bacterial superinfection	50–100 mg orally QID
sulfamethizole *sul-fa-meth'-i-zole*	Thiosulfil Forte	Acute bacterial UTIs	Headache, nausea, vomiting, abdominal pain, crystalluria	0.5–1 g orally TID, QID
trimethoprim (TMP) *trye-meth'-oh-prim*	Proloprim	Acute bacterial UTIs	Rash, pruritus, nausea, vomiting	200 mg/d orally
Urinary Anti-Infective Combinations				
trimethoprim and sulfamethoxazole (TMP-SMZ) *trye-meth'-oh-prim sul-fa-meth-ox'-a-zole*	Bactrim, Bactrim DS, Septra, Septra DS	Acute bacterial UTIs, shigellosis, and acute otitis media	GI disturbances, allergic skin reactions, headache, anorexia, glossitis, hypersensitivity	160 mg TMP/800 SMZ orally q 12h; 8–10 mg/kg/d (based on TMP) IV in 2–4 divided doses
Other Urinary Drugs (Analgesics and Antispasmodics)				
darifenacin HCl *da-ree-fen'-ah-sin*	Enablex	Overactive bladder	Dry mouth, constipation	7.5 mg/d orally
flavoxate *fla-vox'-ate*	Urispas	Urinary symptoms caused by cystitis, prostatitis, and other urinary problems	Dry mouth, drowsiness, blurred vision, headache, urinary retention	100–200 mg orally TID or QID
oxybutynin *ocks-ee-byoo-tie'-nin*	Ditropan	Overactive bladder, neurogenic bladder	Dry mouth, nausea, headache, drowsiness, constipation, urinary retention	5 mg orally BID or TID
solifenacin *sole-ah-fen'-ah-sin*	Vesicare	Overactive bladder	Dry mouth, constipation, blurred vision, dry eyes	5 mg/d orally
tolterodine *toll-tear'-oh-dyne*	Detrol, Detrol LA (long-acting, extended-release)	Overactive bladder	Dry mouth, constipation, headache, dizziness	2 mg orally TID; extended-release: 4 mg/d

GENERIC NAME	TRADE NAME	USES	ADVERSE REACTIONS	DOSAGE RANGES
℞ **trospium** *troz'-pee-um*	Sanctura	Overactive bladder	Dry mouth, constipation, headache	20 mg orally TID
phenazopyridine *fen-az-oh-peer'-i-deen*	Pyridate, Pyridium, Urogesic	Relief of pain associated with irritation of the lower genitourinary tract	Headache, rash, pruritus, GI disturbances, red-orange discoloration of the urine, yellowish discoloration of the skin or sclera	200 mg orally TID

℞ Take this drug at least 1 hour before or 2 hours after meals.
GI, gastrointestinal; UTI, urinary tract infection.

Antispasmodics

Antispasmodics are cholinergic blocking drugs that inhibit bladder contractions and delay the urge to void. These drugs counteract the smooth muscle spasm of the urinary tract by relaxing the detrusor and other muscles through action at the parasympathetic nerve receptors. Flavoxate (Urispas) is used to relieve symptoms of **dysuria** (painful or difficult urination), urinary urgency, **nocturia** (excessive urination during the night), suprapubic pain and frequency, and urge incontinence. The other antispasmodic drugs are also used to treat bladder instability (i.e., urgency, frequency, leakage, incontinence, and painful or difficult urination) caused by a **neurogenic bladder** (impaired bladder function caused by a nervous system abnormality, typically an injury to the spinal cord).

Phenazopyridine is a dye that exerts a topical analgesic effect on the lining of the urinary tract. It does not have anti-infective activity. Phenazopyridine is available as a separate drug but is also included in some urinary tract anti-infective combination drugs.

Adverse Reactions

Anti-Infectives

Adverse reactions are primarily gastrointestinal (GI) disturbances and include

- Anorexia, nausea, vomiting, and diarrhea
- Abdominal pain or stomatitis

Other generalized body system reactions include

- Drowsiness, dizziness, headache, blurred vision, weakness, and peripheral neuropathy
- Rash, pruritus, photosensitivity reactions, and leg cramps

When these drugs are given in large doses, patients may experience burning on urination and bladder irritation;

this should not be mistaken for a continued infection. Nitrofurantoin has been known to cause acute and chronic pulmonary reactions.

Antispasmodics

Adverse reactions to these drugs are similar to those with other cholinergic blocking drugs. They include

- Dry mouth, drowsiness, constipation or diarrhea, decreased production of tears, decreased sweating, GI disturbances, dim vision, and urinary hesitancy

Other generalized body system reactions include

- Nausea and vomiting, nervousness, vertigo, headache, rash, and mental confusion (particularly in older adults)

Patients should be told that both the anti-infective and antispasmodic drugs can discolor the urine (dark orange to brown) and stain undergarments that come in contact with the urine.

Contraindications and Precautions

Anti-Infectives

Anti-infectives are contraindicated in patients with a hypersensitivity to the drugs, and during pregnancy (category C) and lactation. One exception is nitrofurantoin, which is classified as a pregnancy category B drug and is used with caution during pregnancy. Nalidixic acid (NegGram) is contraindicated in patients who have convulsive disorders.

The anti-infectives should be used cautiously in those with renal or hepatic impairment. Patients who are allergic to tartrazine (a food dye) should not take methenamine (Hiprex). This drug is used cautiously in patients with gout because it may cause crystals to form in the urine. Nalidixic acid and nitrofurantoin are used cautiously in patients with cerebral arteriosclerosis, diabetes, or a glucose-6-phosphate dehydrogenase (G6PD) deficiency.

Antispasmodics

Antispasmodic drugs are contraindicated in those patients with known hypersensitivity to the drugs or with glaucoma. Other patients for whom antispasmodics are contraindicated are those with intestinal or gastric blockage, abdominal bleeding, myasthenia gravis, or urinary tract blockage. Phenazopyridine is contraindicated in patients with renal impairment and in undiagnosed urinary tract pain.

The nurse should use these drugs with caution in patients with GI infections, benign prostatic hypertrophy, urinary retention, hyperthyroidism, hepatic or renal disease, and hypertension. The antispasmodic drugs are classified as pregnancy category C drugs and are used only when the benefit to the woman outweighs the risk to the fetus.

Phenazopyridine is used cautiously during pregnancy (category C) and lactation. Phenazopyridine treats the symptom of pain but does not treat the cause of the disorder. No significant interactions have been reported.

Interactions

Anti-Infectives

The following interactions may occur when a specific urinary anti-infective is administered with another agent:

Interacting Drug	Common Use	Effect of Interaction
Nalidixic Acid and Sulfamethoxazole		
oral anticoagulants	Blood thinner	Increased risk for bleeding
Nitrofurantoin		
magnesium trisilicate or magaldrate	Relieve gastric upset	Decreased absorption of anti-infective
anticholinergics	Relieve bladder spasm/ discomfort	Delay in gastric emptying, thereby increasing the absorption of nitrofurantoin
Fosfomycin (Monurol)		
metoclopramide (Reglan)	Relieve gastric upset	Lowers plasma concentration and urinary tract excretion of fosfomycin

An increased urinary pH decreases the effectiveness of methenamine. Therefore, to avoid raising the urine pH when taking methenamine, the patient should not use antacids containing sodium bicarbonate or sodium carbonate.

Antispasmodics

The following interactions may occur when an antispasmodic drug is administered with another agent:

Interacting Drug	Common Use	Effect of Interaction
antibiotics/ antifungals	Fight infection	Decreased effectiveness of anti-infective drug
meperidine, flurazepam, phenothiazines	Preoperative sedation	Increased effect of the antispasmodic
tricyclic antidepressants	Management of depression	Increased effect of the antispasmodic
haloperidol (Haldol)	Antianxiety/ antipsychotic agent	Decreased effectiveness of the antipsychotic drug
digoxin	Management of cardiac problems	Increased serum levels of digoxin

Health Supplement Alert

Cranberry juice has long been recommended for use in treating and preventing UTIs. Clinical studies have confirmed that cranberry juice is beneficial to individuals with frequent UTIs. Cranberry juice inhibits bacteria from attaching to the walls of the urinary tract and prevents certain bacteria from forming dental plaque in the mouth. Cranberry juice is safe for use as a food and for urinary tract health. Cranberry juice and capsules have no contraindications, no known adverse reactions, and no drug interactions. The recommended dosage is 9 to 15 capsules a day (400 to 500 mg/d) or 4 to 8 ounces of juice daily.

NURSING PROCESS

The Patient Receiving a Urinary Tract Anti-Infective or Other Urinary Tract Drug

ASSESSMENT

PREADMINISTRATION ASSESSMENT

When a UTI has been diagnosed, urine culture and sensitivity tests are performed to determine bacterial sensitivity to the drugs (antibiotics and urinary tract anti-infectives) that will control the infection. The nurse questions the patient regarding symptoms of the infection before instituting therapy. The nurse records the color and appearance of the urine. The nurse takes and records the vital signs.

When the miscellaneous drugs are administered, the nurse documents the symptoms the patient is experiencing to provide a baseline for future assessment. The nurse assesses for and documents pain, urinary frequency, bladder distension, and other symptoms associated with the urinary system.

ONGOING ASSESSMENT

Many UTIs are treated on an outpatient basis because hospitalization is seldom required. UTIs may affect the hospitalized patient or nursing home resident with an indwelling urethral catheter or a disorder such as a stone in the urinary tract. The primary nursing intervention to prevent UTIs in the hospitalized patient is good hand hygiene (handwashing).

When caring for a hospitalized patient with a UTI, the nurse monitors the vital signs every 4 hours or as ordered by the primary health care provider. Any significant rise in body temperature is reported to the primary health care provider because intervention to reduce the fever or culture and sensitivity tests may need to be repeated.

The nurse monitors the patient's response to therapy daily. If after several days the symptoms of the UTI do not improve or they become worse, the nurse notifies the primary health care provider as soon as possible. Periodic urinalysis and urine culture and sensitivity tests may be ordered to monitor the effects of drug therapy.

When administering any of the other urinary drugs, such as the antispasmodics, the nurse monitors the patient for a reduction in the symptoms identified in the preadministration assessment, such as dysuria, urinary frequency, urgency, and nocturia, and relief of any pain associated with irritation of the lower genitourinary tract.

NURSING DIAGNOSES

Drug-specific nursing diagnoses are highlighted in the Nursing Diagnoses Checklist. Other nursing diagnoses applicable to these drugs are discussed in depth in Chapter 4.

Nursing Diagnosis Checklist

✓ **Impaired Urinary Elimination** related to discomfort of urinary tract infection

✓ **Ineffective Breathing Pattern** related to adverse reaction to drug

PLANNING

The expected outcomes for the patient may include an optimal response to drug therapy, support of patient needs related to the management of adverse reactions, and an understanding of and compliance with the prescribed therapeutic regimen.

IMPLEMENTATION
PROMOTING AN OPTIMAL RESPONSE TO THERAPY

To promote an optimal response to therapy, the nurse gives urinary tract anti-infectives with food to prevent GI upset. Nitrofurantoin, especially, should be given with food, meals, or milk because this drug is particularly irritating to the stomach. Fosfomycin (Monurol) has special administration requirements; it comes in a 3-g, one-dose packet that must be dissolved in 90 to 120 mL water (not hot water). The nurse administers the drug immediately after dissolving it in water.

Should visual disturbances occur when using nalidixic acid, they are noted after each dose. In many cases, they subside after a few days of therapy.

The dosage of antispasmodic drugs may be reduced when the patient's symptoms improve. Phenazopyridine is administered after meals to prevent GI upset.

Nursing Alert

Phenazopyridine is not administered for more than 2 days when used in combination with an antibacterial drug to treat a UTI. When used for more than 2 days, the drug may mask the symptoms of a more serious disorder.

MONITORING AND MANAGING PATIENT NEEDS

The nurse observes the patient for adverse drug reactions. If an adverse reaction occurs, the nurse contacts the primary health care provider before the next dose of the drug is due. However, serious drug reactions, such as a pulmonary reaction, are reported immediately.

IMPAIRED URINARY ELIMINATION The patient is encouraged to drink at least 2000 mL of fluid daily (if condition permits) to dilute urine and decrease pain on voiding. Drinking extra fluids aids in the physical removal of bacteria from the genitourinary tract and is an important part of UTI treatment (see Patient and Family Teaching Checklist: Preventing and Treating UTIs). The nurse offers fluids, preferably water, to the patient at hourly intervals. Cranberry or prune juice is usually given rather than orange juice or other citrus or vegetable juices. The nurse notifies the primary health care provider if the patient fails to drink extra fluids, if the urine output is low, or if the urine appears concentrated during daytime hours. The urine of those drinking 2000 mL or more daily appears dilute and light in color.

Elderly patients often have a decreased thirst sensation and must be encouraged to increase fluid intake. This is especially true if an antispasmodic drug is also being taken. The nurse offers fluids at regular intervals to older adult patients or those who seem unable to increase their fluid intake without supervision (see Home Care Checklist: Combating Dry Mouth in Chapter 30).

When administering these drugs, the nurse monitors the fluid intake and urinary output for volume and frequency. The nurse measures and records the fluid intake and output every 8 hours, especially when the primary health care provider orders an increase in fluid intake or when a kidney infection is being treated. The primary health care provider may also order daily urinary pH levels when methenamine or nitrofurantoin is administered. These drugs work best in acid urine; failure of the urine to remain acidic may require administration of a urinary acidifier, such as ascorbic acid.

INEFFECTIVE BREATHING PATTERN Pulmonary reactions have been reported with the use of nitrofurantoin and may occur within hours and up to 3 weeks after drug therapy is initiated. Signs and symptoms of an acute pulmonary reaction include dyspnea, chest pain, cough, fever, and chills. If these reactions occur, the nurse immediately notifies the primary health care provider and withholds the next dose of the drug until the patient is seen by a primary health care provider. In addition to the aforementioned signs and symptoms, a nonproductive cough or malaise may indicate a chronic pulmonary reaction, which may occur during prolonged therapy.

PATIENT NEEDS WHEN TAKING ANTISPASMODIC DRUGS Common adverse reactions to cholinergic blocking drugs include dry mouth, dizziness, blurred vision, and constipation (see Chapter 30). For patients with dry mouth, the nurse suggests that the patient not only suck on hard candy, sugarless lozenges, or small pieces of ice but perform frequent mouth care. The dry mouth effect sometimes lessens with continued use of the drug. Hospitalized patients experiencing drowsiness or blurred vision may require assistance when ambulating. For patients with constipation, the nurse encourages fluids, provides a high-fiber diet, and provides times for ambulation or exercise (if the patient's condition allows). If constipation persists, the primary health care provider may prescribe a mild laxative or stool softener.

The nurse informs the patient that phenazopyridine may cause a reddish-orange discoloration of the urine that will stain clothing. In addition, the fluid that lubricates the eyes may change color, causing permanent discoloration of contact lenses. The nurse reassures the patient that this discoloration is normal and will subside when use of the drug is discontinued.

EDUCATING THE PATIENT AND FAMILY
The nurse stresses the importance of increasing fluid intake to at least 2000 mL/d (unless contraindicated) to help remove bacteria from the genitourinary tract (see Patient and Family Teaching Checklist: Preventing and Treating UTIs). In many cases, symptoms are relieved after several days of drug therapy.

Patient and Family Teaching Checklist

Preventing and Treating UTIs
The nurse:

✔ Discusses UTIs and their causes, and the need for fluids and drug therapy.

✔ Reviews the drug therapy regimen, including prescribed drug, dose, and frequency of administration.

✔ Stresses the importance of continued therapy even if patient feels better after a few doses.

✔ Instructs the patient to continue therapy until all of the drug is finished or the primary care provider discontinues therapy.

✔ Explains the rationale for increasing fluid intake to at least 2000 mL/d (unless contraindicated) to aid in physical removal of bacteria.

✔ Urges patient to drink fluids every hour.

✔ Offers suggestions for fluids to drink based on patient's likes and dislikes.

✔ Demonstrates procedure for measuring intake and output using household measures.

✔ Informs patient about urine appearance when intake is increased and describes drug-induced urine color changes that can stain undergarments

✔ Encourages continued increased fluid intake even if symptoms subside.

✔ Instructs the patient to notify primary health care provider if urine output is low, urine appears dark or concentrated during the daytime, or symptoms do not improve after 3 to 4 days.

✔ Reviews signs and symptoms of possible adverse reactions and of new infection or worsening infection, both verbally and in writing.

✔ Emphasizes the importance of follow-up visits and laboratory tests to determine the effectiveness of therapy.

To ensure compliance with the prescribed drug regimen, the nurse stresses the importance of completing the full course of drug therapy even though symptoms have been relieved. A full course of therapy is necessary to ensure that all bacteria have been eliminated from the urinary tract. The nurse should include the following points in a patient and family teaching plan:

ANTI-INFECTIVES

- Take the drug with food or meals (nitrofurantoin must be taken with food or milk). If GI upset occurs despite taking the drug with food, contact the primary health care provider.

- Take the drug at the prescribed intervals and complete the full course of therapy. Do not discontinue taking the drug even though the symptoms have disappeared, unless directed to do so by the primary health care provider.

- If drowsiness or dizziness occurs, avoid driving and performing tasks that require alertness.

- During therapy with this drug, avoid alcoholic beverages and do not take any nonprescription drug unless its use has been approved by the primary health care provider.

- Notify the primary health care provider immediately if symptoms do not improve after 3 or 4 days.

- *Nitrofurantoin*: Take this drug with food or milk to improve absorption. Continue therapy for at least 1 week or for 3 days after the urine shows no signs of infection. Notify the primary health care provider immediately if any of the following occur: fever, chills, cough, shortness of breath, chest pain, or difficulty breathing. Do not take the next dose of the drug until the primary health care provider has been contacted. The urine may appear brown during therapy with this drug; this is not abnormal.

- *Nalidixic acid*: Take this drug with food to prevent GI upset. Avoid prolonged exposure to sunlight or ultraviolet light (tanning beds or lamps) because an exaggerated sunburn may occur.

- *Methenamine*: Avoid excessive intake of citrus products, milk, and milk products.

- *Fosfomycin* comes in dry form as a one-dose packet to be dissolved in 90 to 120 mL water (not hot water). Drink immediately after mixing and take with food to prevent gastric upset.

ANTISPASMODIC AND OTHER DRUGS

- For dry mouth, suck on hard candy, sugarless lozenges, or small pieces of ice and perform frequent mouth care.

- These drugs may cause drowsiness or blurred vision. Do not drive or operate dangerous machinery or participate in any activity that requires full mental alertness until you know how this medication affects you.

- If you experience constipation, drink plenty of fluids, eat a high-fiber diet, and exercise (if your condition allows). If constipation persists, the primary health care provider may prescribe a mild laxative or stool softener.

- *Flavoxate*: Take this drug three to four times daily as prescribed. This drug is used to treat symptoms; other drugs are given to treat the cause.

- *Oxybutynin*: Take this drug with or without food. Oxybutynin (Ditropan XL) contains an outer coating that may not disintegrate and sometimes may be observed in the stool. This is not a cause for concern. If using the transdermal form (patch) of the drug, be sure to apply to a clean, dry area of the hip, abdomen, or buttocks. Remove old patch and rotate sites of new application every 7 days.

- Antispasmodic drugs can cause heat prostration (fever and heat stroke caused by decreased sweating) in high temperatures. If you live in hot climates or will be exposed to high temperatures, take appropriate precautions.

- *Phenazopyridine*: This drug may cause a reddish-orange discoloration of the urine and tears and may stain fabrics or contact lenses. This is normal. Take the drug after meals. Do not take this drug for more than 2 days if you are also taking an antibiotic for the treatment of a UTI.

EVALUATION

- The therapeutic effect is achieved.

- Adverse reactions are identified, reported to the primary health care provider, and managed successfully through appropriate nursing interventions.

- The patient and family demonstrate an understanding of the drug regimen.

- The patient verbalizes the importance of complying with the prescribed therapeutic regimen.

Critical Thinking Exercises

1. Ms. Elliot, aged 42 years, had a UTI 8 weeks ago. She failed to see her primary health care provider for a follow-up urine sample 2 weeks after completing her course of drug therapy. Ms. Elliot is in

Urinary Tract Anti-Infectives, Antispasmodics

to see her primary health care provider because her UTI symptoms have recurred. The primary health care provider suspects that Ms. Elliott may not have followed instructions regarding treatment for her UTI. Analyze the situation to determine what points you would stress in a teaching plan for this patient.

2. Ms. Howard, aged 86 years, has Alzheimer's disease and is a resident in a nursing home. She has a UTI and is prescribed nitrofurantoin (Macrodantin). Discuss specific nursing tasks to include in a nursing care plan for this patient. What potential problems could be anticipated because of the Alzheimer's disease? What drugs might the primary care provider prescribe for the Alzheimer's disease?

Review Questions

1. The nurse correctly administers nitrofurantoin (Macrodantin) _____.

    A. with food

    B. no longer than 7 days

    C. without regard to food

    D. no longer than 2 days

2. To avoid raising the pH when taking methenamine (Hiprex), the nurse advises the patient to _____.

    A. use an antacid before taking the drug

    B. take an antacid immediately after taking the drug

    C. avoid antacids containing sodium bicarbonate or sodium carbonate

    D. avoid the use of antacids 1 hour before or 2 hours after taking the drug

3. What instruction would be most important to give a patient prescribed fosfomycin (Monurol)?

    A. Drink one to two glasses of cranberry juice daily to promote healing of the urinary tract.

    B. You may take the drug without regard to meals.

    C. This drug comes in a one-dose packet that must be dissolved in 90 mL or more of fluids.

    D. This drug may cause mental confusion.

4. What statement(s) would be included in a teaching plan for a patient prescribed phenazopyridine (Pyridium)?

    A. There is a danger of heat prostration or heat stroke when taking phenazopyridine in a hot climate.

    B. This drug may turn the urine dark brown. This is an indication of a serious condition and should be reported immediately.

    C. This drug may cause photosensitivity. Take precautions when out in the sun by wearing sunscreen, a hat, and long-sleeved shirts for protection.

    D. This drug may turn the urine reddish-orange. This is a normal occurrence that will disappear when use of the drug is discontinued.

Medication Dosage Problems

1. Amoxicillin 500 mg is prescribed. The drug is available in 250-mg tablets. The nurse administers _____.

2. Nitrofurantoin oral suspension 50 mg is prescribed. The oral suspension contains 25 mg/5 mL. The nurse administers _____.

To check your answers, see Appendix G.

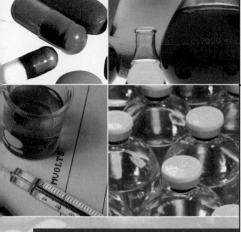

Chapter 47

Drugs That Affect the Upper Gastrointestinal System

Key Terms

chemoreceptor trigger zone (CTZ)
gastric stasis
gastroesophageal reflux disease
Helicobacter pylori
hydrochloric acid
hypersecretory
nausea
paralytic ileus
vertigo
vomiting

Learning Objectives

On completion of this chapter, the student will:

- Discuss the general drug actions, uses, adverse reactions, contraindications, precautions, and interactions of drugs used to treat conditions of the upper gastrointestinal system.
- Discuss important preadministration and ongoing assessment activities the nurse should perform with the patient receiving a drug used to treat conditions of the upper gastrointestinal system.

- List nursing diagnoses particular to a patient receiving a drug used to treat conditions of the upper gastrointestinal system.
- Use the nursing process when administering drugs used to treat conditions of the upper gastrointestinal system.

The gastrointestinal (GI) system is essentially a long tube in the body where ingested food and fluids are processed for absorption of nutrients. The upper GI system consists of the mouth, esophagus, and stomach. The mouth is responsible for breaking down food parts and mixing them with saliva to begin the digestion process. The tubular esophagus connects the mouth to the stomach, where food is mixed with acids and enzymes to become a solution for absorption. Some of the cells of the stomach secrete **hydrochloric acid** (HCl), a substance that aids in the initial digestive process. Problems occur when acids or stomach contents reverse direction and attempt to come back up the GI tract, which can create tissue damage and ulcers. Figure 47-1 illustrates the entire GI system.

Drugs are presented in this chapter according to their function, whether they treat gastric acid production or prevent vomiting. Drugs that neutralize HCl and protect the mucosal lining are called *antacids*. Drugs that reduce the production and release of HCl include histamine H$_2$ antagonists, proton pump inhibitors, and miscellaneous acid-reducing agents. The proton pump inhibitors are particularly important in the treatment of *Helicobacter pylori* infection in patients with active duodenal ulcers. *H. pylori* is believed to cause a type of chronic gastritis and some peptic and duodenal ulcers as well. GI stimulants facilitate emptying of stomach contents into the small intestine, and are used both as ulcer treatments and as antiemetics. Antiemetics are used to treat and prevent nausea and vomiting. Some of the more common drugs are listed in the Summary Drug Table: Drugs Used in Managing Upper Gastrointestinal Disorders.

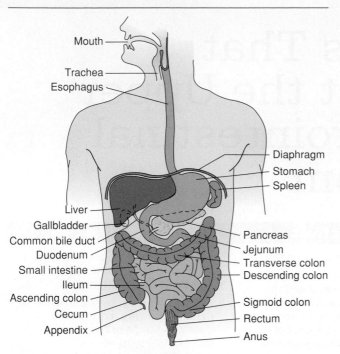

Figure 47.1   The gastrointestinal system. (From Timby, B. K., & Smith, N. E. [2007]. *Introductory medical surgical nursing* [9th ed., p. 810.] Philadelphia: Lippincott Williams & Wilkins.)

ACID NEUTRALIZERS: ANTACIDS

Actions

Antacids ("against acids") are drugs that neutralize or reduce the acidity of stomach and duodenal contents by combining with HCl and increasing the pH of the stomach acid. Antacids do not "coat" the stomach lining, although they may increase the sphincter tone of the lower esophagus. Examples of antacids include aluminum hydroxide gel (Amphojel), magaldrate (Riopan), and magnesium hydroxide (Milk of Magnesia).

Uses

Antacids are used in the treatment of hyperacidity caused by

- Heartburn, acid indigestion, or sour stomach
- **Gastroesophageal reflux disease** (GERD; a reflux or backup of gastric contents into the esophagus)
- Peptic ulcer

Antacids may be used to treat conditions that are not associated with the GI system. For example, aluminum

carbonate is a phosphate-binding agent and is used in treating hyperphosphatemia (often associated with chronic renal failure) or as an adjunct to a low-phosphate diet to prevent formation of phosphate-based urinary stones. Calcium carbonate may be used in treating calcium deficiency states such as menopausal osteoporosis. Magnesium oxide may be used for treating magnesium deficiencies or magnesium depletion from malnutrition, restricted diet, or alcoholism.

Adverse Reactions

The magnesium- and sodium-containing antacids may have a laxative effect and may produce diarrhea. Aluminum- and calcium-containing products tend to produce constipation. Although the antacids have the potential for serious adverse reactions, they have a wide margin of safety, especially when used as prescribed. The less common but more serious adverse reactions include

- Aluminum-containing antacids—constipation, intestinal impaction, anorexia, weakness, tremors, and bone pain
- Magnesium-containing antacids—severe diarrhea, dehydration, and hypermagnesemia (nausea, vomiting, hypotension, decreased respirations)
- Calcium-containing antacids—rebound hyperacidity, metabolic alkalosis, hypercalcemia, vomiting, confusion, headache, renal calculi, and neurologic impairment
- Sodium bicarbonate—systemic alkalosis and rebound hyperacidity

Contraindications and Precautions

The antacids are contraindicated in patients with severe abdominal pain of unknown cause and during lactation. Sodium-containing antacids are contraindicated in patients with cardiovascular problems, such as hypertension or congestive heart failure, and those on sodium-restricted diets. Calcium-containing antacids are contraindicated in patients with renal calculi or hypercalcemia.

Aluminum-containing antacids are used cautiously in patients with gastric outlet obstruction or those with upper GI bleeding. Magnesium- and aluminum-containing antacids are used cautiously in patients with decreased kidney function. The calcium-containing antacids are used cautiously in patients with respiratory insufficiency, renal impairment, or cardiac disease. Antacids are classified as

SUMMARY DRUG TABLE DRUGS USED IN MANAGING UPPER GASTROINTESTINAL DISORDERS

GENERIC NAME	TRADE NAME	USES	ADVERSE REACTIONS	DOSAGE RANGES
Acid Neutralizers				
aluminum carbonate gel, basic *a-loo'-mi-num*	Basaljel	Symptomatic relief of peptic ulcer and stomach hyperacidity, hyperphosphatemia	Constipation, bone softening, neurotoxicity	2 tablets or capsules (10 mL of regular oral suspension) as often as q2h, up to 12 times daily
aluminum hydroxide gel	Alu-Tab, Amphojel, Dialume	Same as aluminum carbonate	Same as aluminum carbonate	500–1500 mg (5–30 mL in oral suspension) 3–6 times daily orally between meals and bedtime
calcium carbonate *kal'-see-um carb-owe-nate*	Tums, Mylanta	Symptomatic relief of peptic ulcer and stomach hyperacidity, calcium deficiencies (osteoporosis)	Acid rebound	0.5–1.5 g orally
magnesia (magnesium hydroxide) *mag-nee'-zee-ah*	Milk of Magnesia, Phillips' MOM	Symptomatic relief of peptic ulcer and stomach hyperacidity, constipation	Diarrhea, bone loss in patients with chronic renal failure	Antacid: 622–1244 mg (5–15 mL in suspension) orally QID Laxative: 15–60 mL orally
magnesium oxide *mag-nee'-zee-um*	Mag-Ox 400, Maox 420, Uro-Mag	Same as magnesia	Same as magnesia	140–800 mg/d orally
sodium bicarbonate *soe-dee'-um*	Bellans	Symptomatic relief of peptic ulcer and stomach hyperacidity	Electrolyte imbalance and metabolic alkalosis	0.3–2 g orally 1–4 times daily
Combined-Product Acid Neutralizer				
magaldrate (hydroxymagnesium aluminate) *mag'-al-drate*	Riopan	Symptomatic relief of peptic ulcer and stomach hyperacidity	Constipation, diarrhea	5–10 mL orally between meals and bedtime
Acid Reducers				
Histamine H$_2$ Antagonists				
cimetidine* *sye-met'-i-deen*	Tagamet	Gastric/duodenal ulcers, GERD, gastric hypersecretory conditions, GI bleeding, heartburn	Headache, somnolence, diarrhea	800–1600 mg/d orally; 300 mg q6h IM or IV
famotidine* *fa-moe'-ti-deen*	Pepcid	Same as cimetidine	Same as cimetidine	20–40 mg orally; IV if unable to take orally
nizatidine *ni-za'-ti-deen*	Axid	Same as cimetidine	Same as cimetidine	150–300 mg/d orally in one dose or divided doses

Drugs That Affect the Upper Gastrointestinal System

⬤ SUMMARY DRUG TABLE *(continued)*

GENERIC NAME	TRADE NAME	USES	ADVERSE REACTIONS	DOSAGE RANGES
ranitidine* *ra-nye'-te-deen*	Zantac	Same as cimetidine, erosive esophagitis	Same as cimetidine	150–600 mg orally in one dose or divided doses orally; 50 mg q6–8h IM, IV (do not exceed 400 mg/d)
Proton Pump Inhibitors				
esomeprazole magnesium *ess-oh-me'-pra-zole*	Nexium	Erosive esophagitis, GERD, *H. pylori* eradication, NSAID-associated gastric ulcers	Headache, nausea, diarrhea	20–40 mg/d orally
lansoprazole *lan-soe'-pra-zole*	Prevacid	Same as esomeprazole, hypersecretory conditions, cystic fibrosis (intestinal malabsorption)	Same as esomeprazole	15–30 mg/d orally
omeprazole *oh-me'-pra-zole*	Prilosec, Zegerid	Same as esomeprazole, hypersecretory conditions, heartburn, reduce risk of upper GI bleeding	Same as esomeprazole	20–60 mg/d orally
pantoprazole sodium *pan-toe'-pra-zole*	Protonix	GERD, erosive esophagitis and hypersecretory conditions	Same as esomeprazole	40 mg/d orally or IV Hypersecretion: 80 mg IV q12h
rabeprazole sodium *rah-beh'-pra-zole*	Aciphex	Same as esomeprazole	Same as esomeprazole	20 mg/d orally
Miscellaneous Acid Reducers				
sucralfate *soo-kral'-fate*	Carafate	Short-term duodenal ulcer treatment	Constipation	1 g/d orally in divided doses
misoprostol *mye-soe-prost'-ole*	Cytotec	Prevention of gastric ulcers in patients taking NSAIDs	Headache, nausea, diarrhea, abdominal pain	100–200 mcg orally QID
GI Stimulants				
dexpanthenol *dex-pan'-the-nole*	Ilopan	Immediate postoperative medication for prevention of paralytic ileus	Itching, tingling, difficulty breathing	250–500 mg IM
Ⓡ **metoclopramide** *met-oh-kloé-pra-mide*	Reglan	Diabetic gastroparesis, GERD, prevention of nausea and vomiting	Restlessness, dizziness, fatigue, extrapyramidal effects	10–15 mg orally; 10–20 mg IM, IV

GENERIC NAME	TRADE NAME	USES	ADVERSE REACTIONS	DOSAGE RANGES
Antiemetics				
Antidopaminergics				
chlorpromazine HCl *klor-proe'-ma-zeen*	Thorazine	Control of nausea and vomiting, intractable hiccoughs	Drowsiness, hypotension, dry mouth, nasal congestion	Nausea and vomiting: 10–25 mg orally q4–6h; 50–100 mg rectal suppository q6–8h; 25–50 mg IM q3–4h Hiccoughs: 25–50 mg orally, IM, slow IV infusion
perphenazine *per-fen'-a-zeen*		Same as chlorpromazine	Same as chlorpromazine	8–16 mg/d orally in divided doses, 5–10 mg IM, IV q6h
prochlorperazine HCl *proe-klor-per'-a-zeen*	Compazine	Control of nausea and vomiting	Same as chlorpromazine	Orally: 5–10 mg TID or QID IM, IV: 5–10 mg Rectal suppository: 25 mg BID Sustained-release: 10–15 mg
promethazine HCl *proe-meth'-a-zeen*	Phenergan	Control of nausea and vomiting associated with anesthesia and surgery, motion sickness	Same as diphenhydramine hydrochloride (Benadryl)	Nausea and vomiting: 12.5–25 mg orally, IM, IV, rectally Motion sickness: 25 mg orally 1–2 h before travel, repeat 8–12 h
thiethylperazine maleate *thye-eth-il-per'-a-zeen*	Torecan	Control of nausea and vomiting	Same as chlorpromazine	10–30 mg orally in divided doses
triflupromazine *trye-flu-proe'-ma-zeen*		Control of severe nausea and vomiting	Same as chlorpromazine	5–15 mg IM q4h; maximum dose, 60 mg/d; 1 mg IV, up to 3 mg/d
Cholinergic Blocking Drug				
trimethobenzamide HCl *trye-meth-oh-ben'-za-mide*	Tigan	Control of nausea and vomiting	Hypotension (IM use), Parkinson-like symptoms, blurred vision, drowsiness, dizziness	250 mg orally or 200 mg IM, rectal suppository TID or QID
5-HT3 Receptor Antagonists				
dolasetron mesylate[†] *doe-laz-ee'-tron*	Anzemet	Prevention of chemotherapy-induced and postoperative nausea, vomiting	Headache, fatigue, fever, abdominal pain	100 mg orally or 1.8 mg/kg IV
granisetron HCl[†] *gran-iz'-ee-tron*	Kytril	Same as dolasetron	Headache, asthenia, diarrhea, constipation	1–2 mg orally or 10 mcg/kg IV
ondansetron HCl[†] *on-dan'-see-tron*	Zofran	Same as dolasetron, bulimia, spinal analgesia–induced pruritus, levodopa-induced psychosis	Headache, fatigue, drowsiness, sedation, constipation, hypoxia	8 mg orally BID or TID; 32 mg IV
palonosetron[†] *pal'-oe-noh'-see-tron*	Aloxi	Same as dolasetron	Same as dolasetron	0.25 mg in a single dose

SUMMARY DRUG TABLE (continued)

GENERIC NAME	TRADE NAME	USES	ADVERSE REACTIONS	DOSAGE RANGES
Miscellaneous Antiemetic				
dronabinol[†] *droe-nab'-ih-nol*	Marinol	Prevention of chemotherapy-induced nausea and vomiting, appetite stimulant for patients with human immunodeficiency virus infection	Drowsiness, somnolence, euphoria, dizziness, vomiting	5 mg/m^2 1–3 h before chemotherapy Appetite stimulant: 2.5 mg orally BID

Ⓡ These drugs are taken at least 30 minutes before meals and at bedtime.
*These drugs are sold over the counter in smaller doses than those listed for therapeutic interventions.
†These drugs are administered according to specific protocols; the nurse should consult the order before administration.
GERD, gastroesophageal reflux disease; GI, gastrointestinal; NSAID, nonsteroidal anti-inflammatory drug.

pregnancy category C drugs and should be used with caution during pregnancy.

Interactions

The following interactions may occur when an antacid is administered with another agent:

Interacting Drug	Common Use	Effect of Interaction
digoxin, isoniazid, phenytoin, and chlorpromazine	Treatment of cardiac problems, infection, seizures, and nausea and vomiting, respectively	Decreased absorption of the interacting drugs results in a decreased effect of those drugs
tetracycline	Anti-infective agent	Decreased effectiveness of anti-infective
corticosteroids	Treatment of inflammation and respiratory problems	Decreased anti-inflammatory properties
salicylates	Pain relief	Pain reliever is excreted more rapidly in the urine
quinidine and amphetamines	Treatment of cardiac problems and central nervous system stimulant, respectively	Interacting drugs are excreted more slowly in the urine

Herbal Alert

Ginger, a pungent root, has been used medicinally for GI problems, such as motion sickness, nausea, vomiting, and digestion. In addition, it is recommended for the pain and inflammation of arthritis, and it may help lower cholesterol. The dosage of the dried form of ginger is 1 g (1000 mg) per day. Adverse reactions are rare, although heartburn has been reported by some individuals. Ginger should be used cautiously in patients with hypertension or gallstones and during pregnancy or lactation. As with any substance, a primary health care provider should be consulted before any ginger remedy is taken, although ginger has been consumed safely as a food by millions of individuals for centuries.

ACID-REDUCING AGENTS

Drugs that reduce the production of HCl include histamine type 2 receptor (H$_2$) antagonists, proton pump inhibitors, and miscellaneous drugs such as pepsin inhibitors, prostaglandins, and cholinergic blockers.

Histamine H$_2$ Antagonists
Actions

These drugs inhibit the action of histamine at H$_2$ receptor cells of the stomach, which then reduces the secretion of gastric acid. Cholinergic blocking drugs typically block the action of histamine throughout the entire body. Histamine H_2 antagonists do not cause the effects of the cholinergic blockers because they are selective only for the H_2 receptors in the stomach, and not the general body H_1 receptors. When ulcers are present, the decrease in acid allows the ulcerated areas to heal. Examples of histamine H_2 antagonists include cimetidine (Tagamet), famotidine (Pepcid), and ranitidine (Zantac).

Uses

These drugs are used prophylactically to treat stress-related ulcers and acute upper GI bleeding in critically ill patients. They are also used for the treatment of

- Heartburn, acid indigestion, and sour stomach
- GERD
- Gastric or duodenal ulcer
- Gastric **hypersecretory** conditions (excessive gastric secretion of HCl)

Adverse Reactions

Histamine H_2 antagonist adverse reactions are usually mild and transient as well as rare (affecting less than 2% of users), and include

- Dizziness, somnolence, headache
- Confusion, hallucinations, diarrhea, and reversible impotence

Contraindications and Precautions

The histamine H_2 antagonists are contraindicated in patients with a known hypersensitivity to the drugs. These drugs are used cautiously in patients with renal or hepatic impairment and in severely ill, elderly, or debilitated patients. Cimetidine is used cautiously in patients with diabetes. Histamine H_2 antagonists are pregnancy category B (cimetidine, famotidine, and ranitidine) and C (nizatidine) drugs and should be used with caution during pregnancy and lactation.

Interactions

The following interactions may occur when a histamine H_2 antagonist is administered with another agent:

Interacting Drug	Common Use	Effect of Interaction
antacids and metoclopramide	GI distress	Decreased absorption of the H_2 antagonists
carmustine	Anticancer therapy	Decreased white blood cell count
opioid analgesics	Pain relief	Increased risk of respiratory depression
oral anticoagulants	Blood thinners	Increased risk of bleeding
digoxin	Cardiac problems	May decrease serum digoxin levels

Proton Pump Inhibitors

Actions

Proton pump inhibitors, such as lansoprazole, omeprazole, pantoprazole, and rabeprazole, are a group of drugs with antisecretory properties. These drugs suppress gastric acid secretion by inhibition of the hydrogen-potassium adenosine triphosphatase (ATPase) enzyme system of the gastric parietal cells. The ATPase enzyme system is also called the acid (proton) pump system. The proton pump inhibitors suppress gastric acid secretion by blocking the final step in the production of gastric acid by the gastric mucosa. Examples of proton pump inhibitors include esomeprazole magnesium (Nexium) and omeprazole (Prilosec).

Uses

The proton pump inhibitors are used for treatment or symptomatic relief of various gastric disorders, including

- Gastric and duodenal ulcers (specifically associated with *H. pylori* infections)
- GERD and erosive esophagitis
- Pathologic hypersecretory conditions

An important use of these drugs is combination therapy for the treatment of *H. pylori* infection in patients with duodenal ulcers. One treatment regimen used to treat infection with *H. pylori* is a triple-drug therapy, such as one of the proton pump inhibitors (e.g., omeprazole or lansoprazole) and two anti-infectives (e.g., amoxicillin and clarithromycin).

Drugs That Affect the Upper Gastrointestinal System

Table 47.1 Agents Used to Eradicate *H. pylori* in Patients With Duodenal Ulcers

Drug	Recommended Usage	Dosage Range
amoxicillin *a-mocks'-ih-sill-in*	In combination with lansoprazole and clarithromycin or lansoprazole alone	1 g BID for 14 d (triple therapy) or 1 g TID (double therapy)
bismuth (Bismatrol) *bis'-muth*	In combination with other products	525 mg QID
clarithromycin (Biaxin) *clair-ith'-roe-my-sin*	In combination with amoxicillin	500 mg TID
lansoprazole (Prevacid) *lan-soe'-pra-zole*	In combination with clarithromycin or amoxicillin	30 mg BID for 14 d (triple therapy) or 30 mg TID for 14 d (double therapy)
metronidazole (Flagyl) *meh-troe-nye'-dah-zoll*	In combination with other products	250 mg QID
omeprazole (Prilosec) *oh-me'-pra-zole*	In combination with clarithromycin	40 mg BID for 4 wk and 20 mg/d for 15–28 d
ranitidine bismuth citrate (Tritec) *rah-nih'-tih-deen*	In combination with clarithromycin	400 mg BID for 4 wk
tetracycline *tet-rah-sye'-cleen*	In combination with other products	500 mg QID
Combination Drugs		
bismuth subsalicylate, metronidazole, tetracycline (Helidac)	*H. pylori* eradication in patients with duodenal ulcer	525-mg chewable tablets, 250 mg metronidazole, 500 mg tetracycline QID orally

Another triple-drug treatment regimen consists of bismuth subsalicylate plus two anti-infective drugs. Helidac, a triple-drug treatment regimen (bismuth subsalicylate, metronidazole, and tetracycline), may be given along with a histamine H_2 antagonist to treat disorders of the GI tract infected with *H. pylori*. Table 47-1 lists various drug combinations used in the treatment of *H. pylori* infection. Additional information concerning anti-infective agents is found in Chapters 6 through 11. The Summary Drug Table: Drugs Used in Managing Upper Gastrointestinal Disorders provides additional information on the proton pump inhibitor drugs used in treating H. pylori infection.

Adverse Reactions

The most common adverse reactions seen with the proton pump inhibitors include headache, nausea, diarrhea, and abdominal pain.

Contraindications and Precautions

The proton pump inhibitors are contraindicated in patients who are hypersensitive to any of the drugs. The proton pump inhibitors are used cautiously in older adults and in patients with hepatic impairment. Prolonged treatment may decrease the body's ability to absorb vitamin B_{12}, resulting in anemia. Omeprazole (pregnancy category C) and lansoprazole, rabeprazole, and pantoprazole (pregnancy category B) are contraindicated during pregnancy and lactation.

Interactions

The following interactions may occur when a proton pump inhibitor is administered with another agent:

Interacting Drug	Common Use	Effect of Interaction
sucralfate	Management of GI distress	Decreased absorption of the proton pump inhibitor
ketoconazole and ampicillin	Anti-infective agent	Decreased absorption of the anti-infective
oral anticoagulants	Blood thinners	Increased risk of bleeding
digoxin	Cardiac problems	Increased absorption of digoxin
benzodiazepines, phenytoin	Management of seizure disorders	Risk for toxic level of antiseizure drugs
clarithromycin (with omeprazole, specifically)	Anti-infective agent	Risk for an increase in plasma levels of both drugs

Miscellaneous Acid Reducers

Three other types of acid-reducing drugs that are less frequently used are the cholinergic blocking drugs (also called *anticholinergic* drugs), a pepsin inhibitor, and a prostaglandin drug. Cholinergic blocking drugs reduce gastric motility and decrease the amount of acid secreted by the stomach. These drugs have been largely replaced by histamine H_2 antagonists, which appear to be more effective and have fewer adverse effects. Examples of cholinergic blocking drugs used for GI disorders include propantheline (Pro-Banthine) and glycopyrrolate (Robinul). For information about specific cholinergic blocking drugs, see Chapter 30.

Sucralfate (Carafate) is known as a pepsin inhibitor or mucosal protective drug. The drug binds with protein molecules to form a viscous substance that buffers acid and protects the mucosal lining. Sucralfate is used in the short-term treatment of duodenal ulcers. The most common adverse reaction is constipation. Drug interactions of sucralfate are similar to those of the proton pump inhibitors.

A prostaglandin drug, misoprostol (Cytotec), has been used to reduce the risk of nonsteroidal anti-inflammatory drug (NSAID)–induced gastric ulcers in high-risk patients, such as older adults or the critically ill. Misoprostol both inhibits the production of gastric acid and has mucosal protective properties. Because this drug can cause abortion or birth defects, it is not recommended for use in ulcer reduction in women who are pregnant or may become pregnant, or who are lactating. Adverse reactions include headache, nausea, diarrhea, and abdominal pain. The drug effects are decreased when it is taken with antacids.

GASTROINTESTINAL STIMULANTS

Actions

Metoclopramide (Reglan) and dexpanthenol (Ilopan) treat delayed gastric emptying and emesis—that is, they increase the motility of the upper GI tract without increasing the production of secretions. By sensitizing tissue to the effects of acetylcholine, the tone and amplitude of gastric contractions are increased, resulting in faster emptying of gastric contents into the small intestine. Stimulation of the **chemoreceptor trigger zone** (CTZ), a group of nerve fibers located on the surface of the fourth ventricle of the brain that sends signals to the vomiting center in the medulla, is also inhibited by metoclopramide.

Uses

The GI stimulants are used in the treatment of

- GERD

- **Gastric stasis** (failure to move food normally out of the stomach) in diabetic patients, in patients with nausea and vomiting associated with cancer chemotherapy, and in patients in the immediate postoperative period

Dexpanthenol may be given intravenously (IV) immediately after major abdominal surgery to reduce the risk of **paralytic ileus** (lack of peristalsis or movement of the intestines).

Adverse Reactions

The adverse reactions associated with metoclopramide are usually mild. Higher doses or prolonged administration may produce central nervous system (CNS) symptoms, such as restlessness, drowsiness, dizziness, extrapyramidal symptoms (tremor, involuntary movements of the limbs, muscle rigidity), facial grimacing, and depression. Dexpanthenol administration may cause itching, difficulty breathing, and urticaria.

Drugs That Affect the Upper Gastrointestinal System

Contraindications and Precautions

The GI stimulants are contraindicated in patients with known hypersensitivity to the drugs, GI obstruction, gastric perforation or hemorrhage, or pheochromocytoma. Patients with Parkinson's disease or a seizure disorder who are taking drugs likely to cause extrapyramidal symptoms should not take these drugs. Dexpanthenol should not be used by patients with hemophilia.

These drugs are used cautiously in patients with diabetes and cardiovascular disease. Metoclopramide is a pregnancy category B drug; dexpanthenol is a pregnancy category C drug. These drugs are secreted in breast milk and should be used with caution during pregnancy and lactation.

Interactions

The following interactions may occur when a GI stimulant is administered with another agent:

Interacting Drug	Common Use	Effect of Interaction
cholinergic blocking drugs or opioid analgesics	Management of GI distress or pain relief	Decreased effectiveness of metoclopramide
cimetidine	Management of GI distress	Decreased absorption of cimetidine
digoxin	Management of cardiac problems	Decreased absorption of digoxin
monoamine oxidase inhibitors	Management of depression	Increased risk of hypertensive episode
levodopa	Management of Parkinson's disease	Decreased effectiveness of metoclopramide and levodopa

ANTIEMETICS

An antiemetic drug is used to treat or prevent **nausea** (unpleasant gastric sensation usually preceding vomiting) or **vomiting** (forceful expulsion of gastric contents through the mouth). The drugs discussed in this section are used to treat severe nausea and vomiting. Individuals may experience

Table 47.2 Examples of Drugs Used for Motion Sickness

Generic Name	Trade Name
buclizine HCl	Bucladin-S
cyclizine	Marezine
dimenhydrinate	Dramamine
diphenhydramine	Benadry1
meclizine HCl	Antivert
scopolamine	Scopace (oral), Transderm-Scop (transdermal path)

nausea due to motion sickness or a condition called **vertigo** (a sensation of spinning or a rotation-type motion). Many of the drugs used to treat motion sickness can be purchased over the counter. Table 47-2 lists examples of drugs used in the treatment of motion sickness or vertigo.

Actions

Vomiting caused by drugs, radiation, and metabolic disorders often occurs because of stimulation of the CTZ, a group of nerve fibers located on the surface of the fourth ventricle of the brain. When these nerves are stimulated by chemicals, such as drugs or toxic substances, impulses are sent to the vomiting center located in the medulla. The vomiting center may also be directly stimulated by disorders such as GI irritation, motion sickness, and vestibular neuritis (inflammation of the vestibular nerve). These drugs appear to act primarily by inhibiting the CTZ and the brain's primary neurotransmitters dopamine and acetylcholine.

A newer classification of antiemetic drugs, the 5-hydroxytryptamine type 3 (5-HT3) receptor antagonists, target serotonin receptors both at the CTZ and peripherally at the nerve endings in the stomach. This action reduces the non-GI adverse effects that are often evident when non-specific cholinergic blocking drugs are used. Because of their localized action in the GI system, these drugs are being tested for use in irritable bowel syndrome as well.

Uses

An antiemetic is used to treat nausea and vomiting, typically by preventive administration (prophylaxis):

- Before surgery to prevent vomiting during surgery
- Immediately after surgery when the patient is recovering from anesthesia

- Before administration of antineoplastic drugs that induce a high degree of nausea and vomiting
- During radiation therapy when the GI tract is in the treatment field

Other causes of nausea and vomiting that may be treated with an antiemetic include bacterial and viral infections and adverse drug reactions. Some antiemetics also are used for motion sickness and vertigo. Dronabinol (Marinol) is the only medically available cannabinoid (marijuana derivative) prescribed for antiemetic use. For a comprehensive listing of antiemetics, see the Summary Drug Table: Drugs Used in Managing Upper Gastrointestinal Disorders.

Adverse Reactions

The most common adverse reactions resulting from these drugs are varying degrees of drowsiness. Additional adverse reactions for each drug are listed in the Summary Drug Table: Drugs Used in Managing Upper Gastrointestinal Disorders.

Contraindications

The antiemetic drugs are contraindicated in patients with known hypersensitivity to these drugs or with severe CNS depression. The 5-HT3 receptor antagonists should not be used by patients with heart block or prolonged QT intervals. In general, these drugs are not recommended during pregnancy and lactation, or for uncomplicated vomiting in young children. Prochlorperazine is contraindicated in patients with bone marrow depression, blood dyscrasia, Parkinson's disease, or severe liver or cardiovascular disease. Thiethylperazine is a pregnancy category X drug and is contraindicated during pregnancy.

Precautions

Severe nausea and vomiting should not be treated with antiemetic drugs alone. The cause of the vomiting must be investigated. Antiemetic drugs may hamper the diagnosis of disorders such as brain tumor or injury, appendicitis, intestinal obstruction, and drug toxicity (e.g., digitalis toxicity). Delayed diagnosis of any of these disorders could have serious consequences for the patient.

Cholinergic blocking antiemetics are used cautiously in patients with glaucoma or obstructive disease of the GI or genitourinary system, those with renal or hepatic dysfunction, and in older men with possible prostatic hypertrophy. Promethazine is used cautiously in patients with hypertension, sleep apnea, or epilepsy. Trimethobenzamide is used cautiously in children with a viral illness because it is thought to increase the risk of Reye's syndrome. The 5-HT3 receptor antagonists should be used cautiously in patients with cardiac conduction problems or electrolyte imbalances.

Perphenazine, prochlorperazine, promethazine, scopolamine, chlorpromazine, and trimethobenzamide are pregnancy category C drugs. Other antiemetics are classified as pregnancy category B (except for thiethylperazine, which is classified as pregnancy category X).

Interactions

The following interactions may occur when an antiemetic is administered with another agent:

Interacting Drug	Common Use	Effect of Interaction
CNS depressants	Analgesia, sedation, or pain relief	Increased risk of sedation
antihistamines	Management of allergy and respiratory distress	Increased adverse cholinergic blocking effects
Antacids	Management of gastric distress	Decreased absorption of antiemetic
Rifampin with 5-HT3 receptor antagonist	Tuberculosis/ human immunodeficiency virus infection management	Decreased effectiveness of 5-HT3 receptor antagonist
Lithium with prochlorperazine	Management of bipolar disorder	Increased risk of extrapyramidal effects

EMETICS

An emetic is a drug that induces vomiting. This is caused by local irritation of the stomach and by stimulation of the vomiting center in the medulla. Emetics are used to empty the stomach rapidly when an individual has accidentally or intentionally ingested a poison or drug overdose. Not all poison ingestions or drug overdoses are treated with emetics. Because more harm can occur from the vomiting of many substances, guidelines were established for the use of syrup of ipecac.*

The U.S. Food and Drug Administration has approved the following warnings for the labeling of syrup of ipecac:

- Do not use in persons who are not fully conscious.

- Do not use this product unless directed by a health care professional. Do not use if turpentine, corrosives, such as alkalis (lye) or strong acids, or petroleum distillates, such as kerosene, paint thinner, cleaning fluid, or furniture polish, have been ingested.

Clinicians have expanded the contraindications for ipecac syrup to include situations in which:

- The patient is comatose or has altered mental status and the risk of aspiration of stomach contents is high.

- The patient is having convulsions.

- The substance ingested is capable of causing altered mental status or convulsions.

- The substance ingested is a caustic or corrosive agent.

- The substance ingested is a low-viscosity petroleum distillate with the potential for pulmonary aspiration and the development of chemical pneumonitis.

- The patient has a medical condition that may be exacerbated by vomiting (e.g., severe hypertension, bradycardia, hemorrhagic diathesis).

Nursing Alert

Before an emetic is given, it is extremely important to know the chemicals or substances that have been ingested, the time they were ingested, and what symptoms were noted before seeking medical treatment. This information will probably be obtained from a family member or friend, but the adult patient may also contribute to the history. The primary health care provider or nurse may also contact the local poison control center to obtain information regarding treatment.

*Manoguerra, A. S. & Cobaugh, D. J. (2005). Guideline on the use of ipecac syrup in the out-of-hospital management of ingested poisons. *Clinical Toxicology* 43(1), 1–10.

The Patient Receiving a Drug for an Upper Gastrointestinal Condition

ASSESSMENT

PREADMINISTRATION ASSESSMENT

The nurse questions the patient regarding the type and intensity of symptoms (e.g., pain, discomfort, nausea, vomiting) to provide a baseline for evaluating the effectiveness of drug therapy. As part of the preadministration assessment for a patient receiving a drug for nausea and vomiting, the nurse documents the number of times the patient has vomited and the approximate amount of fluid lost. Before starting therapy, the nurse takes vital signs and assesses for signs of fluid and electrolyte imbalances.

In the case of preventative administration of an antiemetic, the nurse explains the rationale for preventing an episode of nausea rather than waiting for symptoms to occur when the primary health care provider knows the drugs being given will cause this problem. The nurse questions the patient about any episodes of nausea or vomiting in anticipation of the therapy.

ONGOING ASSESSMENT

The nurse monitors the patient frequently for continued complaints of pain, sour taste, or the production of bloody or coffee-ground emesis. Suction equipment should be kept available in case a nasogastric (NG) tube must be inserted for suctioning to prevent aspiration of emesis. If vomiting is severe, the nurse observes the patient for signs and symptoms of electrolyte imbalance and monitors the blood pressure, pulse, and respiratory rate every 2 to 4 hours or as ordered by the primary health care provider. The nurse carefully measures intake and output (urine, emesis) until vomiting ceases and the patient can take oral fluids in sufficient quantity. The nurse documents in the patient's chart each time the patient vomits. The nurse notifies the primary health care provider if there is blood in the emesis or if vomiting suddenly becomes more severe. The nurse also may need to measure the patient's weight daily to weekly in patients with prolonged and repeated episodes of vomiting (e.g., those receiving chemotherapy for cancer). The nurse assesses the patient at frequent intervals for the effectiveness of the drug in relieving symptoms (e.g., nausea, vomiting, or vertigo) and notifies the primary health care provider if the drug fails to relieve or diminish symptoms.

NURSING DIAGNOSES

Drug-specific nursing diagnoses are highlighted in the Nursing Diagnoses Checklist. Other nursing diagnoses applicable to these drugs are discussed in depth in Chapter 4.

Nursing Diagnosis Checklist

✔ **Risk for Deficient Fluid Volume** related to diarrhea, nausea, and vomiting

✔ **Imbalanced Nutrition: Less Than Body Requirements** related to impaired ability to ingest and retain food and fluids, or offensive tastes and smells

✔ **Individual Effective Therapeutic Regimen Management** related to inability to take oral form of medication

✔ **Risk for Injury** related to adverse drug effects of drowsiness

PLANNING

The expected outcomes for the patient depend on the reason the upper GI drug is administered, but may include an optimal response to drug therapy, support of patient needs related to the management of adverse reactions, and an understanding of the drug regimen.

IMPLEMENTATION

PROMOTING AN OPTIMAL RESPONSE TO THERAPY

ANTACIDS The antacid may be administered hourly for the first 2 weeks when used to treat acute peptic ulcer. After the first 2 weeks, the drug is administered 1 to 2 hours after meals and at bedtime. The primary health care provider may order that the antacid be left at the patient's bedside for self-administration. The nurse ensures that an adequate supply of water and cups for measuring the dose are available.

> ### Nursing Alert
> Because of the possibility of an antacid interfering with the activity of other oral drugs, no oral drug should be administered within 1 to 2 hours of an antacid.

NON-ORAL METHODS OF DRUG ADMINISTRATION Patients taking acid-reducing drugs may not be able to take oral medications because of preparation for an operative procedure, postoperative nausea, or physical condition. Many of these drugs come in forms for both intramuscular (IM) and IV administration. The IV route is typically preferred if the patient has an existing IV line because these drugs are irritating and IM injections need to be given deep into the muscular tissue to minimize harm.

> ### Nursing Alert
> When one of these drugs is given IV, the nurse monitors the rate of infusion at frequent intervals. Too rapid an infusion may induce cardiac arrhythmias.

Patients who are debilitated and require feeding from an NG tube are at risk for gastric ulcer development and may be prescribed acid-reducing drugs. The nurse always checks the medication label to see if the pill can be crushed or the capsule opened before doing so. These can be mixed with 40 mL of apple juice and injected through the NG tube. The tube is flushed with fluid afterward. Many of these drugs come in a liquid form as well as tablet or capsule. The nurse should request the liquid form when administration is in a tube to decrease the chance of a clogged NG tube due to improper flushing.

PREVENTION OF NAUSEA IN PATIENTS UNDERGOING CANCER THERAPY Different protocols for pre-chemotherapy nausea depend on the type of cancer treatment. Some cancer (antineoplastic) drugs rarely cause nausea, and others are highly emetogenic. Granisetron (Kytril), ondansetron (Zofran), and dolasetron (Anzemet) are examples of antiemetics used when cancer chemotherapy drugs are very likely to cause nausea and vomiting. The nurse begins administering these drugs before the chemotherapy is given. The nurse may give the first dose IV during therapy, then ask the patient to take it orally at home for a specified period. It is important for the nurse to explain to the patient that the drug prevents nausea and vomiting and to be sure to take the entire dose prescribed. Administration of antineoplastics and the preadministration of antiemetics should always be performed by a nurse trained in the administration of cancer chemotherapy.

MONITORING AND MANAGING PATIENT NEEDS

RISK FOR DEFICIENT FLUID VOLUME When antacids are given, the nurse keeps a record of the patient's bowel movements because these drugs may cause constipation or diarrhea. If the patient experiences diarrhea, the nurse keeps an accurate record of fluid intake and output along with a description of the diarrhea stool. Changing to a different antacid usually alleviates the problem. Diarrhea may be controlled by combining a magnesium antacid with an antacid containing aluminum or calcium. Uncontrolled diarrhea can lead to fluid loss and dehydration.

Dehydration is a serious concern in the patient experiencing nausea and vomiting. It is important to observe the patient for signs of dehydration, which include poor skin turgor, dry mucous membranes, decrease in or absence of urinary output, concentrated urine, restlessness, irritability, increased respiratory rate, and confusion. The nurse monitors the input and output (urine and emesis) and documents findings every 8 hours. If the patient is able to take and retain small amounts of oral fluids, the nurse offers sips of water at frequent intervals. In addition, it is important to observe the patient for signs of electrolyte imbalance, particularly sodium and potassium deficit (see Chapter 58). If signs of dehydration or electrolyte imbalance are noted, the nurse contacts the primary health care provider because parenteral administration of fluids or fluids with electrolytes may be necessary.

Chronic Care Alert

Observations for fluid and electrolyte disturbances are particularly important in the aged or chronically ill patient in whom severe dehydration may develop quickly. The nurse must immediately report symptoms of dehydration, such as dry mucous membranes, decreased urinary output, concentrated urine, restlessness, or confusion.

IMBALANCED NUTRITION: LESS THAN BODY REQUIREMENTS Nausea, vomiting, vertigo, and dizziness are disagreeable sensations. The nurse provides the patient with an emesis basin and checks the basin at frequent intervals. If vomiting occurs, the nurse empties the emesis basin and measures and documents the volume in the patient's chart. The nurse may give the patient a damp washcloth and a towel to wipe the hands and face as needed. It also is a good idea to give the patient mouthwash or frequent oral rinses to remove the disagreeable taste that accompanies vomiting.

Nausea may make the patient lose his or her appetite and decrease nutritional intake. It is important to make the environment as pleasant as possible to enhance the patient's appetite. The nurse removes items with strong smells and odors. The nurse changes the patient's bedding and clothing or gown as needed because the odor of vomit may intensify the sensations of nausea and further decrease appetite.

INDIVIDUAL EFFECTIVE THERAPEUTIC REGIMEN MANAGEMENT When antacids are given, the nurse instructs the patient to chew the tablets thoroughly before swallowing and then drink a full glass of water or milk. If the patient expresses a dislike for the taste of the antacid or has difficulty chewing the tablet form, the nurse informs the primary health care provider. A flavored antacid may be ordered if the patient finds the taste unpleasant. A liquid form may be ordered if the patient has difficulty chewing a tablet. Liquid antacid preparations must be shaken thoroughly immediately before administration. Liquid antacids are followed by a small amount of water.

If the patient cannot retain the oral form of the drug, the nurse may give it parenterally or as a rectal suppository (if the prescribed drug is available in these forms). If only the oral form has been ordered and the patient cannot retain the drug, the nurse contacts the primary health care provider regarding an order for a parenteral or suppository form of this or another antiemetic drug.

When administering scopolamine for motion sickness, one transdermal system is applied behind the ear approximately 4 hours before the antiemetic effect is needed. Approximately 1 g of scopolamine is administered every 24 hours for 3 days. The nurse advises the individual to discard any disk that becomes detached and to replace it with a fresh disk applied behind the opposite ear. (See Patient and Family Teaching Checklist: Applying Transdermal Scopolamine).

Patient and Family Teaching Checklist

Applying Transdermal Scopolamine
The nurse:

✔ Instructs the patient to apply the transdermal scopolamine system behind the ear.

✔ Explains that after application of the system, the hands are washed *thoroughly* with soap and water and dried. The importance of thorough handwashing to prevent any traces of the drug from coming in contact with the eyes is emphasized.

✔ Teaches that the disk will last about 3 days, at which time the patient may remove the disk and apply another disk, if needed.

✔ Instructs the patient to discard the used disk and throughly wash and dry the hands and previous application site.

✔ Instructs the patient to apply the new disk behind the opposite ear and again thoroughly wash and dry the hands.

✔ Emphasizes that only one disk at a time is used.

✔ Makes sure that the patient has a thorough knowledge of the adverse reactions that may occur with the use of this system: dizziness, dry mouth, and blurred vision.

✔ Stresses the importance of observing caution when driving or performing hazardous tasks.

RISK FOR INJURY Administration of these drugs may result in varying degrees of drowsiness. To prevent accidental falls and other injuries, the nurse assists the patient who is allowed out of bed with ambulatory activities. If extreme drowsiness is noted, the nurse instructs the patient to remain in bed and provides a call light for assistance.

Gerontologic Alert

The older adult is particularly sensitive to the effects of the histamine H_2 antagonists. The nurse must closely monitor older adults for confusion and dizziness. Dizziness increases the risk for falls in the older adult. Assistance is needed for ambulatory activities. The environment is made safe by removing throw rugs, small pieces of furniture, and the like. The nurse reports any change in orientation to the primary health care provider.

The nurse observes patients receiving high or prolonged doses of metoclopramide for adverse reactions related to the CNS (extrapyramidal symptoms or tardive dyskinesia). The nurse reports any sign of extrapyramidal symptoms or tardive dyskinesia to the primary health care provider before the next dose of metoclopramide is administered because the drug therapy may be discontinued. These adverse reactions may be irreversible if therapy is continued.

EDUCATING THE PATIENT AND FAMILY

When a drug to treat the upper GI system is prescribed for outpatient use, the nurse includes the following information in a patient teaching plan:

- Avoid driving or performing other hazardous tasks when taking these drugs because drowsiness may occur with use.

- Do not use an antacid indiscriminately. Check with a primary health care provider before using an antacid if other medical problems, such as a cardiac condition, exist (some laxatives contain sodium).

- Allow effervescent tablets to dissolve completely in water. Allow most of the bubbling to stop before drinking the solution.

- Adhere to the dosage schedule recommended by the primary health care provider. Do not increase the frequency of use or the dose if symptoms become worse; instead, see the primary health care provider as soon as possible.

- Because antacids impair the absorption of some drugs, do not take other drugs within 2 hours before or after taking the antacid unless use of an antacid with a drug is recommended by the primary health care provider.

- If pain or discomfort remains the same or becomes worse, if the stools turn black, or if vomitus resembles coffee grounds, contact the primary health care provider as soon as possible.

- Explain that antacids may change the color of the stool (white, white streaks); this is normal.

- Advise the patient that magnesium-containing products may produce a laxative effect and may cause diarrhea; aluminum- or calcium-containing antacids may cause constipation; magnesium-containing antacids are used to avoid bowel dysfunction.

- Taking too much antacid may cause the stomach to secrete excess stomach acid. Consult the primary health care provider or pharmacist about appropriate dose. Do not use the maximum dose for more than 2 weeks, except under the supervision of a primary health care provider.

- When taking proton pump inhibitors, swallow the tablet whole at least 1 hour before eating. Do not chew, open, or crush.

- When taking metoclopramide, immediately report any of the following signs: difficulty speaking or swallowing; masklike face; shuffling gait; rigidity; tremors; uncontrolled movements of the mouth, face, or extremities; and uncontrolled chewing or unusual movements of the tongue.

- Avoid the use of alcohol and other sedative-type drugs unless use has been approved by the primary health care provider.

- Take antiemetics for cancer chemotherapy as prescribed. Do not omit a dose. Consult the primary health care provider if you have forgotten a dose of the medication.

- When taking rectal suppositories, remove foil wrapper and immediately insert the pointed end into the rectum without using force.

- Take the drug for motion sickness about 1 hour before travel.

- Follow the directions for application of transdermal scopolamine that are supplied with the drug (see Patient and Family Teaching Checklist: Applying Transdermal Scopolamine).

- *Misoprostol:* Because this drug may cause spontaneous abortion, advise women of childbearing age to use a reliable contraceptive. If pregnancy is suspected, discontinue use of the drug and notify the primary health care provider. Report severe menstrual pain, bleeding, or spotting as well.

EVALUATION

- The therapeutic effect is achieved; nausea or pain is controlled.

- Adverse reactions are identified, reported to the primary health care provider, and managed successfully through appropriate nursing interventions.

- No evidence of a fluid volume deficit, nutritional imbalance, or electrolyte imbalance is seen.

- No evidence of injury is apparent.

- The patient verbalizes the importance of complying with the prescribed treatment regimen.

- The patient or family demonstrates an understanding of the drug regimen.

Critical Thinking Exercises

1. The primary health care provider has prescribed cimetidine for the treatment of a duodenal ulcer in Mr. Talley, aged 68 years. A drug history by the nurse reveals that Mr. Talley is also taking digoxin (Lanoxin) 0.5 mg orally each day and a daily aspirin tablet. Analyze this situation. Discuss what you would tell Mr. Talley.

2. Mr. Collins is prescribed transdermal scopolamine to relieve motion sickness. Discuss the rationale you would give him to stress the importance of washing his hands after applying or removing the transdermal system.

3. Discuss the ongoing assessment needs of a patient receiving an antiemetic before chemotherapy for cancer.

4. Ms. Jerkins has four children and wants to keep syrup of ipecac available in case of accidental poisoning. Discuss the information you feel that Ms. Jerkins should know about this drug.

Review Questions

1. When would the nurse most correctly administer an antacid to a patient taking other oral medications?

   A. With the other drugs

   B. 30 minutes before or after administration of other drugs

   C. 2 hours before or after administration of other drugs

   D. In early morning and at bedtime

2. When a histamine H_2 antagonist drug is prescribed for the treatment of a peptic ulcer, the nurse observes the patient for which of the following adverse effects?

   A. Dry mouth, urinary retention

   B. Edema, tachycardia

   C. Constipation, anorexia

   D. Dizziness, somnolence

3. What is the most common adverse reaction the nurse would expect in a patient receiving an antiemetic?

   A. Occipital headache

   B. Drowsiness

   C. Edema

   D. Nausea

4. When explaining how to use transdermal scopolamine, the nurse tells the patient to apply the system to _____.

   A. a nonhairy region of the chest

   B. on the upper back

   C. behind the ear

   D. on the forearm

Medication Dosage Problems

1. Prochlorperazine (Compazine) 10 mg orally is prescribed. Use the drug label below to prepare the correct dosage.

   The nurse would administer _____.

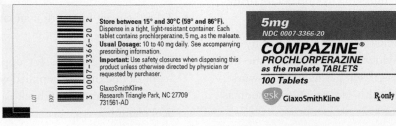

Store between 15°C and 30°C (59° and 86°F). Dispense in a tight, light-resistant container. Each tablet contains prochlorperazine, 5 mg, as the maleate. **Usual Dosage:** 10 to 40 mg daily. See accompanying prescribing information. **Important:** Use safety closures when dispensing this product unless otherwise directed by physician or requested by purchaser.

GlaxoSmithKline
Research Triangle Park, NC 27709
731561-AD

NDC 0007-3366-20

5mg

COMPAZINE®
PROCHLORPERAZINE
as the maleate TABLETS

100 Tablets

gsk GlaxoSmithKline   R̶x only

2. The patient is to receive 400 mg cimetidine (Tagamet) orally. Available for use is the cimetidine
shown below.

The nurse administers _____.

To check your answers, see Appendix G.

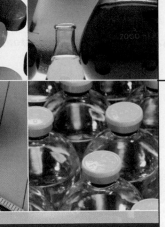

Chapter 48

Drugs That Affect the Lower Gastrointestinal System

Key Terms

antiflatulents
constipation
diarrhea
dyspepsia
inflammatory bowel disease
obstipation

Learning Objectives

On completion of this chapter, the student will:

- Describe how inflammatory bowel disease alters function of the lower gastrointestinal system.
- List the types of drugs prescribed or recommended for lower gastrointestinal disorders.
- Discuss the uses, general drug actions, general adverse reactions, contraindications, precautions, and interactions associated with lower gastrointestinal drugs.

- Discuss important preadministration and ongoing assessment activities the nurse should perform on the patient taking a lower gastrointestinal drug.
- List nursing diagnoses particular to a patient taking a lower gastrointestinal drug.
- Discuss ways to promote an optimal response to therapy, how to manage common adverse reactions, and important points to keep in mind when educating patients about the use of lower gastrointestinal drugs.

The large intestine is responsible for the absorption of water and some of the nutrients from the food and fluids we eat. The speed of transit determines what will be absorbed. Transit of contents rapidly through the bowel is called **diarrhea**. When contents move sluggishly, more water is absorbed, and the fecal material gets harder, resulting in **constipation**. Transit can be triggered by many things. Illness, such as irritable bowel syndrome or ulcerative colitis, bacterial infection, or drugs such as anti-infectives can make transit faster, resulting in diarrhea. Conditions such as Parkinson's disease can slow the bowel, causing constipation. Treatment with opioid drugs and the aftereffects of abdominal surgery can also cause constipation.

Conditions that affect the function of the lower gastrointestinal (GI) system can have a significant impact on activities of daily living; if proper absorption does not occur, people may not have the energy to engage in activities. One such condition that affects function is **inflammatory bowel disease** (IBD). The pain and bloating of a sluggish bowel or fear of stool incontinence may prevent people from socializing, again affecting daily life. The drugs described in this chapter affect the function of the bowel. Antidiarrheals and laxatives, as well as drugs to treat IBD are presented. Some of the more common drugs are listed in the Summary Drug Table: Drugs Used in Managing Lower Gastrointestinal Disorders.

SUMMARY DRUG TABLE DRUGS USED IN MANAGING LOWER GASTROINTESTINAL DISORDERS

GENERIC NAME	TRADE NAME	USES	ADVERSE REACTIONS	DOSAGE RANGES
Drugs Used to Treat Inflammatory Bowel Disease				
Aminosalicylates				
balsalazide disodium *bal-sal'-a-zyde*	Colazal	Active ulcerative colitis	Headache, abdominal pain	2250 mg orally TID for 8 wk
mesalamine *me-sal'-a-meen*	Asacol, Pentasa, Rowasa (enema form)	Active ulcerative colitis, proctosigmoiditis or proctitis	Headache, abdominal pain, nausea	800–1000 mg orally TID or QID Suspension enema: 4 g QD
olsalazine *ole-sal'-a-zeen*	Dipentum	Maintenance of remission of ulcerative colitis	Diarrhea, abdominal pain and cramping	1 g/d orally in two divided doses
sulfasalazine *sul-fa-sal'-a-zeen*	Azulfidine	Ulcerative colitis, rheumatoid arthritis	Headache, nausea, anorexia, vomiting, gastric distress, reduced sperm count	Initial: 3–4 g/d orally in divided doses Maintenance: 2 g orally QID
Miscellaneous Drugs for Bowel Disorders				
infliximab *in-flicks'-ih-mab*	Remicade	Crohn's disease, ulcerative colitis, rheumatoid arthritis	Sore throat, cough, sinus infection, gastric distress	5 mg/kg IV every 2–8 wk
tegaserod maleate *te-gas'-er-odd*	Zelnorm	Irritable bowel syndrome, constipation	Headache, abdominal pain, diarrhea	6 mg orally BID before meals for 4–6 wk
Antidiarrheals				
bismuth subsalicylate	Bismatrol Pepto-Bismol, Pink Bismuth	Nausea, diarrhea, abdominal cramps, *H. pylori* infection with duodenal ulcer	Same as difenoxin	2 tablets or 30 mL orally every 30 min to 1 h, up to 8 doses in 24 h
difenoxin HCl with atropine *dye-fen-ox'-in, a'-troe-peen*	Motofen	Symptomatic relief of acute diarrhea	Dry skin and mucous membranes, nausea, constipation, lightheadedness	Initial dose: 2 tablets orally, then 1 tablet after each loose stool (not to exceed 8 tablets/d)
diphenoxylate HCl with atropine *di-fen-ox'-i-late*	Lomotil, Lonox	Same as difenoxin	Same as difenoxin	5 mg orally QID
loperamide HCl *loe-per'-a-mide*	Imodium, Kaopectate, Maalox Anti-Diarrheal Caplets	Same as difenoxin	Same as difenoxin	Initial dose 4 mg orally; then 2 mg after each loose stool (not to exceed 16 mg/d)
tincture of opium	Paregoric	Severe diarrhea	Somnolence, constipation	0.6 mL orally QID
Antiflatulents				
charcoal	CharcoCaps, Flatulex (combined with simethicone)	Intestinal gas, diarrhea, poisoning antidote	Vomiting, constipation, diarrhea, black stools	520 mg orally after meals (not to exceed 4–16 g/d)
simethicone *sigh-meth'-ih-kohn*	Gas-X, Mylicon, Maalox Anti-Gas, Mylanta Gas	Postoperative distention, dyspepsia, irritable bowel, peptic ulcer	Bloating, constipation, diarrhea, heartburn	40–125 mg orally QID after meals and at bedtime

Drugs That Affect the Lower Gastrointestinal System

SUMMARY DRUG TABLE   (continued)

GENERIC NAME	TRADE NAME	USES	ADVERSE REACTIONS	DOSAGE RANGES
Laxatives				
Bulk-Producing Laxatives				
methylcellulose *meth-ill-cell'-you-los*	Citrucel, Unifiber	Relief of constipation, irritable bowel syndrome, severe watery diarrhea	Diarrhea, nausea, vomiting, bloating, flatulence, cramping, perianal irritation, fainting	Follow directions given on the container
psyllium *sill'-i-um*	Fiberall, Genfiber, Hydrocil, Konsyl, Metamucil, Perdiem	Same as methylcellulose	Same as methylcellulose	Powder, granules, or wafers taken as directed on package
polycarbophil *polly-kar'-boe-fil*	Equalactin, FiberCon, Mitrolan	Same as methylcellulose	Same as methylcellulose	1 g daily to QID or as needed (do not exceed 4 g in 24 h)
Emollients				
mineral oil	Kondremul Plain, Milkinol	Relief of constipation, and fecal impaction	Perianal discomfort and itching due to anal seepage	15–45 mL orally at bedtime
Stool Softeners/Surfactants				
docusate sodium (dioctyl sodium sulfosuccinate; DDS) *dok'-yoo-sate*	Colace, Ex-Lax Stool Softener, Modane Soft	Relief of constipation, prevention of straining during bowel movement	Diarrhea, nausea, vomiting, bloating, flatulence, cramping, perianal irritation, fainting	Follow directions given on the container; comes in enema form
docusate calcium (dioctyl calcium sulfosuccinate)	Surfak Liquigels	Same as docusate sodium	Same as docusate sodium	Follow directions given on the container
Hyperosmotic Agents				
glycerin *gli'-ser-in*	Colace Suppositories, Sani-Supp, Fleet Babylax	Relief of constipation	Same as docusate sodium	Rectal suppository, use as directed
lactulose *lak-tyoo-los*	Cephulac, Chronulac, Constilac, Duphalac	Relief of constipation, hepatic encephalopathy	Same as docusate sodium	Constipation: 15–30 mL/d orally Hepatic encephalopathy: 30–45 mL orally QID, may give enema form
Irritant or Stimulant Laxatives				
cascara sagrada *kas-kar'-asa-grad'-ah*	Aromatic Cascara	Relief of constipation	Same as docusate sodium, darkening of colon mucosa, brownish color to urine	Follow directions given on the container
sennosides *sen'-oh-sides*	Agoral, Ex-Lax, Senokot	Same as cascara	Same as cascara	Follow directions given on the container
bisacodyl *bis-a-koe'-dill*	Bisca-Evac, Dulcolax, Modane, Correctol	Same as cascara	Diarrhea, nausea, vomiting, bloating, flatulence, cramping, perianal irritation	Tablets: 10–15 mg daily orally Rectal suppositories: 10 mg daily; comes in enema form

GENERIC NAME	TRADE NAME	USES	ADVERSE REACTIONS	DOSAGE RANGES
Saline Laxatives				
magnesium preparations *mag-neez'-ee-um*	Milk of Magnesia, Magnesium Citrate, Fleets (enema preparation)	Evacuate colon for endoscopy, relieve constipation	Same as docusate sodium	Follow directions given on the container
Bowel Evacuants				
polyethylene glycol (PEG) solution *polly-eth'-ih-leen*	MiraLax	Relieve constipation	Same as sodium docusate	Follow directions given on the container
polyethylene glycol-electrolyte solution (PEG-ES) *polly-eth'-ih-leen*	CoLyte, GoLYTELY, NuLytely, OCL	Evacuate colon for endoscopy, relieve constipation	Same as sodium docusate	4 L oral solution to be drunk in 3 h

Inflammatory Bowel Disease

According to the Crohn's and Colitis Foundation of America (2005), as many as 1 million Americans have IBD. The term IBD is used collectively for Crohn's disease and ulcerative colitis, diseases that cause inflammation in the intestines. The cause of these diseases is unknown, although it is thought that a virus or bacterial organism interacting with the body's immune system may be the cause. Clinical manifestations of Crohn's disease include abdominal pain and distention. As the disease progresses, other GI symptoms present, such as anorexia, diarrhea, weight loss, dehydration, and nutritional deficiencies. Ulcerative colitis has a more abrupt onset; patients experience the sudden need to defecate, resulting in severe, blood- and mucus-filled diarrhea or no stool at all. Pain and fatigue accompany this disorder as well. No evidence has been found to support the theory that IBD is caused by tension, anxiety, or any other psychological factor or disorder.

Drugs used to treat IBD include antibiotics, corticosteroids, biologic agents, and aminosalicylates. The aminosalicylates are described in this chapter; other drugs used in the treatment of IBD are included in their respective chapters.

AMINOSALICYLATES

Actions and Uses

Aminosalicylates are aspirin-like compounds with anti-inflammatory action. The drugs exert a topical anti-inflammatory effect in the bowel. The exact mechanism of action

of these drugs is unknown. The aminosalicylates are used to treat Crohn's disease and ulcerative colitis as well as other inflammatory diseases.

Adverse Reactions

Because these drugs are topical anti-inflammatory drugs, the most common adverse reactions happen in the GI system and include abdominal pain, nausea, and diarrhea. Other general adverse reactions include headache, dizziness, fever, and weakness.

Contraindications and Precautions

The aminosalicylates are contraindicated in patients with a known hypersensitivity to the drugs or salicylate-containing drugs. In addition, these drugs are contraindicated in patients who have hypersensitivity to the sulfonamides and sulfites or intestinal obstruction, and in children younger than 2 years. The aminosalicylates are pregnancy category B drugs (except olsalazine, which is in pregnancy category C); all are used with caution during pregnancy and lactation (safety has not been established).

Interactions

The following interactions may occur when an aminosalicylate is administered with another agent:

Interacting Drug	Common Use	Effect of Interaction
digoxin	Cardiac problems	Reduced absorption of digoxin
methotrexate	Cancer and autoimmune conditions	Increased risk of immunosuppression
oral hypoglycemic drugs	Diabetes mellitus management	Increased blood glucose level
warfarin	Blood thinner	Increased risk of bleeding

Herbal Alert

Chamomile has several uses in traditional herbal therapy, such as a mild sedative and treatment of digestive upsets, menstrual cramps, and stomach ulcers. It has been used topically for skin irritation and inflammation. Chamomile is on the U.S. Food and Drug Administration list of herbs generally recognized as safe (GRAS). It is one of the most popular teas in Europe. When used as a tea, it appears to produce an antispasmodic effect on the smooth muscle of the GI tract and to protect against the development of stomach ulcers. Although the herb is generally safe and nontoxic, the tea is prepared from the pollen-filled flower heads and has resulted in mild symptoms of contact dermatitis to severe anaphylactic reactions in individuals hypersensitive to ragweed, asters, and chrysanthemums.

ANTIDIARRHEALS

Actions and Uses

Antidiarrheals are used in the treatment of diarrhea. Difenoxin (Motofen) and diphenoxylate (Lomotil) are chemically related to the opioid drugs; therefore, they decrease intestinal peristalsis, which often is increased when the patient has diarrhea. Because these drugs are opioid related they may have sedative and euphoric effects, but no analgesic activity. A drug dependence potential exists; therefore, the drugs are combined with atropine (a cholinergic blocking drug), which causes dry mouth and other mild adverse effects. Abuse potential is reduced because of these unpleasant adverse effects.

Loperamide (Imodium) acts directly on the muscle wall of the bowel to slow motility, and is not related to the opioids. It therefore is also used in treating chronic diarrhea associated with IBD.

Adverse Reactions

Gastrointestinal Reactions

- Anorexia, nausea, vomiting, constipation
- Abdominal discomfort, pain, and distention

Other

- Dizziness, drowsiness, and headache
- Sedation and euphoria
- Rash

Contraindications and Precautions

These drugs are contraindicated in patients whose diarrhea is associated with organisms that can harm the intestinal mucosa (*Escherichia coli*, *Salmonella*, *Shigella*). Patients with pseudomembranous colitis, abdominal pain of unknown origin, and obstructive jaundice also should not take antidiarrheals. The antidiarrheal drugs are contraindicated in children younger than 2 years of age.

Nursing Alert

If diarrhea persists for more than 2 days when over-the-counter antidiarrheal drugs are being used, the patient should discontinue use and seek treatment from the primary health care provider.

The antidiarrheal drugs are used cautiously in patients with severe hepatic impairment or IBD. Antidiarrheals are classified as pregnancy category C drugs and should be used cautiously during pregnancy and lactation. Loperamide is a pregnancy category B drug, yet it is still not recommended for use during pregnancy and lactation.

Interactions

The following interactions may occur when an antidiarrheal drug is administered with another agent:

Interacting Drug	Common Use	Effect of Interaction
antihistamines, opioids, sedatives, or hypnotics	Allergy treatment (antihistamines), sedation, or pain relief	Increased risk of central nervous system (CNS) depression
Antihistamines and general antidepressants	Allergy relief and depression management	Increased cholinergic blocking adverse reactions
monoamine oxidase inhibitor antidepressants	Depression management	Increased risk of hypertensive crisis

ANTIFLATULENTS
Actions

Simethicone (Mylicon) and charcoal are used as **antiflatulents** (drugs that reduce flatus or gas in the intestinal tract). These drugs do not absorb or remove gas; rather, they act to help the body release the gas by belching or flatus. Simethicone has a defoaming action that disperses and prevents the formation of gas pockets in the intestine. Charcoal helps bind gas for expulsion.

Uses

Antiflatulents are used to relieve painful symptoms of excess gas in the digestive tract that may be caused by

- Postoperative gaseous distention and air swallowing
- **Dyspepsia** (fullness or epigastric discomfort)
- Peptic ulcer
- Irritable bowel syndrome or diverticulosis

In addition to its use for the relief of intestinal gas, charcoal may be used in the prevention of nonspecific pruritus associated with kidney dialysis treatment and as an antidote in poisoning. Simethicone is in some antacid products, such as Mylanta Liquid and Di-Gel Liquid.

Adverse Reactions

No adverse reactions have been reported with the use of antiflatulents.

Contraindications and Precautions

The antiflatulents are contraindicated in patients with known hypersensitivity to any components of the drug. The pregnancy category of simethicone has not been determined; because it is not absorbed it may be safe for use during pregnancy, although the primary health care provider should be consulted whenever any drug is to be taken. Charcoal is a pregnancy category C drug.

Interactions

There may be a decreased effectiveness of other drugs because of adsorption by charcoal, which can also adsorb other drugs in the GI tract. There are no known interactions with simethicone.

LAXATIVES
Actions

There are various types of laxatives (see the Summary Drug Table: Drugs Used in Managing Lower Gastrointestinal Disorders). The action of each laxative is somewhat different, yet they produce the same result—the relief of constipation (Display 48-1).

Uses

A laxative is most often prescribed for the short-term relief or prevention of constipation. Specific uses of laxatives include

- Stimulant, emollient, and saline laxatives—evacuate the colon for rectal and bowel examinations
- Stool softeners or mineral oil—prevention of strain during defecation (after anorectal surgery or a myocardial infarction)
- Psyllium and polycarbophil—irritable bowel syndrome and diverticular disease
- Hyperosmotic (lactulose) agents—reduction of blood ammonia levels in hepatic encephalopathy

- Bulk-producing laxatives are not digested by the body and therefore add bulk and water to the contents of the intestines. The added bulk in the intestines stimulates peristalsis, moves the products of digestion through the intestine, and encourages evacuation of the stool. Examples of bulk-forming laxatives are psyllium (Metamucil) and polycarbophil (FiberCon). Sometimes these laxatives are used with severe diarrhea to add bulk to the watery bowel contents and slow transit through the bowel.
- Emollient laxatives lubricate the intestinal walls and soften the stool, thereby enhancing passage of fecal material. Mineral oil is an emollient laxative.
- Stool softeners promote water retention in the fecal mass and soften the stool. One difference between emollient laxatives and stool softeners is that the emollient laxatives do not promote the retention of water in the stool. Examples of stool softeners include docusate sodium (Colace) and docusate calcium (Surfak).
- Hyperosmolar drugs dehydrate local tissues, which causes irritation and increased peristalsis, with consequent evacuation of the fecal mass. Glycerin is a hyperosmolar drug.
- Irritant or stimulant laxatives increase peristalsis by direct action on the intestine. An example of an irritant laxative is cascara sagrada and senna (Senokot).
- Saline laxatives attract or pull water into the intestine, thereby increasing pressure in the intestine, followed by an increase in peristalsis. Magnesium hydroxide (Milk of Magnesia) is a saline laxative.

Adverse Reactions

Constipation may occur as an adverse drug reaction. When the patient has constipation as an adverse reaction to another drug, the primary health care provider may prescribe a stool softener or another laxative to prevent constipation during the drug therapy. Display 48-2 lists some of the drug classifications that may cause constipation.

Laxatives may cause diarrhea and a loss of water and electrolytes, abdominal pain or discomfort, nausea, vomiting, perianal irritation, fainting, bloating, flatulence, cramps, and weakness.

Prolonged use of a laxative can result in serious electrolyte imbalances, as well as the "laxative habit," that is, dependence on a laxative to have a bowel movement.

Some of these products contain tartrazine, which may cause allergic-type reactions (including bronchial asthma) in susceptible individuals. Obstruction of the esophagus, stomach, small intestine, and colon has occurred when bulk-forming laxatives are administered without adequate fluid intake or in patients with intestinal stenosis.

- Anticholinergic (cholinergic blocking drugs)
- Antihistamines
- Phenothiazines
- Tricyclic antidepressants
- Opiates
- Non–potassium-sparing diuretics
- Iron preparations
- Barium sulfate
- Clonidine
- Antacids containing calcium carbonate or aluminum hydroxide

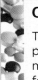

Chronic Care Alert

The very young, the elderly, and debilitated patients are at greatest risk for aspiration of mineral oil into the lungs when it is taken orally for constipation. Aspiration of mineral oil can lead to a lipid pneumonitis.

Contraindications and Precautions

Laxatives are contraindicated in patients with known hypersensitivity and those with persistent abdominal pain, nausea, or vomiting of unknown cause or signs of acute appendicitis, fecal impaction, intestinal obstruction, or acute hepatitis. These drugs are used only as directed because excessive or prolonged use may cause physical dependence on them for normal bowel movements.

Magnesium hydroxide is used cautiously in patients with any degree of renal impairment. Laxatives are used cautiously in patients with rectal bleeding, in pregnant women, and during lactation. The following laxatives are pregnancy category C drugs: cascara sagrada, docusate, glycerin, phenolphthalein, magnesium hydroxide, and senna. These drugs are used during pregnancy only when the benefits clearly outweigh the risks to the fetus.

Interactions

- Mineral oil may impair the GI absorption of fat-soluble vitamins (A, D, E, and K).

- Laxatives may reduce absorption of other drugs present in the GI tract, by combining with them chemically or hastening their passage through the intestinal tract.

- When surfactants are administered with mineral oil, they may increase mineral oil absorption.

- Milk, antacids, histamine H_2 antagonists, and proton pump inhibitors should not be administered 1 to 2 hours before bisacodyl tablets because the enteric coating may dissolve early (before reaching the intestinal tract), resulting in gastric lining irritation or dyspepsia and decreasing the laxative effect of the drug.

NURSING PROCESS

The Patient Receiving a Drug for a Lower Gastrointestinal Disorder

ASSESSMENT

PREADMINISTRATION ASSESSMENT

During the preadministration assessment, the nurse reviews the patient's chart for the medical diagnosis and reason for administration of the prescribed drug. The nurse questions the patient regarding the type and intensity of symptoms (e.g., pain, discomfort, diarrhea, or constipation) to provide a baseline for evaluation of the effectiveness of drug therapy. The nurse listens to bowel sounds and palpates the abdomen, monitoring the patient for signs of guarding or discomfort. Loose stool may indicate diarrhea; however, hypoactive bowel sounds in severe cases of **obstipation** (liquid stool leaked around the fecal mass, presenting as loose stool) are evidence that the patient is constipated, which would indicate very different drug therapy.

ONGOING ASSESSMENT

The nurse assesses the patient receiving one of these drugs for relief of symptoms (e.g., diarrhea, pain, or constipation). The primary health care provider is notified if the drug fails to relieve symptoms. The nurse monitors vital signs daily or more frequently if the patient has severe diarrhea, or another condition that may warrant more frequent observation. The nurse observes the patient for adverse drug reactions associated with the specific GI drug being administered and reports any adverse reactions to the primary health care provider before the next dose is due. The nurse evaluates the effectiveness of drug therapy by a daily comparison of symptoms with those experienced before the initiation of therapy. In some instances, frequent evaluation of the patient's response to therapy may be necessary.

NURSING DIAGNOSES

A key nursing diagnosis applicable to patients with lower GI problems is Risk for Imbalanced Fluid Volume related to diarrhea. Other nursing diagnoses applicable to these drugs are discussed in depth in Chapter 4.

PLANNING

The expected outcomes for the patient depend on the reason for administration of the drug, but may include an optimal response to drug therapy, support of patient needs related to the management of adverse reactions, and an understanding of and compliance with the prescribed therapeutic regimen.

IMPLEMENTATION

PROMOTING AN OPTIMAL RESPONSE TO THERAPY

Ways in which the nurse can help promote an optimal response to therapy when administering lower GI drugs are listed in the following sections.

ANTIDIARRHEALS These drugs may be ordered to be given after each loose bowel movement. The nurse inspects each bowel movement before making a decision to administer the drug.

LAXATIVES The nurse gives bulk-producing or stool-softening laxatives with a full glass of water or juice. The administration of a bulk-producing laxative is followed by an additional full glass of water. Mineral oil preferably is given to the patient with an empty stomach in the evening. Immediately before administration, the nurse thoroughly mixes and stirs laxatives that are in powder, flake, or granule form. If the laxative has an unpleasant or salty taste, the nurse explains this to the patient. The taste of some of these preparations may be disguised by chilling, adding to juice, or pouring over cracked ice.

> **Nursing Alert**
>
> Because activated charcoal can absorb other drugs in the GI tract, when used as an antiflatulent it should not be taken 2 hours before or 1 hour after the administration of other drugs.

MONITORING AND MANAGING PATIENT NEEDS

RISK FOR IMBALANCED FLUID VOLUME The nurse notifies the primary health care provider if the patient experiences an elevation in body temperature, severe abdominal pain, or abdominal rigidity or distention because this may indicate a complication of the disorder, such as infection or intestinal perforation. If diarrhea is severe, additional treatment measures, such as intravenous fluids and electrolyte replacement, may be necessary.

If diarrhea is chronic, the nurse encourages the patient to drink extra fluids. Weak tea, water, bouillon, or a commercial electrolyte preparation may be used.

The nurse closely monitors fluid intake and output. In some instances, the primary health care provider may prescribe an oral electrolyte supplement to replace electrolytes lost by frequent loose stools. Patients with fluid volume losses taking drugs that cause drowsiness or dizziness are at greater risk for injury. The patient may require assistance with ambulatory activities. For perianal irritation caused by loose stools, the nurse cleanses the area with mild soap and water after each bowel movement, dries the area with a soft cloth, and applies an emollient, such as petrolatum.

When a laxative is administered, the nurse records the bowel movement results on the patient's chart. If excessive bowel movements or severe, prolonged diarrhea occur, or if the laxative is ineffective, the nurse notifies the primary health care provider. If a laxative is ordered for constipation, the nurse encourages a liberal fluid intake and an increase in foods high in fiber to prevent a repeat of this problem.

EDUCATING THE PATIENT AND FAMILY

When a lower GI drug must be taken for a long time, there is a possibility that the patient may begin to skip doses or stop taking the drug. The nurse encourages patients to take the prescribed drug as directed by the primary health care provider and emphasizes the importance of not omitting doses or stopping the therapy unless advised to do so by the primary health care provider.

The nurse includes the following information in a patient and family teaching plan:

ANTIDIARRHEALS

- Do not exceed the recommended dosage.
- The drug may cause drowsiness. Observe caution when driving or performing other hazardous tasks.
- Avoid the use of alcohol or other CNS depressants (e.g., tranquilizers, sleeping pills) and other nonprescription drugs unless use has been approved by the primary health care provider.
- Notify the primary health care provider if diarrhea persists or becomes more severe.

ANTIFLATULENTS

- Take simethicone after each meal and at bedtime. Thoroughly chew tablets because complete particle dispersion enhances antiflatulent action.
- Notify the health care provider if symptoms are not relieved within several days.

LAXATIVES

- Avoid long-term use of these products unless use of the product has been recommended by the primary health care provider. Long-term use may result in the "laxative habit," which is dependence on a laxative to have a normal bowel movement. Constipation may also occur with overuse of these drugs. Read and follow the directions on the label.
- Do not use these products in the presence of abdominal pain, nausea, or vomiting.
- Notify the primary health care provider if constipation is not relieved or if rectal bleeding or other symptoms occur.
- To avoid constipation, drink plenty of fluids, get exercise, and eat foods high in bulk or roughage.
- Cascara sagrada or senna—Pink-red, red-violet, red-brown, yellow-brown, or black discoloration of urine may occur.

EVALUATION

- The therapeutic drug effect is achieved.
- Adverse reactions are identified and reported to the primary health care provider.
- The patient and family demonstrate an understanding of the drug regimen.
- The patient verbalizes the importance of complying with the prescribed treatment regimen.
- The patient verbalizes an understanding of treatment modalities and the importance of continued follow-up care.

Critical Thinking Exercises

1. Betty Ross, aged 32 years, has been recently diagnosed with ulcerative colitis. She tells you that her concerns and worries about being a single parent have finally caused her to become sick. Discuss how you would approach her comments about the cause of her illness.

2. Ms. Harris, aged 76 years, tells you that she has been using various laxatives for constipation. She states that a laxative did help, but now she is more constipated than she was before she began taking a laxative. Discuss what advice or suggestions you would give this patient.

3. Mr. Gates, your neighbor, has been given a prescription for diphenoxylate with atropine (Lomotil) to be taken if he should experience diarrhea while he is traveling in a foreign country. Describe the warnings you would give to your neighbor regarding this drug.

Review Questions

1. Which of the following is the best description of the cause of Crohn's disease?

   A. A somatic response to psychological stress

   B. An infection due to bacteria or parasites

   C. An inflammatory response in the colon

   D. A precancerous stage in the bowel

2. The patient asks how stool softeners relieve constipation. Which of the following would be the best response by the nurse? Stool softeners relieve constipation by _____.

   A. stimulating the walls of the intestine

   B. promoting the retention of sodium in the fecal mass

   C. promoting water retention in the fecal mass

   D. lubricating the intestinal walls

3. The nurse administers antidiarrheal drugs _____.

   A. after each loose bowel movement

   B. hourly until diarrhea ceases

   C. with food

   D. twice a day, in the morning and at bedtime

4. The pregnancy category for the antiflatulent drug simethicone is _____.

   A. pregnancy category A

   B. pregnancy category C

   C. pregnancy category X

   D. pregnancy category unknown

Medication Dosage Problems

1. A patient is to drink 4 L of polyethylene glycol-electrolyte solution (GoLYTELY) the night before an outpatient colonoscopy. If the directions state "drink 240 mL every 10 minutes," the nurse tells the patient the solution must be completely drunk in _____ hours.

2. Balsalazide (Colazal) 2250 mg orally TID is prescribed. If the drug comes in 750-mg capsules, the nurse administers _____ capsules with each dose.

To check your answers, see Appendix G.

Drugs That Affect the Endocrine System

The endocrine system consists of a group of glands throughout the body. The work of the endocrine system is to provide hormones (chemicals that assist in function) to various organs in the body. Hormones are produced and circulated through the blood to target receptors on certain cells in specific organs to assist in function. Glands that make up the endocrine system and are discussed in this unit include the pituitary, thyroid, pancreas, adrenal glands, and sex organs.

The pituitary gland sits at the base of the brain and helps with the function of many different organs in the body. Its hormones are secreted and sent to a wide variety of organs to promote and regulate growth and maturation, fluid and electrolyte balance, and metabolism. These hormones and the drugs that affect them are covered in Chapter 50. The adrenal glands are crucial in the secretion of corticosteroids, which are also covered in this chapter.

Located in the lower anterior portion of the neck, the thyroid's purpose is to help control metabolism. Chapter 51 covers the function of the thyroid and its hormones as well as drugs used to supplement function of the thyroid gland.

The pancreas is part of the gastrointestinal system. This organ provides enzymes to assist in the digestion of food, and provides the body with insulin to help cells use the glucose from food sources. As recently as 2006, the American Diabetes Association estimated that 7% (or about 20.8 million people) of the United States population has diabetes. The most up-to-date statistics can be retrieved at www.diabetes.org/about-diabetes.jsp. Diabetes mellitus is a chronic condition characterized by problems with the body's production or use of insulin. Chapter 49 discusses both insulin and the oral antidiabetic drugs used in treating diabetes mellitus.

Hormones play a major role in the development of the reproductive system as people go through puberty. The ovaries in the female and the testes in the male produce hormones that aid in the development of secondary sexual characteristics such as hair, voice, and musculature. Reproduction is controlled by the secretion of hormones. Chapters 52 and 53 describe the function of these hormones and the drugs used to promote optimal reproductive health. Hormones that affect the development of sexual characteristics also can alter the growth of cancer cells; these hormones are covered in Chapter 52.

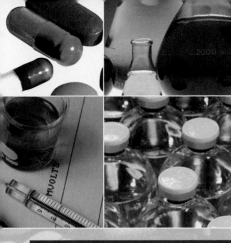

Antidiabetic Drugs

diabetes mellitus
diabetic ketoacidosis
Escherichia coli
glucagon
glucometer
glycosylated hemoglobin
hyperglycemia
hypoglycemia
insulin
lipodystrophy
polydipsia
polyphagia
polyuria
secondary failure

Learning Objectives

On completion of this chapter, the student will:

- Describe the two types of diabetes mellitus.
- Discuss the types, uses, general drug actions, adverse reactions, contraindications, precautions, and interactions of the antidiabetic drugs.
- Discuss important preadministration and ongoing assessment activities

the nurse should perform with the patient taking an antidiabetic drug.

- List nursing diagnoses particular to a patient taking an antidiabetic drug.
- Discuss ways to promote an optimal response to therapy, how to manage common adverse reactions, and important points to keep in mind when educating patients about the use of the antidiabetic drugs.

Insulin, a hormone produced by the pancreas, acts to maintain blood glucose levels within normal limits (60 to 120 mg/dL). This is accomplished by the release of small amounts of insulin into the bloodstream throughout the day in response to changes in blood glucose levels. Insulin is essential for the utilization of glucose in cellular metabolism and for the proper metabolism of protein and fat.

Diabetes mellitus is a complicated, chronic disorder characterized by either insufficient insulin production by the beta cells of the pancreas or by cellular resistance to insulin. Insulin insufficiency results in elevated blood glucose levels, or hyperglycemia. As a result of the disease, individuals with diabetes are at greater risk for a number of disorders, including myocardial infarction, cerebrovascular accident (stroke), blindness, kidney disease, and lower limb amputations.

Insulin and the oral antidiabetic drugs, along with diet and exercise, are the cornerstones of treatment for diabetes mellitus. They are used to prevent episodes of hypoglycemia and normalize carbohydrate metabolism.

There are two major types of diabetes mellitus:

- Type 1—formerly known as insulin-dependent diabetes mellitus or IDDM

- Type 2—formerly known as non–insulin-dependent diabetes mellitus or NIDDM

Those with type 1 diabetes mellitus produce insulin in insufficient amounts and therefore must have insulin supplementation to survive. Type 1 diabetes usually has a rapid onset, occurs before age 20 years, produces more severe symptoms than type 2 diabetes, and is more difficult to control. Major symptoms of type 1 diabetes include hyperglycemia, **polydipsia** (increased thirst), **polyphagia** (increased appetite), **polyuria** (increased urination), and weight loss. Control of type 1 diabetes is particularly difficult because of the lack of insulin production by the pancreas. Treatment requires a strict regimen that typically includes a carefully calculated diet, planned physical activity, home glucose testing several times a day, and multiple daily insulin injections.

Type 2 diabetes mellitus affects about 90% to 95% of individuals with diabetes. Those with type 2 diabetes are affected either by decreased production of insulin by the beta cells of the pancreas or decreased sensitivity of the cells to insulin, making the cells insulin resistant. Although type 2 diabetes mellitus may occur at any age, the disorder occurs most often after age 40 years. The onset of type 2 diabetes is usually insidious. Symptoms are less severe than in type 1 diabetes mellitus, and because it tends to be more stable, type 2 diabetes is easier to control than type 1. Risk factors for type 2 diabetes include

- Obesity
- Older age
- Family history of diabetes
- History of gestational diabetes (diabetes that develops during pregnancy but disappears when pregnancy is over)
- Impaired glucose tolerance
- Minimal or no physical activity
- Race/ethnicity (African Americans, Hispanic/Latino Americans, Native Americans, and some Asian Americans)

Obesity is thought to contribute to type 2 diabetes by placing additional stress on the pancreas, which makes it less able to respond and produce adequate insulin to meet the body's metabolic needs.

In many individuals with type 2 diabetes, the disorder can be controlled with diet, exercise, and oral antidiabetic drugs. However, about 40% of those with type 2 diabetes respond poorly to the oral antidiabetic drugs and require insulin to control the diabetes.

INSULIN

Insulin is a hormone manufactured by the beta cells of the pancreas. It is the principal hormone required for the proper use of glucose (carbohydrate) by the body. Insulin also controls the storage and utilization of amino acids and fatty acids. Insulin lowers blood glucose levels by inhibiting glucose production by the liver.

Pharmaceutical human insulin is derived from a biosynthetic process using strains of *Escherichia coli* (recombinant DNA, rDNA). Human insulin appears to cause fewer allergic reactions than does insulin obtained from animal sources. Insulin analogs, insulin lispro, and insulin aspart are newer forms of human insulin made using recombinant DNA technology and are structurally similar to human insulin.

Insulin that is biologically similar to human insulin is also available as purified extracts from beef and pork pancreas. However, these animal-source insulins are used less frequently today than in the past. They have been replaced by synthetic insulins, such as human insulin or insulin analogs.

Actions

Insulin appears to activate a process that helps glucose molecules enter the cells of striated muscle and adipose tissue. Figure 49-1 depicts normal glucose metabolism. Insulin also stimulates the synthesis of glycogen by the liver. In addition, insulin promotes protein synthesis and helps the body store fat by preventing its breakdown for energy.

Onset, Peak, and Duration of Action

Onset, peak, and duration are three clinically important properties of insulin:

- Onset—when insulin first begins to act in the body
- Peak—when the insulin is exerting maximum action
- Duration—the length of time the insulin remains in effect

To meet the needs of those with diabetes mellitus, various insulin preparations have been developed to delay the onset and prolong the duration of action of insulin. When insulin is combined with protamine (a protein), its absorption from the injection site is slowed and its duration of action is prolonged. The addition of zinc also modifies the onset and duration of action of insulin. Insulin preparations are classified as rapid acting, intermediate acting, or long acting. See the Summary Drug Table: Insulin Preparations for information concerning the onset, peak, and duration of various insulins.

Uses

Insulin is used to

- Control type 1 diabetes
- Control type 2 diabetes when uncontrolled by diet, exercise, or weight reduction
- Treat severe diabetic ketoacidosis (DKA) or diabetic coma
- Treat hypokalemia in combination with glucose

Adverse Reactions

The two major adverse reactions seen with insulin administration are **hypoglycemia** (low blood glucose, or sugar,

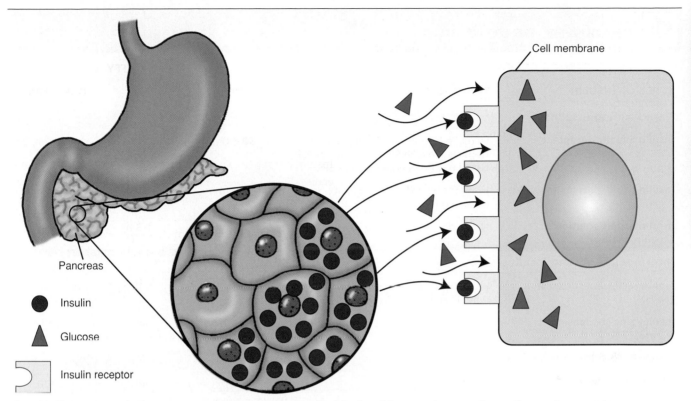

Figure 49.1 Normal glucose metabolism. Once insulin binds with receptors on the cell membrane, glucose can move into the cell, promoting cellular metabolism and energy production.

level) and **hyperglycemia** (elevated blood glucose, or sugar, level). The symptoms of hypoglycemia and hyperglycemia are listed in Table 49-1.

Hypoglycemia may occur when there is too much insulin in the bloodstream in relation to the available glucose (hyperinsulinism). Hypoglycemia may occur when

- The patient eats too little food.

- The insulin dose is incorrectly measured and is greater than that prescribed.

- The patient has drastically increased demands (activity or illness).

Hyperglycemia may occur if there is too little insulin in the bloodstream in relation to the available glucose (hypoinsulinism). Hyperglycemia may occur when

- The patient eats too much food.

- Too little or no insulin is given.

- The patient experiences emotional stress, infection, surgery, pregnancy, or an acute illness.

Another potential adverse reaction may be an allergic reaction to the animal (pig or cow) from which the insulin is obtained or to the protein or zinc added to insulin. To minimize the possibility of an allergic reaction, some health care providers prescribe human insulin or purified insulin. However, on rare occasions, some individuals become allergic to the human and purified insulins.

An individual can also become insulin resistant because antibodies develop against insulin. These patients have impaired receptor function and become so unresponsive to insulin that the dose requirement may be in excess of 500 Units/d, rather than the usual 40 to 60 Units/d. High-potency insulin in a concentrated form (U500) is used for patients requiring more than 200 Units/d.

Contraindications

Insulin is contraindicated in patients with hypersensitivity to any ingredient of the product (e.g., beef or pork) and when the patient is hypoglycemic.

Precautions

Insulin is used cautiously in patients with renal or hepatic impairment and during pregnancy and lactation. The insulins are grouped in pregnancy category B, except for

SUMMARY DRUG TABLE   INSULIN PREPARATIONS

TYPES OF INSULIN	TRADE NAME	ACTIVITY		
		ONSET	PEAK	DURATION
Rapid-Acting Insulins				
insulin injection (regular)	Humulin R, Humulin R Pen, Iletin II Regular, Novolin R, Novolin R PenFill, Novolin R Prefilled, Velosulin BR	30–60 min	2–4 h	8–2 h
insulin lispro (insulin analog)	Humalog, Humalog Mix 50/50, Humalog Mix 75/25	30 min	30 min–1.5 h	2–5 h
insulin aspart solution (insulin analog)	NovoLog	30 min	1–3 h	3–5 h
Intermediate-Acting Insulins				
isophane insulin suspension (NPH)	Humulin N, Novolin N, Novolin N PenFill, Novolin N Prefilled, NPH Iletin II	1.5 h	4–12 h	24 h
insulin zinc suspension (Lente)	Humulin L, Lente Iletin II, Novolin L	1–2.5 h	7–15 h	24 h
Long-Acting Insulins				
insulin glargine solution	Lantus	1 h	none	24 h
extended insulin zinc suspension (Ultralente)	Humulin U	4–8 h	10–30 h	20–36 h
Mixed Insulins				
isophane insulin suspension and insulin injections (NPH)	Humulin 70/30, Humulin 70/30 Pen Novolin 70/30, Novolin 70/30 PenFill, Novolin 70/30 Prefilled	30–60 min, then 1–2 h	2–4 h, then 6–12 h	6–8 h, then 18–24 h
isophane insulin suspension and insulin injection (Reg)	Humulin 50/50	30–60 min, then 1–2 h	2–4 h, then 6–12 h	6–8 h, then 18–24 h

Table 49.1 Hypoglycemia Versus Hyperglycemia

Symptoms	Hypoglycemia (Insulin Reaction)	Hyperglycemia (Diabetic Coma, Ketoacidosis)
Onset	Sudden	Gradual (hours or days)
Blood glucose level	Less than 60 mg/dL	More than 200 mg/dL
Central nervous system	Fatigue, weakness, nervousness, agitation, confusion, headache, diplopia, convulsions, dizziness, unconsciousness	Drowsiness, dim vision
Respirations	Normal to rapid, shallow	Deep, rapid (air hunger)
Gastrointestinal	Hunger, nausea	Thirst, nausea, vomiting, abdominal pain, loss of appetite
Skin	Pale, moist, cool, diaphoretic	Dry, flushed, warm
Pulse	Normal or uncharacteristic	Rapid, weak
Miscellaneous	Numbness, tingling of the lips or tongue	Acetone breath, excessive urination

insulin glargine and insulin aspart, which are in pregnancy category C. Insulin appears to inhibit milk production in lactating women and could interfere with breastfeeding. Lactating women may require adjustment in insulin dose and diet.

Nursing Alert

Pregnancy makes diabetes more difficult to manage. Insulin requirements usually decrease in the first trimester, increase during the second and third trimester, and decrease rapidly after delivery. The patient with diabetes or a history of gestational diabetes must be encouraged to maintain good metabolic control before conception and throughout pregnancy. Frequent monitoring is necessary.

Interactions

When certain drugs are administered with insulin, a resultant decrease or increase in hypoglycemic effect can occur. Display 49-1 identifies selected drugs that decrease and increase the hypoglycemic effect of insulin.

NURSING PROCESS

The Patient Receiving Insulin

ASSESSMENT

PREADMINISTRATION ASSESSMENT

If the patient has recently been diagnosed with diabetes mellitus and has not received insulin, or if the patient is known to have diabetes, the initial physical assessment before administering the first dose of insulin includes taking the blood pressure and pulse and respiratory rates and weighing the patient. The nurse makes a general assessment of the skin, mucous membranes, and extremities, with special attention given to any sores or cuts that appear to be infected or healing poorly, as well as any ulcerations or other skin or mucous membrane changes. The nurse obtains the following information and includes it in the patient's chart:

- Dietary habits
- Family history of diabetes (if any)
- Type and duration of symptoms experienced

The nurse reviews the patient's chart for recent laboratory and diagnostic tests. If the patient has diabetes and has been receiving insulin, the nurse includes the type and dosage of insulin used, the type of diabetic diet, and the average results of glucose testing in the patient's chart. The

---

Display 49.1 Drugs That Alter Insulin Effectiveness

Selected Drugs That Decrease the Effect (More Insulin May Be Required)

acetazolamide	glucagon
albuterol	human immunodeficiency virus (HIV) antivirals
antipsychotics	
asparaginase	
calcitonin	isoniazid
contraceptives, oral	lithium
corticosteroids	morphine sulfate
danazol	niacin
dextrothyroxine	phenothiazines
diazoxide	phenytoin
diltiazem	progestogens
diuretics	protease inhibitors
dobutamine	somatropin
epinephrine	terbutaline
estrogens	thiazide diuretics
ethacrynic acid	thyroid hormones

Drugs That Increase the Effect (Less Insulin May Be Required)

angiotensin-converting enzyme (ACE) inhibitors	lithium
alcohol	monoamine oxidase inhibitors (MAOIs)
anabolic steroids	mebendazole
antidiabetic drugs, oral	pentamidine
beta blocking drugs	pentoxifylline
calcium	phenylbutazone
clofibrate	pyridoxine
clonidine	salicylates
disopyramide	somatostatin analog
fluoxetine	sulfinpyrazone
fibrates	sulfonamides
guanethidine	tetracycline

---

nurse evaluates the patient's past compliance with the prescribed therapeutic regimen, such as diet, weight control, and periodic evaluation by a health care provider.

ONGOING ASSESSMENT

The number and amount of daily insulin doses, times of administration, and diet and exercise requirements require continual assessment. Dosage adjustments may be necessary when changing types of insulin, particularly when changing from the single-peak to the more pure Humulin insulins.

The nurse must assess the patient for signs and symptoms of hypoglycemia and hyperglycemia (see Table 49-1) throughout insulin therapy. The patient is particularly prone to hypoglycemic reactions at the time of peak insulin action (see the Summary Drug Table: Insulin Preparations) or when he or she has not eaten for some time or has skipped a meal. In acute care settings, frequent blood glucose monitoring is routinely done to help detect abnormalities of blood glucose. Testing usually occurs before meals and at bedtime (see the Patient and Family Teaching Checklist: Obtaining a Blood Glucose Reading Using a Glucometer).

Patient and Family Teaching Checklist

Obtaining a Blood Glucose Reading Using a Glucometer

The nurse teaches the patient to:

✔ Carefully follow manufacturer's instructions because blood glucose monitoring devices vary greatly.

✔ Read all of the manufacturer's instructions before using the glucometer.

✔ Prepare the patient's finger by cleansing with warm water to the area. (If the patient cannot prepare the area, the caregiver should wear gloves to comply with Standard Precautions, the guidelines of the Centers for Disease Control and Prevention.)

✔ Most glucometers require a small sample of capillary blood that is obtained from the fingertip using a spring-loaded lancet.

✔ Using the lancet device, perform a finger stick on the side of a finger tip where there are fewer nerve endings and more capillaries.

✔ Milk the finger to produce a large, hanging drop of blood. Using this technique to obtain a blood sample will help prevent inaccurate readings. *Note:* Do not smear the blood or try to obtain an extra drop.

✔ Drop the blood sample on a reagent test strip, wait 45 to 60 seconds, and then wipe off the excess blood with a cotton ball. *Note:* Some glucometers have eliminated the step of excess blood removal from the strip. With these devices, the reagent strip is placed in the glucometer first, allowing all of the blood to remain on the strip for the entire test. Another type of monitoring device uses a sensor cartridge instead of strips to obtain blood glucose levels. The blood is placed on the sensor, and automatic timers provide readings in a shorter time than the traditional glucometer.

✔ Place the test strip in a glucometer that automatically uses the sample to determine a numeric reading representing the current blood glucose level. *The blood glucose level reading should be between 70 and 120 mg/dL.*

Nursing Alert

The nurse must closely observe the patient after administering any insulin, but particularly U500 insulin, because secondary hypoglycemic reactions may occur as long as 24 hours after administration.

Blood glucose levels are monitored frequently in patients with diabetes. Patients in the acute care setting are monitored closely for hyperglycemia. Insulin needs increase in times of stress or illness. The health care provider may order regular insulin as a supplement to the drug regimen to "cover" any episodes of hyperglycemia. For example, blood glucose levels are monitored every 6 hours or before meals and at bedtime, with insulin prescribed to cover any hyperglycemia detected. This coverage is sometimes referred to by the health care providers in a teaching session as a sliding scale, or insulin coverage. The nurse administers supplemental insulin based on blood glucose readings and the amount of insulin prescribed by the primary health care provider in the sliding scale. The nurse must notify the primary health care provider if the blood glucose level is greater than 400 mg/dL.

The primary health care provider may prescribe use of a sliding scale at various times, such as every 4 hours, every 6 hours, or at specified times (e.g., 7:00 AM, 11:00 AM, 4 PM, and 11 PM), depending on the patient's individual needs. Consult your institutional policy; these scales can vary.

NURSING DIAGNOSES

Drug-specific nursing diagnoses are highlighted in the Nursing Diagnoses Checklist. Other nursing diagnoses applicable to these drugs are discussed in depth in Chapter 4.

Nursing Diagnoses Checklist

✔ **Acute Confusion** related to hypoglycemia effects on mentation

✔ **Deficient Fluid Volume** related to fluid loss during DKA

✔ **Anxiety** related to fear of diagnosis, giving own injections, dietary restrictions, other factors (specify)

PLANNING

The expected outcomes of the patient may include an optimal response to therapy, patient needs related to the management of adverse reactions, a reduction in anxiety and fear, improved ability to cope with the diagnosis, and an understanding of and compliance with the prescribed therapeutic regimen.

IMPLEMENTATION

Nursing management of a patient with diabetes requires diligent, skillful, and comprehensive nursing care.

PROMOTING AN OPTIMAL RESPONSE TO THERAPY

There is no standard dose of insulin, as there is for most other drugs. Insulin dosage is highly individualized. Sometimes the health care provider finds that the patient achieves best control with one injection of insulin per day; sometimes the patient requires two or more injections per day. In addition, two different types of insulin may be combined, such as a rapid-acting and a long-acting preparation. The number of insulin injections, dosage, times of administration, and type of insulin are determined by the health care provider after careful evaluation of the patient's metabolic needs and response to therapy. The dosage prescribed for the patient may require changes until the dosage is found that best meets the patient's needs.

> **Nursing Alert**
>
> Insulin requirements may change when the patient experiences any form of stress and with any illness, particularly illnesses resulting in nausea and vomiting.

Insulin is ordered by the generic name (e.g., insulin zinc suspension, extended) or the trade (brand) name (e.g., Humulin U; see the Summary Drug Table: Insulin Preparations). One brand of insulin must never be substituted for another unless the substitution is approved by the primary health care provider because some patients may be sensitive to changes in brands of insulin. In addition, it is important never to substitute one type of insulin for another. For example, do not use insulin zinc suspension instead of the prescribed protamine zinc insulin.

When the nurse or patient is administering insulin, care must be taken to use the correct insulin. Names and packaging are similar and can easily be confused. The nurse carefully reads all drug labels before preparing any insulin preparation. For example, Humalog (insulin lispro) and Humulin R (regular human insulin) are easily confused because of the similar names.

Insulin must be administered by the parenteral route, usually the subcutaneous (SC) route. Insulin cannot be administered orally because it is a protein and readily destroyed in the gastrointestinal (GI) tract. Regular insulin is the only insulin preparation given intravenously (IV). Regular insulin is given 30 to 60 minutes before a meal to achieve optimal results.

Insulin aspart is given immediately before a meal (within 5 to 10 minutes of beginning a meal). Insulin lispro is given 15 minutes before a meal or immediately after a meal. Insulin aspart and lispro make insulin administration more convenient for many patients who find taking a drug 30 to 60 minutes before meals bothersome. In addition, insulin lispro (Humalog) appears to lower the blood glucose level 1 to 2 hours after meals better than does regular human insulin because it more closely mimics the body's natural insulin. It also lowers the risk of low blood glucose reactions from midnight to 6 AM in patients with type 1 diabetes. The longer-acting insulins are given before breakfast or at bedtime (depending on the primary health care provider's instructions). Many patients are maintained on a single dose of intermediate-acting insulin administered SC in the morning.

Insulin glargine is given SC once daily at bedtime. This type of insulin is used in treating adults and children with type 1 diabetes mellitus and in adults with type 2 diabetes who need long-acting insulin for the control of hyperglycemia.

Insulin is available in concentrations of U100 and U500. The nurse must read the label of the insulin bottle carefully for the name, source of insulin (e.g., human, beef, pork, beef and pork, purified beef), and the number of units per milliliter. The dose of insulin is measured in units. U100 insulin has 100 units in each milliliter; U500 has 500 units in each milliliter. Most people with diabetes use the U100 concentration. Patients who are resistant to insulin and require large insulin doses use the U500 concentration.

MIXING INSULINS If the patient is to receive regular insulin and NPH insulin, or regular and Lente insulin, the nurse must clarify with the primary health care provider whether two separate injections are to be given or if the insulins may be mixed in the same syringe. If the two insulins are to be given in the same syringe, the short-acting insulin (regular or lispro) is drawn into the syringe first (Fig. 49-2). Even small amounts of intermediate- or long-acting insulin, if mixed with the short-acting insulin, can bind with the short-acting insulin and delay its onset.

> **Nursing Alert**
>
> Regular insulin is clear, whereas intermediate- and long-acting insulins are cloudy. The clear insulin should be drawn up first. When insulin lispro is mixed with a longer-acting insulin, the insulin lispro is drawn up first.

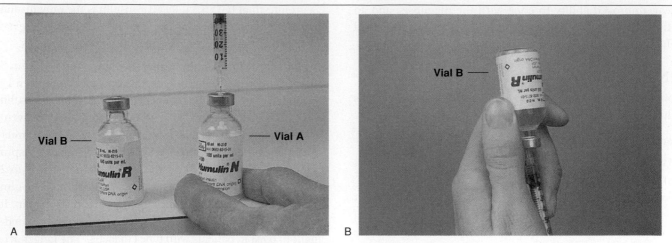

Figure 49.2 (**A**) After cleansing tops of both the Humulin R (regular) insulin and Humulin N (intermediate-acting insulin), with the container upright, the nurse injects air into the Humulin N insulin equal to the prescribed dosage of Humulin N. The nurse removes the needle without touching any fluid, then injects the amount of air into the pre-scribed dosage of the regular insulin and withdraws the prescribed dosage of regular insulin into the syringe. (**B**) After removing any air bubbles and determining what the total combined volume of the two insulins would measure, the nurse inverts the vial with the NPH insulin and carefully withdraws the correct volume of medication. *Note*: The nurse must be sure to check medication and dosage again before returning or discarding vials or administering the insulin.

An unexpected response may be obtained when changing from mixed injections to separate injections or vice versa. If the patient had been using insulin mixtures before admission, the nurse asks whether the insulins were given separately or together.

Several types of premixed insulins are available. These insulins combine regular insulin with the longer-acting NPH insulin. The mixtures are available in ratios of 70/30 and 50/50 of NPH to regular. Although these premixed insulins are helpful for patients who have difficulty drawing up their insulin or seeing the markings on the syringe, they prohibit individualizing the dosage. For patients who have difficulty controlling their diabetes, these premixed insulins may not be effective.

Nursing Alert

Do not mix or dilute insulin glargine with any other insulin or solution because glucose control will be lost and the insulin will not be effective.

PREPARING INSULIN FOR ADMINISTRATION The nurse always checks the expiration date printed on the label of the insulin bottle before withdrawing the insulin. An insulin syringe that matches the concentration of insulin to be given is always used. For example, a syringe labeled as U100 is used only with insulin labeled U100. U500 insulin is given only by the SC or intramuscular (IM) route, and may be administered using a tuberculin syringe if necessary.

When insulin is in a suspension (this can be seen when looking at a vial that has been untouched for about 1 hour), the nurse gently rotates the vial between the palms of the hands and tilts it gently end-to-end immediately before withdrawing the insulin. This ensures even distri-bution of the suspended particles. Care is taken not to shake the insulin vigorously.

The nurse carefully checks the primary health care provider's order for the type and dosage of insulin immedi-ately before withdrawing the insulin from the vial. All air bubbles must be eliminated from the syringe barrel and hub of the needle before withdrawing the syringe from the insulin vial.

Nursing Alert

Accuracy is of the utmost importance when measuring any insulin preparation because of the potential danger of administering an incor-rect dosage. If possible, the nurse should check and consult with another nurse for accuracy of the insulin dosage by comparing the insulin container, the syringe, and the primary health care provider's order before administration.

When regular insulin and another insulin are mixed in the same syringe, the nurse must administer the insulin within 5 minutes of withdrawing the two insulins from the two vials.

ROTATING INJECTION SITES Insulin may be injected into the arms, thighs, abdomen, or buttocks (see Home Care Checklist: Rotating Insulin Injection Sites). Sites of insulin injection are rotated to prevent **lipodystrophy** (atrophy of subcutaneous fat), a problem that can interfere with the absorption of insulin from the injection site. Lipodystrophy appears as a slight dimpling or pitting of the subcutaneous fat. Because absorption rates vary at the different

Home Care Checklist

Rotating Insulin Injection Sites

If your patient must self-administer insulin at home, be sure he or she knows where to inject the insulin and how to rotate the site. Site rotation is crucial to prevent injury to the skin and fatty tissue. Review with the patient appropriate sites, including:

☑ Upper arms, outer aspect

☑ Stomach, except for a 2-inch margin around the umbilicus

☑ Back, right, and left sides just below the waist

☑ Upper thighs, both front and side

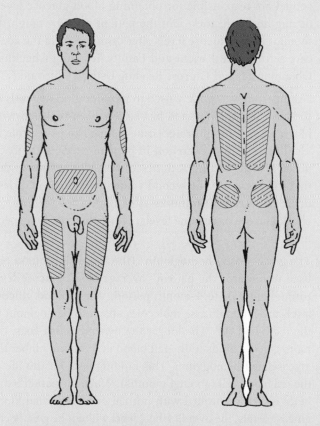

To rotate sites, teach the patient to do the following:

☑ Note the site of the last injection

☑ Place the side of his or her thumb at the old site and measure across its width—about 1 inch

☑ Select a site on the other side of the thumb for the next injection

☑ Repeat the procedure for each subsequent injection

☑ Use the same area for a total of about 10 to 15 injections and then move to another area

sites, with the abdomen having the most rapid rate of absorption, followed by the upper arm, thigh, and buttocks, some health care providers recommend rotating the injection sites within one specific area, rather than rotating areas. For example, all available sites within the abdomen would be used before moving to the thigh.

The nurse carefully plans the injection site rotation pattern and writes this plan in the patient's chart. Before each dose of insulin is given, the nurse checks the patient's chart for the site of the previous injection and uses the next site (according to the rotation plan) for injection. After giving the injection, the nurse records the site used. Each time insulin is given, previous injection sites are inspected for inflammation, which may indicate a localized allergic reaction. The nurse notes any other inflammation or skin reactions. The nurse reports localized allergic reactions, signs of inflammation, or other skin changes to the primary health care provider as soon as possible because a different type of insulin may be necessary.

METHODS OF ADMINISTERING INSULIN Several methods can be used to administer insulin. The most common method is the use of a needle and syringe. Use of microfine needles has reduced the discomfort associated with an injection. Another method is the jet injection system, which uses pressure to deliver a fine stream of insulin below the skin. Another method uses a disposable needle and special syringe. The syringe has a cartridge that is prefilled with a specific type of insulin (e.g., regular human insulin, isophane [NPH] insulin, or a mixture of isophane and regular insulin). The desired units are selected by turning a dial and the locking ring.

Another method of insulin delivery is the insulin pump, which is intended for a select group of individuals, such as the pregnant woman with diabetes with early long-term complications, and those who have undergone, or are candidates for, renal transplantation. This system attempts to mimic the body's normal pancreatic function, uses only regular insulin, is battery powered, and requires insertion of a needle into SC tissue. The needle is changed every 1 to 3 days. The amount of insulin injected can be adjusted according to blood glucose levels, which are monitored four to eight times per day.

The insulin dosage pattern that most closely follows normal insulin production is a multiple-dose plan sometimes called *intensive insulin therapy*. In this regimen, a single dose of intermediate- or long-acting insulin is taken in the morning or at bedtime. Small doses of regular insulin are taken before meals based on the patient's blood glucose levels. This allows for greater flexibility in the patient's lifestyle, but can

also be an inconvenience to the patient (e.g., the need always to carry supplies, the lack of privacy, inconvenient schedules).

Intranasal insulin delivery is being explored. It is designed for administration of rapid-onset and short-duration insulins. Because a small amount of the insulin is actually absorbed, higher doses are needed to obtain the desired effect.

BLOOD AND URINE TESTING Blood glucose levels are monitored often in the patient with diabetes. The primary health care provider may order blood glucose levels to be tested before meals, after meals, and at bedtime. Less frequent monitoring may be performed if the patient's glucose levels are well controlled. The **glucometer** is a device used by the patient with diabetes or the nursing personnel to monitor blood glucose levels. Nursing or laboratory personnel are responsible for obtaining blood glucose levels during hospitalization, but the patient must be taught to monitor blood glucose levels after dismissal from the acute care setting (see Patient and Family Teaching Checklist: Obtaining a Blood Glucose Reading Using a Glucometer).

Urine testing was widely used to monitor glucose levels in the past, but this method has largely been replaced with blood glucose monitoring. Urine testing can play a role in identifying ketone excretion in patients prone to ketoacidosis. If urine testing is done, it is usually recommended that the nurse use the second voided specimen (i.e., fresh urine collected 30 minutes after the initial voiding) to check glucose or acetone levels, rather than the first specimen obtained.

The **glycosylated hemoglobin** (HbA_{1c}) test is a blood test used to monitor the patient's average blood glucose level throughout a 3- to 4-month period. When blood glucose levels are high, glucose molecules attach to hemoglobin in the red blood cell. The longer the hyperglycemia lasts, the more glucose binds to the red blood cell and the higher the glycosylated hemoglobin. This binding lasts for the life of the red blood cell (about 4 months). When the patient's diabetes is well controlled with normal or near-normal blood glucose levels, the overall HbA_{1c} level will not be greatly elevated. However, if blood glucose levels are consistently high, the HbA_{1c} level will be elevated. The test result (expressed as a percentage) refers to the average amount of glucose that has been in the blood throughout the last 4 months. Normal levels vary with the laboratory method used for analysis, but in general levels between 2.5% and 6% indicate good control of diabetes. Results of 10% or greater indicate poor blood glucose control for the last several months. The HbA_{1c} is useful in evaluating the success of diabetes treatment, comparing new treatment regimens with past regimens, and individualizing treatment.

MONITORING AND MANAGING PATIENT NEEDS

ACUTE CONFUSION Close observation of the patient with diabetes is important, especially when diabetes is newly diagnosed, the insulin dosage changes, the patient is pregnant, the patient has a medical illness or surgery, or the patient fails to adhere to the prescribed diet. Episodes of hypoglycemia are corrected as soon as the symptoms are recognized.

Nursing Alert

The nurse should check the patient for hypoglycemia (see Table 49-1) at the peak time of action of the insulin (see Summary Drug Table: Insulin Preparations). Hypoglycemia, which can develop suddenly, may indicate a need for adjustment in the insulin dosage or other changes in treatment, such as a change in diet. Hypoglycemic reactions can occur at any time but are most likely to occur when insulin is at its peak activity.

Methods of terminating a hypoglycemic reaction include the administration of one or more of the following:

- Orange juice or other fruit juice
- Hard candy or honey
- Commercial glucose products
- Glucagon by the SC, IM, or IV route
- Glucose 10% or 50% IV

Selection of any one or more of these methods for terminating a hypoglycemic reaction, as well as other procedures to be followed, such as drawing blood for glucose levels, depends on the written order of the primary health care provider or hospital policy. The nurse should never give oral fluids or substances (such as candy) used to terminate a hypoglycemic reaction to a patient unless the swallowing and gag reflexes are present. Absence of these reflexes may result in aspiration of the oral fluid or substance into the lungs, which can result in extremely serious consequences and even death. If swallowing and gag reflexes are absent, or if the patient is unconscious, glucose or glucagon is given by the parenteral route.

Glucagon is a hormone produced by the alpha cells of the pancreas; it acts to increase blood glucose by stimulating the conversion of glycogen to glucose in the liver. A return of consciousness is observed within 5 to 20 minutes after parenteral administration of glucagon. Glucagon is effective in treating hypoglycemia only if glycogen is available from the liver

The nurse notifies the primary health care provider of any hypoglycemic reaction, the substance and amount used to terminate the reaction, blood samples drawn (if any), the length of time required for the symptoms of hypoglycemia to disappear, and the current status of the patient. After termination of a hypoglycemic reaction, the nurse closely observes the patient for additional hypoglycemic reactions. The length of time close observation is required depends on the peak and duration of the insulin administered.

DEFICIENT FLUID VOLUME Diabetic ketoacidosis (DKA) is a potentially life-threatening deficiency of insulin (hypoinsulinism), resulting in severe hyperglycemia and requiring prompt diagnosis and treatment. Because insulin is unavailable to allow glucose to enter the cell, dangerously high levels of glucose build up in the blood (hyperglycemia). The body, needing energy, begins to break down fat for energy. As fats break down, the liver produces ketones. As more and more fat is used for energy, higher levels of ketones accumulate in the blood. This increase in ketones disrupts the acid–base balance in the body, leading to DKA. DKA is treated with fluids, correction of acidosis and hypotension, and low doses of regular insulin.

Nursing Alert

The nurse immediately reports any of the following symptoms of hyperglycemia: elevated blood glucose levels (over 200 mg/mL), headache, increased thirst, epigastric pain, nausea, vomiting, hot, dry, flushed skin, restlessness, and diaphoresis (sweating).

ANXIETY The patient with newly diagnosed diabetes often has many concerns regarding the diagnosis. For some, initially coping with diabetes and the methods required for controlling the disorder creates many problems. Some of the fears and concerns of these patients may include self-administering an injection, following a diet, weight control, complications associated with diabetes, and changes in eating times and habits. An effective teaching program helps relieve some of this anxiety. The patient in this situation needs time to talk about the disorder, express concerns, and ask questions.

ASSISTING THE PATIENT WITH IMPAIRED ADJUSTMENT, COPING, AND ALTERED HEALTH MAINTENANCE

The patient with newly diagnosed diabetes may have difficulty accepting the diagnosis, and the complexity of the therapeutic regimen can seem overwhelming. Before patients can be expected to carry out treatment, they must accept that they have diabetes and deal with their feelings about having the disorder. The nurse has an important role in helping these patients gradually accept the diagnosis and begin to understand their feelings. Understanding diabetes may help patients work with health care providers and other medical personnel in managing their diabetes.

EDUCATING THE PATIENT AND FAMILY

Noncompliance is a problem in some patients with diabetes, making patient and family teaching vital to the proper management of diabetes. Patients may occasionally lapse in adhering to the prescribed diet, especially around holidays or other special occasions. This slip may not cause a problem if it is brief and not excessive and if the patient immediately returns to the prescribed regimen. However, some patients frequently stray from the prescribed regimen, take extra insulin to cover dietary indiscretions, fast for several days before follow-up blood glucose determinations, and engage in other dangerous behaviors. Although some patients can be convinced that failure to adhere to the prescribed therapeutic regimen is detrimental to their health, others continue to deviate from the prescribed regimen until serious complications develop. Every effort is made to stress the importance of adherence to the prescribed treatment during the initial teaching session and during follow-up office or clinic visits.

The nurse establishes a thorough teaching plan for all patients with newly diagnosed diabetes, for those who have had any change in the management of their diabetes (e.g., diet, insulin type, insulin dosage), and for those whose management has changed because of an illness or disability, such as loss of sight or disabling arthritis. The newly diagnosed patient with diabetes and the family must have an explanation of the disease and methods of treatment as soon as the primary health care provider has revealed the diagnosis to the patient. The nurse should always individualize the teaching plan because the needs of each patient are different.

Self-monitoring of blood glucose levels is an important component in diabetes management (see Patient and Family Teaching Checklist: Obtaining a Blood Glucose Reading Using a Glucometer). It is the preferred method for monitoring glucose by most health care providers for all patients with diabetes, with variations only in the suggested frequency of testing. If the patient is to use a blood glucose monitoring device, the nurse reviews the method of obtaining a small sample of blood from the finger and the use of the device with the patient. Printed instructions

and illustrations are supplied with the device and must be reviewed with the patient. The nurse encourages the patient to purchase the brand recommended by the primary health care provider. Time is allowed for supervised practice. The nurse includes the following information in the teaching plan for a patient with diabetes:

- Blood glucose or urine testing—the testing material recommended by the primary health care provider; a review of the instructions included with the glucometer or the materials used for urine testing; the technique of collecting the specimen; interpreting test results; number of times a day or week the blood or urine is tested (as recommended by the primary health care provider); a record of test results.

- Insulin—types; how dosage is expressed; calculating the insulin dosage; importance of using only the type, source, and brand name recommended by the primary health care provider; importance of not changing brands unless the health care provider approves; keeping a spare vial on hand; prescription for insulin purchase not required.

- Storage of insulin—insulin is kept at room temperature away from heat and direct sunlight if used within 1 month (and up to 3 months if refrigerated); vials not in use are stored in the refrigerator; prefilled insulin in glass or plastic syringes is stable for 1 week under refrigeration. Keep filled syringes in a vertical or oblique position with the needle pointing upward to avoid plugging the needle. Before injection, pull back the plunger and tip the syringe back and forth slightly to agitate and remix the insulins.

- Needle and syringe—purchase the same brand and needle size each time; parts of the syringe; reading the syringe scale. Instruction in proper disposal of used equipment and protection of others from sharp items.

- Preparation for administration—principles of aseptic technique; how to hold the syringe; how to withdraw insulin from the vial; measurement of insulin in the syringe using the syringe scale; mixing insulin in the same syringe (when appropriate); elimination of air in the syringe and needle; what to do if the syringe or needle is contaminated.

- Administration of insulin—sites to be used; rotation of injection sites (see Home Care Checklist: Rotating Insulin Injection Sites); angle of injection; administration at the time of day prescribed by the primary health care provider; disposal of the needle and syringe.

- Insulin needs may change in patients who become ill, especially with vomiting or fever, and during periods of stress or emotional disturbance. Contact the primary health care provider if these situations occur.

- Diet—importance of following the prescribed diet; calories allowed; food exchanges; planning daily menus; establishing meal schedules; selecting food from a restaurant menu; reading food labels; use of artificial sweeteners.

- Traveling—importance of carrying an extra supply of insulin and a prescription for needles and syringes; storage of insulin when traveling; protecting needles and syringes from theft; importance of discussing travel plans (especially foreign travel) with the primary health care provider.

- Hypoglycemia/hyperglycemia—signs and symptoms of hypoglycemia and hyperglycemia; food or fluid used to terminate a hypoglycemic reaction; importance of notifying the primary health care provider immediately if either reaction occurs.

- Personal hygiene—importance of good skin and foot care, personal cleanliness, frequent dental checkups, and routine eye examinations.

- Exercise—importance of following the primary health care provider's recommendations regarding physical activity.

- When to notify the primary health care provider—increase in blood glucose levels; urine positive for ketones; if pregnancy occurs; occurrence of antidiabetic or hyperglycemic episodes; occurrence of illness, infection, or diarrhea (insulin dosage may require adjustment); appearance of new problems (e.g., leg ulcers, numbness of the extremities, significant weight gain or loss).

- Identification—wear identification, such as a MedicAlert bracelet, to inform medical personnel and others of the use of insulin to control the disease.

EVALUATION

- The therapeutic effect is achieved and normal or near-normal blood glucose levels are maintained.

- Adverse reactions are identified, reported to the health care provider, and managed successfully through appropriate nursing interventions.

- Anxiety and fear are reduced.

- The patient demonstrates a beginning ability to cope with the disorder and its required treatment.

- The patient demonstrates a positive outlook and adjustment to the diagnosis.

- The patient verbalizes a willingness to comply with the prescribed therapeutic regimen.

- The patient and family demonstrate an understanding of the drug regimen.

- The patient is able to test blood glucose levels using a glucometer.

- The patient administers insulin correctly.

ORAL ANTIDIABETIC DRUGS

The oral antidiabetic drugs are used to treat patients with type 2 diabetes that is not controlled by diet and exercise alone. These drugs are not effective for treating type 1 diabetes. Five types of oral antidiabetic drugs are currently in use:

- Sulfonylureas
- Biguanides
- Alpha (α)-glucosidase inhibitors
- Meglitinides
- Thiazolidinediones

Additional drugs are listed in the Summary Drug Table: Antidiabetic Drugs.

Uses

The oral antidiabetic drugs are of value only in the treatment of patients with type 2 diabetes mellitus whose condition cannot be controlled by diet alone. These drugs may also be used with insulin in the management of some patients with diabetes. Use of an oral antidiabetic drug with insulin may decrease the insulin dosage in some individuals. Two oral antidiabetic drugs (e.g., a sulfonylurea and metformin) may also be used together when one antidiabetic drug and diet do not control blood glucose levels in type 2 diabetes mellitus. Figure 49-3 indicates the appropriate medication regimen for type 2 diabetes.

Actions

Sulfonylureas

The sulfonylureas appear to lower blood glucose by stimulating the beta cells of the pancreas to release insulin. The sulfonylureas are not effective if the beta cells of the pancreas cannot release a sufficient amount of insulin to meet

SUMMARY DRUG TABLE   ANTIDIABETIC DRUGS

GENERIC NAME	TRADE NAME	USES	ADVERSE REACTIONS	DOSAGE RANGES
Sulfonylureas				
First Generation				
acetohexamide *a-set-oh-hex'-a-mide*		Type 2 diabetes; adjunct to diet and exercise	Nausea, epigastric discomfort, heartburn, hypoglycemia	250 mg–1.5 g/d orally
chlorpropamide *klor-proe'-pa-mide*	Diabinese	Type 2 diabetes; adjunct to diet and exercise, diabetes insipidus	Same as acetohexamide	100–250 mg/d orally
tolazamide *tole-az'-a-mide*	Tolinase	Type 2 diabetes; adjunct to diet and exercise	Same as acetohexamide	100–1000 mg/d orally
tolbutamide *tole-byoo'-ta-mide*		Type 2 diabetes; adjunct to diet and exercise	Same as acetohexamide	0.25–3 g/d orally
Second Generation				
glimepiride *glye-meh'-per-ide*	Amaryl	Type 2 diabetes; adjunct to diet and exercise, may be used in conjunction with insulin	Same as acetohexamide	1–4 mg/d orally
glipizide *glip'-i-zide*	Glucotrol, Glucotrol XL	Type 2 diabetes; adjunct to diet and exercise	Same as acetohexamide	5–40 mg/d orally
glyburide (glibenclamide) *glyé-byoor-ide*	DiaBeta, Micronase, Glynase	Type 2 diabetes; adjunct to diet and exercise	Same as acetohexamide	1.25–20 mg/d orally
α-Glucosidase Inhibitors				
acarbose *aye-kar'-bose*	Precose	Type 2 diabetes; combination therapy with a sulfonylurea to enhance glycemic control	Flatulence, diarrhea, abdominal pain	25–100 mg orally TID
miglitol *mi'-gli-tole*	Glyset	Same as acarbose	Same as acarbose	25–100 mg orally TID
Biguanide				
metformin *met-for'-min*	Glucophage, Glucophage XR	Type 2 diabetes; with a sulfonylurea or insulin to improve glycemic control	Nausea, vomiting, flatulence, diarrhea, asthenia	500–3000 mg/d orally; XR (extended-release): 500–2000 mg/d
Meglitinides				
nateglinide *nah-teg'-lah-nyde*	Starlix	Type 2 diabetes; in combination with metformin to improve glycemic control	Upper respiratory tract infection, back pain, flulike symptoms	60–120 mg orally TID before meals

Antidiabetic Drugs

GENERIC NAME	TRADE NAME	USES	ADVERSE REACTIONS	DOSAGE RANGES
repaglinide *re-pag'-lah-nyde*	Prandin	Same as nateglinide	Hypoglycemia, upper respiratory tract infection, headache	0.5–4 mg orally before meals (maximum dose, 16 mg/d)
Thiazolidinediones				
pioglitazone HCl *pie-oh-glit'-ah-zohn*	Actos	Type 2 diabetes; with sulfonylurea, metformin, or insulin to improve glycemic control	Headache, pain, myalgia, aggravated diabetes, infections, fatigue	15–30 mg/d orally
rosiglitazone maleate *roh-zee-glit'-ah-zohn*	Avandia	Type 2 diabetes; in combination with metformin to improve glycemic control	Headache, pain, diarrhea, hypoglycemia, hyperglycemia, fatigue, infections	4–8 mg/d orally
Antidiabetic Combination Drugs				
glyburide/metformin HCl	Glucovance	Type 2 diabetes	See individual drugs	Starting dose: 1.25 mg/250 mg orally daily or BID Maximum daily dose, 20 mg/2000 mg
glipizide/metformin HCl	Metaglip	Type 2 diabetes	See individual drugs	Individualized; maximum daily dose, 20 mg/2000 mg
rosiglitazone/ metformin HCl	Avandamet	Type 2 diabetes	See individual drugs	Individualized; maximum daily dose, 8 mg/2000 mg
Glucose-Elevating Agents				
diazoxide, oral *die-aze-ox'-ide*	Proglycem	Hypoglycemia due to hyperinsulinism	Sodium and fluid retention, hyperglycemia, glycosuria, tachycardia, congestive heart failure	3–8 mg/kg/d orally in two or three equal doses q8–12 h
glucagon *glue-kuh-gahn*	Glucagon Emergency Kit	Hypoglycemia	Nausea, vomiting, generalized allergic reactions	See instructions on the product

the individual's needs. The first-generation sulfonylureas (e.g., acetohexamide, chlorpropamide, tolazamide, and tolbutamide) are not commonly used today because they have a long duration of action and a higher incidence of adverse reactions, and are more likely to react with other drugs. More commonly used sulfonylureas are the second- and third-generation drugs, such as glimepiride (Amaryl), glipizide (Glucotrol), and glyburide (DiaBeta, Micronase).

Biguanides

Metformin (Glucophage), currently the only biguanide, acts by reducing hepatic glucose production and increasing insulin sensitivity in muscle and fat cells. The liver normally releases glucose by detecting the level of circulating insulin.

When insulin levels are high, glucose is available in the blood, and the liver produces little or no glucose. When insulin levels are low, there is little circulating glucose, so the liver produces more glucose. In type 2 diabetes, the liver may not detect levels of glucose in the blood and, instead of regulating glucose production, releases glucose despite adequate blood glucose levels. Metformin sensitizes the liver to circulating insulin levels and reduces hepatic glucose production.

α-Glucosidase Inhibitors

The α-glucosidase inhibitors, acarbose (Precose) and miglitol (Glyset), lower blood glucose levels by delaying the digestion of carbohydrates and absorption of carbohydrates in the intestine.

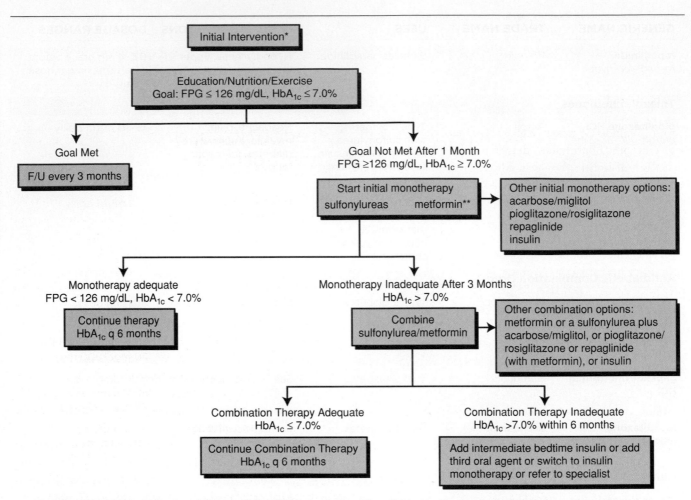

```
                          ┌─────────────────────┐
                          │  Initial Intervention* │
                          └─────────────────────┘
                                    │
                    ┌───────────────────────────────────┐
                    │   Education/Nutrition/Exercise       │
                    │ Goal: FPG ≤ 126 mg/dL, HbA₁c ≤ 7.0%  │
                    └───────────────────────────────────┘
                        │                           │
                   Goal Met                  Goal Not Met After 1 Month
                                             FPG ≥126 mg/dL, HbA₁c ≥ 7.0%
              ┌─────────────────┐
              │ F/U every 3 months │      ┌─────────────────────┐      ┌───────────────────────────┐
              └─────────────────┘      │ Start initial monotherapy│─────▶│ Other initial monotherapy options: │
                                        │ sulfonylureas  metformin**│      │ acarbose/miglitol          │
                                        └─────────────────────┘      │ pioglitazone/rosiglitazone │
                                             │             │          │ repaglinide                │
                                                                      │ insulin                    │
                                                                      └───────────────────────────┘
          Monotherapy adequate              Monotherapy Inadequate After 3 Months
        FPG < 126 mg/dL, HbA₁c < 7.0%                   HbA₁c > 7.0%
        ┌──────────────────┐              ┌──────────────┐      ┌───────────────────────────────┐
        │ Continue therapy  │              │   Combine     │─────▶│ Other combination options:     │
        │ HbA₁c q 6 months  │              │sulfonylurea/metformin│      │ metformin or a sulfonylurea plus │
        └──────────────────┘              └──────────────┘      │ acarbose/miglitol, or pioglitazone/ │
                                             │            │      │ rosiglitazone or repaglinide   │
                                                                 │ (with metformin), or insulin   │
                                                                 └───────────────────────────────┘
              Combination Therapy Adequate           Combination Therapy Inadequate
                     HbA₁c ≤ 7.0%                       HbA₁c >7.0% within 6 months
        ┌──────────────────────────┐        ┌───────────────────────────────┐
        │ Continue Combination Therapy│      │ Add intermediate bedtime insulin or add │
        │    HbA₁c q 6 months        │       │ third oral agent or switch to insulin   │
        └──────────────────────────┘        │ monotherapy or refer to specialist      │
                                             └───────────────────────────────┘
```

*If initial presentation with fasting glucose ≥ 260 mg/dL is a symptomatic patient, consider insulin as initial intervention.
**Preferred in obese or dyslipidemic patients
—Normal HbA₁c = 4-6.1%
—Normal FPG: < 126 mg/dL
—Goals and therapies must be individualized.

Figure 49.3 Pharmacologic algorithm for treating type 2 diabetes. FPG, fasting plasma glucose; HbA₁c, glycosylated hemoglobin.

Meglitinides

Like the sulfonylureas, the meglitinides act to lower blood glucose levels by stimulating the release of insulin from the pancreas. This action depends on the ability of the beta cells in the pancreas to produce some insulin. However, the action of the meglitinides is more rapid than that of the sulfonylureas and their duration of action much shorter. Because of this they must be taken three times a day. Examples of the meglitinides include nateglinide (Starlix) and repaglinide (Prandin).

Thiazolidinediones

The thiazolidinediones, also called glitazones, decrease insulin resistance and increase insulin sensitivity by modifying several processes, resulting in decreased hepatic glucogenesis (formation of glucose from glycogen) and increased insulin-dependent muscle glucose uptake. Examples of the thiazolidinediones are rosiglitazone (Avandia) and pioglitazone (Actos).

Adverse Reactions

Sulfonylureas

Adverse reactions associated with the sulfonylureas include hypoglycemia, anorexia, nausea, vomiting, epigastric discomfort, weight gain, heartburn, and various vague neurologic symptoms, such as weakness and numbness of the extremities. Often, these can be eliminated by reducing the dosage or giving the drug in divided doses. If these reactions become severe, the primary health care provider may try another oral antidiabetic drug or discontinue the use of these drugs. If the drug therapy is discontinued, it may be necessary to control the diabetes with insulin.

Biguanides

Adverse reactions associated with the biguanide, metformin, include GI upset (e.g., abdominal bloating, nausea, cramping, flatulence, diarrhea) and metallic taste (usually self-limiting). These adverse reactions are self-limiting and can be reduced if the patients are started on a low dose with dosage increased slowly, and if the drug is taken with meals. Hypoglycemia rarely occurs when metformin is used alone.

Lactic acidosis (buildup of lactic acid in the blood) may also occur with the administration of metformin. Although lactic acidosis is a rare adverse reaction, its occurrence is serious and can be fatal. Lactic acidosis occurs mainly in patients with kidney dysfunction. Symptoms of lactic acidosis include malaise (vague feeling of bodily discomfort), abdominal pain, rapid respirations, shortness of breath, and muscular pain. In some patients, vitamin B_{12} levels are decreased. This can be reversed with vitamin B_{12} supplements or with discontinuation of the drug therapy. Because weight loss can occur, metformin is sometimes recommended for obese patients or patients with insulin-resistant diabetes.

α-Glucosidase Inhibitors

Because the α-glucosidase inhibitors, acarbose or miglitol, increase the transit time of food in the digestive tract, GI disturbances may occur. The most common adverse reactions are bloating and flatulence. Other adverse reactions, such as abdominal pain and diarrhea, can occur. Although most oral antidiabetic drugs produce hypoglycemia, acarbose and miglitol, when used alone, do not cause hypoglycemia.

Meglitinides

Adverse reactions associated with the administration of the meglitinides include upper respiratory tract infection, headache, rhinitis, bronchitis, headache, back pain, and hypoglycemia.

Thiazolidinediones

Adverse reactions associated with the administration of the thiazolidinediones include aggravated diabetes mellitus, upper respiratory infections, sinusitis, headache, pharyngitis, myalgia, diarrhea, and back pain. When used alone, rosiglitazone and pioglitazone rarely cause hypoglycemia. However, patients receiving these drugs in combination

with insulin or other oral hypoglycemics (e.g., the sulfonylureas) are at greater risk for hypoglycemia. A reduction in the dosage of insulin or the sulfonylurea may be required to prevent episodes of hypoglycemia.

Contraindications, Precautions, and Interactions

Sulfonylureas

The oral antidiabetic drugs are contraindicated in patients with known hypersensitivity to the drugs, DKA, severe infection, or severe endocrine disease. The first-generation sulfonylureas (chlorpropamide, tolazamide, and tolbutamide) are contraindicated in patients with coronary artery disease or liver or renal dysfunction. Other sulfonylureas are used cautiously in patients with impaired liver function because liver dysfunction can prolong the drug's effect. In addition, the sulfonylureas are used cautiously in patients with renal impairment and severe cardiovascular disease. There is a risk for cross-sensitivity with the sulfonylureas and the sulfonamides (sulfa anti-infectives).

Many drugs may affect the action of the sulfonylureas; the nurse must monitor blood glucose carefully when beginning therapy, discontinuing therapy, and any time any change is made in the drug regimen with these drugs. The sulfonylureas may have an increased hypoglycemic effect when administered with the anticoagulants, chloramphenicol, clofibrate, fluconazole, histamine H_2 antagonists, methyldopa, monoamine oxidase inhibitors (MAOIs), salicylates, sulfonamides, and tricyclic antidepressants. The hypoglycemic effect of the sulfonylureas may be decreased when the agents are administered with beta blockers, calcium channel blockers, cholestyramine, corticosteroids, estrogens, hydantoins, isoniazid, oral contraceptives, phenothiazines, rifampin, thiazide diuretics, and thyroid agents.

Biguanides

Metformin is contraindicated in patients with heart failure, renal disease, hypersensitivity to metformin, and acute or chronic metabolic acidosis, including ketoacidosis. The drug is also contraindicated in patients older than 80 years and during pregnancy (pregnancy category B) and lactation.

The drug is used cautiously during surgery. Metformin use is temporarily discontinued for surgical procedures. The drug therapy is restarted when the patient's oral intake has been resumed and renal function is normal.

There is a risk of acute renal failure when iodinated contrast material used for radiologic studies is administered with metformin. Metformin therapy is stopped for 48 hours before and after radiologic studies using iodinated material. Alcohol, amiloride, digoxin, morphine, procainamide, quinidine, quinine, ranitidine, triamterene, trimethoprim, vancomycin, cimetidine, and furosemide all increase the risk of hypoglycemia. There is an increased risk of lactic acidosis when metformin is administered with the glucocorticoids.

α-Glucosidase Inhibitors

The α-glucosidase inhibitors are contraindicated in patients with a hypersensitivity to the drug, DKA, cirrhosis, inflammatory bowel disease, colonic ulceration, partial intestinal obstruction or predisposition to intestinal obstruction, or chronic intestinal diseases. Acarbose and miglitol are used cautiously in patients with renal impairment or preexisting GI problems, such as irritable bowel syndrome or Crohn's disease. These drugs are pregnancy category B drugs and safe use during pregnancy has not been established. Digestive enzymes may reduce the effect of miglitol. Miglitol may decrease absorption of ranitidine and propranolol.

Meglitinides

Theses drugs are contraindicated in patients with hypersensitivity to the drug, type 1 diabetes, and DKA. Both repaglinide and nateglinide are pregnancy category C drugs and are not recommended for use during pregnancy and lactation. These drugs are used cautiously in patients with renal or hepatic impairment. Certain drugs, such as NSAIDs, salicylates, MAOIs, and beta-adrenergic blocking drugs, may potentiate the hypoglycemic action of the meglitinides. Drugs such as the thiazides, corticosteroids, thyroid drugs, and sympathomimetics may decrease the hypoglycemic action of these drugs. The nurse must closely observe the patient receiving one or more of these drugs along with an oral antidiabetic drug.

Thiazolidinediones

The thiazolidinediones are contraindicated in patients with a hypersensitivity to the drug or any component of the drug and severe heart failure. These drugs are pregnancy category C drugs and should not be used during pregnancy unless the potential benefit of therapy outweighs the potential risk to the fetus. The thiazolidinediones are used cautiously in patients with edema, cardiovascular disease, and liver or kidney disease. These drugs may alter the effects of oral contraceptives.

NURSING PROCESS

The Patient Receiving an Oral Antidiabetic Drug

ASSESSMENT

PREADMINISTRATION ASSESSMENT

If the patient has recently been diagnosed with diabetes mellitus and has not received an oral antidiabetic drug, or if the patient is known to have diabetes and has been taking one of these drugs, the nurse should include weight, blood pressure, pulse, and respiratory rate in the initial assessment. The nurse makes a general assessment of the skin, mucous membranes, and extremities, with special attention given to sores or cuts that appear to be healing poorly and ulcerations or other skin or mucous membrane changes. Dietary habits, a family history of diabetes (if any), and an inquiry into the type and duration of symptoms experienced are included in the history. The nurse reviews the patient's chart for recent laboratory and diagnostic tests. If the patient has diabetes and has been receiving an oral antidiabetic drug, the nurse includes the name of the drug and the dosage, the type of diabetic diet, the results of blood glucose testing, and an inquiry into adherence to the dietary and weight control regimen prescribed by the primary health care provider.

ONGOING ASSESSMENT

The most important aspect of the ongoing assessment is observation of the patient every 2 to 4 hours for symptoms of hypoglycemia (see Table 49-1), particularly during initial therapy or after a change in dosage. If both an oral antidiabetic drug and insulin are given, the nurse observes the patient more frequently for hypoglycemic episodes during the initial period of combination therapy. If the patient is receiving only an oral antidiabetic drug and a hypoglycemic reaction occurs, it is often (but not always) less intense than one seen with insulin administration.

The nurse conducts daily ongoing assessments, including monitoring vital signs and observing for adverse drug reactions. The primary health care provider may also order the patient be weighed daily or weekly. The nurse notifies the primary health care provider if an adverse reaction occurs or if there is a significant weight gain or loss.

The best way to monitor long-term glycemic control and response to treatment is with HbA_{1c} levels measured at 3-month intervals. If the first HbA_{1c} indicates that glycemic control during the last 3 months was inadequate, the dosage may be increased for better control.

NURSING DIAGNOSES

Drug-specific nursing diagnoses are highlighted in the Nursing Diagnoses Checklist. Other nursing diagnoses applicable to these drugs are discussed in depth in Chapter 4.

Nursing Diagnoses Checklist

✔ **Acute Confusion** related to hypoglycemic reaction

✔ **Deficient Fluid Volume** related to hyperglycemic reaction (e.g., DKA)

✔ **Anxiety** related to fear of diagnosis, dietary restrictions, other factors (specify)

✔ **Ineffective Breathing Pattern** related to hyperventilation in lactic acidosis

PLANNING

The expected outcomes of the patient may include an optimal response to therapy, support of patient needs related to the management of adverse reactions, a reduction in anxiety, improved ability to cope with the diagnosis, and an understanding of and compliance with the prescribed therapeutic regimen.

IMPLEMENTATION

PROMOTING AN OPTIMAL RESPONSE TO THERAPY

There are no fixed drug dosages in antidiabetic therapy. The drug regimen is individualized on the basis of the effectiveness and tolerance of the drug(s) used and the maximum recommended dose of the drug(s). Glycemic control can often be improved when a second oral medication is added to the drug regimen. The choice of a second medication varies from patient to patient and is prescribed by the primary health care provider. Glucovance, a combination drug, is a mixture of glyburide and metformin. The drug is useful for individuals needing dual therapy and those who are forgetful (only once-daily dosing is required) or mildly confused.

Nursing Alert

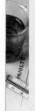

Exposure to stress, such as infection, fever, surgery, or trauma, may cause a loss of control of blood glucose levels in patients who have been stabilized with oral antidiabetic drugs. Should this occur, the primary health care provider may discontinue use of the oral drug and administer insulin.

Oral antidiabetic drugs are given as a single daily dose or in divided doses. The following sections provide specific information for each group of oral antidiabetic drugs.

SULFONYLUREAS Acetohexamide, chlorpropamide (Diabinese), tolazamide (Tolinase), and tolbutamide are given with food to prevent gastrointestinal upset. However, because food delays absorption, the nurse gives glipizide (Glucotrol) 30 minutes before a meal. Glyburide (Micronase) is administered with breakfast or with the first main meal of the day. The primary health care provider orders the meal with which glyburide is given. Glimepiride is given once daily with breakfast or the first main meal of the day.

Gerontologic Alert

Older adults have an increased sensitivity to the sulfonylureas and may require a dosage reduction.

After the patient has been taking sulfonylureas for a period of time, a condition called **secondary failure** may occur, in which the sulfonylurea loses its effectiveness. When the nurse notes that a normally compliant patient has a gradual increase in blood glucose levels, secondary failure may be the cause. This increase in blood glucose levels can be caused by an increase in the severity of the diabetes or a decreased response to the drug. When secondary failure occurs, the primary health care provider may prescribe another sulfonylurea or add an oral antidiabetic drug such as metformin to the drug regimen. See the Summary Drug Table: Antidiabetic Drugs for additional drugs that can be used in combination with the sulfonylureas.

α-GLUCOSIDASE INHIBITORS Acarbose and miglitol are given three times as day with the first bite of the meal because food increases absorption. Some patients begin therapy with a lower dose once daily to minimize gastrointestinal effects such as abdominal discomfort, flatulence, and diarrhea. The dose is then gradually increased to three times daily. The nurse monitors the response to these drugs by periodic testing. Dosage adjustments are made at 4- to 16-week intervals based on 1-hour postprandial blood glucose levels.

BIGUANIDES The nurse administers metformin two or three times a day with meals. If the patient has not experienced a response in 4 weeks using the maximum dose of metformin, the primary health care provider may add an oral sulfonylurea while continuing metformin at the maximum dose. Glucophage XR (metformin, extended-release) is administered once daily with the evening meal.

MEGLITINIDES The nurse usually gives repaglinide 15 minutes before meals but can give it immediately, or up to 30 minutes, before the meal. Nateglinide is taken up to 30 minutes before meals.

THIAZOLIDINEDIONES The thiazolidinediones, pioglitazone and rosiglitazone, are given with or without meals. If the dose is missed at the usual meal, the drug is taken at the next meal. If the dose is missed on one day, it is not doubled the following day. If the drug is taken, the meal must not be delayed. Delay of a meal for as little as 30 minutes can cause hypoglycemia.

MONITORING AND MANAGING PATIENT NEEDS

ACUTE CONFUSION The nurse must immediately terminate a hypoglycemic reaction. The method of terminating a hypoglycemic reaction is the same as for a hypoglycemic reaction occurring with insulin administration, with the following exception: the nurse notifies the primary health care provider as soon as possible if episodes of hypoglycemia occur because the dosage of the oral antidiabetic drug (or insulin, when both insulin and an oral antidiabetic drug are given) may need to be changed.

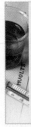

> ### Nursing Alert
>
> When hypoglycemia occurs in a patient taking an α-glucosidase inhibitor (e.g., acarbose or miglitol), the nurse gives the patient an oral form of glucose, such as glucose tablets or dextrose, rather than sugar (sucrose). Absorption of sugar is blocked by acarbose or miglitol.

When oral antidiabetic drugs are combined with other antidiabetic drugs (e.g., sulfonylureas) or insulin, the hypoglycemic effect may be enhanced. Elderly, debilitated, or malnourished patients are more likely to experience hypoglycemia.

> ### Gerontologic Alert
>
> Although older adult patients taking the oral antidiabetic drugs are particularly susceptible to hypoglycemic reactions, these reactions may be difficult to detect in the older patient. The nurse notifies the primary health care provider if blood glucose levels are elevated (consistently above 200 mg/dL) or if ketones are present in the urine.

DEFICIENT FLUID VOLUME Capillary blood specimens are obtained and tested in the same manner as for individuals who take insulin (see Patient and Family Teaching Checklist: Obtaining a Blood Glucose Reading Using a Glucometer). The nurse notifies the health care provider if blood glucose levels are elevated (consistently over 200 mg/dL) or if ketones are present in the urine.

ANXIETY The patient with newly diagnosed diabetes often has many concerns about managing the disease. Some patients, when learning that management of their diabetes can be achieved by diet and an oral drug, may have a tendency to discount the seriousness of the disorder. Without creating additional anxiety, the nurse emphasizes the importance of following the prescribed treatment regimen. Then the nurse encourages the patient to talk about the disorder, express concerns, and ask questions. Allowing these patients time to talk may help them begin to cope with their diabetes.

The patient receiving an oral antidiabetic drug may also express concern about the possibility of having to take insulin in the future. The nurse encourages the patient to discuss this and other concerns with the primary health care provider.

INEFFECTIVE BREATHING PATTERN When taking metformin, the patient is at risk for lactic acidosis. The nurse monitors the patient for symptoms of lactic acidosis, which include unexplained hyperventilation, myalgia, malaise, GI symptoms, or unusual somnolence. If the patient experiences these symptoms, the nurse should contact the primary health care provider at once. Elevated blood lactate levels exceeding 5 mmol/L are associated with lactic acidosis and should be reported immediately. Once a patient's diabetes is stabilized on metformin therapy, the adverse GI reactions that often occur at the beginning of such therapy are unlikely to be related to the drug therapy. A later occurrence of GI symptoms is more likely to be related to lactic acidosis or other serious disease.

EDUCATING THE PATIENT AND FAMILY

Failure to comply with the prescribed treatment regimen may be a problem with patients taking an oral antidiabetic drug because of the erroneous belief that not having to take insulin means that the disease is not serious and therefore does not require strict adherence to the recommended dietary plan. The nurse informs these patients that control of their diabetes is just as important as for patients requiring insulin and that control is achieved only when they adhere to the treatment regimen prescribed by the primary health care provider.

If the diagnosis of diabetes mellitus is new, the nurse discusses the disease and methods of control with the patient and family after the primary health care provider discloses the diagnosis to the patient. Although taking an oral

Antidiabetic Drugs

antidiabetic drug is less complicated than self-administration of insulin, the patient with diabetes taking one of these drugs needs a thorough explanation of the management of the disease. The teaching plan is individualized because the needs of each patient are different. The nurse includes the following information in a teaching plan:

- Take the drug exactly as directed on the container (e.g., with food, 30 minutes before a meal).

- To control diabetes, follow the diet and drug regimen prescribed by the primary health care provider exactly.

- An antidiabetic drug is not oral insulin and cannot be substituted for insulin.

- Never stop taking this drug or increase or decrease the dose unless told to do so by the primary health care provider.

- Take the drug at the same time or times each day.

- Eat meals at about the same time each day. Erratic meal hours or skipped meals may result in difficulty in controlling diabetes with this drug.

- Avoid alcohol, dieting, commercial weight-loss products, and strenuous exercise programs unless use or participation has been approved by the primary health care provider.

- Test blood for glucose and urine for ketones as directed by the primary health care provider. Keep a record of test results and bring this record to each visit to the primary health care provider or clinic.

- Maintain good foot and skin care and routine eye and dental examinations for the early detection of the complications that may occur.

- Exercise should be moderate; avoid strenuous exercise and erratic periods of exercise.

- Wear identification, such as a MedicAlert bracelet, to inform medical personnel and others of diabetes and the drug or drugs currently being used to treat the disease.

- Notify the primary health care provider if any of the following occur: episodes of hypoglycemia, apparent symptoms of hyperglycemia, elevated blood glucose levels, positive results of urine tests for glucose or ketone bodies, or pregnancy. Also notify the primary health care provider of any serious illness not requiring hospitalization.

- Know the symptoms of hypoglycemia and hyperglycemia and the primary health care provider's method for terminating a hypoglycemic reaction.

- *Metformin*—there is a risk of lactic acidosis when using this drug. Discontinue the drug therapy and notify the primary health care provider immediately if any of the following occur: respiratory distress, muscular aches, unusual somnolence, unexplained malaise, or nonspecific abdominal distress.

- *α-Glucosidase inhibitors*—these drugs do not generally cause hypoglycemia. However, if a sulfonylurea or insulin is used in combination with acarbose or miglitol, blood glucose levels can be lowered enough to cause symptoms or even life-threatening hypoglycemia. Have a ready source of glucose to treat symptoms of low blood glucose when taking insulin or a sulfonylurea with these drugs. Adverse reactions usually develop during the first few weeks of therapy and usually involve the gastrointestinal tract: flatulence, diarrhea, or abdominal discomfort.

- *Meglitinides*—if a meal is skipped, do not take the drug. Similarly, if a meal is added, add a dose of the drug for that meal.

EVALUATION

- The therapeutic drug effect is achieved and normal or near-normal blood glucose levels are maintained.

- Hypoglycemic reactions are identified, reported to the primary health care provider, and managed successfully.

- Anxiety is reduced.

- The patient begins to demonstrate the ability to cope with the disorder and its required treatment.

- The patient demonstrates a positive outlook and adjustment to the diagnosis.

- The patient verbalizes a willingness to comply with the prescribed treatment regimen.

- The patient demonstrates an understanding of the drug regimen.

- The patient demonstrates an understanding of the information presented in teaching sessions.

- The patient is able to use the glucometer correctly to monitor blood glucose levels or test urine for glucose and ketones.

Critical Thinking Exercises

1. Ms. Baxter, aged 37 years, has been taking insulin for the past 6 years for type 1 diabetes mellitus. An assessment at the outpatient clinic reveals a blood glucose level of 110 mg/dL. In examining Ms. Baxter's skin, the nurse notices several areas on the thighs that appear scarred and other areas that appear as dimples or pitting in the skin. Analyze this problem. Discuss suggestions you would make to Ms. Baxter for better care.

2. Mr. Goddard, aged 78 years, recently has received a diagnosis of type 2 diabetes mellitus, and the primary health care provider has ordered an oral antidiabetic drug. Mr. Goddard says his friend with diabetes takes insulin and he wonders why insulin was not prescribed for him. How would you help Mr. Goddard understand why he is taking an oral drug and not insulin? What other information does Mr. Goddard, as a patient with newly diagnosed diabetes, need to have?

3. When assessing Jerry Jones, aged 24 years, a patient with recently diagnosed diabetes, you note that he is confused and agitated. His skin is cool and clammy, and he is complaining of hunger. Discuss other assessments you could make and what action, if any, you feel should be taken for Jerry.

Review Questions

1. Which of the following would the nurse mostly likely choose to treat a hypoglycemic reaction?

   A. Regular insulin

   B. NPH insulin

   C. Orange juice

   D. Crackers and milk

2. Which of the following would be the correct method of administering insulin glargine?

   A. Within 10 minutes of meals

   B. Immediately before meals

   C. Any time within 30 minutes before or 30 minutes after a meal

   D. At bedtime

3. Which of the following symptoms would alert the nurse to a possible hyperglycemic reaction?

   A. Fatigue, weakness, confusion

   B. Pale skin, elevated temperature

   C. Thirst, abdominal pain, nausea

   D. Rapid, shallow respirations, headache, nervousness

4. A patient with diabetes received a glycosylated hemoglobin test result of 10%. This indicates _____.

   A. the diabetes is well controlled

   B. poor blood glucose control

   C. the need for an increase in the insulin dosage

   D. the patient is at increased risk for hypoglycemia

5. In patients receiving oral hypoglycemic drugs, the nurse must be aware that hypoglycemic reactions _____.

   A. will most likely occur 1 to 2 hours after a meal

   B. may be more intense than reactions seen with insulin administration

   C. may be less intense than reactions seen with insulin administration

   D. may occur more frequently in patients receiving oral hypoglycemic drugs.

Medication Dosage Problems

1. A patient is prescribed 40 units NPH insulin mixed with 5 units of regular insulin. What is the total insulin dosage? Draw a line on the syringe below showing the total insulin dosage. Describe how you would prepare the insulins.

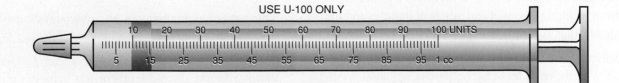

USE U-100 ONLY

2. A patient is prescribed metformin (Glucophage) 1000 mg orally BID. The drug is available in 500-mg tablets. The nurse administers _____. What is the total daily dosage of metformin?_____

3. A patient is prescribed rosiglitazone (Avandia) 8 mg orally daily. Available are 2-mg tablets. The nurse would administer _____.

4. A patient is prescribed insulin Humulin L 32 units. Choose the correct label for the insulin.

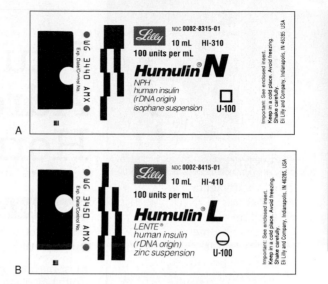

To check your answers, see Appendix G.

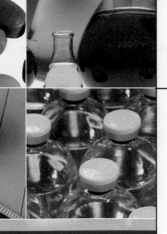

Chapter 50

Pituitary and Adrenocortical Hormones

Key Terms

adrenal insufficiency
corticosteroids
cryptorchism
Cushing's syndrome
diabetes insipidus
feedback mechanism
glucocorticoids
gonadotropins
gonads
hyperstimulation syndrome
mineralocorticoids
rhinyle
somatotropin

Learning Objectives

On completion of this chapter, the student will:

- List the hormones produced by the pituitary gland and the adrenal cortex.

- Discuss general actions, uses, adverse reactions, contraindications, precautions, and interactions of the pituitary and adrenocortical hormones.

- Discuss important preadministration and ongoing assessment activities the nurse should perform with a

patient taking the pituitary and adrenocortical hormones.

- List nursing diagnoses particular to a patient taking a pituitary or adreno-cortical hormone.

- Discuss ways to promote an optimal response to therapy, how to manage common adverse reactions, and important points to keep in mind when educating patients about the use of pituitary or adrenocortical hormones.

The pituitary gland lies deep within the cranial vault, connected to the brain by the infundibular stalk (a downward extension of the floor of the third ventricle) and protected by an indentation of the sphenoid bone called the *sella turcica* (Fig. 50-1). The pituitary gland, a small, gray, rounded structure, has two parts:

- Anterior pituitary (adenohypophysis)

- Posterior pituitary (neurohypophysis)

The gland secretes a number of pituitary hormones that regulate growth, metabolism, the reproductive cycle, electrolyte balance, and water retention or loss. The pituitary gland is often referred to as the "master gland" because it secretes many hormones that regulate numerous vital processes. The hormones secreted by the anterior and posterior pituitary and the organs influenced by these hormones are shown in Figure 50-2.

POSTERIOR PITUITARY HORMONES

The posterior pituitary gland produces two hormones: vasopressin (antidiuretic hormone) and oxytocin (see Chapter 53). Posterior pituitary hormones are summarized in the Summary Drug Table: Posterior and Anterior Pituitary Hormones.

Vasopressin

Actions and Uses

Vasopressin (Pitressin Synthetic) and its derivative, desmopressin (DDAVP), regulate the reabsorption of water by the kidneys. Vasopressin is secreted by the

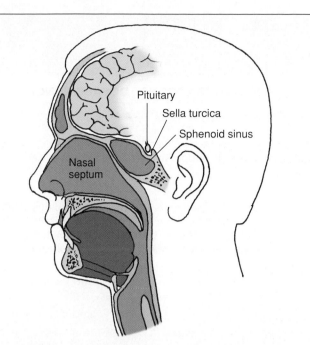

Figure 50.1 Location of the pituitary gland.

pituitary when body fluids must be conserved. This mechanism may be activated, for example, when an individual has severe vomiting and diarrhea with little or no fluid intake. When this and similar conditions are present, the posterior pituitary releases the hormone vasopressin, water in the kidneys is reabsorbed into the blood (i.e., conserved), and the urine becomes concentrated. Vasopressin exhibits its greatest activity on the renal tubular epithelium, where it promotes water resorption and smooth muscle contraction throughout the vascular bed. Vasopressin has some vasopressor activity.

Vasopressin and its derivative are used in treating **diabetes insipidus**, a disease resulting from the failure of the pituitary to secrete vasopressin or from surgical removal of the pituitary. Diabetes insipidus is characterized by marked increase in urination (as much as 10 L in 24 hours) and excessive thirst by inadequate secretion of vasopressin (antidiuretic hormone). Treatment with vasopressin therapy replaces the hormone in the body and restores normal

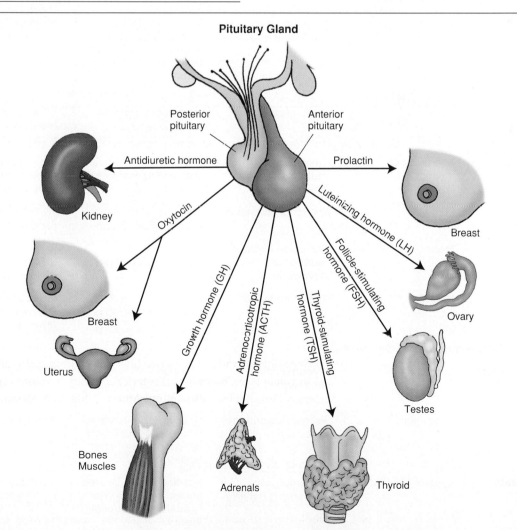

Figure 50.2 The pituitary gland, and the hormones secreted by the anterior pituitary and the posterior pituitary.

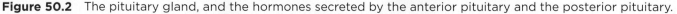

SUMMARY DRUG TABLE — POSTERIOR AND ANTERIOR PITUITARY HORMONES

GENERIC NAME	TRADE NAME	USES	ADVERSE REACTIONS	DOSAGE RANGES
Posterior Pituitary Hormones				
desmopressin acetate *des-moe-press'-in*	DDAVP, Stimate	Diabetes insipidus, hemophilia A, von Willebrand's disease, nocturnal enuresis	Headache, nausea, nasal congestion, abdominal cramps	Doses are individualized, administered orally, intranasally, or SC
vasopressin *vay-soe-press'-in*		Diabetes insipidus, prevention and treatment of postoperative abdominal distention, to dispel gas interfering with abdominal x-ray examination	Tremor, sweating, vertigo, nausea, vomiting, abdominal cramps, headache	Diabetes insipidus: 5–10 units IM, SC q3–4h, parenteral solution may be used intranasally
Anterior Pituitary Hormones and Hormone Inhibitors				
Gonadotropins: Ovarian Stimulants				
choriogonadotropin alfa *kor-ee-oh-goe-nad'-tropin*	Ovidrel	Ovulation induction, follicular maturation	Vasomotor flushes, breast tenderness, abdominal pain, ovarian overstimulation, nausea, vomiting	Injection following follicle stimulation drugs
gonadotropin, follitropins *go-nad'-oh-tropin*	Gonal-f, Gonal-f RFF	Ovulation induction, male infertility	Same as choriogonadotropin	Female: 75 units/d SC for cycle Male: individualized per testosterone levels
gonadotropin, follitropin betas	Follistim AQ	Ovulation induction, multifollicle development	Same as choriogonadotropin	Individualized dosing dependent on follicle stimulation
gonadotropin, lutropin alfas	Luveris	Ovulation induction	Same as choriogonadotropin	75–150 units/d SC for up to 14 d
gonadotropin, menotropin	Menopur, Repronex	Ovulation induction, multifollicle development	Same as choriogonadotropin	Individualized dosing dependent on follicle stimulation
gonadotropin, urofollitropins	Bravelle	Ovulation induction	Same as choriogonadotropin	150 units/d SC or IM for 5 d, may be titrated and repeated
Gonadotropin-Releasing Hormones/Synthetics				
gonadorelin acetate *go-nad-oh-reh'-lin*	Lutrepulse	Hypothalamic amenorrhea	Injection site inflammation, ovarian hyperstimulation	Delivered in mcg/min by infusion pump
histrelin acetate *his-trel'-in*	Supprelin	Precocious puberty	Hot flashes, decreased libido, vaginal dryness, headache, emotional lability	10 mcg/kg SC daily
nafarelin acetate *naf'-a-rel-in*	Synarel	Endometriosis, precocious puberty	Hot flashes, decreased libido, vaginal dryness, headache, emotional lability	400 mcg/d intranasally in 2 doses

GENERIC NAME	TRADE NAME	USES	ADVERSE REACTIONS	DOSAGE RANGES
Gonadotropin-Releasing Hormone Antagonists				
cetrorelix acetate *set-ro'-rel-iks*	Cetrotide	Infertility	Ovarian overstimulation, nausea, vomiting	Dose individualized during cycle
ganirelix acetate *gan-ih-rel'-iks*	Antagon	Infertility	Abdominal pain, fetal death, headache	250 mcg/d SC during cycle
Nonsteroidal Ovarian Stimulant				
clomiphene citrate *klo'-mi-feen*	Clomid, Milophene, Serophene	Ovulatory failure	Vasomotor flushes, breast tenderness, abdominal discomfort, ovarian enlargement, nausea, vomiting	50 mg/d orally for 5 d, may be repeated
Growth Hormone and Hormone Inhibitors				
somatropin *soe-ma-tro'-pin*	Genotropin, Humatrope, Norditropin, Serostim, Nutropin	Growth failure due to deficiency of pituitary growth hormone in children	With injection: diarrhea, arthralgia Long term: growth problems—bone, ear, edema	Doses are individualized, administered by SC injection weekly
octreotide acetate *ok-tree'-oh-tide*	Sandostatin	Reduction of growth hormone in acromegaly and treatment of certain tumors	Nausea, diarrhea, abdominal pain, sinus bradycardia, hypoglycemia, injection site pain	50 mcg SC or IV BID or TID
Adrenocorticotropic Hormone				
adrenocorticotropic hormone (ACTH) *a-dreen-oh-corti-ko-tro'-pic*		Diagnose adrenocortical function, nonsuppurative thyroiditis, hypercalcemia, multiple sclerosis	See Display 50–2	20 units IM, SC QID
Miscellaneous Hormones and Hormone Inhabitors				
aminoglutethimide *ah-meen'-oh-glue-ti-thighmyde*	Cytadren	Suppress adrenal function	Drowsiness, skin rash, nausea, vomiting	1–2 g/d orally
bromocriptine mesylate *bro-moe-cryp'-tin*	Parlodel	Hyperprolactinemia, acromegaly, Parkinson's disease	Headache, dizziness, fatigue, nausea	5–7.5 mg/d orally
cabergoline *ca-ber'-go-leen*	Dostinex	Same as bromocriptine	Same as bromocriptine	1 mg twice weekly orally
cosyntropin	Cortrosyn	Screening for adrenal insufficiency	Dizziness, nausea, vomiting	See package insert
gonadotropin, chorionic (HCG)	Pregnyl	Testicular descent induction, hypogonadism, ovulation induction	Headache, irritability, fluid retention, fatigue, gynecomastia, aggressive behavior	500–5000 units IM up to 3 times weekly depending on results

urination and thirst. Vasopressin may also be used for preventing and treating postoperative abdominal distention and for dispelling gas interfering with abdominal roentgenography (x-ray studies).

Adverse Reactions

Local or systemic hypersensitivity reactions may occur in some patients receiving vasopressin, and the following may also be seen:

- Tremor, sweating, vertigo
- Nasal congestion
- Nausea, vomiting, abdominal cramps
- Water intoxication (overdosage, toxicity)

Contraindications and Precautions

Vasopressin is contraindicated in patients hypersensitive to the drug or its components. Vasopressin is used cautiously in patients with a history of seizures, migraine headaches, asthma, congestive heart failure, or vascular disease (because the substance may precipitate angina or myocardial infarction) and in those with perioperative polyuria. Vasopressin is classified as a pregnancy category C drug. Desmopressin acetate (a pregnancy category B drug) is typically used when diabetes insipidus occurs during pregnancy; however, it still must be used cautiously then and during lactation.

Interactions

Interacting Drug	Common Use	Effect of Interaction
norepinephrine	Neurostimulant	Decreased antidiuretic effect
lithium	Management of psychological problems	Decreased antidiuretic effect
oral anticoagulants	Blood thinners	Decreased antidiuretic effect
carbamazepine	Anticonvulsant	Increased antidiuretic effect
chlorpropamide	Antidiabetic (diabetes mellitus) agent	Increased antidiuretic effect

The Patient Receiving Vasopressin

ASSESSMENT

PREADMINISTRATION ASSESSMENT

Before administering the first dose of vasopressin for managing diabetes insipidus, the nurse takes the patient's blood pressure, pulse, and respiratory rate. The nurse weighs the patient to obtain a baseline weight for future comparison. Serum electrolyte levels and other laboratory tests may be ordered by the primary health care provider.

Before administering vasopressin to relieve abdominal distention, the nurse takes the patient's blood pressure, pulse, and respiratory rate. The nurse auscultates the abdomen and records the findings. The nurse measures and records the patient's abdominal girth.

ONGOING ASSESSMENT

During the ongoing assessment the nurse monitors the blood pressure, pulse, and respiratory rate every 4 hours or as ordered by the primary health care provider. The patient's fluid intake and output are strictly measured. The primary health care provider is notified if there are any significant changes in these vital signs because a dosage adjustment may be necessary.

The dosage of vasopressin or its derivatives may require periodic adjustments. After administration of the drug, the nurse observes the patient every 10 to 15 minutes for signs of an excessive dosage (e.g., blanching of the skin, abdominal cramps, and nausea). If these occur, the nurse reassures the patient that recovery from these effects will occur in a few minutes.

> **Gerontologic Alert**
>
> Older adults are particularly sensitive to the effects of vasopressin and should be monitored closely during administration of the drug.

NURSING DIAGNOSES

Drug-specific nursing diagnoses are highlighted in the Nursing Diagnoses Checklist. Other nursing diagnoses applicable to these drugs are discussed in depth in Chapter 4.

PLANNING

The expected outcomes for the patient may include an optimal response to therapy, support of patient needs

Nursing Diagnoses Checklist

✔ **Deficient Fluid Volume** related to inability to replenish fluid intake secondary to diabetes insipidus

✔ **Acute Pain** related to abdominal distention

Nursing Alert

Excessive dosage is manifested as water intoxication (fluid overload). Symptoms of water intoxication include drowsiness, listlessness, confusion, and headache (which may precede convulsions and coma). If signs of excessive dosage occur, the nurse should notify the primary health care provider before the next dose of the drug is due because a change in the dosage, the restriction of oral or IV fluids, and the administration of a diuretic may be necessary.

related to the management of adverse reactions, and an understanding of the therapeutic regimen.

IMPLEMENTATION

PROMOTING AN OPTIMAL RESPONSE TO THERAPY

Vasopressin may be given intramuscularly (IM) or subcutaneously (SC) to treat diabetes insipidus. The injection (parenteral) solution may also be administered intranasally on cotton pledgets, by nasal spray or dropper. When given parenterally, 5 to 10 Units administered two to three times daily is usually sufficient. To prevent or relieve abdominal distention, 5 Units of the drug is administered initially, which may be increased to 10 Units every 3 or 4 hours IM. When the drug is administered before abdominal roentgenography, the nurse administers two injections of 10 Units each. The first dose is given 2 hours before x-ray examination and the second dose 30 minutes before the testing. An enema may be given before the first dose.

Desmopressin may be given orally, intranasally, SC, or intravenously (IV). The oral dose must be determined for each individual patient and adjusted according to the patient's response to therapy. The drug is available in metered-dose nasal delivery systems. The solution is drawn into a calibrated tube called a **rhinyle**. One end is inserted into the nostril and the patient (if condition allows) blows the other end to deposit solution deep into the nasal cavity. A nasal spray pump may also be used. The nurse instructs the patient to hold the bottle upright with the head in a vertical position when administering the drug. Most adults require 0.2 mL daily in two divided doses to control diabetes insipidus. Patients learn to regulate their dosage based on the frequency of urination and increase of thirst. The drug may also be administered by the SC route or direct IV injection.

MONITORING AND MANAGING PATIENT NEEDS

The adverse reactions associated with vasopressin, such as skin blanching, abdominal cramps, and nausea, may be decreased by administering the agent with one or two glasses of water. If these adverse reactions occur, the nurse informs the patient that they are not serious and should subside within a few minutes.

DEFICIENT FLUID VOLUME The symptoms of diabetes insipidus include the voiding of a large volume of urine at frequent intervals during the day and throughout the night. Accompanied by frequent urination is the need to drink large volumes of fluid because patients with diabetes insipidus are continually thirsty and need to be supplied with large amounts of drinking water. The nurse is careful to refill the water container at frequent intervals. This is especially important when the patient has limited ambulatory activities. Until controlled by a drug, the symptoms of frequent urination and excessive thirst may cause a great deal of anxiety. The nurse reassures the patient that with the proper drug therapy, these symptoms will most likely be reduced or eliminated.

When the patient has diabetes insipidus, the nurse measures the fluid intake and output accurately and observes the patient for signs of dehydration (dry mucous membranes, concentrated urine, poor skin turgor, flushing, dry skin, confusion). This is especially important early in treatment and until such time as the optimum dosage is determined and symptoms have diminished. If the patient's output greatly exceeds intake, the nurse notifies the primary health care provider. In some instances, the primary health care provider may order specific gravity and volume measurements of each voiding or at hourly intervals. The nurse records these results in the chart to aid the primary health care provider in adjusting the dosage to the patient's needs.

ACUTE PAIN If the patient is receiving vasopressin for abdominal distention, the nurse explains in detail the method of treating this problem and the necessity of monitoring drug effectiveness (e.g., auscultation of the abdomen for bowel sounds, insertion of a rectal tube, measurement of the abdomen). If a rectal tube is ordered after administration of vasopressin for abdominal distention, the lubricated end of the tube is inserted past the anal sphincter and taped in place. The tube is left in place for 1 hour or as prescribed by the primary health care provider. The nurse auscultates the abdomen every 15 to 30 minutes and measures abdominal girth hourly, or as ordered by the primary health care provider.

EDUCATING THE PATIENT AND FAMILY

If desmopressin is to be used in the form of a nasal spray or is to be instilled intranasally using the nasal tube delivery system, the nurse ensures that the patient masters the technique of instillation (see Patient and Family Teaching Checklist: Self-Administering Nasal Pituitary Hormones). The nurse includes illustrated patient instructions with the drug and reviews them with the patient. The nurse should discuss the need to take the drug only as directed by the primary health care provider. The patient should not increase the dosage (i.e., the prescribed number or frequency of sprays) unless advised to do so by the primary health care provider.

On occasion, a patient may need to self-administer vasopressin by the parenteral route. If so, the nurse teaches the patient or a family member how to prepare and administer the drug and measure the specific gravity of the urine.

The nurse stresses the importance of adhering to the prescribed treatment program to control symptoms. In addition to instruction in administration, the nurse includes the following in a patient and family teaching plan:

- Drink one or two glasses of water immediately before taking the drug.

- Measure the amount of fluids taken each day.

- Measure the amount of urine excreted at each voiding and then total the amount for each 24-hour period.

- Avoid the use of alcohol while taking these drugs.

- Rotate injection sites for parenteral administration.

- Contact the primary health care provider immediately if any of the following occur: a significant increase or decrease in urine output, abdominal cramps, blanching of the skin, nausea, signs of inflammation or infection at the injection sites, confusion, headache, or drowsiness.

- Wear medical identification naming the disease and the drug regimen.

EVALUATION

- The therapeutic effect is achieved.

- Anxiety is reduced.

- Signs of significant fluid volume loss are absent (diabetes insipidus).

Patient and Family Teaching Checklist

Self-Administering Nasal Pituitary Hormones

Vasopressin

The nurse:

✔ Explains the reason for the drug and prescribed therapy, including drug name, correct dose (number of sprays), and frequency of administration.

✔ Describes equipment to be used for intranasal administration.

✔ Reviews schedule of administration and prescribed number of sprays to each nostril based on signs and symptoms of diabetes insipidus, such as frequency of urination and increased thirst.

✔ Demonstrates step-by-step procedure for instillation and care, with patient performing a return demonstration of procedure.

✔ Provides written instructions for the procedure.

✔ Offers reassurance that symptoms of the disorder will most likely be reduced or eliminated with drug therapy.

✔ Identifies signs and symptoms of fluid overload and explains the need to notify the primary health care provider should any occur.

✔ Reinforces the need for continued follow-up to evaluate therapy.

Desmopressin

The nurse:

✔ Shows how to administer the drug nasally with a nasal tube. The nasal tube delivery system comes with a flexible calibrated plastic tube called a **rhinyle**.

✔ Demonstrates how to draw the prescribed amount of solution is into the rhinyle and assists the patient to insert one end into the nostril and blow into the other end to deposit solution deep into the nasal cavity.

✔ Explains how a nasal spray pump may also be used.

- The patient verbalizes an understanding of the treatment modalities and the importance of continued follow-up care (diabetes insipidus).

- The patient and family demonstrate an understanding of the drug regimen.

- Adverse reactions are identified and reported to the primary health care provider (diabetes insipidus).

- The patient verbalizes the importance of complying with the prescribed therapeutic regimen (diabetes insipidus).

ANTERIOR PITUITARY HORMONES

The hormones of the anterior pituitary include

- Prolactin
- Luteinizing hormone (LH)
- Follicle-stimulating hormone (FSH)
- Thyroid-stimulating hormone (TSH)
- Adrenocorticotropic hormone (ACTH; corticotropin)
- Growth hormone (GH)

The anterior pituitary hormone TSH is discussed in Chapter 51. The remaining hormones can be classified into different groups. FSH and LH are called **gonadotropins** because they influence the **gonads** (the organs of reproduction). GH, also called **somatotropin**, contributes to the growth of the body during childhood, especially the growth of muscles and bones. ACTH is produced by the anterior pituitary and stimulates the adrenal cortex to secrete the corticosteroids. Prolactin, which is also secreted by the anterior pituitary, stimulates the production of breast milk in the postpartum patient. Additional functions of prolactin are not well understood. Prolactin is the only anterior pituitary hormone that is not used medically.

Gonadotropins: Follicle-Stimulating Hormone and Luteinizing Hormone

The gonadotropins (FSH and LH) influence the secretion of sex hormones, development of secondary sex characteristics, and the reproductive cycle in both men and women. The gonadotropins discussed in this chapter include menotropins, urofollitropin, clomiphene, and chorionic gonadotropin.

Action and Uses

These drugs are purified preparations of the gonadotropins (FSH and LH) extracted from the urine of postmenopausal women or produced by a recombinant form of DNA. Gonadotropins are used to induce ovulation and pregnancy in anovulatory women (women whose bodies fail to produce an ovum or fail to ovulate). Menotropin (Menopur) is also used in assisted reproductive technology (ART) programs to stimulate multiple follicles for in vitro fertilization. Besides their use in treating female infertility, some of these drugs are used in men. Human chorionic gonadotropin (HCG) is extracted from human placentas. The actions of HCG are identical to those of the pituitary LH. This drug is also used in boys to treat prepubertal **cryptorchism** (failure of the testes to descend into the scrotum) and in men to treat selected cases of hypogonadotropic hypogonadism. Follitropin is used to induce sperm production (spermatogenesis). For additional information on the gonadotropins, see the Summary Drug Table: Posterior and Anterior Pituitary Hormones.

Clomiphene (Clomid) and ganirelix acetate (Antagon) are synthetic nonsteroidal compounds that bind to estrogen receptors, decreasing the amount of available estrogen receptors and causing the anterior pituitary to increase secretion of FSH and LH. These drugs are used to induce ovulation in anovulatory (nonovulating) women.

Adverse Reactions

Hormone-Associated Reactions

- Vasomotor flushes (which are like the hot flashes of menopause)
- Breast tenderness
- Abdominal discomfort, ovarian enlargement
- Hemoperitoneum (blood in the peritoneal cavity)

Generalized Reactions

- Nausea, vomiting
- Headache, irritability, restlessness, fatigue
- Edema and irritation at the injection site

> ### Nursing Alert
>
> Fetal effects have been demonstrated in animal studies when gonadotropins have been administered. Birth defects have been reported in human studies; therefore, gonadotropins should not be administered to women known to be pregnant.

Contraindications, Precautions, and Interactions

These drugs are contraindicated in patients who are hypersensitive to the drug or any component of the drug. The gonadotropins are contraindicated in patients with high gonadotropin levels, thyroid dysfunction, adrenal dysfunction, liver disease, abnormal bleeding, ovarian cysts, or sex hormone–dependent tumors, or those with an organic intracranial lesion (pituitary tumor). Gonadotropins are contraindicated during pregnancy (category X).

These drugs are used cautiously in patients with epilepsy, migraine headaches, asthma, or cardiac or renal dysfunction, and during lactation. There are no known clinically significant interactions with the gonadotropins.

NURSING PROCESS

The Patient Receiving a Gonadotropin

ASSESSMENT

PREADMINISTRATION ASSESSMENT

These drugs are almost always administered on an outpatient basis. Before prescribing any of these drugs, the primary health care provider takes a thorough medical history and performs a physical examination. Additional laboratory and diagnostic tests for ovarian function and tubal patency may also be performed. The nurse takes and records the patient's vital signs and weight before therapy begins. A pelvic examination may be performed by the primary health care provider to rule out ovarian enlargement, pregnancy, or uterine problems.

ONGOING ASSESSMENT

At the time of each office or clinic visit, the nurse questions the patient regarding the occurrence of adverse reactions and records the patient's vital signs and weight.

NURSING DIAGNOSES

Drug-specific nursing diagnoses are highlighted in the Nursing Diagnoses Checklist. Other nursing diagnoses applicable to these drugs are discussed in depth in Chapter 4.

PLANNING

The expected outcomes of the patient may include an optimal response to drug therapy, support of patient needs related to the management of adverse reactions, reduction in anxiety, and an understanding of the therapeutic regimen.

Nursing Diagnoses Checklist

✔ **Acute Pain** related to adverse reactions (ovarian enlargement, irritation at the injection site)

✔ **Anxiety** related to inability to conceive, treatment outcome, other factors

---

IMPLEMENTATION
PROMOTING AN OPTIMAL RESPONSE TO THERAPY

Clomiphene is an oral tablet prescribed for 5 days and is self-administered in the outpatient setting.

Nursing Alert

If the patient complains of visual disturbances, the drug therapy is discontinued and the primary health care provider notified. An examination by an ophthalmologist is usually indicated.

The patient is observed for symptoms of ovarian stimulation (abdominal pain, distention, sudden ovarian enlargement, ascites). Therapy is discontinued and the primary health care provider notified if symptoms occur.

MONITORING AND MANAGING PATIENT NEEDS

ACUTE PAIN Menotropins, urofollitropin, and HCG injections are given in the primary health care provider's office or clinic. These drugs are administered IM or SC because they are destroyed in the gastrointestinal (GI) tract. The nurse should rotate sites and examine previous sites for redness and irritation. Female patients taking these drugs are usually examined by the primary health care provider every other day during treatment and at 2-week intervals to detect excessive ovarian stimulation, called **hyperstimulation syndrome** (sudden ovarian enlargement with ascites). The patient may or may not report pain. This syndrome usually develops quickly, within 3 to 4 days.

Nursing Alert

The patient is checked for signs of excessive ovarian enlargement (abdominal distention, pain, ascites [with serious cases]). The drug is discontinued at the first sign of ovarian stimulation or enlargement. The patient is usually admitted to the hospital for supportive measures.

ANXIETY Patients wishing to become pregnant often experience a great deal of anxiety. In addition, when taking these drugs, the patient faces the possibility of multiple births. The success rate of these drugs varies and depends on many factors. The primary health care provider usually discusses the value of this, as well as other approaches, with the patient and her sexual partner. The nurse allows the patient time to talk about her problems or concerns about the proposed treatment program.

EDUCATING THE PATIENT AND FAMILY

Patients are instructed by the primary health care provider about the frequency of sexual intercourse. The nurse should assess whether the patient understands the directions given by the primary health care provider. When a gonadotropin is prescribed, the nurse should instruct the patient taking the hormone to keep all primary health care provider appointments and to report adverse reactions to the nurse or primary health care provider. The nurse includes the following information when a gonadotropin is prescribed:

HORMONAL OVARIAN STIMULANTS

- Before beginning therapy, be aware of the possibility of multiple births and birth defects.

- It is a good idea to use a calendar to track the treatment schedule and ovulation.

- Report bloating, abdominal pain, flushing, breast tenderness, and pain at the injection site.

NONHORMONAL OVARIAN STIMULANTS

- Take the drug as prescribed (5 days) and do not stop taking the drug before the course of therapy is finished unless told to do so by the primary health care provider.

- Notify the primary health care provider if bloating, stomach or pelvic pain, jaundice, blurred vision, hot flashes, breast discomfort, headache, nausea, or vomiting occurs.

- Keep in mind that if ovulation does not occur after the first course of therapy, a second or third course may be used. If therapy does not succeed after three courses, the drug is considered unsuccessful and is discontinued.

EVALUATION

- The therapeutic effect is achieved.

- Adverse reactions are identified and reported to the primary health care provider.

- Anxiety is reduced.

- The patient demonstrates knowledge of treatment and dosage regimen, adverse drug reactions, risks of treatment, and importance of complying with the primary health care provider's recommendations.

Growth Hormone

Growth hormone, also called *somatotropic hormone*, is secreted by the anterior pituitary. This hormone regulates the growth of the individual until approximately early adulthood or the time when the person no longer gains height.

Action and Uses

Growth hormone is available as the synthetic product somatropin. Of recombinant DNA origin, somatropin is identical to human GH and produces skeletal growth in children. This drug is administered to children who have not grown because of a deficiency of pituitary GH; it must be used before closure of the child's bone epiphyses. Bone epiphyses are the ends of bones. They are separated from the main bone but joined to it by cartilage, which allows for growth or lengthening of the bone. GH is ineffective in patients with closed epiphyses because when the epiphyses close, growth (in length) can no longer occur.

Adverse Reactions

Somatropin causes few adverse reactions when administered as directed. Antibodies to somatropin may develop in a small number of patients, resulting in a failure to experience response to therapy, namely, failure of the drug to produce growth in the child. Some patients may experience hypothyroidism or insulin resistance. Swelling, joint pain, and muscle pain may also occur.

Contraindications, Precautions, and Interactions

Somatropin is contraindicated in patients with known hypersensitivity to somatropin or sensitivity to benzyl alcohol, and those with epiphyseal closure or underlying cranial lesions (e.g., pituitary tumor). The drug is used cautiously in patients with thyroid disease or diabetes, and during pregnancy (category C) and lactation. Excessive amounts of glucocorticoids may decrease the response to somatropin.

NURSING PROCESS

The Patient Receiving Growth Hormone

ASSESSMENT

PREADMINISTRATION ASSESSMENT

A thorough physical examination and laboratory and diagnostic tests are performed before a child is accepted into a growth hormone program. Before therapy starts, the nurse takes and records the patient's vital signs, height, and weight.

ONGOING ASSESSMENT

Children may increase their growth rate from 3.5 to 4 cm/year before treatment to 8 to 10 cm/year during the first year of treatment. Each time the child visits the primary health care provider's office or clinic (usually every 3 to 6 months), the nurse measures and records the child's height and weight to evaluate the response to therapy. Bone age is monitored periodically for growth and to detect epiphyseal closure, at which time therapy must stop.

NURSING DIAGNOSES

A key nursing diagnosis for patients receiving growth hormone therapy is Disturbed Body Image related to changes in appearance, physical size, or failure to grow. Other nursing diagnoses applicable to these drugs are discussed in depth in Chapter 4.

PLANNING

The expected outcomes of the patient may include an optimal response to drug therapy, support of patient needs related to the management of adverse reactions, reduction in anxiety, and an understanding of the therapeutic regimen.

IMPLEMENTATION

PROMOTING AN OPTIMAL RESPONSE TO THERAPY

Growth hormone is administered SC. The vial containing the hormone is not shaken but swirled to mix. The solution is clear; the nurse should not administer it if it is cloudy. The weekly dosage is divided and given in three to seven doses throughout the week. The drug may (if possible) be given at bedtime to adhere most closely to the body's natural release of the hormone. Periodic testing of growth hormone levels, glucose tolerance, and thyroid function may be done during treatment.

MONITORING AND MANAGING PATIENT NEEDS

DISTURBED BODY IMAGE Children requiring treatment are usually of short stature. The parents, and sometimes the children, may be concerned about the success or possible failure of treatment with GH. The child is provided with the opportunity to share fears, concerns, or anger. The nurse acknowledges these feelings as normal and corrects any misconceptions the child or parents may have concerning treatment. Time is allowed for the parents and children to ask questions not only before therapy is started but during the months of treatment.

EDUCATING THE PATIENT AND FAMILY

When the patient is receiving GH, the primary health care provider discusses in detail the therapeutic regimen for increasing growth (height) with the child's parents or guardians. If the drug is to be given at bedtime and not in the outpatient clinic, the nurse instructs the parents on the proper injection technique. The parents are encouraged to keep all clinic or office visits with the child. The nurse explains that the child may experience sudden growth and increase in appetite and instructs the parents to report lack of growth, symptoms of diabetes (e.g., increased hunger, increased thirst, or frequent voiding) or symptoms of hypothyroidism (e.g., fatigue, dry skin, intolerance to cold).

EVALUATION

- The therapeutic effect is achieved and the child grows in height.

- Adverse reactions are identified and reported to the primary health care provider.

- Anxiety is reduced.

- The parents verbalize understanding of the treatment program.

- The child maintains a positive body image.

Adrenocorticotropic Hormone (ACTH): Corticotropin

Actions and Uses

Corticotropin (ACTH) is an anterior pituitary hormone that stimulates the adrenal cortex to produce and secrete adrenocortical hormones, primarily the glucocorticoids. Corticotropin is used for diagnostic testing of adrenocortical function. This drug may also be used for managing acute exacerbations of multiple sclerosis, nonsuppurative thyroiditis, and hypercalcemia associated with cancer. It is also used as an anti-inflammatory and immunosuppressant drug when conventional glucocorticoid therapy has not been effective (Display 50-1).

Adverse Reactions

Because ACTH stimulates the release of glucocorticoids from the adrenal gland, adverse reactions seen with the administration of this hormone are similar to those seen with the glucocorticoids (Display 50-2) and affect many body systems.

Contraindications and Precautions

ACTH is contraindicated in patients with adrenocortical insufficiency or hyperfunction, allergy to pork or pork

Display 50.1 Uses of Glucocorticoids

- **Endocrine disorders:** Primary or secondary adrenal cortical insufficiency, congenital adrenal hyperplasia, nonsuppurative thyroiditis, hypercalcemia associated with cancer
- **Rheumatic disorders:** Short-term management of acute ankylosing spondylitis, acute and subacute bursitis, acute nonspecific tenosynovitis, acute gouty arthritis, psoriatic arthritis, rheumatoid arthritis, post-traumatic osteoarthritis, synovitis of osteoarthritis, epicondylitis
- **Collagen diseases:** Systemic lupus erythematosus, acute rheumatic carditis, systemic dermatomyositis
- **Dermatologic disorders:** Pemphigus, bullous dermatitis herpetiformis, severe erythema multiforme (Stevens-Johnson syndrome), exfoliative dermatitis, mycosis fungoides, severe psoriasis, severe seborrheic dermatitis, angioedema, urticaria, various skin disorders (e.g., lichen planus or keloids)
- **Allergic states:** Control of severe or incapacitating allergic conditions not controlled by other methods, bronchial asthma (including status asthmaticus), contact dermatitis, atopic dermatitis, serum sickness, drug hypersensitivity reactions
- **Ophthalmic diseases:** Severe acute and chronic allergic and inflammatory processes, keratitis, allergic corneal marginal ulcers, herpes zoster of the eye, iritis, iridocyclitis, chorioretinitis, diffuse posterior uveitis, optic neuritis, sympathetic ophthalmia, anterior segment inflammation
- **Respiratory diseases:** Seasonal allergic rhinitis, berylliosis, fulminating or disseminating pulmonary tuberculosis, aspiration pneumonia
- **Hematologic disorders:** Idiopathic or secondary thrombocytopenic purpura, hemolytic anemia, red blood cell anemia, congenital hypoplastic anemia
- **Neoplastic diseases:** Leukemia, lymphomas
- **Edematous states:** Induction of diuresis or remission of proteinuria in nephrotic syndrome
- **Gastrointestinal diseases:** During critical period of ulcerative colitis, regional enteritis, intractable sprue
- **Nervous system disorders:** Acute exacerbations of multiple sclerosis

Display 50.2 Adverse Reactions Associated With Glucocorticoids

- **Fluid and electrolyte disturbances:** Sodium and fluid retention, potassium loss, hypokalemic alkalosis, hypertension, hypocalcemia, hypotension or shocklike reactions
- **Musculoskeletal disturbances:** Muscle weakness, loss of muscle mass, tendon rupture, osteoporosis, aseptic necrosis of femoral and humeral heads, spontaneous fractures
- **Cardiovascular disturbances:** Thromboembolism or fat embolism, thrombophlebitis, necrotizing angiitis, syncopal episodes, cardiac arrhythmias, aggravation of hypertension, fatal cardiac arrhythmias with rapid, high-dose IV methylprednisolone administration, congestive heart failure in susceptible patients
- **Gastrointestinal disturbances:** Pancreatitis, abdominal distention, ulcerative esophagitis, nausea, vomiting, increased appetite and weight gain, possible peptic ulcer or bowel perforation, hemorrhage
- **Dermatologic disturbances:** Impaired wound healing, thin, fragile skin, petechiae, ecchymoses, erythema, increased sweating, suppression of skin test reactions, subcutaneous fat atrophy, purpura, striae, hirsutism, acneiform eruptions, urticaria, angioneurotic edema, perineal itch
- **Neurologic disturbances:** Convulsions, increased intracranial pressure with papilledema (usually after treatment is discontinued), vertigo, headache, neuritis or paresthesia, steroid psychosis, insomnia
- **Endocrine disturbances:** Amenorrhea, other menstrual irregularities, development of cushingoid state, suppression of growth in children, secondary adrenocortical and pituitary unresponsive (particularly in times of stress), decreased carbohydrate tolerance, manifestation of latent diabetes mellitus, increased requirements for insulin or oral hypoglycemic agents (in diabetic patients)
- **Ophthalmic disturbances:** Posterior subcapsular cataracts, increased intraocular pressure, glaucoma, exophthalmos
- **Metabolic disturbances:** Negative nitrogen balance (due to protein catabolism)
- **Other disturbances:** Anaphylactoid or hypersensitivity reactions, aggravation of existing infections, malaise, increase or decrease in sperm motility and number

products (corticotropin is obtained from porcine pituitaries), systemic fungal infections, ocular herpes simplex, scleroderma, osteoporosis, and hypertension. Patients taking ACTH also should avoid any vaccinations with live virus.

ACTH is used cautiously in patients with diabetes, diverticulosis, renal insufficiency, myasthenia gravis, tuberculosis (may reactivate the disease), hypothyroidism, cirrhosis, nonspecific ulcerative colitis, heart failure, seizures, or febrile infections. The drug is classified as a pregnancy category C drug and is used cautiously during pregnancy and lactation. ACTH also is used cautiously in children because it can inhibit skeletal growth.

Interactions

Interacting Drug	Common Use	Effect of Interaction
amphotericin B	Anti-infective	Increased risk of hypokalemia
diuretics	Fluid retention/ cardiac problems	Increased risk of hypokalemia
insulin or oral antidiabetic	Diabetes management	Increased need for antidiabetic medication
barbiturates	Sedation	Decreased effect of ACTH
cholinergic blockers	Decrease of spasms or secretions; treatment of Parkinson's disease	Decreased muscle function

Live virus vaccines received while the patient is taking ACTH may potentiate virus replication, increase any adverse reaction to the vaccine, and decrease the patient's antibody response to the vaccine.

NURSING PROCESS

The Patient Receiving Corticotropin (ACTH)

ASSESSMENT

PREADMINISTRATION ASSESSMENT

Before administering ACTH, the nurse reviews the patient's chart for the diagnosis, laboratory tests, and other pertinent information. The nurse obtains the patient's weight and assesses skin integrity, lungs, and mental status. The nurse takes and records vital signs. Additional assessments depend on the patient's condition and diagnosis. The primary health care provider may order baseline diagnostic tests, such as chest or upper GI x-ray studies and serum electrolytes, urinalysis, or complete blood count.

ONGOING ASSESSMENT

The nurse monitors the patient's weight and fluid intake and output daily during therapy. The nurse observes for and reports any evidence of edema, such as weight gain, rales, increased pulse or dyspnea, or swollen extremities. The nurse monitors blood glucose levels for a rise in blood glucose concentration. In addition, the nurse checks stools for evidence of bleeding (dark or tarry in color, positive guaiac test result). Patients receiving prolonged therapy should have periodic hematologic, serum electrolyte, and serum glucose studies.

Nursing Diagnoses Checklist

✔ **Risk for Infection** related to masking of signs of infection
✔ **Disturbed Thought Processes** related to adverse drug reactions

NURSING DIAGNOSES

Drug-specific nursing diagnoses are highlighted in the Nursing Diagnoses Checklist. Other nursing diagnoses applicable to these drugs are discussed in depth in Chapter 4.

PLANNING

The expected outcomes of the patient may include an optimal response to therapy, support of patient needs related to the management of adverse reactions, and an understanding of the therapeutic regimen.

IMPLEMENTATION

PROMOTING AN OPTIMAL RESPONSE TO THERAPY

Nursing management depends on the patient's diagnosis and physical status and the reason for use of the drug. The nurse may need to assess vital signs every 4 hours and observe for the adverse reactions that occur with glucocorticoid administration.

This drug may be given by the IV, SC, or IM route. During parenteral administration of ACTH, the nurse observes the patient for hypersensitivity reactions. Symptoms of hypersensitivity include rash, urticaria, hypotension, tachycardia, or difficulty breathing. If the drug is given IM or SC, the nurse observes the patient for hypersensitivity reactions immediately and for about 2 hours after the drug is given. If a hypersensitivity reaction occurs, the nurse notifies the primary health care provider immediately. Long-term use increases the risk of hypersensitivity.

MONITORING AND MANAGING PATIENT NEEDS

RISK FOR INFECTION Corticotropin may mask signs of infection, including fungal or viral eye infections.

Nursing Alert

The nurse reports any complaints of sore throat, cough, fever, malaise, sores that do not heal, or redness or irritation of the eyes in the patient taking ACTH.

There may be a decreased resistance and inability to identify the source of the infection. The nurse observes the skin daily for localized signs of infection, especially at injection sites or IV access sites. Visitors are monitored to protect the patient against those with infectious illness.

DISTURBED THOUGHT PROCESSES Corticotropin can also cause disturbances in the psyche. The nurse must report any evidence of behavior change, such as mental depression, insomnia, euphoria, mood swings, or nervousness. If disturbances occur, the nurse encourages communication with the staff and family members, provides a quiet, nonthreatening environment, and spends time actively listening as the patient talks. It is important to encourage verbalization of fears and concerns. Anxiety usually decreases with understanding of the therapeutic regimen. The nurse allows time for a thorough explanation of the drug regimen and answering of questions.

EDUCATING THE PATIENT AND FAMILY

The nurse includes the following in a teaching plan for the patient receiving ACTH:

- Report any adverse reactions.

- Avoid contact with those who have an infection because resistance to infection may be decreased.

- Report any symptoms of infection immediately (e.g., sore throat, fever, cough, or sores that do not heal).

- *Patients with diabetes*—Monitor blood glucose (if self-monitoring is being done) or urine closely and notify the primary health care provider if glucose appears in the urine or the blood glucose level increases significantly. An increase in the dosage of the oral antidiabetic drug or insulin may be needed.

- Notify the primary health care provider of a marked weight gain, swelling in the extremities, muscle weakness, persistent headache, visual disturbances, or behavior change.

EVALUATION

- The therapeutic effect is achieved.

- Adverse reactions are identified, reported to the primary health care provider, and managed using appropriate nursing interventions.

- The patient verbalizes an understanding of the therapeutic regimen and adverse effects requiring notification of the primary health care provider.

ADRENOCORTICAL HORMONES

The adrenal gland lies on the superior surface of each kidney. It is a double organ composed of an outer cortex and an inner medulla. In response to ACTH secreted by the anterior pituitary, the adrenal cortex secretes several hormones (the glucocorticoids, the mineralocorticoids, and small amounts of sex hormones).

This section of the chapter discusses the hormones produced by the adrenal cortex or the adrenocortical hormones, which are the glucocorticoids and mineralocorticoids. These hormones are essential to life and influence many organs and structures of the body. The **glucocorticoids** and **mineralocorticoids** are collectively called **corticosteroids**.

Glucocorticoids

The glucocorticoids influence or regulate functions such as the immune response, glucose, fat, and protein metabolism, and the anti-inflammatory response. Table 50-1 describes the activity of the glucocorticoids in the body.

Actions

The glucocorticoids enter target cells and bind to receptors, initiating many complex reactions in the body. Some of the actions are considered undesirable, depending on the indication for which these drugs are used. Examples of the glucocorticoids include cortisone, hydrocortisone (Cortef), prednisone, prednisolone (Prelone), and triamcinolone (Aristocort). The Summary Drug Table: Adrenocortical Hormones: Glucocorticoids and Mineralocorticoids provides information concerning these hormones.

Uses

The glucocorticoids are used to treat

- Adrenocortical insufficiency (replacement therapy)

- Allergic reactions

- Collagen diseases (e.g., systemic lupus erythematosus)

- Dermatologic conditions

- Rheumatic disorders

- Shock

- Multiple other conditions (see Display 50-1)

The anti-inflammatory activity of these hormones makes them valuable for suppressing inflammation and modifying the immune response.

Adverse Reactions

The adverse reactions that may result from the administration of the glucocorticoids are given in Display 50-2. Long-

Table 50.1 Activity of Glucocorticoids in the Body

Function Within the Body	Description of Bodily Activity
Anti-inflammatory	Stabilizes lysosomal membrane and prevents the release of proteolytic enzymes during the inflammatory process.
Regulation of blood pressure	Potentiates vasoconstrictor action of norepinephrine. Without glucocorticoids the vasoconstricting action is decreased, and blood pressure falls.
Metabolism of carbohydrates and protein	Facilitates the breakdown of protein in the muscle, leading to increased plasma amino acid levels. Increases activity of enzymes necessary for glucogenesis, producing hyperglycemia, which can aggravate diabetes, precipitate latent diabetes, and cause insulin resistance.
Metabolism of fat	A complex phenomenon that promotes the use of fat for energy (a positive effect) and permits fat stores to accumulate in the body, causing buffalo hump and moon-shaped or round face (a negative effect).
Interference with the immune response	Decreases the production of lymphocytes and eosinophils in the blood by causing atrophy of the thymus gland; blocks the release of cytokines, resulting in a decreased performance of T and B monocytes in the immune response. (This action, coupled with the anti-inflammatory action, makes the corticosteroids useful in delaying organ rejection in patients with transplants.)
Protection during stress	As a protective mechanism, the corticosteroids are released during periods of stress (e.g., injury or surgery). The release of epinephrine or norepinephrine by the adrenal medulla during stress has a synergistic effect along with the corticosteroids.
Central nervous system responses	Affects mood and possibly causes neuronal or brain excitability, causing euphoria, anxiety, depression, psychosis, and an increase in motor activity in some individuals.

or short-term high-dose therapy may also produce many of the signs and symptoms seen with **Cushing's syndrome**, a disease caused by the overproduction of endogenous glucocorticoids. Some of the signs and symptoms of this Cushing-like (cushingoid) state include a buffalo hump (a hump on the back of the neck), moon face, oily skin and acne, osteoporosis, purple striae on the abdomen and hips, altered skin pigmentation, and weight gain. When a serious disease or disorder is treated, it is often necessary to allow these effects to occur because therapy with these drugs is absolutely necessary.

Contraindications, Precautions, and Interactions

The glucocorticoids are contraindicated in patients with serious infections, such as tuberculosis and fungal and antibiotic-resistant infections. The glucocorticoids are administered with caution to patients with renal or hepatic disease, hypothyroidism, ulcerative colitis, diverticulitis, peptic ulcer disease, inflammatory bowel disease, hypertension, osteoporosis, convulsive disorders, or diabetes. The glucocorticoids are classified as pregnancy category C

drugs and should be used with caution during pregnancy and lactation.

Multiple drug interactions may occur with the glucocorticoids. Table 50-2 identifies selected clinically significant interactions.

Mineralocorticoids
Actions and Uses

The mineralocorticoids consist of aldosterone and desoxycorticosterone and play an important role in conserving sodium and increasing potassium excretion. Because of these activities, the mineralocorticoids are important in controlling salt and water balance. Aldosterone is the more potent of these two hormones. Deficiencies of the mineralocorticoids result in a loss of sodium and water and a retention of potassium. Fludrocortisone (Florinef) is a drug that has both glucocorticoid and mineralocorticoid activity and is the only currently available mineralocorticoid drug. Fludrocortisone is used for replacement therapy for primary and secondary adrenocortical deficiency. Even though this drug has both mineralocorticoid and glucocorticoid activity, it is used only for its mineralocorticoid effects.

SUMMARY DRUG TABLE	ADRENOCORTICAL HORMONES: GLUCO-CORTICOIDS AND MINERALOCORTICOIDS			
GENERIC NAME	**TRADE NAME**	**USES**	**ADVERSE REACTIONS**	**DOSAGE RANGES**
Glucocorticoids				
betamethasone *bay-ta-meth'-a-zone*	Celestone	See Display 50-1	See Display 50-2	Individualize dosage; syrup or injectable, see package insert
budesonide *bue-des'-oh-nide*	Entocort EC	Crohn's disease	See Display 50-2	9 mg QD in AM for 8 wk
cortisone *kor'-ti-sone*		See Display 50-1	See Display 50-2	25–300 mg/d orally
dexamethasone *dex-a-meth'-a-sone*	Decadron, Hexadrol	Cerebral edema, other conditions listed in Display 50-1	See Display 50-2	Individualize dosage based on severity of condition and response
hydrocortisone (cortisol) *hye-droe-kor'-ti-zone*	Cortef, Solu-Cortef, A-hydroCort	See Display 50-1	See Display 50-2	Individualize dosage based on severity of condition and response
methylprednisolone *meth-ill-pred-niss'-oh-lone*	Medrol, Depo-Medrol, Solu-Medrol	See Display 50-1	See Display 50-2	Individualize dosage based on severity of condition and response
prednisolone *pred-niss'-oh-lone*	Prelone	Multiple sclerosis	See Display 50-2	200 mg/d for 1 wk, then 80 mg every other day
prednisone *pred'-ni-sone*		See Display 50-1	See Display 50-2	Individualize dosage: initial dose usually between 5 and 60 mg/d orally
triamcinolone *trye-am-sin'-oh-lone*	Aristocort, Kenacort	See Display 50-1	See Display 50-2	4–60 mg/d orally
Mineralocorticoid				
fludrocortisone acetate *floo-droe-kor'-te-sone*	Florinef	Partial replacement therapy for Addison's disease, salt-losing adrenogenital syndrome	See Display 50-2	0.1 mg 3 times a week to 0.2 mg/d orally

Adverse Reactions

Adverse reactions may occur if the dosage is too high or prolonged or if withdrawal is too rapid. Administration of fludrocortisone may cause

- Edema, hypertension, congestive heart failure, enlargement of the heart
- Increased sweating, allergic skin rash
- Hypokalemia, muscular weakness, headache, hypersensitivity reactions

Because this drug has glucocorticoid and mineralocorticoid activity and is often given with the glucocorticoids, adverse reactions of the glucocorticoids must be closely monitored as well (see Display 50-2).

Contraindications, Precautions, and Interactions

Fludrocortisone is contraindicated in patients with hypersensitivity to fludrocortisone and those with systemic fungal

Table 50.2 Selected Drug Interactions of Glucocorticoids

Precipitant drug	Object drug	Description
barbiturates	corticosteroids	Decreased pharmacologic effects of the corticosteroid may be observed.
cholestyramine	hydrocortisone	The effects of hydrocortisone may be decreased.
oral contraceptives	corticosteroids	Corticosteroid concentration may be increased and clearance decreased.
estrogens	corticosteroids	Corticosteroid clearance may be decreased.
hydantoins	corticosteroids	Corticosteroid clearance may be increased, resulting in reduced therapeutic effects.
ketoconazole	corticosteroids	Corticosteroid clearance may be decreased.
rifampin	corticosteroids	Corticosteroid clearance may be increased, resulting in decreased therapeutic effects.
corticosteroids	anticholinesterases	Anticholinesterase effects may be antagonized in myasthenia gravis.
corticosteroids	oral anticoagulants	Anticoagulant dose requirements may be reduced. Corticosteroids may decrease the anticoagulant action.
corticosteroids	digitalis glycosides	Coadministration may enhance the possibility of digitalis toxicity associated with hypokalemia.
corticosteroids	isoniazid	Isoniazid serum concentrations may be decreased.
corticosteroids	potassium-depleting diuretics	Hypokalemia may occur.
corticosteroids	salicylates	Corticosteroids will reduce serum salicylate levels and may decrease their effectiveness.
corticosteroids	somatrem	Growth-promoting effect of somatrem may be inhibited.
corticosteroids	theophyllines	Alterations in the pharmacologic activity of either agent may occur.

infections. Fludrocortisone is used cautiously in patients with Addison's disease or infection, and during pregnancy (category C) and lactation. Fludrocortisone decreases the effects of the barbiturates, hydantoins, and rifampin. There is a decrease in serum levels of the salicylates when those agents are administered with fludrocortisone.

NURSING PROCESS

The Patient Receiving a Glucocorticoid or Mineralocorticoid

ASSESSMENT

PREADMINISTRATION ASSESSMENT

Before administering a glucocorticoid or mineralocorticoid, the nurse takes and records the patient's blood pressure, pulse, and respiratory rate. Additional physical assessments depend on the reason for use and the general condition of the patient. When feasible, the nurse performs an assessment of the area of disease involvement, such as the respiratory tract or skin, and records the findings in the patient's record. These findings provide baseline data for evaluating the patient's response to drug therapy. The nurse weighs patients who are acutely ill and those with a serious systemic disease before starting therapy.

ONGOING ASSESSMENT

Ongoing assessments of the patient receiving a glucocorticoid, and the frequency of these assessments, depend largely on the disease being treated. The nurse should take and record vital signs every 4 to 8 hours. The nurse also weighs the patient daily to weekly, depending on the diagnosis and the primary health care provider's orders. The patient's response to the drug is assessed by daily evaluations. More frequent assessment may be necessary if a glucocorticoid is used for emergency situations. Because these drugs are used to treat a great many diseases and conditions, an evaluation of drug response is based on the patient's diagnosis and the signs and symptoms of disease.

The nurse assesses for signs of adverse effects of the mineralocorticoid or glucocorticoid, particularly signs of electrolyte imbalance, such as hypocalcemia, hypokalemia, and hypernatremia (see Chapter 58). The nurse assesses the patient's mental status for any change, especially if there is a history of depression or other psychiatric problems or if high doses of the drug are prescribed. The nurse also monitors for signs of an infection, which may be masked by glucocorticoid therapy. The blood of the patient without diabetes is checked weekly for glucose levels because glucocorticoids may aggravate latent diabetes. Those with diabetes must be checked more frequently.

When administering fludrocortisone, the nurse monitors the patient's blood pressure at frequent intervals. Hypotension may indicate insufficient dosage. The nurse weighs the patient daily and assesses for edema, particularly swelling of the feet and hands. The lungs are auscultated for adventitious sounds (e.g., rales/crackles).

NURSING DIAGNOSES

Drug-specific nursing diagnoses are highlighted in the Nursing Diagnoses Checklist. Other nursing diagnoses applicable to these drugs are discussed in depth in Chapter 4.

PLANNING

The expected outcomes of the patient include an optimal response to therapy, support of patient needs related to the management of adverse reactions, and an understanding of the therapeutic regimen.

Nursing Diagnoses Checklist

✔ **Risk for Infection** related to immune suppression or impaired wound healing

✔ **Risk for Injury** related to muscle atrophy, osteoporosis, or spontaneous fractures

✔ **Acute Pain** related to epigastric distress of gastric ulcer formation

✔ **Excess Fluid Volume** related to adverse reactions (sodium and water retention)

✔ **Disturbed Body Image** related to adverse reactions (cushingoid appearance)

✔ **Disturbed Thought Processes** related to adverse reactions (depression, psychosis, other changes in mental status)

IMPLEMENTATION

PROMOTING AN OPTIMAL RESPONSE TO THERAPY

The glucocorticoids may be administered orally, IM, SC, IV, topically, or as an inhalant. The primary health care provider may also inject the drug into a joint (intra-articular), a lesion (intralesional), soft tissue, or bursa. The drug dosage is individualized and based on the severity of the condition and the patient's response.

Nursing Alert

The nurse must never omit the dose of a glucocorticoid. If the patient cannot take the drug orally because of nausea or vomiting, the nurse must notify the primary health care provider immediately because the drug needs to be ordered given by the parenteral route. Patients who are receiving nothing by mouth for any reason must have the glucocorticoid given by the parenteral route.

Daily oral doses are usually given before 9:00 AM to minimize adrenal suppression and to coincide with normal adrenal function. However, alternate-day therapy may be prescribed for patients receiving long-term therapy (see later). Fludrocortisone is given orally and is well tolerated in the GI tract.

Gerontologic Alert

The corticosteroids are administered with caution in older adults because they are more likely to have preexisting conditions, such as congestive heart failure, hypertension, osteoporosis, and arthritis, that may be worsened by the use of such agents. The nurse monitors older adults for exacerbation of existing conditions during corticosteroid therapy. In addition, lower dosages may be needed because of the effects of aging, such as decreases in muscle mass, renal function, and plasma volume.

ALTERNATE-DAY THERAPY The alternate-day therapy approach to glucocorticoid administration is used in treating diseases and disorders requiring long-term therapy, especially the arthritic disorders. This regimen involves giving twice the daily dose of the glucocorticoid every other day. The drug is given only once on the alternate day and before 9 AM. The purpose of alternate-day administration is to provide the patient requiring long-term glucocorticoid therapy with the beneficial effects of the drug while minimizing certain undesirable reactions (see Display 50-2).

Plasma levels of the endogenous adrenocortical hormones vary throughout the day and nighttime hours. They are normally higher between 2 AM and 8 AM, and lower between 4 PM and midnight. When plasma levels are lower, the anterior pituitary releases ACTH, which in turn stimulates the adrenal cortex to manufacture and release glucocorticoids. When plasma levels are high, the pituitary gland does not release ACTH. The response of the pituitary to high or low plasma levels of glucocorticoids and the resulting release or nonrelease of ACTH is an example of the feedback mechanism, which may also be seen in other glands of the body, such as the thyroid gland.

The **feedback mechanism** (also called the *feedback control*) is the method by which the body maintains most hormones at relatively constant levels in the bloodstream. When the hormone concentration falls, the rate of production of that hormone increases. Likewise, when the hormone level becomes too high, the body decreases production of that hormone.

Administration of a short-acting glucocorticoid on alternate days and before 9 AM, when glucocorticoid plasma levels are still relatively high, does not affect the release of ACTH later in the day, yet it gives the patient the benefit of exogenous glucocorticoid therapy.

THE PATIENT WITH DIABETES Patients with diabetes who are receiving a glucocorticoid may require frequent adjustment of their insulin or oral hypoglycemic drug dosage. The nurse monitors blood glucose levels several times daily or as prescribed by the primary health care provider. If the blood glucose levels increase or urine is positive for glucose or ketones, the nurse notifies the primary health care provider. Some patients may have latent (hidden) diabetes. In these cases, the corticosteroid may precipitate hyperglycemia. Therefore, all patients, those with diabetes and those without, should have blood glucose levels checked frequently.

ADRENAL INSUFFICIENCY Administration of the glucocorticoids poses the threat of adrenal gland insufficiency (particularly if the alternate-day therapy is not prescribed). Administration of glucocorticoids several times a day and during a short time (as little as 5 to 10 days) results in shutting off the pituitary release of ACTH because there are always high levels of the glucocorticoids in the plasma (caused by the body's own glucocorticoid production plus the administration of a glucocorticoid drug). Ultimately, the pituitary atrophies and ceases to release ACTH. Without ACTH, the adrenals fail to manufacture and release (endogenous) glucocorticoids. When this happens, the patient has acute adrenal insufficiency, which is a life-threatening situation until corrected with the administration of an exogenous glucocorticoid.

Adrenal insufficiency is a critical deficiency of the mineralocorticoids and the glucocorticoids; the disorder requires immediate treatment. Symptoms of adrenal insufficiency include fever, myalgia, arthralgia, malaise, anorexia, nausea, orthostatic hypotension, dizziness, fainting, dyspnea, and hypoglycemia. Death due to circulatory collapse will result unless the condition is treated promptly. Situations producing stress (e.g., trauma, surgery, severe illness) may precipitate the need for an increase in dosage of the corticosteroids until the crisis or stressful situation is resolved.

Nursing Alert

Glucocorticoid therapy must never be discontinued suddenly. When administration of a glucocorticoid extends beyond 5 days and the drug therapy is to be discontinued, the dosage must be reduced gradually (tapered) over several days. In some instances, it may be necessary to taper the dose over 7 to 10 or more days. Abrupt discontinuation of glucocorticoid therapy usually results in acute adrenal insufficiency, which, if not recognized in time, can result in death. Tapering the dosage allows normal adrenal function to return gradually, thereby preventing adrenal insufficiency.

MONITORING AND MANAGING PATIENT NEEDS

RISK FOR INFECTION The nurse should report any slight rise in temperature, sore throat, or other signs of infection to the primary health care provider as soon as possible because of a possible decreased resistance to infection during glucocorticoid therapy. Nursing personnel and visitors with any type of infection or recent exposure to an infectious disease should avoid patient contact.

RISK FOR INJURY The nurse observes patients receiving long-term glucocorticoid therapy, especially those allowed limited activity, for signs of compression fractures of the vertebrae and pathologic fractures of the long bones. If the patient reports back or bone pain, the nurse notifies the primary health care provider. Extra care is also necessary to prevent falls and other injuries when the patient is confused or is allowed out of bed. If the patient is weak, the nurse assists the patient to the bathroom or when ambulating. Edematous extremities are handled with care to prevent trauma.

ACUTE PAIN Peptic ulcer has been associated with glucocorticoid therapy. The nurse reports to the primary health care provider any patient complaints of epigastric burning or pain, bloody or coffee-ground emesis, or the passing of tarry stools. Giving oral corticosteroids with food or a full glass of water may minimize gastric irritation.

EXCESS FLUID VOLUME Fluid and electrolyte imbalances, particularly excess fluid volume, are common with corticosteroid therapy. The nurse checks the patient for visible edema, keeps an accurate fluid intake and output record, obtains a daily weight, and restricts sodium if indicated by the primary health care provider. Edematous extremities are elevated and the patient's position is changed frequently. The nurse informs the primary health care provider if signs of electrolyte imbalance or glucocorticoid drug effects are noted. Dietary adjustments are made for the increased potassium loss and sodium retention if necessary. Consultation with a dietitian may be indicated.

DISTURBED BODY IMAGE A body image disturbance may occur, especially if the patient experiences cushingoid effects (e.g., buffalo hump, moon face), acne, or hirsutism. If continuation of drug therapy is necessary, the nurse thoroughly explains the cushingoid appearance reaction and emphasizes the necessity of continuing the drug regimen. The nurse assesses the patient's emotional state and helps the patient express feelings and concerns. The nurse offers positive reinforcement, when possible. The nurse instructs the patient with acne to keep the affected areas clean and use over-the-counter acne drugs and water-based cosmetics or creams.

DISTURBED THOUGHT PROCESSES Mental and emotional changes may occur when the glucocorticoids are administered. The nurse accurately documents mental changes and informs the primary health care provider of their occurrence. Patients who appear extremely depressed must be closely observed. The nurse evaluates mental status, memory, and impaired thinking (e.g., changes in orientation, impaired judgment, thoughts of hopelessness, guilt). The nurse allows time for the patient to express feeling and concerns.

EDUCATING THE PATIENT AND FAMILY

To prevent noncompliance, the nurse must provide the patient and family with thorough instructions and warnings about the drug regimen:

- These drugs may cause GI upset. To decrease GI effects, take the oral drug with meals or snacks.

- Take antacids between meals to help prevent peptic ulcer.

SHORT-TERM GLUCOCORTICOID THERAPY

- Take the drug exactly as directed in the prescription container. Do not increase, decrease, or omit a dose unless advised to do so by the primary health care provider.

- Take single daily doses before 9:00 AM.

- Follow the instructions for tapering the dose because they are extremely important.

- If the problem does not improve, contact the primary health care provider.

ALTERNATE-DAY ORAL GLUCOCORTICOID THERAPY

- Take this drug before 9 AM once every other day. Use a calendar or some other method to identify the days of each week to take the drug.

- Do not stop taking the drug unless advised to do so by the primary health care provider.

- If the problem becomes worse, especially on the days the drug is not taken, contact the primary health care provider.

Most of the following teaching points may also apply to alternate-day therapy, especially when higher doses are used and therapy extends over many months.

LONG-TERM OR HIGH-DOSE GLUCOCORTICOID THERAPY

- Do not omit this drug or increase or decrease the dosage except on the advice of the primary health care provider.

- Inform other primary health care providers, dentists, and all medical personnel of therapy with this drug. Wear medical identification or another form of identification to alert medical personnel of long-term therapy with a glucocorticoid.

- Do not take any nonprescription drug unless its use has been approved by the primary health care provider.

- Do not receive live virus vaccines because of the risk for a lack of antibody response. (This does not include patients receiving the corticosteroids as replacement therapy.)

- Whenever possible, avoid exposure to infections. Contact the primary health care provider if minor cuts or abrasions fail to heal, persistent joint swelling or tenderness is noted, or fever, sore throat, upper respiratory infection, or other signs of infection occur.

- If the drug cannot be taken orally for any reason or if diarrhea occurs, contact the primary health care provider immediately. If you are unable to contact the primary health care provider before the next dose is due, go to the nearest hospital emergency department (preferably where the original treatment was started or where the primary health care provider is on the hospital staff) because the drug must be given by injection.

- Weigh yourself weekly. If significant weight gain or swelling of the extremities is noted, contact the primary health care provider.

- Remember that dietary recommendations made by the primary health care provider are an important part of therapy and must be followed.

- Follow the primary health care provider's recommendations regarding periodic eye examinations and laboratory tests.

INTRA-ARTICULAR OR INTRALESIONAL ADMINISTRATION

- Do not overuse the injected joint, even if the pain is gone.

- Follow the primary health care provider's instructions concerning rest and exercise.

MINERALOCORTICOID (FLUDROCORTISONE) THERAPY

- Take the drug as directed. Do not increase or decrease the dosage except as instructed to do so by the primary health care provider.

- Do not discontinue use of the drug abruptly.

- Inform the primary health care provider if the following adverse reactions occur: edema, muscle weakness, weight gain, anorexia, swelling of the extremities, dizziness, severe headache, or shortness of breath.

- Carry patient identification, such as a MedicAlert tag, so that drug therapy will be known to medical personnel during an emergency situation.

- Keep follow-up appointments to determine if a dosage adjustment is necessary.

EVALUATION

- The therapeutic effect is achieved.

- Adverse reactions are identified, reported to the primary health care provider, and managed appropriately.

- The patient verbalizes an understanding of the dosage regimen.

- The patient verbalizes the importance of complying with the prescribed therapeutic regimen and importance of continued follow-up care.

- The patient and family demonstrate an understanding of the drug regimen.

- The patient demonstrates an understanding of the importance of not suddenly discontinuing therapy (long-term or high-dose therapy).

Critical Thinking Exercises

1. Clomiphene has been prescribed for Judy Cowan, aged 28 years, to induce ovulation and pregnancy. Judy is very anxious and wants desperately to become pregnant. Her husband, Jim, has come to the clinic with her. Discuss assessments the nurse would consider important before treatment with clomiphene is initiated. Discuss information the nurse would include in a teaching plan for Jim and Judy.

2. Plan a team conference to discuss the administration of ACTH (corticotropin). Identify three critical points that would be essential to discuss. Explain your rationale for choosing each point.

3. Discuss the rationale for administering oral prednisone at 7 AM every other day.

Review Questions

1. Which of the following adverse reactions would the nurse expect with the administration of clomiphene?

   A. Edema

   B. Vasomotor flushes

   C. Sedation

   D. Hypertension

2. Which of the following assessments would be most important for the nurse to make when a child receiving growth hormone comes to the primary health care provider's office?

   A. Blood pressure, pulse, and respiration

   B. Diet history

   C. Height and weight

   D. Measurement of abdominal girth

3. Which of the following signs would lead the nurse to suspect a cushingoid appearance adverse reaction in a patient taking a corticosteroid?

   A. Moon face, hirsutism

   B. Kyphosis, periorbital edema

   C. Pallor of the skin, acne

   D. Exophthalmos

4. Which of the following statements, if made by the patient, would indicate a possible adverse reaction to the administration of vasopressin?

   A. "I am unable to see well at night."

   B. "My stomach is cramping."

   C. "I have a sore throat."

   D. "I am hungry all the time."

5. Adverse reactions to the administration of fludro-cortisone include _____.

   A. hyperactivity and headache

   B. sedation, lethargy

   C. edema, hypertension

   D. dyspnea, confusion

Medication Dosage Problems

1. Methylprednisolone 40 mg IM is prescribed. The drug is available in a suspension for injections in a solution of 20 mg/mL. The nurse prepares to administer _____.

2. Prednisolone 60 mg orally is prescribed. The drug is available as syrup of prednisolone 15 mg/5 mL. The nurse administers _____.

To check your answers, see Appendix G.

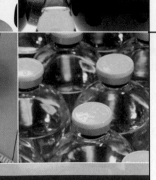

Thyroid and Antithyroid Drugs

Learning Objectives

On completion of this chapter, the student will:

- Identify the hormones produced by the thyroid gland.
- Discuss the uses, general drug actions, adverse reactions, contraindications, precautions, and interactions of thyroid and antithyroid drugs.
- Discuss important preadministration and ongoing assessment activities the

nurse should perform with the patient taking thyroid and antithyroid drugs.

- List the signs and symptoms of iodism (too much iodine) and iodine allergy.
- Discuss ways to promote an optimal response to therapy, how to manage adverse reactions, and important points to keep in mind when educating patients about the use of thyroid and antithyroid drugs.

The thyroid gland is located in the neck in front of the trachea. This highly vascular gland manufactures and secretes two hormones: thyroxine (T_4) and triiodothyronine (T_3). Iodine is an essential element for the manufacture of both of these hormones. The activity of the thyroid gland is regulated by thyroid-stimulating hormone, produced by the anterior pituitary gland (see Fig. 50-2 in Chapter 50). When the level of circulating thyroid hormones decreases, the anterior pituitary secretes thyroid-stimulating hormone, which then activates the cells of the thyroid to release stored thyroid hormones. This is an example of the feedback mechanism described in the nursing process section of Chapter 50.

Two diseases are related to the hormone-producing activity of the thyroid gland:

- **Hypothyroidism**—a decrease in the amount of thyroid hormones manufactured and secreted
- **Hyperthyroidism**—an increase in the amount of thyroid hormones manufactured and secreted

The symptoms of hypothyroidism and hyperthyroidism are given in Table 51-1. Thyroid hormones are used as replacement therapy when the patient is hypothyroid. By supplementing the decreased endogenous thyroid production and secretion with exogenous thyroid hormones, an attempt is made to create a **euthyroid** (normal thyroid) state.

Myxedema is a severe hypothyroidism manifested by lethargy, apathy, and memory impairment; emotional changes; slow speech and deep, coarse voice; thick, dry skin; cold intolerance; slow pulse; constipation; weight gain; and absence of menses. A severe form of hyperthyroidism, called **thyrotoxicosis** or **thyroid storm**, is characterized by high fever, extreme tachycardia, and altered mental status. Thyroid hormones are used to treat hypothyroidism and antithyroid drugs and radioactive iodine are used to treat hyperthyroidism.

Table 51.1 Signs and Symptoms of Thyroid Dysfunction

Body System or Function	Hypothyroidism	Hyperthyroidism
Metabolism	Decreased with anorexia, intolerance to cold, low body temperature, weight gain despite anorexia	Increased with increased appetite, intolerance to heat, elevated body temperature, weight loss despite increased appetite
Cardiovascular	Bradycardia, moderate hypotension	Tachycardia, moderate hypertension
Central nervous system	Lethargy, sleepiness	Nervousness, anxiety, insomnia, tremors, exophthalmos
Skin, skin structures	Pale, cool, dry skin; face appears puffy; coarse hair; nails thick and hard	Flushed, warm, moist skin, thinning hair, goiter
Ovarian function	Heavy menses, may be unable to conceive, loss of fetus possible	Irregular or scant menses
Testicular function	Low sperm count	

THYROID HORMONES

Thyroid hormones used in medicine include both the natural and synthetic hormones. The synthetic hormones are generally preferred because they are more uniform in potency than are the natural hormones obtained from animals. Thyroid hormones are listed in the Summary Drug Table: Thyroid and Antithyroid Drugs.

Actions

The thyroid hormones influence every organ and tissue of the body. These hormones are principally concerned with increasing the metabolic rate of tissues, which results in increases in the heart and respiratory rate, body temperature, cardiac output, oxygen consumption, and the metabolism of fats, proteins, and carbohydrates. The exact mechanisms by which the thyroid hormones exert their influence on body organs and tissues are not well understood.

Uses

Thyroid hormones are also used in the treatment or prevention of

- Euthyroid **goiter** (enlargement of a normal thyroid gland)
- Thyroid nodules and multinodular goiter
- Subacute or chronic lymphocytic thyroiditis (Hashimoto's disease)
- Thyroid cancer

Levothyroxine (Synthroid) is the drug of choice for hypothyroidism because it is relatively inexpensive, requires once-a-day dosage, and has a more uniform potency than do other thyroid hormone replacement drugs. The hormone may be used with the antithyroid drugs to treat thyrotoxicosis. Thyroid hormones also may be used as a diagnostic measure to differentiate suspected hyperthyroidism from euthyroidism.

Nursing Alert

All thyroid hormone replacement drugs are not equivalent. Patients should not change brands or types of thyroid hormone without first checking with their primary health care provider. The primary health care provider needs to determine the equivalent dosages when changing medication brands.

Adverse Reactions

Treatment of hypothyroidism is based on individualized doses of the hormone. During initial therapy, the most common adverse reactions are signs of overdose and hyperthyroidism as titration of the drug is being attempted (see Table 51-1). Adverse reactions other than symptoms of hyperthyroidism are rare.

Contraindications and Precautions

These drugs are contraindicated in patients with known hypersensitivity to the drug, an uncorrected adrenal cortical

SUMMARY DRUG TABLE   THYROID AND ANTITHYROID DRUGS

GENERIC NAME	TRADE NAME	USES	ADVERSE REACTIONS	DOSAGE RANGES
Thyroid Hormones				
levothyroxine sodium (T$_4$) *lee-voe-thye-rox'-een*	Levothroid, Levoxyl, Synthroid, Unithroid	Hypothyroidism, thyroid-stimulating hormone suppression, thyrotoxicosis, thyroid diagnostic testing	Palpitations, tachycardia, headache, nervousness, insomnia, diarrhea, vomiting, weight loss, fatigue, sweating, flushing	100–125 mcg/d orally
liothyronine sodium (T$_3$) *lye'-oh-thye'-roe-neen*	Cytomel, Trio stat	Same as levothyroxine	Same as levothyroxine	25–75 mcg/d orally
liotrix (T$_3$, T$_4$) *lye'-oh-trix*	Thyrolar	Same as levothyroxine	Same as levothyroxine	Initial: 1 Thyrolar half-grain tablet/d orally Maintenance: 1 Thyrolar, 1-grain or 2-grain tablet/d orally
thyroid USP desiccated		Same as levothyroxine	Same as levothyroxine	Initial: 30 mg/d orally Maintenance: 60–120 mg/d orally
Antithyroid Preparations				
methimazole *meth-im'-a-zole*	Tapazole	Hyperthyroidism	Numbness, headache, loss of hair, skin rash, nausea, vomiting, agranulocytosis	5–40 mg/d orally, divided doses at 8-h intervals
propylthiouracil (PTU) *proe-pill-thye-oh-yoor'-a-sill*		Same as methimazole	Same as methimazole	300–900 mg/d orally, divided doses at 8-h intervals
Iodine Products				
sodium iodide (^{131}I) *eye'-oh-dide*	Iodotope	Eradicate hyperthyroidism, selected cases of thyroid cancer	Bone marrow depression, nausea, vomiting, tachycardia, itching, rash, hives	Measured by a radioactivity calibration system before administering orally 4–10 microcuries Thyroid cancer: 50–150 mCi

insufficiency, or thyrotoxicosis. These drugs should not be used as a treatment for obesity or infertility. Thyroid hormone should not be used after a recent myocardial infarction. When hypothyroidism is a cause or contributing factor to a myocardial infarction or heart disease, the physician may prescribe small doses of thyroid hormone.

These drugs are used cautiously in patients with cardiac disease and during lactation. The thyroid hormones are classified as pregnancy category A and should be continued by hypothyroid women during pregnancy.

Interactions

The following interactions may occur with the thyroid hormones:

Interacting Drug	Common Use	Effect of Interaction
digoxin, beta blockers	Management of cardiac problems	Decreased effectiveness of cardiac drug
oral hypoglycemics and insulin	Treatment of diabetes	Increased risk of hypoglycemia
oral anticoagulants	Blood thinners	Prolonged bleeding
Selective serotonin reuptake inhibitors (SSRIs), antidepressants	Treatment of depression	Decreased effectiveness of thyroid drug
All other antidepressant drug categories	Treatment of depression	Increased effectiveness of thyroid drug

NURSING PROCESS

The Patient Receiving a Thyroid Hormone

ASSESSMENT

PREADMINISTRATION ASSESSMENT

After a patient receives a diagnosis of hypothyroidism and before therapy starts, the nurse takes vital signs and weighs the patient. A history of the patient's signs and symptoms is obtained. The nurse performs a general physical assessment to determine outward signs of hypothyroidism.

Gerontologic Alert

The symptoms of hypothyroidism may be confused with symptoms associated with aging, such as depression, cold intolerance, weight gain, confusion, or unsteady gait. The presence of these symptoms should be thoroughly evaluated and documented in the preadministration assessment and periodically throughout therapy.

ONGOING ASSESSMENT

The full effects of thyroid hormone replacement therapy may not be apparent for several weeks or more, but early effects may be apparent in as little as 48 hours. During the ongoing assessment, the nurse monitors the vital signs as ordered and observes the patient for signs of hyperthyroidism, which may signal excessive drug dosage. Signs of a therapeutic response include weight loss, mild diuresis, increased appetite, an increased pulse rate, and decreased puffiness of the face, hands, and feet. The patient may also report an increased sense of well-being and increased mental activity.

NURSING DIAGNOSES

Drug-specific nursing diagnoses are highlighted in the Nursing Diagnoses Checklist. Other nursing diagnoses applicable to these drugs are discussed in depth in Chapter 4.

Nursing Diagnoses Checklist

✓ **Risk for Ineffective Therapeutic Regimen Management** related to discomfort of adverse reactions during titration of individualized dosing

✓ **Anxiety** related to symptoms, adverse reactions, treatment regimen, other (specify)

PLANNING

The expected outcomes of the patient may include an optimal response to therapy, support of patient needs related to the management of adverse reactions, and an understanding of and compliance with the prescribed therapeutic regimen.

IMPLEMENTATION

PROMOTING AN OPTIMAL RESPONSE TO THERAPY

Thyroid hormones are administered once a day, early in the morning and preferably before breakfast. An empty stomach increases the absorption of the oral preparation. Levothyroxine (Synthroid) and liothyronine (Triostat) also can be given intravenously and are prepared for administration immediately before use.

MONITORING AND MANAGING PATIENT NEEDS

RISK FOR INEFFECTIVE THERAPEUTIC REGIMEN MANAGEMENT The dosage is individualized to the needs of the patient. The nurse monitors the patient for any adverse reactions, especially during the initial stages of dosage adjustment. If the dosage is inadequate, the patient will continue to experience signs of hypothyroidism (see Table 51-1). If the dosage is excessive, the patient will exhibit signs of hyperthyroidism. It is important for the nurse to monitor reactions and document them well to provide information for correct dosing. The primary health care provider makes dose adjustments carefully based on the patient's hormone responses. At times, several upward or downward dosage adjustments must be made until the optimal therapeutic dosage is reached and the patient becomes euthyroid.

ANXIETY Some patients may exhibit anxiety related to the symptoms of their disorder, as well as concern about relief of their symptoms. The patient should be reassured that although relief may not be immediate, symptoms should begin to decrease or even disappear in a few weeks.

Thyroid hormone replacement therapy in patients with diabetes may increase the intensity of the symptoms or the diabetes. The nurse closely monitors the patient with diabetes during thyroid hormone replacement therapy for signs of hyperglycemia (see Chapter 49) and notifies the primary health care provider if this problem occurs.

The nurse carefully observes patients who have cardiovascular disease and who take the thyroid hormones. The development of chest pain or worsening of cardiovascular disease should be reported to the primary health care provider immediately because the patient may require a reduction in the dosage of the thyroid hormone.

EDUCATING THE PATIENT AND FAMILY

Thyroid hormones are usually given on an outpatient basis. The nurse emphasizes the importance of taking the drug exactly as directed and not stopping the drug even though symptoms have improved. The nurse provides the following information to the patient and family when thyroid hormone replacement therapy is prescribed:

- Replacement therapy is for life, with the exception of transient hypothyroidism seen in those with thyroiditis.
- Do not increase, decrease, or skip a dose unless advised to do so by the primary health care provider.
- Take this drug in the morning, preferably before breakfast, unless advised by the primary health care provider to take it at a different time of day.
- Notify the primary health care provider if any of the following occur: headache, nervousness, palpitations, diarrhea, excessive sweating, heat intolerance, chest pain, increased pulse rate, or any unusual physical change or event.
- Normally, the dosage of this drug may require periodic adjustments. Dosage changes are based on a response to therapy and thyroid function tests.
- Therapy needs to be evaluated at periodic intervals, which may vary from every 2 weeks during the beginning of therapy to every 6 to 12 months once symptoms are controlled. Periodic thyroid function tests will be needed.
- Weigh yourself weekly and report any significant weight gain or loss to the primary health care provider.
- Do not change from one brand of this drug to another without consulting the primary health care provider.

EVALUATION

- The therapeutic effect is achieved.
- Adverse reactions are identified and reported to the primary health care provider.
- The patient verbalizes the importance of complying with the prescribed treatment regimen.
- The patient verbalizes an understanding of the treatment modalities and importance of continued follow-up care.
- The patient and family demonstrate an understanding of the drug regimen.

ANTITHYROID DRUGS

Antithyroid drugs or thyroid antagonists are used to treat hyperthyroidism. In addition to the antithyroid drugs, hyperthyroidism may be treated by the use of radioactive iodine (^{131}I), or by surgical removal of some or almost all of the thyroid gland (subtotal thyroidectomy).

Actions

Antithyroid drugs inhibit the manufacture of thyroid hormones. They do not affect existing thyroid hormones that are circulating in the blood or stored in the thyroid gland. For this reason, therapeutic effects of the antithyroid drugs may not be observed for 3 to 4 weeks. Antithyroid drugs are listed in the Summary Drug Table: Thyroid and Antithyroid Drugs.

Radioactive iodine is used because the thyroid has an affinity for iodine. The radioactive isotope accumulates in the cells of the thyroid gland, where destruction of thyroid cells occurs without damaging other cells throughout the body.

Not all patients respond adequately to antithyroid drugs; therefore, a thyroidectomy may be necessary. Antithyroid drugs may be administered before surgery to return the patient temporarily to an euthyroid state. When used for this reason, the vascularity of the thyroid gland is reduced typically using potassium iodide, and the tendency to bleed excessively during and immediately after surgery is decreased.

Uses

Methimazole (Tapazole) and propylthiouracil (PTU) are used for the medical management of hyperthyroidism. Potassium iodide may be given orally with methimazole or propylthiouracil to prepare for thyroid surgery. Radioactive iodine (^{131}I) may be used for treatment of hyperthyroidism and selected cases of cancer of the thyroid. The drug is given orally either as a solution or in a gelatin capsule.

Adverse Reactions

Generalized System Reactions

- Hay fever, sore throat, skin rash, fever, headache
- Nausea, vomiting, paresthesias

Severe System Reactions

- Agranulocytosis (decrease in the number of white blood cells)
- Exfoliative dermatitis, granulocytopenia, hypoprothrombinemia

Contraindications, Precautions, and Interactions

The antithyroid drugs are contraindicated in patients with hypersensitivity to the drug or any constituent of the drug.

Mothers taking methimazole or propylthiouracil should not breastfeed their children. Radioactive iodine (pregnancy category X) is contraindicated during pregnancy and lactation.

Methimazole and propylthiouracil are used with extreme caution during pregnancy (category D) because they can cause hypothyroidism in the fetus. However, if an antithyroid drug is necessary during pregnancy, propylthiouracil is the preferred drug because it does not cross the placenta. The potential for bleeding increases when these products are taken with oral anticoagulants.

NURSING PROCESS

The Patient Receiving an Antithyroid Drug

ASSESSMENT

PREADMINISTRATION ASSESSMENT

Before a patient starts therapy with an antithyroid drug, the nurse obtains a history of the symptoms of hyperthyroidism. It is important to include vital signs, weight, and a notation regarding the outward symptoms of the hyperthyroidism (see Table 51-1) in the physical assessment. If the patient is prescribed an iodine procedure, it is essential that the nurse take a careful allergy history, particularly to iodine or seafood (which contains iodine).

ONGOING ASSESSMENT

During the ongoing assessment, the nurse observes the patient for adverse drug effects. During short-term therapy before surgery, adverse drug reactions are usually minimal. Long-term therapy is usually on an outpatient basis. The nurse questions the patient regarding relief of symptoms, as well as signs or symptoms indicating an adverse reaction related to a decrease in blood cells, such as fatigue, fever, sore throat, easy bruising or bleeding, fever, cough, or any other signs of infection. As the patient becomes euthyroid, signs and symptoms of hyperthyroidism become less obvious. The nurse monitors the patient for signs of thyroid storm (high fever, extreme tachycardia, and altered mental status), which can occur in patients whose hyperthyroidism is inadequately treated.

NURSING DIAGNOSES

Drug-specific nursing diagnoses are highlighted in the Nursing Diagnoses Checklist. Other nursing diagnoses applicable to these drugs are discussed in depth in Chapter 4.

PLANNING

The expected outcomes of the patient may include an optimal response to therapy, support of patient needs related to the management of adverse reactions, and an understanding of and compliance with the prescribed drug regimen.

IMPLEMENTATION

PROMOTING AN OPTIMAL RESPONSE TO THERAPY

The patient with an enlarged thyroid gland may have difficulty swallowing the tablet. If this occurs, the nurse discusses the problem with the primary health care provider. Radioactive iodine is given by the primary health care provider, orally as a single dose. The effects of iodides are evident within 24 hours, with maximum effects attained after 10 to 15 days of continuous therapy. If the patient is hospitalized, radiation safety precautions identified by the hospital's department of nuclear medicine are followed.

Once an euthyroid state is achieved, the primary health care provider may add a thyroid hormone to the therapeutic regimen to prevent or treat hypothyroidism, which may develop slowly during long-term antithyroid drug therapy or after administration of ^{131}I.

The patient with hyperthyroidism is likely to have cardiac symptoms such as tachycardia or palpitations. Propranolol, an adrenergic blocking drug (see Chapter 28), may be prescribed by the primary health care provider as adjunctive treatment for several weeks until the therapeutic effects of the antithyroid drug are obtained.

MONITORING AND MANAGING PATIENT NEEDS

RISK FOR INEFFECTIVE THERAPEUTIC REGIMEN MANAGEMENT The patient with hyperthyroidism may be concerned with the results of medical treatment and with the problem of taking the drug at regular intervals around the clock (usually every 8 hours). Whereas some patients may be awake early in the morning and retire late at night, others may experience difficulty in an 8-hour dosage schedule. Another concern may be a tendency to forget the first dose early in the morning, thus causing a problem with the two following doses.

If the patient expresses a concern about the dosage schedule, the nurse may be able to offer suggestions. For example, the nurse may suggest the following 8-hour interval schedule: 7 AM, 3 PM, and 11 PM. The nurse may also suggest posting a notice on a bathroom mirror to remind the individual that the first dose is due immediately after rising. After a week or more of therapy, most patients remember to take their morning dose on time. If the first or last dose interferes with sleep, the nurse should suggest the patient discuss this with the primary health care provider.

RISK FOR INFECTION The nurse monitors the patient throughout therapy for adverse drug reactions. The nurse monitors the patient frequently for signs of agranulocytosis. It is important that the patient be protected from individuals with infectious disease because if agranulocytosis is present, the patient is at increased risk of contracting any infection, particularly an upper respiratory tract infection. The nurse monitors for signs of infection, particularly upper respiratory infection, in visitors and other health care personnel.

Nursing Alert

Agranulocytosis is potentially the most serious adverse reaction to methimazole and propylthiouracil. The nurse notifies the primary health care provider if shortness of breath, fever, sore throat, rash, headache, hay fever, yellow discoloration of the skin, or vomiting occurs.

RISK FOR IMPAIRED SKIN INTEGRITY If the patient experiences a rash while taking methimazole or propylthiouracil, the nurse carefully documents the affected areas, noting size, texture, and extent of the rash, and reports the occurrence of the rash to the primary health care provider. Soothing creams or lubricants may be applied, and soap is used sparingly, if at all, until the rash subsides.

EDUCATING THE PATIENT AND FAMILY

The nurse reviews with the patient and family the dosage and times the drug is to be taken. The following additional teaching points are included in a teaching plan:

METHIMAZOLE AND PROPYLTHIOURACIL

- Take these drugs at regular intervals around the clock (e.g., every 8 hours) unless directed otherwise by the primary health care provider.

- Do not take these drugs in larger doses or more frequently than as directed on the prescription container.

- Notify the primary health care provider promptly if any of the following occur: sore throat, fever, cough, easy bleeding or bruising, headache, or a general feeling of malaise.

- Record weight twice a week and notify the primary health care provider if there is any sudden weight gain or loss. (Note: the primary health care provider may also want the patient to monitor pulse rate. If this is recommended, the patient needs instruction in the proper technique and a recommendation to record the pulse rate and bring the record to the primary health care provider's office or clinic.)

- Avoid the use of nonprescription drugs unless the primary health care provider has approved the use of a specific drug.

RADIOACTIVE IODINE

- Follow the directions of the department of nuclear medicine regarding precautions to be taken. (*Note:* In some instances, the dosage is small and no special precautions may be necessary.)

- Keep in mind that tenderness and swelling of the neck, sore throat, and cough may occur in 2 to 3 days after the procedure

- Also keep in mind that thyroid hormone replacement therapy may be necessary if hypothyroidism develops.

- Schedule necessary follow-up evaluations to review the thyroid gland and the effectiveness of treatment.

EVALUATION

- The therapeutic effect is achieved.

- Adverse reactions are identified and reported to the primary health care provider.

- Anxiety is reduced.

- The patient verbalizes an understanding of the dosage regimen.

- The patient verbalizes the importance of complying with the prescribed treatment regimen.

- The patient and family demonstrate an understanding of the drug regimen.

Critical Thinking Exercises

1. Ms. Hartman, aged 47 years, has been prescribed levothyroxine (Synthroid) for hypothyroidism. Develop a teaching plan for Ms. Hartman that would provide her with the knowledge she needs to maintain a therapeutic treatment regimen.

2. Mr. Conrad will receive a dose of radioactive iodine from the primary health care provider. Discuss how you would prepare Mr. Conrad before the drug is administered. In preparation for dismissal, analyze

the most important points to stress to Mr. Conrad about radioactive iodine.

3. Ms. Coker, aged 38 years, is prescribed methimazole for hyperthyroidism. Discuss important preadministration assessments for Ms. Coker.

Review Questions

1. What adverse reaction is most likely to occur in the early days of therapy in a patient taking a thyroid hormone?

   A. Congestive heart failure

   B. Hyperthyroidism

   C. Hypothyroidism

   D. Euthyroidism

2. The nurse informs the patient that therapy with a thyroid hormone may not produce a therapeutic response for _____.

   A. 24 to 48 days

   B. 1 to 3 days

   C. several weeks or more

   D. 8 to 12 months

3. Which of the following symptoms best indicates that serious adverse reactions are developing in a patient receiving methimazole (Tapazole)?

   A. Fever, sore throat, bleeding from an injection site

   B. Cough, periorbital edema, constipation

   C. Constipation, anorexia, blurred vision

   D. Unsteady gait, blurred vision, insomnia

4. Which of the following statements made by a patient would indicate to the nurse that the patient is experiencing an adverse reaction to radioactive iodine?

   A. "I am sleepy most of the day."

   B. "I am unable to sleep at night."

   C. "My throat hurts when I swallow."

   D. "My body aches all over."

Medication Dosage Problems

1. Methimazole 40 mg is prescribed. The drug is available in 10-mg tablets. The nurse administers _____.

2. Levothyroxine 0.2 mg orally is prescribed. Available are 0.1-mg tablets. The nurse administers _____.

To check your answers, see Appendix G.

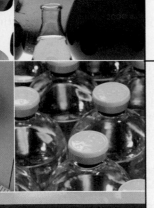

Chapter 52

Male and Female Hormones

Key Terms

anabolism
androgens
catabolism
endogenous
estradiol
estriol
estrogen
estrone
gynecomastia
menarche
progesterone
progestins
testosterone
virilization

Learning Objectives

On completion of this chapter, the student will:

- Discuss the medical uses, actions, adverse reactions, contraindications, precautions, and interactions of the male and female hormones.
- Discuss important preadministration and ongoing assessment activities the nurse should perform with the patient taking male or female hormones.

- List nursing diagnoses particular to a patient taking male or female hormones.
- Discuss ways to promote an optimal response to therapy, how to manage adverse reactions, and important points to keep in mind when educating the patient about the use of male or female hormones.

Male and female hormones play a vital role in the development and maintenance of secondary sex characteristics; they are necessary for human reproduction. Although hormones are naturally produced by the body, administration of a male or female hormone may be indicated in the treatment of certain disorders, such as an advanced-stage cancer, male hypogonadism, and male or female hormone deficiency. Hormones also are used as contraceptives and for treating the symptoms of menopause. Drugs to inhibit the activity of hormones are also used to treat cancers.

MALE HORMONES

Male hormones—**testosterone** and its derivatives—are collectively called **androgens**. Androgen secretion is under the influence of the anterior pituitary gland. Small amounts of male and female hormones are also produced by the adrenal cortex (see Chapter 50). The anabolic steroids are closely related to the androgen testosterone and have both androgenic and anabolic (stimulate cellular growth and repair) activity. Androgen hormone inhibitors inhibit the conversion of testosterone into a potent androgen.

Actions

Androgens

The male hormone testosterone and its derivatives actuate the reproductive potential in the adolescent boy. From puberty onward, androgens continue to aid in the development and maintenance of secondary sex characteristics: facial hair, deep voice, body hair, body fat distribution, and muscle development. Testosterone also stimulates the growth in size of the accessory sex organs (penis, testes, vas deferens, prostate) at the time of puberty. The androgens also promote tissue-building processes (**anabolism**) and reverse tissue-depleting processes (**catabolism**). Examples of androgens are fluoxymesterone (Halotestin), methyltestosterone (Testred), and testosterone. Additional examples of androgens are given in the Summary Drug Table: Male Hormones.

SUMMARY DRUG TABLE   MALE HORMONES

GENERIC NAME	TRADE NAME	USES	ADVERSE REACTIONS	DOSAGE RANGES
Androgens				
fluoxymesterone *floo-oxi-mes'-te-rone*	Halotestin	Males: hypogonadism, delayed puberty Females: inoperable advanced breast cancer	Nausea, vomiting, acne, hair thinning, headache, libido changes, anxiety, mood changes, hematopoietic and electrolyte imbalances Males: gynecomastia, testicular atrophy, erectile dysfunction Females: amenorrhea, virilization	Males: 5–20 mg/d orally Females: 10–40 mg/d orally
methyltestosterone *meth-ill-tess-toss'-ter-one*	Android, Testred	Same as fluoxymesterone	Same as fluoxymesterone	Males: 10–50 mg/d orally Females: 50–200 mg/d orally
testosterone *tess-toss'-ter-one*	Androderm, Androgel (Transdermal) Delatestryl, Depo-Testosterone (injectable), Striant (oral, buccal)	Primary or hypogonadotropic hypogonadism, delayed puberty	Same as fluoxymesterone	Buccal: 30 mg BID Gel: apply daily Injectable: 50–400 mg every 2–4 wk Pellet: 150–450 mg SC every 3–6 mo Transdermal 6 mg/d, apply patch daily
Anabolic Steroids				
nandrolone decanoate *nan'-droe-lone*		Anemia of renal insufficiency	Nausea, vomiting, diarrhea, acne, hair thinning, libido changes, anxiety, mood changes, edema, anemia, electrolyte imbalances Males: gynecomastia, testicular atrophy, sexual dysfunction Females: amenorrhea, virilization	50–200 mg/wk IM
oxymetholone	Anadrol-50	Anemia	Same as nandrolone decanoate	1–5 mg/kg/d orally
oxandrolone *oks-an'-droe-lone*	Oxandrin	Bone pain, weight gain, protein catabolism	Acne, hair thinning, libido changes, anxiety, mood changes, edema, electrolyte imbalances Males: gynecomastia, testicular atrophy, sexual dysfunction Females: amenorrhea, virilization	2.5–20 mg/d orally in divided doses
Androgen Hormone Inhibitors				
dutasteride	Avodart	Benign prostatic hypertrophy	Impotence, decreased libido	0.5 mg/d orally
finasteride *fin-as'-teh-ride*	Propecia, Proscar	Male-pattern baldness, benign prostatic hypertrophy	Impotence, decreased libido, asthenia, dizziness, postural hypotension	1–5 mg/d orally

Male and Female Hormones

Anabolic Steroids

The anabolic steroids are synthetic drugs chemically related to the androgens. Like the androgens, they promote tissue-building processes. Given in normal doses, they have a minimal effect on the accessory sex organs and secondary sex characteristics. Examples of anabolic steroids are given in the Summary Drug Table: Male Hormones.

Androgen Hormone Inhibitor

The androgen hormone inhibitors are synthetic compound drugs that inhibit the conversion of testosterone into the potent androgen 5-alpha (α)-dihydrotestosterone (DHT). The development of the prostate gland is dependent on DHT. The lowering of serum levels of DHT reduces the effect of this hormone on the prostate gland, resulting in a decrease in the size of the gland and the symptoms associated with prostatic gland enlargement. Examples of androgen hormone inhibitors include finasteride (Proscar) and dutasteride (Avodart).

Uses

Androgen therapy may be given as replacement therapy for
- Testosterone deficiency
- Hypogonadism (failure of the testes to develop)
- Delayed puberty
- Development of testosterone deficiency after puberty

In the female patient, androgen therapy may be used for
- Postmenopausal, metastatic breast carcinoma
- Premenopausal, hormone-dependent metastatic breast carcinoma

The transdermal testosterone system is used as replacement therapy when endogenous testosterone is deficient or absent.

Anabolic steroid use includes
- Management of anemia of renal insufficiency
- Control of metastatic breast cancer in women
- Promotion of weight gain in those with weight loss after surgery, trauma, or infections

Androgen hormone inhibitors are used in the treatment of
- Prevention of male pattern baldness
- Symptoms associated with benign prostatic hypertrophy (BPH), which include difficulty starting the urinary stream, frequent passage of small amounts of urine, and having to urinate during the night (nocturia). Several months of therapy may be required before a significant improvement is noted and symptoms of BPH decrease.

Nursing Alert

The use of anabolic steroids to promote an increase in muscle mass and strength has become a serious problem. Anabolic steroids are not intended for this use. Unfortunately, deaths in young, healthy individuals have been directly attributed to the use of these drugs. Nurses should discourage the illegal use of anabolic steroids to increase muscle mass.

Adverse Reactions

Androgens

In men, administration of an androgen may result in breast enlargement (**gynecomastia**), testicular atrophy, inhibition of testicular function, impotence, enlargement of the penis, nausea, vomiting, jaundice, headache, anxiety, male pattern baldness, acne, and depression. Fluid and electrolyte imbalances, which include sodium, water, chloride, potassium, calcium, and phosphate retention, may also occur.

In women receiving an androgen preparation for breast carcinoma, the most common adverse reactions are amenorrhea, other menstrual irregularities, and **virilization** (acquisition of male sexual characteristics by a woman). Virilization produces facial hair, a deepening of the voice, and enlargement of the clitoris. Male pattern baldness and acne may also result.

Anabolic Steroids

Virilization in the woman is the most common reaction associated with anabolic steroids, especially when higher doses are used. Acne occurs frequently in all age groups and both sexes. Nausea, vomiting, diarrhea, fluid and electrolyte imbalances (the same as for the androgens, discussed previously), testicular atrophy, jaundice, anorexia, and muscle cramps may also be seen. Blood-filled cysts of the liver and sometimes the spleen, malignant and benign liver tumors, an increased risk of atherosclerosis, and mental changes are the most serious adverse reactions that may occur during prolonged use.

Many serious adverse drug reactions are being reported in healthy individuals using anabolic steroids. There is some indication that prolonged high-dose use has resulted in psychological and possibly physical dependence, and some individuals have required treatment in drug abuse centers. Severe mental changes, such as uncontrolled rage, severe depression, suicidal tendencies, malignant and benign liver tumors, aggressive behavior, increased risk of atherosclerosis, inability to concentrate, and personality

---

Display 52.1 Drugs for Erectile Dysfunction

Erectile dysfunction results from a failure of the penile corpus cavernosum to become engorged with blood, preventing sexual intercourse. This condition can be a result of age-related, neurologic, or vascular changes in the tissue. A number of oral drugs are now on the market that can facilitate blood flow into the penis, resulting in an erection.

Generic Name	Trade Name	Duration of Action
sildenafil	Viagra	30 minutes to 4 hours before sexual activity
tadalafil	Cialis	Up to 36 hours before sexual activity
vardenafil	Levitra	1 hour before sexual activity

Because these drugs affect smooth muscle, patients with preexisting cardiac problems should discuss use with their primary health care provider before using the drug. Medical attention should be sought for erections sustained for more than 4 hours. Ocular problems may occur when using these drugs; again, the primary health care provider should be consulted before use.

---

changes are not uncommon. In addition, the incidence of the severe adverse reactions cited earlier appears to be increased in those using anabolic steroids for this purpose.

Androgen Hormone Inhibitor

Adverse reactions usually are mild and do not require discontinuing use of the drug. Adverse reactions, when they occur, are related to the sexual drive and include impotence, decreased libido, and a decreased volume of ejaculate. For more information, see Display 52-1.

Contraindications and Precautions

The male hormones and hormone inhibitors are contraindicated in patients with known hypersensitivity to the drugs, liver disorders, or serious cardiac disease, and in men with prostate gland disorders (e.g., prostate carcinoma and prostate enlargement). These drugs are classified as pregnancy category X drugs and should not be administered during pregnancy and lactation. Anabolic steroids are contraindicated for use to enhance physical appearance or athletic performance. Anabolic steroids should be used cautiously in older men because of increased risk of prostate enlargement and prostate cancer.

Interactions

The following interactions may occur with the male hormones and male hormone inhibitors:

Interacting Drug	Common Use	Effect of Interaction
oral anticoagulants	Blood thinners	Increased antidiuretic effect
imipramine and androgen	Treatment of depression	Increased risk of paranoid behavior
sulfonylureas and anabolic steroids	Anti-infective	Increased risk of hypoglycemia

Herbal Alert

Saw palmetto is used to relieve the symptoms of BPH. The herb reduces urinary frequency, increases the flow of urine, and decreases the incidence of nocturia. Saw palmetto may delay the need for prostate surgery. The dosage of the herb is

- 160 mg twice daily of standardized extract
- One 585-mg capsule or tablet up to three times daily
- 20 to 30 drops up to four times a day (tincture, 1:2 liquid extract)

It is not recommended to take saw palmetto as a tea because the active constituents are not water soluble. Improvement can be seen after 1 to 3 months of therapy. It is usually recommended that the herb be taken for 6 months, followed by evaluation by a primary health care provider.

NURSING PROCESS

The Patient Receiving a Male Hormone

ASSESSMENT

PREADMINISTRATION ASSESSMENT

Assessment of the patient receiving an androgen or anabolic steroid depends on the drug, the patient, and the reason for administration.

ANDROGENS In most instances, androgens are administered to the man on an outpatient basis. Before and during therapy, the primary health care provider may order electrolyte studies because use of these drugs can result in fluid and electrolyte imbalances.

When these drugs are given to the female patient with advanced breast carcinoma, the nurse evaluates the patient's current status (physical, emotional, and nutritional) carefully and records the findings in the patient's chart. Problem areas, such as pain, any limitation of motion, and the ability to participate in the activities of daily living, are carefully evaluated and recorded in the patient's record. The nurse takes and records vital signs and weight. Baseline laboratory tests may include a complete blood count, hepatic function tests, serum electrolytes, and serum and urinary calcium levels. The nurse reviews these tests and notes any abnormalities.

ANABOLIC STEROIDS The nurse evaluates and records the patient's physical and nutritional status before starting therapy with anabolic steroids. The nurse takes the patient's weight, blood pressure, pulse, and respiratory rate. Baseline laboratory studies may include a complete blood count, hepatic function tests, and serum electrolytes and serum lipid levels. The nurse reviews these studies and notes any abnormalities.

ANDROGEN HORMONE INHIBITOR The nurse questions the patient at length about symptoms of BPH, such as frequency of voiding during the day and night and difficulty starting the urinary stream. The nurse records all symptoms in the patient's chart.

> ### Nursing Alert
>
> Women who are pregnant or may become pregnant should not handle crushed or broken finasteride (Propecia, Proscar) or dutasteride (Avodart) tablets or capsules. Absorption of the drug poses substantial risk for abnormal growth to a male fetus.

ONGOING ASSESSMENT

The ongoing assessment depends on the reason the drug was prescribed and the condition of the patient. Men receiving an androgen or anabolic steroid are questioned by the primary health care provider or nurse regarding the effectiveness of drug therapy.

The nurse weighs the patient with advanced breast carcinoma daily or as ordered by the primary health care provider. If the patient is on complete bed rest, the nurse may measure weight every 3 to 4 days (or as ordered)

using a bed scale. The nurse notifies the primary health care provider if there is a significant (5-lb) increase or decrease in the weight. The nurse checks the lower extremities daily for signs of edema.

> ### Nursing Alert
>
> The nurse observes the patient each day for adverse drug reactions, especially signs of fluid and electrolyte imbalance, jaundice (which may indicate hepatotoxicity), and virilization. The primary health care provider must be alerted to any signs of fluid and electrolyte imbalance or jaundice.

The nurse takes vital signs every 4 to 8 hours, depending on the patient's condition, and then evaluates the patient's response to drug therapy based on original assessment findings. Possible responses include a decrease in pain, an increase in appetite, and a feeling of well-being.

> ### Chronic Care Alert
> When the androgens are administered to a patient with diabetes, blood glucose levels should be measured frequently because glucose tolerance may be altered. Adjustments may need to be made in insulin dosage, oral antidiabetic drugs, or diet. The nurse monitors the patient for signs for hypoglycemia and hyperglycemia (see Chapter 49).

When anabolic steroids are used for weight gain, the nurse weighs the patient at intervals ranging from daily to weekly. A good dietary regimen is necessary to promote weight gain. The nurse consults the dietitian if the patient eats poorly.

NURSING DIAGNOSES

Drug-specific nursing diagnoses are highlighted in the Nursing Diagnoses Checklist. Other nursing diagnoses applicable to these drugs are discussed in depth in Chapter 4.

> ### Nursing Diagnoses Checklist
> ✓ **Excess Fluid Volume** related to adverse reactions (sodium and water retention)
> ✓ **Disturbed Body Image** (in the female) related to adverse reactions (virilization)

PLANNING

The expected outcomes of the patient may include an optimal response to therapy, support of patient needs related to the management of adverse reactions, and an understanding of and compliance with the prescribed therapeutic regimen.

IMPLEMENTATION

PROMOTING AN OPTIMAL RESPONSE TO THERAPY

If the androgen is to be administered as a buccal tablet, the nurse demonstrates the placement of the tablet and warns the patient not to swallow the tablet but to allow it to dissolve in the mouth. The nurse reminds the patient not to smoke or drink water until the tablet is dissolved. Oral and parenteral androgens are often taken or given by injection on an outpatient basis. When given by injection, the injection is administered deep intramuscularly (IM) into the gluteal muscle. Alternatively, a pellet dose is placed under the skin and repeated every 3 to 6 months. Oral testosterone is given with or before meals to decrease gastrointestinal (GI) upset.

Androderm is a transdermal system that is applied nightly to clean, dry skin on the abdomen, thigh, back, or upper arm. This system is not applied to the scrotum. Sites are rotated, with 7 days between applications to any specific site. The system is applied immediately after opening the pouch and removing the protective covering. If the patient has not exhibited a therapeutic response after 8 weeks of therapy, another form of testosterone replacement therapy should be considered.

Testosterone gel (Androgel) is applied once daily (preferably in the morning) to clean, dry, intact skin of the shoulders and upper arms or abdomen. After the packet is opened, the contents are squeezed into the palm of the hand and immediately applied to the application sites. The application sites are allowed to dry before the patient gets dressed. The gel is not applied to the genitals.

MONITORING AND MANAGING PATIENT NEEDS

The nurse observes the patient receiving an androgen or anabolic steroid for signs of adverse drug reactions.

EXCESS FLUID VOLUME Sodium and water retention may also occur with androgen or anabolic steroid administration, causing the patient to become edematous. In addition, other electrolyte imbalances, such as hypercalcemia, may occur. The nurse monitors the patient for fluid and electrolyte disturbances (see Chapter 58 for signs and symptoms of electrolyte disturbance).

Gerontologic Alert

Older adults with cardiac problems or kidney disease are at increased risk for sodium and water retention when taking the androgens or anabolic steroids.

The nurse makes a daily comparison of the patient's preadministration weight with current weights and makes sure to note the appearance of puffy eyelids and dependent swelling of the hands or feet (if the patient is ambulatory) or the sacral area (if the patient is nonambulatory) and reports any findings to the primary health care provider. The nurse monitors the daily fluid intake and output to calculate fluid balance.

DISTURBED BODY IMAGE With long-term administration of a male hormone, the female patient may experience mild to moderate masculine changes (virilization), namely, facial hair, a deepening of the voice, and enlargement of the clitoris. Male-pattern baldness, patchy hair loss, skin pigmentation, and acne may also result. Although these adverse effects are not life-threatening, they often are distressing and only add to the patient's discomfort and anxiety. These problems may be easy to identify, but they are not always easy to solve. If hair loss occurs, the nurse can suggest wearing a wig; mild skin pigmentation may be covered with makeup, but severe and widespread pigmented areas and acne are often difficult to conceal. Each patient is different, and the emotional responses to these outward changes may range from severe depression to a positive attitude and acceptance. The nurse works with the patient as an individual, first identifying the problems, and then helping the patient, when possible, to deal with these changes.

EDUCATING THE PATIENT AND THE FAMILY

The nurse explains the dosage regimen and possible adverse drug reactions to the patient and family and develops a teaching plan to include the following points:

ANDROGENS

- Notify the primary health care provider if any of the following occur: nausea, vomiting, swelling of the legs, or jaundice. Women should report any signs of virilization to the primary health care provider.

- Oral tablets—Take with food or a snack to avoid GI upset.

- Buccal tablets—Place the tablet between the cheek and molars and allow it to dissolve in the mouth. Do not smoke or drink water until the tablet is dissolved.

- Testosterone transdermal system—Apply according to the directions supplied with the product. Be sure the skin is clean and dry and the placement area is free of hair. Do not store outside the pouch or use damaged systems. Discard systems in household trash in a safe manner to prevent ingestion by children or pets.

ANABOLIC STEROIDS

- Anabolic steroids may cause nausea and GI upset. Take this drug with food or meals.

- Keep all primary health care provider or clinic visits because close monitoring of therapy is essential.

- *Female patients*: Notify the primary health care provider if signs of virilization occur.

ANDROGEN HORMONE INHIBITOR

- Take this drug without regard to meals.

- Inform the primary health care provider immediately if sexual partner is or may become pregnant because additional measures, such as discontinuing the drug or use of a condom, may be necessary.

- Women who are or may become pregnant should not handle this medication.

EVALUATION

- The therapeutic response is achieved.

- Adverse reactions are identified and reported to the primary health care provider.

- The patient verbalizes the importance of complying with the prescribed treatment regimen.

- The patient and family demonstrate an understanding of the drug regimen.

- The patient verbalizes an understanding of treatment modalities and importance of continued follow-up care.

FEMALE HORMONES

The two **endogenous** (produced by the body) female hormones are **estrogen** and **progesterone**. Like the androgens, their production is under the influence of the anterior pituitary gland. The endogenous estrogens are **estradiol**, **estrone**, and **estriol**. The most potent of these three estrogens is estradiol. Examples of estrogens used as drugs include estropipate (Ortho-Est) and estradiol (Estrace).

There are natural and synthetic progesterones, which are collectively called **progestins**. Examples of progestins used as drugs include medroxyprogesterone (Provera) and norethindrone (Aygestin). Examples of estrogens and progestins are given in the Summary Drug Table: Female Hormones.

Actions

Estrogens

The estrogens are secreted by the ovarian follicle and in smaller amounts by the adrenal cortex. Estrogens are important in the development and maintenance of the female reproductive system and the primary and secondary sex characteristics. At puberty, they promote growth and development of the vagina, uterus, fallopian tubes, and breasts. They also affect the release of pituitary gonadotropins (see Chapter 50).

Other actions of estrogen include fluid retention, protein anabolism, thinning of the cervical mucus, and the inhibition or facilitation of ovulation. Estrogens contribute to the conservation of calcium and phosphorus, the growth of pubic and axillary hair, and pigmentation of the breast nipples and genitals. Estrogens also stimulate contraction of the fallopian tubes (which promotes movement of the ovum). They modify the physical and chemical properties of the cervical mucus, and restore the endometrium after menstruation.

Progestins

Progesterone is secreted by the corpus luteum, placenta, and in small amounts by the adrenal cortex. Progesterone and its derivatives (i.e., the progestins) transform the proliferative endometrium into a secretory endometrium. Progestins are necessary for the development of the placenta and inhibit the secretion of pituitary gonadotropins, which in turn prevents maturation of the ovarian follicle and ovulation. The synthetic progestins are usually preferred for medical use because of the decreased effectiveness of progesterone when administered orally.

Uses

Estrogens

Estrogen is most commonly used in combination with progesterones as a contraceptive agent or as estrogen replacement therapy (ERT) in postmenopausal women. In addition, the estrogens are used in

- Relief of moderate to severe vasomotor symptoms of menopause (flushing, sweating)

- Treatment of female hypogonadism

- Treatment of atrophic vaginitis

- Treatment of osteoporosis in women past menopause

- Palliative treatment of advanced prostatic carcinoma

- Selected cases of advanced breast carcinoma

SUMMARY DRUG TABLE   FEMALE HORMONES

GENERIC NAME	TRADE NAME	USES	ADVERSE REACTIONS	DOSAGE RANGES
Estrogens				
estrogens, conjugated *ess'-troe-jens*	Premarin	Oral: vasomotor symptoms associated with menopause, atrophic vaginitis, osteoporosis, hypogonadism, primary ovarian failure, breast and prostate cancer palliation Parenteral: abnormal uterine bleeding from hormonal imbalance	Headache, dizziness, melasma, venous thromboembolism, nausea, vomiting, abdominal bloating and cramps, breakthrough bleeding/ spotting, vaginal changes, rhinitis, changes in libido, breast enlargement and tenderness, weight changes, generalized pain	0.3–2.5 mg/d orally; IM: 25 mg/injection
estrogens, esterified	Menest	Same as conjugated estrogens	Same as conjugated estrogens	0.3–1.25 mg/d orally
estrogens, topical	Estrogel	Vaginal atrophy and vasomotor symptoms associated with menopause	Rare: minor vaginal irritation or itching	Metered dose for daily application
estrogens, vaginal	Estring, Femring; Estrace, Ogen, and Premarin Vaginal Creams	Vaginal atrophy and vasomotor symptoms associated with menopause	Rare: minor vaginal irritation or itching	See package insert; used weekly or monthly
estradiol, oral *ess-troe-dye'-ole*	Estrace, Femtrace, Gynodiol	Vasomotor symptoms associated with menopause, osteoporosis prevention, hypoestrogenism palliative therapy for breast and prostate cancer	Same as conjugated estrogens	0.5–10 mg/d orally
estradiol cypionate *ess-troe-dye'-ole 'sip-ee-oh-nate*	Depo-Estradiol	Moderate to severe vasomotor symptoms associated with menopause, female hypogonadism	Same as conjugated estrogens; pain at injection site	1–5 mg IM, every 3–4 wk
estradiol hemihydrate	Vagifem	Atrophic vaginitis	Same as conjugated estrogens	I tablet vaginally daily
estradiol transdermal system	Alora, Climara, Estraderm, Menostar, Vivelle	Same as conjugated estrogens	Same as conjugated estrogens	Variable doses, applied to skin weekly
estradiol topical emulsion	Estrasorb	Vasomotor symptoms of menopause		Two prepackaged pouches/d
estradol valerate *ess-troc-dye'-ole val'-eh-rate*	Delestrogen	Same as estradiol cypionate	Same as conjugated estrogens; pain at injection site	10–20 mg IM monthly
estropipate *ess-troe-pi'-pate*	Ogen (cream), Ortho-Est (tablet)	Moderate to severe vasomotor symptoms associated with menopause, female hypogonadism, ovarian failure, osteoporosis	Same as conjugated estrogens	0.625–9 mg/d orally

SUMMARY DRUG TABLE (*continued*)

GENERIC NAME	TRADE NAME	USES	ADVERSE REACTIONS	DOSAGE RANGES
synthetic conjugated estrogens, A	Cenestin	Moderate to severe vasomotor symptoms associated with menopause, vaginal atrophy	Same as conjugated estrogens	0.45 mg/d orally, then adjust according to symptoms
synthetic conjugated estrogens, B	Enjuvia	Moderate to severe vasomotor symptoms associated with menopause	Same as conjugated estrogens	0.3 mg/d orally, then adjust according to symptoms
Progestins				
progesterone *pro-jess'-te-rone*	Crinone, Prometrium	Endometrial hyperplasia (oral), amenorrhea, abnormal uterine bleeding (injection), infertilty (gel)	Breakthrough bleeding, spotting, change in menstrual flow, amenorrhea, breast tenderness, weight gain or loss, melasma, insomnia	Orally: 200 mg for 12 d of cycle IM: 5–10 mg/d for 6–8 d Gel: 90 mg/d
medroxy-progesterone acetate *me-drox'-ee-proe-jess'-te-rone*	Provera	Amenorrhea, abnormal uterine bleeding, endometrial hypoplasia	Same as progesterone	5–10 mg/d orally
norethinerone acetate *nor-eth-in'-drone*	Aygestin	Amenorhea, abnormal uterine bleeding, endometriosis	Same as hydroxyprogesterone caproate	2.5–10 mg/d for 5–10 d of cycle
Combination Products				
estrogens and progestins combined	ClimaraPro, CombiPatch, Femhrt, Prefest, Premphase, Prempro	Treatment of moderate to severe vasomotor symptoms associated with menopause, treatment of vulval and vaginal atrophy, osteoporosis	Adverse reactions of both hormones; same as synthetic conjugated estrogens and progesterone	Oral or transdermal, variable dosing, used daily or weekly. See package insert.
Miscellanous Drug				
raloxifene	Evista	Osteoporosis prevention and treatment	Hot flashes, flulike symptoms, arthralgia, rhinitis, increased cough	60 mg/d orally

The estradiol transdermal system is also used after removal of the ovaries in premenopausal women (female castration) and primary ovarian failure.

Estrogen is given IM or intravenously (IV) to treat uterine bleeding caused by hormonal imbalance. When estrogen is used to treat menopausal symptoms in a woman with an intact uterus, concurrent use of progestin is recommended to decrease the risk of endometrial cancer. After a hysterectomy, estrogen alone may be used for ERT.

The estrogens, in combination with a progestin, are also used as oral contraceptives (Table 52-1). The uses of individual estrogens are given in the Summary Drug Table: Female Hormones.

Progestins

The progestins are used in the treatment of amenorrhea, endometriosis, and functional uterine bleeding. Progestins are also used as oral contraceptives, either alone or in combination with an estrogen (see the Summary Drug Table: Female Hormones; see also Table 52-1).

Contraceptive Hormones

Combination estrogens and progestins are used as oral contraceptives. There are three types of estrogen and progestin combination oral contraceptives: monophasic, biphasic, and triphasic. The monophasic oral contraceptives provide a fixed dose of estrogen and progestin

Table 52.1 Oral Contraceptives

Generic Name	Trade Name
Monophasic Oral Contraceptives	
50 mcg ethinyl estradiol acetate, 1 mg norethindrone	Norinyl 1 + 50, Ortho-Novum 1/50
50 mcg ethinyl estradiol, 1 mg ethynodiol diacetate	Demulen 1/50, Zovia 1/50E
35 mcg ethinyl estradiol, 1 mg norethindrone	Norinyl 1 + 135, Ortho-Novum 1/35
35 mcg ethinyl estradiol, 0.5 mg norethindrone	Brevicon, Modicon
35 mcg ethinyl estradiol, 0.4 mg norethindrone	Ovcon-35
35 mcg ethinyl estradiol, 0.25 mg norgestimate	Ortho-Cyclen, Sprintec
35 mcg ethinyl estradiol, 1 mg ethynodiol diacetate	Demulen 1/35, Zovia 1/35E
30 mcg ethinyl estradiol, 1.5 mg norethindrone acetate	Loestrin 21 1.5/30, Loestrin Fe 1.5/30, Microgestin Fe 1.5/30
30 mcg ethinyl estradiol, 0.3 mg norgestrel	Lo/Ovral, Low-Ogestrel, Cryselle
30 mcg ethinyl estradiol, 0.15 mg desogestrel	Desogen
30 mcg ethinyl estradiol, 0.15 mg levonorgestrel	Levora, Nordette, Portia
30 mcg ethinyl estradiol, 3 mg drospirenone	Yasmin
20 mcg ethinyl estradiol, 1 mg norethindrone acetate	Loestrin 21 1/20, Loestrin Fe 1/20, Microgestin Fe 1/20
20 mcg ethinyl estradiol, 0.1 mg levonorgestrel	Alesse, Aviane, Lessina, Levlite
50 mcg mestranol, 1 mg norethindrone acetate	Norinyl 1 + 50, Ortho-Novum 1/50
Biphasic Oral Contraceptives	
Phase one: 35 mcg ethinyl estradiol, 0.5 mg norethindrone Phase two: 35 mcg ethinyl estradiol, 1 mg norethindrone	Necon 10/11, Ortho-Novum 10/11
Triphasic Oral Contraceptives	
Phase one: 35 mcg ethinyl estradiol, 0.5 mg norethindrone Phase two: 35 mcg ethinyl estradiol, 1 mg norethindrone Phase three: 35 mcg ethinyl estradiol, 0.5 mg norethindrone	Tri-Norinyl
Phase one: 35 mcg ethinyl estradiol, 0.5 mg norethindrone Phase two: 35 mcg ethinyl estradiol, 0.75 mg norethindrone Phase three: 35 mcg ethinyl estradiol, 1 mg norethindrone	Ortho-Novum 7/7/7
Phase one: 30 mcg ethinyl estradiol, 0.05 mg levonorgestrel Phase two: 40 mcg ethinyl estradiol, 0.075 mg levonorgestrel Phase three: 30 mcg ethinyl estradiol, 0.125 mg levonorgestrel	Triphasil, Trivora, Enpresse
Phase one: 35 mcg ethinyl estradiol, 0.18 mg norgestimate Phase two: 35 mcg ethinyl estradiol, 0.215 mg norgestimate Phase three: 35 mcg ethinyl estradiol, 0.25 mg norgestimate	Ortho Tri-Cyclen, Tri-Sprintec, Tri-Previfem
Phase one: 25 mcg ethinyl estradiol, 0.18 mg norgestimate Phase two: 25 mcg ethinyl estradiol, 0.215 mg norgestimate Phase three: 25 mcg ethinyl estradiol, 0.25 mg norgestimate	Ortho Tri-Cyclen Lo
Phase one: 1 mg norethindrone acetate, 20 mcg ethinyl estradiol Phase two: 30 mcg ethinyl estradiol, 1 mg norethindrone acetate Phase three: 35 mcg ethinyl estradiol, 1 mg norethindrone acetate	Estrostep Fe

Table 52.1 (continued)

Generic Name	Trade Name
Triphasic Oral Contraceptives	
Phase one: 25 mcg ethinyl estradiol, 0.1 mg desogestrel	Cyclessa
Phase two: 25 mcg ethinyl estradiol, 0.125 mg norgestimate	
Phase three: 25 mcg ethinyl estradiol, 0.15 mg norgestimate	
Progestin-Only Contraceptive	
0.35 mg norethindrone	Camila, Errin, Nor-QD

throughout the cycle. The biphasic and triphasic oral contraceptives deliver hormones similar to the levels naturally produced by the body (see Table 52-1). The oral contraceptives have changed a great deal since their introduction in the 1960s. Today, lower hormone dosages provide reduced levels of hormones compared with the older formulations, while retaining the same degree of effectiveness (more than 99% when used as prescribed).

Taking the contraceptive hormones provides health benefits not related to contraception, such as regulating the menstrual cycle and decreasing menstrual blood loss, the incidence of iron deficiency anemia, and dysmenorrhea. Health benefits related to the inhibition of ovulation include a decrease in ovarian cysts and ectopic pregnancies. In addition, there is a decrease in fibrocystic breast disease, acute pelvic inflammatory disease, endometrial cancer, and ovarian cancer, improved maintenance of bone density, and a decrease in symptoms related to endometriosis in women taking contraceptive hormones. Newer combination contraceptives such as norgestimate and ethinyl estradiol combinations (Ortho Tri-Cyclen) have been shown to help reduce moderate acne and maintain clear skin in women 15 years of age or older (who menstruate, want contraception, and have no response to topical antiacne medications).

Adverse Reactions: Estrogens

Administration of estrogens by any route may result in many adverse reactions, although the incidence and intensity of these reactions vary. Some of the adverse reactions seen with the administration of estrogens follow.

Central Nervous System Reactions

- Headache, migraine
- Dizziness, mental depression

Dermatologic Reactions

- Dermatitis, pruritus
- Chloasma (pigmentation of the skin) or melasma (discoloration of the skin), which may continue when use of the drug is discontinued

Gastrointestinal Reactions

- Nausea, vomiting
- Abdominal bloating and cramps

Genitourinary Reactions

- Breakthrough bleeding, withdrawal bleeding, spotting, change in menstrual flow
- Dysmenorrheal, premenstrual-like syndrome, amenorrhea
- Vaginal candidiasis, cervical erosion, vaginitis

Local Reactions

- Pain at injection site or sterile abscess with parenteral form of the drug
- Redness and irritation at the application site with transdermal system

Ophthalmic Reactions

- Steepening of corneal curvature
- Intolerance to contact lenses

Miscellaneous Reactions

- Edema, rhinitis, changes in libido
- Breast pain, enlargement, and tenderness
- Reduced carbohydrate tolerance
- Venous thromboembolism, pulmonary embolism
- Weight gain or loss
- Generalized and skeletal pain

Warnings associated with the administration of estrogen include an increased risk of endometrial cancer, gallbladder disease, hypertension, hepatic adenoma (a benign tumor of the liver), cardiovascular disease, and thromboembolic disease, and hypercalcemia in those with breast cancer and bone metastases.

Adverse Reactions: Progestins

Administration of the progestins by any route may result in many adverse reactions, although the incidence and intensity of these reactions vary. Progestin administration may result in

- Breakthrough bleeding, spotting, change in the menstrual flow, amenorrhea

- Breast tenderness, edema, weight increase or decrease

- Acne, chloasma or melasma, insomnia, mental depression

In addition to the adverse reactions seen with progestins, the use of a levonorgestrel implant system may result in bruising after insertion, scar tissue formation at the site of insertion, and hyperpigmentation at the implant site. The use of medroxyprogesterone acetate contraceptive injection may result in the same adverse reactions as those associated with administration of any progestin.

Adverse Reactions: Contraceptive Hormones

When estrogen–progestin combinations are used as oral contraceptives, these drugs may exhibit adverse reactions that vary depending on their estrogen or progestin content, so the adverse reactions of each must be considered. Table 52-2 identifies the symptoms of estrogen and progestin excess or deficiency. The adverse effects are minimized by adjusting the estrogen–progestin balance or dosage.

Contraindications and Precautions

Estrogen and progestin therapy is contraindicated in patients with known hypersensitivity to the drugs, breast cancer (except for metastatic disease), estrogen-dependent neoplasms, undiagnosed abnormal genital bleeding, and thromboembolic disorders. The progestins also are contraindicated in patients with cerebral hemorrhage or impaired liver function. Both the estrogens and progestins are classified as pregnancy category X drugs and are contraindicated during pregnancy.

The estrogens are used cautiously in patients with gallbladder disease, hypercalcemia (may lead to severe hypercalcemia in patients with breast cancer and bone metastasis), cardiovascular disease, and liver impairment. Cardiovascular complications are greater in women who smoke and use estrogen. The progestins are used cautiously in patients with a history of migraine headaches, epilepsy, asthma, and cardiac or renal impairment.

The warnings associated with the use of oral contraceptives are the same as those for the estrogens and progestins and include cigarette smoking, which increases the risk of cardiovascular side effects, such as venous and arterial thromboembolism, myocardial infarction, and thrombotic and hemorrhagic stroke. Also reported with oral contraceptive use are hepatic adenomas and other tumors, visual disturbances, gallbladder disease, hypertension, and fetal abnormalities.

Table 52.2 Estrogen and Progestin: Excess and Deficiency

Hormone*	Signs of Excess	Signs of Deficiency
estrogen	Nausea, bloating, cervical mucorrhea (increased cervical discharge), polyposis (numerous polyps), melasma (discoloration of the skin), hypertension, migraine headache, breast fullness or tenderness, edema	Early or midcycle breakthrough bleeding, increased spotting, hypomenorrhea
progestin	Increased appetite, weight gain, tiredness, fatigue, hypomenorrhea, acne, oily scalp, hair loss, hirsutism (excessive growth of hair), depression, monilial vaginitis, breast regression	Late breakthrough bleeding, amenorrhea, hypermenorrhea

*Hormonal balance is achieved by adjusting the estrogen/progestin dosage. Oral contraceptives have different amounts of progestin and estrogen, varying the estrogenic and progestational activity in each product.

Interactions

The following interactions may occur with the female hormones:

Interacting Drug	Common Use	Effect of Interaction
Estrogens		
oral anticoagulants	Blood thinners	Decreased anticoagulant effect
tricyclic antidepressants	Treatment of depression	Increased effectiveness of antidepressant
barbiturates or rifampin	Sedation or anti-infective, respectively	Increased risk of breakthrough bleeding
hydantoins	Seizure control	Increased risk of breakthrough bleeding and pregnancy
Progestins		
anticonvulsants, barbiturates, or rifampin	Seizure control, sedation, or anti-infective, respectively	Decreased effectiveness of progestin
penicillins or tetracyclines	Anti-infective agents	Decreased effectiveness of oral contraceptives

Herbal Alert

Black cohosh, an herb reported to be beneficial in managing symptoms of menopause, is generally regarded as safe when used as directed. Black cohosh is a member of the buttercup flower family. The dosage of standardized extract is 2 tablets twice a day, or 40 drops of standardized tincture twice a day, or one 500- to 600-mg tablet or capsule three times daily. Black cohosh tea is not considered as effective as other forms. Boiling the root releases only a portion of the therapeutic constituents.

The benefits of black cohosh (not to be confused with blue cohosh) include

- Reduction in physical symptoms of menopause: hot flashes, night sweats, headaches, heart palpitations, dizziness, vaginal atrophy, and tinnitus (ringing in the ears)

- Decrease in psychological symptoms of menopause: insomnia, nervousness, irritability, and depression
- Improvement in menstrual cycle regularity by balancing the hormones and reducing uterine spasms

Adverse reactions are rare when using the recommended dosage. The most common adverse reaction is nausea. Black cohosh is contraindicated during pregnancy. Toxic effects include dizziness, headache, nausea, impaired vision, and vomiting. This herb is purported to be an alternative to hormone replacement therapy (HART). Women who choose HART may increase their risk for endometrial cancer (cancer of the membrane lining the uterus), along with gallbladder disease, breast tenderness, high blood pressure, depression, and weight gain. Patients desiring to use any herbal remedy should consult with the primary health care provider before beginning therapy. Although no specific drug interactions have been reported, it is important that women taking HART should consult with their primary health care provider. In addition to its popularity as an herb for women's hormonal balance, black cohosh has been used for muscular and arthritic pain, headache, and eyestrain.

NURSING PROCESS

The Patient Receiving a Female Hormone

ASSESSMENT

PREADMINISTRATION ASSESSMENT

Before administering an estrogen or progestin, the nurse obtains a complete patient health history, including a menstrual history, which includes the **menarche** (age of onset of first menstruation), menstrual pattern, and any changes in the menstrual pattern (including a menopause history when applicable). In patients prescribed an estrogen (including oral contraceptives), the nurse obtains a history of thrombophlebitis or other vascular disorders, a smoking history, and a history of liver diseases. Blood pressure, pulse, and respiratory rate are taken and recorded. The primary health care provider usually performs a breast and pelvic examination and a Papanicolaou (Pap) test before starting therapy. Liver function tests may also be ordered.

If the male or female patient is being treated for a cancer, the nurse enters in the patient's record a general evaluation of the patient's physical and mental status. The primary health care provider may also order laboratory tests, such as serum electrolytes and liver function tests.

ONGOING ASSESSMENTS

OUTPATIENTS At the time of each office or clinic visit, the nurse obtains the blood pressure, pulse, respiratory rate, and weight. The nurse questions the patient regarding any adverse drug effects, as well as the result of drug therapy. For example, if the patient is receiving an estrogen for the symptoms of menopause, the nurse asks her to compare her original symptoms with the symptoms she is currently experiencing, if any. The nurse weighs the patient and reports a steady weight gain or loss. A periodic (usually annual) physical examination is performed by the primary health care provider and may include a pelvic examination, breast examination, Pap test, and laboratory tests. The patient with a prostatic or breast carcinoma usually requires more frequent evaluations of response to drug therapy.

HOSPITALIZED PATIENTS The hospitalized patient receiving a female hormone requires careful monitoring. The nurse takes the vital signs daily or more often, depending on the patient's physical condition and the reason for drug use. The nurse observes the patient for adverse drug reactions, especially those related to the liver (the development of jaundice) or the cardiovascular system (thromboembolism). The nurse weighs the patient weekly or as ordered by the primary health care provider. The nurse reports any significant weight gain or loss to the primary health care provider.

In patients with breast or prostate cancer, the nurse observes for and evaluates signs indicating a response to therapy, including relief of pain, an increase in appetite, and a feeling of well-being. Patients with prostate cancer may respond rapidly to therapy, but patients with breast cancer usually respond slowly.

NURSING DIAGNOSES

Drug-specific nursing diagnoses are highlighted in the Nursing Diagnoses Checklist. Other nursing diagnoses applicable to these drugs are discussed in depth in Chapter 4.

Nursing Diagnoses Checklist

✓ **Effective Therapeutic Regimen Management** related to administration of medications routinely despite adverse reactions

✓ **Excess Fluid Volume** related to adverse reactions (sodium and water retention)

✓ **Ineffective Tissue Perfusion** related to adverse reactions (thromboembolic effects)

✓ **Imbalanced Nutrition: More or Less Than Body Requirements** related to adverse reactions (weight gain or loss)

✓ **Anxiety** related to diagnosis, use of estrogen replacement therapy, or other factors

PLANNING

The expected outcomes of the patient may include an optimal response to therapy, support of patient needs related to the management of adverse reactions, a reduction in anxiety, and an understanding of and compliance with the prescribed therapeutic regimen.

IMPLEMENTATION
PROMOTING AN OPTIMAL RESPONSE TO THERAPY

ESTROGENS Estrogens may be administered orally, IM, IV, or intravaginally. Oral estrogens are administered with food or immediately after eating to reduce GI upset. When estrogens are given vaginally for atrophic vaginitis, the nurse gives the patient instructions on proper use.

CONTRACEPTIVE HORMONES The monophasic oral contraceptives are administered on a 21-day regimen, with the first tablet taken on the first Sunday after the menses begin or on the day the menses begin if the menses begin on Sunday. After the 21-day regimen, the next 7 days are skipped, then the cycle is begun again. With the biphasic oral contraceptives, the first phase is 10 days of a smaller dosage of progestin, and the second phase is a larger amount of progestin. The estrogen dosage remains constant for 21 days, followed by no estrogen for 7 days. Some regimens contain seven placebo tablets for easier management of the therapeutic regimen. With the triphasic oral contraceptives, the estrogen amount stays the same or may vary and the progestin amount varies throughout the 21-day cycle. Progestin-only oral contraceptives are taken daily and continuously.

CONTRACEPTIVE IMPLANT SYSTEM Levonorgestrel, a progestin, is available as an implant contraceptive system (Norplant System). Six capsules, each containing levonorgestrel, are implanted under local anesthesia in the subdermal (below the skin) tissues of the mid-portion of the upper arm. The capsules provide contraceptive protection for 5 years but may be removed at any time at the request of the patient. See Display 52-2 for more information on ways to promote an optimal response when taking the contraceptive hormones.

Nursing Alert

If the interval is greater than 14 weeks between the IM injections of medroxyprogesterone acetate, the nurse must be certain that the patient is not pregnant before administering the next injection.

Display 52.2 Alternatives to Oral Contraceptive Hormones

Patients who choose to use contraceptive hormone preparations need to be fully informed of their benefits and drawbacks. Nurses can be instrumental in educating patients about these drugs. Included here are contraceptive methods used by women in place of the traditional oral contraceptive pills.

Emergency Contraceptives (Plan B)

These preparations are used for emergency contraception after unprotected intercourse or known contraceptive failure. They prevent pregnancy; they do not work if the patient is already pregnant.

- When using high-dose levonorgestrel (Plan B), take one tablet within 72 hours after unprotected intercourse. Take the second dose of Plan B 12 hours later.
- This drug can be used any time during the menstrual cycle.
- If vomiting occurs within 1 hour after taking either dose, notify the primary health care provider.
- Emergency contraceptives are not effective in terminating an existing pregnancy.
- Emergency contraceptives should not be used as a routine form of contraception.

Etonogestrel/Ethinyl Estradiol Vaginal Ring (Nuvaring)

- The woman inserts the vaginal ring into the vagina, where it remains continuously for 3 weeks. It is removed for 1 week, during which bleeding usually occurs (usually 2 to 3 days after removal).
- Insert a new ring 1 week after the last ring was removed, on the same day of the week as it was inserted in the previous cycle. Do this even if bleeding is not finished.
- *Insertion*: Position for insertion by the woman may be standing with one leg up, squatting, or lying down. Compress the ring and insert into the vagina. (The exact position of the vaginal ring inside the vagina is not critical to its effectiveness.)
- The vaginal ring is removed after 3 weeks on the same day of the week as it was started. Removal is accomplished by hooking the index finger under the forward rim or by grasping the rim between the thumb and index finger and pulling it out. Discard the used ring in the foil pouch in a waste receptacle out of the reach of children or pets. (Do not flush the ring down the toilet.)
- Consider the menstrual cycle, timing of ovulation, and the possibility of pregnancy before beginning treatment.

- The vaginal ring may be accidentally expelled (e.g., when it was not inserted properly, during straining for defecation, while removing a tampon, or with severe constipation). If this occurs, rinse the vaginal ring with lukewarm water and reinsert promptly. (If the ring has been out of the vagina for more than 3 hours, contraceptive effectiveness may be reduced and an alternative contraceptive must be used for the next 7 days.
- The most common adverse effects leading to discontinuation of contraceptive use involve device-related problems, such as foreign body sensations, coital problems, and device expulsion.
- Other adverse effects include vaginitis, headache, upper respiratory tract infection, leukorrhea, sinusitis, weight gain, and nausea.

Levonorgestrel Implants (Norplant System)

This is a long-term (5-year) reversible contraceptive system, and an informed consent may be required in some institutions before implementing this procedure. The patient needs to know that a surgical incision is required to insert six capsules and that removal also requires surgical intervention.

Levonorgestrel-Releasing Intrauterine System (Mirena)

The capsules of the levonorgestrel-releasing intrauterine system (LRIS) are inserted during the first 7 days of the menstrual cycle or immediately after a first trimester abortion. LRIS is an intrauterine contraception device for use for not more than 5 years. Before insertion, provide the patient with the patient package insert. Also before insertion, a complete medical and social history, including that of the partner, is obtained to determine conditions that might influence the use of an intrauterine device (IUD). Several patient teaching points follow:

- Irregular menstrual bleeding, spotting, prolonged episodes of bleeding, and amenorrhea may occur. These symptoms diminish with continued use. The patient should check after each menstrual period to ensure that the thread attached to the LRIS still protrudes from the cervix. Caution her not to pull the thread.
- If pregnancy occurs with the LRIS in place, the LRIS should be removed. If the LRIS is not removed there is an increased risk of miscarriage/abortion, sepsis, premature labor, and premature delivery.

Display 52.2 Alternatives to Oral Contraceptive Hormones (continued)

- The patient should self-monitor for flulike symptoms, fever, chills, cramping, pain, bleeding, vaginal discharge, or leakage of fluid.
- Reexamination and evaluation are done shortly after the first menses or within the first 3 months after insertion.
- Menstrual flow usually decreases after the first 3 to 6 months of LRIS use; therefore, an increase of menstrual flow may indicate expulsion of the device.
- Symptoms of partial or complete expulsion include pain and bleeding. However, the LRIS also can be expelled without any noticeable effects.

Medroxyprogesterone Contraceptive Injection (Depo-Provera)

Medroxyprogesterone is available as a long-term injectable contraceptive administered IM every 3 months. The injection is given only during the first 5 days after the onset of a normal menstrual period, within 5 days postpartum if the woman is not breastfeeding, or at 6 weeks postpartum. Patient teaching points include the following:

- Bleeding irregularities may occur (i.e., irregular or unpredictable bleeding or spotting, or heavy continuous bleeding). Bleeding usually decreases to amenorrhea as treatment continues.
- Women tend to gain weight while using this form of contraception.
- The drug is not readministered if there is a sudden partial or complete loss of vision or if the patient experiences ptosis, diplopia, depression, or migraine.

Norelgestromin/Ethinyl Estradiol Transdermal System (Ortho Evra)

- The system is designed around a 28-day cycle, with a new patch applied each week for 3 weeks. Week 4 is patch free.

- Apply the new patch on the same day each week (note patch change day on the calendar).
- Discard used patch (only wear one patch at a time).
- Use no creams or lotions on area where patch is to be applied. Apply patch to clean, dry, intact, healthy skin on the buttock, abdomen, upper outer arm, or upper torso in a place where the patch will not be rubbed by clothing. Patch should not be placed on the breast or on areas that are red or irritated.
- *Beginning treatment*: First day start (apply first patch on the first day of the menstrual cycle) or Sunday start (apply first patch on the first Sunday after the menstrual period begins).
- A backup contraceptive should be used for the first week of the *first* treatment cycle.
- If the patch partially or completely detaches for less than 24 hours, reapply to the same place or replace with a new patch immediately (no backup contraception needed).
- If the patch detaches for more than 24 hours, apply new patch immediately (new patch change day). Backup contraception needed for the first week (7 days) of the new cycle.
- If the patch change is forgotten, begin again immediately, making this day the new patch change day. (Backup contraception needed for the first 7 days.)
- If breakthrough bleeding continues longer than a few cycles, a cause other than the patch should be considered. Do not stop patch if bleeding occurs.
- Bleeding should occur during the patch-free week. If no bleeding occurs, consider the possibility of pregnancy.
- If pregnancy is confirmed, discontinue treatment.

MEDROXYPROGESTERONE ACETATE CONTRACEPTIVE INJECTION Medroxyprogesterone acetate (Depo-Provera), a synthetic progestin used in the treatment of abnormal uterine bleeding and secondary amenorrhea, is also used as a contraceptive. This drug is given IM every 3 months, and the initial dosage is given within the first 5 days of menstruation or within 5 days postpartum. When this drug is given IM, the solution must be shaken vigorously before use to ensure uniform suspension, and the drug is given deep IM into the gluteal or deltoid muscle.

MONITORING AND MANAGING PATIENT NEEDS

EFFECTIVE THERAPEUTIC REGIMEN MANAGEMENT The patient prescribed the female hormones usually takes them for several months or years. Throughout that time, the patient must be monitored for adverse reactions. These drugs are self-administered at home. Patients may decide to regulate their own drug doses to alleviate adverse reactions; this can lead to ineffective dosing and more unwanted reactions such as pregnancy. Therefore, patient education is an important avenue for detecting and managing adverse reactions.

With the estrogens it is important to monitor for breakthrough bleeding. If breakthrough bleeding occurs with either the estrogens or progestin, the patient notifies the primary health care provider. A dosage change may be necessary.

Gastrointestinal upsets such as nausea, vomiting, abdominal cramps, and bloating may also occur. Nausea usually decreases or subsides within 1 to 2 months of therapy. However, until then the discomfort may be decreased if the drug is taken with food. If nausea is continual, frequent small meals may help. If nausea and vomiting persist, an antiemetic may be prescribed. Bloating may be alleviated with light to moderate exercise or by limiting fluid intake with meals.

The nurse carefully monitors the patient with diabetes who is taking female hormones. The primary health care provider is notified if blood glucose levels are elevated or the urine is positive for glucose or ketone bodies because a change in the dosage of insulin or the oral hypoglycemic drug may be required. See Chapter 49 for the management of hypoglycemic and hyperglycemic episodes.

EXCESS FLUID VOLUME Sodium and water retention may occur during female hormone therapy. In addition to reporting any swelling of the hands, ankles, or feet to the primary health care provider, the nurse weighs the hospitalized patient daily, keeps an accurate record of the intake and output, encourages ambulation (if not on bed rest), and helps the patient to eat a diet low in sodium (if prescribed by the primary health care provider).

INEFFECTIVE TISSUE PERFUSION The nurse monitors the patient for signs of thromboembolic effects, such as pain, swelling, tenderness in the extremities, headache, chest pain, and blurred vision. These adverse effects are reported to the primary health care provider. Patients with previous venous insufficiency, who are on bed rest for other medical reasons, or who smoke are at increased risk for thromboembolic effects. The nurse encourages the patient to elevate the lower extremities when sitting, if possible, and to exercise the lower extremities by walking.

> **Nursing Alert**
>
> There is an increased risk of postoperative thromboembolic complications in women taking oral contraceptives. If possible, use of the drug is discontinued at least 4 weeks before a surgical procedure associated with thromboembolism or during prolonged immobilization.

IMBALANCED NUTRITION: MORE OR LESS THAN BODY REQUIREMENTS Alterations in nutrition can occur, resulting in significant weight gain or loss. Weight gain occurs more frequently than weight loss. The nurse encourages a daily diet that includes adequate amounts of protein and carbohydrates and is low in fats. A variety of nutritious foods (fruits, vegetables, grains, cereals, meats, and poultry) should be included in the daily diet, with portion sizes decreased to meet individual needs. A dietitian may be consulted if necessary. An exercise program is helpful in both losing weight and maintaining weight loss.

Weight loss is often as difficult to manage as weight gain. When a patient taking the female hormones has a decrease in appetite and loses weight, the nurse encourages the individual to increase protein, carbohydrates, and calories in the diet. Small feedings with several daily snacks are usually better tolerated in those with a loss of appetite than are three larger meals. Patients are encouraged to eat foods they like. Dietary supplements may be necessary if a significant weight loss occurs. A dietitian may be consulted if necessary. Weights are usually taken on a weekly, rather than daily, basis.

ANXIETY The woman taking female hormones may have many concerns about therapy with these drugs. Some concerns may be based on inaccurate knowledge, such as the woman who hears incorrect facts about certain dangers associated with female hormones. Although there are dangers associated with long-term use of female hormones, many of these adverse reactions occur in a small number of patients. When the patient is closely followed by the primary health care provider, the dangers associated with long-term use are often minimized.

Some women may be anxious because of a fear of experiencing uterine cancer as the result of ERT. The nurse explains that taking progestin, which counteracts the negative effect of estrogen, can prevent estrogen-induced cancer of the uterus. Other women may fear the development of breast cancer. Most research studies find that there is little risk for breast cancer developing and that the benefits of ERT often outweigh the risk of breast cancer. Newer studies question the effectiveness of ERT, and this worries some women about whether they have made correct decisions regarding their health.

The nurse encourages the patient to ask questions about her therapy. Information that is inaccurate is clarified before therapy is started. The nurse refers to the primary health care provider questions that cannot or should not be answered by a nurse.

The male patient with advanced prostatic carcinoma also may have concerns about taking a female hormone. The nurse assures the patient that the dosage is carefully regulated and that feminizing effects, if they occur, are usually minimal.

EDUCATING THE PATIENT AND FAMILY

The instructions for starting oral contraceptive therapy vary with the product used. Each product has detailed patient instruction sheets regarding starting oral contraceptive therapy, and the nurse reviews them with the patient. The instructions for missed doses also are included in the package insert and are reviewed with the patient.

The nurse gives the patient a thorough explanation of the dosage regimen and adverse reactions that may result from the prescribed drug therapy. The nurse advises those taking oral contraceptives that skipping a dose could result in pregnancy. See Display 52-2 for more information to include in a teaching plan for a woman taking the contraceptive hormones.

In most instances, the primary health care provider performs periodic examinations, such as laboratory analyses, a pelvic examination, or a Pap test. The patient is encouraged to keep all appointments for follow-up evaluation of therapy. The nurse includes several points in a teaching plan:

ESTROGENS AND PROGESTINS

- Carefully read the patient package insert available with the drug. If there are any questions about this information, discuss them with the primary health care provider.

- If GI upset occurs, take the drug with food.

- Notify the primary health care provider if any of the following occurs: pain in the legs or groin area, sharp chest pain or sudden shortness of breath, lumps in the breast, sudden severe headache, dizziness or fainting, vision or speech disturbances, weakness or numbness in the arms or legs, severe abdominal pain, depression, or yellowing of the skin or eyes.

- *Female patient*: If pregnancy is suspected or abnormal vaginal bleeding occurs, stop taking the drug and contact the primary health care provider immediately.

- *Patient with diabetes*: Check the blood glucose or urine daily, or more often. Contact the primary health care provider if the blood glucose is elevated or if the urine is positive for glucose or ketones. An elevated blood glucose level or urine positive for glucose or ketones may require a change in diabetic therapy (insulin, oral hypoglycemic drug) or diet; these changes must be made by the primary health care provider.

ORAL CONTRACEPTIVES

- A patient package insert is available with the drug. Read the information carefully. Begin the first dose as directed in the package insert or as directed by the primary health care provider. If there are any questions about this information, discuss them with the primary health care provider.

- To obtain a maximum effect, take this drug as prescribed and at intervals not exceeding once every 24 hours. An oral contraceptive is best taken with the evening meal or at bedtime. The effectiveness of this drug depends on following the prescribed dosage schedule. Failure to comply with the dosage schedule may result in a pregnancy.

- Use an additional method of birth control (as recommended by the primary health care provider) until after the first week in the next cycle.

- If one day's dose is missed, take the missed dose as soon as remembered or take two tablets the next day. If 2 days are missed, take two tablets for the next 2 days and continue on with the normal dosing schedule. However, another form of birth control must be used until the cycle is completed and a new cycle is begun. If 3 days in a row or more are missed, discontinue use of the drug and use another form of birth control until a new cycle can begin. Before restarting the dosage regimen, make sure a pregnancy did not result from the break in the dosage regimen.

- If there are any questions regarding what to do about a missed dose, discuss the procedure with the primary health care provider.

- Avoid smoking or excessive exposure to second-hand smoke while taking these drugs; cigarette smoking during estrogen therapy may increase the risk of cardiovascular effects.

- Report adverse reactions such as fluid retention or edema to the extremities; weight gain; pain, swelling, or tenderness in the legs; blurred vision; chest pain; yellowed skin or eyes; dark urine; or abnormal vaginal bleeding.

- Remember that while taking these drugs, patients need periodic examinations by the primary health care provider and laboratory tests.

ESTRADIOL TRANSDERMAL SYSTEM

- Alora, Estraderm, Menostar, and Vivelle are applied twice weekly; Climara is applied every 7 days.

- Apply the system immediately after opening the pouch, with the adhesive side down (Fig. 52-1). Apply to

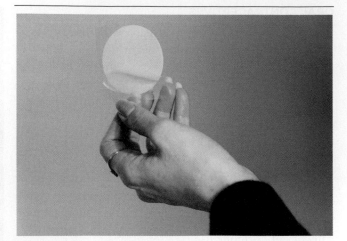

Figure 52.1 This low-dose estrogen transdermal patch, available as the trade name Estraderm (Estradiol Transdermal System), is transparent and about the size of a silver dollar. It releases small amounts of estrogen directly into the bloodstream at a constant and controlled rate to a woman requiring estrogen replacement therapy for postmenopausal symptoms.

clean, dry skin of the trunk, buttocks, abdomen, upper inner thigh, or upper arm. Do not apply to breasts, waistline, or a site exposed to sunlight. The area should not be oily or irritated.

- Press the system firmly in place with the palm of the hand for about 10 seconds. The application site is rotated, with at least 1-week intervals between applications to a particular site.

- Avoid areas that may be exposed to rubbing or where clothing may rub the system off or loosen the edges.

- Remove the old system before applying a new system unless the primary health care provider directs otherwise. Rotate application sites to prevent skin irritation.

- Follow the directions of the primary health care provider regarding application of the system (e.g., continuous, 3 weeks use followed by 1 week off, changed weekly, or applied twice weekly).

- If the system falls off, reapply it or apply a new system. Continue the original treatment schedule.

INTRAVAGINAL APPLICATION

- Use the applicator correctly. Refer to the package insert for correct procedure. The applicator is marked with the correct dosage and accompanies the drug when purchased.

- Wash the applicator after each use in warm water with a mild soap and rinse well.

- Maintain a recumbent position for at least 30 minutes after instillation.

- Use a sanitary napkin or panty liner to protect clothing if necessary.

- Do not double the dosage if a dose is missed. Instead, skip the dose and resume treatment the next day (see Patient and Family Teaching Checklist: Self-Administering Intravaginal Estrogen).

- When using the vaginal ring, press the ring into an oval and insert into the upper third of the vaginal vault.

EVALUATION

- The therapeutic effect is achieved.

- Adverse reactions are identified, reported to the primary health care provider, and managed using appropriate nursing interventions.

Patient and Family Teaching Checklist

Self-Administering Intravaginal Estrogen
The nurse:

✔ Explains the reason for the drug and prescribed therapy, including drug name, correct dosage, and frequency of administration.

✔ Describes the equipment to be used.

✔ Reinforces the need to empty the bladder and wash hands before administration.

✔ Demonstrates step-by-step procedure for filling applicator with drug and administration.

✔ Recommends a relaxed, supine position with knees flexed and legs spread.

✔ Instructs patient to insert applicator into vagina, angling it toward the tailbone and advancing it about 2 inches.

✔ Warns that drug may feel cold when inserted.

✔ Urges patient to remain recumbent for about 30 minutes after inserting drug.

✔ Suggests use of panty liner to prevent staining of clothes.

✔ Advises patient to wash applicator with mild soap and warm water, rinse well, and dry with paper towel after use.

✔ Cautions patient not to double dose if dose is missed but to skip dose and resume treatment the next day.

✔ Encourages daily inspection of perineal area for irritation or signs of allergic reaction.

- Anxiety is reduced.

- The patient verbalizes an understanding of the dosage regimen and the importance of continued follow-up care.

- The patient verbalizes the importance of complying with the prescribed therapeutic regimen.

HORMONES FOR CANCER TREATMENT

Hormones are used in cancer therapy because the receptors for specific hormones that are needed for cell growth are found on the surface of some tumor cells. By stopping the production of a hormone, blocking hormone receptors, or substituting a drug for the actual hormone, cancer cells can be killed or their growth slowed. These drugs also appear to counteract the effect of male or female hormones in hormone-dependent tumors. Hormones are not used as curative drugs in cancer treatment; rather, they have an adjuvant role because of their ability to slow or reverse tumor growth.

Examples of hormones used as antineoplastic drugs include the androgen testolactone (Teslac), conjugate estrogen, and the progestin megestrol (Megace). Gonadotropin-releasing hormone analogs, such as goserelin (Zoladex), appear to act by inhibiting the anterior pituitary secretion of gonadotropins, thus suppressing the release of pituitary gonadotropins. Consult the specific chapters in this book to learn the uses, cautions, adverse reactions, and nursing care associated with each category of hormone used in cancer treatment. For a listing of names, categories, and typical adverse reactions, see the Summary Drug Table: Hormonal Therapy for Cancer.

SUMMARY DRUG TABLE HORMONAL THERAPY FOR CANCER

GENERIC NAME	TRADE NAME	USES	ADVERSE REACTIONS	DOSAGES
Adrenal Steroid Inhibitors				
mitotane *mye'-toe-tane*	Lysodren	Adrenal cortical cancer	Leukocytosis, gastrointestinal symptoms (nausea, vomiting, diarrhea, abdominal pain), fatigue, edema, hyperglycemia, dyspnea, cough, rash or itching, headaches, dizziness	2–10 g/d in divided doses
Gonadotropin-Releasing Hormone Antagonists				
abarelix	Plenaxis	Prostate cancer	Hot flashes, pain, sleep distubances, breast enlargement and tenderness, constipation	Regulated use, see package insert
Gonadotropin-Releasing Hormone Analogs				
goserelin acetate *goe'-se-rel-in*	Zoladex	Prostate and breast cancer, endometriosis, endometrial thinning	Headache, emotional lability, depression, sweating, acne, breast atrophy, sexual dysfunction, vaginitis, hot flashes, pain, edema	3.6 mg monthly implant, 10.8 mg every 3 mo implant
histrelin acetate *hys'-trell-in*	Vantas	Prostate cancer	Hot flashes, fatigue, implant site irritation	50–60 mcg/d delivered e.g., implant changed yearly
leuprolide acetate *loo-proe'-lide*	Lupron, Viadur	Prostate cancer, endometriosis, precocious puberty, uterine leiomyomata	Hot flashes, edema, bone pain, electrocardiographic changes, hypertension	1 mg/d SC, provided in monthly injection form and implant
triptorelin pamoate *trip-toe-rell'-in*	Trelstar Depot, LA	Prostate cancer	Hot flashes, skeletal pain, headache, impotence	3.75 mg IM every 28 d

GENERIC NAME	TRADE NAME	USES	ADVERSE REACTIONS	DOSAGES
Antiandrogens				
bicalutamide bye-cal-loo'-ta-mide	Casodex	Prostate cancer	Hot flashes, dizziness, constipation, nausea, diarrhea, nocturia, hematuria, peripheral edema, general pain, asthenia, infection	50 mg/d orally
flutamide flu'-ta-mide	Eulexin	Prostate cancer	Hot flashes, loss of libido, impotence, diarrhea, nausea, vomiting, gynecomastia	250 mg/orally TID
nilutamide nah-loo'-ta-mide	Nilandron	Prostate cancer	Pain, headache, asthenia, flulike symptoms, insomnia, nausea, constipation, testicular atrophy, dyspnea	300 mg/d for 1 mo, then 150 mg/d orally
Estrogen				
estramustine phosphate sodium	Emcyt	Prostate cancer	Breast tenderness and enlargement, nausea, diarrhea, edema	14 mg/kg/d orally in divided doses
Androgen				
testolactone tess-toe-lak'-tone	Teslac	Palliative treatment: breast cancer	Paresthesia, glossitis, anorexia, nausea, vomiting, maculopapular erythema, aches, alopecia, edema of the extremities, increase in blood pressure	250 mg orally QID
Aromatase Inhibitors				
anastrazole an-ahs'-troh-zole	Arimidex	Breast cancer	Vasodilation, mood disturbances, nausea, hot flashes, pharyngitis, asthenia, pain	1 mg/d orally
exemestane ex-ah'-mess-tane	Aromasin	Breast cancer	Same as anastrazole	25 mg/d orally
letrozole le'-tro-zole	Femara	Breast cancer	Same as anastrazole	2.5 mg/d orally
Progestins				
medroxyprog-esterone me-drox'-ee-proe-jess'-te-rone	Depo-Provera	Endometrial or renal cancer	Fatigue, nervousness, rash, pruritus, acne, edema	400–1000 mg/wk IM
megestrol acetate me-jess'-trole	Megace	Breast or endometrial cancer, appetite stimulant in human immunodeficiency virus infection	Weight gain, nausea, vomiting, edema, breakthrough bleeding	40–320 mg/d orally in divided doses
Antiestrogens				
fulvestrant full-ves'-trant	Faslodex	Breast cancer	Nausea, vomiting, asthenia, pain, pharyngitis, headache	250 mg IM once monthly
tamoxifen citrate ta-moks'-i-fen	Nolvadex	Breast cancer, prophylactic therapy for women at high risk for breast cancer	Hot flashes, rashes, headaches, vaginal bleeding and discharge	20–40 mg/d orally
toremifene citrate tore-em'-ih-feen	Fareston	Breast cancer	Hot flashes, sweating, nausea, dizziness, edema, vaginal bleeding, and discharge	60 mg/d orally

Critical Thinking Exercises

1. Ms. Burton calls the office where you work, concerned about her mother. She has read that hormones can put a woman at risk for cancer, so she cannot understand why the primary health care provider is starting her mother on hormone therapy for her cancer. Explain how you can discuss her fears and help her to understand hormone therapy.

2. John, a friend of your brother, has started to use anabolic steroids to increase his strength and muscle mass to improve his chances of getting a football scholarship. Your brother tells you that this is acceptable because his friend wants an education. Discuss how you would approach your brother with concerns about John's choices.

3. Susan Parker, a mother of three young children, calls the health clinic where you work, stating that she has missed 3 days of oral contraceptives when she was ill. She wants to know if she can continue with the oral contraceptive. Discuss what information Susan needs to know to protect herself from becoming pregnant.

Review Questions

1. The nurse monitors the patient taking an anabolic steroid for the more severe adverse reactions, which include _____.

   A. anorexia

   B. nausea and vomiting

   C. severe mental changes

   D. acne

2. The nurse must be aware that older men taking the androgens are _____.

   A. prone to urinary problems

   B. at greater risk for hypertension

   C. at increased risk for confusion

   D. at increased risk for prostate cancer

3. When monitoring a patient taking an oral contraceptive, the nurse would observe the patient for signs of excess progestin. Which of the following reactions would indicate to the nurse that a patient has an excess of progestin?

   A. Increased appetite, hair loss

   B. Virilization, constipation

   C. Nausea, early breakthrough bleeding

   D. Deepening of the voice, lightheadedness

4. A patient calls the outpatient clinic and says that she missed 1 day's dose of her "birth control pills." Which of the following statements would be most appropriate for the nurse to make to the patient?

   A. Do not take an additional tablet but resume the regular schedule today.

   B. Discontinue use of the drug and use another type of contraceptive until after your next menstrual period.

   C. Take two tablets today; then resume the regular daily schedule.

   D. Come into the office immediately for a pregnancy test.

5. When teaching the patient taking an oral contraceptive for the first time, the nurse emphasizes the importance of taking _____.

   A. two tablets per day at the first sign of ovulation

   B. the drug at the same time each day

   C. the drug early in the morning before arising

   D. the drug each day for 20 days beginning on the first of the month

Medication Dosage Problems

1. Medroxyprogesterone 650 mg IM is prescribed. The drug is available in a solution of 400 mg/mL. The nurse administers _____.

2. The physician prescribes estrone 0.5 mg IM for a postmenopausal woman with vasomotor symptoms. On hand is a vial of estrone with a solution containing 0.5 mg/mL. The nurse administers _____.

To check your answers, see Appendix G.

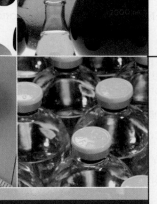

Chapter 53

Drugs Acting on the Uterus

Key Terms

ergotism
oxytocic
uterine atony
water intoxication

Learning Objectives

On completion of this chapter, the student will:

- Discuss the actions, uses, adverse reactions, contraindications, precautions, and interactions of drugs acting on the uterus.
- Discuss important preadministration and ongoing assessment activities the nurse should perform with the patient taking an oxytocic or tocolytic drug.

- List some nursing diagnoses particular to a patient taking an oxytocic or tocolytic drug.
- Discuss ways to promote an optimal response to therapy, how to manage adverse reactions, and important points to keep in mind when educating patients about the use of an oxytocic or tocolytic drug.

D rug therapy is beneficial for use in labor and delivery to promote the well-being of the woman and fetus. Depending on the patient's need, drugs may be used to stimulate, intensify, or inhibit uterine contractions. The two types of drugs discussed in this chapter for their effect on the uterus are the oxytocics and the tocolytics. Drugs acting on the uterus are listed in the Summary Drug Table: Drugs Acting on the Uterus.

OXYTOCIC DRUGS

Oxytocic drugs are used antepartum (before birth of the neonate) to induce uterine contractions similar to those of normal labor. These drugs are desirable when early vaginal delivery is in the best interest of the woman and the fetus. An oxytocic drug is one that stimulates the uterus. Included in this group of drugs are ergonovine, methylergonovine (Methergine), and oxytocin (Pitocin).

Action and Uses

Oxytocin

Oxytocin is an endogenous hormone produced by the posterior pituitary gland (see Chapter 50). This hormone has uterus-stimulating properties, acting on the smooth muscle of the uterus, especially on the pregnant uterus. As pregnancy progresses, the sensitivity of the uterus to oxytocin increases, reaching a peak immediately before the birth of the infant. This sensitivity enables oxytocic drugs to exert their full therapeutic effect on the uterus and produce the desired results. Oxytocin also has antidiuretic and vasopressor effects.

Oxytocin is administered intravenously (IV) for starting or improving labor contractions to obtain an early vaginal delivery of the fetus. An early vaginal delivery may be indicated when there are fetal or maternal problems, such as a woman with diabetes and a large fetus, Rh problems, premature rupture of the membranes, uterine inertia, and eclampsia or preeclampsia (also called *pregnancy-induced hypertension*).

SUMMARY DRUG TABLE — DRUGS ACTING ON THE UTERUS

GENERIC NAME	TRADE NAME	USES	ADVERSE REACTIONS	DOSAGE RANGES
Oxytocics				
ergonovine maleate *er-goe-noe'-veen*		Postpartum uterine atony and hemorrhage	Elevated blood pressure when spinal analgesia used	0.2 mg IM, orally q2-4h
methylergonovine maleate *meth-ill-er-goe-noe'-veen*	Methergine	Control of postpartum bleeding and hemorrhage, uterine atony	Dizziness, headache, nausea, vomiting, elevated blood pressure	0.2 mg IM, IV after delivery of the placenta; 0.2 mg orally TID, QID
oxytocin *ox-i-toe'-sin*	Pitocin	Antepartum: to initiate or improve uterine contractions Postpartum: control of postpartum bleeding and hemorrhage	Nausea, vomiting, pelvic hematoma, postpartum bleeding, cardiac arrhythmias, anaphylactic reactions	Induction of labor: individualize dose not to exceed 10 units/min Postpartum bleeding: IV infusion of 10-40 units in 1000 mL IV solution or 10 Units IM after placenta delivery
Tocolytics				
indomethacin *in-doe-meth'-ah-sin*	Indocin	Preterm labor before 31 weeks' gestation	Headache, dizziness, nausea, vomiting, stomach upset or heartburn, prolonged vaginal bleeding	100 mg rectally, then 50 mg orally q6h for a total of 8 doses
magnesium sulfate *mag-nee'-zee-um*		Preterm labor, seizure control	Fatigue, headaches, flushing, diplopia	4-6 g IV over 2 min, then infuse 1-4 g/h
ritodrine HCl *ri'-toe-dreen*		Preterm labor	Alterations in fetal and maternal heart rates and maternal blood pressure, palpitations, headache, nausea, vomiting	IV: 0.05-0.35 mg/min depending on patient response
terbutaline *ter-byoo'-ta-leen*	Brethine	Preterm labor	Nervousness, restlessness, tremor, headache, anxiety, hypertension, palpitations, arrhythmias, hypokalemia, pulmonary edema	SC: 250 mcg hourly until contractions stop Orally: 2.5 mg q4-6h until delivery

Preeclampsia is a condition of pregnancy characterized by hypertension, headache, albuminuria, and edema of the lower extremities occurring at, or near, term. The condition may progressively worsen until eclampsia (a serious condition occurring between the 20th week of pregnancy and the end of the 1st week postpartum and characterized by convulsive seizures and coma) occurs. Oxytocin may also be used in managing inevitable or incomplete abortion. Oxytocin is given intramuscularly (IM) during the third stage of labor (period from the time the neonate is expelled until the placenta is expelled) to produce uterine contractions and control postpartum bleeding and hemorrhage. It may also be administered intranasally to stimulate the milk ejection (milk letdown) reflex.

Ergonovine and Methylergonovine

Ergonovine and methylergonovine are uterine stimulants that increase the strength, duration, and frequency of uterine contractions and decrease the incidence of uterine bleeding. They are given after the delivery of the placenta and are used to prevent postpartum and postabortal hemorrhage caused by **uterine atony** (marked relaxation of the uterine muscle).

Adverse Reactions

Oxytocin

Administration of oxytocin may result in

- Fetal bradycardia, uterine rupture, uterine hypertonicity
- Nausea, vomiting, cardiac arrhythmias, anaphylactic reactions

Because of its antidiuretic effect, serious **water intoxication** (fluid overload, fluid volume excess) may occur, particularly when the drug is administered by continuous infusion and the patient is receiving fluids by mouth. When oxytocin is used as a nasal spray, adverse reactions are rare.

Ergonovine and Methylergonovine

The adverse reactions associated with ergonovine and methylergonovine include

- Nausea, vomiting
- Elevated blood pressure, temporary chest pain
- Dizziness, water intoxication, headache

Allergic reactions may also occur. In some instances hypertension associated with seizure or headache may occur. **Ergotism** (overdosage of ergonovine) is manifested by nausea, vomiting, abdominal pain, numbness, tingling of the extremities, and an increase in blood pressure. In severe cases, these symptoms are followed by hypotension, respiratory depression, hypothermia, gangrene of the fingers and toes, convulsions, hallucinations, and coma.

Contraindications, Precautions, and Interactions

Oxytocin

Oxytocin is contraindicated in patients with known hypersensitivity to the drug, cephalopelvic disproportion, and unfavorable fetal position or presentation. It is also contraindicated in obstetric emergencies, situations of fetal distress when delivery is not imminent, severe toxemia (preeclampsia, eclampsia), and hypertonic uterus, as well as during pregnancy (intranasal administration) when there is

total placenta previa. It is contraindicated as an agent to induce labor when vaginal delivery is contraindicated. Oxytocin is not expected to be a risk to the fetus when administered as indicated. When oxytocin is administered with vasopressors, however, severe maternal hypertension may occur.

Ergonovine and Methylergonovine

Ergonovine is contraindicated in those with known hypersensitivity to the drug or hypertension, and before the delivery of the placenta. Ergonovine is used cautiously in patients with heart disease, obliterative vascular disease, renal or hepatic disease, and during lactation.

Methylergonovine is contraindicated in patients with a known hypersensitivity to the drug, hypertension, and preeclampsia and should not be used to induce labor (pregnancy category C). Methylergonovine is used cautiously in patients with renal or hepatic impairment. When methylergonovine is administered concurrently with vasopressors, or to patients who are heavy cigarette smokers, excessive vasoconstriction may occur.

NURSING PROCESS

The Patient Receiving an Oxytocic Drug
ASSESSMENT
PREADMINISTRATION ASSESSMENT

Before starting an IV infusion of oxytocin to induce labor, the nurse obtains an obstetric history (e.g., parity, gravidity, previous obstetric problems, type of labor, stillbirths, abortions, live-birth infant abnormalities) and a general health history. Immediately before starting the IV infusion of oxytocin, the nurse assesses the fetal heart rate (FHR) and the patient's blood pressure, pulse, and respiratory rate.

In addition, the nurse assesses and records the activity of the uterus (strength, duration, and frequency of contractions, if any). Monitoring uterine contractions for strength and length of the contractions can be done with an external monitor or by an internal uterine catheter with an electronic monitor. A fetal monitor is placed to assess the FHR.

Ergonovine and methylergonovine may be given orally during the postpartum period to reduce the possibility of postpartum hemorrhage and to prevent relaxation of the uterus. When the patient is to receive either of these drugs after delivery, it is important to take the blood pressure, pulse, and respiratory rate before administration.

ONGOING ASSESSMENT

After injecting an oxytocic drug, the nurse monitors the patient's blood pressure, pulse, and respiratory rate at the intervals ordered by the primary health care provider.

Drugs Acting on the Uterus

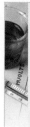

Nursing Alert

All patients receiving IV oxytocin must be under constant observation to identify complications. A one-to-one nurse–patient ratio is recommended when monitoring a patient receiving an oxytocin infusion. In addition, the primary health care provider should be immediately available at all times.

The nurse assesses the patient's blood pressure, pulse, and respiratory rate every 30 minutes. The FHR and uterine contractions are assessed every 15 minutes or as ordered by the primary health care provider. Three to four firm uterine contractions should occur every 10 minutes, followed by a palpable relaxation of the uterus.

Nursing Alert

Hyperstimulation of the uterus during labor may lead to uterine tetany with marked impairment of the uteroplacental blood flow, uterine rupture, cervical rupture, amniotic fluid embolism, and trauma to the infant. Over-stimulation of the uterus is dangerous to both the fetus and the mother and may occur even when the drug is administered properly in a uterus that is hypersensitive to oxytocin.

When monitoring uterine contractions, the nurse notifies the primary health care provider immediately if any of the following occurs:

- A significant change in the FHR or rhythm

- A marked change in the frequency, rate, or rhythm of uterine contractions; uterine contractions lasting more than 60 seconds; or contractions occurring more frequently than every 2 to 3 minutes, or no palpable relaxation of the uterus

- A marked increase or decrease in the patient's blood pressure or pulse or any significant change in the patient's general condition

If any of these conditions are noted, the nurse should immediately discontinue the oxytocin infusion and run the primary IV line at the rate prescribed by the primary health care provider until the primary health care provider examines the patient.

The nurse immediately reports any signs of water intoxication or fluid overload (e.g., drowsiness, confusion, headache, listlessness, and wheezing, coughing, rapid breathing) to the primary health care provider.

Oxytocin may be given IM after delivery of the placenta. After administering the drug, the nurse obtains the patient's blood pressure, pulse, and respiratory rate every 5 to 10 minutes. Then the nurse palpates the patient's uterine fundus for firmness and position. The nurse immediately reports any excess bleeding to the primary health care provider.

When administering ergonovine and methylergonovine after delivery, the nurse monitors vital signs every 4 hours and also notes the character and amount of vaginal bleeding. The patient may report abdominal cramping with the administration of these drugs. If cramping is moderately severe to severe, the nurse notifies the primary health care provider because it may be necessary to discontinue use of the drug.

NURSING DIAGNOSES

Drug-specific nursing diagnoses are highlighted in the Nursing Diagnoses Checklist. Other nursing diagnoses applicable to these drugs are discussed in depth in Chapter 4.

PLANNING

The expected patient outcomes may include an optimal response to drug therapy (e.g., initiation of the normal labor process), adverse reactions (e.g., absence of a fluid volume excess with oxytocin administration) identified and reported to the primary health care provider, and an understanding of the treatment regimen.

IMPLEMENTATION

PROMOTING AN OPTIMAL RESPONSE TO THERAPY

OXYTOCIN When oxytocin is prescribed, the primary health care provider orders the type and amount of IV fluid, the number of units of oxytocin added to the IV solution, and the IV infusion rate. An electronic infusion device is used to control the infusion rate. The primary

Nursing Diagnoses Checklist

☑ **Anxiety** related to fears associated with the process of labor and delivery

☑ **Risk for Injury** (fetal) related to adverse drug effects of oxytocin on the fetus (fetal bradycardia)

☑ **Excess Fluid Volume** related to administration of IV fluids and the antidiuretic effects associated with oxytocin.

☑ **Acute Pain** related to adverse reactions (abdominal cramping, nausea, headache)

health care provider establishes guidelines for administering the oxytocin solution and for increasing or decreasing the flow rate or discontinuing the administration of oxytocin. Usually, the flow rate is increased every 20 to 30 minutes, but this may vary according to the patient's response. The strength, frequency, and duration of contractions and the FHR are monitored closely.

When administering oxytocin intranasally to facilitate the letdown of milk, the nurse places the patient in an upright position, and with the squeeze bottle held upright, administers the prescribed number of sprays to one or both nostrils. The patient then waits 2 to 3 minutes before breastfeeding the infant or pumping the breasts. If the patient uses a breast pump, the nurse records the amount of milk pumped from the breasts.

The nurse notifies the primary health care provider if milk drips from the breast before or after breastfeeding or if milk drips from the opposite breast during breastfeeding because there would be no need to continue drug therapy. The primary health care provider is notified if nasal irritation, palpitations, or uterine cramping occurs.

ERGONOVINE AND METHYLERGONOVINE The nurse administers ergonovine and methylergonovine at the direction of the primary health care provider. Ergonovine is usually given during the third stage of labor after the placenta has been delivered. Ergonovine is primarily administered IM, but in emergencies when a quicker response is needed, the drug may be administered IV.

Methylergonovine is usually given IM at the time of the delivery of the anterior shoulder or after the delivery of the placenta. The drug is not given routinely IV because it may produce sudden hypertension and stroke. If the drug is given IV, the nurse administers the drug slowly over a period of 1 minute or more with close monitoring of the patient's blood pressure.

When ergonovine or methylergonovine is administered in the delivery room, the nurse briefly explains the purpose of the injection to the patient. If either of these drugs is given after delivery of the infant, the nurse explains the purpose of the drug, which is to improve the tone of the uterus and help the uterus to return to its (near) normal size.

MONITORING AND MANAGING PATIENT NEEDS

ANXIETY The patient receiving oxytocin to induce labor may have concern over the use of the drug to produce contractions. When given to induce or stimulate contractions, oxytocin may be given IV only. The nurse explains the purpose of the IV infusion and the expected results to the patient. Because the patient receiving oxytocin must be closely supervised, the nurse spends time with the patient and offers encouragement and reassurance to help reduce anxiety.

RISK FOR INJURY (FETAL) When oxytocin is administered, some adverse reactions must be tolerated or treated symptomatically until therapy is discontinued. For example, if the patient is nauseated, the nurse provides an emesis basin and perhaps a cool towel for the forehead. If vomiting occurs, the nurse notifies the primary health care provider.

If contractions are frequent, prolonged, or excessive, the infusion is stopped to prevent fetal anoxia or trauma to the uterus. Excessive stimulation of the uterus can cause uterine hypertonicity and possible uterine rupture. The nurse places the patient on her left side and provides supplemental oxygen. The effects of the drug diminish rapidly because oxytocin is a short-acting drug.

EXCESS FLUID VOLUME When oxytocin is administered IV, there is a danger of an excessive fluid volume (water intoxication) because oxytocin has an antidiuretic effect. The nurse measures the fluid intake and output. In some instances, hourly measurements of output are necessary. The nurse observes the patient for signs of fluid overload (see Chapter 58). If any of these signs or symptoms is noted, the nurse should immediately discontinue the oxytocin infusion but let the primary IV line run at the rate prescribed by the primary health care provider until the primary health care provider examines the patient.

ACUTE PAIN When ergonovine or methylergonovine is administered for uterine atony and hemorrhage, abdominal cramping can occur and is usually an indication of drug effectiveness. The uterus is palpated in the lower abdomen as small, firm, and round. However, the nurse should report persistent or severe cramping to the primary health care provider.

> **Nursing Alert**
>
> In some patients who are calcium deficient, the uterus may not respond to ergonovine. The nurse immediately reports a lack of response to ergonovine. Administration of calcium by IV injection usually restores response to the drug.

Although rare, ergotism or ergot poisoning can occur with the administration of excessive amounts of ergonovine or methylergonovine.

Nursing Alert

Symptoms of ergotism that must be reported immediately include coolness, numbness and tingling of extremities, dyspnea, nausea, confusion, tachycardia or bradycardia, chest pain, hallucinations, and convulsions. If these reactions occur, the nurse immediately reports them to the primary health care provider because use of the drug must be discontinued.

EDUCATING THE PATIENT AND FAMILY

The treatment regimen is explained to the patient and family (when appropriate). The nurse answers any questions the patient may have regarding treatment and instructs the patient to report any adverse reactions. The nurse also informs the patient and family about the therapeutic response during administration of the drug, and if nasal spray is to be used, teaches the patient the proper technique.

EVALUATION

- The therapeutic effect is achieved, and normal labor is initiated.
- Adverse reactions are managed effectively.
- No evidence of fluid volume excess (oxytocin administration) is seen.
- The patient is knowledgeable regarding the therapeutic regimen.

TOCOLYTICS

Drugs used to prevent uterine contractions are called *tocolytics*. They are useful in the management of preterm labor. These drugs decrease uterine activity and prolong the pregnancy to allow the fetus to develop more fully, thereby increasing the chance of neonatal survival. Magnesium sulfate is the most commonly used drug to decrease uterine muscle contractions, followed by the nonsteroidal anti-inflammatory drugs (NSAIDs) such as indomethacin. Ritodrine and terbutaline (Brethine) are used as second line therapies because of the greater risks these drugs pose to the mother.

Actions and Uses

Magnesium sulfate is a calcium antagonist that works to decrease the force of uterine contractions. Typically, infusions last less than 48 hours to prevent preterm delivery until steroid prophylaxis (for fetal lung maturation) can be initiated. Magnesium sulfate is used to manage preterm labor in pregnancies of greater than 27 weeks' gestation. Magnesium sulfate administration requires hospitalization. Indomethacin is an NSAID that blocks the production of substances called *prostaglandins* (see Chapter 18), which contribute to uterine contractions.

Adverse Reactions

Adverse reactions to magnesium sulfate include
- Fatigue, flushing, headache, diplopia
- Sweating, hypotension, depressed reflexes, and flaccid paralysis are other adverse reactions associated with IV administration. They are related to hypocalcemia induced by the therapy.

Adverse reactions observed with indomethacin include
- Headaches, dizziness
- Nausea, vomiting, stomach upset or heartburn
- Prolonged vaginal bleeding

Contraindications, Precautions, and Interactions

Magnesium sulfate is contraindicated in patients with known hypersensitivity to the drug, heart block or myocardial damage, or eclampsia or severe preeclampsia, and within 2 hours of delivery. Magnesium sulfate is classified as a pregnancy category A drug and indomethacin is a pregnancy category B drug. Although these drugs are given for preterm labor, they still should be given cautiously during pregnancy.

There is an increased effectiveness of central nervous system depressants (e.g., opioids, analgesics, and sedatives) when magnesium sulfate is administered. The effectiveness of neuromuscular blocking agents is enhanced as well. See Chapter 18 for drug interactions with indomethacin.

NURSING PROCESS

The Patient Receiving a Tocolytic Agent

ASSESSMENT
PREADMINISTRATION ASSESSMENT

Before starting an IV infusion containing a tocolytic drug, the nurse obtains the patient's vital signs. The nurse auscultates lung sounds to provide a baseline assessment. The patient has a monitoring device in place to determine uterine contractions and the FHR before and during administration.

Before magnesium sulfate is initiated, baseline blood tests (e.g., complete blood count and creatinine level) are performed. Because magnesium sulfate affects the neuromuscular system, a neurologic examination is performed as well. Mentation, cranial nerve function, and deep tendon reflexes are assessed. When indomethacin is used as the tocolytic drug, additional tests include liver function tests and amniotic fluid index (AFI).

ONGOING ASSESSMENT

During the ongoing assessment of a patient receiving a tocolytic drug, nursing activities include the following at 15- to 30-minute intervals:

- Obtaining blood pressure, pulse, and respiratory rate
- Monitoring FHR
- Checking the IV infusion rate
- Examining the area around the IV needle insertion site for signs of infiltration
- Monitoring uterine contractions (frequency, intensity, length)
- Measuring maternal intake and output

NURSING DIAGNOSES

Drug-specific nursing diagnoses are highlighted in the Nursing Diagnoses Checklist. Other nursing diagnoses applicable to these drugs are discussed in depth in Chapter 4.

PLANNING

The expected outcomes of the patient may include an optimal response to therapy, a reduction in anxiety, and an understanding of the treatment of preterm labor.

IMPLEMENTATION

PROMOTING AN OPTIMAL RESPONSE TO THERAPY

Nursing management for a patient receiving magnesium sulfate, ritodrine, or terbutaline is similar. For IV administration, the nurse prepares the solution according to the primary health care provider's instructions. An infusion pump is used to control the flow rate. Magnesium sulfate,

ritodrine, or terbutaline may be piggybacked to the primary line, allowing the primary line to maintain patency should it become necessary temporarily to discontinue infusion of the drug. In some cases, the primary health care provider may prescribe indomethacin for administration by the rectal or oral route throughout the treatment, rather than by the IV route. Terbutaline may be given orally or by subcutaneous (SC) injection. In any case, the nurse places a cardiac monitor on the patient and, to minimize hypotension, the nurse positions the patient in a left lateral position unless the primary health care provider orders a different position.

The primary health care provider is kept informed of the patient's response to the drug because a dosage change may be necessary. The primary health care provider establishes guidelines for the regulation of the IV infusion rate, as well as the blood pressure and pulse ranges that require stopping the IV infusion.

MONITORING AND MANAGING PATIENT NEEDS

During administration of the drug, the nurse monitors maternal and fetal vital signs every 15 minutes and uterine contractions frequently throughout the infusion.

ANXIETY The patient in preterm labor may have many concerns about her pregnancy as well as the effectiveness of drug therapy. The woman is encouraged to verbalize any fears or concerns. The nurse listens to the patient's concerns and carefully and accurately answers any questions she may have concerning drug therapy. In addition, the nurse offers emotional support and encouragement while the drug is being administered. If allowed by the institution, the presence of family members may decrease anxiety in the woman experiencing preterm labor.

IMPAIRED GAS EXCHANGE The nurse reports to the primary care provider a pulse rate of 140 bpm, persistent elevation of pulse rate, irregular pulse, or increase in respiratory rate of more than 20 respirations/min. The nurse assesses the respiratory status for symptoms of pulmonary edema (e.g., dyspnea, tachycardia, increased respiratory rate, rales, and frothy sputum). If these reactions occur, the primary health care provider is notified immediately because use of the drug may be discontinued or the dosage may be decreased. After contractions cease, the nurse tapers the dosage to the lowest effective dose by decreasing the drug infusion rate at regular intervals prescribed by the primary health care provider. The infusion continues for at least 12 hours after uterine contractions cease. Because treatment duration is brief, mild adverse reactions must be tolerated. If adverse reactions are severe, use of the drug is discontinued or the dosage decreased.

Nursing Diagnoses Checklist

✓ **Anxiety** related to fears concerning preterm labor

✓ **Impaired Gas Exchange** related to pulmonary edema from drug therapy and IV fluids

EDUCATING THE PATIENT AND FAMILY

The nurse carefully explains the treatment regimen to the patient. The primary health care provider usually discusses the expected outcome of treatment with the patient and answers any questions regarding therapy. Although the patient is monitored closely during therapy, the patient is instructed to notify the nurse immediately if any of the following occur: nausea, vomiting, palpitations, or shortness of breath. If a patient is taking ritodrine, the nurse discusses the importance of lying on the left side during IV administration.

If oral indomethacin or terbutaline is prescribed for preterm labor, the patient is instructed on use of the drug and adverse reactions to report (excessive tremor, nervousness, drowsiness, headache, nausea, dizziness, yellow coloration of skin or eyes). If contractions resume during oral therapy, the patient is instructed to notify the primary health care provider if four to six contractions per hour occur.

EVALUATION

- The therapeutic drug effect is achieved.
- Adverse reactions are identified and reported to the primary health care provider.
- Anxiety is reduced.
- The patient demonstrates an understanding of in-hospital treatment.

Critical Thinking Exercises

1. Develop a nursing care plan for Ms. Morris, a 28-year-old woman who is admitted to the obstetric unit with premature labor during her third trimester. This is her second child, and she has had two miscarriages. She is prescribed ritodrine for preterm labor. Analyze what nursing diagnoses would have the highest priority. Discuss how you would explore and plan to meet her emotional needs.

2. Judith Watson, aged 28 years, is admitted to the obstetric unit and is to receive oxytocin to induce labor. This is her first child, and she is extremely anxious. Analyze what information would be necessary for her to receive from the nurse before the administration of oxytocin. What assessments would be important for the nurse to make during treatment with oxytocin?

Review Questions

1. When oxytocin is administered over a prolonged time, which of the following adverse reactions would be most likely to occur?

   A. Hyperglycemia

   B. Renal impairment

   C. Increased intracranial pressure

   D. Water intoxication

2. When the patient is receiving oxytocin, the nurse would notify the primary health care provider in which of the following conditions?

   A. Uterine contractions occur every 5 to 10 minutes.

   B. Uterine contractions last more than 60 seconds or contractions occur more frequently than every 2 to 3 minutes.

   C. Patient experiences pain during a uterine contraction.

   D. Patient experiences increased thirst.

3. Which of the following adverse reactions is most indicative of ergotism?

   A. Numbness, tingling of the extremities

   B. Headache, blurred vision

   C. Tachycardia and cardiac arrhythmias

   D. Diaphoresis, increased respirations

4. During administration of ritodrine, in what position would the nurse most probably place the patient?

   A. Supine

   B. Prone

   C. On the left side

   D. On the right side

Medication Dosage Problems

1. Terbutaline 2.5 mg is prescribed. The drug is available in 5-mg tablets. The nurse administers _____.

2. Methylergonovine 0.2 mg IM is prescribed. The drug is available as 0.2 mg/mL. The nurse administers _____.

To check your answers, see Appendix G.

Drugs That Affect the Immune System

The immune system is not located in any single portion of the body. Rather, it flows through the entire body as a set of cells and fluid designed to recognize and respond to invasion. The chapters in this unit describe the drugs used to support the immune system in either recognizing invasion of an outside pathogen or by identifying the body's own cells growing out of control.

The lymphatic system plays a major role in the immune system. Cells called *T lymphocytes (T cells)* circulate in the bloodstream and lymphatics, prepared to protect the body. The various kinds of T cells include

- Helper T4 cells—function in the bloodstream to identify and destroy antigens

- Helper T1 cells—increase B-lymphocyte antibody production

- Helper T2 cells—increase activity of cytotoxic (killer) T cells, which attack cells directly by altering the cell membrane and causing cell lysis (destruction)

- Suppressor T cells—suppress the immune response

- Memory T lymphocytes—recognize previous contact with antigens and activate an immune response

Immunizations, covered in Chapter 54, are individual drugs or a series of drugs given to help the body identify a pathogenic invader. In the past, communicable diseases and injuries were the primary illnesses health care providers treated. Today, some communicable diseases, such as smallpox and polio, have been almost eradicated because of the ability to immunize large populations of people at or near birth. All nurses play an important role in the continued immunization and protection of the population from easily preventable diseases.

Cancer is still a dreaded disease in our culture. At one time, a diagnosis of cancer was akin to a death sentence. With the advent of numerous drugs, known as *chemotherapy*, cancer is now viewed as a chronic illness in which people may be diagnosed and treated, then monitored for the remainder of their lives and treated again should cancer cells re-emerge. The information provided in Chapter 55 about antineoplastic drugs is meant to inform the nursing student about these medications—not to prepare students to administer them. Most hospitals and clinics require that nurses receive specialized training and standardized educational preparation before they are permitted to administer antineoplastic drugs. The Oncology Nursing Society has developed guidelines and educational tools for credentialing nurses for certification in administering chemotherapy.

The information in Chapter 55 is based on the need of all nurses to be able to assess and treat patients undergoing chemotherapy, whether they present with adverse reactions in the primary health care provider's outpatient office or hospital emergency department, or are being treated in the acute care setting for other illnesses or injuries.

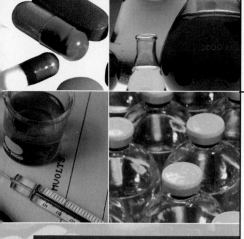

Immunologic Agents

Learning Objectives

On completion of this chapter, the student will:

- Discuss humoral immunity and cell-mediated immunity.
- Distinguish between and define the different types of immunity.
- Discuss the use of vaccines, toxoids, immune globulins, and antivenins to provide immunity against disease.
- Discuss preadministration and ongoing assessments the nurse should perform with the patient receiving an immunologic agent.
- Identify nursing diagnoses particular to a patient receiving an immunologic agent.
- Discuss ways to promote an optimal response, management of common adverse reactions, special considerations, and important points to keep in mind when educating a patient taking an immunologic agent.

Immunity refers to the ability of the body to identify and resist microorganisms that are potentially harmful. This ability enables the body to fight or prevent infectious disease and inhibit tissue and organ damage. The immune system is not confined to any one part of the body. Immune stem cells, formed in the bone marrow, may remain in the bone marrow until maturation, or they may migrate to different body sites for maturation. After maturation, most immune cells circulate in the body and exert specific effects. The immune system has two distinct, but overlapping, mechanisms with which to fight invading organisms:

- Cell-mediated defenses (cellular immunity)
- Antibody-mediated defenses (humoral immunity)

Cell-Mediated Immunity

Cell-mediated immunity (CMI) results from the activity of many leukocyte actions, reactions, and interactions that range from simple to complex. This type of immunity depends on the actions of the T lymphocytes, which are responsible for a delayed type of immune response. The T lymphocyte becomes sensitized by its first contact with a specific antigen. Subsequent exposure to an antigen stimulates multiple reactions aimed at destroying or inactivating the offending antigen. T lymphocytes and macrophages (large cells that surround, engulf, and digest microorganisms and cellular debris) work together in CMI to destroy the antigen. T lymphocytes attack the antigens directly, rather than produce antibodies (as is done in humoral immunity). Cellular reactions may also occur without macrophages.

The T lymphocytes defend against viral infections, fungal infections, and some bacterial infections. If CMI is reduced, as in the case of acquired immunodeficiency syndrome (AIDS), the body is unable to protect itself against many viral, bacterial, and fungal infections.

Humoral Immunity

In **humoral immunity**, special lymphocytes (white blood cells), called *B lymphocytes*, produce circulating antibodies to act against a foreign substance. This type of immunity is based on the antigen–antibody response. An **antigen** is a substance, usually a protein, that stimulates the body to produce antibodies. An **antibody** is a globulin (protein) produced by the B lymphocytes as a defense against an antigen. Humoral immunity protects the body against bacterial and viral infections.

Specific antibodies are formed for a specific antigen—that is, chickenpox antibodies are formed when the person is exposed to the chickenpox virus (the antigen). This is called an **antigen–antibody response**. Once manufactured, antibodies circulate in the bloodstream, sometimes only for a short time, and at other times for the lifetime of the person. When an antigen enters the body, specific antibodies neutralize the specific invading antigen; this condition is called *immunity*. Thus, the individual with specific circulating antibodies is immune (or has immunity) to a specific antigen. Immunity is the resistance that an individual has against disease.

Cell-mediated and humoral immunity are interdependent; CMI influences the function of the B lymphocytes, and humoral immunity influences the function of the T lymphocytes.

Active and Passive Immunity

Active and passive immunity involve the use of agents that stimulate antibody formation (active immunity) or the injection of ready-made antibodies found in the serum of immune individuals or animals (passive immunity).

Active Immunity

When a person is exposed to certain infectious microorganisms (antigens), the body begins to form antibodies (or build an immunity) to the invading microorganism. This is called **active immunity**. The two types of active immunity are naturally acquired active immunity and artificially acquired active immunity. The Summary Drug Table: Agents for Active Immunization identifies agents that produce active immunity.

Naturally Acquired Active Immunity

Naturally acquired active immunity occurs when the person is exposed to and experiences a disease, and the body manufactures antibodies to provide future immunity to the disease. It is called *active* immunity because the antibodies are produced by the person who had the disease (Fig. 54-1). Thus, having the disease produces immunity. Display 54-1 provides an example of naturally acquired active immunity.

Artificially Acquired Active Immunity

Artificially acquired active immunity occurs when an individual is given a killed or weakened antigen, which stimulates the formation of antibodies against the antigen. The antigen does not cause the disease, but the individual still manufactures specific antibodies against the disease. When a vaccine containing an **attenuated** (weakened) antigen is given, the individual may experience a few minor symptoms of the disease or even a mild form of the disease, but the symptoms are almost always milder than the disease itself and usually last for a short time.

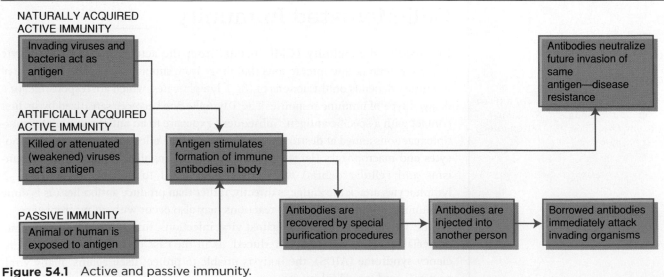

Figure 54.1 Active and passive immunity.

SUMMARY DRUG TABLE   AGENTS FOR ACTIVE IMMUNIZATION

GENERIC DRUG	TRADE NAME	USES	ADVERSE REACTIONS	DOSAGE RANGES
Vaccines, Bacterial (Routine Immunizations)				
Hemophilus influenzae type B conjugate vaccine *he'-maw-fil-us in-flu-en'-zah kon'-jew-gate*	ActHIB, HibTITER, PedvaxHIB	Routine immunization of children	Rare; minor local reactions such as local tenderness, pain at injection site, anorexia, fever, myalgia	0.5 mL IM, see immunization schedule
meningococcal polysaccharide vaccine *men-in-jo'-kok'-al po-ly-sack'-a-ride*	Menomune	Routine immunization of adolescents	Same as *H. influenzae* vaccine	0.5 mL SC only
pneumococcal vaccine (PCV), polysaccharide (PPV) *new-mo-kok'-kal*	Pneumovax 23	Routine immunization of children, PPV is recommended for certain high-risk groups who can not take PCV	Same as *H. influenzae* vaccine	0.5 mL SC or IM, see immunization schedule
Vaccines, Bacterial (Special Populations)				
BCG vaccine		Prevention of pulmonary TB in negative, high-risk populations (health care workers, infants and children in high-TB areas)	Same as *H. influenzae* vaccine	0.2–0.3 mL percutaneous, repeat in 2–3 mo
pneumococcal 7-valent conjugate vaccine	Prevnar	Active immunization against *Streptococcus pneumoniae* for infants and toddlers, prevention of otitis media	Rare; minor local reactions such as local tenderness, pain at injection site, decreased appetite, irritability, drowsiness, fever	0.5 mL IM
typhoid vaccine *tye'-foid*	Typhim Vi, Vivotif Berna	Immunization against typhoid	Same as *H. influenzae* vaccine	Oral: total of 4 capsules 1 wk before exposure Parenteral: adults and children 2 y and older, 1 dose of 0.5 mL IM
Vaccines, Viral (Routine Immunizations)				
measles (rubeola), mumps and rubella virus vaccine *me'-zuls, ru-be'-o-la, ru-bell'-ah*	MMR II (live) ProQuad (attenuated)	Routine immunization of children	Mild fever, rash, cough, rhinitis	0.5 mL SC
hepatitis A vaccine, inactivated *hep-ah-tie'-tis A*	Havrix, Vaqta	Routine immunization of children	Same as measles vaccine	Administered IM; dosage varies with product; see package insert for specific dosages

● SUMMARY DRUG TABLE *(continued)*

GENERIC DRUG	TRADE NAME	USES	ADVERSE REACTIONS	DOSAGE RANGES
hepatitis B vaccine, recombinant	Engerix-B, Recombivax HB	Routine immunization of children	Minor local reactions such as local tenderness, pain at injection site, anorexia, fever, myalgia	3–4 doses of 0.5–2 mL IM
poliovirus vaccine, inactivated (IPV) *po'-lee-o-vi'-rus*	IPOL	Routine immunization of children	Rare; malaise, nausea, diarrhea, fever	0.5 mL IM or SC; see immunization schedule
varicella virus vaccine *var-i-sel'-a*	Varivax	Routine immunization of children	Minor local reactions, such as local tenderness, pain at injection site, rash, fever, cough, irritability	0.5 mL SC; see immunization schedule
Vaccines, Viral (Special Populations)				
measles virus vaccine, live, attenuated*	Attenuvax	Selective active immunization against measles	Mild fever, rash, cough, rhinitis	0.5 mL SC
mumps virus vaccine, live*	Mumpsvax	Selective active immunization against mumps	Same as measles vaccine	0.5 mL SC
rubella virus vaccine, live*	Meruvax II	Selective active immunization against rubella	Same as measles vaccine	0.5 mL SC
rubella and mumps virus vaccine, live*	Biavax-II	Selective active immunization against rubella and mumps	Same as measles vaccine	0.5 mL SC
influenza virus vaccine *in-flu-en'-za*	FluMist, Fluvirin, Fluzone	Active immunization against the specific influenza virus strains contained in the formulation	Same as measles vaccine	One dose 0.5 mL IM Nasal: 1–2 doses (FluMist only)
rotavirus vaccine *row'-ta-vye'-rus*	RotaShield	Prevention of gastroenteritis caused by rotavirus serotypes contained in the vaccines	Fever, decreased appetite, abdominal cramping, irritability, decreased activity	Three 2.5-mL doses given orally
rabies vaccine *ray'-bees*	Imovax Rabies Vaccine, RabAvert	Prevention of rabies in people with greater risk (e.g., veterinarians, animal handlers, forest rangers); postexposure prophylaxis: bite by an animal suspected of carrying rabies	Transient pain, erythema, swelling or itching at the injection site, headache, nausea, abdominal pain, muscle aches, dizziness	Pre-exposure prophylaxis: 1 mL IM, see package insert for dosing Postexposure: give vaccine IM after initial immune globulin injection

GENERIC DRUG	TRADE NAME	USES	ADVERSE REACTIONS	DOSAGE RANGES
Toxoids (Routine Immunizations)				
diphtheria and tetanus toxoids and acellular pertussis vaccine, (DTaP) *dif-ther'-ee-ah, tet-ah-nus toks'-oyds, a-sell'-u-lar per-tuss'-us*	Daptacel, Infanrix, Tripedia	Active immunization against diphtheria, tetanus, and pertussis	Headache, dizziness, rash, itching, nausea, fever	0.5 mL IM; see immunization schedule
Toxoids (Special Populations)				
diphtheria and tetanus toxoids, combined (DTTd)		Booster immunization against diphtheria and tetanus	Headache, dizziness, rash, itching, nausea, fever	0.5 mL IM, caution with site rotation; see package insert and immunization schedule
Combination Products (Viral/Bacterial Vaccine or Toxoid Together)				
hepatitis A and B combination vaccine	Twinrix	Twinrix for those over 18 y traveling to endemic areas	See individual vaccines	See package insert for specific dosing
diphtheria, tetanus toxoids, acellular pertussis, and *H. influenzae* type B	TriHIBit	See individual vaccines	See individual vaccines	See package insert for specific dosing
vaccine combined Pediarix (diphtheria, tetanus toxoids and acellular pertussis, hepatitis B [recombinant], and inactivated poliovirus)		See individual vaccines	See individual vaccines	See package insert for specific dosing

TB, tuberculosis.
*The trivalent measles-mumps-rubella (MMR) vaccine is the preferred immunizing agent for most children and adults.

Display 54.1 Example of Naturally Acquired Active Immunity

Naturally acquired active immunity is exemplified by an individual who is exposed to chickenpox for the first time and who has no immunity to the disease. The body immediately begins to manufacture antibodies against the chickenpox virus. However, the production of a sufficient quantity of antibodies takes time, and the individual gets the disease. At the time of exposure and while the individual still has chickenpox, the body continues to manufacture antibodies. These antibodies circulate in the individual's bloodstream for life. In the future, any exposure to the chickenpox virus results in the antibodies mobilizing to destroy the invading antigen.

The decision to use an attenuated, rather than a killed, virus as a vaccine to provide immunity is based on research. For example, many antigens, when killed, produce a poor antibody response, whereas when the antigen is merely weakened, a good antibody response occurs. Immunization against a specific disease provides artificially acquired active immunity. Display 54-2 gives an example of artificially acquired active immunity.

Artificially acquired immunity against some diseases may require periodic booster injections to keep an adequate antibody level (or antibody titer) circulating in the blood. A **booster** injection is the administration of an additional dose of the vaccine to "boost" the production of antibodies to a level that will maintain the desired immunity. The booster is given months or years after the initial

Display 54.2 Example of Artificially Acquired Active Immunity

Although chickenpox may seem like a minor illness, it can cause herpes zoster (shingles) later in life, which is a painful condition. An example of the use of an attenuated virus is the administration of the varicella virus vaccine to an individual who has not had chickenpox. The varicella (chickenpox) vaccine contains the live, attenuated varicella virus. The individual receiving the vaccine develops a mild or modified chickenpox infection, which then produces immunity against the varicella virus. The varicella vaccine protects the recipient for several years or, for some individuals, for life. An example of a killed virus used for immunization is the yearly influenza vaccine. These vaccines protect those who receive the vaccine for about 3 to 6 months.

Display 54.3 Examples of Diseases Preventable by Vaccination

Diseases Prevented by Routine Vaccination

- *Hemophilus influenzae* type B
- Hepatitis A
- Hepatitis B
- Influenza
- Mumps
- Measles
- Pertussis
- Pneumococcal disease
- Poliomyelitis
- Rubella
- Tetanus
- Varicella

Diseases Preventable by Vaccination Before Travel to Endemic Areas

- Cholera
- Diphtheria
- Japanese encephalitis
- Lyme disease
- Smallpox
- Typhoid
- Yellow fever

vaccine and may be needed because the life of some antibodies is short.

The measles vaccine is considered an immunization. Immunization is a form of artificial active immunity and an important method of controlling some of the infectious diseases that are capable of causing serious and sometimes fatal consequences. The immunization schedule for children is given in Figure 54-2. Currently, many infectious diseases may be prevented by **vaccine** (artificial active immunity). Examples of some of these diseases can be found in Display 54-3.

Passive Immunity

Passive immunity is obtained from the administration of immune globulins or antivenins. This type of immunity provides the individual with ready-made antibodies from another human or an animal (see Fig. 54-1). Passive immunity provides immediate immunity to the invading antigen, but lasts for only a short time. The Summary Drug Table: Agents for Passive Immunity identifies agents for passive immunizations. Display 54-4 provides an example of passive immunity.

IMMUNOLOGIC AGENTS

Some immunologic agents capitalize on the body's natural defenses by stimulating the immune response, thereby creating protection to a specific disease within the body. Other immunologic agents supply ready-made antibodies to provide passive immunity. Examples of immunologic agents include vaccines, toxoids, and immune globulins.

Actions and Uses

Vaccines and Toxoids

Antibody-producing tissues cannot distinguish between an antigen that is capable of causing disease (a live antigen), an attenuated antigen, or a killed antigen. Because of this phenomenon, vaccines, which contain either an attenuated or a killed antigen, have been developed to create immunity to certain diseases. The live antigens are either killed or weakened during the manufacturing process. The weakened or killed antigens contained in the vaccine do not have sufficient strength to cause disease. Although it is a rare occurrence, vaccination with any vaccine may not result in a protective antibody response in all individuals given the vaccine.

Display 54.4 Example of Passive Immunity

An example of passive immunity is the administration of immune globulins (see Summary Drug Table: Agents for Passive Immunity) to prevent organ rejection in patients after organ transplantation surgery.

DEPARTMENT OF HEALTH AND HUMAN SERVICES • CENTERS FOR DISEASE CONTROL AND PREVENTION

Recommended Childhood and Adolescent Immunization Schedule UNITED STATES • 2006

Vaccine ▼ / Age ▶	Birth	1 month	2 months	4 months	6 months	12 months	15 months	18 months	24 months	4–6 years	11–12 years	13–14 years	15 years	16–18 years
Hepatitis B[1]	HepB	HepB		HepB[1]	HepB	HepB				HepB Series				
Diphtheria, Tetanus, Pertussis[2]			DTaP	DTaP	DTaP		DTaP			DTaP	Tdap	Tdap		
Haemophilus influenzae type b[3]			Hib	Hib	Hib[3]	Hib								
Inactivated Poliovirus			IPV	IPV	IPV					IPV				
Measles, Mumps, Rubella[4]						MMR				MMR	MMR			
Varicella[5]						Varicella				Varicella				
Meningococcal[6]							*Vaccines within broken line are for selected populations*		MPSV4		MCV4	MCV4	MCV4	
Pneumococcal[7]			PCV	PCV	PCV	PCV			PCV	PPV				
Influenza[8]					Influenza (Yearly)					Influenza (Yearly)				
Hepatitis A[9]						HepA Series								

This schedule indicates the recommended ages for routine administration of currently licensed childhood vaccines, as of December 1, 2005, for children through age 18 years. Any dose not administered at the recommended age should be administered at any subsequent visit when indicated and feasible. ▓ Indicates age groups that warrant special effort to administer those vaccines not previously administered. Additional vaccines may be licensed and recommended during the year. Licensed combination vaccines may be used whenever any components of the combination are indicated and other components of the vaccine are not contraindicated and if approved by the Food and Drug Administration for that dose of the series. Providers should consult the respective ACIP statement for detailed recommendations. Clinically significant adverse events that follow immunization should be reported to the Vaccine Adverse Event Reporting System (VAERS). Guidance about how to obtain and complete a VAERS form is available at www.vaers.hhs.gov or by telephone, 800-822-7967.

▓ Range of recommended ages   ▓ Catch-up immunization   ▓ 11–12 year old assessment

1. Hepatitis B vaccine (HepB). *AT BIRTH:* All newborns should receive monovalent HepB soon after birth and before hospital discharge. **Infants born to mothers who are HBsAg-positive** should receive HepB and 0.5 mL of hepatitis B immune globulin (HBIG) within 12 hours of birth. **Infants born to mothers whose HBsAg status is unknown** should receive HepB within 12 hours of birth. The mother should have blood drawn as soon as possible to determine her HBsAg status; if HBsAg-positive, the infant should receive HBIG as soon as possible (no later than age 1 week). **For infants born to HBsAg-negative mothers,** the birth dose can be delayed in rare circumstances but only if a physician's order to withhold the vaccine and a copy of the mother's original HBsAg-negative laboratory report are documented in the infant's medical record. *FOLLOWING THE BIRTHDOSE:* The HepB series should be completed with either monovalent HepB or a combination vaccine containing HepB. The second dose should be administered at age 1–2 months. The final dose should be administered at age ≥24 weeks. It is permissible to administer 4 doses of HepB (e.g., when combination vaccines are given after the birth dose); however, if monovalent HepB is used, a dose at age 4 months is not needed. **Infants born to HBsAg-positive mothers** should be tested for HBsAg and antibody to HBsAg after completion of the HepB series, at age 9–18 months (generally at the next well-child visit after completion of the vaccine series).

2. Diphtheria and tetanus toxoids and acellular pertussis vaccine (DTaP). The fourth dose of DTaP may be administered as early as age 12 months, provided 6 months have elapsed since the third dose and the child is unlikely to return at age 15–18 months. The final dose in the series should be given at age ≥4 years.

Tetanus and diphtheria toxoids and acellular pertussis vaccine (Tdap – adolescent preparation) is recommended at age 11–12 years for those who have completed the recommended childhood DTP/DTaP vaccination series and have not received a Td booster dose. Adolescents 13–18 years who missed the 11–12-year Td/Tdap booster dose should also receive a single dose of Tdap if they have completed the recommended childhood DTP/DTaP vaccination series. Subsequent **tetanus and diphtheria toxoids (Td)** are recommended every 10 years.

3. *Haemophilus influenzae* **type b conjugate vaccine (Hib).** Three Hib conjugate vaccines are licensed for infant use. If PRP-OMP (PedvaxHIB® or ComVax® [Merck]) is administered at ages 2 and 4 months, a dose at age 6 months is not required. DTaP/Hib combination products should not be used for primary immunization in infants at ages 2, 4 or 6 months but can be used as boosters after any Hib vaccine. The final dose in the series should be administered at age ≥12 months.

4. Measles, mumps, and rubella vaccine (MMR). The second dose of MMR is recommended routinely at age 4–6 years but may be administered during any visit, provided at least 4 weeks have elapsed since the first dose and both doses are administered beginning at or after age 12 months. Those who have not previously received the second dose should complete the schedule by age 11–12 years.

5. Varicella vaccine. Varicella vaccine is recommended at any visit at or after age 12 months for susceptible children (i.e., those who lack a reliable history of chickenpox). Susceptible persons aged ≥13 years should receive 2 doses administered at least 4 weeks apart.

6. Meningococcal vaccine (MCV4). Meningococcal conjugate vaccine (MCV4) should be given to all children at the 11–12 year old visit as well as to unvaccinated adolescents at high school entry (15 years of age). Other adolescents who wish to decrease their risk for meningococcal disease may also be vaccinated. All college freshmen living in dormitories should also be vaccinated, preferably with MCV4, although **meningococcal polysaccharide vaccine (MPSV4)** is an acceptable alternative. Vaccination against invasive meningococcal disease is recommended for children and adolescents aged ≥2 years with terminal complement deficiencies or anatomic or functional asplenia and certain other high risk groups (see *MMWR* 2005;54 [RR-7]:1-21); use MPSV4 for children aged 2–10 years and MCV4 for older children, although MPSV4 is an acceptable alternative.

7. Pneumococcal vaccine. The heptavalent **pneumococcal conjugate vaccine (PCV)** is recommended for all children aged 2–23 months and for certain children aged 24–59 months. The final dose in the series should be given at age ≥12 months. **Pneumococcal polysaccharide vaccine (PPV)** is recommended in addition to PCV for certain high-risk groups. See *MMWR* 2000; 49(RR-9):1-35.

8. Influenza vaccine. Influenza vaccine is recommended annually for children aged ≥6 months with certain risk factors (including, but not limited to, asthma, cardiac disease, sickle cell disease, human immunodeficiency virus [HIV], diabetes, and conditions that can compromise respiratory function or handling of respiratory secretions or that can increase the risk for aspiration), healthcare workers, and other persons (including household members) in close contact with persons in groups at high risk (see *MMWR* 2005;54[RR-8]:1-55). In addition, healthy children aged 6–23 months and close contacts of healthy children aged 0–5 months are recommended to receive influenza vaccine because children in this age group are at substantially increased risk for influenza-related hospitalizations. For healthy persons aged 5–49 years, the intranasally administered, live, attenuated influenza vaccine (LAIV) is an acceptable alternative to the intramuscular trivalent inactivated influenza vaccine (TIV). See *MMWR* 2005;54(RR-8):1-55. Children receiving TIV should be administered a dosage appropriate for their age (0.25 mL if aged 6–35 months or 0.5 mL if aged ≥3 years). Children aged ≤8 years who are receiving influenza vaccine for the first time should receive 2 doses (separated by at least 4 weeks for TIV and at least 6 weeks for LAIV).

9. Hepatitis A vaccine (HepA). HepA is recommended for all children at 1 year of age (i.e., 12–23 months). The 2 doses in the series should be administered at least 6 months apart. States, counties, and communities with existing HepA vaccination programs for children 2–18 years of age are encouraged to maintain these programs. In these areas, new efforts focused on routine vaccination of 1-year-old children should enhance, not replace, ongoing programs directed at a broader population of children. HepA is also recommended for certain high risk groups (see *MMWR* 1999; 48[RR-12]1-37).

The Childhood and Adolescent Immunization Schedule is approved by:
Advisory Committee on Immunization Practices www.cdc.gov/nip/acip • American Academy of Pediatrics www.aap.org • American Academy of Family Physicians www.aafp.org

Figure 54.2 Recommended childhood immunization schedule, Centers for Disease Control and Prevention, 2006. Available at www.cdc.gov/nip/recs/child-schedule.htm#printable.

Immunologic Agents

Recommended Immunization Schedule
for Children and Adolescents Who Start Late or Who Are More Than 1 Month Behind

UNITED STATES • 2006

The tables below give catch-up schedules and minimum intervals between doses for children who have delayed immunizations.
There is no need to restart a vaccine series regardless of the time that has elapsed between doses. Use the chart appropriate for the child's age.

CATCH-UP SCHEDULE FOR CHILDREN AGED 4 MONTHS THROUGH 6 YEARS

Vaccine	Minimum Age for Dose 1	Minimum Interval Between Doses			
		Dose 1 to Dose 2	Dose 2 to Dose 3	Dose 3 to Dose 4	Dose 4 to Dose 5
Diphtheria, Tetanus, Pertussis	6 wks	4 weeks	4 weeks	6 months	6 months[1]
Inactivated Poliovirus	6 wks	4 weeks	4 weeks	4 weeks[2]	
Hepatitis B[3]	Birth	4 weeks	8 weeks (and 16 weeks after first dose)		
Measles, Mumps, Rubella	12 mo	4 weeks[4]			
Varicella	12 mo				
Haemophilus influenzae type b[5]	6 wks	4 weeks if first dose given at age <12 months / 8 weeks (as final dose) if first dose given at age 12-14 months / No further doses needed if first dose given at age ≥15 months	4 weeks[6] if current age <12 months / 8 weeks (as final dose)[6] if current age ≥12 months and second dose given at age <15 months / No further doses needed if previous dose given at age ≥15 mo	8 weeks (as final dose) This dose only necessary for children aged 12 months–5 years who received 3 doses before age 12 months	
Pneumococcal[7]	6 wks	4 weeks if first dose given at age <12 months and current age <24 months / 8 weeks (as final dose) if first dose given at age <12 months or current age 24–59 months / No further doses needed for healthy children if first dose given at age ≥24 months	4 weeks if current age <12 months / 8 weeks (as final dose) if current age ≥12 months / No further doses needed for healthy children if previous dose given at age ≥24 months	8 weeks (as final dose) This dose only necessary for children aged 12 months–5 years who received 3 doses before age 12 months	

CATCH-UP SCHEDULE FOR CHILDREN AGED 7 YEARS THROUGH 18 YEARS

Vaccine	Minimum Interval Between Doses		
	Dose 1 to Dose 2	Dose 2 to Dose 3	Dose 3 to Booster Dose
Tetanus, Diphtheria[8]	4 weeks	6 months	6 months if first dose given at age <12 months and current age <11 years; otherwise 5 years
Inactivated Poliovirus[9]	4 weeks	4 weeks	IPV[2,9]
Hepatitis B	4 weeks	8 weeks (and 16 weeks after first dose)	
Measles, Mumps, Rubella	4 weeks		
Varicella[10]	4 weeks		

1. **DTaP.** The fifth dose is not necessary if the fourth dose was administered after the fourth birthday.
2. **IPV.** For children who received an all-IPV or all-oral poliovirus (OPV) series, a fourth dose is not necessary if third dose was administered at age ≥4 years. If both OPV and IPV were administered as part of a series, a total of 4 doses should be given, regardless of the child's current age.
3. **HepB.** Administer the 3-dose series to all children and adolescents<19 years of age if they were not previously vaccinated.
4. **MMR.** The second dose of MMR is recommended routinely at age 4–6 years but may be administered earlier if desired.
5. **Hib.** Vaccine is not generally recommended for children aged ≥5 years.

6. **Hib.** If current age <12 months and the first 2 doses were PRP-OMP (PedvaxHIB® or ComVax® [Merck]), the third (and final) dose should be administered at age 12–15 months and at least 8 weeks after the second dose.
7. **PCV.** Vaccine is not generally recommended for children aged ≥5 years.
8. **Td.** Adolescent tetanus, diphtheria, and pertussis vaccine (Tdap) may be substituted for any dose in a primary catch-up series or as a booster if age appropriate for Tdap. A five-year interval from the last Td dose is encouraged when Tdap is used as a booster dose. See ACIP recommendations for further information.
9. **IPV.** Vaccine is not generally recommended for persons aged ≥18 years.
10. **Varicella.** Administer the 2-dose series to all susceptible adolescents aged ≥13 years.

Report adverse reactions to vaccines through the federal Vaccine Adverse Event Reporting System. For information on reporting reactions following immunization, please visit www.vaers.hhs.gov or call the 24-hour national toll-free information line 800-822-7967. Report suspected cases of vaccine-preventable diseases to your state or local health department.

For additional information about vaccines, including precautions and contraindications for immunization and vaccine shortages, please visit the National Immunization Program Website at www.cdc.gov/nip or contact 800-CDC-INFO (800-232-4636) (In English, En Español — 24/7)

Figure 54.2 (continued)

SUMMARY DRUG TABLE   AGENTS FOR PASSIVE IMMUNITY

GENERIC NAME	TRADE NAME	USES	ADVERSE REACTIONS	DOSAGE RANGES
Immune Globulins				
botulism immune globulin (BIG-IV) *botch'-oo-lizm i-mune' glob'-u-lin*	BabyBIG	Treatment of infant botulism	Headache, chills, fever	IV administration only; see dosing schedule
cytomegalovirus immune globulin (CMV-IGIV) *sy'-toe-meg'-a-lo-vi-rus*	CytoGam	Prevention of CMV post-organ transplantation	Injection site: tenderness, pain, muscle stiffness Systemic: headache, chills, fever	See dosing schedule, varies weeks out from transplantation
hepatitis B immune globulin (HBIG) *hep-ah-ti'- tus*	BayHep B, Nabi-HB	Prevention of hepatitis B after exposure to the disease (use if not previously immunized)	Same as CMV-IGIV	0.06 mL/kg (3–5 mL) IM
immune globulin (gamma globulin; IgG)	BayGam	Prevention of disease after exposure (use if not previously immunized); hepatitis A, measles (rubeola), Varicella, Rubella, immunoglobulin deficiency	Same as CMV-IGIV	See dosing schedule, varies for disease
immune globulin intravenous (IGIV)	Gamimune N, Gamunex, Polygam S/D, Venoglobulin	Immunodeficiency syndrome, ITP, chronic lymphocytic leukemia, bone marrow transplanta-tion, pediatric human immunodefficiency virus infection	Headache, chills, fever	IV administration only; see dosing schedule, varies for disease
lymphocyte immune globulin* *lymph'-o-site*	Atgam	Treatment of rejection post-organ transplantation, aplastic anemia	Chills, fever, arthralgia	After skin test dose, IV administration only; see dosing schedule, varies for disease
antithymocyte globulin*	Thymoglobulin	Treatment of acute rejection post kidney transplantation, aplastic anemia	Chills, fever, arthralgia	IV administration only; see dosing schedule
rabies immune globulin (RIG) *ray'-bees*	Bay Rab, Imogam	Prevention of rabies after exposure to the disease (use if not previously immunized)	Same as CMV-IGIV	See dosing schedule
Rh immune globulin (IGIM)	BayRho-D, RhoGAM	Prevention of Rh hemolytic disease after birth	Same as CMV-IGIV	300 mcg (1 vial) IM within 72 h of delivery

Immunologic Agents

SUMMARY DRUG TABLE *(continued)*

GENERIC NAME	TRADE NAME	USES	ADVERSE REACTIONS	DOSAGE RANGES
Rh immune globulin (IGIV)	WinRho SDF	Suppression of Rh isoimmunization after termination of pregnancy; ITP	Headache, chills, fever	IV administration only; see dosing schedule
Rh immune globulin microdose (IG-microdose)	BayRho-D Mini Dose, MICRho GAM	Suppression of Rh isoimmunization after termination of pregnancy before 12 weeks gestation	Same as CMV-IGIV	50 mcg (1 vial) IM
Respiratory syncytial virus immune globulin (RSV-IGIV) *sin-sish'-al vi'-rus*	RespiGam	Respiratory syncytial virus	Headache, chills, fever	IV administration only; see dosing schedule
tetanus immune globulin (TIG) *tet'-ah-nus*	BayTet	Tetanus prophylaxis after injury in patients whose immunization is incomplete or uncertain	Same as CMV-IGIV	250 units IM
varicella-zoster immune globulin (VZIG) *var-i-sel'-a zos'-ter*		Prevention of varicella in compromised patients after exposure to the disease (use if not previously immunized)	Same as CMV-IGIV	IM administration only; see dosing schedule
Antivenins				
crotalidae polyvalent immune Fab *kro-tal'-i-day pol-ee-va'-lent*	CroFab	For treatment of mild to moderate North American rattlesnake bites	Urticaria, rash	See package insert for mixing and administration
antivenin (*Micrurus fulvius*) *an-tee-ven'-in*		Passive transient protection for toxic effects of venoms of coral snake in United States	Urticaria, rash	See package insert for mixing and administration

ITP, idiopathic thrombocytopenic purpura.
*Must be prescribed and administered by specialized physicians.

A **toxin** is a poisonous substance produced by some bacteria, such as *Clostridium tetani*, the bacterium that cause tetanus. A toxin is capable of stimulating the body to produce antitoxins, which are substances that act in the same manner as antibodies. Toxins are powerful substances, and like other antigens, they can be attenuated. A toxin that is attenuated (or weakened) but still capable of stimulating the formation of antitoxins is called a **toxoid**.

Both vaccines and toxoids are administered to stimulate the body's immune response to specific antigens or toxins. These agents must be administered before exposure to the disease-causing organism. The initiation of the immune response, in turn, produces resistance to a specific infectious disease. The immunity produced in this manner is active immunity.

Vaccines and toxoids are used for

- Routine immunization of infants and children (see Fig. 54-1)

- Immunization of adults against tetanus
- Immunization of adults at high risk for certain diseases (e.g., pneumococcal and influenza vaccines)
- Immunization of children or adults at risk for exposure to a particular disease (e.g., hepatitis A for those going to endemic areas)
- Immunization of prepubertal girls or nonpregnant women of childbearing age against rubella

Immune Globulins and Antivenins

Globulins are proteins present in blood serum or plasma that contain antibodies. **Immune globulins** are solutions obtained from human or animal blood containing antibodies that have been formed by the body to specific antigens. Because they contain ready-made antibodies, they are given for passive immunity against disease. The immune globulins are administered to provide passive immunization to one or more infectious diseases. Those receiving immune globulins receive antibodies only to the diseases to which the donor blood is immune. The onset of protection is rapid but of short duration (1 to 3 months).

Antivenins are used for passive, transient protection from the toxic effects of bites by spiders (black widow and similar spiders) and snakes (rattlesnakes, copperhead and cottonmouth, and coral). The most effective response is obtained when the drug is administered within 4 hours after exposure.

Adverse Reactions

Vaccines and Toxoids

Adverse reactions from the administration of vaccines or toxoids are usually mild. Chills, fever, muscular aches and pains, rash, and lethargy may be present. Pain and tenderness at the injection site may also occur. Although rare, a hypersensitivity reaction may occur. The Summary Drug Table: Agents for Active Immunization provides a listing of the typical adverse reactions.

Immune Globulins and Antivenins

Adverse reactions to immune globulins are rare. However, local tenderness and pain at the injection site may occur. The most common adverse reactions include urticaria, angioedema, erythema, malaise, nausea, diarrhea, headache, chills, and fever. Adverse reactions, if they occur, usually last for several hours. Systemic reactions are extremely rare, with the exception of immune globulins given to prevent post-transplantation rejection. These immune globulins are made from equine (horse) or rabbit serum and can produce anaphylactic reactions. They should be administered only under the direction of a physician specializing in transplantation medicine.

The antivenins may cause various reactions, with hypersensitivity being the most severe. Some antivenins are prepared from equine serum, and if a patient is sensitive to equine serum, serious reactions or death may result. The immediate reactions usually occur within 30 minutes after administration of the antivenin. Symptoms include apprehension; flushing; itching; urticaria; edema of the face, tongue, and throat; cough; dyspnea; vomiting; cyanosis; and collapse. Other adverse reactions are included in the Summary Drug Table: Agents for Passive Immunity.

Contraindications and Precautions

Vaccines and Toxoids

Immunologic agents are contraindicated in patients with known hypersensitivity to the agent or any component of it. The measles, mumps, rubella, and varicella vaccines are contraindicated in patients who have had an allergic reaction to gelatin, neomycin, or a previous dose of one of the vaccines. The measles, mumps, rubella, and varicella vaccines are contraindicated during pregnancy, especially during the first trimester, because of the danger of birth defects. Women are instructed to avoid becoming pregnant at least 3 months after receiving these vaccines. Vaccines and toxoids are contraindicated during acute febrile illnesses, leukemia, lymphoma, immunosuppressive illness or drug therapy, and nonlocalized cancer. See Display 54-5 for additional information on the contraindications to immunologic agents.

Display 54.5 Contraindications to Immunization

- Moderate or severe illness, with or without fever
- Anaphylactoid reactions (e.g., hives, swelling of the mouth and throat, difficulty breathing [dyspnea], hypotension, and shock)
- Known allergy to vaccine or vaccine constituents, particularly gelatin, eggs, or neomycin
- Individuals with an immunologic deficiency should not receive a vaccine (virus is transmissible to the immunocompromised individual).
- Immunizations are postponed during the administration of steroids, radiation therapy, and antineoplastic (anticancer) drug therapy.
- Virus vaccines against measles, rubella, and mumps should not be given to pregnant women.
- Patients who experience severe systemic or neurologic reactions after a previous dose of the vaccine should not be given any additional doses.

The immunologic agents are used with extreme caution in individuals with a history of allergies. Sensitivity testing may be performed in individuals with a history of allergies. No adequate studies have been conducted in pregnant women, and it is not known whether these agents are excreted in breast milk. Thus, the immunologic agents (pregnancy category C) are used with caution in pregnant women and during lactation.

Immune Globulins and Antivenins

The immune globulins are contraindicated in patients with a history of allergic reactions after administration of human immunoglobulin preparations and in individuals with isolated immunoglobulin A (IgA) deficiency (individuals could have an anaphylactic reaction to subsequent administration of blood products that contain IgA).

Nursing Alert

Human immune globulin intravenous (IGIV) products have been associated with renal impairment, acute renal failure, osmotic nephrosis, and death. Individuals with a predisposition to acute renal failure (e.g., those with preexisting renal disease), those with diabetes mellitus, individuals older than 65 years of age, or patients receiving nephrotoxic drugs should not be given human IGIV products.

The antivenins are contraindicated in patients with hypersensitivity to equine serum or any other component of the serum.

The immune globulins and antivenins are administered cautiously during pregnancy and lactation (pregnancy category C) and in children.

Interactions

Vaccines and Toxoids

Vaccinations containing live organisms are not administered within 3 months of immune globulin administration because antibodies in the globulin preparation may interfere with the immune response to the vaccination. Corticosteroids, antineoplastic drugs, and radiation therapy depress the immune system to such a degree that insufficient numbers of antibodies are produced to prevent the disease. When the salicylates are administered with the varicella vaccination, there is an increased risk of Reye's syndrome developing.

Immune Globulins and Antivenins

Antibodies in the immune globulin preparations may interfere with the immune response to live virus vaccines, particularly measles, but including others such as mumps and rubella. It is recommended that the live virus vaccines be administered 14 to 30 days before or 6 to 12 weeks after administration of immune globulins. No known interactions have been reported with antivenins.

NURSING PROCESS

The Patient Receiving an Immunologic Agent

ASSESSMENT

PREADMINISTRATION ASSESSMENT

Before the administration of any vaccine, the nurse obtains an allergy history. If the individual is known or thought to have allergies of any kind, the nurse tells the primary health care provider before the vaccine is given. Some vaccines contain antibodies obtained from animals, whereas other vaccines may contain proteins or preservatives to which the individual may be allergic. A highly allergic person may have an allergic reaction that could be serious and even fatal. If the patient has an allergy history, the primary health care provider may decide to perform skin tests for allergy to one or more of the components or proteins in the vaccine. The nurse also determines whether the patient has any conditions that contraindicate the administration of the agent (e.g., cancer, leukemia, lymphoma, immunosuppressive drug therapy).

ONGOING ASSESSMENT

The patient is usually not hospitalized after administration of an immunologic agent (with the exception of transplant recipients). However, the patient may be asked to stay in the clinic or office for observation for about 30 minutes after the injection to observe for any signs of hypersensitivity (e.g., laryngeal edema, hives, pruritus, angioneurotic edema, and severe dyspnea [see Chapter 2 for additional information]). Emergency resuscitation equipment is kept available to be used in the event of a severe hypersensitivity reaction.

NURSING DIAGNOSES

Drug-specific nursing diagnoses are highlighted in the Nursing Diagnoses Checklist. Other nursing diagnoses applicable to these drugs are discussed in depth in Chapter 4.

PLANNING

The expected outcomes of the patient may include an optimal response to the immunologic agent, support of patient needs related to the management of common adverse drug

Nursing Diagnoses Checklist

✓ **Acute Pain** related to adverse reactions (pain and discomfort at the injection site, muscular aches and pain)

✓ **Individual Effective Therapeutic Regimen Management** related to timing of immunization schedule

effects, and an understanding of and compliance with the prescribed immunization schedule.

IMPLEMENTATION
PROMOTING AN OPTIMAL RESPONSE TO THERAPY

If a vaccine is not in liquid form and must be reconstituted, the nurse must read the directions enclosed with the vaccine. It is important to follow the enclosed directions carefully. Package inserts also contain information regarding dosage, adverse reactions, method of administration, administration sites (when appropriate), and, when needed, recommended booster schedules.

Nursing Alert

The American Academy of Family Physicians states that children 12 to 15 months of age may receive up to seven injections during a single office visit. Many manufacturers are preparing combination products to reduce the number of injections during the vaccination process. Examples include the measle, mumps, and rubella (MMR) vaccine and the diphtheria, tetanus, pertussis, and *Hemophilus* B (TriHIBit) vaccine.

On occasion, it may be necessary to postpone the regular immunization schedule, particularly for children. This is of special concern to parents. The decision to delay immunization because of illness or for other reasons must be discussed with the primary health care provider. However, the decision to administer or delay vaccination because of febrile illness (illness causing an elevated temperature) depends on the severity of the symptoms and the specific disorder. In general, all vaccines can be administered to those with minor illness, such as a cold, and to those with a low-grade fever. However, moderate or severe febrile illness is a contraindication. In instances of moderate or severe febrile illness, vaccination is done as soon as the acute phase of the illness is over. Display 54-5 lists general contraindications to immunizations. Specific contraindications and precautions may be found in the package insert that comes with the drug.

The nurse documents the following information in the patient's chart or form provided by the institution:

- Date of vaccination
- Route and site, vaccine type, manufacturer
- Lot number and expiration date
- Name, address, and title of individual administering vaccine

MONITORING AND MANAGING PATIENT NEEDS

Minor adverse reactions, such as fever, rashes, and aching joints, are possible with the administration of a vaccine. In most cases, these reactions subside within 48 hours.

ACUTE PAIN General interventions, such as increasing the fluids in the diet, allowing for adequate rest, and keeping the atmosphere quiet and nonstimulating, may be beneficial. The primary health care provider may prescribe acetaminophen, every 4 hours, to control these reactions. Local irritation at the injection site may be treated with warm or cool compresses, depending on the patient's preference. A lump may be palpated at the injection site after a diphtheria, pertussis, and tetanus (DPT) vaccination or other immunization. This is not abnormal and resolves itself within several days to several months.

INDIVIDUAL EFFECTIVE THERAPEUTIC REGIMEN MANAGEMENT Because of the effectiveness of various types of vaccines in the prevention of disease, nurses must inform the public about the advantages of immunization. Parents are encouraged to have infants and young children receive the immunizations suggested by the primary health care provider. The nurse should provide the parents with a copy of the record of immunizations. This is especially helpful if multiple providers will be involved in the immunization schedule. Because evidence of immunization is required by schools (even at the college level), the record provided to parents by the provider is even more important. The nurse can download both information about immunizations and copies of blank record-keeping sheets from the Centers for Disease Control and Prevention website at www.cdc.gov/nip. This helps to empower the parent in the care of the child, making compliance with the routine immunization schedule likely.

Nursing Alert

In most cases, the risk of serious adverse reactions from an immunization is much smaller than the risk of contracting the disease for which the immunizing agent is given.

Serious viral infections of the central nervous system and fatalities have been associated with the use of vaccines. Although the number of these incidents is small, a risk factor still remains when some vaccines are given. It is also important for the parents to understand that a risk is also associated with not receiving immunization against some infectious diseases. That risk may be higher than and just as serious as the risk associated with the use of vaccines. Keep in mind that when a large segment of the population is immunized, the few not immunized are less likely to be exposed to and be infected with the disease-producing microorganism. However, when large numbers of the population are not immunized, there is a great increase in the chances of exposure to the infectious disease and a significant increase in the probability that the individual will experience the disease.

EDUCATING THE PATIENT AND FAMILY

When an adult or child is receiving a vaccine for immunization, the nurse explains to the patient or a family member the possible reactions that may occur, such as soreness at the injection site or fever.

The nurse advises those traveling to a foreign country to contact their primary health care provider or local health department well in advance of their departure date for information about the immunizations that will be needed. Immunizations should be given well in advance of departure because it may take several weeks to produce adequate immunity.

The nurse encourages the parents or guardians to report any adverse reactions or serious adverse events occurring after administration of a vaccine. It may be necessary to report the event to the Vaccine Adverse Event Reporting System (VAERS) (Display 54-6).

Display 54.6 Vaccine Adverse Event Reporting System

The Vaccine Adverse Event Reporting System (VAERS) is a national vaccine safety surveillance program cosponsored by the Centers for Disease Control and Prevention (CDC) and the U.S. Food and Drug Administration (FDA). VAERS collects and analyzes information from reports of adverse reactions after immunization. Anyone can report to VAERS. Reports are sent in by vaccine manufacturers, health care providers, and vaccine recipients and their parents or guardians. An example of the VAERS and instructions for completing the form are found in Appendix E. Any clinically significant adverse event that occurs after the administration of any vaccine should be reported. Individuals are encouraged to provide the information on the form even if the individual is uncertain if the event was related to the immunization. A copy of the form can be obtained by calling 1-800-822-7967 or by submitting the information by the Internet at www.vaers.hhs.gov.

The following list summarizes the information to be included when educating the parents of a child receiving a vaccination:

- Discuss briefly the risks of contracting vaccine-preventable diseases and the benefits of immunization.

- Instruct the parents to bring immunization records to all visits.

- Provide the date for return for the next vaccination.

- Discuss common adverse reactions (e.g., fever, soreness at the injection site) and methods to combat these reactions (e.g., acetaminophen, warm compresses).

- Instruct the parents to report any unusual or severe adverse reactions after the administration of a vaccination.

EVALUATION

- The therapeutic effect is achieved and the disease for which immunization is given does not present itself.

- Adverse drug reactions are managed successfully.

- The patient or parents/guardians comply with the immunization schedule.

- The patient and family express an understanding of the need for immunizations.

Herbal Alert

The *shiitake mushroom*, an edible variety of mushroom, is associated with general health maintenance but not with any severe adverse reactions. Mild side effects, such as skin rashes and gastrointestinal upset, have been reported. The recommended dosages follow:

- 3 to 4 fresh shiitake mushrooms
- 1 to 5 capsules/day
- 1 dropper two to three times a day

Lentinan, a derivative of the shiitake mushroom, is proving to be valuable in boosting the body's immune system and may prolong the survival time of patients with cancer by supporting immunity. In Japan, lentinan is commonly used to treat cancer. Additional possible benefits of this herb include lowering cholesterol levels by increasing the rate at which cholesterol is excreted from the body. Under no circumstances should shiitake or lentinan be used for cancer or any serious illness without consulting a primary health care provider.

Critical Thinking Exercises

1. Ms. Wilson has brought her 2-month-old daughter, Michelle, to the clinic for the first of the series of three DPT and one polio vaccine (IPV) immunizations. Ms. Wilson asks you to explain how a vaccination will keep her daughter from getting sick and why she has to have two injections. Discuss how you would address these topics with Ms. Wilson.

2. Jimmy, aged 4 months, has a slight cold with a "runny nose" when he comes for his regular well-baby checkup. His mother tells the nurse that because Jimmy is sick, she does not think he needs his DPT injection at this time. She says that she will bring him in next month for this immunization. Analyze the situation to determine the best response to Jimmy's mother. Discuss any assessments that you think would be important to make before giving your response.

Review Questions

1. When discussing the possibility of adverse reactions after receiving a vaccine, the nurse tells the parents of a young child that _____.

   A. adverse reactions may be severe, and the child should be monitored closely for 24 hours

   B. adverse reactions are usually mild

   C. the child will likely experience a hypersensitivity reaction

   D. the most common adverse reaction is a severe headache

2. Which of the following statements made by the patient would alert the nurse to a possibility of an allergy to the measles vaccine? My daughter is allergic to _____.

   A. gelatin

   B. peanut butter

   C. sugar

   D. corn

3. What type of immunity does an antivenin produce?

   A. Artificially acquired active immunity

   B. Naturally acquired active immunity

   C. Passive immunity

   D. Cell-mediated immunity

4. What type of immunity is produced by the hepatitis B vaccine recombinant?

   A. Artificially acquired active immunity

   B. Naturally acquired active immunity

   C. Passive immunity

   D. Cell-mediated immunity

To check your answers, see Appendix G.

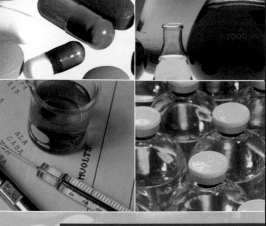

Chapter 55

Antineoplastic Drugs

Key Terms

- alopecia
- anemia
- anorexia
- antineoplastic
- bone marrow suppression
- cell cycle nonspecific
- cell cycle specific
- chemotherapy
- extravasation
- leukopenia
- metastasis
- myelosuppression
- neutropenia
- oral mucositis
- palliation
- stomatitis
- thrombocytopenia
- vesicants

Learning Objectives

On completion of this chapter, the student will:

- List the types of drugs used in the treatment of neoplastic diseases.
- Discuss the uses, general drug actions, general adverse reactions, contraindications, precautions, and interactions of the antineoplastic drugs.
- Discuss important preadministration and ongoing assessment activities

the nurse should perform with the patient taking antineoplastic drugs.

- List nursing diagnoses particular to a patient taking antineoplastic drugs.
- Discuss ways to promote an optimal response to therapy, how to manage common adverse reactions, and important points to keep in mind when educating patients about the use of an antineoplastic drug.

Antineoplastic drugs are used as one of the tools in the treatment of malignant diseases (cancer). The term **chemotherapy** is often used to refer to therapy with antineoplastic drugs. Although these drugs may not always lead to a complete cure of the cancer, they often slow the rate of tumor growth and delay **metastasis** (spreading of the cancer to other sites). These drugs can be used for cure, control, or **palliation** (comfort care, the relief of symptoms at the end of life).

THE CELL CYCLE

All cells grow in a specific pattern of growth called the *cell cycle* (Fig. 55-1). During the cell cycle, different components of a cell are synthesized, and the cell divides into two new cells. Listed are the five phases of cell growth:

G_1—RNA (ribonucleic acid) and proteins are built

S—DNA (deoxyribonucleic acid) is made from the components of the G_1 phase

G_2—RNA and protein synthesis preparing for cell division

M—mitotic cell division (the cell has doubled its contents and splits into two separate cells)

G_0—the dormant or resting phase.

CONCEPTSin action**ANIMATION**

When the cell goes into a resting phase, the cell completes its intended work (e.g., a white blood cell might fight infection) or it prepares to start the cycle of cell division again. Some cells, such as blood cells, rapidly reproduce in a matter of hours. Other cells, such as nerve cells, complete their cell division and then go into the resting phase for years. Some cells tend to stay in the resting phase but quickly divide if the tissue is injured. Liver cells are a good example; they do not replicate unless there is damage to the liver.

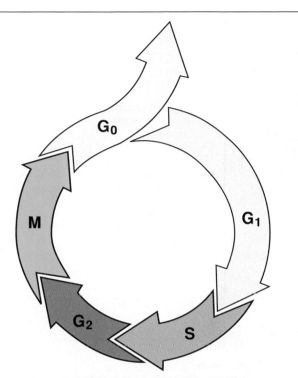

Figure 55.1 The cell cycle: G_1, RNA and protein synthesis; S, DNA synthesis; G_2, RNA and protein synthesis; M, mitotic cell division; G_0, cell resting phase, during which the cell differentiates to perform its function, or dies.

Antineoplastic drugs are designed to attack a cell during one or many of the phases of cell division. Drugs are categorized as **cell cycle specific** (meaning they target the cell in one of the phases of cell division) or as **cell cycle nonspecific** (they can target the cell at any phase of the cycle). Many subcategories of antineoplastic drugs are available to treat malignancies. The antineoplastic drugs covered in this chapter include the cell cycle nonspecific and cell cycle specific drugs. Other drugs, such as biologic and chemoprotective agents, are listed in various tables. Many hormones and antihormones are used in treating cancers associated with the sex organs (see Chapter 52), and new agents are on the horizon (Display 55-1).

The purpose of antineoplastic drug therapy is to affect cells that rapidly divide and reproduce. Malignant neoplasms or cancerous tumors usually consist of rapidly growing (abnormal) cells. Cancer cells have no biologic feedback controls to stop their growth or proliferation. Cancer cells are more sensitive to antineoplastic drugs when the cells are in the process of growing and dividing. Chemotherapy is administered at the time the cell population is dividing as part of a strategy to optimize cell death.

Display 55.1 New Frontiers in Cancer Treatment: Targeted Therapies

Used in conjunction with conventional antineoplastic drugs, targeted therapies, as the term implies, are agents used to target specific malignant cell components without hurting normal cells.

Specific Targeting Agents

Signal Transduction Inhibitors

cetuximab (Erbitux)
erlotinib (Tarceva)
gefitinib (Iressa)
imatinib mesylate (Gleevec)

Biologic Response Modifiers

aldesleukin (Proleukin)
BCG
denileukin diftitox (Ontak)

Proteasome Inhibitor

bortezomib (Velcade)

Monoclonal Antibodies

alemtuzumab (Campath)
gemtuzumab ozogamicin (Mylotarg)
ibritumomab tioxetan (Zevalin)
rituximab (Rituxan)
trastuzumab (Herceptin)

Angiogenesis Inhibitors

bevacizumab (Avastin)
interferon-alpha
thalidomide

Because the drugs are given systemically (i.e., they circulate through the entire body), other rapidly growing cells are usually affected by these drugs. The normal cells that line the oral cavity and gastrointestinal (GI) tract, and cells of the gonads, bone marrow, hair follicles, and lymph tissue are also rapidly dividing cells. Thus, antineoplastic drugs may affect normal as well as malignant cells, causing unpleasant adverse reactions.

Chemotherapy is administered in a series of cycles to allow for recovery of the normal cells and to destroy more of the malignant cells (Fig. 55-2). According to the cell kill theory, a drug regimen is intended to kill about 90% of the cancer cells during the first course of treatment. The second course, according to this theory, targets the remaining cancer cells and reduces those cells by another 90%. Each cycle of treatment with the antineoplastic drugs kills some, but by no means all, of the

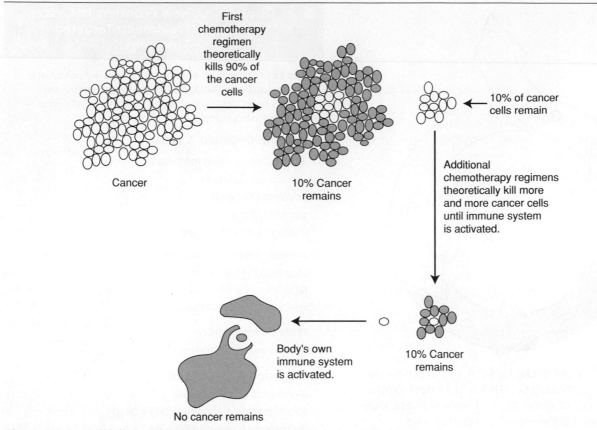

Figure 55.2 Cell kill theory of the activity of repeated chemotherapy regimens.

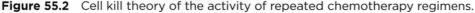

cancer cells. Theoretically, when few cells remain, the body's own immune system will be triggered and destroy what is left. By understanding the cell kill theory and the cell cycle, one can appreciate the rationale for using repeated doses of chemotherapy with different antineo-

---

Herbal Alert

Green tea and black teas come from the same plant. The difference is in the processing. Green tea is simply dried tea leaves, whereas black tea is fermented, giving it the dark color, stronger flavor, and the lowest amount of tannins and polyphenols. The beneficial effects of green tea lie in the polyphenols, or flavonoids, which have antioxidant properties. Antioxidants are thought to play a major role in preventing disease (e.g., colon cancer) and reducing the effects of aging. Green tea polyphenols are powerful antioxidants. The polyphenols are thought to act by inhibiting the reactions of free radicals in the body that are believed to play a role in aging. The benefits of green tea include an overall sense of well-being, cancer prevention, dental health, and maintenance of heart and liver health. Green tea taken as directed is safe and well tolerated. It contains as much as 50 mg of caffeine per cup. Decaffeinated green tea retains all of the polyphenol content. The recommended dosage is 2 to 5 cups a day. Standardized green tea extracts vary in strength, so dosages may need to be adjusted. The recommended dosage is 250 to 400 mg/d of extract standardized to 90% polyphenols. Because green tea contains caffeine, nervousness, restlessness, insomnia, and GI upset may occur. Green tea should be avoided during pregnancy because of its caffeine content. Patients with hypertension, cardiac conditions, anxiety, insomnia, diabetes, and ulcers should use green tea with caution.

---

plastic drugs. Different drugs that target cancer cells at various phases of the cell cycle are administered in order to kill as many cells as possible. Therefore, repeated courses of chemotherapy are used to kill an ever greater proportion of the malignant cells, until theoretically no cells are left.

CELL CYCLE–SPECIFIC DRUGS

Actions and Uses

Cell cycle–specific drugs act on the cell in one specific phase of the process of cell division, affecting both malignant and normal cells. A combination of these drugs, all acting at different phases of cell division, is typically used to treat leukemias, lymphomas, and a variety of solid tumors. The site of action of each drug depends on the drug subcategory. See the Summary Drug Table: Cell Cycle–Specific Drugs for more information.

Plant Alkaloids

Drugs that are derived from plant alkaloids include the vinca alkaloids, taxanes, podophyllotoxins, and the camptothecin analog drugs. The vinca alkaloids interfere with amino acid production in the S phase and formation of microtubules in the M phase. Taxanes also interfere in the M phase with microtubules. Cells are stopped during the S and G_2 phases by the podophyllotoxins and thus are unable to divide. DNA synthesis during the S phase is inhibited by camptothecin analog drugs such as topotecan (Hycamtin).

Antimetabolites

The antimetabolite drugs are substances that incorporate themselves into the cellular components during the S phase of cell division. This interferes with the synthesis of RNA and DNA, making it impossible for the cancerous cell to divide into two daughter cells. These drugs are used for many of the leukemias, lymphomas, and solid tumors as well as autoimmune diseases. Methotrexate is an example of the antimetabolite drugs.

CELL CYCLE–NONSPECIFIC DRUGS

Actions and Uses

Cell cycle–nonspecific drugs interfere with the process of cell division of malignant and normal cells. Because they do not exert action specifically on one portion of the cell cycle, they are called *nonspecific* drugs. These drugs are used to cure, control, or provide palliation in the treatment of leukemias, lymphomas, and many different solid tumors, and are also used in the treatment of certain autoimmune diseases.

Alkylating Agents

The alkylating agents make the cell a more alkaline environment, which in turn damages the cell. Malignant cells appear to be more susceptible to the effects of the alkylating drugs than normal cells. A number of subcategories are included in this group of cell cycle–nonspecifc drugs. Nitrogen mustard derivatives, ethylenimines, and the platinum-based drugs all break or interfere with the crosslinks in the DNA structure. The alkyl sulfonate drug, busulfan, interferes with DNA of granulocytes and is used primarily for leukemias. The hydrazine group interferes with multiple phases in the synthesis of RNA, DNA, and protein. Nitrosoureas are unique in that they can cross the blood–brain barrier, and therefore are used in treating brain tumors.

Antineoplastic Antibiotics

The antineoplastic antibiotics, unlike their anti-infective antibiotic relatives, do not fight infection. Rather, their action is similar to the alkylating drugs. Antineoplastic antibiotics appear to interfere with DNA and RNA synthesis, thereby delaying or inhibiting cell division and blocking the reproductive ability of malignant cells. An example of an antineoplastic antibiotic is doxorubicin (Adriamycin), which is used in the treatment of many solid tumors.

Miscellaneous Antineoplastic Drugs

A number of drugs are used for their antineoplastic actions, but they do not belong to any one category. The mechanism of action of many of the drugs in this unrelated group is not entirely clear. Examples of miscellaneous antineoplastics are provided in the Summary Drug Table: Cell Cycle–Nonspecific Drugs.

Adverse Reactions

Adverse reactions to antineoplastic drugs can be viewed in three different time frames: immediate (during the actual administration), during therapy cycles, and long term (many years later, during survivorship). Immediate adverse reactions occur as a result of administration. These include nausea and vomiting from highly emetic drugs or the potential of intravenous (IV) extravasation of irritating solutions. Antineoplastic drugs are potentially toxic and their administration is often associated with serious adverse reactions. At times, some of these adverse effects are allowed because the only alternative is to stop treatment of the cancer. A treatment plan is developed that will prevent, lessen, or treat most or all of the symptoms of a specific adverse reaction. An example of prevention is giving an antiemetic before administering an antineoplastic drug known to cause severe nausea and vomiting. Display 55-2 provides a list of those drugs most likely to cause nausea and vomiting.

An example of a treatment for an adverse reaction is the administration of an antiemetic and IV fluids with

SUMMARY DRUG TABLE   CELL CYCLE–SPECIFIC DRUGS

GENERIC NAME	TRADE NAME	USES	ADVERSE REACTIONS
Plant Alkaloids			
Vinca Alkaloids			
vinblastine sulfate *vin-blas'-teen*	Velban	Leukemia/lymphomas: Hodgkin's disease, other lymphomas Solid tumors: testicular, breast, KS Nonmalignant: mycosis fungoides	Immediate: extravasation potential During therapy cycles: alopecia, anemia, leukopenia, paresthesias, nausea, vomiting, constipation Long term: fertility problems
vincristine sulfate *vin-kris'-teen*	Oncovin, Vincasar	Leukemia/lymphomas: acute leukemia, other lymphomas Solid tumors: rhabdomyosarcoma, bladder, breast, KS Nonmalignant: idiopathic thrombocytopenic purpura	Immediate: extravasation potential During therapy cycles: alopecia, anemia, leukopenia, paresthesias, nausea, vomiting, stomatitis, constipation Long term: renal, adrenal, fertility problems
vinorelbine *vin-no'-rell-bean*	Navelbine	Solid tumors: NSCLC Unlabeled use: other solid tumors, KS	Immediate: extravasation potential During therapy cycles: leukopenia, paresthesias, nausea, constipation, alopecia, radiation recall
Taxanes			
docetaxel *dohs-eh-tax'-el*	Taxotere	Solid tumors: breast, NSCLC, prostate Unlabeled use: other solid tumors	Immediate: extravasation potential During therapy cycles: nausea, peripheral neuropathy, alopecia, cutaneous changes, fever, anemia, leukopenia, vomiting, diarrhea, stomatitis, fluid retention Long term: fertility problems
paclitaxel *pack-leh-tax'-el*	Taxol, Abraxane	Solid tumors: ovary, breast, NSCLC, KS Unlabeled use: other solid tumors	Immediate: cardiac changes, hypotension, extravasation potential During therapy cycles: nausea, vomiting, peripheral neuropathy, alopecia, fever, anemia, leukopenia, diarrhea, stomatitis Long term: fertility problems
Podophyllotoxins			
etoposide *e-toe'-poe-side*	Toposar, VePesid	Solid tumors: testicular, SCLC Unlabeled use: other solid tumors, leukemias and lymphomas	During therapy cycles: anemia, leukopenia, thrombocytopenia, alopecia, nausea, vomiting
teniposide (VM-26) *teh-nip-oh-side*	Vumon	Leukemia/lymphomas: ALL	Immediate: extravasation potential During therapy cycles: anemia, leukopenia, thrombocytopenia, alopecia, nausea, vomiting
Camptothecin Analogs			
irinotecan HCl *eye-rin-oh-tea'-kan*	Camptosar	Solid tumors: metastatic colon or rectal	Immediate: nausea, vomiting, diarrhea, inflammation potential (IV site) During therapy cycles: diarrhea, anemia, leukopenia, thrombocytopenia, asthenia, alopecia

GENERIC NAME	TRADE NAME	USES	ADVERSE REACTIONS
topotecan HCl *toe-poh -te'-kan*	Hycamtin	Solid tumors: metastatic ovarian, SCLC	During therapy cycles: anemia, leukopenia, thrombocytopenia, alopecia, nausea, vomiting, diarrhea, constipation

Antimetabolites

Folic Acid Antagonist

methotrexate *meth-o-trex'- ate*	Rheumatrex, Trexall	Leukemia/lymphomas; ALL, non-Hodgkin's lymphoma Solid tumors: breast, head/neck, choriocarcinomas, osteosarcomas Nonmalignant: mycosis fungoides, severe psoriasis, rheumatoid arthritis Unlabeled use: multiple sclerosis, inflammatory bowel disease	Immediate: nausea, vomiting (high dose) During therapy cycles: anemia, leukopenia, thrombocytopenia, stomatitis, diarrhea, renal damage Long term: hepatotoxicity
pemetrexed *pem-ah-trex'-ed*	Alimta	Solid tumors: NSCLC, malignant pleural mesothelioma	During therapy cycles: anemia, leukopenia, thrombocytopenia, skin rashes

Pyrimidine Antagonists

capecitabine *kap-ah-seat'-ah-bean*	Xeloda	Solid tumors: breast, colon	During therapy cycles: anemia, leukopenia, thrombocytopenia, diarrhea, hand and foot syndrome
cytarabine (ara-C) *sye-tare'-a-bean*	Cytosar-U, DepoCyt (liposomal)	Leukemia/lymphomas: ALL, AML	Immediate: nausea, vomiting During therapy cycles: anemia, leukopenia, thrombocytopenia
fluorouracil (5-FU) *flure-oh-yoor'-a-sil*	Adrucil	Palliative treatment for solid tumors: breast, stomach, pancreas, colon, rectum	During therapy cycles: anemia, leukopenia, thrombocytopenia, nausea, vomiting, stomatitis, diarrhea, alopecia
gemcitabine HCl *jem-site'-ah-bean*	Gemzar	Solid tumors: pancreatic, NSCLC	During therapy cycles: anemia, leukopenia, thrombocytopenia, fever, rash nausea, vomiting, diarrhea, proteinuria

Purine Antagonists

mercaptopurine (6-MP) *mer-kap-toe-pyoor'-een*	Purinethol	Leukemia/lymphomas: ALL, AML Unlabeled use: inflammatory bowel disease	During therapy cycles: anemia, leukopenia, thrombocytopenia, hyperuricemia
thioguanine *thye-oh-gwon'-een*	Tabloid	Acute leukemias Unlabeled use: severe psoriasis, inflammatory bowel disease	During therapy cycles: anemia, leukopenia, thrombocytopenia, hyperuricemia

Adenosine Deaminase Inhibitors

cladribine *kla'-dri-bean*	Leustatin	Leukemia/lymphomas: hairy cell leukemia Unlabeled use: other leukemias and lymphomas	During therapy cycles: anemia, leukopenia, thrombocytopenia, fever, nausea, rash
fludarabine *floo-ar'-a-bean*	Fludara	Leukemia/lymphomas: chronic lymphocytic leukemia Unlabeled use: other leukemias and lymphomas	During therapy cycles: anemia, leukopenia, thrombocytopenia

Antineoplastic Drugs

SUMMARY DRUG TABLE   *(continued)*

GENERIC NAME	TRADE NAME	USES	ADVERSE REACTIONS
nelarabine *nella-ra'-ben*	Arranon	Leukemia/lymphomas: T-cell acute lymphoblastic leukemia and T-cell lymphoblastic lymphoma	During therapy cycles: fatigue, neurologic toxicity
pentostatin *pen'-toe-stat-in*	Nipent	Leukemia/lymphomas: hairy cell leukemia Unlabeled use: other leukemias and lymphomas	During therapy cycles: anemia, leukopenia, thrombocytopenia, rash, itching, nausea, vomiting, diarrhea

ALL, acute lymphocytic leukemia; AML, acute myelogenous leukemia; KS, Kaposi's saccoma; NSCLC, non–small cell lung cancer; SCLC, small cell lung cancer.

electrolytes when severe vomiting is anticipated. When the drugs listed in Display 55-2 are given, antiemetic protocols should always be followed to reduce adverse reactions. Some drugs, such as platinum-based agents, may damage certain organs during administration. Again, prechemotherapy protocols for IV fluid administration are initiated to prevent adverse reactions.

Some of these reactions are dose dependent; that is, their occurrence is more common or their intensity is more severe when multiple doses (or cycles) are used. Because the antineoplastic drugs affect cancer cells and rapidly proliferating normal cells (i.e., cells in the bone marrow, GI tract, reproductive tract, and hair follicles), adverse reactions occur as the result of action on these cells.

Adverse reactions common to many of the antineoplastic drugs include bone marrow suppression (anemia, leukopenia, thrombocytopenia), stomatitis, diarrhea, and hair loss.

Display 55.2 Emetic Potential of Antineoplastic Drugs

The following drugs have a 60% or greater chance of causing nausea and vomiting when administered to patients.

Alkylating Agents
carboplatin
carmustine
cisplatin
cyclophosphamide
dacarbazine
ifosfamide
lomustine
mechlorethamine
melphalan
procarbazine
streptozocin

Antibiotics
dactinomycin
daunorubicin
doxorubicin
mitoxantrone

Antimetabolites
cytarabine
methotrexate

Plant Alkaloid
irinotecan

The most common reactions are leukopenia and thrombocytopenia, which may cause cycles of chemotherapy to be delayed until blood cell counts can be raised. Some drugs, especially the alkaloids, affect the nervous system. These adverse reactions can range from a peripheral tingling sensation to hand and foot syndrome (tiny capillary leaks in extremities causing skin color changes to numbness).

Because the drugs used to treat cancer are effective, many people are living with the disease either cured or in remission. Some of the adverse reactions to antineoplastic drugs can have long-lasting effects. These include damage to the gonads, causing fertility problems, and to other specific organ systems, leading to cardiac, pulmonary, or neurologic problems. In addition, secondary cancers like leukemia can be caused by the original cancer treatment. These problems are listed in the Summary Drug Tables. Appropriate references should be consulted when administering these drugs because there are a variety of uses and dose ranges and, in some instances, many adverse reactions.

Contraindications and Precautions

The information discussed in this section is general, and the contraindications, precautions, and interactions for each antineoplastic drug vary. The nurse should consult appropriate sources before administering any antineoplastic drug.

The antineoplastic drugs are contraindicated in patients with leukopenia, thrombocytopenia, anemia, serious infections, serious renal disease, or known hypersensitivity to the drug, and during pregnancy (see Display 55-3 for pregnancy classifications of selected antineoplastic drugs) or lactation.

Antineoplastic drugs are used cautiously in patients with renal or hepatic impairment, active infection, or other debilitating illnesses, or in those who have recently completed treatment with other antineoplastic drugs or radiation therapy.

SUMMARY DRUG TABLE   CELL CYCLE–NONSPECIFIC DRUGS

GENERIC NAME	TRADE NAME	USES	ADVERSE REACTIONS
Alkylating Drugs			
Nitrogen Mustard Derivatives			
chlorambucil *klor-am'-byoo-still*	Leukeran	Leukemia/lymphomas: CLL, lymphomas, Hodgkin's disease	During therapy cycles: anemia, leukopenia, thrombocytopenia Long term: fertility problems
cyclophosphamide *sye-klo-foss'-fam-ide*	Cytoxan, Neosar	Leukemia/lymphomas: ALL, AML, CLL, advanced lymphomas, Hodgkin's disease Solid tumors: breast, ovary, neuroblastoma, retinoblastoma, Nonmalignant: mycosis fungoides nephrotic syndrome (children), rheumatoid arthritis, systemic lupus erythematosus, multiple sclerosis	Immediate: nausea, vomiting During therapy cycles: leukopenia, hemorrhagic cystitis, thrombocytopenia Long term: fertility problems, secondary cancers
ifosfamide *eye-fos'-fam-ide*	Ifex	Leukemia/lymphomas: unlabeled use (except AML) Solid tumors: testicular; Unlabeled use: lung, breast, ovary, gastric, pancreatic	Immediate: nausea, vomiting During therapy cycles: leukopenia, thrombocytopenia, hemorrhagic cystitis, alopecia, somnolence, confusion
mechlorethamine *me-klor-eth'-a-meen*	Mustargen	Palliative treatment for CLL, CML, advanced lymphomas, Hodgkin's disease Solid tumors: lung, metastatic disease, mycosis fungoides	Immediate: nausea, vomiting, extravasation potential, lymphocytopenia During therapy cycles: anemia, leukopenia, thrombocytopenia, hyperuremia, diarrhea Long term: fertility problems, secondary cancers
melphalan *mel'-fa-lan*	Alkeran	Palliative treatment for multiple myeloma Solid tumors: ovary Unlabeled use: testicular, breast, bone marrow transplantation	Immediate: nausea, vomiting During therapy cycles: leukopenia, thrombocytopenia, diarrhea, alopecia Long term: fertility problems, secondary cancers
Ethyleneimines			
altretamine (hexamethyl melamine) *al-tret'-ah-meen*	Hexalen	Palliative treatment for solid tumors: ovary	During therapy cycles: anemia, leukopenia, thrombocytopenia, nausea, vomiting, peripheral neuropathy, dizziness
thiotepa *thye-oh-tep'-a*	Thioplex	Solid tumors: breast, ovary, bladder	During therapy cycles: anemia, leukopenia, thrombocytopenia, alopecia Long term: fertility problems
Alkyl Sulfonate			
busulfan *byoo-sul'-fan*	Busulfex, Myleran	Palliative treatment for CML	Immediate: induce seizures During therapy cycles: anemia, leukopenia, thrombocytopenia, hyperuremia, graft-versus-host disease Long term: fertility problems

Antineoplastic Drugs

SUMMARY DRUG TABLE *(continued)*

GENERIC NAME	TRADE NAME	USES	ADVERSE REACTIONS
Hydrazines			
dacarbazine *da-kar'-ba-zeen*	DTIC	Leukemia/lymphomas: Hodgkin's disease Solid tumors: melanoma Unlabeled use: pheochromocytoma, KS	Immediate: nausea, vomiting During therapy cycles: anemia, leukopenia, thrombocytopenia
procarbazine HCl *proe-kar'-ba-zeen*	Matulane	Leukemia/lymphomas: Hodgkin's disease Unlabeled use: other lymphomas, brain, small cell lung cancer, melanoma	Immediate: nausea, vomiting During therapy cycles: anemia, leukopenia, thrombocytopenia, peripheral neuropathy, alopecia
temozolomide *tem-oh-zoll'-oh-myde*	Temodar	Solid tumors: glioblastoma, astrocytoma Unlabeled use: melanoma	During therapy cycles: leukopenia, thrombocytopenia, headache, nausea, vomiting, alopecia
Nitrosoureas			
carmustine (BCNU) *car-mus'-teen*	Gliadel	Palliative treatment for Hodgkin's disease, multiple myeloma, various brain tumors Unlabeled use: T-cell lymphoma, melanoma	Immediate: nausea, vomiting During therapy cycles: leukopenia, thrombocytopenia Long term: pulmonary fibrosis
lomustine (CCNU) *loe-mus'-teen*	CeeNU	Leukemia/lymphomas: secondary treatment for Hodgkin's disease Solid tumors: brain	Immediate: nausea, vomiting During therapy cycles: leukopenia, thrombocytopenia, alopecia, stomatitis Long term: pulmonary fibrosis, fertility problems
streptozocin *strep'-toe-zoe-sin*	Zanosar	Solid tumors: pancreatic	Immediate: nausea, vomiting During therapy cycles: azotemia, proteinuria, stomatitis
Platinum-Based Drugs			
cisplatin *sis-pla'-tin*	Platinol-AQ	Solid tumors: ovarian, testicular, bladder	Immediate: nausea, vomiting, renal damage During therapy cycles: anemia, leukopenia, thrombocytopenia tinnitus, hyperuricemia
oxaliplatin *ox-al'-ih-pla-tin*	Eloxatin	Solid tumors: colon, rectal	During therapy cycles: leukopenia, thrombocytopenia, peripheral neuropathy
carboplatin *kar'-boe-pla-tin*	Paraplatin	Solid tumors: ovarian Unlabeled use: lung, head and neck, testicular	During therapy cycles: anemia, leukopenia, thrombocytopenia
Antibiotics			
Anthracyclines			
daunorubicin HCl *daw-noe-roo'-bi-sin*	DaunoXome	Leukemia/lymphomas: ALL, AML Solid tumors: KS	Immediate: nausea, vomiting, extravasation potential During therapy cycles: anemia, leukopenia, thrombocytopenia, alopecia, stomatitis, hyperuricemia, urine discoloration Long term: cardiotoxicity

GENERIC NAME	TRADE NAME	USES	ADVERSE REACTIONS
doxorubicin HCl *dox-oh-roo'-bi-sin*	Adriamycin, Doxil	Leukemia/lymphomas; ALL, AML, and various lymphomas Solid tumors: Wilms' tumor, neuroblastoma, KS, various sarcomas, breast, lung, ovary, bladder, thyroid, gastric	Immediate: nausea, vomiting, extravasation potential During therapy cycles: anemia, leukopenia, thrombocytopenia, alopecia, cutaneous changes, stomatitis, hyperuricemia, urine discoloration, radiation recall, hand and foot syndrome Long term: cardiotoxicity
epirubicin *ep-ee-roo'-bi-sin*	Ellence	Solid tumors: breast Unlabeled use: advanced esophageal	Immediate: extravasation potential During therapy cycles: anemia, leukopenia, thrombocytopenia, nausea, vomiting, alopecia, stomatitis, diarrhea, urine discoloration, radiation recall Long term: cardiotoxicity, fertility problems
idarubicin HCl *eye-da-roo'-bi-sin*	Idamycin	Leukemia/lymphomas: AML	Immediate: extravasation potential During therapy cycles: anemia, leukopenia, thrombocytopenia, alopecia, nausea, vomiting, stomatitis, diarrhea, hyperuricemia, urine discoloration Long term: cardiotoxicity
mitoxantrone HCl *mye-toe-zan'-trone*	Novantrone	Leukemia/lymphomas: acute non-lymphocytic leukemia, Solid tumors: advanced prostate Nonmalignant: multiple sclerosis	Immediate: nausea, vomiting, extravasation potential During therapy cycles: leukopenia, nausea, alopecia Long term: cardiotoxicity, AML

Chromomycins

GENERIC NAME	TRADE NAME	USES	ADVERSE REACTIONS
dactinomycin *dak-ti-no-my'-sin*	Cosmegen	Solid tumors: various sarcomas, Wilms' tumor, gestational neoplasia, testicular	Immediate: nausea, vomiting, extravasation potential During therapy cycles: anemia, leukopenia, thrombocytopenia, alopecia, skin erythema Long term: fertility problems

Miscellaneous Antibiotics

GENERIC NAME	TRADE NAME	USES	ADVERSE REACTIONS
bleomycin sulfate *blee-oh-my'-sin*	Blenoxane	Palliative treatment for lymphomas, pleural effusion Solid tumors: testicular, various types Unlabeled use: mycosis fungoides, KS	During therapy cycles: anemia, leukopenia, thrombocytopenia, vomiting, alopecia, skin erythema, cutaneous changes Long term: pneumonitis, pulmonary fibrosis
mitomycin *mye-toe-my'-sin*	Mutamycin	Solid tumors: stomach, pancreas	Immediate: extravasation potential During therapy cycles: anemia, leukopenia, thrombocytopenia, hyperuricemia

Miscellaneous Agents

DNA Inhibitor

GENERIC NAME	TRADE NAME	USES	ADVERSE REACTIONS
hydroxyurea *hye-drox-ee-yoor-ee'-ah*	Hydrea, Mylocel	Solid tumors: melanoma Unlabeled use: thrombocythemia, human immunodeficiency virus infection, psoriasis	During therapy cycles: anemia, leukopenia, thrombocytopenia, radiation recall

⬤ **SUMMARY DRUG TABLE** *(continued)*

GENERIC NAME	TRADE NAME	USES	ADVERSE REACTIONS
Adrenocortical Inhibitor			
mitotane *mye'-toe-tane*	Lysodren	Solid tumors: adrenal cortex Unlabeled use: Cushing's disease	During therapy cycles: nausea, vomiting, diarrhea
Enzymes			
asparaginase *a-spare'-a-gi-nase*	Elspar	Leukemia/lymphomas: ALL	During therapy cycles: anemia, leukopenia, thrombocytopenia, hyperuricemia, rash, urticaria, acute anaphylaxis
pegaspargase *peg-ah-spar'-gaze*	Oncaspar	Same as asparaginase	Same as asparaginase
Antimicrotubule Agent			
estramustine phosphate sodium (estradiol/nitrogen mustard) *ess-tra-muss'-teen*	Emcyt	Palliative treatment for solid tumors e.g., prostate	Immediate: nausea, diarrhea During therapy cycles: breast tenderness, thrombophlebitis, fluid retention Long term: gynecomastia, impotence
Retinoids			
tretinoin *tret'-i-noyn*	Vesanoid	Leukemia/lymphomas: acute promyelocytic leukemia	During therapy cycles: headache, fever, weakness, fatigue, edema, retinoic acid–acute promyelocytic leukemia (RA-APL) syndrome (acute anaphylactic reaction)
bexarotene *bex-air'-oh-teen*	Targretin	Leukemia/lymphomas: cutaneous T-cell lymphoma	During therapy cycles: elevated blood lipids, rash, leukopenia, dry skin

ALL, acute lymphocytic leukemia; AML, acute myelocytic leukemia; CLL, chronic lymphocytic leukemia; CML, chronic myelocytic leukemia; KS, Kaposi's sarcoma.

Interactions

A number of antineoplastic drugs are harmful to normal cells as well as cancer cells. Cytoprotective agents are drugs used with the antineoplastic drug to protect the normal cells or organs of the body. In this way, enough of the chemotherapeutic drug can be given to eradicate the cancer without irreversible harm to the patient. Cytoprotective agents used with antineoplastic drugs are listed in Display 55-4.

The following table lists selected interactions of the plant alkaloids, antimetabolites, alkylating drugs, antibiotics, and miscellaneous antineoplastic drugs. Typically, additive bone marrow depressive effects occur when any category of antineoplastic drug is administered with another chemotherapy drug or radiation therapy. The nurse should consult appropriate sources for a more complete listing of interactions before any antineoplastic drug is administered.

Interacting Drug	Common Use	Effect of Interaction
Plant Alkaloids		
digoxin	Cardiac problems	Decrease serum level of digoxin
phenytoin	Seizure disorders	Increased risk of seizures
oral anticoagulants	Blood thinners	Prolonged bleeding
Antimetabolites		
digoxin	Cardiac problems	Decrease serum level of digoxin
phenytoin	Seizure disorders	Decreased need for antiseizure medication

Interacting Drug	Common Use	Effect of Interaction
Nonsteroidal anti-inflammatory drugs (NSAIDs)	Pain relief	methotrexate toxicity
Alkylating Drugs		
aminoglycosides	Anti-infective agents	Increased risk of nephrotoxicity and ototoxicity
loop diuretics	Heart problems and edema	Increased risk of ototoxicity
phenytoin	Seizure disorder	Increased risk of seizure
Antineoplastic Antibiotics		
digoxin	Cardiac problems	Decrease serum level of digoxin
Miscellaneous Antineoplastic Drugs		
insulin and oral hypoglycemics	Diabetes management	Increased risk of hyperglycemia
oral anticoagulants	Blood thinners	Prolonged bleeding
antidepressants, antihistamines, opiates, or the sedatives	Depression, allergy, pain relief, or sedation, respectively	Increased risk of central nervous system depression

The Patient Receiving an Antineoplastic Drug

ASSESSMENT

PREADMINISTRATION ASSESSMENT

The extent of the preadministration assessment depends on the type of cancer and the patient's general physical condition. The initial assessment of the patient scheduled for chemotherapy may include

- The type and location of the neoplastic lesion (as stated on the patient's chart)

- The stage of the disease, for example, early, metastatic, or terminal

- The patient's general physical condition

- The patient's emotional response to the disease

- The anxiety or fears the patient may have regarding chemotherapy treatments

- Previous or concurrent treatments (if any), such as surgery, radiation therapy, other antineoplastic drugs

- Other current nonmalignant disease or disorder, such as congestive heart failure or peptic ulcer, that may or may not be related to the malignant disease

- The patient's knowledge or understanding of the proposed chemotherapy regimen

- Other factors, such as the patient's age, financial problems that may be associated with a long-term illness, family cooperation and interest in the patient, and the adequacy of health insurance coverage (which may be of great concern to the patient)

Immediately before administering the first dose of an antineoplastic drug, the nurse takes the patient's vital signs and obtains a current weight because the dose of some antineoplastic drugs is based on the patient's weight in kilograms or pounds. The dosages of some antineoplastic drugs also may be based on body surface measurements and are stated as a specific amount of drug per square meter (m^2) of body surface. When an antineoplastic drug has a depressing effect on the bone marrow, laboratory tests, such as a complete blood count, are ordered to determine the effect of the previous drug dosage. Before the first dose of the drug is administered, pretreatment laboratory tests provide baseline data for future reference. The administration route of chemotherapy is routinely monitored; examples include assessment of vessel integrity for IV access or patency of venous access devices.

Some antineoplastic drugs require treatment measures before administration. An example of preadministration treatment is hydration of the patient with 1 to 2 L of IV fluid infused before administration of cisplatin (Platinol) or administration of an antiemetic before the administration of irinotecan (Camptosar). These measures are ordered by the primary health care provider and, in some instances, may vary slightly from the manufacturer's recommendations.

ONGOING ASSESSMENT

The patient who is acutely ill with many physical problems requires different ongoing assessment activities than does one who is ambulating and able to participate in the activities of daily living. Once the patient's general condition is assessed and needs identified, the nurse develops a care plan to meet those needs. Patients receiving chemotherapy can be at different stages of their disease; therefore, nurses must individualize the nursing care of

Display 55.3 Pregnancy Classification for Selected Antineoplastic Drugs

Pregnancy Category C

asparaginase	mitotane	streptozocin
dacarbazine	pegaspargase	

Pregnancy Category D

altretamine	doxorubicin	mitoxantrone
bleomycin	epirubicin	nelarabine
busulfan	etoposide	oxaliplatin
capecitabine	fludarabine	paclitaxel
carboplatin	fluorouracil	pemetrexed
carmustine	gemcitabine	pentostatin
chlorambucil	hydroxyurea	procarbazine
cisplatin	idarubicin	temozolomide
cladribine	ifosfamide	thioguanine
cyclophos- phamide	irinotecan lomustine	thiotepa topotecan
cytarabine	mechlorethamine	vinblastine
dactinomycin	melphalan	vincristine
daunorubicin	mercaptopurine	vinorelbine
docetaxel	mitomycin	

Pregnancy Category X

methotrexate

---

each patient based on the patient's needs, and not just on the type of drug administered.

In general, after the administration of an antineoplastic drug, the nurse bases the ongoing assessment on the following factors:

Display 55.4 Cytoprotective Agents

The following drugs function to protect cells or counteract adverse reactions resulting from therapeutic doses of the antineoplastic drugs.

- allopurinol, rasburicase (Elitek): Counteract the increase in uric acid and subsequent hyperuricemia resulting from the metabolic waste buildup from rapid tumor lysis (cell destruction)
- amifostine (Ethyol): Binds with metabolites of cisplatin to protect the kidneys from nephrotoxic effects
- dexrazoxane (Zinecard): Cardioprotective agent used with doxorubicin
- leucovorin (Wellcovorin): Provides folic acid to cells after methotrexate administration
- mesna (Mesnex): Binds with metabolites of ifosfamide to protect the bladder from hemorrhagic cystitis

- The patient's general condition
- The patient's individual response to the drug
- Adverse reactions that may occur
- Guidelines established by the primary health care provider or hospital
- Results of periodic laboratory tests and radiographic scans

Different types of laboratory tests may be used to monitor the patient's response to therapy. Some of these tests, such as a complete blood count, may be used to determine the response of the bone marrow to an antineoplastic drug. Other tests, such as kidney function tests, may be used to detect nephrotoxicity, an adverse reaction that sometimes occurs with the administration of some of these drugs. Abnormal laboratory test results may also require a change in the nursing care plan. For example, a significant drop in the neutrophil count may require a delay in treatment, administration of colony-stimulating factors (see Chapter 44), and patient teaching about ways to recognize and prevent infection and sepsis.

The nurse reviews the results of all laboratory tests at the time they are reported. The primary health care provider is

Nursing Diagnoses Checklist

✓ **Imbalanced Nutrition: Less Than Body Requirements** related to anorexia, nausea, vomiting, and stomatitis

✓ **Fatigue** related to anemia and myelosuppression

✓ **Risk for Injury** related to thrombocytopenia and myelosuppression

✓ **Risk for Infection** related to neutropenia, leukopenia, and myelosuppression

✓ **Disturbed Body Image** related to adverse reactions of antineoplastic drugs (e.g., alopecia, weight loss)

✓ **Anxiety** related to diagnosis, necessary treatment measures, the occurrence of adverse reactions, other factors

✓ **Impaired Tissue Integrity** related to adverse reactions of the antineoplastic drugs (radiation recall and extravasation)

notified of the results before the administration of successive doses of an antineoplastic drug. If these tests indicate a severe depressant effect on the bone marrow or other test abnormalities, the primary health care provider may reduce the next drug dose or temporarily stop chemotherapy to allow the affected body systems to recover.

NURSING DIAGNOSES

The nursing diagnoses for the patient with cancer are usually extensive and are based on many factors, such as the patient's physical and emotional condition, the adverse reactions resulting from antineoplastic drug therapy, and the stage of the disease. Drug-specific nursing diagnoses are highlighted in the Nursing Diagnoses Checklist. Other nursing diagnoses applicable to these drugs are discussed in depth in Chapter 4.

PLANNING

The expected outcomes of the patient may include an optimal response to therapy, support of patient needs related to the management of adverse reactions, and an understanding of the prescribed treatment modalities.

IMPLEMENTATION
PROMOTING AN OPTIMAL RESPONSE TO THERAPY

Care of the patient receiving an antineoplastic drug depends on factors such as the drug or combination of drugs given, the dosage of the drugs, the route of administration, the patient's physical response to therapy, the response of the tumor to chemotherapy, and the type and

severity of adverse reactions. Some drugs may be administered by various routes, depending on the cancer being treated. For example, thiotepa may be administered by the IV route for breast cancer, intravesicular route for superficial bladder cancer, intrapleural route for malignant pleural effusions, and by the intraperitoneal route for ovarian cancer. As the methods of administration have changed, so has the location for administration. Once given as long IV infusions over days or a week in the hospital, many of the antineoplastic drugs are still given IV but as push or small-volume infusions, and they are delivered in an outpatient setting by highly skilled nurses.

GUIDELINES ESTABLISHED BY THE SETTING FOR CARE
In these settings (hospital, outpatient chemotherapy clinics, or office), policies are established to provide nursing personnel with specific guidelines for the assessment and care of patients receiving a single or combination chemotherapeutic drug regimen. During chemotherapy, the primary health care provider may write orders for certain nursing procedures, such as measuring fluid intake and output, monitoring the vital signs at specific intervals, and increasing the fluid intake to a certain amount. Even when orders are written, the nurse should increase the frequency of certain assessments, such as monitoring vital signs, if the patient's condition changes. Some settings have written guidelines for nursing management when the patient is receiving a specific antineoplastic drug. The nurse incorporates these guidelines into the nursing care plan with nursing observations and assessments geared to the individual. The nurse adds further assessments to the nursing care plan when the patient's condition changes.

If treatment is given in a setting where guidelines are not provided, it is important for the nurse to review the drugs being given before their administration. These drugs should not be prescribed by a generalist health care provider; rather, antineoplastics should be prescribed only by a provider trained specifically in the care of oncology patients. The nurse consults appropriate references to obtain information regarding the preparation and administration of a particular drug, the average dose ranges, all the known adverse reactions, and the warnings and precautions given by the manufacturer.

PROTECTION OF THE PROVIDER Those involved in the administration of antineoplastic drugs are at risk for many adverse reactions from accidental absorption of the drugs. Because so many of the drugs are given in the outpatient setting, personnel in clinics and offices are at high risk for exposure. It is important to follow the directions of the manufacturer regarding the type of solution to be used for

Table 55.1 Personal Protective Equipment for Safe Handling of Antineoplastic Drugs

Route of Potential Exposure	Safety Equipment
Skin	Gowns—single-use, disposable gowns with closed front and cuffs and made of impermeable or minimally permeable fabric (to the agents in use) Gloves—powder-free; made of latex, nitrile, or neoprene; labeled and tested for use with chemotherapeutic drugs
Ingestion	Safety goggles—to protect face and eyes from possible splashes
Inhalation	NIOSH-approved respirator—when a spill must be cleaned up

Adapted from Polovich, M. (2004) Safe handling of hazardous drugs. *Online Journal of Issues in Nursing,* 9(3), Manuscript 5. Available at www.nursingworld.org/ojin/topic25/tpc25_5.htm.

preparation, dilution, or administration. The Occupational Safety and Health Administration (OSHA) guidelines state that antineoplastic drug preparation is to be performed in a biologic safety cabinet (BSC) in a designated area. This is to prevent accidental inhalation and exposure to the person preparing the drugs. In addition, nurses need to be protected during administration and cleanup from accidental ingestion, inhalation, or absorption of the drugs. Table 55-1 outlines the protective items that should be available to staff working with antineoplastic drugs.

ORAL ADMINISTRATION A number of antineoplastic drugs are administered orally. The oral route is convenient and noninvasive. Most oral drugs are well absorbed when the GI tract is functioning normally. Antineoplastic drugs such as capecitabine (Xeloda) or temozolomide (Temodar) are given orally. Most oral drugs are administered by the patient in a home setting. The section on Educating the Patient and Family, later, provides information to include in a teaching plan.

PARENTERAL ADMINISTRATION Although some of these drugs are given orally, others are given by the parenteral route. Antineoplastic drugs may be administered subcutaneously (SC), intramuscularly (IM), and IV. When giving these drugs IM, the nurse gives the injection into the large muscles using the Z-track method (see Chapter 2) because administration can cause stinging or burning. When the SC method of administration is used, the injection should contain no more than 1 mL, and injections are given in the usual SC injection sites (see Chapter 2). If the injections

are given frequently, the sites should be rotated and charted appropriately.

Intravenous administration may be accomplished using a vascular access device, an Angiocath, or a butterfly needle. These devices have become common methods of drug delivery and, depending on the patient's individual treatment regimen, may be inserted before therapy. Selection of the device depends on the type of therapy the patient is to receive, the condition of the veins, and how long the treatment regimen is to be continued. Special directions for administration, stated by either the primary health care provider or manufacturer, are also important. For example, cisplatin cannot be prepared or administered with needles or IV administration sets containing aluminum because aluminum reacts with cisplatin, causing formation of a precipitate and loss of potency.

Nurses who are certified in chemotherapy drug administration administer these drugs, but any nurse may be involved in monitoring patients receiving antineoplastic drugs. Antineoplastic drugs are potentially toxic drugs that can cause a variety of effects during and after their administration. Display 55-5 summarizes important points

Display 55.5 Points to Keep in Mind About Antineoplastic Drug Administration

Great care and accuracy are important in preparing and administering these drugs. Important points to keep in mind during drug administration follow:

- Wear personal protective equipment when preparing any of these drugs for parenteral administration.
- Administer any prophylactic medications or fluids in a timely manner to prevent reactions.
- Observe the patient closely before, during, and after the administration of an antineoplastic drug.
- Observe the IV site closely to detect any signs of **extravasation** (leakage into the surrounding tissues). Tissue necrosis can be a serious complication. Discontinue the infusion and notify the primary health care provider if discomfort, redness along the pathway of the vein, or infiltration occurs.
- Continually update nursing assessments, nursing diagnoses, and nursing care plans to meet the changing needs of the patient.
- Notify the primary health care provider of all changes in the patient's general condition, the appearance of adverse reactions, and changes in laboratory test results.
- Provide the patient and family with both physical and emotional support during treatment.

to keep in mind when administering an antineoplastic drug.

MONITORING AND MANAGING PATIENT NEEDS

Not all patients have the same response to a specific antineoplastic drug. For example, an antineoplastic drug may cause vomiting, but the amount of fluid and electrolytes lost through vomiting may vary from patient to patient. One patient may require additional sips of water once nausea and vomiting have subsided, whereas another may require IV fluid and electrolyte replacement. Nursing management is focused not only on what may or what did happen, but on the effects produced by a particular adverse reaction.

IMBALANCED NUTRITION: LESS THAN BODY REQUIREMENTS Patients may not eat because they are tired or not hungry. **Anorexia** (loss of appetite resulting in the inability to eat) is a common occurrence with the antineoplastic drugs. This may be due to nausea, taste alterations, or sores in the GI system. Nausea and vomiting are common adverse reactions to some of the highly emetic antineoplastic drugs. To minimize this adverse reaction, the primary health care provider may order an antiemetic, such as ondansetron (Zofran), to be given before treatment and continued for a few days after administration of the chemotherapy. Because this is an expensive drug, other protocols may include different (and less expensive) antiemetics. Some of these have adverse effects, such as a sedative action, which might add to the patient's lack of desire to eat. In the example of the patient who is vomiting, it is important to measure accurately all fluid intake and all output from the GI and urinary tracts, as well as to observe the patient for signs of dehydration and electrolyte imbalances. These measurements and observations aid the primary health care provider in determining if fluid replacement is necessary. The nurse assesses the nutritional status of the patient before and during treatment.

To stimulate appetite, the nurse provides small, frequent meals to coincide with the patient's tolerance for food. Greasy or fatty foods and unpleasant sights, smells, and tastes are avoided. Cold foods, dry foods, and salty foods may be better tolerated. It is a good idea to provide diversional activities, such as music, television, and books. Relaxation, visualization, guided imagery, hypnosis, and other nonpharmacologic measures have been helpful to some patients.

It is not uncommon for the patient to report alterations in the sense of taste during the course of chemotherapy. Some drugs give protein foods such as beef a bitter, metallic taste. Small, frequent meals (five to six meals daily) are usually better tolerated than are three large meals. Breakfast is often the best-tolerated meal of the day. The nurse stresses the importance of eating meals high in nutritive value, particularly protein (e.g., eggs, milk products, tuna, beans, peas, and lentils). Some patients prefer to have available high-protein finger foods such as cheese or peanut butter and crackers. Nutritional supplements may also be prescribed. The nurse monitors the patient's body weight weekly (or more often if necessary) and reports any weight loss. If the patient continues to lose weight, a feeding tube or total parenteral nutrition (TPN) may be used to supplement nutritional needs. Although this is not ideal, the patient who is malnourished and weak may benefit from this intervention.

Because the cells in the mouth grow rapidly, they are particularly sensitive to the effects of the antineoplastic drugs. **Stomatitis** (inflammation of the mouth) or **oral mucositis** (inflammation of the oral mucous membranes) may appear 5 to 7 days after chemotherapy is started and continue up to 10 days after therapy. This adverse reaction is particularly uncomfortable because irritation of the oral mucous membranes affects the nutritional aspects of care. The patient must avoid any foods or products that are irritating to the mouth, such as alcoholic beverages, spices, alcohol-based mouthwash or toothpaste. The nurse provides soft or liquid food high in nutritive value. The oral cavity is inspected for increased irritation. The nurse reports any white patches on the tongue, throat, or gums; any burning sensation; and bleeding from the mouth or gums. Mouth care is encouraged every 4 hours with normal saline solution. Lemon/glycerin swabs are avoided because they tend to irritate the oral mucosa and complicate stomatitis. The primary health care provider may order a topical viscous anesthetic, such as lidocaine viscous, to decrease discomfort.

FATIGUE, RISK FOR INJURY, AND RISK FOR INFECTION: MYELOSUPPRESSION Many antineoplastic drugs interfere with the bone marrow's ability to make new cells. This interference is called **bone marrow suppression** or **myelosuppression** and is a potentially dangerous adverse reaction. Bone marrow suppression is manifested by abnormal laboratory test results and clinical evidence of leukopenia, thrombocytopenia, or anemia. For example, there is a decrease in the white blood cells or leukocytes (**leukopenia**), a decrease in the thrombocytes (**thrombocytopenia**), and a decrease in the red blood cells, resulting in anemia.

Anemia occurs as the result of a decreased production of red blood cells in the bone marrow and is characterized by fatigue, dizziness, shortness of breath, and palpitations. The nurse helps the patient learn to prioritize activity to conserve energy. Permission is given to the active patient to slow down and even take daytime naps. In some cases, the administration of blood transfusions may be necessary to correct the anemia.

Patients with **neutropenia** (reduction in the neutrophil type of white blood cells) have a decreased resistance to infection, and the nurse must monitor them closely for any signs of infection. Combined therapy, such as chemotherapy and radiation together, can have an additive effect on the reduction of blood cells.

> ### Nursing Alert
>
> Because of the severity of leukopenia when taking temozolomide (Temodar) in conjunction with radiation to the brain, patients should be started on prophylactic therapy to prevent *Pneumocystis carinii* pneumonia (PCP).

Patients are instructed to stay away from crowds or ill individuals while receiving myelosuppressive drugs. Sepsis, without the typical signs of infection, can affect patients because they lack neutrophils. The primary health care provider may prescribe colony-stimulating factor injections to promote the production of blood cells between the chemotherapy cycles. Low blood counts are one of the primary reasons a chemotherapy treatment may be delayed.

> ### Nursing Alert
>
> The nurse should report any of the following signs of infection to the health care provider immediately: temperature of 100.4°F (38°C) or higher, cough, sore throat, chills, frequent urination, or a white blood cell count of less than 2500/mm³.

Thrombocytopenia is characterized by a decrease in the platelet count (less than 100,000/mm³). The nurse monitors patients with thrombocytopenia for bleeding tendencies and takes precautions to prevent bleeding. Injections and multiple blood draws are avoided but, if necessary, the nurse applies pressure to the injection site for 3 to 5 minutes to prevent bleeding into the tissue and the formation of a hematoma. The nurse informs the patient to avoid the use of disposable razors, nail trimmers, dental floss, firm toothbrushes, or any sharp objects. The patient is taught to refrain from contact and highly physical activities at this time. The patient is monitored closely for easy bruising, skin lesions, and bleeding from any orifice (opening) of the body.

> ### Nursing Alert
>
> The nurse reports any of the following to the health care provider immediately: bleeding gums, easy bruising, petechiae (pinpoint hemorrhages), increased menstrual bleeding, tarry stools, bloody urine, or coffee-ground emesis.

DISTURBED BODY IMAGE Adverse reactions seen with the administration of these drugs may range from very mild to life-threatening. Some of these reactions, such as the loss of hair (**alopecia**), may have little effect on the physical status of the patient but certainly may have a serious effect on the patient's mental health. Because nursing is concerned with the whole patient, such physically altering reactions that can have a profound effect on the patient must be considered when planning nursing management.

Some drugs cause severe hair loss, whereas others cause gradual thinning. Examples of drugs commonly associated with severe hair loss are doxorubicin and vinblastine. If hair loss is associated with the antineoplastic drug being given, the nurse informs the patient that hair loss may occur. This problem may occur 10 to 21 days after the first treatment cycle. Hair loss is usually temporary, and hair will grow again when the drug therapy is completed. The nurse forewarns the patient that hair loss may occur suddenly and in large amounts. Hair will be lost not only from the head but from the entire body. Although it is not life-threatening, alopecia can have an impact on both self-esteem and body image, serving as a reminder that the individual is undergoing treatment for cancer.

Depending on the patient, the nurse may need to assist in making plans for the purchase of a wig or cap to disguise the hair loss until the hair grows back. The nurse should be aware that this might be as great a problem to a male patient as it is to a female patient. The patient is reminded about the importance of a head covering because of the amount of body heat that can be lost with the hair gone.

ANXIETY The word *cancer* still evokes dread in people. Patients and family members are usually devastated by the diagnosis of cancer. Patients have to absorb much information and make quick, critical decisions about treatment. The emphasis on the safety requirements of chemotherapy administration adds to the demands and fears placed on patients. The emotional impact of the disease may be forgotten or put aside by members of the health care team as they plan and institute therapy to control the disease. Because cancer treatment happens over time, the nurse has the opportunity to offer consistent and empathetic emotional support to the patient and family members. This support can help reduce some of the fear and anxiety experienced by the patient and family during treatment.

IMPAIRED TISSUE INTEGRITY Erythema consists of a red, warm, and sometimes painful area on the skin. Because the skin cells are rapidly growing cells, the integument is at risk for breakdown during antineoplastic drug therapy. Care should be taken by patients to avoid the sun, wear loose, protective clothing, and to watch areas of skinfolds for breakdown. Some antineoplastic drugs have the ability to sensitize skin that has previously been irradiated. The nurse makes sure to instruct the patient about this adverse reaction because it can be both surprising and painful.

> **Nursing Alert**
>
> Radiation recall is a skin reaction in which an area that was previously irradiated becomes reddened when a patient is administered chemotherapy drugs. This is well differentiated from a reaction exclusive to the drugs because of the defined outline of the previous radiation treatment field on the body.

Some antineoplastic drugs are **vesicants** (i.e., they cause tissue necrosis if they infiltrate or extravasate out of the blood vessel and into the soft tissue). If extravasation occurs, underlying tissue is damaged. The damage can be severe, causing physical deformity or loss of vascularity or tendon function. If the damage is severe, skin grafting may be necessary to preserve function. Examples of vesicant drugs are daunorubicin, doxorubicin, and vinblastine.

> **Nursing Alert**
>
> Patients at risk for extravasation are those unable to communicate to the nurse about the pain of extravasation, the elderly, debilitated, or confused patient, and any patient with fragile veins.

When the patient is receiving a vesicant, the nurse ensures that extravasation protocol orders are signed and that an extravasation kit is on the unit before vesicant drugs are administered. The nurse monitors the IV site continuously and checks for blood return frequently during IV push procedures (every 1 to 2 mL). If a vesicant is prescribed as an infusion, it is given through a central line only and checked every 1 to 2 hours. The nurse keeps an extravasation kit containing all materials necessary to manage an extravasation available, along with the extravasation policy and procedure guidelines.

Extravasation may occur without warning, or signs may be detected by an alert nurse. The earlier the extravasation is detected, the less likely soft tissue damage will occur.

> **Nursing Alert**
>
> Signs of extravasation include
> - Swelling (most common)
> - Stinging, burning, or pain at the injection site (not always present)
> - Redness
> - Lack of blood return (if this is the only symptom, the IV line should be reevaluated; a lack of blood return alone is not always indicative of extravasation, and extravasation can occur even if a blood return is present)
>
> If extravasation is suspected, the infusion is stopped immediately, antidotal procedures initiated, and the extravasation reported to the primary health care provider.

EDUCATING THE PATIENT AND FAMILY

The nurse explains all treatments and possible adverse effects to the patient before the initiation of therapy. The primary health care provider usually discusses the proposed treatment and possible adverse drug reactions with the patient and family members. The nurse briefly reviews these explanations immediately before parenteral administration of a drug.

Some antineoplastic drugs are taken orally at home. The areas included in a patient and family teaching plan for this type of treatment regimen are based on the drug prescribed, the primary health care provider's explanation of the chemotherapy regimen and instructions for taking the drug, and the needs of the individual. Some hospitals, clinics, or primary health care providers give printed instructions to the patient. The nurse reviews these instructions after the patient has read them and allows time for the patient or family member to ask questions. The patient has a right to know the dangers associated with these drugs and the adverse effects that may occur.

In some instances, a drug to prevent nausea may be prescribed to be taken at home before administration of the antineoplastic drugs in the outpatient setting. To obtain the best possible effects, the nurse stresses to the patient that the drug must be taken at the time specified by the primary health care provider. It is important for the patient to comply with the treatment regimen to maximize therapeutic effect. Most patients are compliant with antineoplastic therapy; however, some of the drugs have modified schedules, such as when given in conjunction with radiation therapy with certain weeks on therapy and others off therapy, and these administration schedules can become confusing. The nurse must stress the importance of maintaining the dosing schedule exactly as prescribed. A calendar indicating the doses to take and dates the drug is to be taken, with space to record each dose, is often given to the patient. The patient is instructed to bring the treatment calendar to each appointment, and he or she is questioned about any omitted or delayed doses. In general, one course of therapy is prescribed at a time to avoid inadvertent overdosing that could be life-threatening.

The nurse includes the following points in a patient and family teaching plan when oral therapy is prescribed:

- Take the drug only as directed on the prescription container. Unless otherwise indicated, take the drug on an empty stomach with water to enhance absorption. However, the patient should follow specific directions, such as "take on an empty stomach" or "take at the same time each day"; they are extremely important.

- Familiarize yourself with the brand or trade name and the generic name to avoid confusion. If you live with another person at home, ask them to help you verify the correct drug and dose of the drug before you take it.

- Never increase, decrease, or omit a dose unless advised to do so by the primary health care provider.

- If any problems (adverse reactions) occur, no matter how minor, contact the primary health care provider immediately.

- All recommendations given by the primary health care provider, such as increasing the fluid intake or eating or avoiding certain foods, are important.

- The effectiveness or action of the drug could be altered if these directions are ignored. Other recommendations, such as checking the mouth for sores, rinsing the mouth thoroughly after eating or drinking, or drinking extra fluids, are given to identify or minimize some of the effects these drugs have on the body. It is important to follow these recommendations.

- Keep all appointments for chemotherapy. These drugs must be given at certain intervals to be effective.

- Do not take any nonprescription drug unless the use of a specific drug has been approved by the primary health care provider.

- Avoid drinking alcoholic beverages unless the primary health care provider has approved their use.

- Always inform other physicians, dentists, and medical personnel of therapy with this drug.

- Keep all appointments for the laboratory tests ordered by the primary health care provider. If you are unable to keep a laboratory appointment, notify the primary health care provider immediately.

EVALUATION

- The therapeutic effect is achieved.

- Adverse reactions are identified, reported to the primary health care provider, and managed using nursing interventions.

- Anxiety is reduced.

- The patient verbalizes an understanding of the dosage regimen.

- The patient verbalizes an understanding of treatment modalities and the importance of continued follow-up care.

- The patient verbalizes the importance of complying with the prescribed therapeutic regimen.

Critical Thinking Exercises

1. Dennis, aged 10 years, has leukemia and is to begin chemotherapy with chlorambucil (Leukeran). What information would be important to discuss with Dennis and his parents before beginning the treatment regimen?

2. Ms. Thompson has cancer of the lung and will begin a treatment regimen with methotrexate. Discuss important preadministration assessments you would perform before beginning therapy with methotrexate.

3. Patients with a malignant disease need special consideration, understanding, and emotional support. On occasion, these needs are unrecognized by members of the health care profession. Suppose you recently received a diagnosis of cancer. Discuss some of the feelings you would experience at this time. Describe what you would want the nurse to do for you at this time. Analyze your thoughts about your future. Discuss what you would want to know or not know. As you think about this or discuss these questions, remember that any patient may have these same emotional responses and need the same things you would expect from the nurse or other members of the medical profession.

Review Questions

1. Which of the following findings would be most indicative to the nurse that the patient has thrombocytopenia?

   A. Nausea

   B. Blurred vision

   C. Headaches

   D. Easy bruising

2. Which of the following is the most common symptom of extravasation?

   A. Swelling around the injection site

   B. Redness along the vein and around the injection site

   C. Pain at the injection site

   D. Tenderness along the path of the vein

3. Which of the following adverse reactions to the antineoplastic drugs is most likely to affect the patient's body image?

   A. Hematuria

   B. Alopecia

   C. Nausea

   D. Diarrhea

4. When assessing the patient for leukopenia, the nurse _____.

   A. checks the patient every 8 hours for hematuria

   B. monitors the patient for fever, sore throat, chills

   C. checks female patients for increased menstrual bleeding

   D. reports a white blood cell count of 5000/mm³

5. Which of the following interventions would be most helpful for a patient with stomatitis?

   A. Mouth care should be provided at least once daily.

   B. Swab the mouth with lemon glycerin swabs every 4 hours.

   C. Provide frequent mouth care with normal saline.

   D. Use a hard-bristle toothbrush to cleanse the mouth and teeth of debris.

Medication Dosage Problems

1. Chlorambucil (Leukeran) dosage is calculated based on the patient's body weight. Mrs. Garcia weighs 142 pounds. The prescribed dosage of chlorambucil is 0.2 mg/kg of body weight per day. What is the correct daily dosage for Mrs. Garcia?

2. A patient weighing 120 pounds is to receive bleomycin sulfate (Blenoxane) 0.25 units/kg of body weight. What is the correct dosage of bleomycin?

To check your answers, see Appendix G.

Drugs That Affect Other Body Systems

This unit covers a variety of drugs affecting various body systems, including topical drugs used to treat skin disorders, otic (ear) and ophthalmic (eye) preparations, and fluids and electrolytes. Chapter 56 discusses topical drugs used in the treatment of skin disorders. The skin forms a barrier between the outside environment and the structures located beneath the skin. The **epidermis** is the outermost layer of the skin. Immediately below the epidermis is the **dermis**, which contains small capillaries that supply nourishment to the dermis and epidermis, sebaceous (oil-secreting) glands, sweat glands, nerve fibers, and hair follicles. Because of the skin's proximity to the outside environment, it is subject to various types of injury and trauma, as well as to changes in the skin itself. Topical drugs discussed include anti-infectives, corticosteroids, antipsoriatics, enzymes, keratolytics, and anesthetics.

Chapter 57 discusses drugs used to treat disorders of the eye and ear. Ophthalmic drugs are used for diagnostic and therapeutic purposes. As a diagnostic tool, ophthalmic drugs are used to anesthetize the eye, dilate the pupil, and stain the cornea to identify anomalies. Therapeutic purposes include the treatment of infection, allergy, and eye disorders such as glaucoma. Ophthalmic drugs discussed include an alpha₂-adrenergic agonist, sympathomimetics, alpha-adrenergic blocking drugs, beta-adrenergic blocking drugs, miotics (direct acting and cholinesterase inhibitors), carbonic anhydrase inhibitors, prostaglandin agonists, mast cell stabilizers, nonsteroidal anti-inflammatory drugs, corticosteroids, cycloplegics, mydriatics, artificial tears, and various anti-infectives. Otic drugs may be used to treat infection and inflammation of the ear or to soften and remove cerumen (wax).

The composition of body fluids remains relatively constant despite the many demands placed on the body each day. On occasion, these demands cannot be met, and electrolytes and fluids must be given in an attempt to restore equilibrium. The solutions used in managing body fluids discussed in Chapter 58 include blood plasma, plasma protein fractions, protein substrates, energy substrates, plasma proteins, electrolytes, and miscellaneous replacement fluids.

Electrolytes are electrically charged particles (ions) that are essential for normal cell function and are involved in various metabolic activities. The major electrolytes discussed include potassium, calcium, magnesium, sodium, and bicarbonate. Chapter 58 discusses the use of electrolytes to replace one or more electrolytes that may be lost by the body. The last section of this chapter gives a brief overview of total parenteral nutrition (TPN). Parenteral nutrients are used to correct nutritional or fluid deficiencies, as well as to treat certain diseases and conditions.

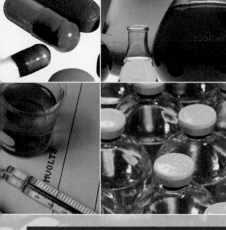

Chapter 56

Topical Drugs Used in the Treatment of Skin Disorders

Learning Objectives

On completion of this chapter, the student will:

- List the types of drugs used in the treatment of skin disorders.

- Discuss the general drug actions, uses, and reactions to and any contraindications, precautions, and interactions associated with drugs used in treating skin disorders.

- Discuss important preadministration and ongoing assessment activities

the nurse should perform on patients receiving a drug used to treat skin disorders.

- List nursing diagnoses particular to a patient using a drug to treat a skin disorder.

- Discuss ways to promote an optimal response to therapy and important points to keep in mind when educating the patient about a skin disorder.

T his chapter discusses the following types of topical drugs: anti-infectives, corticosteroids, antipsoriatics, enzymes, keratolytics, and anesthetics. Each of the following sections discusses only select topical drugs. See the Summary Drug Table: Dermatologic Drugs for a more complete listing of the drugs and additional information.

TOPICAL ANTI-INFECTIVES

Localized skin infections may require the use of a topical anti-infective. The topical anti-infectives include antibiotic, antifungal, and antiviral drugs.

Actions and Uses

Topical Antibiotic Drugs

Topical antibiotics exert a direct local effect on specific microorganisms and may be **bactericidal** (i.e., lethal to bacteria) or **bacteriostatic** (i.e., inhibit bacterial growth). Bacitracin inhibits cell wall synthesis. Bacitracin, gentamicin, and erythromycin are examples of topical antibiotics.

These drugs are used to

- Treat primary and secondary skin infections

- Prevent infection in minor cuts, wounds, scrapes, and minor burns

- Treat acne vulgaris

SUMMARY DRUG TABLE   DERMATOLOGIC DRUGS

GENERIC NAME	TRADE NAME	USES	ADVERSE REACTIONS	DOSAGE RANGES
Antibiotic Drugs				
azelaic acid *ah-zeh-lay-c*	Azelex, Finacea	Acne vulgaris, rosacea	Mild and transient pruritus, burning, stinging, erythema	Apply BID
bacitracin *ba-ci-tray'-sin*	Various brand names	Relief of skin infections, to help prevent infections in minor cuts and burns	Rare; occasionally redness, burning, pruritus, stinging	Apply daily to TID
benzoyl peroxide *ben'-zoyl per-ox'-ide*	Various brand names	Mild to moderate acne vulgaris and oily skin	Excessive drying, stinging, peeling, erythema, possible edema, allergic dermatitis	Use daily or BID
clindamycin, topical *clin-da-my-sin*	Cleocin T, Clinda Max, Clindets, Clindagel	Acne vulgaris	Dryness, erythema, burning, itching, peeling, oily skin, diarrhea, bloody diarrhea, abdominal pain, colitis	Apply a thin film daily (Clindagel) or BID to affected area
erythromycin *ee-rith-ro-mye'-sin*	Akne-Mycin, Emgel, Erygel	Acne vulgaris	Skin irritation, tenderness, pruritus, erythema, peeling, oiliness, burning sensation	Clean and apply to affected area BID
gentamicin *jen-ta-mye'-sin*	Various brand names	Relief of primary and secondary skin infections	Mild and transient pruritus, burning, stinging, erythema, photosensitivity	Apply TID or QID to affected area
metronidazole *meh-trow-ney'-dah-zole*	Metro-Gel, Metrolotion, Noritate	Rosacea	Watery (tearing) eyes, transient redness, mild dryness, burning, skin irritation, nausea, tingling/numbness of extremities	Apply a thin film daily or BID to affected areas
mupirocin *mew-peer'-oh-sin*	Bactroban, Bactroban Nasal	Impetigo infections caused by *Staphylococcus aureus* and *Streptococcus pyogenes* Nasal: eradication of MRSA as part of an infection control program to reduce the risk of institutional outbreaks of MRSA	Ointment: burning, stinging, pain, itching, rash, nausea, erythema, dry skin Cream: headache, rash, nausea, abdominal pain, burning at application site, dermatitis Nasal: headache, rhinitis, respiratory disorders (e.g., pharyngitis), taste perversion, burning, stinging, cough	Ointment: apply TID for 3–5 d Cream: apply TID for 10 d Nasal: divide the single-use tube between nostrils and apply BID for 5 d

GENERIC NAME	TRADE NAME	USES	ADVERSE REACTIONS	DOSAGE RANGES
Antifungal Drugs				
butenafine HCl *byoo-ten'-ah-feen*	Mentax, Lotrimin Ultra	Dermatologic infections, tinea versicolor, tinea	Burning, stinging, itching, worsening of the condition, contact dermatis, erythema, irritation corporis (ringworm), tinea cruris (jockitch)	Apply daily or BID for 2–4 wk
ciclopirox *sic-lo-peer'-ox*	Loprox, Penlac Nail Lacquer	Loprox, cream and suspension: tinea pedis (athlete's foot), tinea cruris, tinea corporis, cutaneous candidiasis Gel: interdigital tinea pedis and tinea corporis, seborrheic dermatitis of the scalp Penlac: mild to moderate onychomycosis of fingernails and toenails	Cream: pruritus at the application site, worsening of clinical signs and symptoms, burning Loprox Gel: burning sensation on application, contact dermatitis, pruritus, dry skin, acne, rash, alopecia, eye pain, facial edema Loprox shampoo: increased itching, burning, erythema, itching, rash, headache Penlac: periungual erythema, nail disorders, irritation, ingrown toenail, burning of the skin	Apply to affected areas daily or BID Shampoo: wet hair and apply approx. 1 teaspoon (5 mL) of shampoo to the scalp. Up to 10 mL may be used for long hair. Lather and leave on hair and scalp for 3 min. Avoid contact with eyes. Rinse and repeat treatment twice weekly for 4 wk with a minimum of 3 d between applications. Penlac: Apply QD preferably at bedtime or 8 h before washing
clotrimazole *kloe-trim'-a-zole*	Cruex, Lotrimin AF, Desenex	Tinea pedis, tinea cruris, and other skin infections caused by ringworm	Burning, itching, erythema, peeling, edema, general skin irritation	Apply thin layer to affected areas BID for 2–4 wk
econazole nitrate *ee-kon'-a-zole*	Spectazole	Tinea pedis, tinea cruris, tinea corporis, tinea versicolor, cutaneous candidiasis	Local burning, itching, stinging, erythema, pruritic rash	Apply to affected areas daily or BID
gentian violet *jen'-shun*		External treatment of abrasions, minor cuts, surface injuries, superficial fungal infections of the skin	Local irritation or sensitivity reactions	Apply locally BID Do not bandage
haloprogin *ha-lo-pro'-jin*	Halotex	Tinea pedis, tinea cruris, tinea corporis, tinea manuum	Local irritation, burning sensation, vesicle formation, erythema, scaling, itching, pruritus	Apply liberally BID for 2–4 wk
ketoconazole *kee-toe-koe'-na-zole*	Nizoral	Cream: tinea cruris, tinea corporis, tinea versicolor Shampoo: reduction of scaling due to dandruff	Cream: Severe itching, pruritus, stinging Shampoo: increase in hair loss, abnormal hair texture, scalp pustules, mild dryness of the skin, itching, oiliness/dryness of the hair	Cream: apply daily to affected areas for 2–6 wk Shampoo: twice a week for 4 wk with at least 3 d between each shampoo
miconazole niteate *mi-kon'-a-zole*	Tetterine, Micatin, Monistat-Derm, Micatin, Fungold Tincture	Tinea pedis, tinea cruris, tinea corporis, cutaneous candidiasis	Local irritation, burning, maceration, allergic contact dermatitis	Cover affected areas BID

⬤ SUMMARY DRUG TABLE *(continued)*

GENERIC NAME	TRADE NAME	USES	ADVERSE REACTIONS	DOSAGE RANGES
naftifine HCl *naf'-ti-feen*	Naftin	Topical treatment of tinea pedis, tinea cruris, tinea corporis	Burning, stinging, erythema, itching, local irritation, rash, tenderness	Apply BID for 4 wk
nystatin *nye-stat'-in*	Mycostatin, Nystex	Mycotic infections caused by *Candida albicans* and other *Candida* species	Virtually nontoxic and nonsensitizing; well tolerated by all age groups, even with prolonged administration; if irritation occurs, discontinue use	Apply BID or TID until healing is complete
oxiconazole *ox-ee-kon'-ah-zole*	Oxistat	Tinea pedis, tinea cruris, tinea corporis	Pruritus, burning, stinging, irritation, contact dermatitis, scaling, tingling	Apply daily or BID for 1 mo
suconazole nitrate *sue-kon'-ah-zole*	Exelderm	Same as oxiconazole	Pruritus, burning, stinging, irritation	Apply daily or BID for 3–6 wk
terbinafine HCl *ter-ben'-a-feen*	Lamisil	Same as oxiconazole	Same as oxiconazole	Apply BID until infection clears (1–4 wk)
tolnaftate *tole-naf'-tate*	Aftate, Genaspor, Tinactin, Ting	Same as oxiconazole	Same as oxiconazole	Apply BID for 2–3 wk (4–6 wk may be needed)
Antiviral Drugs				
acyclovir *ay-sye'-kloe-veer*	Zovirax	Ointment: herpes genitalis, herpes simplex virus infections Cream: recurrent herpes labialis (cold sores) in adults and adolescents 12 y of age and older	Ointment: Mild pain with transient burning/stinging Cream: pruritus, rash, vulvitis, edema or pain at application site	Onintment: apply to all lesions q3h 6 times daily for 7 d Cream: apply 5 times daily for 4 d
penciclovir *pen-sye'-kloe-veer*	Denavir	Herpes labialis	Irritation at application site, local anesthesia, taste perversion, headache, mild erythema, rash	Apply q2h (while awake) for 4 d
Antiseptics and Germicides				
chlorhexidine gluconate *klor-hex'-e-deen*	Bacto Shield 2, Betasept, Exidine-2 Scrub, Hibiclens	Surgical scrub, skin cleanser, preoperative skin preparation, skin wound cleanser, preoperative showering and bathing	Irritation, dermatitis, photosensitivity (rare), deafness, mild sensitivity reactions	Varies, depending on administration
hexachlorophene *hex-a-klor'-oh-feen*	pHisoHex, Septisol	Surgical scrub and bacteriostatic skin cleanser, control of an outbreak of gram-positive infection when other procedures are unsuccessful	Dermatitis, photosensitivity, sensitivity to hexachlorophene, redness or mild scaling or dryness	Surgical wash or scrub: as indicated Bacteriostatic cleansing: wet hand with water and squeeze approx. 5 mL into palm, add water and work up lather, apply to area to be cleansed, rinse thoroughly
povidone-iodine *poe'-vi-done*	Acu-Dyne, Aerodine, Betadine	Microbicidal against bacteria, fungi, viruses, spores, protozoa, yeasts	Dermatitis, irritation, burning, sensitivity reactions	Varies, depending on administration

GENERIC NAME	TRADE NAME	USES	ADVERSE REACTIONS	DOSAGE RANGES
triclosan *trye'-klo-san*	Clearasil Daily Face Wash	Skin cleanser and degermer	None significant	Apply 5 mL on hands or face and rub thoroughly for 30 sec, rinse thoroughly, pat dry
Corticosteroids, Topical				
alclometasone dipropionate *al-kloe-met'-a-sone* *die-pro'-pee-oh-nate*	Aclovate	Treatment of various allergic/immunologic skin problems	Allergic contact dermatitis, burning, dryness, edema, irritation	Apply 1–6 times daily according to directions
amcinonide *am-sin'-oh-nide*	Cyclocort	Same as alclometasone	Same as alclometasone	Apply 1–6 times daily according to directions
augmented betamethasone dipropionate *bay-ta-meth'-a-sone*	Diprolene	Same as alclometasone	Same as alclometasone	Apply 1–4 times daily according to directions
betamethasone dipropionate	Alphatrex, Diprosone, Maxivate	Same as alclometasone	Same as alclometasone	Apply 1–4 times daily according to directions
betamethasone valerate *val'-eh-rate*	Betatrex	Same as alclometasone	Same as alclometasone	Apply 1–4 times daily according to directions
desoximetasone *dess-ox-i-met'-a-sone*	Topicort	Same as alclometasone	Same as alclometasone	Apply 1–4 times daily according to directions
dexamethasone sodium phosphate *dex-a-meth'-a-sone*	Decadron Phosphate	Same as alclometasone	Same as alclometasone	Apply 1–4 times daily according to directions
diflorasone diacetate *dye-flor'-a-sone*	Florone, Maxiflor	Same as alclometasone	Same as alclometasone	Apply 1–4 times daily according to directions
fluocinolone acetonide *floo-oh-sin'-oh-lone*	Fluonid, Flurosyn, Synalar	Same as alclometasone	Same as alclometasone	Apply 1–4 times daily according to directions
fluocinonide *floo-oh-sin'-oh-nide*	Lidex	Same as alclometasone	Same as alclometasone	Apply 1–4 times daily according to directions
flurandrenolide *floor-an-dren'-oh-lide*	Cordran	Same as alclometasone	Same as alclometasone	Apply 1–4 times daily according to directions
hydrocortisone *hye-droe-kor'-ti-sone*	Bactine, Cort-Dome, Hytone	Same as alclometasone	Same as alclometasone	Apply 1–4 times daily according to directions
hydrocortisone buteprate	Pandel	Psoriasis and other deep-seated dermatoses	Same as alclometasone	Apply daily or BID
hydrocortisone butyrate	Locoid	Same as alclometasone	Same as alclometasone	Apply BID or TID
triamcinolone acetonide *trye-am-sin'-oh-lone*	Aristocort, Flutex, Kenalog, Triacet	Same as alclometasone	Same as alclometasone	Apply 1–4 times daily according to directions
Antipsoriatic Drugs				
ammoniated mercury *ah-mo'-ne-at-ed* *mer'-ku-re*	Emersal	Psoriasis	Ammoniated mercury is a potential sensitizer that can cause allergic reactions	Apply daily or BID

SUMMARY DRUG TABLE   *(continued)*

GENERIC NAME	TRADE NAME	USES	ADVERSE REACTIONS	DOSAGE RANGES
anthralin *an-thra'-lin*	Anthraderm Drithocreme, Miconal	Psoriasis	Few; transient irritation of normal skin or uninvolved skin	Apply daily
calcipotriene *cal-cip-o-try'-een*	Dovonex	Psoriasis	Burning, itching, skin irritation, erythema, dry skin, peeling, rash, worsening of psoriasis, dermatitis, hyperpigmentation	Apply BID
selenium sulfide *se-le'-ne-um*	Exsel Head and Shoulders Intensive Treatment Dandruff Shampoo, Selsun Blue	Treatment of dandruff, seborrheic dermatitis of the scalp, and tinea versicolor	Skin irritation, greater than normal hair loss, hair discoloration, oiliness or dryness of hair	Massage 5–10 mL into wet scalp and allow to remain on scalp for 2–3 min, rinse
Enzyme Preparations				
collagenase *koll-ah'-gen-ase*	Santyl	For debriding chronic dermal ulcers and severely burned areas	Well tolerated and nonirritating; transient burning sensation may occur	Apply daily according to directions
enzyme combinations	Accuzyme, Granul-Derm Granulex, Panafil	Debridement of necrotic tissue and liqueaction of slough in acute and chronic lesions such as pressure ulcers, varicose and diabetic ulcers, burns, wounds, pilonidal cyst wounds, and miscellaneous traumatic or infected wounds	Well tolerated and nonirritating; transient burning sensation may occur	Aerosol: apply BID or TID according to directions Ointment: apply daily or BID according to directions
Keratolytic Drugs				
masoprocol *ma-so'-pro-kole*	Actinex	Actinic keratoses	Erythema, flaking, dryness, itching, edema, burning, soreness, bleeding, crusting, skin roughness	Apply BID
Salicylic acid *sal-i-sill'-ik*	Duofilm, Wart Remover, Fostex, Fung-O, Mosco, Panscol	Aids in the removal of excessive keratin in hyperkeratotic skin disorders, including warts, psoriasis, calluses, and corns	Local irritation	Apply as directed in individual product labeling
Local Anesthetics				
benzocaine *benz'-o-kane*	Lanacane	Topical anesthesia in local skin disorders	Rare; hypersensitivity, local burning, stinging, tenderness, sloughing	Apply to affected area
dibucaine *di'-bu-kane*	Nupercainal	Topical anesthesia in local skin disorders, local anesthesia of accessible mucous membranes	Same as benzocaine	Topical: apply to affected area as needed Mucous membranes: dosage varies and depends on the area to be anesthetized

GENERIC NAME	TRADE NAME	USES	ADVERSE REACTIONS	DOSAGE RANGES
lidocaine *lie'-doe-kane*	ELA-Max, Lidocaine Viscous, Xylocaine	Same as dibucaine	Same as benzocaine	Topical: apply to affected area as needed Mucous membranes: dosage varies and depends on the area to be anesthetized
lidocaine HCl	DentiPatch	Topical anesthesia of accessible mucous membranes of the mouth before dental procedures	Rare; local burning, stinging, tenderness	Apply to affected area
butamben picrate *byoo'-tam-ben*		Topical anesthesia	Rare; local burning, stinging, tenderness	Apply to affected area

MRSA, methicillin-resistant *S. aureus*.

Topical Antifungal Drugs

Antifungal drugs exert a local effect by inhibiting growth of fungi. Examples of antifungal drugs include miconazole, ketoconazole, and ciclopirox. Antifungal drugs are used for treating

- Tinea pedis (athlete's foot), tinea cruris (jock itch), tinea corporis (ringworm)
- Cutaneous candidiasis
- Other superficial fungal infections of the skin

Topical Antiviral Drugs

Acyclovir and penciclovir are the only topical antiviral drugs currently available. These drugs inhibit viral replication. Acyclovir is used in treating

- Initial episodes of genital herpes
- Herpes simplex virus infections in **immunocompromised** patients (patients with an immune system incapable of fighting infection)

Penciclovir is used for treating recurrent herpes labialis (cold sores) in adults.

Adverse Reactions

Adverse reactions to topical anti-infectives are usually mild. Occasionally, the patient may experience a rash, itching, urticaria (hives), dermatitis, irritation, or redness, which may indicate a **hypersensitivity** (allergic) reaction to the drug. Prolonged use of topical antibiotic preparations may result in a superficial **superinfection** (an overgrowth of bacterial or fungal microorganisms not affected by the antibiotic being administered).

Contraindications, Precautions, and Interactions

These drugs are contraindicated in patients with known hypersensitivity to the drugs or any components of the drug.

The topical antibiotics are pregnancy category C drugs and are used cautiously during pregnancy and lactation. Acyclovir and penciclovir are pregnancy category B drugs and are used cautiously during pregnancy and lactation. The pregnancy categories of the antifungals are unknown except for econazole nitrate, which is in pregnancy category C, and ciclopirox, which is in pregnancy category B; both are used with caution during pregnancy and lactation. There are no significant interactions for the topical anti-infectives.

Herbal Alert

Aloe vera is used to prevent infection and promote healing of minor burns (e.g., sunburn) and wounds. When used externally, aloe helps to repair skin tissue and reduce inflammation. Aloe gel is naturally thick when taken from the leaf but quickly becomes watery because of the action of enzymes in the plant. Commercially available preparations have additive thickeners to make the aloe appear like the fresh gel. The agent can be applied directly from the fresh leaf by cutting the leaf in half lengthwise and gently rubbing the inner gel directly onto the skin. Commercially prepared products are applied externally as needed. Rare reports of

Topical Drugs Used in the Treatment of Skin Disorders

Herbal Alert *(continued)*

allergy have been reported with the external use of aloe. Although aloe vera is available as an oral juice, its benefits have not been confirmed. Some individuals have reported the oral juice effective in healing and preventing stomach ulcers.

TOPICAL ANTISEPTICS AND GERMICIDES

An **antiseptic** is a drug that stops, slows, or prevents the growth of microorganisms. A **germicide** is a drug that kills bacteria.

Actions

The exact mechanism of action of topical antiseptics and germicides is not well understood. These drugs affect a variety of microorganisms. Some of these drugs have a short duration of action, whereas others have a long duration of action. The action of these drugs may depend on the strength used and the time the drug is in contact with the skin or mucous membrane.

Chlorhexidine

Chlorhexidine gluconate affects a wide range of microorganisms, including gram-positive and gram-negative bacteria.

Hexachlorophene

Hexachlorophene (pHisoHex) is a bacteriostatic drug that acts against staphylococci and other gram-positive bacteria. Cumulative antibacterial action develops with repeated use.

Iodine

Iodine has anti-infective action against many bacteria, fungi, viruses, yeasts, and protozoa. Povidone–iodine (Betadine) is a combination of iodine and povidone that liberates free iodine. Povidone–iodine is often preferred over iodine solution or tincture because it is less irritating to the skin and treated areas may be bandaged or taped. For more information, see the Home Care Checklist: Using an Occlusive Dressing.

Home Care Checklist

Using an Occlusive Dressing

In certain circumstances, the patient who requires a topical drug must also apply an occlusive dressing to enhance the drug's effectiveness. Although commercial occlusive dressings are available, they are expensive, especially if your patient requires frequent dressing changes at home. So, if appropriate, suggest these less costly home alternatives:

☑ Plastic food wrap such as Saran wrap

☑ Plastic food storage bags

After your patient gathers the necessary supplies, instruct him or her to do the following:

☑ Wash hands before beginning care.

☑ Remove the old dressing.

☑ Cleanse the area as directed.

☑ Apply the topical drug as ordered.

☑ Cover the area with a dry gauze dressing.

☑ Apply a skin adhesive to the area around the gauze dressing.

☑ Cover the gauze dressing with the occlusive dressing, making sure that the occlusive dressing is approximately 1 inch larger than the gauze dressing on all sides. For example, if the gauze dressing is 4 inches × 4 inches, then the occlusive dressing should be 5 inches × 5 inches.

☑ Check to make sure that the occlusive dressing lies flat without wrinkles.

☑ Run fingers around all the edges of the occlusive dressing to ensure good adhesion.

☑ Tape the edges of the occlusive dressing on all sides, preferably with paper tape, to secure it.

Uses

Topical antiseptics and germicides are used

- To reduce the number of bacteria on skin surfaces
- As a surgical scrub and preoperative skin cleanser
- For washing the hands before and after caring for patients
- In the home to cleanse the skin
- On minor cuts and abrasions to prevent infection

Adverse Reactions

Topical antiseptics and germicides provoke few adverse reactions. Occasionally, an individual may be allergic to the drug, and a skin rash or itching may occur. If an allergic reaction is noted, use of the topical drug is discontinued.

Contraindications, Precautions, and Interactions

These drugs are contraindicated in patients with known hypersensitivity to the individual drug or any component of the preparation. There are no significant precautions or interactions when the drugs are used as directed.

TOPICAL CORTICOSTEROIDS

Topical corticosteroids vary in potency, depending on the concentration (percentage) of the drug, the vehicle (lotion, cream, aerosol spray) in which the drug is suspended, and the area (open or denuded skin, unbroken skin, thickness of the skin over the treated area) to which the drug is applied. Examples of topical corticosteroids include amcinonide, betamethasone dipropionate, fluocinolone acetonide, hydrocortisone, and triamcinolone acetate.

Actions and Uses

Topical corticosteroids exert localized anti-inflammatory activity. When applied to inflamed skin, they reduce itching, redness, and swelling. These drugs are use in treating skin disorders such as

- Psoriasis
- Dermatitis

- Rashes
- Eczema
- Insect bites
- First- and second-degree burns, including sunburn

Adverse Reactions

Localized reactions may include burning, itching, irritation, redness, dryness of the skin, allergic contact dermatitis, and secondary infection. These reactions are more likely to occur if occlusive dressings are used. Systemic reactions may also occur with hypothalamic-pituitary-adrenal axis suppression, Cushing's syndrome, hyperglycemia, and glycosuria.

Contraindications, Precautions, and Interactions

The topical corticosteroids are contraindicated in patients with known hypersensitivity to the drug or any component of the drug; as monotherapy for bacterial skin infections; for use on the face, groin, or axilla (only the high-potency corticosteroids); and for ophthalmic use (may cause steroid-induced glaucoma or cataracts). The topical corticosteroids are not used as sole therapy in widespread plaque psoriasis. The topical corticosteroids are pregnancy category C drugs and are used cautiously during pregnancy and lactation. There are no significant interactions when these drugs are administered as directed.

TOPICAL ANTIPSORIATICS

Action and Uses

Topical **antipsoriatics** are drugs used to treat psoriasis (a chronic skin disease manifested by bright red patches covered with silvery scales or plaques) by helping to remove the plaques associated with the disorder. Examples of antipsoriatics include anthralin and calcipotriene.

Adverse Reactions

These drugs may cause burning, itching, and skin irritation. Anthralin may cause skin irritation, as well as temporary discoloration of the hair and fingernails.

Contraindications, Precautions, and Interactions

Topical antipsoriatics are contraindicated in patients with known hypersensitivity to the drugs. Anthralin and calcipotriene, pregnancy category C drugs, are used cautiously during pregnancy and lactation.

TOPICAL ENZYMES
Actions and Uses

A topical enzyme is used to help remove necrotic tissue from
- Chronic dermal ulcers
- Severely burned areas

These enzymes aid in the removal of dead soft tissues by hastening the reduction of proteins into simpler substances. The process is called **proteolysis** or a **proteolytic** action. The components of certain types of wounds, namely **necrotic** (dead) tissues and **purulent exudates** (pus-containing fluid), prevent proper wound healing. Removal of this type of debris by application of a topical enzyme aids in healing. Examples of conditions that may respond to application of a topical enzyme include second- and third-degree burns, pressure ulcers, and ulcers caused by peripheral vascular disease. An example of a topical enzyme is collagenase.

Adverse Reactions

The application of collagenase may cause mild, transient pain and possibly numbness and dermatitis. There is a low incidence of adverse reactions to collagenase.

Contraindications, Precautions, and Interactions

The topical enzyme preparations are contraindicated in patients with known hypersensitivity to the drugs, in wounds in contact with major body cavities or where nerves are exposed, and in fungating neoplastic ulcers. These drugs are pregnancy category B drugs and are used cautiously during pregnancy and lactation. Enzymatic activity may be impaired by certain detergents and heavy metal ions, such as mercury and silver, which are used in some antiseptics. The optimal pH for collagenase is 6 to 8. Higher or lower pH conditions decrease the enzyme's activity.

KERATOLYTICS
Actions and Uses

A **keratolytic** is a drug that removes excess growth of the epidermis (top layer of skin) in disorders such as warts. These drugs are used to remove
- Warts
- Calluses
- Corns
- Seborrheic keratoses (benign, variously colored skin growths arising from oil glands of the skin)

Examples of keratolytics include salicylic acid and masoprocol. Some strengths of salicylic acid are available as nonprescription products for the removal of warts on the hands and feet.

Adverse Reactions

These drugs are usually well tolerated. Occasionally a transient burning sensation, rash, dry skin, scaling, or flu-like syndrome may occur.

Contraindications, Precautions, and Interactions

The keratolytics are contraindicated in patients with known hypersensitivity to the drugs and for use on moles, birthmarks, or warts with hair growing from them, on genital or facial warts, on warts on mucous membranes, or on infected skin. Prolonged use of the keratolytics in infants and in patients with diabetes or impaired circulation is contraindicated. Salicylic acid may cause salicylate toxicity with prolonged use (see Chapter 17). These drugs are pregnancy category C drugs and are used cautiously during pregnancy and lactation. See Chapter 17 for a listing of the drug interactions with the salicylates.

TOPICAL LOCAL ANESTHETICS

A topical anesthetic may be applied to the skin or mucous membranes.

Actions and Uses

Topical anesthetics temporarily inhibit the conduction of impulses from sensory nerve fibers. These drugs may be used to relieve itching and pain due to skin conditions, such as minor burns, fungal infections, insect bites, rashes, sunburn, and plant poisoning (e.g., poison ivy). Some are applied to mucous membranes as local anesthetics. Examples of local anesthetics include benzocaine, dibucaine, and lidocaine.

Adverse Reactions

Occasionally, local irritation, dermatitis, rash, burning, stinging, and tenderness may be noted.

Contraindications, Precautions, and Interactions

These drugs are contraindicated in those with a known hypersensitivity to any component of the preparation. The topical anesthetics are used cautiously in patients receiving class I antiarrhythmic drugs such as tocainide and mexiletine because the toxic effects are additive and potentially synergistic.

NURSING PROCESS

The Patient Receiving a Topical Drug for a Skin Disorder

ASSESSMENT

PREADMINISTRATION ASSESSMENT

The preadministration assessment involves a visual inspection and palpation of the involved area(s). The nurse carefully records the areas of involvement, including the size, color, and appearance. A specific description is important so that changes indicating worsening or improvement of the lesions can be readily identified. Terms used to describe skin lesions are found in Table 56-1. The nurse notes the presence of scales, crusting, or drainage and any complaint of itching. Some agencies may provide a figure on which the lesions can be drawn, indicating the shape and distribution of the involved areas.

ONGOING ASSESSMENT

At the time of each application, the nurse inspects the affected area for changes (e.g., signs of improvement or

Table 56.1 Terms Used to Describe Skin Lesions

Lesion	Description
Macule	Flat spot on the skin
Papule	Raised spot on the skin
Nodule	Small solid swelling on the skin
Pustule	Lesion containing pus
Petechia	Pinpoint hemorrhagic areas of the skin
Erythema	Redness
Ecchymosis	Bruised area
Vesicle	Fluid-filled swelling (blister)

worsening of the infection) and for adverse reactions, such as redness or rash. The nurse contacts the primary health care provider, and the drug is not applied if these or other changes are noted or if the patient reports new problems, such as itching, pain, or soreness at the site. The nurse may be responsible for checking the treatment sites 1 day or more after application and should inform the primary health care provider of any signs of extreme redness or infection at the application site.

Pediatric Alert

Because infants and children have a high ratio of skin surface area to body mass, they are at greater risk than adults for systemic adverse effects when treated with topical medication.

NURSING DIAGNOSES

Drug-specific nursing diagnoses are highlighted in the Nursing Diagnoses Checklist. Other nursing diagnoses applicable to these drugs are discussed in depth in Chapter 4.

Nursing Diagnoses Checklist

✓ **Impaired Skin Integrity** related to the inflammatory process (increased sensitivity to the drug)

✓ **Acute Pain** related to skin condition or increased sensitivity to drug therapy

✓ **Risk for Infection** related to entry of pathogens into affected areas

✓ **Risk for Disturbed Body Image** related to the presence of skin lesions

PLANNING

The expected outcomes of the patient may include an optimal response to drug therapy and an understanding of the application or the reason for use of a topical drug.

IMPLEMENTATION
PROMOTING AN OPTIMAL RESPONSE TO THERAPY

TOPICAL ANTI-INFECTIVES Before each application, the nurse cleanses the skin with soap and warm water unless the primary health care provider orders a different method. The nurse applies the anti-infective as prescribed (e.g., thin layer or applied liberally) and the area is either covered or left exposed as prescribed.

> ### Nursing Alert
>
> The nurse must exercise care when applying anti-infectives or any topical drug near or around the eyes.

TOPICAL ANTISEPTICS AND GERMICIDES The nurse uses, instills, or applies antiseptics and germicides as directed by the primary health care provider or by the label on the product. Topical antiseptics and germicides are not a substitute for clean or aseptic techniques. Occlusive dressings are not to be used after application of these products unless a dressing is specifically ordered by the primary health care provider. Iodine permanently stains clothing and temporarily stains the skin. The nurse should remove or protect the patient's personal clothing when applying iodine solution or tincture.

Antiseptic and germicidal drugs kept at the patient's bedside must be clearly labeled with the name of the product, the strength, and, when applicable, the date of preparation of the solution. The nurse replaces hard-to-read or soiled, stained labels as needed. These solutions are not kept at the bedside of any patient who is confused or disoriented because the solution may be mistaken for water or another beverage.

TOPICAL CORTICOSTEROIDS Before drug application, the nurse washes the area with soap and warm water unless the primary health care provider directs otherwise. Topical corticosteroids are usually ordered to be applied sparingly. The primary health care provider also may order the area of application to be covered or left exposed to the air. Some corticosteroids are applied with an occlusive dressing. The nurse applies the drug while the skin is still moist after washing with soap and water and applies a dressing if ordered by the primary health care provider.

> ### Pediatric Alert
>
> Do not use tight-fitting diapers or pants on a child treated in the diaper area. These types of clothing may work like an occlusive dressing and cause more of the drug to be absorbed into the child's body, resulting in a greater risk for adverse reactions.

TOPICAL ENZYMES Certain types of wounds may require special preparations before applying the topical enzyme. The nurse cleanses or prepares the area and applies the topical enzyme as directed by the primary health care provider.

TOPICAL ANTIPSORIATICS The nurse may be responsible for applying the product and inspecting the areas of application. Care is exercised so that the product is applied only to the psoriatic lesions and not to surrounding skin. The nurse brings signs of excessive irritation to the attention of the primary health care provider.

> ### Gerontologic Alert
>
> Adults older than 65 years have more skin-related adverse reactions to calcipotriene. The nurse should use calcipotriene cautiously in older adults.

TOPICAL ANESTHETICS The nurse applies the anesthetic as directed by the primary health care provider. Before the first application, the nurse cleanses and dries the area. For subsequent applications, the nurse removes all previous residue.

When a topical gel, such as lidocaine viscous, is used for oral anesthesia, the nurse instructs the patient not to eat food for 1 hour after use because local anesthesia of the mouth or throat may impair swallowing and increase the possibility of aspiration.

MONITORING AND MANAGING PATIENT NEEDS

Most topical drugs cause few adverse reactions and, if they occur, discontinuing use of the drug may be all that is necessary to relieve the symptoms.

IMPAIRED SKIN INTEGRITY Dry skin increases the risk of skin breakdown from scratching. The nurse can advise the patient to keep nails short, use warm water with mild soap for cleaning the skin, and rinse and dry the skin thoroughly.

ACUTE PAIN Occasionally, increased skin sensitivity occurs, causing greater redness, discomfort, and itching. With itching and rash the nurse may use cool, wet compresses or a bath to relieve the itching. Keeping the environment cool may also make the patient more comfortable.

RISK FOR INFECTION Bath oils, creams, and lotions may be used, if necessary, as long as the primary health care provider is consulted before use. Dry, flaky skin is subject to breakdown and infection. The nurse observes the skin for signs of infection (e.g., redness, heat, pus, and elevated temperature and pulse) and immediately reports any sign of infection.

RISK FOR DISTURBED BODY IMAGE Some patients may experience anxiety about the appearance of certain skin lesions or the symptoms of a specific dermatologic disorder. This may cause a negative body image. The nurse must allow time for the patient to verbalize concerns or ask questions concerning therapy. The nurse reassures the patient that the lesions are temporary and will diminish or disappear with treatment (if that is true).

EDUCATING THE PATIENT AND FAMILY

If the primary health care provider has prescribed or recommended the use of a topical drug, the nurse includes the following in a teaching plan.

GENERAL TEACHING POINTS

- Wash the hands thoroughly before and after applying the product.

- If the enclosed directions state that the product will stain clothing, be sure clothing is moved away from the treated area. If the product stains the skin, wear disposable gloves when applying the drug.

- Follow the directions on the label or use as directed by the primary health care provider. Read any enclosed directions for use of the product carefully.

- Prepare the area to be treated as recommended by the primary health care provider or as described in the directions supplied with the product.

- Do not apply to areas other than those specified by the primary health care provider. Apply the drug as directed (e.g., thin layer or apply liberally).

- Follow the directions of the primary health care provider regarding covering the treated area or leaving it exposed to air. The effectiveness of certain drugs depends on keeping the area covered or leaving it open (see Home Care Checklist: Using an Occlusive Dressing).

- Keep the product away from the eyes (unless use in or around the eye has been recommended or prescribed). Do not rub or put the fingers near the eyes unless the hands have been thoroughly washed and all remnants of the drug removed from the fingers. If the product is accidentally spilled, sprayed, or splashed in the eye, wash the eye immediately with copious amounts of running water. Contact the primary health care provider immediately if burning, pain, redness, discomfort, or blurred vision persists for more than a few minutes.

- The drug may cause momentary stinging or burning when applied.

- Discontinue use of the drug and contact the primary health care provider if rash, burning, itching, redness, pain, or other skin problems occur.

ANTI-INFECTIVES

- Gentamicin may cause photosensitivity. Take measures to protect the skin from ultraviolet rays (e.g., wear protective clothing and use a sunscreen when out in the sun).

- Topical clindamycin can be absorbed in sufficient amounts to cause systemic effects. If severe diarrhea, stomach cramps, or bloody stools occur, contact the primary health care provider immediately.

ANTIVIRAL AGENT (ACYCLOVIR)

- Acyclovir is most effective when used early at the start of herpes simplex virus infection.

- When applying ointment, use a finger cot or glove to prevent autoinoculation of other body sites.

- This product will not prevent transmission of infection to others.

- Transient burning, itching, and rash may occur.

TOPICAL CORTICOSTEROIDS

- Apply ointments, creams, or gels sparingly in a light film; rub in gently.

- Use only as directed. Do not use bandages, dressings, cosmetics, or other skin products over the treated area unless so directed by the primary health care provider.

ENZYME PREPARATIONS

- If, for any reason, it becomes necessary to inactivate collagenase, this can be accomplished by washing the area with povidone–iodine.

EVALUATION

- The therapeutic drug response is achieved.

- The patient or family member demonstrates an understanding of the use and application of the prescribed or recommended drug.

Critical Thinking Exercises

1. A nurse tells you that she is upset because she was reprimanded about the labeling of a topical antiseptic used for cleaning a pressure ulcer and for leaving the solution at the patient's bedside. She

thinks her supervisor is unfair and that the situation is not as serious as the supervisor contends. Analyze the situation to determine what you would say to this nurse.

2. Discuss the ongoing assessment activities you would include in the daily assessment of a patient prescribed a topical drug.

3. Describe important preadministration assessments that the nurse would make before administering a topical corticosteroid.

Review Questions

1. What reaction could occur with prolonged use of the topical antibiotics?

   A. Water intoxication

   B. Superficial superinfection

   C. An outbreak of eczema

   D. Cellulitis

2. Which of the following drugs has a proteolytic action?

   A. amcinonide

   B. collagenase

   C. bacitracin

   D. ciclopirox

3. A keratolytic agent would be safe to use on which of the following skin conditions?

   A. Moles

   B. Birthmarks

   C. Facial warts

   D. Calluses

4. What type of action do the corticosteroids have when used topically?

   A. Bactericidal activity

   B. Anti-inflammatory activity

   C. Antifungal activity

   D. Antiviral activity

5. Which of the following drugs is best suited to be used as a topical antiseptic?

   A. amphotericin B

   B. benzocaine

   C. iodine

   D. povidone–iodine

To check your answers, see Appendix G.

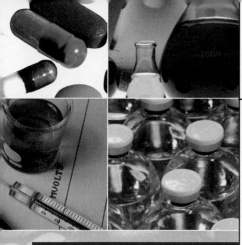

Otic and Ophthalmic Preparations

Learning Objectives

On completion of this chapter, the student will:

- Discuss the general actions, uses, adverse reactions, contraindications, precautions, and interactions of otic and ophthalmic preparations.

- Discuss important preadministration and ongoing assessment activities the nurse should perform on a patient receiving otic and ophthalmic preparations.

- List nursing diagnoses particular to a patient taking an otic or ophthalmic preparation.

- Discuss ways to promote an optimal response to therapy, how to administer the preparations, and important points to keep in mind when educating patients about the use of otic or ophthalmic preparations.

The eyes and ears are subject to various disorders that range from mild to serious. Because the eyes and ears are among the interpreters of our outside environment, any disease or injury that has the potential for partial or total loss of function of these organs must be treated.

OTIC PREPARATIONS

Disorders of the ear are categorized according to the part of the ear affected: the outer, the middle, or the inner ear. The disorders most often treated with the preparations discussed in this chapter are of the outer and middle ear. **Otitis media**, by far the most common disorder of the middle ear, is fluid in the middle ear accompanied by symptoms of intense local or systemic infection. The most common causes are viruses and bacteria. Symptoms include pain in the ear, drainage of fluid from the ear canal, and hearing loss. Other symptoms that may be present if the disorder becomes systemic include fever, irritability, headache, and anorexia.

Actions

Various types of preparations are used for treating **otic** disorders. Otic preparations can be divided into three categories: antibiotics; antibiotic and steroid combinations; and miscellaneous preparations. The miscellaneous preparations usually contain one or more of the following ingredients:

- Benzocaine—a local anesthetic used to temporally relieve pain

- Phenylephrine—a vasoconstrictor decongestant

- Hydrocortisone, desonide—corticosteroids for anti-inflammatory and antipruritic effects

- Glycerin—an emollient and a solvent
- Antipyrine—an analgesic
- Acetic acid, boric acid, benzalkonium chloride, aluminum acetate, benzethonium chloride—provide antifungal or antibacterial action
- Carbamide peroxide—aids in removing **cerumen** (yellowish or brownish ear wax) by softening and breaking up the wax

    Examples of otic preparations are given in the Summary Drug Table: Selected Otic Preparations.

Uses

Otic preparations are instilled in the external auditory canal and may be used to

- Relieve pain
- Treat infection and inflammation
- Aid in the removal of cerumen

When the patient has an inner ear infection, systemic antibiotic therapy is indicated.

Adverse Reactions

When otic drugs are applied topically, the amount of drug that enters the systemic circulation usually is not sufficient to produce adverse reactions. Prolonged use of otic preparations containing an antibiotic, such as ofloxacin, may result in a **superinfection** (an overgrowth of bacterial or fungal microorganisms not affected by the antibiotic being administered). Local adverse reactions that may occur include

- Ear irritation
- Itching
- Burning

Contraindications, Precautions, and Interactions

These drugs are contraindicated in patients with a known hypersensitivity to the drugs. The otic drugs are used with caution during pregnancy and lactation. The pregnancy category of most of these drugs is unknown when they are used as otic drugs. Otic drugs available in dropper bottles may be dangerous if ingested. Therefore, the drugs are stored safely out of the reach of children and pets. Drugs to remove cerumen are not used if ear drainage, discharge, pain, or irritation is present; if the eardrum is perforated; or after ear surgery.

If an allergy is suspected, the drug is not administered. Ofloxacin is a pregnancy category C drug and should be administered in pregnancy only if the potential benefit justifies the risk to the fetus. No significant interactions have been reported with use of the otic preparations.

NURSING PROCESS

The Patient Receiving an Otic Preparation

ASSESSMENT
PREADMINISTRATION ASSESSMENT

Before administration of an otic preparation, the primary health care provider examines the ear and external structures surrounding the ear and prescribes the drug indicated to treat the disorder. The nurse may be responsible for examining the outer structures of the ear (i.e., the earlobe and the skin around the ear). The nurse documents a description of any drainage or impacted cerumen. Perforated eardrums may be a contraindication to some of the otic preparations. The nurse must check with the primary health care provider before administering an otic preparation to a patient with a perforated ear drum.

ONGOING ASSESSMENT

The nurse assesses the patient's response to therapy. For example, a decrease in pain or inflammation should occur. The nurse examines the outer ear and ear canal for any local redness or irritation that may indicate sensitivity to the drug.

> **Pediatric Alert**
>
> When assessing the infant, the nurse looks for the infant to pull, grab, or tug at his or her ears. This may be a sign that the child's ear hurts. (However, infants do pull their ears for all kinds of reasons or for no reason at all, so if the infant seems fine otherwise, an ear infection need not be suspected). In addition, the infant may have a change in behavior, cry, be fussy or irritable, or have a fever.

NURSING DIAGNOSES

Drug-specific nursing diagnoses are highlighted in the Nursing Diagnoses Checklist. Other nursing diagnoses applicable to these drugs are discussed in depth in Chapter 4.

> **Nursing Diagnoses Checklist**
>
> ✓ **Risk for Infection (superinfection)** related to prolonged use of the anti-infective otic drug
>
> ✓ **Anxiety** related to ear pain or discomfort, changes in hearing, diagnosis, or other factors

SUMMARY DRUG TABLE SELECTED OTIC PREPARATIONS

GENERIC COMBINATIONS	TRADE NAME	USES	ADVERSE REACTIONS	DOSAGE RANGES
Corticosteroid and Antibiotic Combinations, Solutions				
1% hydrocortisone, 5 mg neomycin sulfate, 10,000 units polymyxin B	Antibiotic Ear Solution, AntibiOtic, Cortisporin Otic, Drotic, Ear-Eze, Otic-Care, OticairOtic, Otocort, Otosporin	Bacterial infections of the external auditory canal	Few; can cause ear irritation, burning, or itching; when used for prolonged periods there is a danger of a superinfection	4 gtt instilled TID or QID
0.5% hydrocortisone, 10,000 units polymyxin B	Otobiotic Otic	Same as 1% hydrocortisone solution	Same as 1% hydrocortisone solution	4 gtt instilled TID or QID
Corticosteroid and Antibiotic Combinations, Suspensions				
1% hydrocortisone, 5 mg neomycin sulfate, 10,000 units polymyxin B	AK-Spore, AntibiOtic, Antibiotic Ear Suspension, Otocort, UAD Otic, Pediotic	Same as 1% hydrocortisone solution	Same as 1% hydrocortisone solution	4 gtt instilled TID or QID
1% hydrocortisone, 4.71 mg neomycin sulfate	Coly-Mycin S Otic	Same as 1% hydrocortisone solution	Same as 1% hydrocortisone solution	4 gtt instilled TID or QID
1% hydrocortisone, 3.3 mg neomycin sulfate	Cortisporin-TC Otic	Same as 1% hydrocortisone solution	Same as 1% hydrocortisone solution	4 gtt instilled TID or QID
2 mg ciprofloxacin, 10 mg hydrocortisone/mL	Cipro HC Otic	Same as 1% hydrocortisone solution	Same as 1% hydrocortisone solution	4 gtt instilled TID or QID
Otic Antibiotic				
ofloxacin (otic)	Floxin Otic	Otitis externa, chronic suppurative otitis media, acute otitis media	Local irritation, itching, burning, earache	Ages 1–12 y: 5 gtt BID into affected ear for 10 d Ages 12 y and older: 10 gtt BID into affected ear for 10–14 d
Select Miscellaneous Preparations				
1% hydrocortisone, 2% acetic acid, 3% propylene glycol diacetate, 0.015% sodium acetate, 0.02% benzethonium chloride	Acetasol HC, VoSoL HC Otic	Relieve pain, inflammation, and irritation in the external auditory canal	Local irritation, itching, burning	Insert saturated wick into ear; leave for 24 h, keeping moist with 3–5 gtt q4–6h. Keep moist for 24 h; remove wick and instill 5 gtt TID or QID
1% hydrocortisone, 1% pramoxine HCl, 0.1% chloroxylenol, 3% propylene glycol diacetate and benzalkonium chloride	Cortic	Same as 1% hydrocortisone solution	Same as 1% hydrocortisone solution	Insert saturated wick into ear; leave in for 24 h, keeping moist with 3–5 gtt q4–6h; remove wick and instill 5 gtt TID or QID

Otic and Ophthalmic Preparations

SUMMARY DRUG TABLE   (*continued*)

GENERIC COMBINATIONS	TRADE NAME	USES	ADVERSE REACTIONS	DOSAGE RANGES
1% hydrocortisone, 2% acetic acid glacial, 3% propylene glycol diacetate, 0.02% benzethonium chloride, 0.015% sodium acetate, 0.2% citric acid	AA-HC Otic	Same as 1% hydrocortisone solution	Same as 1% hydrocortisone solution	Insert saturated wick into the ear; leave in for 24 h, keeping moist with 3–5 gtt q4–6h; remove wick and instill 5 gtt TID or QID
1.4% benzocaine, 5.4% antipyrine glycerin	Allergen Ear Drops, Auralgan Otic, Auroto Otic Ear Drops, Otocalm Ear	Relieve ear pain	Local irritation, itching, burning	Fill ear canal with 2–4 gtt; insert saturated cotton pledget; repeat TID or QID or q1–2h
20% benzocaine, 0.1% benzethoniwn chloride, 1% glycerin, PEG 300	Americaine Otic, Otocain	Relieve ear pain temporarily	Local irritation, itching, burning	Instill 4–5 gtt; insert cotton pledget; repeat q1–2h
10% triethanolamine polypeptide oleate-condensate, 0.5% chlorobutanol, propylene glycol	Cerumenex Drops	Aid in the removal of ear wax	Local irritation, itching, burning	Fill ear canal, insert cotton plug, allow to remain 15–30 min, flush ear
1 mg chloroxylenol, 10 mg hydrocortisone, 10 mg/mL pramoxine HCl	Otomar-HC	Relieve pain and irritation in the external auditory canal	Local irritation, itching, burning	Instill 5 gtt into affected ear TID or QID
2% acetic acid in aluminum acetate solution	Burow's Otic, Otic Domeboro	Relieve pain and irritation in the external auditory canal	Local irritation, itching, burning	Insert saturated wick; keep moist for 24 h; instill 4–6 gtt q2–3h

PLANNING

The expected outcomes of the patient depend on the reason for administering the drug and may include an optimal response to the drug, support of patient needs related to the management of adverse reactions, a reduction in anxiety, and an understanding of the application and use of an otic preparation.

IMPLEMENTATION

PROMOTING AN OPTIMAL RESPONSE TO THERAPY

Ear disorders may result in symptoms such as pain, a feeling of fullness in the ear, tinnitus, dizziness, or a change in hearing. Before instilling an otic solution, the nurse informs the patient that a feeling of fullness may be felt in the ear and that hearing in the treated ear may be impaired while the solution remains in the ear canal.

Before instillation of otic preparations, the nurse holds the container in the hand for a few minutes to warm it to body temperature. Cold and warm (above body temperature) preparations may cause dizziness or other sensations after being instilled into the ear.

Nursing Alert

Only preparations labeled as "otic" are instilled in the ear. The nurse must check the label of the preparation carefully for the name of the drug and a statement indicating that the preparation is for otic use.

Special instructions for specific ear preparations are found in the Summary Drug Table: Selected Otic Preparations. When instilling ear drops, the nurse has the patient lie on his or her side with the affected ear toward the ceiling. If the patient wishes to remain in an upright position, the head is tilted toward the untreated side with the ear toward the ceiling (Fig. 57-1). When administering an otic

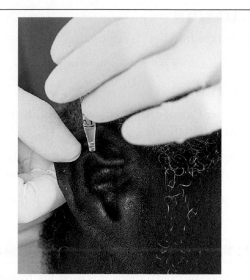

Figure 57.1 Instilling ear drops. With the head turned toward the unaffected side, the nurse pulls the cartilaginous portion of the outer ear (pinna) up and back in the adult and instills the prescribed number of drops on the side of the auditory canal.

drug the ear canal should be straightened. To straighten the ear canal in the adult and children age 3 years and older, the cartilaginous portion of the outer ear is gently pulled up and back. Be particularly gentle because some conditions make the ear canal very sensitive. Never insert the dropper or applicator tip into the ear canal.

Pediatric Alert

In children younger than 3 years of age, the ear canal is straighter and needs less manipulation. The cartilaginous portion of the outer ear is gently pulled down and back. The nurse instills the prescribed number of drops into the ear canal. If the child struggles, the nurse can gently secure the head by using the hand holding the dropper. When the child stops struggling, the nurse can administer the drops.

The patient is kept lying on the untreated side after the medication is instilled for approximately 5 minutes to facilitate the penetration of the drops into the ear canal. If medication is needed in the other ear, it is best to wait at least 5 minutes after instillation of the first ear drops before administering drops to the other ear. Once the patient is upright, the solution running out of the ear may be gently removed with gauze. If ordered, a piece of cotton can be loosely inserted into the ear canal to prevent the medication from flowing out. The cotton is not inserted too deeply because it may cause increased pressure within the ear canal.

Cerumen is a natural product of the ear and is produced by modified sweat glands in the auditory canal. Sometimes too much cerumen is produced, particularly in older adults. Drugs that loosen cerumen, such as Cerumenex, work by softening the dried ear wax inside the ear canal. Cerumenex is available by prescription and is not allowed to stay in the ear canal more than 30 minutes before irrigation. When Cerumenex is administered, the ear canal is filled with the solution and a cotton plug is inserted. The drug is allowed to remain in the ear for 15 to 30 minutes, and then the ear is flushed with warm water using a soft rubber bulb ear syringe.

Gerontologic Alert

The older adult is especially prone to hearing loss from excess cerumen, especially the patient who is mentally impaired or debilitated. Cerumen is thicker in the elderly, making the accumulation of excess cerumen more likely. It is important for nurses in the community setting or in the nursing home to assess patients for excess cerumen.

MONITORING AND MANAGING PATIENT NEEDS

RISK FOR INFECTION When using the otic antibiotics there is a danger of a superinfection, or another infection on top of the original one, from prolonged use of the drug (see Chapter 7 for a discussion of superinfection). If, after administering the drops as directed for 1 week, the infection does not improve, the primary health care provider should be notified.

ANXIETY Patients with an ear disorder or injury usually have great concern over the effect the problem will have on their hearing. The nurse reassures the patient that every effort is being made to treat the disorder and relieve the symptoms.

EDUCATING THE PATIENT AND FAMILY

The nurse gives the patient or a family member instructions or a demonstration of the instillation technique of an otic preparation.

Pediatric Alert

Because some children are prone to recurrent attacks of acute otitis media, parents should be taught to identify signs and symptoms of otitis media and seek medical attention early when their child exhibits these symptoms. If acute or chronic otitis media is not treated, spontaneous rupture of the ear drum may occur, resulting in temporary or permanent hearing loss. The nurse needs to stress that medication should be used exactly as prescribed for the entire course of therapy.

Otic and Ophthalmic Preparations

The following information may be given to the patient when an ear ointment or solution is prescribed:

- Wash the hands thoroughly before cleansing the area around the ear (when necessary) and instilling ear drops or ointment.

- If the solution is cool or cold, warm to room temperature by holding solution in the hand for 1 to 2 minutes before administering.

- Instill the prescribed number of drops in the ear. Do not put the applicator or dropper tip in the ear or allow the tip to become contaminated from the fingers or other sources.

- Immediately after use, replace the cap or dropper and refrigerate the solution if so stated on the label.

- If the drops are in a suspension form, shake the container well for 10 seconds before using.

- Keep the head tilted or lie on the untreated side for approximately 5 minutes to allow the solution to remain in contact with the ear. Excess solution and solution running out of the ear can be wiped off with a tissue.

- Do not insert anything into the ear canal before or after applying the prescribed drug unless advised to do so by the primary health care provider. At times a soft cotton plug may be inserted into the affected ear.

- Complete a full course of treatment with the prescribed drug to achieve satisfactory results.

- Do not use nonprescription ear products during or after treatment unless such use has been approved by the primary health care provider.

- Remember that temporary changes in hearing or a feeling of fullness in the ear may occur for a short time after the drug has been instilled.

- Notify the primary health care provider if symptoms do not improve or become worse.

DRUGS USED TO REMOVE CERUMEN

- Do not use if ear drainage, discharge, pain, or irritation occurs.

- Do not use for more than 4 days. If excessive cerumen remains, consult the primary health care provider.

- Any wax remaining after the treatment may be removed by gently flushing the ear with warm water using a soft rubber bulb ear syringe.

- If dizziness occurs, consult the primary health care provider.

EVALUATION

- The therapeutic effect is achieved.

- The patient does not have a superinfection.

- Anxiety is reduced.

- The patient demonstrates the ability to instill an otic preparation in the ear.

- The patient verbalizes knowledge of and the importance of complying with the therapeutic regimen.

- The patient and family demonstrate an understanding of the drug regimen.

OPHTHALMIC PREPARATIONS

Various types of preparations are used for treating **ophthalmic** (eye) disorders, such as glaucoma, to lower the **intraocular pressure** (IOP; the pressure within the eye); and to treat bacterial or viral infections of the eye, inflammatory conditions, and symptoms of allergy related to the eye.

Glaucoma is a condition of the eye in which there is an increase in the IOP, causing progressive atrophy of the optic nerve with deterioration of vision and, if untreated, blindness. The higher the IOP, the greater the risk of optic nerve damage, visual loss, and blindness. There are two types of glaucoma: angle-closure glaucoma and open-angle, or chronic, glaucoma. Display 57-1 describes the two types of glaucoma.

Most of the drug classifications used to treat ophthalmic conditions have been discussed in previous chapters. The following sections provide a short summary of these classifications and their implications for ophthalmic use. When appropriate, the student is referred to the specific chapter where additional information can be found. The Summary Drug Table: Selected Ophthalmic Preparations provides examples of the drugs used to treat ophthalmic problems.

The incidence of adverse reactions associated with the ophthalmic drugs is usually low. Because small amounts of the ophthalmic preparation may be absorbed systemically, some of the adverse effects associated with systemic administration of the particular drug may be observed. Some ophthalmic preparations produce momentary stinging or burning on instillation.

Actions and Uses

Alpha₂-Adrenergic Drugs

Brimonidine tartrate is an alpha$_2$ (α_2)-adrenergic receptor agonist used to lower IOP in patients with open-angle

Display 57.1 Glaucoma

The eye's lens, iris, and cornea are continuously bathed and nourished by a fluid called *aqueous humor*. As aqueous humor is produced, excess fluid normally flows out through a complex network of tissue called *trabecular meshwork*. An angle is formed where the trabeculum and iris meet. This forms a filtration angle that maintains the normal pressure within the eye by allowing excess aqueous humor to leave the anterior chamber of the eye.

In chronic or open-angle glaucoma, the angle that permits the drainage of aqueous humor appears to be normal but does not function properly. In angle-closure glaucoma, the iris blocks the trabecular meshwork and limits the flow of aqueous humor from the anterior chamber of the eye. This limitation of outflow causes an accumulation of intraocular fluid, followed by increased IOP. Some individuals have an anatomic defect that causes the angle to be more narrow than normal, but do not have any symptoms and do not develop glaucoma under normal circumstances. However, certain situations, such as medication that causes dilation of the eye, fear, or pain, may precipitate an attack. The aim of treatment in glaucoma is to lower the IOP. For more information on glaucoma, see Chapter 29.

glaucoma or ocular hypertension. This drug acts to reduce production of aqueous humor and increase the outflow of aqueous humor.

Sympathomimetic Drugs

Sympathomimetics have α- and beta (β)-adrenergic activity (see Chapter 27 for a detailed discussion of adrenergic drugs). These drugs lower the IOP by increasing the outflow of aqueous humor in the eye and are used to treat glaucoma. Apraclonidine is used to control or prevent postoperative elevations in IOP. The Summary Drug Table: Selected Ophthalmic Preparations provides additional information about these drugs.

Alpha-Adrenergic Blocking Drugs

Dapiprazole acts by blocking the alpha-adrenergic receptor in smooth muscle and produces **miosis** (constriction of the pupil) through an effect on the dilator muscle of the iris. The drug is used primarily after ophthalmic examinations to reverse the diagnostic **mydriasis** (dilation of the pupil).

Beta-Adrenergic Blocking Drugs

The β-adrenergic blocking drugs decrease the rate of production of aqueous humor and thereby lower the IOP. These drugs are used to treat glaucoma.

Miotics, Direct Acting

Miotics contract the pupil of the eye (miosis), resulting in an increase in the space through which the aqueous humor flows. This increased space and improved flow results in a decrease in the IOP. Miotics may be used in the treatment of glaucoma (see Chapter 27). The miotics were, for a number of years, the drug of choice for glaucoma. These drugs have lost that first choice treatment status to the β-adrenergic blocking drugs.

Miotics, Cholinesterase Inhibitors

The cholinesterase inhibitors are more potent and longer acting than the direct-acting miotics and are used to treat open-angle glaucoma. When administered into the eye, these drugs produce intense miosis and muscle contractions, causing a decreased resistance to aqueous outflow.

Carbonic Anhydrase Inhibitors

Except for dorzolamide and brinzolamide, carbonic anhydrase inhibitors are administered systemically. Carbonic anhydrase is an enzyme found in many tissues of the body, including the eye. Inhibition of carbonic anhydrase in the eye decreases aqueous humor secretion, resulting in a decrease of IOP. These drugs are used in the treatment of elevated IOP seen in open-angle glaucoma.

Prostaglandin Agonists

The prostaglandin agonists are used to lower IOP in patients with open-angle glaucoma and ocular hypertension in patients who do not tolerate other IOP-lowering medications or have an insufficient response to these medications. These drugs act to lower IOP by increasing the outflow of aqueous humor through the trabecular meshwork.

Mast Cell Stabilizers

The mast cell stabilizers currently approved for ophthalmic use are nedocromil and pemirolast. These drugs are used to prevent itching of the eyes caused by allergic conjunctivitis. The mast cell stabilizers act by inhibiting the antigen-induced release of inflammatory mediators (e.g., histamine) from human mast cells.

Nonsteroidal Anti-Inflammatory Drugs

The nonsteroidal anti-inflammatory drugs (NSAIDs) inhibit prostaglandin synthesis (see Chapter 18 for a discussion of the NSAIDs), thereby exerting anti-inflammatory action. These drugs are used to treat postoperative inflammation after cataract surgery (diclofenac), for the relief of itching of the eyes caused by seasonal allergies (ketorolac), and during eye surgery to prevent miosis (flurbiprofen).

SUMMARY DRUG TABLE   SELECTED OPHTHALMIC PREPARATIONS

GENERIC NAME	TRADE NAME	USES	DOSAGE RANGES
Alpha₂-Adrenergic Agonist			
brimonidine tartrate *brih-moe'-nih-deen*	Alphagan	Lowers IOP in patients with open-angle (chronic) glaucoma	1 gtt in affected eye(s) TID
Sympathomimetics			
apraclonidine HCl *app-rah-kloe'-nih-deen*	Iopidine	1% Solution: control or prevention of postoperative elevations in IOP 5% Solution: short-term therapy in patients receiving maximal medical therapy who require additional IOP reduction	1% Solution: 1 gtt in operative eye 1 h before surgery and 1 gtt immediately after surgery 5% Solution: 1–2 gtt in the affected eye(s) TID
dipivefrin HCl (**dipivalyl epinephrine**) *die-pihv'-eh-frin*	Propine, AKPro	Open-angle glaucoma	1 gtt into affected eye(s) q12h
epinephrine *epp-ih-neff'-rin*	Epifrin, Glaucon Solution	Open-angle (chronic) glaucoma; may be used in combination with miotics, beta blockers, or carbonic anhydrase inhibitors	1–2 gtt into affected eye(s) daily or BID
Alpha-Adrenergic Blocking Drugs			
dapiprazole HCl *dap-ih-pray'-zole*	Rev-Eyes	Reverse diagnostic mydriasis after ophthalmic examination	2 gtt into the conjunctiva of each eye, followed 5 min later by an additional 2 gtt
Beta-Adrenergic Blocking Drugs			
betaxolol *bay-tax'-oh-lahl*	Betoptic, Betoptic S	Chronic open-angle glaucoma, ocular hypertension	1–2 gtt in the affected eye(s) BID
carteolol HCl *car'-tee-oh-lahl*	Ocupress	Same as betaxolol	1 gtt in affected eye(s) TID
levobetaxolol HCl *lee'-voe-beh-tax'-oh-lahl*	Betaxon	Same as betaxolol	1 gtt in affected eye(s) BID
levobunolol HCl *lee'-voe-byoo'-no-lahl*	AkBeta, Betagan Liquifilm	Same as betaxolol	0.5% Solution: 1–2 gtt in affected eye(s) daily 0.25% Solution: 1–2 gtt in affected eye(s) BID
metipranolol HCl *meh-tih-pran'-oh-lahl*	OptiPranolol	Treatment of elevated IOP in patients with ocular hypertension or open-angle glaucoma	1 gtt in affected eye(s) BID
timolol *ti'-moe-lahl*	Betimol, Timoptic, Timoptic-XE	Reduces IOP in ocular hypertension or open-angle glaucoma	1 gtt in affected eye(s) daily or BID Gel: invert the closed container and shake once before each use; administer 1 gtt/d
Miotics, Direct Acting			
carbachol *car'-bah-kole*	Carboptic, Isopto Carbachol	Glaucoma	1–2 gtt up to TID
pilocarpine HCl *pie-low-car'-peen*	Isopto Carpine, Pilopine HS	Glaucoma, preoperative and postoperative intraocular hypertension	Solution: 1–2 gtt in affected eye(s) Gel: apply a 0.5-in ribbon in the lower conjunctival sac of affected eye(s) daily at bedtime

GENERIC NAME	TRADE NAME	USES	DOSAGE RANGES
pilocarpine nitrate	Pilagan	Lowers elevated IOP, emergency relief of acute glaucoma, reverse mydriasis caused by cycloplegic agents	1–2 gtt in affected eye(s) BID–QID
pilocarpine ocular therapeutic system	Ocusert Pilo-20, Ocusert Pilo-40	Open-angle glaucoma	See package insert
Miotic, Cholinesterase Inhibitor			
echothiophate iodide *eck-oh-thigh'-oh-fate eyé-oh-dide*	Phospholine iodide	Chronic open-angle glaucoma, accommodative esotropia	Glaucoma: 2 doses/d in the morning and at bedtime or 1 dose every other day Esotropia: 1 gtt daily
Carbonic Anhydrase Inhibitors			
brinzolamide *brin-zolé-ah-mide*	Azopt	Open-angle glaucoma, ocular hypertension	1 gtt in affected eye(s) TID
dorzolamide HCl *dore-zolé-ah-mide*	Trusopt	Open-angle glaucoma, ocular hypertension	1 gtt in affected eye(s) TID
Prostaglandin Agonists			
latanoprost *lah-tan'-oh-prahst*	Xalatan	First-line treatment of open-angle glaucoma, ocular hypertension	1 gtt in affected eye(s) daily in the evening
travoprost *trav'-oh-prahst*	Travatan	Reduction of increased IOP in patients with glaucoma who do not respond to or cannot take other drugs to lower IOP	1 gtt in affected eye(s) daily in the evening
bimatoprost *bi-mat'-oh-prahst*	Lumigan	Same as travoprost	1 gtt in affected eye(s) daily in the evening
unoprostone isopropyl *yoo-noh-prost'-ohn*	Rescula	Same as travoprost	1 gtt in affected eye(s) BID
Combinations Used to Treat Glaucoma			
pilocarpine and epinephrine	E-Pilo-1, E-Pilo-2, E-Pilo-4, E-Pilo-6, P_1E_1, P_4E_1	Glaucoma	1–2 gtt in the affected eye(s) 1–4 times daily
dorzolamide HCl and timolol maleate *dore-zolé-ah-mide*	Cosopt	Open-angle glaucoma and ocular hypertension	1 gtt into the affected eye(s) BID
Mast Cell Stabilizers			
nedocromil sodium *neh-doé-roe-mill*	Alocril	Allergic conjunctivitis	1–2 gtt in each eye BID
pemirolast potassium *peh-meer'-oh-last*	Alamast	Allergic conjunctivitis	1–2 gtt in each eye QID
Nonsteroidal Anti-inflammatory Drugs			
diclofenac sodium *di-klo'-fen-ak*	Voltaren	Postoperative inflammation after cataract surgery	1 gtt QID
flurbiprofen sodium *flure-bi'-pro-fen*	Ocufen	Inhibition of intraoperative miosis	1 gtt q30min beginning 2 h before surgery (total of 4 gtt)
ketorolac tromethamine *ke-tor'-o-lac*	Acular	Relief of ocular itching due to seasonal allergies, pain after corneal refractive surgery	Allergies: 1 drop QID Postoperative pain: 1 gtt in operated eye

SUMMARY DRUG TABLE *(continued)*

GENERIC NAME	TRADE NAME	USES	DOSAGE RANGES
Corticosteroids			
dexamethasone phosphate *dex-a-meth'-a-some*	AK-Dex, Maxidex	Treatment of inflammatory conditions of the conjunctiva, eyelid, cornea, anterior segment of the eye	Solution: 1–2 gtt qh during the day and q2h at night, reduced to 1 gtt q4h when response noted, then 1 gtt TID or QID Ointment: thin coating in lower conjunctival sac TID or QID
fluorometholone *flure-oh-meth'-oh-lone*	Flarex, Fluor-Op	Treatment of inflammatory conditions of the conjunctiva, lid, cornea, anterior segment of the eye	Suspension: 1–2 gtt BID–QID, may increase to 2 gtt q2h Ointment: thin coating in lower conjunctival sac 1 to 3 times daily (up to 1 application q4h)
loteprednol etabonate *low-teh-pred'-nol ett-ab'-ohn-ate*	Alrex, Lotemax	Allergic conjunctivitis	1–2 gtt QID
prednisolone *pred-niss'-oh-lone*	AK-Pred, Pred Forte, Pred Mild	Treatment of inflammatory conditions of the conjunctiva, lid, cornea, anterior segment of the eye	1–2 gtt/h during the day and q2h at night, reduced to 1 gtt q4h, then 1 gtt TID or QID Suspensions: 1–2 gtt BID–QID
Antibiotics			
bacitracin *bass-i-tray'-sin*	AK-Tracin	Treatment of eye infections	See package insert
chloramphenicol *klor-am-fen'-i-kole*	Chloromycetin	Same as bacitracin	See package insert
ciprofloxacin *sih-proe-flox'-a-sin*	Ciloxan	Same as bacitracin	See package insert
erythromycin *er-ith-roe-mye'-sin*	Ilotycin	Same as bacitracin	See package insert
gatifloxacin *ga-tah-flox'-a-sin*	Zymar	Treatment of bacterial conjunctivitis caused by susceptible organisms	Days 1 and 2: instill 1 gtt in affected eye(s) q2h while awake, up to 8 times daily Days 3–7: instill 1 gtt in affected eye up to QID while awake
gentamicin sulfate *jen-ta-mye'-sin*	Garamycin, Gentacidin, Gentak	Same as bacitracin	See package insert
levofloxacin *lee-voe-flox'-a-sin*	Quixin	Same as gatifloxacin	Days 1 and 2: instill 1–2 gtt in affected eye(s) q2h while awake, up to 8 times daily Days 3–7: instill 1–2 gtt in affected eye up to QID while awake
moxifloxacin HCl *mocks-ah-flox'-a-sin*	Vigamox	Same as bacitracin	Adults and children at least 1 year of age: 1 drop in affected eye TID for 7 days

GENERIC NAME	TRADE NAME	USES	DOSAGE RANGES
norfloxacin *nor-flox'-a-sin*	Chibroxin	Same as gatifloxacin	Adults and children age 1 year and older: 1 or 2 gtt applied topically in the affected eye(s) QID for up to 7 d; dosage may be 1 or 2 gtt q2h during waking hours the first day of treatment if the infection is severe
ofloxacin *oe-flox'-a-sin*	Ocuflox	Same as gatifloxacin, corneal ulcers	Bacterial conjunctivitis: days 1 and 2: 1–2 gtt q2–4h in the affected eye(s) Days 3–7: 1–2 gtt QID Bacterial corneal ulcer: Days 1 and 2: 1–2 gtt into the affected eye q30min while awake; awaken approximately q4–6h and instill 1–2 gtt Days 3 through 7–9: instill 1–2 drops QID
polymyxin B sulfate *paw-lee-mix'-in*		Same as bacitracin	See package insert
tobramycin *toe-bra-mye'-sin*	Tobrex, Defy	Same as bacitracin	See package insert
sulfacetamide sodium *sul-fah-see'-tah-myde*	Sulster, AK-Sulf, Bleph-10, Ocusulf-10	Ocular infections, trachoma	Ocular infections: 1–2 gtt q1–4h Trachoma: 2 gtt q2h Ointments: 0.5 in into lower conjunctival sac TID or QID
sulfisoxazole diolamine *sul-fah-socks'-a-zole*	Gantrisin	Ocular infections, trachoma	Ocular infections: 1–2 gtt q1–4h Trachoma: 2 gtt q2h

Silver Compound

GENERIC NAME	TRADE NAME	USES	DOSAGE RANGES
silver nitrate *nyé-trate*		Prevention of ophthalmia neonatorum	2 gtt of 1% solution in each eye

Antiviral Drugs

GENERIC NAME	TRADE NAME	USES	DOSAGE RANGES
idoxuridine *eye-dox-yoor'-i-deen*	Herplex	Herpes simplex keratitis	1 gtt qh during the day and q2h at night
trifluridine *tri-flur'-i-deen*	Viroptic	Keratoconjunctivitis keratitis, epithelial keratitis	Adults and children over 6 years: 1 gtt onto the corners of affected eye(s) while awake Maximum daily dose: 9 gtt until corneal ulcer has completely re-epithelialized, treat for an additional 7 d with 1 gtt q4h for a maximum of 5 gtt/d
vidarabine *vye-dare'-a-been*	Vira-A	Treatment of herpes simplex keratitis and conjunctivitis	0.5 in of ointment into lower conjunctival sac 5 times daily at 3-h intervals

Antifungal Drug

GENERIC NAME	TRADE NAME	USES	DOSAGE RANGES
natamycin *na-ta-mye'-sin*	Natacyn	Fungal infections of the eye	1 gtt q1–2h

Vasoconstrictors/Mydriatics

GENERIC NAME	TRADE NAME	USES	DOSAGE RANGES
oxymetazoline HCl *ox-i-met-az'-oh-leen*	OcuClear, Visine LR	Relief of redness of eye due to minor irritation	1–2 gtt q6h

Otic and Ophthalmic Preparations

SUMMARY DRUG TABLE *(continued)*

GENERIC NAME	TRADE NAME	USES	DOSAGE RANGES
phenylephrine HCl *fen-ill-eff'-rin*	AK-Dilate 2.5%, Neo-Synephrine 10%, AK-Nephrin	0.12% for relief of redness of eye due to minor irritation; 2.5% and 10% for treatment of uveitis, glaucoma; refraction procedures, before eye surgery	0.12%: 1–2 gtt up to QID 2.5% and 10%: 1–2 gtt in the eye up to QID (may have up to 8 gtt/d)
tetrahydrozoline HCl *tet-ra-hye-drozz'-a-leen*	Murine Plus Eye Drops, Visine	Relief of eye redness due to minor irritation	1–2 gtt up to QID
Cycloplegics/Mydriatics			
atropine sulfate *a'-troe-peen*	Isopto-Atropine	Mydriasis/cycloplegia	1–2 gtt up to TID
homatropine hydrobromide *hoe-ma'-troe-peen*	Isopto Homatropine	Mydriasis/cycloplegia	1–2 gtt q3–4h
Ocular Lubricants			
benzalkonium chloride *benz-al-koe'-nee-um*	Artificial Tears	Treatment of dry eyes	1–2 gtt TID or QID
0.25% glycerin, EDTA sodium chloride, benzalkonium chloride	Eye-Lube-A	Treatment of dry eyes	1–2 gtt TID or QID

IOP, intraocular pressure.

Corticosteroids

These drugs possess anti-inflammatory activity and are used for inflammatory conditions, such as allergic conjunctivitis, keratitis, herpes zoster keratitis, and inflammation of the iris. Corticosteroids also may be used after injury to the cornea or after corneal transplantation to prevent rejection.

Antibiotics and Sulfonamides

Antibiotics possess antibacterial activity and are used in the treatment of eye infections. Sulfonamides possess a bacteriostatic effect against a wide range of gram-positive and gram-negative microorganisms. They are used in treating conjunctivitis, corneal ulcer, and other superficial infections of the eye. See the Summary Drug Table: Selected Ophthalmic Preparations and Chapter 6 for additional information on the sulfonamides.

Silver

Silver possesses antibacterial activity against gram-positive and gram-negative microorganisms. Silver protein, mild, is occasionally used in the treatment of eye infections. Silver nitrate is occasionally used to prevent gonorrheal ophthalmia neonatorum (gonorrheal infection of the newborn's eyes). Ophthalmic tetracycline and erythromycin have largely replaced the use of silver nitrate in newborns.

Antiviral Drugs

Antiviral drugs interfere with viral reproduction by altering DNA synthesis. These drugs are used in the treatment of herpes simplex infections of the eye, treatment of immunocompromised patients with cytomegalovirus (CMV) retinitis, and for the prevention of CMV retinitis in patients undergoing transplantation.

Antifungal Drugs

Natamycin is the only ophthalmic antifungal in use. This drug possesses antifungal activity against a variety of yeast and other fungi.

Vasoconstrictors/Mydriatics

Mydriatics are drugs that dilate the pupil (mydriasis), constrict superficial blood vessels of the sclera, and decrease the formation of aqueous humor. Depending on the specific drug and strength, these drugs may be used before eye surgery in the treatment of glaucoma, for relief of minor eye irritation, and to dilate the pupil for examination of the eye.

Cycloplegic Mydriatics

Cycloplegic mydriatics cause mydriasis and **cycloplegia** (paralysis of the ciliary muscle, resulting in an inability to focus the eye). These drugs (see Chapter 30) are used in the treatment of inflammatory conditions of the iris and uveal tract of the eye and for examination of the eye.

Artificial Tear Solutions

These products lubricate the eyes and are used for conditions such as dry eyes and eye irritation caused by inadequate tear production. Inactive ingredients may be found in some preparations. Examples of these inactive ingredients include preservatives, antioxidants, which prevent deterioration of the product, and drugs that slow drainage of the drug from the eye into the tear duct. Examples of the types of eye preparations are found in the Summary Drug Table: Selected Ophthalmic Preparations.

Adverse Reactions

Alpha₂-Adrenergic Drugs

Although side effects are usually mild, treatment with brimonidine tartrate includes local and systemic effects:

- Local effects include ocular hyperemia, burning and stinging, headache, visual blurring, foreign body sensation, ocular allergic reactions, and ocular pruritus.

- Systemic effects include fatigue and drowsiness.

Sympathomimetic Drugs

These drugs may cause transient local reactions and systemic reactions.

- Transient local reactions may be burning and stinging, eye pain, brow ache, headache, allergic lip reactions, and ocular irritation. With prolonged use, adrenochrome (a red pigment contained in epinephrine) deposits may occur in the conjunctiva and cornea.

- Rare systemic reactions may occur, including palpitations, tachycardia, extrasystoles, cardiac arrhythmia, hypertension, and faintness.

Note: Dipivefrin appears to be better tolerated and is associated with fewer adverse effects than the other sympathomimetic drugs used to lower IOP.

Alpha-Adrenergic Blocking Drugs

α-Adrenergic blockers may cause local effects, such as burning in the eye, ptosis (drooping of the upper eyelid), eyelid edema, itching, corneal edema, brow ache, dryness of the eye, tearing, and blurred vision.

Beta-Adrenergic Blocking Drugs

- Local adverse reactions associated with the β-adrenergic blocking drugs include eye irritation, burning, tearing, conjunctivitis, decreased night vision, ptosis, abnormal corneal staining, and corneal sensitivity.

- Systemic reactions, although rare, include arrhythmias, palpitation, headache, nausea, and dizziness (see Chapter 28 for additional systemic adverse reactions).

Miotics, Direct Acting

- The direct-acting miotics may cause local reactions, such as stinging on instillation, transient burning, tearing, headache, brow ache, and decreased night vision.

- Systemic adverse reactions include hypotension, flushing, breathing difficulties, nausea, vomiting, diarrhea, cardiac arrhythmias, and frequent urge to urinate.

Miotics, Cholinesterase Inhibitors

Adverse reactions and systemic toxicity are more common in the cholinesterase inhibitor ophthalmic preparations than in the direct-acting miotics.

- Ophthalmic adverse reactions include iris cysts, burning, lacrimation, eyelid muscle twitching, conjunctivitis, ciliary redness, brow ache, headache, activation of latent iritis or uveitis (an inner eye inflammation), and conjunctival thickening.

- Systemic adverse reactions include nausea, vomiting, abdominal cramps, diarrhea, urinary incontinence, fainting, salivation, difficulty breathing, and cardiac irregularities.

Iris cysts may form, enlarge, and obstruct vision. The iris cyst usually shrinks with discontinuation of the drug, or after a reduction in strength of the drops or frequency of instillation.

Carbonic Anhydrase Inhibitors

- Local adverse reactions associated with use of the carbonic anhydrase inhibitors include ocular burning, stinging, or discomfort immediately after administration, ocular allergic reaction, blurred vision, tearing, dryness, foreign body sensation, ocular discomfort, and headache.

- Systemic reactions include bitter taste, dermatitis, and photophobia.

Prostaglandin Agonists

- Local adverse reactions associated with the prostaglandin agonists include blurred vision, burning and stinging, foreign body sensation, itching, increased pigmentation of the iris, dry eye, excessive tearing, and eyelid discomfort and pain.

- Systemic reaction involves photophobia.

Mast Cell Stabilizers

- These drugs may cause local reactions such as ocular burning or irritation, dry eye, eye redness, foreign body sensation, and ocular discomfort.

- Although mild, the systemic adverse reactions associated with the mast cell inhibitors include headache, rhinitis, unpleasant taste, asthma, and cold- or flu-like symptoms.

Nonsteroidal Anti-Inflammatory Drugs

The most common adverse reactions associated with the NSAIDs are local and include transient burning and stinging on instillation and other minor ocular irritations.

Corticosteroids

Local adverse reactions associated with administration of the corticosteroid ophthalmic preparations include elevated IOP with optic nerve damage, loss of visual acuity, cataract formation, delayed wound healing, secondary ocular infection, exacerbation of corneal infections, dry eyes, ptosis, blurred vision, discharge, ocular pain, foreign body sensation, and pruritus.

Antibiotics, Sulfonamides, and Silver

The antibiotic and sulfonamide ophthalmics are usually well tolerated, and few adverse reactions are seen. Local adverse reactions include occasional transient irritation, burning, itching, stinging, inflammation, and blurred vision. With prolonged or repeated use, a superinfection may occur.

Antiviral Drugs

- Administration of the antiviral ophthalmics may cause local reactions such as irritation, pain, pruritus, inflammation, edema of the eyes or eyelids, foreign body sensation, and corneal clouding.

- Systemic reactions include photophobia and allergic reactions.

Antifungal Drugs

Adverse reactions are rare. Occasional local irritation to the eye may occur.

Vasoconstrictors/Mydriatics

- Local adverse reactions include transitory stinging on initial instillation, blurring of vision, mydriasis, increased redness, irritation and discomfort, and increased IOP.

- Systemic adverse reactions include headache, brow ache, palpitations, tachycardia, arrhythmias, hypertension, myocardial infarction, and stroke.

Cycloplegic Mydriatics

- Local adverse reactions associated with administration of the cycloplegic mydriatics include increased IOP, transient stinging or burning, and irritation with prolonged use (e.g., conjunctivitis, edema, exudates).

- Systemic adverse reactions include dryness of the mouth and skin, blurred vision, photophobia, corneal staining, tachycardia, headache, parasympathetic stimulation, and somnolence.

Artificial Tear Solutions

Adverse reactions are rare, but on occasion redness or irritation may occur.

Contraindications, Precautions, and Interactions

Alpha₂-Adrenergic Drugs

α_2-Adrenergic agonists are contraindicated in patients with hypersensitivity to the drug or any component of the drug and in patients taking the monoamine oxidase inhibitors (MAOIs). Patients should wait at least 15 minutes after instilling brimonidine before inserting soft contact lenses because the preservative in the drug may be absorbed by soft contact lenses. The drug is used cautiously during pregnancy (category B) and lactation and in patients with cardiovascular disease, depression, cerebral or coronary insufficiency, orthostatic hypotension, or Raynaud's phenomenon. When brimonidine is used with central nervous system (CNS) depressants, such as alcohol, barbiturates, opiates, sedatives, or anesthetics, there is a risk for an additive CNS depressant effect. Use the drug cautiously in combination with antihypertensive drugs and cardiac glycosides because a synergistic effect may occur.

Sympathomimetic Drugs

These drugs are contraindicated in patients with hypersensitivity to the drug or any component of the drug. Epinephrine is contraindicated in patients with narrow-angle glaucoma, or patients with a narrow angle but no glaucoma, and aphakia (absence of the crystalline lens of the eye). Epinephrine should not be used while wearing soft contact lenses (discoloration of the lenses may occur).

These drugs are used cautiously during pregnancy (epinephrine and apraclonidine, pregnancy category C; dipivefrin, pregnancy category B) and lactation and in patients with hypertension, diabetes, hyperthyroidism, heart disease, cerebral arteriosclerosis, or bronchial asthma. Some of these drugs contain sulfites that may cause allergic-like reactions (hives, wheezing, anaphylaxis) in patients with sulfite sensitivity. See Chapter 27 for information on interactions.

Alpha-Adrenergic Blocking Drugs

Dapiprazole is contraindicated in patients with hypersensitivity to the drug or any component of the drug; in conditions in which pupil constriction is not desirable, such as in acute iritis (inflammation of the iris); and in the treatment of IOP in open-angle glaucoma. This drug is used cautiously during pregnancy (category B) and lactation. No significant drug interactions have been reported.

Beta-Adrenergic Blocking Drugs

The β-adrenergic blocking drugs are contraindicated in patients with bronchial asthma, obstructive pulmonary disease, sinus bradycardia, heart block, cardiac failure, or cardiogenic shock and in patients with hypersensitivity to the drug or any components of the drug. These drugs are in pregnancy category C and are used cautiously during pregnancy and lactation and in patients with cardiovascular disease, diabetes (may mask the symptoms of hypoglycemia), and hyperthyroidism (may mask symptoms of hyperthyroidism). The patient taking β-adrenergic blocking drugs for ophthalmic reasons may experience increased or additive effects when the drugs are administered with the oral β-adrenergic blockers. Coadministration of timolol maleate and calcium antagonists may cause hypotension, left ventricular failure, and condition disturbances within the heart. There is a potential additive hypotensive effect when the β-adrenergic blocking ophthalmic drugs are administered with the phenothiazines.

Miotics, Direct Acting

These drugs are contraindicated in patients with hypersensitivity to the drug or any component of the drug and in conditions where constriction is undesirable (e.g., iritis, uveitis, and acute inflammatory disease of the anterior chamber). The drugs are used cautiously in patients with corneal abrasion, pregnancy (category C), lactation, cardiac failure, bronchial asthma, peptic ulcer, hyperthy-

roidism, gastrointestinal spasm, urinary tract infection, Parkinson's disease, recent myocardial infarction, hypotension, or hypertension. These drugs are also used cautiously in patients with angle-closure glaucoma because miotics occasionally can precipitate angle-closure glaucoma by increasing the resistance to aqueous flow from posterior to anterior chamber. See Chapter 29 for information on interactions.

Miotics, Cholinesterase Inhibitors

The cholinesterase inhibitors are contraindicated in patients with hypersensitivity to the drug or any components of the drug. Some of these products contain sulfites, and patients with sulfite sensitivity may experience allergic-type reactions. The drugs are also contraindicated in patients with any active inflammatory disease of the eye and during pregnancy (echothiophate iodine, pregnancy category C) and lactation.

The cholinesterase inhibitors are used cautiously in patients with myasthenia gravis (may cause additive adverse effects), before and after surgery, and in patients with chronic angle-closure (narrow-angle) glaucoma or those with anatomically narrow angles (may cause papillary block and increase the angle blockage). When the cholinesterase inhibitors are administered with systemic anticholinesterase drugs, there is a risk for additive effects. Individuals such as farmers, warehouse workers, or gardeners working with carbamate–organophosphate insecticides or pesticides are at risk for systemic effects of the cholinesterase inhibitors from absorption of the pesticide or insecticide through the respiratory tract or the skin. Individuals working with pesticides or insecticides containing carbamate–organophosphate and taking a cholinesterase inhibitor should be advised to wear respiratory masks, change clothes frequently, and wash exposed clothes thoroughly.

Carbonic Anhydrase Inhibitors

Use of the carbonic anhydrase inhibitors is contraindicated in patients with hypersensitivity to the drug or any components of the drug and during pregnancy (category C) and lactation. The drugs are used cautiously in patients with renal or hepatic impairment. When high doses of the salicylates are administered concurrently, toxic levels of the carbonic anhydrase inhibitors have been reported. See Chapter 45 for more information on interactions when administering the carbonic anhydrase inhibitors.

Prostaglandin Agonists

These drugs are contraindicated in patients with hypersensitivity to the drug or any component of the drug and

Otic and Ophthalmic Preparations

during pregnancy (category C). The drugs are used cautiously in lactating women and in patients with active intraocular inflammation, those wearing contact lenses (contact lenses must be removed and left out for at least 15 minutes after administration of the drug), and those with macular edema.

Mast Cell Stabilizers

These drugs are contraindicated in patients with hypersensitivity to the drug or any component of the drug. The mast cell stabilizers are used cautiously in patients who wear contact lenses (preservative may be absorbed by the soft contact lenses) and during pregnancy (pemirolast, pregnancy category C; nedocromil, pregnancy category B) and lactation. There have been no significant drug–drug interactions associated with these drugs.

Nonsteroidal Anti-inflammatory Drugs

These drugs are contraindicated in individuals with known hypersensitivity to an individual drug or any components of the drug. The NSAID flurbiprofen is contraindicated in patients with herpes simplex keratitis. Diclofenac and ketorolac are contraindicated in patients who wear soft contact lenses (may cause ocular irritation). The NSAIDs are used cautiously during pregnancy (pregnancy category C, flurbiprofen, ketorolac; pregnancy category B, diclofenac) and lactation.

The NSAIDs are used cautiously in patients with bleeding tendencies. When used topically there is less risk of interactions with drugs or other substances. There is a possibility of a cross-sensitivity reaction when the NSAIDs are administered to patients allergic to the salicylates. The corticosteroids and the antibiotics are used cautiously in patients with sulfite sensitivity because an allergic-type reaction may result. Coadministration of idoxuridine with solutions containing boric acid may cause irritation. The sulfonamides are incompatible with silver nitrate.

Corticosteroids

The corticosteroid ophthalmic preparations are contraindicated in patients with acute superficial herpes simplex keratitis or other viral or fungal diseases of the eye, and after removal of a superficial corneal foreign body.

The corticosteroid ophthalmic preparations are used cautiously in patients with infectious conditions of the eye. These drugs are pregnancy category C drugs and are used cautiously during pregnancy and lactation. Prolonged use of the corticosteroids may result in elevated IOP and optic nerve damage.

Antibiotics and Sulfonamides

The antibiotic and sulfonamide ophthalmics are contraindicated in patients with a hypersensitivity to the drug or any component of the drug. These drugs are also contraindicated in patients with epithelial herpes simplex keratitis, varicella, mycobacterial infection of the eye, and fungal diseases of the eye. There are no significant precautions or interactions when the drugs are administered as directed by the primary health care provider.

Antiviral Drugs

These drugs are contraindicated in patients with hypersensitivity to the drug or any component of the drug. These drugs are used cautiously in immunocompromised patients and during pregnancy and lactation. Some of these solutions contain boric acid and may form a precipitate that causes irritation.

Antifungal Drugs

Natamycin is contraindicated in patients with hypersensitivity to the drug or any component of the drug. The drug is a pregnancy category C drug and is used cautiously during pregnancy and lactation. If use of the drug for 7 to 10 days does not result in improvement, the infection may be attributable to another microorganism not susceptible to natamycin.

Vasoconstrictors/Mydriatics

These drugs are contraindicated in individuals with hypersensitivity to the drug or any component of the drug and in patients with narrow-angle glaucoma or anatomically narrow angle and in patients with a sulfite sensitivity (some of these products contain sulfites). The drugs are used cautiously in patients with hypertension, diabetes, hyperthyroidism, cardiovascular disease, and arteriosclerosis. Local anesthetics can increase absorption of topical drugs. Systemic adverse reactions may occur more frequently when these drugs are administered with the β-adrenergic blocking drugs. When the mydriatics (drugs that dilate the pupil) are administered with the MAOIs or as long as 21 days after MAOI administration, exaggerated adrenergic effects may occur.

Cycloplegic Mydriatics

These drugs are contraindicated in patients with a hypersensitivity to the drug or any component of the drug and in patients with glaucoma. Some of these preparations contain sulfites, and individuals who are allergic to sulfites may exhibit allergic-like symptoms. The cycloplegic mydriatics are used cautiously in elderly patients and during pregnancy (category C) and lactation. No significant interactions have been reported when the drugs are applied topically.

Artificial Tear Solutions

Artificial tears are contraindicated in patients who are allergic to any component of the solution. No precautions or interactions have been reported.

Herbal Alert

Bilberry, also known as whortleberry, blueberry, trackleberry, and huckleberry, is a shrub with bluish flowers that appear in early spring and ripen in July and August. A beneficial use appears to be in promoting healthy eyes. Other benefits reportedly include improved visual acuity, improved night vision, prevention of free radical damage, and promotion of capillary blood flow in the eyes, hands, and feet. Bilberry extract has been used in treating nonspecific, mild diarrhea and as a mouthwash or gargle for inflammation of the mouth and throat.

Bilberry fruit is a safe substance with no known adverse reactions or toxicity. There are no known contraindications to its use as directed unless the individual has an allergy to bilberry. The dosage of standard extract is 80 to 160 mg per day.

NURSING PROCESS

The Patient Receiving an Ophthalmic Preparation

ASSESSMENT

PREADMINISTRATION ASSESSMENT

The primary health care provider examines the eye and external structures surrounding the eye and prescribes the drug indicated to treat the disorder. The nurse performs a baseline assessment by examining the eye for irritation, redness, and the presence of any exudate and carefully documents the findings in the patient's record. A purulent discharge is often found with infection of the eye. Pruritus (itching) is often present with allergic conditions of the eye. It is also important to determine if any visual impairment is present because this would indicate the need for assistance with ambulation and possibly activities of daily living. The nurse also assesses the patient for any hypersensitivities to the specific medication being administered and notes any cautions to the drug as well.

ONGOING ASSESSMENT

During the ongoing assessment the nurse observes for a therapeutic drug effect and reports any increase in symptoms and the presence of any redness, irritation, or pain in the eye. Patients admitted for treatment of acute glaucoma

Nursing Diagnoses Checklist

✓ **Disturbed Sensory Perception: Visual** related to adverse drug effects or disease condition

✓ **Risk for Injury** related to adverse reactions to drug therapy (blurring of the vision)

✓ **Acute Pain** related to eye disorder or adverse reaction to medication

✓ **Anxiety** related to eye pain or discomfort, diagnosis, other factors

should be assessed every 2 hours for relief of pain. Pain in the eye may indicate increased IOP.

NURSING DIAGNOSES

Drug-specific nursing diagnoses are highlighted in the Nursing Diagnoses Checklist. Other nursing diagnoses applicable to these drugs are discussed in depth in Chapter 4.

PLANNING

The expected outcomes of the patient depend on the reason for administration but may include an optimal response to therapy, support of patient needs related to the management of adverse reactions, minimized anxiety, and an understanding of the application and use of an ophthalmic preparation (see the Home Care Checklist: Instilling an Ophthalmic Preparation).

IMPLEMENTATION

PROMOTING AN OPTIMAL RESPONSE TO THERAPY

Before instillation, ophthalmic solutions and ointments can be warmed in the hand for a few minutes. The nurse checks the medication to make sure the solution is clear and not discolored. Ophthalmic ointments are applied to the eyelids or dropped into the lower conjunctival sac; ophthalmic solutions are dropped into the middle of the lower conjunctival sac (Fig. 57-2). The nurse avoids touching the eye with the tip of the dropper or container to prevent contamination of the product. When eye solutions are instilled, the nurse applies gentle pressure on the inner canthus to delay drainage of the drug down the tear duct. This prevents the drug from being absorbed systemically.

Gerontologic Alert

Older adults, in particular, are at risk for exacerbation of existing disorders such as hypertension, tachycardia, or arrhythmias if systemic absorption of sympathomimetic ophthalmic drugs occurs.

Home Care Checklist

Instilling an Ophthalmic Preparation

Because of shortened hospital stays and increases in the number of ambulatory surgeries for many eye problems, the patient may be required to instill eye drops or ointment at home. If the patient is unable to do so, a family member or friend may have to instill the preparation. The nurse uses the following guide to evaluate whether the patient or caregiver can properly instill the eye drops or ointment.

The patient or caregiver:

☑ Washes hands thoroughly before beginning.

☑ Holds bottle (drops) or tube (ointment) in hand for a few minutes before using.

☑ Cleanses the area around the eye of any secretions.

☑ Squeezes the eye dropper bulb to release and then refill the dropper, squeezes the bottle to fill the drop chamber, or squeezes ointment to tip of the tube.

☑ Tilts head slightly backward and toward the eye to be treated.

☑ Pulls affected lower lid down.

☑ Positions dropper, bottle, or tube over lower conjunctival sac.

☑ Steadies hand by resting fingers against cheek or by resting base of hand on cheek.

☑ Looks up at ceiling and squeezes dropper, bottle, or tube.

☑ Drops ordered number of drops into the middle of lower conjunctival sac; instills prescribed amount of ointment to eyelid or lower conjunctival sac.

☑ Closes eye briefly and gently and releases lower lid (does not squeeze eyes shut after instilling the drug).

☑ Places finger on inner canthus to avoid absorption through the tear duct (when instilling drops and only if ordered).

☑ Repeats procedure with other eye (if ordered).

☑ If more than one type of ophthalmic preparation is being instilled, waits the recommended time before instilling the second drug (usually 5 minutes for drops and 10–15 minutes for ointment).

☑ Replaces the cap of the eye preparation immediately after instilling the eye drops or ointment. Does not touch the tip of the dropper, bottle, or tube.

The primary health care provider is consulted regarding use of this technique before the first dose is instilled because this technique can be potentially dangerous in some eye conditions—for example, after recent eye surgery. When two eye drops are prescribed for use at the same time, the nurse waits at least 5 minutes before instilling the second drug. This helps prevent dilution of the drug and loss of some therapeutic effect from tearing.

Patients using the pilocarpine ocular therapeutic system must have the system replaced every 7 days. The system is inserted at bedtime because **myopia** (nearsightedness) occurs for several hours after insertion.

When a patient is scheduled for eye surgery, it is most important that the eye drops ordered by the primary health care provider are instilled at the correct time. This is espe-cially important when the purpose of the drug is to change the size of the pupil.

Nursing Alert

Only preparations labeled as "ophthalmic" are instilled in the eye. The nurse must check the label of the preparation carefully for the name of the drug, the percentage of the preparation, and a statement indicating that the preparation is for ophthalmic use.

MONITORING AND MANAGING PATIENT NEEDS

DISTURBED SENSORY PERCEPTION: VISUAL Although adverse reactions are rare, these drugs can cause visual impairment such as blurring of vision and local irritation

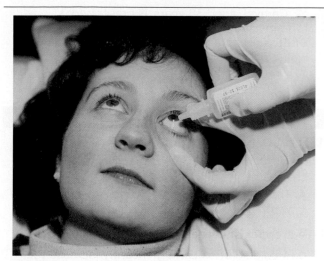

Figure 57.2 Instilling eye medication. While the patient looks upward, the nurse gently pulls the lower lid down and instills the correct number of drops into the lower conjunctival sac.

and burning. These reactions are most often self-limiting and resolve if the patient waits a few minutes. Visual impairment that does not clear within 30 minutes after therapy should be reported to the primary health care provider.

RISK FOR INJURY When the ophthalmic drugs produce blurring of vision, this can result in falls and other injuries. The nurse warns patients to exercise care when getting out of bed when the vision is impaired by these drugs. If needed, the nurse provides assistance with ambulation to prevent injury from falls.

ACUTE PAIN Pain can occur with eye conditions such as glaucoma and eye infections. Patients with acute glaucoma are assessed for relief of pain. Pain in the eye may indicate increased IOP and should be reported to the primary health care provider. Pain associated with infection should decrease with administration of medication. Any increase in pain or no decrease in the symptoms after 1 to 2 days of treatment should be reported to the primary health care provider. Headache and brow ache are associated with adverse reactions of some of the ophthalmic agents and are usually self-limiting.

ANXIETY Eye injuries and some eye infections are very painful. Other eye conditions may result in discomfort or a loss of or change in vision. The patient with an eye disorder or injury usually has great concern about the effect the problem will have on his or her vision. The nurse reassures the patient that every effort is being made to treat the disorder.

EDUCATING THE PATIENT AND FAMILY

The patient or a family member will require instruction in the technique of instilling an ophthalmic preparation (see

Home Care Checklist: Instilling an Ophthalmic Preparation). In addition, the nurse may give the following information to the patient and family member when an eye ointment or solution is prescribed:

- Eye preparations may cause a momentary stinging or burning sensation; this is normal.

- Temporary blurring of vision may occur. Avoid activities requiring visual acuity until vision returns to normal.

- If more than one topical ophthalmic drug is being used, administer the drugs at least 5 to 10 minutes apart or as directed by the physician.

- Complete a full course of treatment with the prescribed drug to achieve satisfactory results.

- Do not rub the eyes, and keep hands away from the eyes.

- Do not use nonprescription eye products during or after treatment unless such use has been approved by the primary health care provider.

- Some of these preparations cause sensitivity (photophobia) to light; to minimize this, wear sunglasses.

- Notify the primary health care provider if symptoms do not improve or if they worsen.

ALPHA₂-ADRENERGIC AGONISTS

- Patients wearing contact lenses should wait at least 15 minutes after instilling brimonidine to insert soft contact lenses.

- Brimonidine may cause fatigue or drowsiness in some patients. Use caution when engaging in activities requiring mental alertness.

SYMPATHOMIMETICS

- Do not use if solution is brown or contains a precipitate.

- Do not use while wearing soft contact lenses.

- Headache or brow ache may occur.

- Report any decrease in visual acuity.

ALPHA-ADRENERGIC BLOCKING AGENTS

- Dapiprazole may cause difficulty in dark adaptation and may reduce field of vision. Use caution when driving at night or performing activities in poor illumination.

- Do not use any solution that is not clear and colorless.

MIOTICS, DIRECT ACTING

- May sting on instillation, especially the first few doses.

- May cause headache, brow ache, and decreased night vision. Use caution while night driving or performing hazardous tasks in poor light.

- If using the ocular therapeutic system, check the system before retiring at night and on arising. Follow instructions in package insert.

PROSTAGLANDIN AGONISTS

- Remove contact lenses before administration and leave out at least 15 minutes before reinserting them.
- If more than one ophthalmic drug is being used, administer the drugs 5 minutes apart.
- Advise patient that changes may occur to the lashes—length, thickness, pigmentation, and number—in the eye being treated.
- The color of the iris may change because of an increase in the brown pigment. This may be more noticeable in patients with blue, green, gray-brown, or other light-colored eyes. This discoloration may be permanent.

CORTICOSTEROIDS

- If improvement in the condition being treated does not occur within 2 days, or pain, redness, itching, or swelling of the eye occurs, notify the primary health care provider.

EVALUATION

- The therapeutic effect is achieved.
- Adverse reactions are managed.
- The patient has improved visual acuity.
- The patient does not fall.
- The patient has minimal to no pain.
- Anxiety is reduced.
- The patient demonstrates the ability to instill an ophthalmic preparation in the eye.
- The patient and family demonstrate an understanding of the drug regimen.
- The patient verbalizes knowledge of the treatment regimen and its importance.

Critical Thinking Exercises

1. Prepare a teaching plan for a patient prescribed Cerumenex for removal of earwax.

2. Ms. Stone, aged 76 years, has glaucoma and is prescribed timolol eye drops. Your initial assessment reveals that she has severe arthritis and appears to have difficulty following instructions. Discuss any further investigations you feel are important to make before developing a teaching plan for this patient.

3. Mr. Caravel, aged 38 years, is prescribed tobramycin ophthalmic for bacterial conjunctivitis. Discuss preadministration assessments the nurse would perform before instilling the drug.

Review Questions

1. What is the rationale for warming an otic solution that has been refrigerated before instilling the drops into the patient's ear?

   A. The drug becomes thick when refrigerated, and warming liquefies the solution.

   B. It helps to prevent dizziness on instillation.

   C. A cold solution can significantly increase the patient's blood pressure.

   D. A cold solution could damage the tympanic membrane.

2. Which of the following adverse reactions would the nurse suspect in a patient receiving prolonged treatment with an antibiotic otic drug?

   A. Congestive heart failure

   B. Superinfection

   C. Anemia

   D. Hypersensitivity reactions

3. When administering an ophthalmic solution the drug is instilled into the ____.

   A. inner canthus

   B. upper conjunctival sac

   C. lower conjunctival sac

   D. upper canthus

4. Which of the following instructions would be included in a teaching plan for the patient prescribed an ophthalmic solution?

   A. Squeeze the eyes tightly after the solution is instilled.

   B. Immediately wipe the eye using pressure to squeeze out excess medication.

   C. After the drug is instilled, remain upright with the head bent slightly forward for about 2 minutes.

   D. A temporary stinging or burning may be felt at the time the drug is instilled.

To check your answers, see Appendix G.

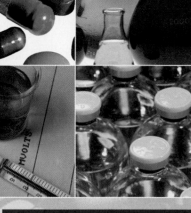

Fluids and Electrolytes

Learning Objectives

On completion of this chapter, the student will:

- List the types and uses of solutions used in the management of body fluids.

- Discuss the adverse reactions associated with the administration of a solution or electrolyte used in the management of body fluids.

- List the types and uses of electrolytes used in the management of electrolyte imbalances.

- Discuss the more common signs and symptoms of electrolyte imbalance.

- Discuss preadministration and ongoing assessment activities the nurse should perform with the patient taking an electrolyte or a solution to manage body fluids.

- List nursing diagnoses particular to a patient receiving an electrolyte or a solution to manage body fluids.

- Discuss ways to promote an optimal response to therapy and important points to keep in mind when educating patients about the use of an electrolyte or a solution to manage body fluids.

- Discuss the use of total parenteral nutrition (TPN).

Various solutions are used in the management of body fluids. These solutions are used when the body cannot sustain the fluid or electrolyte balance needed for normal functioning.

SOLUTIONS USED IN THE MANAGEMENT OF BODY FLUIDS

The next section gives a brief overview of the following solutions: blood plasma, plasma protein fractions, protein substrates, plasma expanders, and intravenous (IV) replacement fluids.

Actions and Uses

Blood Plasma

Blood plasma is the liquid part of blood, containing water, sugar, electrolytes, fats, gases, proteins, bile pigment, and clotting factors. Human plasma, also called human pooled plasma, is obtained from donated blood. Although whole blood must be typed and crossmatched because it contains red blood cells carrying blood type and Rh factors, human plasma does not require this procedure. Because of this, plasma can be given in acute emergencies.

Plasma administered IV is used

- To increase blood volume when severe hemorrhage has occurred and it is necessary partially to restore blood volume while waiting for whole blood to be typed and crossmatched.

- In treating conditions when plasma alone has been lost, as may be seen in severe burns.

Plasma Protein Fractions

Plasma protein fractions include human plasma protein fraction 5% and normal serum albumin 5% (Albuminar-5, Buminate 5%) and 25% (Albuminar-25, Buminate 25%). Plasma protein fraction 5% is an IV solution containing 5% human plasma proteins. Serum albumin is obtained from donated whole blood and is a protein found in plasma. The albumin fraction of human blood acts to maintain plasma colloid osmotic pressure and as a carrier of intermediate metabolites in the transport and exchange of tissue products. It is critical in regulating the volume of circulating blood. When blood is lost from shock, such as in hemorrhage, there is a reduced plasma volume. When blood volume is reduced, albumin quickly restores the volume in most situations.

Plasma protein fractions are used to treat

- Hypovolemic (low blood volume) shock that occurs as the result of burns, trauma, surgery, and infections, or in conditions where shock is not currently present but likely to occur

- Hypoproteinemia (a deficiency of protein in the blood), as might be seen in patients with nephrotic syndrome and hepatic cirrhosis, as well as other diseases or disorders

As with human pooled plasma, blood type and crossmatch are not needed when plasma protein fractions are given.

Protein Substrates

A **substrate** is a substance that is the basic component of a compound or organism. Protein substrates are amino acids, which are essential to life. **Protein substrates** are amino acid preparations that act to promote the production of proteins (anabolism). Amino acids are necessary to promote synthesis of structural components, reduce the rate of protein breakdown (catabolism), promote wound healing, and act as buffers in the extracellular and intracellular fluids. Crystalline amino acid preparations are hypertonic solutions of balanced essential and nonessential amino acid concentrations that provide substrates for protein synthesis or act to conserve existing body protein.

Amino acids promote the production of proteins, enhance tissue repair and wound healing, and reduce the rate of protein breakdown. Amino acids are used in

- Certain disease states, such as severe kidney and liver disease

- Total parenteral nutrition (TPN) solutions in patients with impaired gastrointestinal (GI) absorption of protein; those with an increased requirement for protein, as seen in patients with extensive burns or infections; and patients with no available oral route for nutritional intake

Energy Substrates

Energy substrates include dextrose solutions and fat emulsion. Solutions used to supply energy and fluid include dextrose (glucose) in water or sodium chloride, alcohol in dextrose, and IV fat emulsion. Dextrose is a carbohydrate used to provide a source of calories and fluid. Alcohol (as alcohol in dextrose) also provides calories. Dextrose is available in various strengths (or percentages of the carbohydrate) in a fluid, which may be water or sodium chloride (saline). Dextrose and dextrose in alcohol are available in various strengths (or percentages of the carbohydrate and percent of the alcohol) in water. Dextrose solutions also are available with electrolytes, such as Plasma-Lyte 56 and 5% Dextrose.

An IV fat emulsion contains soybean or safflower oil and a mixture of natural triglycerides, predominantly unsaturated fatty acids. It is used in the prevention and treatment of essential fatty acid deficiency. It also provides nonprotein calories for those receiving TPN when calorie requirements cannot be met by glucose. Examples of IV fat emulsion include Intralipid 10% and 20%, Liposyn II 10% and 20%, and Liposyn III 10% and 20%. Fat emulsion is used as a source of calories and essential fatty acids for patients requiring parenteral nutrition for extended periods (usually more than 5 days). No more than 60% of the patient's total caloric intake should come from fat emulsion, with carbohydrates and amino acids comprising the remaining 40% or more of caloric intake.

Plasma Expanders

The IV solutions of plasma expanders include hetastarch (Hespan), low–molecular-weight dextran (Dextran 40), and high–molecular-weight dextran (Dextran 70, Dextran 75).

Plasma expanders are used

- To expand plasma volume when shock is caused by burns, hemorrhage, surgery, and other trauma

- For prophylaxis of venous thrombosis and thromboembolism

When used in the treatment of shock, plasma expanders are not a substitute for whole blood or plasma, but they are of value as emergency measures until the latter substances can be used.

Intravenous Replacement Solutions

Intravenous replacement solutions are used

- As a source of electrolytes and water for hydration (Normosol M Ringer's Injection, Lactated Ringer's, Plasma-Lyte R)

- To facilitate amino acid utilization and maintain electrolyte balance (Lypholyte, Multilyte, TPN Electrolytes)

- As a parenteral source of electrolytes, calories, or water for hydration (Dextrose and electrolyte solutions such as Plasma-Lyte R and 5% Dextrose)
- As a source of calories and hydration (sugar–electrolyte solutions, such as Multiple Electrolytes and Travert 5% and 10%)

Adverse Reactions

Fluid Overload

One adverse reaction commonly associated with all solutions administered by the parenteral route is fluid overload, that is, the administration of more fluid than the body is able to handle.

The term **fluid overload** (circulatory overload) describes a condition when the body's fluid requirements are met and the administration of fluid occurs at a rate that is greater than the rate at which the body can use or eliminate the fluid. Thus, the amount of fluid and the rate of administration of fluid that will cause fluid overload depend on several factors, such as the patient's cardiac status and adequacy of renal function. The signs and symptoms of fluid overload are listed in Display 58-1.

Reactions to Plasma Protein Fractions

Adverse reactions are rare when plasma protein fractions are administered, but nausea, chills, fever, urticaria, and hypotensive episodes may occasionally be seen.

Display 58.1 Signs and Symptoms of Fluid Overload

- Headache
- Weakness
- Blurred vision
- Behavioral changes (confusion, disorientation, delirium, drowsiness)
- Weight gain
- Isolated muscle twitching
- Hyponatremia
- Rapid breathing
- Wheezing
- Coughing
- Rise in blood pressure
- Distended neck veins
- Elevated central venous pressure
- Convulsions

Reactions to Protein Substrates

Administration of protein substrates (amino acids) may result in nausea, fever, flushing of the skin, metabolic acidosis or alkalosis, and decreased phosphorus and calcium blood levels.

Reactions to Energy Substrates

Low– or high–molecular-weight dextran administration may result in allergic reactions, which are evidenced by urticaria, hypotension, nausea, vomiting, headache, dyspnea, fever, tightness of the chest, and wheezing. Hyperglycemia and phlebitis may be seen with administration of glucose.

Reactions to Fat Emulsions

The most common adverse reaction associated with the administration of fat emulsion is sepsis caused by administration equipment and thrombophlebitis caused by venous irritation from concurrently administering hypertonic solutions. Less frequent adverse reactions include dyspnea, cyanosis, hyperlipidemia, hypercoagulability, nausea, vomiting, headache, flushing, increased body temperature, sweating, sleepiness, chest and back pain, slight pressure over the eyes, and dizziness.

Reactions to Plasma Expanders

Administration of hetastarch, a plasma expander, may be accompanied by vomiting, a mild temperature elevation, itching, and allergic reactions. Allergic reactions are evidenced by wheezing, swelling around the eyes (periorbital edema), and urticaria. Other plasma expanders may result in mild cutaneous eruptions, generalized urticaria, hypotension, nausea, vomiting, headache, dyspnea, fever, tightness of the chest, bronchospasm, wheezing, and, rarely, anaphylactic shock.

Contraindications, Precautions, and Interactions

Blood Plasma

Solutions used in the management of body fluids are contraindicated in patients with hypersensitivity to any component of the solution. All solutions used to manage body fluids discussed in this chapter are pregnancy category C drugs and are used cautiously during pregnancy and lactation. No interactions have been reported.

Plasma Protein Fractions

Plasma proteins are contraindicated in those with a history of allergic reactions to albumin, severe anemia, or cardiac failure; in the presence of normal or increased intravascular volume; and in patients on cardiopulmonary bypass. Plasma protein fractions are used cautiously in patients who are in shock or dehydrated and in those with congestive heart failure (CHF) or hepatic or renal failure. These solutions are pregnancy category C drugs and are used cautiously during pregnancy and lactation.

Most IV solutions should not be combined with any other solutions or drugs but should be administered alone. The nurse should consult the drug insert or other appropriate sources before combining any drug with any plasma protein fraction.

Protein Substrates

Solutions used in managing body fluids are contraindicated in patients with hypersensitivity to any component of the solution. Plasma expanders are used cautiously in patients with renal disease, CHF, pulmonary edema, and severe bleeding disorders. These solutions are pregnancy category C drugs and are used cautiously during pregnancy and lactation. Protein substrates should not be combined with any other solutions or drugs without consulting the drug insert or other appropriate sources.

Energy Substrates

The energy substrates are contraindicated in patients with hypersensitivity to any component of the solution. Dextrose solutions are contraindicated in patients in diabetic coma with excessively high blood sugar. Concentrated dextrose solutions are contraindicated in patients with increased intracranial pressure, delirium tremens (if patient is dehydrated), hepatic coma, or glucose–galactose malabsorption syndrome. Alcohol dextrose solutions are contraindicated in patients with epilepsy, urinary tract infections, alcoholism, or diabetic coma.

Alcohol dextrose solutions are used cautiously in patients with hepatic or renal impairment, vitamin deficiency (may cause or potentate vitamin deficiency), diabetes, or shock; during postpartum hemorrhage; and after cranial surgery.

The nurse should consult the drug insert or other appropriate sources before combining any drug with an IV solution. Dextrose solutions are used cautiously in patients receiving a corticosteroid or corticotropin.

Intravenous fat emulsions are contraindicated in conditions that interfere with normal fat metabolism (e.g., acute pancreatitis) and in patients allergic to eggs. IV fat emulsions are used with caution in those with severe liver impairment, pulmonary disease, anemia, and blood coagulation disorders. These solutions are pregnancy category C drugs and are used cautiously during pregnancy and lactation.

In general, fat emulsions should not be combined with any other solutions or drugs except when combined in TPN. The nurse should consult appropriate sources before combining any drug with a fat emulsion.

Plasma Expanders

Plasma expanders are contraindicated in patients with hypersensitivity to any component of the solution and those with severe bleeding disorders, severe cardiac failure, renal failure with oliguria, or anuria. Plasma expanders are used cautiously in patients with renal disease, CHF, pulmonary edema, and severe bleeding disorders. Plasma expanders are pregnancy category C drugs and are used cautiously during pregnancy and lactation. The nurse should consult the drug insert or other appropriate sources before combining a plasma expander with another drug for IV administration.

NURSING PROCESS

The Patient Receiving a Solution for Management of Body Fluids
ASSESSMENT
PREADMINISTRATION ASSESSMENT

Solutions used to manage body fluids are usually administered IV. Before administering an IV solution, the nurse assesses the patient's general status, reviews recent laboratory test results (when appropriate), weighs the patient (when appropriate), and takes the vital signs. Blood pressure, pulse, and respiratory rate provide a baseline, which is especially important when the patient is receiving blood plasma, plasma expanders, or plasma protein fractions for shock or other serious disorders.

ONGOING ASSESSMENT

During the ongoing assessment, the nurse checks the needle site every 15 to 30 minutes or more frequently if the patient is restless or confused. When one of these preparations is given with a regular IV infusion set, the nurse checks the infusion rate every 15 minutes. The needle site is inspected for signs of **extravasation** (escape of fluid from a blood vessel into surrounding tissues) or **infiltration** (the collection of fluid into tissues). If signs of extravasation or infiltration are apparent, the nurse restarts the infusion in another vein.

When these solutions are given, a central venous pressure line may be inserted to monitor the patient's response to therapy. Central venous pressure readings are taken as ordered. During administration, the nurse takes the blood pressure, pulse, and respiratory rate as ordered or at intervals determined by the patient's clinical condition. For example, a patient in shock and receiving a plasma expander may require monitoring of the blood pressure and pulse rate every 5 to 15 minutes, whereas the patient receiving dextrose 3 days after surgery may require monitoring every 30 to 60 minutes.

FAT EMULSIONS When a fat emulsion is administered, the nurse must monitor the patient's ability to eliminate the infused fat from the circulation because the lipidemia must clear between daily infusions. The nurse monitors for lipidemia by assessing the results of the following laboratory examinations: hemogram, blood coagulation, liver function tests, plasma lipid profile, and platelet count. The nurse reports an increase in the results of any of these laboratory examinations as abnormal.

NURSING DIAGNOSES

Drug-specific nursing diagnoses are highlighted in the Nursing Diagnoses Checklist. Other nursing diagnoses applicable to these drugs are discussed in depth in Chapter 4.

Nursing Diagnoses Checklist

✔ **Excess Fluid Volume** related to adverse effects resulting from too rapid intravenous infusion

✔ **Deficient Fluid Volume** related to inability to take oral fluids, abnormal fluid loss, other factors (specify cause of deficient fluid volume)

✔ **Imbalanced Nutrition: Less Than Body Requirments** related to inability to eat, recent surgery, other factors (specify cause of altered nutrition)

PLANNING

The expected outcomes of the patient may depend on the reason for administration, but may include an optimal response to therapy, prevention of fluid overload, correction of the fluid volume deficit (where appropriate), improved oral nutrition (where appropriate), and an understanding of the administration procedure.

IMPLEMENTATION

PROMOTING AN OPTIMAL RESPONSE TO THERAPY

Patients receiving an IV fluid should be made as comfortable as possible, although under some circumstances this may be difficult. The extremity used for administration

should be made comfortable and supported as needed by a small pillow or other device. An IV infusion pump may be ordered for the administration of these solutions. The nurse sets the alarm of the infusion pump and checks the functioning of the unit at frequent intervals.

Nursing Alert

The nurse must administer all IV solutions with great care. At no time should any IV solution be infused at a rapid rate, unless there is a specific written order to do so.

Unless otherwise directed, the IV solution should be administered at room temperature. If the solution is refrigerated, the nurse allows the solution to warm by exposing it to room temperature 30 to 45 minutes before use. The average length of time for infusion of 1000 mL of an IV solution is 4 to 8 hours. One exception is when there is a written or verbal order by the primary health care provider to give the solution at a rapid rate because of an emergency. In this instance, the order must specifically state the rate of administration as drops per minute, milliliters per minute, or the period of time over which a specific amount of fluid is to be infused (e.g., 125 mL/h or 1000 mL in 8 hours). Calculation of IV flow rates is discussed in Chapter 3.

LIPID SOLUTIONS Fat solutions (emulsions) should be handled with care to decrease the risk of separation or "breaking out of the oil." Separation can be identified by yellowish streaking or the accumulation of yellowish droplets in the emulsion. Fat solutions are administered to adults at a rate no greater than 1 to 2 mL/min.

Nursing Alert

During the first 30 minutes of infusion of a fat solution, the nurse carefully observes the patient for difficulty in breathing, headache, flushing, nausea, vomiting, or signs of a hypersensitivity reaction. If any of these reactions occur, the nurse discontinues the infusion and immediately notifies the primary health care provider.

AMINO ACIDS A microscopic filter is attached to the IV line when amino acid solutions are administered. The filter prevents microscopic aggregates (particles that may form in the IV bag) from entering the bloodstream, where they could cause massive emboli.

MONITORING AND MANAGING PATIENT NEEDS

EXCESS FLUID VOLUME The nurse monitors patients receiving IV solutions at frequent intervals for signs of fluid overload. If signs of fluid overload (see Display 58-1) are observed, the nurse slows the IV infusion rate and immediately notifies the primary health care provider.

Gerontologic Alert

Older adults are at increased risk for fluid overload because of the increased incidence of cardiac disease and decreased renal function that may accompany old age. Careful monitoring for signs and symptoms of fluid overload (see Display 58-1) is extremely important when administering fluids to older adults.

DEFICIENT FLUID VOLUME AND IMBALANCED NUTRITION: LESS THAN BODY REQUIREMENTS Often, the solutions used in the management of body fluids are given to correct a fluid volume deficit and to supply carbohydrates (nutrition). The nurse reviews the patient's chart for a full understanding of the rationale for administration of the specific solution.

When appropriate, nursing measures that may be instituted to correct a fluid volume and carbohydrate deficit may be included in a plan of care. Examples of these measures include offering oral fluids at frequent intervals and encouraging the patient to take small amounts of nourishment between meals and to eat as much as possible at mealtime.

EDUCATING THE PATIENT AND FAMILY

The nurse gives the patient or family a brief explanation of the reason for and the method of administration of an IV solution. Sometimes, patients and families tamper with or adjust the rate of flow of IV administration sets. The nurse emphasizes the importance of not touching the IV administration set or the equipment used to administer IV fluids.

EVALUATION

- The therapeutic effect of the drug is achieved.
- The fluid volume deficit is corrected.
- The nutrition deficit is corrected.
- The patient and family demonstrate an understanding of the procedure.

ELECTROLYTES

Along with a disturbance in fluid volume (e.g., loss of plasma, blood, or water) or a need to provide parenteral nutrition with the previously discussed solutions, an electrolyte imbalance may exist. An **electrolyte** is an electrically

charged substance essential to the normal functioning of all cells. Intracellular and extracellular fluids have specific chemical compositions of electrolytes. Major electrolytes in intracellular fluid include

- Potassium
- Magnesium

Major electrolytes in extracellular fluid include

- Calcium
- Sodium

Electrolytes circulate in the blood at specific levels, where they are available for use when needed by the cells. An electrolyte imbalance occurs when the concentration of an electrolyte in the blood is either too high or too low. In some instances, an electrolyte imbalance may be present without an appreciable disturbance in fluid balance. An electrolyte imbalance can profoundly affect a patient's physiologic functioning, the body's water distribution, neuromuscular activity, and acid-base balance. An electrolyte imbalance can occur from any disorder that alters electrolyte levels in the body's fluid compartments. An imbalance can also occur from vomiting, surgery, diagnostic tests, or drug administration. For example, a patient taking a diuretic is able to maintain fluid balance by an adequate oral intake of water, which replaces the water lost through diuresis. However, the patient is likely to be unable to replace the potassium that is also lost during diuresis. When the potassium concentration in the blood is too low, as may occur with the administration of a diuretic, an imbalance may occur that requires the addition of potassium. Electrolyte replacement drugs are inorganic or organic salts that increase deficient electrolyte levels that help to maintain homeostasis. Commonly used electrolyte replacement drugs are listed in the Summary Drug Table: Electrolytes.

Actions and Uses

Calcium (Ca^{++})

Calcium is necessary for the functioning of nerves and muscles, the clotting of blood (see Chapter 43), the building of bones and teeth, and other physiologic processes. Examples of calcium salts are calcium gluconate and calcium carbonate. Calcium may be given for the treatment of **hypocalcemia** (low blood calcium), which may be seen in those with parathyroid disease or after accidental removal of the parathyroid glands during surgery of the thyroid gland. Calcium may also be given

SUMMARY DRUG TABLE   ELECTROLYTES

GENERIC NAME	TRADE NAME	USES	ADVERSE REACTIONS	DOSAGE RANGES
calcium acetate	PhosLo	Control of hyperphosphatemia in end-stage renal failure	See Display 58-2	3–4 tablets orally with each meal
calcium carbonate	Calcium-600, Apo-Cal, Caltrate, Oyster Shell Calcium Tums, Rolaids, Calcium Rich, Tums E-X	Dietary supplement for prevention or treatment of calcium deficiency for conditions such as pregnancy and lactation, chronic diarrhea, osteoporosis, osteomalacia, rickets, and latent tetany, and to reduce the symptoms of premenstrual syndrome	Rare; see Display 58-2 for signs of hypercalcemia	500–2000 mg/d orally
calcium citrate	Citracal, Citracal Liquitab	Same as calcium carbonate	Same as calcium carbonate	500–2000 mg/d orally
calcium gluconate		Hypocalcemic tetany, hyperkalemia with secondary cardiac toxicity, magnesium intoxication, exchange transfusion	Same as calcium carbonate	Adults: dosage range 1.35–70 mEq/d IV Children: 2.3 mEq/kg/d well diluted; give slowly in divided doses
calcium lactate	Cal-Lac	Same as calcium carbonate	Same as calcium carbonate	500–2000 mg/d orally
magnesium	Magonate, Mag-Ox 400, Magtrate, Mag-200, Slow-Mag	Dietary supplement, hypomagnesemia	Rare; see Display 58-2 for signs of hypermagnesemia	54–483 mg/d orally
magnesium sulfate		Mild to severe hypomagnesemia, seizures	Toxicity, weak or absent deep tendon reflexes, flaccid paralysis, drowsiness, stupor, weak pulse, arrhythmias, hypotension, circulatory collapse, respiratory paralysis	Hypomagnesemia: 2–5 g IV in 1 L of solution; 4–5 g over 3 h Seizures: 4–5 g magnesium sulfate in 250 mL $D_5 W$; simultaneously give 4–5 g magnesium sulfate (undiluted) IM to each buttock for initial dose of 10–14 g; followed by 1–2 g/h IV infusion until seizure controlled
oral electrolyte mixtures	Infalyte Oral Solution, Naturalyte, Pedialyte, Pedialyte Electrolyte, Pedialyte Freezer Pops, Rehydralyte, Resol Solution	Maintenance of water and electrolytes after corrective parenteral therapy of severe diarrhea; maintenance to replace mild to moderate fluid losses when food and liquid intake are discontinued, to restore fluid and minerals lost in diarrhea and vomiting in infants and children	Rare	Individualize dosage following the guidelines on the product labeling

Fluids and Electrolytes

SUMMARY DRUG TABLE (*continued*)

GENERIC NAME	TRADE NAME	USES	ADVERSE REACTIONS	DOSAGE RANGES
potassium replacements	Effer K, K Norm, Kaon Cl, K-Dur, Klor-Con, K-Lyte, K-Tab, Micro-K, Slow-K	Hypokalemia	See Display 58-2; most common: nausea, vomiting, diarrhea, flatulence, abdominal discomfort, skin rash	40–100 mEq/d orally
sodium chloride	Slo-Salt	Prevention or treatment of extracellular volume depletion, dehydration, sodium depletion, aid in the prevention of heat prostration	Nausea, vomiting, diarrhea, abdominal cramps, edema, irritability, restlessness, weakness, hypertension, tachycardia, fluid accumulation, pulmonary edema, respiratory arrest (see Display 58-2)	Individualize dosage
Alkalinizing Drugs				
bicarbonate		Metabolic acidosis, cardiac arrest, systemic and urinary alkalinization	Tetany, edema, gastric distention, flatulence, belching, hypokalemia, metabolic alkalosis	Metabolic acidosis and cardiac arrest: dosage varies depending on laboratory results and patient's condition Urinary alkalinization: 4 g orally initially, followed by 1–2 g orally q6h
tromethamine	Tham	Metabolic acidosis during cardiac bypass surgery or cardiac arrest	Fever, hypoglycemia, hyperkalemia, respiratory depression, hemorrhagic hepatic necrosis, venospasm, vein necrosis	9 ml /kg (not to exceed total single dose of 500 mL)
Acidifying Drug				
ammonium chloride		Metabolic alkalosis	Loss of electrolytes, especially potassium, metabolic acidosis	Varies depending on patient's tolerance and condition

during cardiopulmonary resuscitation, particularly after open heart surgery, when epinephrine fails to improve weak or ineffective myocardial contractions. Calcium may be used as adjunct therapy of insect bites or stings to reduce muscle cramping, such as occurs with black widow spider bites. Calcium may also be recommended for those eating a diet low in calcium or as a dietary supplement when there is an increased need for calcium, such as during pregnancy.

Magnesium (Mg^{++})

Magnesium plays an important role in the transmission of nerve impulses. It is also important in the activity of many enzyme reactions, such as carbohydrate metabolism. Magnesium sulfate ($MgSO_4$) is used as replacement therapy in hypomagnesemia. Magnesium sulfate is also used in the

prevention and control of seizures in obstetric patients with pregnancy-induced hypertension (PIH; also referred to as *eclampsia* and *preeclampsia*). It may also be added to TPN mixtures.

Potassium (K$^+$)

Potassium is the major electrolyte in intracellular fluid and must be consumed daily because it cannot be stored. It is necessary for the transmission of impulses; the contraction of smooth, cardiac, and skeletal muscles; and other important physiologic processes. Potassium may be given to correct **hypokalemia** (low blood potassium) resulting from increased potassium excretion or depletion. Examples of causes of hypokalemia are a marked loss of GI fluids (severe vomiting, diarrhea, nasogastric suction, draining intestinal fistulas), diabetic acidosis, marked diuresis, severe malnutrition, use of a potassium-depleting diuretic, excess antidiuretic hormone, and excessive urination. Potassium as a drug is available as potassium chloride (KCl) and potassium gluconate, and is measured in milliequivalents (mEq)—for example, 40 mEq in 20 mL or 8 mEq controlled-release tablet.

Sodium (Na$^+$)

Sodium is a major electrolyte in extracellular fluid and is important in maintaining acid-base balance and normal heart action, and in the regulation of osmotic pressure in body cells (water balance). Sodium is administered for **hyponatremia** (low blood sodium). Examples of causes of hyponatremia are excessive diaphoresis, severe vomiting or diarrhea, excessive diuresis, diuretic use, wound drainage, and draining intestinal fistulas.

Sodium, as sodium chloride (NaCl), may be given IV. A solution containing 0.9% NaCl is called **normal saline**, and a solution containing 0.45% NaCl is called **half-normal saline**. Sodium also is available combined with dextrose, such as dextrose 5% and sodium chloride 0.9%.

Combined Electrolyte Solutions

Combined electrolyte solutions are available for oral and IV administration. The IV solutions contain various electrolytes and dextrose. The amount of electrolytes, given as milliequivalents per liter (mEq/L), also varies. The IV solutions are used to replace fluid and electrolytes that have been lost and to provide calories through their carbohydrate content. Examples of IV electrolyte solutions are dextrose 5% with 0.9% NaCl, lactated Ringer's, and Plasma-Lyte. The primary health care provider selects the type of combined electrolyte solution that will meet the patient's needs.

Oral electrolyte solutions contain a carbohydrate and various electrolytes. Examples of combined oral electrolyte solutions are Pedialyte and Rehydralyte. Oral electrolyte solutions are most often used to replace lost electrolytes and fluids in conditions such as severe vomiting or diarrhea.

Adverse Reactions

Reactions to Calcium (Ca^{++})

Irritation of the vein used for administration, tingling, a metallic or chalky taste, and "heat waves" may occur when calcium is given IV. Rapid IV administration (calcium gluconate) may result in bradycardia, vasodilation, decreased blood pressure, cardiac arrhythmias, and cardiac arrest. Oral administration may result in GI disturbances. Administration of calcium chloride may cause peripheral vasodilation, a temporary fall in blood pressure, and a local burn-

ing. Display 58-2 lists adverse reactions associated with hypercalcemia and hypocalcemia.

Reactions to Magnesium (Mg^{++})

Adverse reactions from magnesium administration are most likely related to overdose and may include flushing, sweating, hypotension, depressed reflexes, muscle weakness, respiratory failure, and circulatory collapse (see Display 58-2).

Reactions to Potassium (K$^+$)

Nausea, vomiting, diarrhea, abdominal pain, and phlebitis have been seen with oral and IV administration of potassium. Adverse reactions related to hypokalemia or hyperkalemia are listed in Display 58-2.

If extravasation of the IV solution should occur, local tissue necrosis (death of tissue) may be seen. If extravasation occurs, the primary health care provider is contacted immediately and the infusion slowed to a rate that keeps the vein open.

Reactions to Sodium (Na$^+$)

Sodium as the salt (e.g., NaCl) has no adverse reactions except those related to overdose (see Display 58-2). In some instances, excessive oral use may produce nausea and vomiting.

Contraindications, Precautions, and Interactions

Calcium (Ca^{++})

Calcium is contraindicated in patients with hypercalcemia or ventricular fibrillation and in patients taking digitalis. Calcium is used cautiously in patients with cardiac disease. Hypercalcemia may occur when calcium is administered with the thiazide diuretics. When calcium is administered with atenolol there is a decrease in the effect of atenolol, possibly resulting in decreased beta blockade. There is an increased risk of digitalis toxicity when digitalis preparations are administered with calcium. The clinical effect of verapamil may be decreased when the drug is administered with calcium. Concurrent ingestion of spinach or cereal may decrease the absorption of calcium supplements.

Magnesium (Mg^{++})

Magnesium sulfate is contraindicated in patients with heart block or myocardial damage and in women with PIH during the 2 hours before delivery. Magnesium is a pregnancy category A drug, and studies indicate no increased risk of fetal

Display 58.2 Signs and Symptoms of Electrolyte Imbalances

Calcium

Normal laboratory values: 4.5–5.3 mEq/L or 9–11 mg/dL*

Hypocalcemia

Hyperactive reflexes, carpopedal spasm, perioral paresthesias, positive Trousseau's sign, positive Chvostek's sign, muscle twitching, muscle cramps, tetany (numbness, tingling, and muscular twitching usually of the extremities), laryngospasm, cardiac arrhythmias, nausea, vomiting, anxiety, confusion, emotional lability, convulsions

Hypercalcemia

Anorexia, nausea, vomiting, lethargy, bone tenderness or pain, polyuria, polydipsia, constipation, dehydration, muscle weakness and atrophy, stupor, coma, cardiac arrest

Magnesium

Normal laboratory values: 1.5–2.5 mEq/L or 1.8–3 mg/dL*

Hypomagnesemia

Leg and foot cramps, hypertension, tachycardia, neuromuscular irritability, tremor, hyperactive deep tendon reflexes, confusion, disorientation, visual or auditory hallucinations, painful paresthesias, positive Trousseau's sign, positive Chvostek's sign, convulsions

Hypermagnesemia

Lethargy, drowsiness, impaired respiration, flushing, sweating, hypotension, weak to absent deep tendon reflexes

Potassium

Normal laboratory values: 3.5–5 mEq/L*

Hypokalemia

Anorexia, nausea, vomiting, mental depression, confusion, delayed or impaired thought processes, drowsiness, abdominal distention, decreased bowel sounds, paralytic ileus, muscle weakness or fatigue, flaccid paralysis, absent or diminished deep tendon reflexes, weak, irregular pulse, paresthesias, leg cramps, ECG changes

Hyperkalemia

Irritability, anxiety, listlessness, mental confusion, nausea, diarrhea, abdominal distress, gastrointestinal hyperactivity, paresthesias, weakness and heaviness of the legs, flaccid paralysis, hypotension, cardiac arrhythmias, ECG changes

Sodium

Normal laboratory values: 132–145 mEq/L*

Hyponatremia

Cold, clammy skin, decreased skin turgor, apprehension, confusion, irritability, anxiety, hypotension, postural hypotension, tachycardia, headache, tremors, convulsions, abdominal cramps, nausea, vomiting, diarrhea

Hypernatremia

Fever; hot, dry skin; dry, sticky mucous membranes; rough, dry tongue; edema, weight gain, intense thirst, excitement, restlessness, agitation, oliguria or anuria

ECG, electrocardiographic
*These laboratory values may not concur with the normal range of values in all hospitals and laboratories. The hospital policy manual or laboratory values sheet should be consulted for the normal ranges of all laboratory tests.

---

abnormalities if the agent is used during pregnancy. Nevertheless, caution is used when administering magnesium during pregnancy. Magnesium sulfate is used with caution in patients with renal function impairment. When magnesium sulfate is used with alcohol, antidepressants, antipsychotics, barbiturates, hypnotics, general anesthetics, and narcotics, an increase in central nervous system depression may occur. Prolonged respiratory depression and apnea may occur when magnesium is administered with the neuromuscular blocking agents. When magnesium is used with digoxin, heart block may occur.

Potassium (K$^+$)

Potassium is contraindicated in patients who are at risk for hyperkalemia, such as those with renal failure, oliguria, azotemia (the presence of nitrogen-containing compounds

in the blood), anuria, severe hemolytic reactions, untreated Addison's disease (see Chapter 50), acute dehydration, heat cramps, and any form of hyperkalemia. Potassium is used cautiously in patients with renal impairment or adrenal insufficiency, heart disease, metabolic acidosis, or prolonged or severe diarrhea.

Concurrent use of potassium with angiotensin-converting enzyme (ACE) inhibitors may result in an elevated serum potassium level. Potassium-sparing diuretics and salt substitutes used with potassium can produce severe hyperkalemia. The use of digitalis with potassium increases the risk of digoxin toxicity.

Sodium (Na$^+$)

Sodium is contraindicated in patients with hypernatremia or fluid retention, and when the administration of sodium or chloride could be detrimental. Sodium is used cautiously in surgical patients and those with circulatory insufficiency, hypoproteinemia, urinary tract obstruction, CHF, edema, or renal impairment. Sodium is a pregnancy category C drug and is used cautiously during pregnancy.

ALKALINIZING AND ACIDIFYING DRUGS

Alkalinizing and acidifying drugs are used to correct an acid-base imbalance in the blood. The acid-base imbalances are

- Metabolic acidosis—decrease in the blood pH caused by an excess of hydrogen ions in the extracellular fluid (treated with alkalinizing drugs)
- Metabolic alkalosis—increase in the blood pH caused by an excess of bicarbonate in the extracellular fluid (treated with acidifying drugs)

Alkalinizing Drug: Bicarbonate (HCO_3^-)

Action and Uses

Bicarbonate (HCO_3^-) plays a vital role in the acid-base balance of the body. Alkalinizing drugs are used to treat metabolic acidosis and to increase blood pH. Bicarbonate may be given IV as sodium bicarbonate ($NaHCO_3$) in the treatment of metabolic acidosis, a state of imbalance that may be seen in diseases or conditions such as severe shock, diabetic acidosis, severe diarrhea, extracorporeal circulation of blood, severe renal disease, and cardiac arrest. Oral sodium bicarbonate is used as a gastric and urinary alkalinizer. It may be used as a single drug or may be found as one of the ingredients in some antacid preparations. It is also useful in treating severe diarrhea accompanied by bicarbonate loss.

A low blood pH means the body is in an acidic condition, and a high blood pH indicates an alkaline condition. To raise the pH, an alkalinizing drug must be administered. Sodium bicarbonate, an alkalinizing drug, separates in the blood and the bicarbonate functions as a buffer to decrease the hydrogen ion concentration and raise the blood pH.

Adverse Reactions

In some instances, excessive oral use of bicarbonate may produce nausea and vomiting. Some individuals may use sodium bicarbonate (baking soda) for the relief of GI disturbances such as pain, discomfort, symptoms of indigestion, and gas. Prolonged use of oral sodium bicarbonate or excessive doses of IV sodium bicarbonate may result in systemic alkalosis.

Contraindications, Precautions, and Interactions

Bicarbonate is contraindicated in patients losing chloride by continuous GI suction or through vomiting, in patients with metabolic or respiratory alkalosis, hypocalcemia, renal failure, or severe abdominal pain of unknown cause, and in those on sodium-restricted diets.

Bicarbonate is used cautiously in patients with CHF or renal impairment and those receiving glucocorticoid therapy. Bicarbonate is a pregnancy category C drug and is used cautiously during pregnancy.

Oral administration of bicarbonate may decrease the absorption of ketoconazole. Increased blood levels of quinidine, flecainide, or sympathomimetics may occur when these agents are administered with bicarbonate. There is an increased risk of crystalluria when bicarbonate is administered with the fluoroquinolones. Possible decreased effects of lithium, methotrexate, chlorpropamide, salicylates, and tetracyclines may occur when these drugs are administered with sodium bicarbonate. Sodium bicarbonate is not administered within 2 hours of enteric-coated drugs because the protective enteric coating may disintegrate before the drug reaches the intestine.

Acidifying Drug: Ammonium Chloride

Actions and Uses

Ammonium chloride lowers the blood pH by being metabolized first into urea, then to hydrochloric acid, which is further metabolized to hydrogen ions to acidify the blood.

Adverse Reactions and Interactions

Adverse reactions to ammonium chloride include metabolic acidosis and loss of electrolytes, especially potassium. Use of ammonium chloride and spironolactone may increase systemic acidosis.

NURSING PROCESS

The Patient Receiving an Electrolyte

ASSESSMENT

PREADMINISTRATION ASSESSMENT

Before administering any electrolyte, electrolyte salt, or a combined electrolyte solution, the nurse assesses the patient for signs of an electrolyte imbalance (see Display 58-2). All recent laboratory and diagnostic tests appropriate to the imbalance are reviewed. The nurse obtains vital signs to provide a database.

ONGOING ASSESSMENT

During therapy, the nurse periodically obtains (daily or more frequently) serum electrolyte or bicarbonate studies to monitor therapy.

CALCIUM Before, during, and after the administration of IV calcium, the nurse monitors the blood pressure, pulse, and respiratory rate every 30 minutes until the patient's condition has stabilized. After administration of calcium, the nurse observes the patient for signs of hypercalcemia (see Display 58-2).

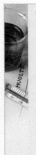

> ### Nursing Alert
>
> Systemic overloading of calcium ions in the systemic circulation results in acute hypercalcemic syndrome. Symptoms of hypercalcemic syndrome include elevated plasma calcium, weakness, lethargy, severe nausea and vomiting, coma, and, if left untreated, death. The nurse reports any signs of hypercalcemic syndrome immediately to the primary health care provider.

To combat hypercalcemic syndrome, the primary health care provider may prescribe IV sodium chloride and a potent diuretic, such as furosemide. When used together, these two drugs markedly increase calcium renal clearance and reduce hypercalcemia.

POTASSIUM Patients receiving oral potassium should have their blood pressure and pulse monitored every 4 hours, especially during early therapy. The nurse also observes the patient for signs of hyperkalemia (see Display 58-2), which would indicate that the dose of potassium is too high. Signs of hypokalemia may also occur during therapy and may indicate that the dose of potassium is too low and must be increased. If signs of hypokalemia or hyperkalemia are apparent or suspected, the nurse notifies the primary health care provider. In some instances, frequent laboratory monitoring of the serum potassium may be ordered.

The nurse inspects the IV needle site every 30 minutes for signs of extravasation. Potassium is irritating to the tissues. If extravasation occurs, the nurse discontinues the IV immediately and notifies the primary health care provider. The acutely ill patient and the patient with severe hypokalemia require monitoring of the blood pressure and pulse rate every 15 to 30 minutes during the IV infusion. The nurse measures the intake and output every 8 hours. The infusion rate is slowed to keep the vein open, and the primary health care provider is notified if an irregular pulse is noted.

MAGNESIUM When magnesium sulfate is ordered to treat convulsions or severe hypomagnesemia, the patient requires constant observation. The nurse obtains the patient's blood pressure, pulse, and respiratory rate immediately before the drug is administered, as well as every 5 to 10 minutes during the time of IV infusion or place the patient on a device for continuous monitoring. The nurse continues monitoring these vital signs at frequent intervals until the patient's condition has stabilized. Because magnesium is eliminated by the kidneys, it is used with caution in patients with renal impairment. The nurse monitors the urine output to verify an output of at least 100 mL every 4 hours. Voiding less than 100 mL of urine every 4 hours is reported to the primary health care provider.

SODIUM When NaCl is administered by IV infusion, the nurse observes the patient during and after administration for signs of hypernatremia (see Display 58-2). The nurse checks the rate of IV infusion as ordered by the primary health care provider, usually every 15 to 30 minutes. More frequent monitoring of the infusion rate may be necessary when the patient is restless or confused. To minimize venous irritation during administration of sodium or any electrolyte solution, the nurse uses a small-bore needle placed well within the lumen of a large vein.

Patients receiving a 3% or 5% NaCl solution by IV infusion are observed closely for signs of pulmonary edema (i.e., dyspnea, cough, restlessness, bradycardia). If any one or more of these symptoms occurs, the IV infusion is slowed to keep the vein open and the primary health care provider is contacted immediately. Patients receiving NaCl by the IV route have their intake and output measured every 8 hours. The nurse observes the patient for signs of hypernatremia every 3 to 4 hours and contacts the primary health care provider if this condition is suspected.

BICARBONATE When given in the treatment of metabolic acidosis, the drug may be added to the IV fluid or given as a prepared IV sodium bicarbonate solution. Frequent laboratory monitoring of the blood pH and blood gases is usually ordered because dosage and length of therapy depend on test results. The nurse frequently observes the patient for signs of clinical improvement and monitors the blood pressure, pulse, and respiratory rate every 15 to 30 minutes or as ordered by the primary health care provider. Extravasation of the drug requires selection of another needle site because the drug is irritating to the tissues.

NURSING DIAGNOSES

Drug-specific nursing diagnoses are highlighted in the Nursing Diagnoses Checklist. Other nursing diagnoses applicable to these drugs are discussed in depth in Chapter 4.

Nursing Diagnoses Checklist

✓ **Imbalanced Nutrition: Less Than Body Requirements** related to adverse drug reaction (nausea, vomiting)

✓ **Risk for Injury** related to adverse drug effects (muscular weakness)

✓ **Disturbed Thought Processes** related to adverse drug effects

✓ **Risk for Decreased Cardiac Output** related to adverse drug effects (cardiac arrhythmias)

PLANNING

The expected outcomes of the patient depend on the specific drug, dose, route of administration, and reason for administration of an electrolyte, but may include an optimal response to therapy, compliance with the prescribed therapeutic regimen, and an understanding of the drug regimen and adverse drug effects.

IMPLEMENTATION

PROMOTING AN OPTIMAL RESPONSE TO THERAPY

In some situations, electrolytes are administered when an electrolyte imbalance may potentially occur. For example, the patient with nasogastric suction is prescribed one or more electrolytes added to an IV solution, such as 5% dextrose or a combined electrolyte solution, to be given IV to make up for the electrolytes that are lost through nasogastric suction. In other instances, electrolytes are given to replace those already lost, such as the patient admitted to the hospital with severe vomiting and diarrhea of several days' duration.

When electrolytes are administered parenterally, the dosage is expressed in milliequivalents (mEq)—for example, calcium gluconate 7 mEq IV. When administered orally, sodium bicarbonate, calcium, and magnesium

dosages are expressed in milligrams (mg). Potassium liquids and effervescent tablet dosages are expressed in milliequivalents; capsule or tablet dosages may be expressed as milliequivalents or milligrams.

Electrolyte disturbances can cause varying degrees of confusion, muscular weakness, nausea, vomiting, and cardiac irregularities (see Display 58-2 for specific symptoms). Serum electrolyte blood levels have a very narrow therapeutic range. Careful monitoring is needed to determine if blood levels fall above or below normal. Normal values may vary with the laboratory, but a general range of normal values for each electrolyte is found in Display 58-2. Adverse reactions are usually controlled by maintaining blood levels of the various electrolytes within the normal range.

ADMINISTERING CALCIUM When calcium is administered IV, the solution is warmed to body temperature immediately before administration, and the drug is administered slowly. In some clinical situations, the primary health care provider may order cardiac monitoring because additional drug administration may be determined by electrocardiographic changes.

ADMINISTERING POTASSIUM When given orally, potassium may cause GI distress. Therefore, it is given immediately after meals or with food and a full glass of water. Oral potassium must not be crushed or chewed. If the patient has difficulty swallowing, the nurse consults the primary health care provider regarding the use of a solution or an effervescent tablet, which fizzes and dissolves on contact with water. Potassium in the form of effervescent tablets, powder, or liquid must be thoroughly mixed with 4 to 8 oz of cold water, juice, or other beverage. Effervescent tablets must stop fizzing before the solution is sipped slowly during a period of 5 to 15 minutes. Oral liquids and soluble powders that have been mixed and dissolved in cold water or juice are also sipped slowly over a period of 5 to 15 minutes. The nurse advises patients that liquid potassium solutions have a salty taste. Some of these products are flavored to make the solution more palatable.

The primary health care provider orders the dose of the potassium salt (in milliequivalents) and the amount and type of IV solution, as well as the interval during which the solution is to be infused. After the drug is added to the IV container, the container is gently rotated to ensure mixture of the solution. A large vein is used for administration; the veins on the back of the hand should be avoided. An IV containing potassium should infuse in no less than 3 to 4 hours. This necessitates frequent monitoring of the IV infusion rate, even when an IV infusion pump is used.

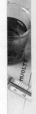

Nursing Alert

Concentrated potassium solutions are for IV mixtures only and should never be used undiluted. Direct IV injection of potassium could result in sudden death. When potassium is given IV, it is always diluted in 500 to 1000 mL of an IV solution. The maximum recommended concentration of potassium is 80 mEq in 1000 mL of IV solution (although in acute emergency situations a higher concentration of potassium may be required).

ADMINISTERING MAGNESIUM Magnesium sulfate may be ordered intramuscularly (IM), IV, or by IV infusion diluted in a specified type and amount of IV solution. When ordered to be given IM, this drug is given undiluted as a 50% solution for adults and a 20% solution for children. Magnesium sulfate is given deep IM in a large muscle mass, such as the gluteus muscle.

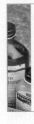

Gerontologic Alert

Older adults may need a reduced dosage of magnesium because of decreased renal function. The nurse should closely monitor serum magnesium levels when magnesium is administered to older adults.

The nurse observes the patient for early signs of hypermagnesemia (see Display 58-2) and contacts the primary health care provider immediately if this imbalance is suspected. Frequent plasma magnesium levels are usually ordered. The nurse notifies the primary health care provider if the magnesium level is higher or lower than the normal range.

Nursing Alert

As plasma magnesium levels rise above 4 mEq/L, the deep tendon reflexes are first decreased and then disappear as the plasma levels reach 10 mEq/L. The knee jerk reflex is tested before each dose of magnesium sulfate. If the reflex is absent or a slow response is obtained, the nurse withholds the dosage and notifies the primary health care provider. IV calcium is kept available to reverse the respiratory depression and heart block that may occur with magnesium overdose.

ADMINISTERING BICARBONATE The nurse gives oral sodium bicarbonate tablets with a full glass of water; the powdered form is dissolved in a full glass of water. If oral sodium bicarbonate is used to alkalinize the urine, the nurse checks the urine pH two or three times a day or as ordered by the primary health care provider. If the urine remains acidic, the nurse notifies the primary health care provider because an increase in the dose of the drug may be necessary. IV sodium bicarbonate is given in emergency situations, such as metabolic acidosis or certain types of drug overdose, when alkalinization of the urine is necessary to hasten drug elimination.

MONITORING AND MANAGING PATIENT NEEDS

When electrolyte solutions are administered, adverse reactions are most often related to overdose. Correcting the imbalance by decreasing the dosage or discontinuing the solution usually works, and the adverse reactions subside quickly. Frequent serum electrolyte levels are used to monitor blood levels.

IMBALANCED NUTRITION: LESS THAN BODY REQUIREMENTS Electrolyte imbalances may cause nausea, vomiting, and other GI disturbances. If GI disturbances occur from oral administration, taking the drug with meals may decrease the nausea. Offering smaller, more frequent meals may help to stabilize nutritional status. Correcting the electrolyte imbalance usually solves the problem of nausea and vomiting.

RISK FOR INJURY The patient is at increased risk of falling because of weakness or muscular cramping. Frequent observation and quickly answering the call light helps to maintain the patient's safety. If weakness or muscular cramping occurs, the nurse assists the patient when ambulating to prevent falls or other injury.

DISTURBED THOUGHT PROCESSES The patient with an electrolyte imbalance may be confused or disoriented. The nurse approaches the patient in a calm and nurturing manner. The nurse gently reorients the individual and explains any procedures carefully before performing any procedures with the patient. The nurse reassures the patient that these symptoms are part of the imbalance but can recede as the imbalance improves (if applicable).

RISK FOR DECREASED CARDIAC OUTPUT Some electrolytes may cause cardiac irregularities. The nurse checks the pulse rate at regular intervals, usually every 4 hours or more often if an irregularity in the heart rate is observed. Depending on the patient's condition, cardiac monitoring may be indicated when administering the electrolytes (particularly when administering potassium or calcium). For example, if potassium is administered to a patient with cardiac disease, a cardiac monitor is needed to monitor the heart rate and rhythm continuously during therapy.

Nursing Alert

Mild (5.5 to 6.5 mEq/L) to moderate (6.5 to 8 mEq/L) potassium blood level increases may be asymptomatic and manifested only by increased serum potassium concentrations and characteristic electrocardiographic changes, such as disappearance of P waves or spreading (widening) of the QRS complex.

EDUCATING THE PATIENT AND FAMILY

To ensure accurate compliance with the prescribed drug regimen, the nurse carefully explains the dose and time intervals to the patient or a family member. Because overdose (which can be serious) may occur if the patient does not adhere to the prescribed dosage and schedule, it is most important that the patient completely understands how much and when to take the drug. The nurse stresses the importance of adhering to the prescribed dosage schedule during patient teaching.

The primary health care provider may order periodic laboratory and diagnostic tests for some patients receiving oral electrolytes. The nurse encourages the patient to keep all appointments for these tests, as well as primary health care provider or clinic visits. Persons with a history of using sodium bicarbonate (baking soda) as an antacid are warned that overuse can result in alkalosis and could disguise a more serious problem. Those with a history of using salt tablets (NaCl) are advised not to do so during hot weather unless it is recommended by a primary health care provider. Excessive use of salt tablets can result in a serious electrolyte imbalance.

The nurse includes the following points for specific electrolytes in a patient teaching plan:

CALCIUM

- Contact the primary health care provider if the following occur: nausea, vomiting, anorexia, constipation, abdominal pain, dry mouth, thirst, or polyuria (symptoms of hypercalcemia).
- Do not exceed the dosage recommendations.
- Take oral calcium with a full glass of water.
- The following substances interfere with calcium absorption: rhubarb and spinach (contain oxalic acid), bran and whole-grain cereals, and dairy products. Avoid taking calcium with these products.
- Take oral calcium 1 to 1.5 hours after meals if GI upset occurs.

POTASSIUM

- Take the drug exactly as directed on the prescription container. Do not increase, decrease, or omit doses of the drug unless advised to do so by the primary health care provider.
- Take the drug immediately after meals or with food and a full glass of water.
- Avoid the use of nonprescription drugs and salt substitutes (many contain potassium) unless use of a specific drug or product has been approved by the primary health care provider.
- Contact the primary health care provider if tingling of the hands or feet, a feeling of heaviness in the legs, vomiting, nausea, abdominal pain, or black stools occur.
- If the tablet has an enteric coating, swallow it whole. Do not chew or crush the tablet.
- If effervescent tablets are prescribed, place the tablet in 4 to 8 oz of cold water or juice. Wait until the fizzing stops before drinking. Sip the liquid during a period of 5 to 10 minutes.
- If an oral liquid or a powder is prescribed, add the dose to 4 to 8 oz of cold water or juice and sip slowly during a period of 5 to 10 minutes. Measure the dose accurately.

MAGNESIUM

- Do not take oral magnesium when abdominal pain, nausea, or vomiting is present. If diarrhea and abdominal cramping occur, discontinue the drug.

EVALUATION

- The therapeutic effect of the drug is achieved.
- The patient complies with the prescribed drug regimen.
- The patient and family demonstrate an understanding of the drug regimen.
- The patient verbalizes the importance of complying with the prescribed therapeutic regimen.

TOTAL PARENTERAL NUTRITION

When normal enteral feeding in not possible or is inadequate to meet an individual's nutritional needs, IV nutritional therapy or **total parenteral nutrition** (TPN) is required. TPN is a method of administering nutrients to the body by an IV route. TPN is a very complex admixture of chemicals combined in a single container. The components of the TPN mixture may include proteins (amino acids), fats, glucose, electrolytes, vitamins, minerals, and sterile water. Products used to meet the IV nutritional requirements of the patient include protein substrates (amino acids), energy substrates (dextrose and fat emulsions), fluids, electrolytes, and trace minerals.

Total parenteral nutrition is used to prevent nitrogen and weight loss or to treat negative nitrogen balance (a situation in which more nitrogen is used by the body than is taken in) in the following situations:

- The oral, gastrostomy, or jejunostomy route cannot or should not be used.

- GI absorption of protein is impaired by obstruction.

- Inflammatory disease or antineoplastic therapy prevents normal GI functioning.

- Bowel rest is needed (e.g., after bowel surgery).

- Metabolic requirements for protein are significantly increased (e.g., in hypermetabolic states such as serious burns, infections, or trauma).

- Morbidity and mortality may be reduced by replacing amino acids lost from tissue breakdown (e.g., renal failure).

- Tube feeding alone cannot provide adequate nutrition.

If a patient's intake of protein nutrients is significantly less than is required by the body to meet energy expenditures, a state of negative nitrogen balance occurs. The body begins to convert protein from the muscle into carbohydrate for energy to be used by the body. This results in weight loss and muscle wasting. In these situations, traditional IV fluids do not provide sufficient calories or nitrogen to meet the body's daily requirements. TPN may be administered through a peripheral vein or a central venous catheter in a highly concentrated form to improve nutritional status, establish a positive nitrogen balance, and enhance the healing process. Peripheral TPN is used for relatively short periods (no more than 5 to 7 days) and when the central venous route is not possible or necessary. An example of a solution used in TPN is amino acids with electrolytes. These solutions may be used alone or combined with dextrose (5% or 10%) solutions.

Total parenteral nutrition through a central vein is indicated to promote protein synthesis in patients who are severely hypercatabolic or severely depleted of nutrients, or who require long-term parenteral nutrition. For example, amino acids combined with hypertonic dextrose and IV fat emulsions are infused through a central venous catheter to promote protein synthesis. Vitamins, trace minerals, and electrolytes may be added to the TPN mixture to meet the patient's individual needs. The daily dose depends on the patient's daily protein requirement and his or her metabolic state and clinical responses.

The preferred method of delivering TPN is with an infusion pump. The pump infuses a small amount (0.1 to 10 mL/h) continuously to keep the vein open. Feeding schedules vary; one example is administration of the feeding continuously over a few hours, leveling off the rate for several hours, and then increasing the rate of administration for several hours to simulate a normal set of meal times.

Nursing Alert

Hyperglycemia is a common metabolic complication. A too-rapid infusion of amino acid–carbohydrate mixtures may result in hyperglycemia, glycosuria, mental confusion, and loss of consciousness. Blood glucose levels may be assessed every 4 to 6 hours to monitor for hyperglycemia and guide the dosage of dextrose and insulin (if required). To minimize these complications, the primary health care provider may decrease the rate of administration, reduce the dextrose concentration, or administer insulin.

To prevent a rebound hypoglycemic reaction from the sudden withdrawal of TPN containing a concentrated dose of dextrose, the rate of administration is slowly reduced or the concentration of dextrose gradually decreased. If TPN must be abruptly withdrawn, a solution of 5% or 10% dextrose is begun to reduce gradually the amount of dextrose administered. The primary health care provider is notified if the patient exhibits symptoms of hypoglycemia, including weakness, tremors, diaphoresis, headache, hunger, and apprehension. Other complications of TPN include bacterial infection, sepsis, embolism, metabolic problems, and hemothorax or pneumothorax.

Critical Thinking Exercises

1. Ms. Land is receiving 20 mEq of potassium chloride (KCl) added to 1000 mL of 5% dextrose and water. Discuss preadministration and ongoing assessments you would make while her IV is infusing.

2. Mr. Kendall is prescribed an oral potassium chloride liquid. Discuss the instructions you should give to Mr. Kendall regarding preparing and taking the drug.

3. Ms. Hartsel is to receive an IV fat emulsion. Discuss special precautions the nurse should take when administering the solution.

Review Questions

1. Which of the following is a symptom of fluid over-load?

   A. Tinnitus

   B. Hypotension

   C. Decreased body temperature

   D. Behavioral changes

2. Which of the following symptoms would indicate hypocalcemia?

   A. Tetany

   B. Constipation

   C. Muscle weakness

   D. Hypertension

3. Which of the following potassium plasma concentration laboratory results would the nurse report immediately to the physician?

   A. 3.5 mEq/L

   B. 4.0 mEq/L

   C. 4.5 mEq/L

   D. 5.5 mEq/mL

4. Which of the following symptoms would most likely indicate hypernatremia?

   A. Fever, increased thirst

   B. Cold, clammy skin

   C. Decreased skin turgor

   D. Hypotension

5. Which of the following is a common metabolic complication of TPN?

   A. Hypomagnesemia

   B. Hypermagnesemia

   C. Hypoglycemia

   D. Hyperglycemia

Medication Dosage Problems

1. Mr. Parker is to receive 1000 mL of 5% dextrose and water during a period of 10 hours. Calculate how many milliliters should be infused each hour (see Chapter 3 for additional information on calculation).

2. The patient is prescribed potassium 40 mEq orally. The drug is available from the pharmacy in a solution of 20 mEq/15mL. The nurse administers _____.

To check your answers, see Appendix G.

Fluids and Electrolytes

Glossary

A

abstinence syndrome: symptoms that occur if a drug causing physical or psychological dependence is suddenly discontinued

acetylcholine: neurotransmitter that transmits impulses across the parasympathetic branch of the autonomic nervous system

acetylcholinesterase: enzyme that can inactivate the neurotransmitter acetylcholine

achalasia: failure to relax; usually referring to the smooth muscle fibers of the gastrointestinal tract, especially failure of the lower esophagus to relax, causing difficulty swallowing and a feeling of fullness in the sternal region

action potential: electrical impulse that passes from cell to cell in the myocardium of the heart and stimulates the fibers to shorten, causing heart muscle to contract

active immunity: type of immunity that occurs when the person is exposed to a disease and develops the disease, and the body makes antibodies to provide future protection against the disease

acute pain: pain with duration of fewer than 6 months

addiction: a compulsive desire or craving to use a drug or chemical with a resultant physical dependence

additive drug reaction: the combined effect of two drugs equals the sum of the effects of each drug given alone

adjunctive treatment: therapy used in addition to the primary treatment

adrenal insufficiency: deficiency in corticosteroids

adrenergic: pertaining to the sympathetic branch of the nervous system, which controls heart rate, breathing rate, and ability to divert blood to the skeletal muscles

adrenergic drug: a drug that acts like or mimics the actions of the sympathetic nervous system

adverse reaction: undesirable drug effect

aerobic: organisms that require oxygen to live

affective domain: in regard to patient teaching, the patient's or caregiver's attitudes, feelings, beliefs, and opinions

afferent nerve fiber: a sensory nerve that carries an impulse toward the brain

aggregation: clumping of blood elements

agonist: drug that binds with a receptor to produce a therapeutic response

agonist-antagonist: drug with both agonist and antagonist properties

agranulocytosis: a decrease or lack of granulocytes (a type of white blood cell)

akathisia: extreme restlessness and increased motor activity

alanine aminotransferase: liver enzyme

aldosterone: hormone secreted by the adrenal cortex and contributing to a rise in blood pressure

allergic reaction: adverse effects, such as itching, hives, swelling, difficulty breathing; see *hypersensitivity*; see also *anaphylactic shock*

alopecia: abnormal loss of hair; baldness

alpha-adrenergic blocking drugs: drugs use to block neurotransmission in the sympathetic nervous system

alpha/beta-adrenergic blocking drugs: drugs that block both alpha- and beta-adrenergic receptors

Alzheimer's disease: progressive disorder that affects cognition, emotion, and movement

amebiasis: invasion by single-cell parasites

amenorrhea: absence or suppression of menstruation

anabolism: tissue-building process

anaerobic: organisms that do not require oxygen to live

analeptics: drugs that stimulate respiratory center of the brain

analgesia: absence of pain

analgesic: a drug that relieves pain

analysis: using data to determine patient need or nursing diagnosis

anaphylactic shock (also called *anaphylactic* reaction or *anaphylactoid reaction*): a sudden, severe hypersensitivity reaction with symptoms that progress rapidly and may result in death if not treated

anaphylactoid reactions: unusual or exaggerated allergic reactions; see *anaphylactic shock*

androgen: male hormone, testosterone and its derivatives

anemia: a decrease in the number of red blood cells and hemoglobin value below normal

anesthesia: loss of feeling or sensation

anesthesiologist: a physician with special training in administering anesthesia

anesthetist: a nurse with special training who administers anesthesia; also called *nurse anesthetist*

angina (angina pectoris): acute pain in the chest resulting from decreased blood supply to the heart muscle

angioedema: localized wheals or swellings in subcutaneous tissues or mucous membranes, which may be due to an allergic response; also called *angioneurotic edema*

angiotensin vasopressor: produced when renin is released from the kidney

anhedonia: finding no pleasure in activities

anorexia: loss of appetite

anorexiants: drugs used to suppress the appetite

antagonist: drugs that join with a receptor to prevent the action of an agonist

anthelmintic: a drug used to treat helminthiasis (worms)

antiadrenergic drugs: see *adrenergic blocking drugs*; also called *sympatholytic drugs*

antianxiety drugs: drugs that diminish anxious feelings

antibacterial: active against bacteria

antibody: molecule with the ability to bind to a specific antigen; responsible for the immune response

anticholinergic effects: blockage of parasympathetic nervous system

anticholinergics: see *cholinergic blocking drugs*; also called *cholinergic blockers* or *parasympatholytic drugs*

anticonvulsants: drugs used to manage seizure disorders

antiemetic: drug used to treat or prevent nausea

antiflatulents: drugs that work against flatus (gas)

antigen: substance that is capable of inducing a specific immune response

antigen–antibody response: antibodies formed in response to exposure to a specific antigen

antihistamine: drug used to counteract the effects of histamine on body organs and structures

anti-infective: a drug used to treat infection

antineoplastic: a drug used to treat neoplasia (cancer)

antipyretic: fever-reducing agent

antipsoriatics: drugs used to treat psoriasis

antiseptic: an agent that stops, slows, or prevents the growth of microorganisms

antitussive: drug used to relieve coughing

anuria: cessation of urine production

anxiety: feelings of apprehension, worry, or uneasiness

anxiolytics: drugs used to treat anxiety

aplastic anemia: a blood disorder caused by damage to the bone marrow resulting in a marked reduction in the number of red blood cells and some white blood cells

apothecaries' system: old system of measure developed for use by pharmacists (apothecaries)

arrhythmia: abnormal heart rate or rhythm; also called *dysrhythmia*

assessment: the collection of subjective and objective data

asthenia: weakness; loss of strength

asthma: respiratory disorder characterized by bronchospasm and difficulty in breathing, especially exhaling

ataxia: unsteady gait; muscular incoordination

atherosclerosis: a disease characterized by deposits of fatty plaques on the inner walls of arteries

atrial fibrillation: quivering of the atria of the heart

attention deficit hyperactivity disorder (ADHD): disorder characterized by inattention, hyperactivity, and impulsivity

attenuate: weaken

aura: sense preceding a sudden attack or convulsion

auscultation: the process of listening for sounds within the body

autonomic nervous system: a division of the peripheral nervous system concerned with functions essential to the life of the organism and not consciously controlled (e.g., blood pressure, heart rate, gastrointestinal activity)

azotemia: retention of excessive amounts of nitrogenous compounds in the blood caused by failure of the kidney to remove urea from the blood

B

bacterial resistance: phenomenon by which a bacteria-produced substance inactivates or destroys an antibiotic drug

bactericidal: a drug or agent that destroys or kills bacteria

bacteriostatic: a drug or agent that slows or retards the multiplication of bacteria

beta-adrenergic blocking drugs: drugs that decrease stimulation of the sympathetic nervous system on certain tissues in order to decrease heart rate and cardiac workload and dilate blood vessels; also called *beta blockers*

beta-lactam ring: portion of the penicillin drug molecule

bigeminy: an irregular pulse rate consisting or two beats followed by a pause before the next paired beats

biliary colic: pain caused by the pressure of passing gallstones

bile acid sequestrants: drugs used to treat hyperlipidemia and pruritus associated with partial biliary obstruction

biotransformation: the process by which the body changes a drug to a more or less active form that can be excreted

bipolar disorder: mental health disorder characterized by severe mood swings from extreme hyperactivity to depression

blepharospasm: a twitching or spasm of the eyelid

blood–brain barrier: ability of the nervous system to prohibit large and potentially harmful molecules from crossing from the blood into the brain

blood dyscrasias: abnormality of blood cell structure

blood pressure: the force of blood against artery walls

bone marrow suppression: a decreased production of all blood cells

booster: an immunogen injected after a specified interval; often after the primary immunization to stimulate and sustain the immune response

botanical medicine: type of complementary/alternative therapy that uses plants or herbs to treat various disorders; also called *herbal therapy*

bowel preparation: treatment protocol to cleanse the bowel of bacteria before surgery or other procedures

brachial plexus: a network of spinal nerves affecting the arm, forearm, and hand

brachial plexus block: type of regional anesthesia produced by injection of a local anesthetic into the brachial plexus

bradycardia: slow heart rate, usually below 60 beats per minute

bradykinesia: slow movement

broad spectrum: describes an antibiotic that affects a large number of different strains of bacteria

bronchodilator: drug that dilates the bronchioles of the lung to ease breathing

bronchospasm: spasm or constriction of the bronchi resulting in difficulty breathing

buccal: space in the mouth between the gum and the cheek in either the upper or lower jaw

bulla: blister or skin vesicle filled with fluid

bursa: padlike sac found in connecting tissue, usually located in the joint area

C

cachectic: malnourished, in poor health, physically wasted

candidiasis: infection of the skin or mucous membrane with the yeast *Candida albicans*

cardiac arrhythmia: abnormal rhythm of the heart

cardiac glycosides: cardiotonic drugs derived from the leaves of digitalis plants

cardiac output: volume of blood discharged from the left or right ventricle per minute

catabolism: tissue-depleting process

catalyst: substance that accelerates a chemical reaction without itself undergoing a change

cell cycle nonspecific: pertaining to a drug used in cancer treatment, effective in any phase of cell division

cell cycle specific: pertaining to a drug used in cancer treatment, affecting a specific phase of cell division

cell-mediated immunity: immune reaction caused by white blood cells

Celsius (C): temperature scale, synonymous with *centigrade*, in which water freezes at 0° and boils at 100°

centigrade: scale of temperature, synonymous with *Celsius*

central nervous system: one of two main divisions of the nervous system, consisting of the brain and spinal cord

cerumen: ear wax

cervical mucorrhea: increased cervical discharge

cheilosis: cracking of the edges of the lips

chelating agent: a substance that selectively and chemically binds the ion of a metal to itself, thus aiding in the elimination of the metallic ion from the body

chemoreceptor trigger zone: a group of nerve fibers located on the surface of the fourth ventricle of the brain that, when stimulated, results in vomiting

chemotherapy: drug therapy with a chemical, often used when referring to treatment with an antineoplastic drug

cholesterol: a fatlike substance produced mostly in the liver of animals

cholinergic blocking drugs: affect the parasympathetic branch of the autonomic nervous system; also called *anticholinergics*

cholinergic crisis: cholinergic drug toxicity

chorea: continuous, rapid, jerky, involuntary movements

choreiform movements: involuntary muscular twitching of the limbs or facial muscles

chronic pain: a pain that lasts more than 6 months

chylomicrons: small particles of fat in the blood

cinchonism: quinidine toxicity or poisoning

circumoral: encircling the mouth

cognitive domain: intellectual activities such as thought, recall, decision making, and drawing conclusions

conduction block: type of regional anesthesia produced by injection of a local anesthetic drug into or near a nerve trunk

conjunctivitis: inflammation of the conjunctiva (mucous membrane lining the inner surfaces of the eye)

constipation: hardened fecal material that is difficult to pass

controlled substances: drugs that have the potential for abuse and dependency, both physical and psychological

convulsion: paroxysm (occurring suddenly) of involuntary muscular contractions and relaxations

corticosteroids: glucocorticoid and mineralocorticoid hormones

coughing: forceful expulsion of air from the lungs

Crohn's disease: inflammation of the terminal portion of the ileum

cross-allergenicity: allergy to drugs in the same or related groups

cross-sensitivity: see *cross-allergenicity*

cryptorchism: failure of the testes to descend into the scrotum

crystalluria: formation of crystals in the urine

culture and sensitivity test: culture of bacteria to determine to which antibiotic the microorganism is sensitive

cumulative drug effect: when the body is unable to metabolize and excrete one dose of a drug before the next is given

Cushing's syndrome: a disease caused by the overproduction of endogenous glucocorticoids

cyanosis: bluish, grayish, or dark purple discoloration of the skin due to abnormal amounts of reduced hemoglobin in the blood

cyclooxygenase: the enzyme responsible for prostaglandin synthesis

cyclooxygenase-1 (COX-1): enzyme that helps to maintain the stomach lining

cyclooxygenase-2 (COX-2): enzyme that triggers pain and inflammation

cycloplegia: paralysis of the ciliary muscle, resulting in an inability to focus the eye

cytomegalovirus (CMV): any of a group of herpes viruses infecting humans, monkeys, or rodents; the human CMV is found in the salivary glands and causes cytomegalic inclusion disease

cystinuria: presence of cystine, an amino acid, in urine

cystitis: inflammation of the bladder

D

debridement: removal of all foreign material and dead or damaged tissue from a wound or infected lesion

decaliter: 10 L or 10,000 mL

decimal: *in the metric system of measure,* a fraction in which the denominator is 10 or a power of 10

decimal fraction: number that falls to the right of the decimal point

decongestant: drug that reduces swelling of the nasal passages, which promotes drainage of the nasal sinuses

delirium tremens: signs and symptoms of withdrawal from a drug or chemical, including tremors, weakness, anxiety, restlessness, excessive perspiration, nausea, and vomiting

delusion: false belief that cannot be changed with reason

dementia: decrease in cognitive function

denominator: part of a fraction (the number under the line)

dependency: the compulsive need to use a substance repeatedly to achieve a pleasurable sensation or to avoid undesirable symptoms related to disuse of the substance

depolarization: movement of ions in a nerve cell from inside to outside and vice versa

depression: feeling sad, unhappy, down in the dumps, hopeless

dermis: a layer of skin immediately below the epidermis

diabetes insipidus: a disease caused by failure of the pituitary gland to secrete vasopressin or by surgical removal of the pituitary

diabetes mellitus: a disease caused by insufficient insulin production

diabetic ketoacidosis: life-threatening deficiency of insulin resulting in severe hyperglycemia and excessively high levels of ketones in the blood

diaphoresis: increased sweating or perspiration

diarrhea: loose, watery stool

digitalis glycosides: see *cardiac glycosides*

digitalis toxicity: toxic drug effects from administration of digoxin

digitalization: administration of digitalis at intervals to produce and maintain a therapeutic blood level

diluent: a fluid that dilutes

dimensional analysis: a method of calculating drug dosages based on fractions

diplopia: double vision

directly observed therapy (DOT): drug dose taken in front of the administrator

disulfiram-like: pertaining to a reaction, usually to alcohol, characterized by flushing, throbbing head, vomiting, sweating, chills, and hypotension

diuretic: drug that produces urine excretion

dividend: the number to be divided

divisor: the number that is divided into the dividend

dram: *in the apothecary system,* unit of measure equal to 60 grains

drug error: any event or activity that can cause a patient to receive the wrong dose, the wrong drug, a drug by the wrong route, or a drug given at the wrong time

drug idiosyncrasy: any unusual or abnormal response that differs from the response normally expected to a specific drug and dosage

drug tolerance: decreased response to a drug, requiring an increase in dosage to achieve the desired effect

dyscrasia: disease or disorder; abnormality

dyskinesia: impairment of voluntary movement

dyspepsia: fullness or epigastric discomfort

dysphoric: characterized by extreme or exaggerated sadness, anxiety, or unhappiness

dyspnea: labored or difficult breathing

dystonia: prolonged muscle contractions that may cause twisting and repetitive movements of abnormal posture

dysuria: painful or difficult urination

E

edema: accumulation of excess water in the body

efferent nerve fiber: carries nerve impulse away from brain

electrolyte: electrically charged substance essential to the normal functioning of all cells

embolus: thrombus that detaches from a blood vessel wall and travels through the bloodstream

emetic: drug that induces vomiting

endogenous: pertaining to something that normally occurs or is produced within the organism

enteric coating: special coating on drug that prevents absorption until drug reaches the small bowel

epidermis: outermost layer of the skin

epidural: outside or above the dura mater

epidural block: type of regional anesthesia produced by injection of a local anesthetic into the space surrounding the dura of the spinal cord

epilepsy: a permanent, recurring seizure disorder

epiphysis: a center of ossification (conversion of tissue to bone) at each extremity of long bone

epistaxis: nosebleed

ergotism: overdose of an ergot drug

erythema: marked reddening of skin; may be accompanied by warmth, pain, or blistering

erythrocytes: red blood cells; one of several formed elements in the blood

erythropoiesis: process of making red blood cells

Escherichia coli: a nonpathogenic colon bacillus; may cause infection outside the colon

essential hypertension: hypertension that has no known cause

estradiol: an endogenous estrogen

estriol: an endogenous estrogen

estrogens: female hormones

estrone: an endogenous estrogen

euthyroid: normal thyroid function

evaluation: a decision-making process determining the effectiveness of nursing actions or interventions

exacerbation: increase in severity

exfoliative dermatitis: reddish rash in which the erythema is followed by scaling

exogenous: pertaining to something that normally occurs or is produced outside of the organism or community

expected outcomes: define the expected behavior and physical and mental state of the patient after a therapeutic intervention

expectorant: drug that aids in raising thick, tenacious mucus from the respiratory tract

extended release: formulation in which drug is released over time

extrapulmonary: occurring outside of the lungs in the respiratory system

extrapyramidal syndrome: a group of adverse reactions involving the extrapyramidal portion of the nervous system causing abnormal muscle movements, especially akathisia and dystonia

extravasation: escape of fluid from a blood vessel into surrounding tissue

F

Fahrenheit (F): temperature scale in which water freezes at 32 degrees and boils at 212 degrees

fat soluble: dissolves in fat

febrile: related to fever (elevated body temperature)

feedback mechanism: method to control output

fibrolytic: a drug that dissolves clots already formed within blood vessel walls

first-dose effect: marked adverse reaction with the first dose

first-pass effect: action by which an oral drug is absorbed and carried directly to the liver, where it is inactivated by enzymes before it enters the general bloodstream

flattened affect: absence of emotion

fluid drams: units of volume in the apothecary system of measurement

fluid ounces: units of volume in the household system of measurement

fluid overload: condition in which the body's fluid requirements are met and the administration of fluid occurs at a rate that is greater than the rate at which the body can use or eliminate the fluid; also called *circulatory overload*

folinic acid rescue: *in chemotherapy,* the technique of administering leucovorin after a large dose of methotrexate, thereby allowing normal cells to survive; also called *leucovorin rescue*

fungicidal: deadly to fungi

fungistatic: pertaining to agents that retard growth of fungi

fungus: a single-cell, colorless plant that lacks chlorophyll, such as yeast or mold

G

gastric stasis: failure of the body to remove stomach contents normally

gastroesophageal reflux disease (GERD): reflux or backup of gastric contents into the esophagus

general anesthesia: sensation-free state of entire body

generalized seizure: loss of consciousness during seizure

germicide: an agent that kills bacteria

gingival hyperplasia: overgrowth of gum tissue

gingivitis: inflammation of the gums

glaucoma: a group of diseases of the eye characterized by increased intraocular pressure; results in changes within the eye, visual field defects, and eventually blindness (if left untreated)

globulins: plasma proteins that are insoluble in water

glossitis: inflammation of the tongue

glucagon: hormone secreted by the alpha cells of the pancreas that increases the concentration of glucose in the blood

glucocorticoid: hormone produced by adrenal gland

glucometer: device to monitor blood glucose level

glycosylated hemoglobin: blood test that monitors average blood glucose level over a 3- to 4-month period

goiter: enlargement of the thyroid gland causing a swelling in the front part of the neck, usually caused by a lack of iodine in the diet

gonadotropin: hormone that stimulates the sex glands (gonads)

gonads: glands responsible for sexual activity and characteristics

gout: uric acid accumulation in joints

grain: basic unit of mass measure in the apothecaries' system of measure

gram: mass metric measure equivalent to one thousandth of a kilogram

granulocytopenia: a reduction or decrease in the number of granulocytes (a type of white blood cell)

gynecomastia: male breast enlargement

H

HAART: highly active antiretroviral therapy; multiple drugs used together for treatment of HIV infection

habituation: continual use of a drug for the desired effect with no physical, but some psychological, dependence

half-life: the time required for the body to eliminate 50% of a drug

half-normal saline: solution containing 0.45% sodium chloride (salt) and water

hallucination: false perception of reality

hallucinogen: drug capable of producing a state of delirium characterized by visual or sensory disturbances

heart failure: a condition in which the heart cannot pump enough blood to meet the tissue needs of the body

Helicobacter pylori: stomach bacterium that causes peptic ulcer

helminthiasis: invasion by helminths (worms)

hematuria: blood in the urine

hemolysis: destruction of red blood cells

hemolytic anemia: disorder characterized by chronic premature destruction of red blood cells

hemostasis: complex process by which fibrin forms and blood clots

heparin lock: equipment consisting of an adapter and tubing introduced into a vein to maintain access to circulation

hepatic coma: coma induced by liver disease

herb: plant used as medicine or food seasoning

high-density lipoproteins (HDL): macromolecules that carry cholesterol from the body cells to the liver to be excreted

highly active antiretroviral therapy: see HAART

hirsutism: excessive growth of hair or hair growth in unusual places, usually in women

histamine: a substance found in various parts of the body (i.e., liver, lungs, intestines, skin) and produced from the animo acid histidine in response to injury to trigger the inflammatory response

HMG-CoA reductase inhibitors: drugs that inhibit the manufacture or promote breakdown of cholesterol

household measurement: system of measure based on household utensils, such as teaspoons and cups

humoral immunity: antibody-mediated immune response of the body

hydrochloric acid (HCl): stomach acid that aids in digestion

hyperglycemia: high blood glucose (sugar) level

hyperinsulinism: elevated levels of insulin in the body

hyperkalemia: increase in potassium levels in the blood

hyperlipidemia: an increase in the lipids in the blood

hypersecretory: characterized by excessive secretion of a substance

hypersensitivity: allergic reaction to a drug or other substance

hyperstimulation syndrome: sudden ovarian enlargement caused by overstimulation

hypertension: high blood pressure

hypertensive emergency: extremely high blood pressure that must be lowered immediately to prevent damage to target organs (i.e., heart, kidneys, eyes)

hyperthyroidism: overactive thyroid function

hypnotic: drug that induces sleep

hypocalcemia: low blood calcium level

hypoglycemia: low blood glucose (sugar) level

hypoinsulinism: low levels of insulin in the body

hypokalemia: low blood potassium level

hyponatremia: low blood sodium level

hypotension: abnormally low blood pressure

hypotension, orthostatic: a decrease in blood pressure occurring after standing in one place for an extended period

hypotension, postural: a decrease in blood pressure after a sudden change in body position

hypothyroidism: underactive thyroid function

hypoxia: inadequate oxygen at the cellular level

I

idiosyncrasy: unusual or abnormal drug response

immune globulin: solution obtained from human or animal blood containing antibodies that have been formed by the body to specific antigens; administered to provide passive immunity to one or more infectious diseases

immune suppressed: state in which number or activity of cells of the immune system is reduced

immunity: resistance to infection

immunocompromised: having an immune system incapable of fighting infection

implementation: the carrying out of a plan of action

improper fraction: fraction having a numerator that is the same as or larger than the denominator (e.g., 6/3)

independent nursing actions: actions that do not require a physician's orders

infiltration: the collection of fluid into tissue

inflammatory bowel disease: inflammation of the bowel (e.g., Crohn's disease and ulcerative colitis)

inhalation: drug administration route in which the patient inhales the drug orally or nasally

initial assessment: gathering of baseline data

inotropic: affecting the force of muscular contractions

insulin: hormone secreted by the pancreas; necessary for the metabolism of carbohydrates and fats (conversion of glucose to glycogen to regulate blood glucose level)

intermittent claudication: group of symptoms characterized by pain in the calf muscle of one or both legs, caused by walking and relieved by rest

intradermal: pertaining to the area within the upper layers of the skin

intramuscular: area within a muscle

intraocular pressure: the pressure within the eye

intravenous: area within a vein

intrinsic factor: substance produced by the cells in the stomach and necessary for the absorption of vitamin B_{12}

iritis: inflammation of the ocular iris

iron deficiency anemia: condition resulting when the body does not have enough iron to meet its need for iron

isolated systolic hypertension: systolic blood pressure over 140 mm Hg with diastolic blood pressure under 90 mm Hg

J

jaundice: yellow discoloration of the skin

K

keratolytic: an agent that removes excessive growth of the epidermis (top layer of skin)

ketoacidosis: a type of metabolic acidosis caused by an accumulation of ketone bodies in the blood

ketonuria: presence of ketones in the blood

L

laryngospasm: spasm of the larynx resulting in dyspnea and noisy respirations

learning: acquisition of new knowledge or skills; outcome of learning is change in behavior, thinking, or both

left ventricular dysfunction: a condition characterized by shortness of breath and moist cough in heart failure

leprosy: a chronic, communicable disease cause by *Mycobacterium leprae*; also called *Hansen's disease*

lethargic: sluggish, difficult to rouse

leucovorin rescue: see *folinic acid rescue*

leukopenia: a decrease in the number of leukocytes (white blood cells)

leukotriene: bronchoconstrictive substances released by the body during the inflammatory process

lipids: a group of fats or fatlike substances

lipodystrophy: atrophy of subcutaneous fat

lipoprotein: macromolecule consisting of lipid (fat) and protein; how fats are transported in the blood

liter: metric measure of volume, roughly equivalent to a quart in household measure

local anesthesia: provision of a pain-free state in a specific body area

low-density lipoproteins (LDL): macromolecules that carry cholesterol from the liver to the body cells

lumen: inner diameter of a tube; the space or opening within an artery

lupus erythematosus: A chronic inflammatory connective tissue disease affecting the skin, joints, kidneys, nervous system, and mucous membranes; a butterfly rash or erythema may be seen on the face, particularly across the nose

lysis: dissolution or destruction of cells

M

macrocytic anemia: anemia resulting from abnormal formation (enlargement) of erythrocytes

malaise: discomfort, uneasiness

megacolon: dilation and hypertrophy of the colon

megaloblastic anemia: anemia characterized by large, abnormal, immature erythrocytes circulating in the blood; results from folic acid deficiency

melasma: discoloration of the skin

melena: blood in the stools

menarche: age of onset of first menstruation

merozoites: cells formed as the result of asexual reproduction

metabolite: inactive form of the original drug

metastasis: spread of cancer outside the original organ or tissue

meter: metric measure of distance

methemoglobinemia: clinical condition in which more than 1% of hemoglobin in the blood has been oxidized to the ferric form

methicillin-resistant *Staphylococcus aureus* (MRSA): bacterium that is resistant to methicillin

metric system: system of measurement based on units of 10

micturition: voiding of urine

mineralocorticoids: hormones produced by the adrenal gland

minim: basic unit of liquid measure in the apothecaries' system

miosis: constriction of the pupil

miotic: drug that constricts the pupil

mixed decimal fraction: a number consisting of numbers to the right and left of the decimal point (e.g., 8.25)

mixed number: a number consisting of a whole number and a fraction (e.g., 1 2/3)

motor seizure: uncontrolled muscle stiffening

mucolytic: drug that loosens and thins respiratory secretions (lowers the viscosity of the secretions)

mucositis: inflammation of the mucous membranes

muscarinic receptors: neurologic receptors that stimulate smooth muscle

musculoskeletal: pertaining to the bones and muscles

myasthenia gravis: condition characterized by weakness and fatigability of the muscles

Mycobacterium leprae: the bacterium that causes leprosy (Hansen's disease)

Mycobacterium tuberculosis: the bacterium that causes tuberculosis (TB)

mycotic: pertaining to a fungus or fungal infection

mycotic infection: infection caused by fungi

mydriasis: dilation of the pupil

mydriatic: drug that dilates the pupil

myelosuppression: bone marrow suppression

myocardial infarction: heart attack

myoclonic seizure: sudden, forceful muscular contraction myopia: nearsightedness

myxedema: condition caused by hypothyroidism or deficiency of thyroxine and characterized by swelling of the face, periorbital tissues, hands, and feet

N

narcolepsy: a chronic disorder that results in recurrent attacks of drowsiness and sleep during daytime

narcotic: properties of a drug producing numbness or a stupor-like state

narrow spectrum: describes an antibiotic that affects only one or a few strains of bacteria

nausea: an unpleasant and uncomfortable feeling in the stomach, sometimes followed by vomiting

necrotic: pertaining to death of tissue (n. *necrosis*)

nephrotoxic: harmful to the kidney

nephrotoxicity: damage to the kidneys by a toxic substance

neurogenic bladder: altered bladder function caused by abnormality in nervous system

neurohormonal activity: *in heart failure*, increased secretions of epinephrine and norepinephrine, resulting in increased heart rate and vasoconstriction that trigger a worsening of heart failure and reduced ability of the heart to contract effectively

neurohormones: secreted rather than transmitted neurosubstances

neurohypophysis: posterior lobe of the pituitary gland

neuroleptanalgesia: altered state of consciousness or sensation

neuroleptic malignant syndrome: rare reaction to antipsychotic drug; includes extrapyramidal syndrome, hypothermia, and autonomic disturbances

neuromuscular blockade: acute muscle paralysis and apnea

neurotoxicity: damage to the nervous system by a toxic substance

neurotransmitter: chemical substances released at the nerve ending that facilitate the transmission of nerve impulses

neutropenia: abnormally small number of neutrophils (type of white blood cell)

nicotinic receptors: neurologic receptors that stimulate skeletal muscles

nocturia: excessive urination at night

nonpathogenic: not disease causing

nonprescription drugs: drugs that are designated by the U.S. Food and Drug Administration (FDA) to be safe (if taken as directed) and obtainable without a prescription, also called *over-the-counter* (OTC) drugs; may be purchased in various settings, such as a pharmacy, drugstore, or supermarket

nonproductive cough: dry, hacking cough that produces no secretions

nonsteroidal: not a steroid

normal flora: nonpathogenic microorganisms in the body

normal saline: a solution of 0.9% sodium chloride and water, which is the proportion of salt and water normally circulating in body fluid

numerator: part of a fraction (the numeral above the line)

nurse anesthetist: nurse with advanced education and training that qualifies her or him to administer anesthetic agents

nursing diagnosis: description of a patient problem

nursing process: a framework for nursing action, consisting of a series of problem-solving steps, that helps members of the health care team provide effective and consistent patient care

nystagmus: an involuntary and constant movement of the eyeball

O

objective data: information obtained through a physical assessment or physical examination

obstipation: watery stool leakage around a hard fecal impaction

oliguria: a decrease in urinary output

ongoing assessment: the continuing assessment activities that proceed from the initial nursing assessment

on-off phenomenon: levodopa therapy problem characterized by alternating improved status and loss of therapeutic effect

onychomycosis: finger or toenail fungal infection

ophthalmic: pertaining to the eye

opioid: drug having opiate properties but not necessarily derived from opium; used to relieve moderate to severe pain

opioid naive: no previous use or infrequent use of opioid medications

opportunistic infection: infection resulting from microorganisms commonly found in the environment that normally do not cause an infection unless there is an impaired immune system

optic neuritis: inflammation of the optic nerve

oral mucositis: inflammation of the oral mucous membranes

orthostatic hypotension: see *hypotension, orthostatic*

osteoarthritis: noninflammatory degeneration of joints and cartilage

osteomalacia: a softening of the bones

osteoporosis: a loss of calcium from the bones, resulting in a decrease in bone density

otic: pertaining to the ear

otitis media: infection of the middle ear

ototoxic: harmful to the ear

ototoxicity: damage to the organs of hearing by a toxic substance

ounce: measure of weight (16 solid ounces = 1 pound) or volume (32 fluid ounces = 1 quart) in the household system of measure

overactive bladder: condition characterized by involuntary contraction of bladder muscles

overt: not hidden, clearly evident

over-the-counter: pertaining to drugs or other substances sold without a prescription; see *nonprescription*

oxytocic: agent that stimulates contractions of the uterus, resulting in labor

P

pain: an unpleasant sensory or emotional perception

palliation: therapy designed to treat symptoms, not to produce a cure

pancytopenia: a reduction in all cellular elements of the blood

paralytic ileus: paralysis of the bowel resulting in lack of movement of bowel contents

parasite: organism living in or on another organism (host) without contributing to the survival or well-being of the host

parasympathetic: pertaining to the part of the autonomic nervous system concerned with conserving body energy (i.e., slowing the heart rate, digesting food, and eliminating waste)

parasympatholytic: blocking the parasympathetic nervous system

parasympathomimetic drugs: mimic the activity of the parasympathetic nervous system; also called *cholinergic drugs*

parenteral: administration of a substance, such as a drug, by any route other than through the gastrointestinal system (e.g., oral or rectal route)

paresthesia: an abnormal sensation such as numbness, tingling, prickling, or heightened sensitivity

parkinsonism: referring to the symptoms of Parkinson's disease (i.e., fine tremors, slowing of voluntary movements, muscular weakness)

Parkinson's disease: a degenerative disorder caused by an imbalance of dopamine and acetylcholine in the central nervous system

partial agonist: agent that binds to a receptor but produces a limited response

partial seizure: localized seizure in the brain

passive immunity: a type of immunity occurring from the administration of ready-made antibodies from another individual or animal

pathogenic: disease producing

patient-controlled analgesia: drug pump and delivery system that allows patients to administer their own analgesic medication intravenously within a preset protocol

penicillinase: enzyme produced by bacteria that deactivates penicillin

perioperative: pertaining to the preoperative, intraoperative, or postoperative period

peripheral: pertaining to the outward surface; away from the center

peripheral nervous system: all nerves outside of brain and spinal cord

peripheral neuropathy: numbness and tingling of the extremities

petechiae: tiny purple or red spots that appear on the skin as a result of pinpoint hemorrhages in the outer layers of the skin

pharmaceutic: pertaining to the phase during which a drug dissolves in the body

pharmacodynamics: study of the drug mechanisms that produce biochemical or physiologic changes in the body

pharmacogenetic disorder: genetically determined abnormal response to normal doses of a drug

pharmacokinetics: the study of body mechanisms (or activity) after a drug is administered; these mechanisms include absorption, distribution, metabolism, and excretion

pharmacology: the study of drugs and their action on living organisms

phenylketonuria: genetic disorder in which the body lacks the enzyme necessary to metabolize phenylalanine; without treatment, the disorder results in mental retardation

pheochromocytoma: tumor of the adrenal medulla characterized by hypersecretion of epinephrine and norepinephrine

phlebitis: inflammation of a vein

photophobia: an aversion to or intolerance of light

photosensitivity: exaggerated sunburn reaction when the skin is exposed to sunlight or ultraviolet light

physical dependence: compulsive need to use a substance repeatedly to avoid withdrawal symptoms

planning: design of steps to carry out nursing actions

plasma expanders: intravenous solutions used to expand plasma volume in shock due to burns, hemorrhage, or other trauma

polarization: the status of a nerve cell at rest, with positive ions on the outside of the cell membrane and negative ions on the inside

polydipsia: excessive thirst

polyphagia: eating large amounts of food

polypharmacy: taking a large number of drugs (may be prescribed or over-the-counter drugs)

polyposis: numerous polyps

polyuria: increased urination

positive inotropic action: increase in the force of cardiac contraction

postural hypotension: see *hypotension, postural*

preanesthetic: pertaining to status before administration of an anesthetic agent

prehypertension: systolic blood pressure between 120 and 139 mm Hg or diastolic pressure between 80 and 89 mm Hg

prepubertal: before puberty

prescription drugs: drugs the federal government has designated as potentially harmful unless their use is supervised by a licensed health care provider, such as a nurse practitioner, physician, or dentist

priapism: painful, persistent penile erection

proarrhythmic effect: creation of new arrhythmia or worsening of existing arrhythmia, resulting from administration of an antiarrhythmic drug

productive cough: cough by which secretions from the lower respiratory tract are expelled

progesterone: a female hormone produced by the corpus luteum that works in the uterus (along with estrogen) to prepare the uterus for possible conception

progestins: natural and synthetic progesterones

proper fraction: part of a whole or any number less than a whole number

prophylactic: preventive

prophylaxis: prevention

prostaglandins: a fatty acid derivative found in almost every tissue and fluid of the body that affects the uterus and other smooth muscles; also thought to increase the sensitivity of peripheral pain receptors to painful stimuli

prostatic hypertrophy: abnormal enlargement of the prostate gland

prostatitis: inflammation of the prostate gland

protein substrates: amino acids essential to life

proteinuria: protein in the urine

proteolysis: enzymatic action that helps remove dead soft tissues by reducing proteins to simpler substances

proteolytic: pertaining to proteolysis (see *proteolysis*)

prothrombin: substance that is essential for the clotting of blood; clotting factor II

pruritus: itching

pseudomembranous colitis: a severe, life-threatening form of diarrhea

psychological dependence: compulsion to use a substance to obtain a pleasurable experience

psychomotor domain: in education, the area concerned with teaching and learning physical skills and tasks ptosis: drooping of the upper eyelid

purpura: condition characterized by various degrees of hemorrhaging into the skin or mucous membranes, producing ecchymoses (bruises) and petechiae (small red patches) on the skin

purulent exudates: pus-containing fluids

pyelonephritis: inflammation of the kidney nephron

Q

quiescent: having no symptoms

quotient: the number that results from dividing one number by another (example: when 10 is divided by 2, the quotient is 5)

R

rales: abnormal lung sounds often described as "crackles"

ratio: relationship in degree or number of one value or "thing" compared with another

receptor: *in pharmacology*, a reactive site on the surface of a cell; when a drug binds to and interacts with the receptor, a pharmacologic response occurs

red-man syndrome: a severe adverse drug reaction characterized by a sudden and profound fall in blood pressure, fever, chills, paresthesias, and erythema (redness) of the neck and back

refractory period: the quiet period between the transmission of nerve impulses along a nerve fiber

regional anesthesia: injection of a local anesthetic around nerves to block sensation

REM (rapid eye movement): the dreaming stage of sleep

remainder: the value or part that remains after subtracting one number from another or after dividing one number by another

remission: periods of partial or complete disappearance of signs and symptoms

repolarization: return of positive and negative ions to their original place on the nerve cell after an impulse has passed along the nerve fiber (see *polarization*)

retinitis: inflammation of the retina

retrovirus: virus that uses RNA as its primary component instead of DNA

Reye's syndrome: acute and potentially fatal disease of childhood; associated with a previous viral infection

rhinyle: tube used to instill drug deep into nasal cavity

S

salicylates: drugs derived from salicylic acid

salicylism: adverse reaction to a salicylate characterized by dizziness, impaired hearing, nausea, vomiting, flushing, sweating, rapid, deep breathing, tachycardia, diarrhea, mental confusion, lassitude, drowsiness, respiratory depression, and possibly coma

secondary failure: *in diabetes mellitus*, loss of the effectiveness of sulfonylurea, an oral antidiabetic drug

secondary hypertension: hypertension with a known cause, such as kidney disease

sedative: a drug producing a relaxing, calming effect

seizure: periodic electrical activity in brain

shock: inadequate blood flow to the bodily tissues

solvent: the fluid in which a solid dissolves

somatotropic hormone: growth hormone (see *somatotropin*)

somatosensory: change in sensation due to a seizure

somatotropin: hormone produced by the anterior pituitary gland that contributes to the growth of muscles and bones; also called *growth hormone*

somnolence: prolonged drowsiness; sleepiness

spinal anesthesia: type of regional anesthesia produced by injection of a local anesthetic drug into the subarachnoid space of the spinal cord

sprue: disease characterized by weakness, anemia, weight loss, and malabsorption of essential nutrients

Standard Precautions: the recommendation that gloves and/or other protective gear be worn when touching blood or body fluids, mucous membranes, or any broken skin area; also see *Universal Precautions*

status epilepticus: an emergency situation characterized by continual seizure activity

Stevens-Johnson syndrome: fever, cough, muscular aches and pains, headache, and lesions of the skin, mucous membranes, and eyes; the lesions appear as red wheals or blisters, often starting on the face, in the mouth, or on the lips, neck, and extremities

stomatitis: inflammation of a cavity opening

striae: lines or bands elevated above or depressed below surrounding tissue, or differing in color or texture

subcutaneous: under the skin

subjective data: information supplied by the patient or family

sublingual: under the tongue

substrate: substance that is the basic component of an organism—for example, amino acids

sulfonylurea: an oral drug used to lower blood sugar in persons with diabetes mellitus

superinfection: an overgrowth of bacterial or fungal microorganisms not affected by the antibiotic being administered

sympathetic: pertaining to the sympathetic nervous system

sympathetic nervous system: part of the autonomic nervous system concerned with mobilizing body systems

sympatholytic: blocking the sympathetic nervous system

sympathomimetic: acting like the sympathetic nervous system

synergism: action that occurs when two substances (drugs) interact to produce an effect that is greater than the sum of their separate actions

T

tachycardia: heart rate above 100 beats/minute

tardive dyskinesia: rhythmic, involuntary movements of the tongue, face, mouth, jaw, and sometimes the extremities

teaching: an interactive process that promotes learning

teratogen: a drug or substance that causes abnormal development of the fetus, leading to deformities

testosterone: the primary male sex hormone; acts to stimulate development of the male reproductive organs and secondary sex characteristics

tetany: nervous condition characterized by sharp flexion of the wrist and ankle joints, muscle twitching, cramps, and possible convulsions, usually caused by abnormal levels of calcium, vitamin D, and alkalosis

theophyllinization: delivery of a high enough dose of theophylline to bring blood levels to a therapeutic range more quickly than over several days

threshold: term applied to any stimulus of the lowest intensity that will give rise to a response in a nerve fiber

thrombocytopenia: low number of platelets in the blood

thrombolytic: drug that helps to eliminate blood clots

thrombophlebitis: inflammation of a vein with clot formation

thrombosis: formation of a blood clot

thrombus: a blood clot (pl. *thrombi*)

thrush: candidiasis (candidal infection) of the mouth

thyroid storm: see *thyrotoxicosis*

thyrotoxicosis: severe hyperthyroidism characterized by high fever, extreme tachycardia, and altered mental status (also called *thyroid storm*)

tinea corporis: superficial fungal infection, commonly called *ringworm*

tinea cruris: superficial fungal infection of the groin region, commonly called *jock itch*

tinea pedis: superficial fungal infection of the foot, commonly called *athlete's foot*

tinnitus: ringing in the ears

tonic-clonic seizure: generalized seizure activity consisting of alternating contraction (tonic) and relaxation of muscles (clonic)

topical: pertaining to a substance applied directly to the skin by patch, ointment, gel, or other formulation

toxic: poisonous or harmful

toxic epidermal necrolysis (TEN): toxic skin reaction with sloughing of skin and mucous membranes

toxin: poisonous substance

toxoid: an attenuated toxin that is capable of stimulating the formation of antitoxins

transdermal: through the skin

transdermal system: drug delivery system by which the drug is applied to and absorbed through the skin

transient ischemic attack (TIA): temporary interference with blood supply to the brain causing symptoms related to the portion of the brain affected (i.e., temporary blindness, aphasia, dizziness, numbness, difficulty swallowing, or paresthesias); may last a few moments to several hours, after which no residual neurologic damage is evident

transsacral block: anesthesia of caudal region of spinal cord and canal

trigeminy: an irregular pulse rate consisting of three beats followed by a pause before the next three beats

triglycerides: types of lipids that circulate in the blood

tuberculosis: infection caused by *Mycobacterium tuberculosis*

tyramine: an amino acid; substance found in most cheeses and in beer, bean pods, yeast, wine, and chicken liver

U

unit dose: system of drug delivery by which a drug order is filled and medication dispensed to fill each medication order(s) for a 24-hour period; each drug dose (unit) is dispensed in a package labeled with the drug name and dosage

Universal Precautions: guidelines set forth by the Centers for Disease Control and Prevention (CDC) to control the spread of disease

unlabeled use: use of a drug not officially approved by the U.S. Food and Drug Administration (FDA)

urge incontinence: involuntary passage of urine

urinary tract infection (UTI): infection by pathogenic microorganisms of one or more structures of the urinary tract

urinary urgency: immediate sensation of need to void

urticaria: hives; itchy wheals on the skin resulting from contact with or ingestion of an allergenic substance or food

uterine atony: marked relaxation of the uterine muscle

uveitis: a nonspecific term for any intraocular inflammatory disorder

V

vaccine: substance containing either weakened or killed antigens developed for the purpose of creating resistance to disease

vancomycin-resistant enterococci (VRE): bacteria resistant to the drug vancomycin

vasodilation: an increase in the diameter of the blood vessels that, when widespread, results in a drop in blood pressure

vasopressors: drugs that raise the blood pressure

venous: pertaining to the veins

vertigo: a feeling of a spinning or rotational motion; dizziness

vesicant: caustic drug substance

virilization: acquisition of male sexual characteristics by a woman

vitamin: organic substance needed by the body in small amounts for normal growth and nutrition

volatile liquids: anesthetic agents that are flammable

vomiting: spasmodic ejection of stomach contents through the mouth

von Willebrand's disease: a congenital bleeding disorder manifested at an early age by epistaxis and easy bruising; symptoms usually decrease in severity with age

W

water intoxication: fluid overload in the body when electrolytes are imbalanced

water soluble: dissolves in water

X-Y-Z

xanthine derivatives: drugs that stimulate the central nervous system to promote bronchodilation

xerostomia: drying of oral secretions

Z-track: method of intramuscular drug injection used when a drug is highly irritating to subcutaneous tissues or has the ability permanently to stain the skin

Appendix A

U.S. Department of Health and Human Services

MEDWATCH

The FDA Safety Information and
Adverse Event Reporting Program

For VOLUNTARY reporting of
adverse events, product problems and
product use errors

Page _____ of _____

Form Approved: OMB No. 0910-0291, Expires: 10/31/08
See OMB statement on reverse.

FDA USE ONLY

Triage unit
sequence #

A. PATIENT INFORMATION

1. Patient Identifier	2. Age at Time of Event, or Date of Birth:	3. Sex	4. Weight
In confidence		☐ Female ☐ Male	_____ lb or _____ kg

B. ADVERSE EVENT, PRODUCT PROBLEM OR ERROR

Check all that apply:

1. ☐ Adverse Event   ☐ Product Problem (e.g., defects/malfunctions)
   ☐ Product Use Error   ☐ Problem with Different Manufacturer of Same Medicine

2. **Outcomes Attributed to Adverse Event**
   (Check all that apply)

   ☐ Death: _____ (mm/dd/yyyy)
   ☐ Life-threatening
   ☐ Hospitalization - initial or prolonged
   ☐ Required Intervention to Prevent Permanent Impairment/Damage (Devices)
   ☐ Disability or Permanent Damage
   ☐ Congenital Anomaly/Birth Defect
   ☐ Other Serious (Important Medical Events)

3. **Date of Event** (mm/dd/yyyy)   4. **Date of this Report** (mm/dd/yyyy)

5. **Describe Event, Problem or Product Use Error**

6. **Relevant Tests/Laboratory Data, Including Dates**

7. **Other Relevant History, Including Preexisting Medical Conditions** (e.g., allergies, race, pregnancy, smoking and alcohol use, liver/kidney problems, etc.)

C. PRODUCT AVAILABILITY

Product Available for Evaluation? (Do not send product to FDA)

☐ Yes   ☐ No   ☐ Returned to Manufacturer on: _____ (mm/dd/yyyy)

PLEASE TYPE OR USE BLACK INK

D. SUSPECT PRODUCT(S)

1. **Name, Strength, Manufacturer** (from product label)

   #1
   #2

2. | | Dose or Amount | Frequency | Route |
   |---|---|---|---|
   | #1 | | | |
   | #2 | | | |

3. **Dates of Use** (If unknown, give duration) from/to (or best estimate)

   #1
   #2

4. **Diagnosis or Reason for Use** (Indication)

   #1
   #2

6. **Lot #**   7. **Expiration Date**
   #1   #1
   #2   #2

5. **Event Abated After Use Stopped or Dose Reduced?**
   #1 ☐ Yes ☐ No ☐ Doesn't Apply
   #2 ☐ Yes ☐ No ☐ Doesn't Apply

8. **Event Reappeared After Reintroduction?**
   #1 ☐ Yes ☐ No ☐ Doesn't Apply
   #2 ☐ Yes ☐ No ☐ Doesn't Apply

9. **NDC # or Unique ID**

E. SUSPECT MEDICAL DEVICE

1. **Brand Name**

2. **Common Device Name**

3. **Manufacturer Name, City and State**

4. **Model #** | **Lot #** | 5. **Operator of Device**
   Catalog # | Expiration Date (mm/dd/yyyy) | ☐ Health Professional
   Serial # | Other # | ☐ Lay User/Patient ☐ Other:

6. **If Implanted, Give Date** (mm/dd/yyyy)   7. **If Explanted, Give Date** (mm/dd/yyyy)

8. **Is this a Single-use Device that was Reprocessed and Reused on a Patient?**
   ☐ Yes   ☐ No

9. **If Yes to Item No. 8, Enter Name and Address of Reprocessor**

F. OTHER (CONCOMITANT) MEDICAL PRODUCTS

Product names and therapy dates (exclude treatment of event)

G. REPORTER (See confidentiality section on back)

1. **Name and Address**

   Phone # | E-mail

2. **Health Professional?** ☐ Yes ☐ No   3. **Occupation**   4. **Also Reported to:**
   ☐ Manufacturer
   ☐ User Facility
   ☐ Distributor/Importer

5. **If you do NOT want your identity disclosed to the manufacturer, place an "X" in this box:** ☐

FORM FDA 3500 (10/05)   Submission of a report does not constitute an admission that medical personnel or the product caused or contributed to the event.

ADVICE ABOUT VOLUNTARY REPORTING

Detailed instructions available at: http://www.fda.gov/medwatch/report/consumer/instruct.htm

Report adverse events, product problems or product use errors with:

- Medications *(drugs or biologics)*
- Medical devices *(including in-vitro diagnostics)*
- Combination products *(medication & medical devices)*
- Human cells, tissues, and cellular and tissue-based products
- Special nutritional products *(dietary supplements, medical foods, infant formulas)*
- Cosmetics

Report product problems - quality, performance or safety concerns such as:

- Suspected counterfeit product
- Suspected contamination
- Questionable stability
- Defective components
- Poor packaging or labeling
- Therapeutic failures (product didn't work)

Report SERIOUS adverse events. An event is serious when the patient outcome is:

- Death
- Life-threatening
- Hospitalization - initial or prolonged
- Disability or permanent damage
- Congenital anomaly/birth defect
- Required intervention to prevent permanent impairment or damage
- Other serious (important medical events)

Report even if:

- You're not certain the product caused the event
- You don't have all the details

How to report:

- Just fill in the sections that apply to your report
- Use section D for all products except medical devices
- Attach additional pages if needed
- Use a separate form for each patient
- Report either to FDA or the manufacturer *(or both)*

Other methods of reporting:

- 1-800-FDA-0178 -- To FAX report
- 1-800-FDA-1088 -- To report by phone
- www.fda.gov/medwatch/report.htm -- To report online

If your report involves a serious adverse event with a device and it occurred in a facility outside a doctor's office, that facility may be legally required to report to FDA and/or the manufacturer. Please notify the person in that facility who would handle such reporting.

If your report involves a serious adverse event with a vaccine call 1-800-822-7967 to report.

Confidentiality: The patient's identity is held in strict confidence by FDA and protected to the fullest extent of the law. FDA will not disclose the reporter's identity in response to a request from the public, pursuant to the Freedom of Information Act. The reporter's identity, including the identity of a self-reporter, may be shared with the manufacturer unless requested otherwise.

-Fold Here-

-Fold Here-

The public reporting burden for this collection of information has been estimated to average 36 minutes per response, including the time for reviewing instructions, searching existing data sources, gathering and maintaining the data needed, and completing and reviewing the collection of information. Send comments regarding this burden estimate or any other aspect of this collection of information, including suggestions for reducing this burden to:

Department of Health and Human Services
Food and Drug Administration - MedWatch
10903 New Hampshire Avenue
Building 22, Mail Stop 4447
Silver Spring, MD 20993-0002

Please DO NOT
RETURN this form
to this address.

OMB statement:
"An agency may not conduct or sponsor, and a person is not required to respond to, a collection of information unless it displays a currently valid OMB control number."

U.S. DEPARTMENT OF HEALTH AND HUMAN SERVICES
Food and Drug Administration

FORM FDA 3500 (10/05) (Back)   Please Use Address Provided Below -- Fold in Thirds, Tape and Mail

---

DEPARTMENT OF
HEALTH & HUMAN SERVICES

Public Health Service
Food and Drug Administration
Rockville, MD 20857

Official Business
Penalty for Private Use $300

NO POSTAGE
NECESSARY
IF MAILED
IN THE
UNITED STATES
OR APO/FPO

BUSINESS REPLY MAIL
FIRST CLASS MAIL   PERMIT NO. 946   ROCKVILLE MD

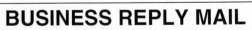

MEDWATCH
The FDA Safety Information and Adverse Event Reporting Program
Food and Drug Administration
5600 Fishers Lane
Rockville, MD 20852-9787

Appendix B: Select Herbs and Natural Products Used for Medicinal Purposes

Common Name(s)	Scientific Name	Uses	Adverse Reactions	Significant Considerations
Aloe vera	*Aloe vera*	Inhibits infection and promotes healing of minor burns and wounds; laxative	None significant if used as directed; may cause burning sensation in wound	Rare reports of delayed healing when used in the gel form on a wound. If taken internally as a laxative, do not take longer than 1–3 wk without consulting primary health care provider. Decrease dosage if cramping occurs.
Bilberry	*Vaccinium myrtillus*	Vision enhancement and eye health, microcirculation, spider veins and varicose veins, capillary strengthening before surgery	No adverse effects have been reported in clinical studies	None significant
Black cohosh (black snakeroot, squawroot)	*Cimicifuga racemosa*	Management of some symptoms of menopause and as an alternative to hormone replacement therapy; may be beneficial for hypercholesterolemia or peripheral vascular disease	Overdose causes nausea, dizziness, nervous system and visual disturbances, decreased pulse rate and increased perspiration	Should not be used during pregnancy. Possible interactions with hormone therapy.
Chamomile	*Matricaria chamomilla*	As a tea for gastrointestinal disturbances (e.g., diarrhea, flatulence, stomatitis), as a sedative, and as an anti-inflammatory agent	Possible contact dermatitis and, in rare instances, anaphylaxis	Chamomile is a member of the ragweed family and those allergic to ragweed should not take the herb. Avoid use during pregnancy. May enhance anticoagulant effect when administered with anticoagulants. Do not administer to a child without checking with primary health care provider.
Chondroitin	Chondroitin sulfate, chondroitin sulfuric acid, chonsurid	Arthritis	None significant if used as directed	Because chondroitin is concentrated in cartilage, theoretically it produces no toxic or teratogenic effects.

Common Name(s)	Scientific Name	Uses	Adverse Reactions	Significant Considerations
Cranberry	*Vaccinium macrocarpon*	Prevents urinary tract infection (UTI)	Large doses can produce gastrointestinal (GI) symptoms (e.g., diarrhea)	None significant. Safe for use during pregnancy and while breastfeeding. Inform patient that sugar-free cranberry juice or supplements are available if the patient has diabetes mellitus. Antibiotic is usually needed to treat active UTI.
Echinacea (American coneflower, black-eyed susans)	*Echinacea angustifolia*	Prevents and shortens symptoms and duration of upper respiratory infections (URIs), including colds	Rare; nausea and mild GI upsets	Should not be used by individuals with autoimmune diseases such as tuberculosis, collagenosis, multiple sclerosis, AIDS, and HIV infection. Advise patient not to delay obtaining medical attention if symptoms do not improve. Take herb at the first sign of illness and continue for up to 14 d. Do not use this herb in place of antibiotics.
Feverfew	*Tanacetum parthenium*	Migraine headaches, antipyretic, asthma, arthritis, relief of menstrual cramps	Most are mild; rash or contact dermatitis may indicate allergy and herb should be withdrawn	Possible interaction with anticoagulants. Patient should be observed for abnormal bleeding. Do not use during pregnancy or lactation.
Flax	*Linum usitatissimum*	Topical emollient, laxative, diverticulitis, irritable bowel syndrome	Few when taken as directed	Advise patient to drink adequate water while taking flax. Advise patient not to take any drug for at least 2 hours after taking flax. Advise patient not to take during pregnancy.
Garlic	*Allium sativum*	Lowers blood glucose, cholesterol, and lipid levels	May cause abnormal blood glucose levels	Increased risk of bleeding in patients taking the coumarins, salicylates, or antiplatelet drugs.
Ginger (ginger root, black ginger)	*Zingiber officinale*	Antiemetic, cardiotonic, antithrombotic, antibacterial, antioxidant, antitussive, anti-inflammatory, GI disturbances, lower cholesterol, prophylaxis for nausea and vomiting, colic	Excessive doses may cause CNS depression and interfere with cardiac functioning or anticoagulant activity.	Theoretically, ginger could enhance the effects of the antiplatelet drugs, such as coumarin Observe for excessive bleeding (e.g., nose bleeding, easy bruising) Consult primary health care provider for use during pregnancy.

Common Name(s)	Scientific Name	Uses	Adverse Reactions	Significant Considerations
Ginkgo (maiden hair tree, kew tree)	*Ginkgo biloba*	Cerebral insufficiency dementias, circulatory problems, headaches, macular degeneration, diabetic retinopathy, premenstrual syndrome	Rare if used as directed; possible effects include headache, dizziness, heart palpitations, GI effects, rash, allergic dermatitis	Do not take with antidepressant drugs, such as the MAOIs, or the antiplatelet drugs such as coumarin, unless advised to do so by the primary health care provider. Discontinue use at least 2 wk before surgery.
Ginseng	*Panax quinquefolius* *Panax ginseng*	Fatigue, lack of concentration, atherosclerosis, improves cardiovascular or CNS function	Most common: nervousness, excitation, hypoglycemia Rare: diffuse mammary nodularity, vaginal bleeding	Taking ginseng in combination with stimulants such as caffeine is not advised. Do not use for longer than 3 mo. (Some herbalists recommend use for 1 mo followed by nonuse for 2 mo.)
Goldenseal	*Hydrastis canadensis*	Antiseptic for skin (topical), astringent for mucous membranes (mouthwash), wash for inflamed eyes	Large doses may cause dry or irritated mucous membranes and injury to the GI system	Should not be taken for more than 3-7 d. Contraindicated in pregnancy and hypertension.
Glucosamine (chitosamine)	2-Amino-2-deoxy-glucose	Antiarthritic in osteoarthritis	Usually well tolerated. Mild adverse reactions such as heartburn, diarrhea, nausea, and itching have been reported	No direct toxic effects have been reported. Cautious use is recommended in diabetes because there is a potential for altering blood glucose levels.
Green tea	*Camellia sinensis*	Reduces cancer risk, lowers lipid levels, helps prevent dental caries, antimicrobial and antioxidative effects	Well tolerated; contains caffeine (may cause mild stimulant effects such as anxiety, nervousness, heart irregularities, restlessness, insomnia, and digestive irritation)	No direct toxic effects have been reported. Contains caffeine and should be avoided during pregnancy and by individuals with hypertension, anxiety, eating disorders, insomnia, diabetes, and ulcers. Inform patient to avoid taking green tea with iron supplements because green tea interferes with iron absorption.
Hawthorne	*Crataegus oxyacantha*	Regulation of blood pressure and heart rhythm, treat atherosclerosis and angina pectoris, sedative	Hypotension and sedation (in high doses)	May interfere with serum digoxin effects. Notify primary health care provider and pharmacist if taking the herb.
Kava (kawa, kava-kava, awa yangona)	*Piper methysticum*	Mild to moderate anxiety, sedative	Scaly skin rash, disturbances in visual accommodation, habituation	Limit use to no more than 3 mo.

Common Name(s)	Scientific Name	Uses	Adverse Reactions	Significant Considerations
Lemon balm (balm, melissa, sweet balm)	*Melissa officinalis*	Graves' disease, sedative, antispasmodic, cold sores (topical)	None significant	None significant
melatonin	*melatonin*	Insomnia, topically to protect against ultraviolet light	Headache, depression, possible additive effects when taken with alcohol	Avoid hazardous activities until the CNS effects of this supplement are known. Do not take for prolonged periods because effects of prolonged use are not known. May interfere with conception.
Milk thistle	*Silyburn marianum*	Treatment for liver damage, dyspnea	Few adverse reactions have been reported; GI disturbances and mild allergic reactions.	Do not to take this herb while pregnant or breastfeeding.
Passion flower (passion fruit, granadilla, water lemon, apricot vine)	*Passiflora incarnata*	Promotes sleep, treatment for pain and nervous exhaustion	None if used as directed. Excessively large doses may cause CNS depression.	May interact with anticoagulants and MAOIs.
Saw palmetto (cabbage palm, fan palm, scrub palm)	*Serenoa repens*	Symptoms of benign prostatic hypertrophy	Generally well tolerated; occasional GI effects	May interact with hormones such as oral contraceptive drugs and hormone replacement therapy.
St. John's wort (Klamath weed, goatweed, rosin rose)	*Hypericum perforatum*	Antidepressant and antiviral	Usually mild. May cause dry mouth, dizziness, constipation, other GI symptoms, photosensitivity	May decrease efficacy of theophylline, warfarin, and digoxin; use with other prescriptions is not recommended.
Tea tree oil	*Melaleuca alternifolia*	Topical antimicrobial	Contact dermatitis	For topical use only; do not take orally.
Valerian	*Valeriana officinalis*	Restlessness, sleep disorders	Rare if used as directed	May interact with the barbiturates (e.g., phenobarbital), the benzodiazepines (e.g., diazepam) and the opiates, (e.g., morphine).
Willow bark (weidenrinde, white willow, purple osier willow, crack willow)	*Salix alba, S. purpurea, S. fragilis*	Analgesic	Adverse reactions are those associated with the salicylates	Do not use with aspirin or other NSAIDs. Do not use in patients with peptic ulcers and other medical conditions in which the salicylates are contraindicated.

Appendix C

USP MEDICATION ERRORS REPORTING PROGRAM
Presented in cooperation with the Institute for Safe Medication Practices

USP is an FDA MEDWATCH partner

Reporters should not provide any individually identifiable health information, including names of practitioners, names of patients, names of healthcare facilities, or dates of birth (age is acceptable).

Date and time of event:

Please describe the error. Include description/sequence of events, type of staff involved, and work environment (e.g., code situation, change of shift, short staffing, no 24-hr. pharmacy, floor stock). If more space is needed, please attach a separate page.

_____
_____
_____

Did the error reach the patient? ❑ Yes ❑ No

Was the incorrect medication, dose, or dosage form administered to or taken by the patient?   ❑ Yes ❑ No

Circle the appropriate Error Outcome Category (select one—see back for details): A B C D E F G H I

Describe the direct result of the error on the patient (e.g., death, type of harm, additional patient monitoring). _____

Indicate the possible error cause(s) and contributing factor(s) (e.g., abbreviation, similar names, distractions, etc.). _____

Indicate the location of the error (e.g., hospital, outpatient or community pharmacy, clinic, nursing home, patient's home, etc.). _____

What type of staff or healthcare practitioner made the initial error? _____

Indicate if other practitioner(s) were also involved in the error (type of staff perpetuating error). _____

What type of staff or healthcare practitioner discovered the error or recognized the potential for error? _____

How was the error (or potential for error) discovered/intercepted? _____

If available, provide patient age, gender, diagnosis. Do not provide any patient identifiers. _____

Please complete the following for the product(s) involved. (If more space is needed for additional products, please attach a separate page.)

	Product #1	Product #2
Brand/Product Name (If Applicable)		
Generic Name		
Manufacturer		
Labeler		
Dosage Form		
Strength/Concentration		
Type and Size of Container		

Reports are most useful when relevant materials such as product label, copy of prescription/order, etc., can be reviewed.

Can these materials be provided? ❑ Yes ❑ No   Please specify: _____

Suggest any recommendations to prevent recurrence of this error, or describe policies or procedures you instituted or plan to institute to prevent future similar errors. _____

Name and Title/Profession	Telephone Number ( )	Fax Number ( )
Facility/Address and Zip		E-mail
Address/Zip (where correspondence should be sent)		

Your name, contact information, and a copy of this report are routinely shared with the Institute for Safe Medication Practices (ISMP). Copies of reports will be sent to third parties such as the manufacturer/labeler, and to the Food and Drug Administration (FDA). You have the option of including your name on these copies.

In addition to releasing my name and contact information to ISMP, USP may release my identity to these third parties as follows (check boxes that apply):

❑ The manufacturer and/or labeler as listed above   ❑ FDA   ❑ Other persons requesting a copy of this report   ❑ Anonymous to all third parties

Signature	Date

Return to:
USP CAPS
12601 Twinbrook Parkway
Rockville, MD 20852-1790

Submit via the Web at www.usp.org/mer
Call Toll Free: 800-23-ERROR (800-233-7767)
or FAX: 301-816-8532

Date Received by USP	File Access Number

NCC MERP Index for Categorizing Medication Errors	NCC MERP Index for Categorizing Medication Errors Algorithm

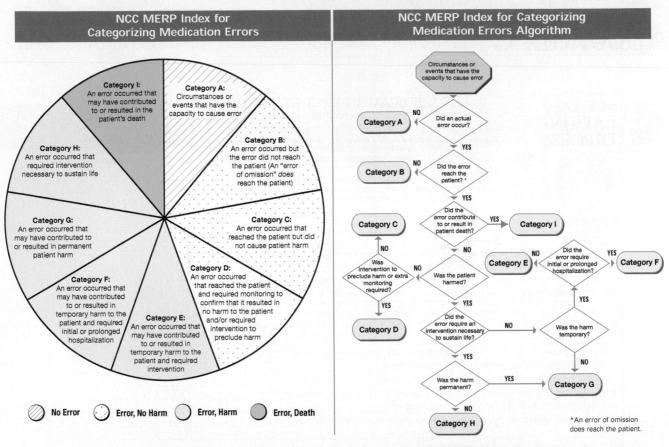

© 2003 National Coordinating Council for Medication Error Reporting and Prevention

Full-size copies are available: **INDEX**—www.nccmerp.org/010612_color_index.pdf; **ALGORITHM**—www.nccmerp.org/010612_color_algo.pdf

National Coordinating Council for Medication Error Reporting and Prevention Definitions

Harm
Impairment of the physical, emotional, or psychological function or structure of the body and/or pain resulting therefrom.

Monitoring
To observe or record relevant physiological or psychological signs.

Intervention
May include change in therapy or active medical/surgical treatment.

Intervention Necessary to Sustain Life
Includes cardiovascular and respiratory support (e.g., CPR, defibrillation, intubation, etc.).

U.S. Pharmacopeia
12601 Twinbrook Parkway
Rockville, MD 20852-1790

NO POSTAGE
NECESSARY
IF MAILED
IN THE
UNITED STATES

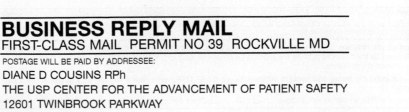

BUSINESS REPLY MAIL
FIRST-CLASS MAIL PERMIT NO 39 ROCKVILLE MD

POSTAGE WILL BE PAID BY ADDRESSEE:
DIANE D COUSINS RPh
THE USP CENTER FOR THE ADVANCEMENT OF PATIENT SAFETY
12601 TWINBROOK PARKWAY
ROCKVILLE MD 20897-5211

Appendix D: Body Surface Area Nomograms

Nomogram for Estimating Body Surface Area of Infants and Young Children

HEIGHT	SURFACE AREA	WEIGHT
feet centimeters	in square meters	pounds kilograms

To determine the surface area of the patient, draw a straight line between the point representing his height on the left vertical scale to the point representing his weight on the right vertical scale. The point at which this line intersects the middle vertical scale represents the patient's surface area in square meters. (Courtesy of Abbott Laboratories)

Nomogram for Estimating Body Surface Area of Older Children and Adults

HEIGHT	SURFACE AREA	WEIGHT
feet centimeters	in square meters	pounds kilograms

(Courtesy of Abbott Laboratories)

Appendix E: Vaccine Adverse Event Reporting

VACCINE ADVERSE EVENT REPORTING SYSTEM
24 Hour Toll-Free Information 1-800-822-7967
P.O. Box 1100, Rockville, MD 20849-1100
PATIENT IDENTITY KEPT CONFIDENTIAL

VAERS

For CDC/FDA Use Only
VAERS Number _____
Date Received _____

Patient Name: _____

Last	First	M.I.

Address
_____
_____
_____

City	State	Zip

Telephone no. (____) _____

Vaccine administered by (Name): _____

Responsible
Physician _____
Facility Name/Address
_____
_____
_____

City	State	Zip

Telephone no. (____) _____

Form completed by (Name): _____

Relation ☐ Vaccine Provider ☐ Patient/Parent
to Patient ☐ Manufacturer ☐ Other
Address *(if different from patient or provider)*
_____
_____
_____

City	State	Zip

Telephone no. (____) _____

1. State	2. County where administered	3. Date of birth ___/___/___ mm dd yy	4. Patient age	5. Sex ☐ M ☐ F	6. Date form completed ___/___/___ mm dd yy

7. Describe adverse events(s) (symptoms, signs, time course) and treatment, if any

8. Check all appropriate:
☐ Patient died   (date ___/___/___ mm dd yy)
☐ Life threatening illness
☐ Required emergency room/doctor visit
☐ Required hospitalization (_____days)
☐ Resulted in prolongation of hospitalization
☐ Resulted in permanent disability
☐ None of the above

9. Patient recovered ☐ YES ☐ NO ☐ UNKNOWN	10. Date of vaccination ___/___/___ mm dd yy Time _____ AM PM	11. Adverse event onset ___/___/___ mm dd yy Time _____ AM PM

12. Relevant diagnostic tests/laboratory data

13. Enter all vaccines given on date listed in no. 10

	Vaccine (type)	Manufacturer	Lot number	Route/Site	No. Previous Doses
a.					
b.					
c.					
d.					

14. Any other vaccinations within 4 weeks prior to the date listed in no. 10

	Vaccine (type)	Manufacturer	Lot number	Route/Site	No. Previous doses	Date given
a.						
b.						

15. Vaccinated at: ☐ Private doctor's office/hospital ☐ Military clinic/hospital ☐ Public health clinic/hospital ☐ Other/unknown	16. Vaccine purchased with: ☐ Private funds ☐ Military funds ☐ Public funds ☐ Other/unknown	17. Other medications

18. Illness at time of vaccination (specify)	19. Pre-existing physician-diagnosed allergies, birth defects, medical conditions (specify)

20. Have you reported this adverse event previously? ☐ No ☐ To health department ☐ To doctor ☐ To manufacturer	**Only for children 5 and under**
	22. Birth weight _____ lb. _____ oz.	23. No. of brothers and sisters

21. Adverse event following prior vaccination (check all applicable, specify)	**Only for reports submitted by manufacturer/immunization project**

	Adverse Event	Onset Age	Type Vaccine	Dose no. in series
☐ In patient				
☐ In brother or sister				

24. Mfr./imm. proj. report no.	25. Date received by mfr./imm.proj.
26. 15 day report? ☐ Yes ☐ No	27. Report type ☐ Initial ☐ Follow-Up

Health care providers and manufacturers are required by law (42 USC 300aa-25) to report reactions to vaccines listed in the Table of Reportable Events Following Immunization. Reports for reactions to other vaccines are voluntary except when required as a condition of immunization grant awards.

Form VAERS-1(FDA)

"Fold in thirds, tape & mail — DO NOT STAPLE FORM"

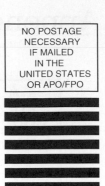

BUSINESS REPLY MAIL
FIRST-CLASS MAIL   PERMIT NO. 1895   ROCKVILLE, MD

POSTAGE WILL BE PAID BY ADDRESSEE

VAERS
P.O. Box 1100
Rockville MD 20849-1100

DIRECTIONS FOR COMPLETING FORM
(Additional pages may be attached if more space is needed.)

GENERAL

- Use a separate form for each patient. Complete the form to the best of your abilities. Items 3, 4, 7, 8, 10, 11, and 13 are considered essential and should be completed whenever possible. Parents/Guardians may need to consult the facility where the vaccine was administered for some of the information (such as manufacturer, lot number or laboratory data.)
- Refer to the Reportable Events Table (RET) for events mandated for reporting by law. Reporting for other serious events felt to be related but not on the RET is encouraged.
- Health care providers other than the vaccine administrator (VA) treating a patient for a suspected adverse event should notify the VA and provide the information about the adverse event to allow the VA to complete the form to meet the VA's legal responsibility.
- These data will be used to increase understanding of adverse events following vaccination and will become part of CDC Privacy Act System 09-20-0136, "Epidemiologic Studies and Surveillance of Disease Problems". Information identifying the person who received the vaccine or that person's legal representative will not be made available to the public, but may be available to the vaccinee or legal representative.
- Postage will be paid by addressee. Forms may be photocopied (must be front & back on same sheet).

SPECIFIC INSTRUCTIONS

Form Completed By: To be used by parents/guardians, vaccine manufacturers/distributors, vaccine administrators, and/or the person completing the form on behalf of the patient or the health professional who administered the vaccine.

Item 7:	Describe the suspected adverse event. Such things as temperature, local and general signs and symptoms, time course, duration of symptoms, diagnosis, treatment and recovery should be noted.
Item 9:	Check "YES" if the patient's health condition is the same as it was prior to the vaccine, "NO" if the patient has not returned to the pre-vaccination state of health, or "UNKNOWN" if the patient's condition is not known.
Item 10: and 11:	Give dates and times as specifically as you can remember. If you do not know the exact time, please indicate "AM" or "PM" when possible if this information is known. If more than one adverse event, give the onset date and time for the most serious event.
Item 12:	Include "negative" or "normal" results of any relevant tests performed as well as abnormal findings.
Item 13:	List ONLY those vaccines given on the day listed in Item 10.
Item 14:	List any other vaccines that the patient received within 4 weeks prior to the date listed in Item 10.
Item 16:	This section refers to how the person who gave the vaccine purchased it, not to the patient's insurance.
Item 17:	List any prescription or non-prescription medications the patient was taking when the vaccine(s) was given.
Item 18:	List any short term illnesses the patient had on the date the vaccine(s) was given (i.e., cold, flu, ear infection).
Item 19:	List any pre-existing physician-diagnosed allergies, birth defects, medical conditions (including developmental and/or neurologic disorders) for the patient.
Item 21:	List any suspected adverse events the patient, or the patient's brothers or sisters, may have had to previous vaccinations. If more than one brother or sister, or if the patient has reacted to more than one prior vaccine, use additional pages to explain completely. For the onset age of a patient, provide the age in months if less than two years old.
Item 26:	This space is for manufacturers' use only.

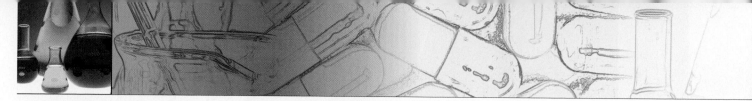

Appendix F: Key to Abbreviations

The following abbreviations appear in the Summary Drug Tables in this textbook..

BID	twice daily
d	day
g	gram
gtt	drops
h	hour
IM	intramuscular
IV	intravenous
kg	kilogram
min	minute
mcg	microgram
mg	milligram
mg/kg/d	milligrams per kilogram of body weight per day
mL	milliliter
prn	as needed
qh	every hour (q2h = every 2 hours, q3h = every 3 hours, etc.)
QID	four times daily
SC	subcutaneous
sec	second
TID	three times daily
wk	week

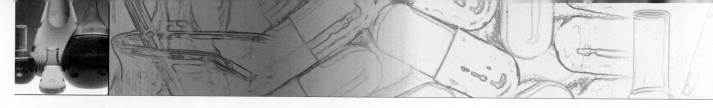

Appendix G: Answers to Review Questions and Medication Dosage Problems

UNIT I Foundations of Clinical Pharmacology

Chapter 1 General Principles of Pharmacology

Review Questions
1. a
2. b
3. b
4. d
5. a

Chapter 2 Administration of Drugs

Review Questions
1. c
2. c
3. d
4. b
5. b

Chapter 3 Review of Arithmetic and Calculation of Drug Dosages

Answers are in the chapter.

Chapter 4 The Nursing Process

Review Questions
1. d
2. c
3. a

Chapter 5 Patient and Family Teaching

Review Questions
1. d
2. a
3. b
4. c
5. b

UNIT II Anti-Infectives

Chapter 6 Sulfonamides

Review Questions
1. b
2. d
3. c
4. b

Medication Dosage Problems
1. 10 mL or 2 teaspoons
2. 2 tablets

Chapter 7 Penicillins

Review Questions
1. b
2. b
3. b
4. d

Medication Dosage Problems
1. 1 teaspoon (t) = 250 mg of amoxicillin (1 t = 5 mL). The nurse will administer 2 teaspoons (t) or 10 mL of amoxicillin.
2. a. Ninety milliliters (90 mL) of water needed for reconstitution.

   b. Directions for reconstitution: Tap bottle until all powder flows freely. Add approximately 2/3 of the 90 mL of water; shake vigorously to wet powder. Add remaining water and shake vigorously again.

   c. Strength of reconstituted solution is 125 mg/5 mL. (The nurse would administer 20 mL.)

Chapter 8 Cephalosporins

Review Questions
1. b
2. a
3. d
4. c

Medication Dosage Problems
1. 2 capsules
2. 4 mL

Chapter 9 Tetracyclines, Macrolides, and Lincosamides

Review Questions
1. c
2. b
3. d
4. a

Medication Dosage Problems
1. 2 tablets, 1 tablet
2. 2 mL
3. 20 mL

Chapter 10 Fluoroquinolones and Aminoglycosides

Review Questions
1. c
2. c
3. b
4. a
5. c

Medication Dosage Problems
1. 1 mL
2. 2 tablets

Chapter 11 Miscellaneous Anti-Infectives

Review Questions
1. b
2. c
3. a
4. b

Medication Dosage Problems
1. 1 tablet
2. 15 mL
3. 20 mL

Chapter 12 Antitubercular Drugs

Review Questions
1. a
2. d
3. c

4. b
5. d

Medication Dosage Problems
1. 6 mL
2. 4 tablets

Chapter 13 Leprostatic Drugs

Review Questions
1. d
2. c
3. a
4. b

Medication Dosage Problems
1. 6 tablets
2. 2 tablets

Chapter 14 Antiviral Drugs

Review Questions
1. a
2. a
3. a
4. b

Medication Dosage Problems
1. 2 tablets
2. 10 mg
3. 10 mL

Chapter 15 Antifungal Drugs

Review Questions
1. a
2. c
3. a
4. d

Medication Dosage Problems
1. (140 lbs = 63.6 kg) 95.4 mg, or 95 if rounded to the nearest whole number
2. 2 tablets

Chapter 16 Antiparasitic Drugs

Review Questions
1. b
2. b
3. c
4. a

Medication Dosage Problems

1. 2 capsules

2. 2 tablets

UNIT III Drugs Used to Manage Pain

Chapter 17 Nonopioid Analgesics: Salicylates and Nonsalicylates

Review Questions

1. c

2. a

3. c

4. c

5. c

6. b

Medication Dosage Problems

1. 1.5 or 1½ mL

2. 2 tablets

Chapter 18 Nonopioid Analgesics: Nonsteroidal Anti-Inflammatory Drugs (NSAIDs)

Review Questions

1. a

2. a

3. d

4. b

Medication Dosage Problems

1. 10 mL

2. 2 tablets

Chapter 19 Opioid Analgesics

Review Questions

1. d

2. c

3. b

4. c

5. a

Medication Dosage Problems

1. 1.2 mL

2. 1 mL

Chapter 20 Opioid Antagonists

Review Questions

1. b

2. c

Medication Dosage Problems

1. 0.8 mL

2. 4 injections

UNIT IV Drugs That Affect the Neuromuscular System

Chapter 21 Anesthetic Drugs

Review Questions

1. b

2. c

3. a

4. b

Medication Dosage Problems

1. 1 mL

2. 0.3 mg

Chapter 22 Antianxiety Drugs

Review Questions

1. a

2. d

3. b

4. c

Medication Dosage Problems

1. 1 mL

2. 2 tablets, 3 times

Chapter 23 Sedatives and Hypnotics

Review Questions

1. a

2. c

3. a

4. d

5. c

Medication Dosage Problems

1. 1 tablet

2. 2 tablets

Chapter 24 Antidepressant Drugs

Review Questions

1. d

2. c

3. c

4. b

Medication Dosage Problems

1. 3 tablets
2. 25 mL

Chapter 25 Central Nervous System Stimulants

Review Questions

1. c
2. a
3. d
4. d

Medication Dosage Problems

1. 24 mg, yes
2. 2 tablets

Chapter 26 Antipsychotic Drugs

Review Questions

1. c
2. b
3. c
4. b

Medication Dosage Problems

1. 1.5 mL
2. 2 tablets
3. 2 tablets

Chapter 27 Adrenergic Drugs

Review Questions

1. b
2. a
3. d
4. d

Medication Dosage Problems

1. 0.6 mg
2. 1/2 mL

Chapter 28 Adrenergic Blocking Drugs

Review Questions

1. d
2. d
3. a
4. b

Medication Dosage Problems

1. 15 mL
2. 4 tablets

Chapter 29 Cholinergic Drugs

Review Questions

1. a
2. b
3. b

Medication Dosage Problems

1. 10 tablets
2. ½ mL

Chapter 30 Cholinergic Blocking Drugs

Review Questions

1. b
2. b
3. d
4. b

Medication Dosage Problems

1. ½ mL
2. 10 mL

Chapter 31 Anticonvulsants

Review Questions

1. d
2. b
3. a
4. c
5. b

Medication Dosage Problems

1. 3.3 mL
2. 2 tablets
3. 10 mL

Chapter 32 Antiparkinsonism Drugs

Review Questions

1. a
2. b
3. d
4. b

Medication Dosage Problems

1. one 500-mg tablet and one 250-mg tablet
2. 3 tablets

Chapter 33 Cholinesterase Inhibitors

Review Questions

1. b
2. c
3. a
4. d

Medication Dosage Problems

1. 3 mL

2. 2 tablets

Chapter 34 Drugs Used to Treat Disorders of the Musculoskeletal System

Review Questions

1. c

2. a

3. c

4. d

5. d

Medication Dosage Problems

1. 3 tablets

2. 3 tablets

UNIT V Drugs That Affect the Respiratory System

Chapter 35 Antitussives, Mucolytics, and Expectorants

Review Questions

1. b

2. a

3. d

4. a

5. a

Medication Dosage Problems

1. 5 mL

2. 5 mL

Chapter 36 Antihistamines and Decongestants

Review Questions

1. a

2. c

3. b

4. c

5. a

Medication Dosage Problems

1. 10 mL

2. 2 tablets

Chapter 37 Bronchodilators and Antiasthma Drugs

Review Questions

1. d

2. d

3. d

4. a

5. a

Medication Dosage Problems

1. 0.25 mL

2. 2 tablets, 40 mg each day

UNIT VI Drugs That Affect the Cardiovascular System

Chapter 38 Cardiotonics and Miscellaneous Inotropic Drugs

Review Questions

1. b

2. d

3. a

4. a

5. c

Medication Dosage Problems

1. one 0.5-mg tablet and one 0.25-mg tablet

2. ½ mL

Chapter 39 Antiarrhythmic Drugs

Review Questions

1. a

2. d

3. a

4. d

5. c

Medication Dosage Problems

1. 2 tablets

2. 2 tablets

Chapter 40 Antianginal and Peripheral Vasodilating Drugs

Review Questions

1. b

2. b

3. c

4. b

5. a

6. d

Medication Dosage Problems

1. 3 tablets

2. 2 tablets

Chapter 41 Antihypertensive Drugs

Review Questions

1. c

2. c

3. d

4. b

5. b

Medication Dosage Problems

1. 4 tablets

2. 90-mg tablets and give 2 tablets

Chapter 42 Antihyperlipidemic Drugs

Review Questions

1. c

2. a

3. a

4. b

5. c

Medication Dosage Problems

1. 2 tablets

2. Yes, 200 mg is an appropriate dosage. However, if the patient requires 200 mg, it is preferable to give a 200-mg capsule rather than three 67-mg capsules. The nurse should notify the primary health care provider that only 67-mg capsules are available.

UNIT VII Drugs That Affect the Hematologic System

Chapter 43 Anticoagulant and Thrombolytic Drugs

Review Questions

1. d

2. d

3. b

4. a

5. b

Medication Dosage Problems

1. 0.67 mL or 0.7 mL

2. 2 tablets

Chapter 44 Agents Used in the Treatment of Anemia

Review Questions

1. a

2. a

3. c

4. a

5. c

Medication Dosage Problems

1. ½ mL

2. 0.2 mL

UNIT VIII Drugs That Affect the Gastrointestinal and Urinary Systems

Chapter 45 Diuretics

Review Questions

1. b

2. b

3. c

4. b

5. d

6. c

Medication Dosage Problems

1. 2 tablets

2. 2.5 mL

Chapter 46 Urinary Tract Anti-Infectives, Antispasmodics, and Other Urinary Drugs

Review Questions

1. a

2. d

3. c

4. d

Medication Dosage Problems

1. 2 tablets

2. 10 mL

Chapter 47 Drugs That Affect the Upper Gastrointestinal System

Review Questions

1. c

2. d

3. b

4. c

Medication Dosage Problems

1. 2 tablets

2. 1 tablet

Chapter 48 Drugs That Affect the Lower Gastrointestinal System

Review Questions

1. c

2. c

3. a

4. d

Medication Dosage Problems

1. 3 hours

2. 3 capsules

UNIT IX Drugs That Affect the Endocrine System

Chapter 49 Antidiabetic Drugs

Review Questions

1. c

2. d

3. c

4. b

5. c

Medication Dosage Problems

1. Draw an arrow to the number 45.

2. 2 tablets at each dose; total daily dose 2000 mg

3. 4 tablets

4. Label B

Chapter 50 Pituitary and Adrenocortical Hormones

Review Questions

1. b

2. c

3. a

4. b

5. c

Medication Dosage Problems

1. 2 mL

2. 20 mL

Chapter 51 Thyroid and Antithyroid Drugs

Review Questions

1. b

2. c

3. a

4. c

Medication Dosage Problems

1. 4 tablets

2. 2 tablets

Chapter 52 Male and Female Hormones

Review Questions

1. c

2. d

3. c

4. a

5. b

Medication Dosage Problems

1. 1.6 mL

2. 1 mL

Chapter 53 Drugs Acting on the Uterus

Review Questions

1. d

2. b

3. a

4. c

Medication Dosage Problems

1. ½ tablet

2. 1 mL

UNIT X Drugs That Affect the Immune System

Chapter 54 Immunologic Agents

Review Questions

1. b

2. a

3. c

4. a

Chapter 55 Antineoplastic Drugs

Review Questions

1. d

2. a

3. b

4. b

5. c

Medication Dosage Problems

1. 13.7 mg/d

2. 1.375 or 1.4 units

UNIT XI Drugs That Affect Other Body Systems

Chapter 56 Topical Drugs Used in the Treatment of Skin Disorders

Review Questions

1. b
2. b
3. d
4. b
5. d

Chapter 57 Otic and Ophthalmic Preparations

Review Questions

1. b
2. b

3. c
4. d

Chapter 58 Fluids and Electrolytes

Review Questions

1. d
2. a
3. d
4. a
5. d

Medication Dosage Problems

1. 100 mL/hour
2. 30 mL

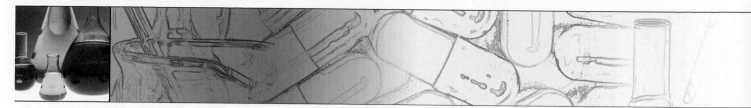

Index

Page numbers followed by f, t, and d, indicate figures, tables, and display material, respectively

Benzonatate, 357t
Benzoyl peroxide, 668t
Benzphetamine HCl, 258t
Benztropine mesylate, 324t
Bepridil HCl, 422t, 426, 446
Beta-adrenergic blocking drugs,
    288–289
    antihypertensive use, 439t–440t
    definition, 284
    drug summary, 285t–286t, 439t–440t
    elderly use, 288
    nursing process for, 290–294
    ophthalmic uses, 687, 688t, 693, 695
Beta blockers. *see* Beta-adrenergic
    blocking drugs
Betadine. *see* Povidone-iodine
Betagan Liquifilm. *see* Levobunolol HCl
Beta-lactam ring, 93
Betamethasone, 581t
Betamethasone dipropionate, 671t
Betamethasone valerate, 671t
Betapace. *see* Sotalol HCl
Betapen. *see* Penicillin V
Betasept. *see* Chlorhexidine gluconate
Betatrex. *see* Betamethasone valerate
Betaxolol HCl, 285t, 286t, 288, 439t,
    688t
Betaxon. *see* Levobetaxolol HCl
Bethanechol chloride, 297t, 298
Betimol. *see* Timolol
Betoptic. *see* Betaxolol HCl
Bexarotene, 654t
Biavax-II. *see* Rubella and mumps virus
    vaccine
Biaxin. *see* Clarithromycin
Bicalutamide, 615t
Bicarbonate, 708t, 711, 712–713, 714
Bicillin C-R. *see* Penicillin G benzathine
Bicillin L-A. *see* Penicillin G benzathine
Bidhist. *see* Brompheniramine
BIG-IV. *see* Botulism immune globulin
Biguanides
    action, 557
    administration, 561
    adverse reactions, 559
    contraindications, precautions, inter-
        actions, 559–560
    drug summary, 556t
Bilberry, 697
Bile acid sequestrants, 452, 453t, 455,
    460–461
Bimatoprost, 689t
Biocef. *see* Cephalexin
Biotransformation, 9
Biperiden, 324t
Bipolar disorder, 263
Birth defects, 7, 573
Bisacodyl, 532t
Bisca-Evac. *see* Bisacodyl
Bismatrol. *see* Bismuth subsalicylate

Bismuth subsalicylate, 520t, 531t
Bismuth subsalicylate metronidazole
    tetracycline, 520t
Bisoprolol fumarate, 285t, 439t
Bisphosphonates, 341–342, 343t, 348, 349
Bitolterol mesylate, 373t
Black cohosh, 608
Bladder
    neurogenic, 507
    overactive, 504–505
Bleeding, 467, 475, 476
Blenoxane. *see* Bleomycin sulfate
Bleomycin sulfate, 653t
Bleph-10. *see* Sulfacetamide sodium
Blocadren. *see* Timolol maleate
Blood-brain barrier, 325, 326f
Blood glucose. *see* Glucose
Blood plasma, 701, 703
Blood pressure, 433, 434t
Blood thinners. *see* Anticoagulants
B lymphocytes, 630
Body fluid solutions
    blood plasma, 701, 703
    energy substrates, 702, 703, 704
    fat emulsions, 702, 703, 704, 705
    fluid overload, 703, 705–706
    intravenous replacement solutions,
        702–703
    nursing process for, 704–706
    plasma expanders, 702, 703, 704
    plasma protein fractions, 702,
        703–704
    protein substrates, 702, 703, 704
Body image
    and cushingoid effects, 585
    and fungal infections, 160
    and growth hormone, 576
    and leprosy, 139
    and male hormones, 601
    and protease inhibitors, 150
Body surface area, 49, 51
Bone marrow suppression, 659
Bone resorption inhibitors,
    341–342, 343t
Boniva. *see* Ibandronate
Bontril. *see* Phendimetrazine tartrate
Booster injection, 633–634
Botanical medicine, 15
Botulism immune globulin, 637t
Bowel evacuants, 533t
Bowel preparation, 112, 116
Brachial plexus block, 220
Bradykinesia, 323
Bravelle. *see* Urofollitropins
Breathing pattern, ineffective, 370,
    510, 562
Brethine. *see* Terbutaline sulfate
Bretylium tosylate, 409t, 415
Brevibloc. *see* Esmolol HCl
Brevital. *see* Methohexital

Brimonidine tartrate, 686–687, 688t, 694
Brinzolamide, 689t
Broad spectrum drugs, 69, 109
Bromocriptine mesylate, 324t, 569t
Brompheniramine, 365t
Brompton's mixture, 206
Bronchodilators
    administration, 383–384, 385
    cholinergic blocking drugs, 372
    definition, 372
    drug summary, 373t–374t
    educating patient/family, 385, 386,
        387, 389
    nursing process for, 382–390
    sympathomimetic, 372, 375
    xanthine derivatives, 375–376
Bronchospasm, 386
BroveX. *see* Brompheniramine
Buccal administration, 25, 425, 428
Budesonide, 379t, 581t
Buffered aspirin, 183t
Bufferin. *see* Buffered aspirin; Magne-
    sium salicylate
Bulk-producing laxatives, 532t, 536d
Bumetanide, 492t, 494, 500t
Bumex. *see* Bumetanide
Buprenex. *see* Buprenorphine
Buprenorphine, 201t
Bupropion HCl, 247, 249t
Burns, 75
Burow's otic. *see* 2% acetic acid in alu-
    minum acetate solution
BuSpar. *see* Buspirone HCl
Buspirone HCl, 227, 228, 229t, 231
Busulfan, 651t
Busulfex. *see* Busulfan
Butamben picrate, 673t
Butenafine HCl, 156t, 669t
Butoconazole nitrate, 157t
Butorphanol, 201t

C

Cabergoline, 569t
Cachectic patients, 205
Cafcit. *see* Caffeine
Caffeine, 255, 257t, 260
Calan. *see* Verapamil HCl
Calcipotriene, 672t, 678
Calcium
    assessment of, 712
    hypercalcemia, 341t, 710d
    hypocalcemia, 706, 710d
    normal values, 710d
    replacements, 707t
        actions and uses, 706–708
        administration, 713
        adverse reactions, 706
        contraindications, precautions,
            interactions, 709
        educating patient/family, 715

benzethonium chloride, 0.015% sodium acetate, 0.2% citric acid, 684t

1% hydrocortisone, 3.3 mg neomycin sulfate, 683t

1% hydrocortisone, 4.71 mg neomycin sulfate, 683t

1% hydrocortisone, 5 mg neomycin sulfate, 10,000 Units polymyxin B, 683t

1% hydrocortisone, 1% pramoxine HCl, 0.1% chloroxylenol, 3% propylene glycol diacetate and benzalkonium chloride, 683t

Hydrocortisone buteprate, 671t

Hydrocortisone butyrate, 671t

HydroDIURIL. see Hydrochlorothiazide

Hydroflumethiazide, 494t

Hydromorphone, 200t

Hydroxychloroquine sulfate, 343t

Hydroxymagnesium aluminate, 515t

Hydroxyurea, 653t

Hydroxyzine, 222t, 227, 230t, 365t

Hylorel. see Guanadrel

Hypercalcemia, 341t, 710d

Hyperglycemia, 545, 546t, 553, 716

Hyperkalemia, 495, 499, 499d, 710d

Hyperlipidemia, 394, 451. see also Antihyperlipidemic drugs

Hypermagnesemia, 710d

Hypernatremia, 710d

Hyperosmotic agents, 532t, 536d

Hypersecretory conditions, 519

Hypersensitivity reactions
  to cephalosporins, 93–94, 95
  definition, 10–11
  to penicillins, 83–84, 85
  to sulfonamides, 73
  to topical anti-infectives, 673

Hyperstat IV. see Diazoxide

Hyperstimulation syndrome, 574

Hypertension. See also Antihypertensive drugs
  adrenergic blocking drugs for, 287
  algorithm for treatment of, 436f
  definition, 394, 433, 434t
  drug administration for, 498
  drug therapy for, 434–435
  educating patient/family, 293–394
  essential, 433
  isolated systolic, 434d
  nondrug management of, 434
  risks and effects of, 433–434
  secondary, 434
  supine, 279

Hypertensive emergency
  definition, 437
  drugs used for, 443t–444t, 446–447
  and MAOIs, 244, 245

Hyperthyroidism, 588, 589t

Hypnotics. see Sedatives and hypnotics

Hypocalcemia, 706, 710d

Hypoglycemia, 544–545, 546t, 553

Hypoglycemic reaction, 553, 562

Hypokalemia
  definition, 708
  and digitalis toxicity, 400
  and diuretics, 447, 495, 498–499, 499d, 500
  signs and symptoms, 710d

Hypomagnesemia, 400, 499d, 710d

Hyponatremia, 447, 499d, 709, 710d

Hypotension
  adrenergic drugs for, 281–282
  orthostatic
  and adrenergic blocking drugs, 293
  and adrenergic drugs, 279, 282
  and antidepressants, 251
  and antihypertensives, 437, 447, 448
  postural, 293, 426

Hypothyroidism, 588, 589t, 591

Hypovolemic shock, 278t

Hytone. see Hydrocortisone

Hytrin. see Terazosin

Hytuss. see Guaifenesin

I

Ibandronate, 343t

Ibuprofen, 192t, 194, 195

Ibutilide fumarate, 410t

Idamycin. see Idarubicin HCl

Idarubicin HCl, 653t

Identification of patients, 19–20, 21

Idoxuridine, 691t

Ifex. see Ifosfamide

Ifosfamide, 651t

IgG. see Immune globulin

IGIV. see Immune globulin, intravenous

IG-microdose. see Rh (D) immune globulin microdose

Iletin II Regular. see Insulin

Ilopan. see Dexpanthenol

Ilotycin. see Erythromycin

Imdur. see Isosorbide mononitrate

Imipenem-cilastatin, 120, 121t, 123–125

Imipramine, 248t

Imiquimod, 143t

Immune globulin, intravenous, 637t, 640

Immune Globulins
  actions and uses, 639
  adverse reactions, 639
  contraindications and precautions, 640
  definition, 639
  interactions, 640
  summary of, 637t–638t

Immune system, 627

Immunity
  active, 630, 634
  cell-mediated, 629
  definition of, 629, 630
  humoral, 630
  passive, 634

Immunizations. see Vaccines

Immunocompromised patients, 673

Immunologic agents
  actions and uses, 634, 638–639
  adverse reactions, 639, 641–642
  contraindications and precautions, 639–640
  interactions, 640
  nursing process for, 640–642
  recommended schedules for, 635f–636f
  summary of, 637t–638t

Immunosuppression, 70

Imodium. see Loperamide HCl

Imogam. see Rabies immune globulin

Imovax Rabies vaccine. see Rabies vaccine

Implant contraceptive system, 609

Implementation
  and administration of medication, 54f
  and deficient knowledge, 57, 63
  definition of, 56
  in nursing process, 56–58
  in patient teaching, 65
  and therapeutic regimen management, 56–57

Improper fraction, 35

Imuran. see Azathioprine

Inamrinone lactate, 397t, 398–399

Inapsine. see Droperidol

Incontinence, 505

Indapamide, 494t

Independent nursing actions, 55

Inderal. see Propranolol HCl

Indinavir, 144t, 148, 150

Indocin. see Indomethacin

Indomethacin, 192t, 619t, 623, 624, 625

Infalyte Oral Solution. see Oral electrolyte mixtures

Infanrix. see Diphtheria and tetanus toxoids and acellular pertussis vaccine

Infants. see Children

Infections. see also Anti-infectives; Superinfections
  and antiarrhythmic drugs, 415–416
  and antithyroid drugs, 594
  and clozapine, 270–271
  and corticotropins, 578–579
  and glucocorticoid therapy, 584
  overview of, 69–70
  secondary, 70, 75
  viral, 141

InFeD. see Iron dextran

Infiltration, 30, 704

Inflammatory bowel disease, 530, 531t, 533–534

Infliximab, 344t, 345, 531t

Influenza, 146d

Influenza virus vaccine, 632t

Infusion controllers and pumps, 29, 30

INH. see Isoniazid